W9-BYK-767

Cystic Fibrosis

Cystic Fibrosis

Third edition

Margaret Hodson
Professor of Respiratory Medicine and Consultant Physician,
Department of Cystic Fibrosis,
Royal Brompton & Harefield NHS Trust, London, UK

Duncan Geddes
Professor of Respiratory Medicine and Consultant Physician,
Royal Brompton & Harefield NHS Trust, London, UK

Andrew Bush
Professor of Paediatric Respirology and Consultant Paediatric Chest Physician,
Royal Brompton & Harefield NHS Trust, London, UK

Hodder Arnold

A MEMBER OF THE HODDER HEADLINE GROUP

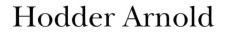

First published in Great Britain in 1995
Second edition 2000
This third edition published in 2007 by
Hodder Arnold, an imprint of Hodder Education and a member of the
Hodder Headline Group, an Hachette Livre UK company,
338 Euston Road, London NW1 3BH

http://www.hoddereducation.com

Whilst the advice and information in this book are believed to be true and
accurate at the date of going to press, neither the author[s] nor the publisher can
accept any legal responsibility or liability for any errors or omissions that
may be made. In particular (but without limiting the generality of the preceding
disclaimer) every effort has been made to check drug dosages; however it is
still possible that errors have been missed. Furthermore, dosage schedules
are constantly being revised and new side-effects recognized. For these reasons
the reader is strongly urged to consult the drug companies' printed instructions
before administering any of the drugs recommended in this book.

British Library Cataloguing in Publication Data
A catalogue record for this book is available from the British Library

Library of Congress Cataloging-in-Publication Data
A catalog record for this book is available from the Library of Congress

ISBN   978 0 340 90758 0

1 2 3 4 5 6 7 8 9 10

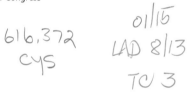

Commissioning Editor: Philip Shaw
Project Editor: Heather Fyfe
Production Controller: Karen Tate
Cover Designer: Andrew Campling

Typeset in 10/12 pts Minion by Charon Tec Ltd (A Macmillan Company), Chennai, India
www.charontec.com
Printed and bound in Great Britain by CPI Bath

What do you think about this book? Or any other Hodder Arnold title?
Please visit our website: **www.hoddereducation.com**

Contents

Color plates appear between pages 259 and 260.

Contributors   ix
Preface   xiii

PART 1   INTRODUCTION: WHAT IS CYSTIC FIBROSIS?

1   History of cystic fibrosis   3
    James M. Littlewood
2   Epidemiology of cystic fibrosis   21
    Sarah Walters and Anil Mehta

PART 2   BASIC SCIENCE FOR THE CLINICIAN

3   Molecular biology of cystic fibrosis: *CFTR* processing and functions, and classes of mutations   49
    Malka Nissim-Rafinia, Batsheva Kerem and Eitan Kerem
4   Pathophysiology: epithelial cell biology and ion channel function in the lung, sweat gland and pancreas   59
    Raymond D. Coakley and Richard C. Boucher
5   Immunology of cystic fibrosis   69
    Gerd Döring and Felix Ratjen
6a   Genotype–phenotype correlations and modifier genes   81
    Jane C. Davies
6b   Variability of clinical course in cystic fibrosis   87
    Michael Schechter

PART 3   DIAGNOSTIC ASPECTS OF CYSTIC FIBROSIS

7   Diagnosis of cystic fibrosis   99
    Colin Wallis
8a   The challenge of screening newborn infants for cystic fibrosis   109
    Kevin W. Southern
8b   How to manage the screened patient   117
    Philip Robinson
9   Microbiology of cystic fibrosis: role of the clinical microbiology laboratory, susceptibility and synergy studies and infection control   123
    Samiya Razvi and Lisa Saiman

PART 4   CLINICAL ASPECTS OF CYSTIC FIBROSIS

10   Respiratory disease: infection   137
    Ian M. Balfour-Lynn and J. Stuart Elborn
11   Respiratory disease: non-infectious complications   159
    Margaret Hodson and Andrew Bush

12   Sleep, lung mechanics and work of breathing, including NIPPV   175
     Brigitte Fauroux and Annick Clément
13   Delivery of therapy to the cystic fibrosis lung   185
     Harm A. W. M. Tiddens and Sunalene G. Devadason
14   The upper airway in cystic fibrosis   199
     William E. Grant
15a Gastrointestinal disease in cystic fibrosis   209
     Ian Gooding and David Westaby
15b Liver, biliary and pancreatic disease   225
     Vicky Dondos and David Westaby
16   Insulin deficiency and diabetes related to cystic fibrosis   241
     Christopher D. Sheldon and Lee Dobson
17   Growth and puberty   253
     Nicola Bridges
18   Cystic-fibrosis-related low bone mineral density   261
     Sarah L. Elkin and Charles S. Haworth
19   Other system disorders in cystic fibrosis   269
     Khin Ma Gyi
20   Sexual and reproductive health   279
     Susan M. Sawyer
21   Transplantation   291
     Paul Aurora, Khin Gyi and Martin Carby

PART 5   MONITORING

22   Using databases to improve care   311
     Sheila G. McKenzie and Margaret E. Hodson
23a Infant and pre-school children: lung function   321
     Sarath Ranganathan
23b Infant and pre-school children: role of bronchoscopy   331
     Gary Connett
23c Infant and pre-school children: imaging the lungs   337
     Samatha Sonnappa and Catherine M. Owens
24   Physiological monitoring of older children and adults   345
     Mark Rosenthal
25a Exercise: testing   353
     David M. Orenstein and Wolfgang Gruber
25b Exercise: use in therapy   361
     David M. Orenstein and Linda W. Higgins
26   Clinical outcome measures to assess new treatments for CF lung disease   375
     Jane C. Davies and Eric W.F.W. Alton on behalf of the UK CF Gene Therapy Consortium

PART 6   MULTIDISCIPLINARY CARE

27   Cystic fibrosis center care   387
     Penny Agent and Susan Madge
28   Nursing care   399
     Susan Madge and Christine Hockings
29   Physiotherapy   407
     Craig Lapin, Anne Lapin and Jennifer A. Pryor
30   Nutritional aspects   421
     Sue Wolfe and Sarah Collins
31   Psychological aspects of cystic fibrosis   431
     Alistair J. A. Duff and Helen Oxley
32   Palliative care in cystic fibrosis   441
     Catherine E. Urch and Margaret E. Hodson

PART 7   CYSTIC FIBROSIS: THE FUTURE

33a   Gene and stem cell therapy   453
      Uta Griesenbach and Eric W. F. W. Alton on behalf of the UK CF Gene Therapy Consortium
33b   Non-gene therapy treatments: what will they deliver?   463
      Adam Jaffé and Pierre Barker
34   The future: how will management change?   471
      Andrew Bush and Duncan Geddes

APPENDICES

Appendix 1   Transition form   479
      Susan Madge and Jacqueline Francis
Appendix 2   Practical nursing care required by the cystic fibrosis patient and its delivery   483
      Frances Duncan–Skingle and Tracey Catling

Index   487

Contributors

Penny Agent BSc PgDMS
Service Lead, Superintendent Physiotherapist, Department of Physiotherapy, Royal Brompton Hospital, London, UK

Eric W. F. W. Alton MD FRCP FMedSci
Professor of Gene Therapy and Respiratory Medicine, Department of Gene Therapy, National Heart & Lung Institute, Imperial College, London, UK

Paul Aurora MBBS MRCP PhD
Cardiothoracic Transplant and Respiratory Units, Great Ormond Street Hospital for Children, and Portex Respiratory Unit, Institute of Child Health, University College London, London, UK

Ian M. Balfour-Lynn BSc MBBS MD FRCP FRCPCH FRCS(Ed) DHMSA
Consultant in Pediatric Respiratory Medicine, Department of Pediatric Respiratory Medicine, Royal Brompton Hospital, London, UK

Pierre Barker MD FAAP MRCP
Associate Professor of Pediatrics, University of North Carolina, NC, USA

Richard C. Boucher MD
William R. Kenan Professor of Medicine and Director, CF Research and Treatment Center, University of North Carolina at Chapel Hill, NC, USA

Nicola Bridges DM MRCP FRCPCH
Consultant Pediatric Endocrinologist, Chelsea & Westminster Hospital, London, UK

Andrew Bush MD FRCP FRPCH
Professor of Pediatric Respirology and Consultant Paediatric Chest Physician, Royal Brompton & Harefield NHS Trust, London, UK

Martin Carby BSc MBBS MRCP
Consultant Respiratory and Transplant Physician, Cardiothoracic Transplant Unit, Harefield Hospital, Harefield, Middlesex, UK

Tracey Catling RGN
Clinical Nurse Specialist, Royal Brompton Hospital, London, UK

Annick Clément MD PhD
Professor of Pediatrics, Pediatric Pulmonology Department and Research Unit INSERM U719, Armand Trousseau Hospital, Hôpitaux de Paris, Paris, France

Raymond D. Coakley MD
Assistant Professor of Medicine, CF Research and Treatment Center, University of North Carolina at Chapel Hill, NC, USA

Sarah Collins BSc MSc RD
Senior Dietitian (Adult CF), Dietetic Department, Royal Brompton Hospital, London, UK

Gary Connett MB ChB MRCP FRCPCH MD
Consultant Pediatrician, Department of Pediatrics, Southampton University Hospitals Trust, Southampton, UK

Jane C. Davies MB MD ChB MRCP MRCPCH
Senior Lecturer in Gene Therapy & Honorary Consultant in Pediatric Respiratory Medicine, Department of Gene Therapy, National Heart & Lung Institute, Imperial College, London, and Department of Pediatric Respiratory Medicine, Royal Brompton Hospital, London, UK

Sunalene G. Devadason PhD
Senior Research Fellow, School of Paediatrics and Child Health, University of Western Australia, Perth, Australia

Lee Dobson MBChB MRCP
Consultant Physician, Department of Respiratory Medicine, Torbay Hospital, Torquay, UK

Vicky Dondos
Research fellow, The Royal Brompton Hospital, London, UK

Gerd Döring PhD
Professor for Experimental Hygeine and Microbiology, Institute für Medizinische Mikrobiologie und Hygiene, Tübingen, Germany

Alistair J. A. Duff MA MSc DClinPsych
Consultant Clinical Psychologist & Head of Pediatric Psychology Services, Department of Clinical & Health Psychology, St James' University Hospital, Leeds, UK

Frances Duncan-Skingle RGN NDNCert HVCert
Nurse Consultant (retired), Royal Brompton Hospital, London, UK

J. Stuart Elborn MD FRCP
Professor of Respiratory Medicine, Department of Respiratory Medicine, Belfast City Hospital, and Queen's University, Belfast, NI

Sarah L. Elkin MCSP MD MRCP
Consultant Physician, Respiratory and General Medicine, St Mary's Hospital, London, UK

Brigitte Fauroux MD PhD
Professor of Pediatrics, Pediatric Pulmonology Department and
Research Unit INSERM U719, Armand Trousseau Hospital,
Hôpitaux de Paris, Paris, France

Jacqueline Francis EN(G) RGN RSCN BSc(Hons)
Pediatric Cystic Fibrosis Care Coordinator, Royal Brompton
Hospital, London, UK

Duncan Geddes MA MBBS MD FRCP
Professor of Respiratory Medicine and Consultant Physician, Royal
Brompton & Harefield NHS Trust, London, UK

Ian Gooding MA MB BChir MRCP
Specialist Registrar, Department of Gastroenterology,
Charing Cross Hospital, London, UK

William E. Grant MCh FRCSI FRCSEd FRCS(ORL)
Consultant Ear, Nose & Throat Surgeon, Ear, Nose and Throat
Department, Chelsea & Westminster and Charing Cross Hospitals,
London, UK

Uta Griesenbach PhD
Senior Lecturer in Gene Therapy, Department of Gene Therapy,
National Heart & Lung Institute, Imperial College, London, UK

Wolfgang Gruber PhD MSc
Department of Sports Therapy, Fachklinik Sattelduene,
Nebel/Amrum, Germany

Khin Ma Gyi MBBS DTMRH FRCP (Glasgow)
Consultant and Honorary Senior Lecturer in Respiratory Medicine,
Department of Cystic Fibrosis, Royal Brompton Hospital,
London, UK

Charles S. Haworth MD MRCP
Adult Cystic Fibrosis Centre, Papworth Hospital, Cambridge, UK

Linda W. Higgins PhD RN
Research Associate, Antonio J. and Janet Palumbo Cystic Fibrosis
Center, Children's Hospital of Pittsburgh; Adjunct Assistant
Professor of Health and Community Systems, School of Nursing,
University of Pittsburgh, PA, USA

Christine Hockings BA RN
Clinical Nurse Specialist, Royal Brompton Hospital, London, UK

Margaret E. Hodson MD MSc FRCP Dmed Ed
Professor of Respiratory Medicine and Consultant Physician,
Department of Cystic Fibrosis, Royal Brompton & Harefield Trust,
London, UK

Adam Jaffé MD FRCP FRCPCH
Consultant and Honorary Senior Lecturer in Respiratory Medicine,
Portex Anaesthesia, Intensive Therapy & Respiratory Medicine
Unit, Great Ormond Street Hospital for Children and Institute for
Child Health, London, UK

Batsheva Kerem PhD
Professor in Genetics, Department of Genetics, The Life Sciences
Institute, Hebrew University, Jerusalem, Israel

Eitan Kerem MD
Professor in Pediatrics, Head, Department of Pediatrics and CF
Center, Hadassah-Hebrew University Hospital, Jerusalem, Israel

Anne Lapin MCSP PT
Physiotherapist, Central Connecticut Cystic Fibrosis Center,
Connecticut Children's Medical Center, Hartford; Adjunct Faculty,
Department of Physical Therapy, University of Connecticut, Storrs,
CT, USA

Craig Lapin MD
Director, Central Connecticut Cystic Fibrosis Center, Connecticut
Children's Medical Center, Hartford; Associate Professor of
Pediatrics, University of Connecticut, Farmington,
CT, USA

James M. Littlewood OBE MB ChB MD FRCP FRCPE FRCPCH DCH
Chairman, UK Cystic Fibrosis Trust; and Regional Paediatric Cystic
Fibrosis Unit, St James' University Hospital, Leeds, UK

Sheila G. McKenzie BSc PhD
Pharmacology Consultant, Victoria, British Columbia, Canada

Susan Madge SRN RSCN MSc MCGI PhD
Consultant Nurse, Royal Brompton Hospital, London, UK

Anil Mehta MSc FRCPCH FRCP (Edin)
Tayside Institute of Child Health, Ninewells Hospital & Medical
School, Dundee, UK

Malka Nissim-Rafinia PhD
Department of Genetics, The Life Sciences Institute,
Hebrew University, Jerusalem, Israel

David M. Orenstein MD
Antonio J. and Janet Palumbo Professor of Cystic Fibrosis;
Director, Antonio J. and Janet Palumbo Cystic Fibrosis Center,
Children's Hospital of Pittsburgh; Professor of Pediatrics,
School of Medicine; Professor of Health and Physical Activity,
School of Education, University of Pittsburgh, Pittsburgh,
PA, USA

Catherine M. Owens BSc MBBS MRCP FRCR
Consultant Pediatric Radiologist, Great Ormond Street Hospital
for Children, London, UK

Helen Oxley BSc MSc
Consultant Clinical Psychologist, Manchester Adult Cystic Fibrosis
Centre, Wythenshawe Hospital, Manchester, UK

Jennifer A. Pryor PhD MBA FNZSP MCSP
Honorary Lecturer, University College London; Senior Research
Fellow in Physiotherapy, Royal Brompton Hospital, London, UK

Sarath Ranganathan MB ChB MRCP PhD FRCPCH FRACP
Consultant in Respiratory Medicine, Royal Children's Hospital
Melbourne; Senior Fellow, Department of Pediatrics, University
of Melbourne and Honorary Fellow, Infection, Immunity and
Environment Theme, Murdoch Children's Research Institute,
Melbourne, Australia

Felix Ratjen MD FRCP(C)
Head, Division of Respiratory Medicine, Sellers Chair of Cystic Fibrosis, Professor, University of Toronto, Hospital for Sick Children, Toronto, Ontario, Canada

Samiya Razvi MD
Pediatric Pulmonary Fellow, Department of Pediatric Pulmonary Medicine, Morgan-Stanley Children's Hospital Of New York-Presbyterian, NY, USA

Philip Robinson BMedSc PhD MD MBBS FRACP
Director, Cystic Fibrosis Unit, Department of Respiratory Medicine, Royal Children's Hospital, Melbourne, Australia

Mark Rosenthal MD FRCP FRCPCH
Consultant in Pediatric Respiratory Medicine, Royal Brompton Hospital, London, UK

Lisa Saiman MD MPH
Professor of Clinical Pediatrics, Department of Pediatrics, University of Columbia, NY, USA

Susan M. Sawyer MBBS MD FRACP
Professor of Adolescent Health, The University of Melbourne; Director, Centre for Adolescent Health and Consultant Respiratory Paediatrician, Royal Children's Hospital, Melbourne, Australia

Michael S. Schechter MD MPH
Associate Professor of Paediatrics, CF Center Director, Associate Director, Division of Pediatric Pulmonology, Allergy/Immunology, Cystic Fibrosis and Sleep, Emory University School of Medicine, Atlanta, GA, USA

Christopher D. Sheldon DM FRCP
Consultant Physician, Department of Respiratory Medicine, Royal Devon & Exeter Hospital, Exeter, UK

Samatha Sonnappa MD DCH MRCP FRCPH
Research Fellow and Honorary Consultant in Respiratory Medicine, Portex Anaesthesia, Intensive Therapy and Respiratory Medicine Unit, Great Ormond Street Hospital for Children and Institute of Child Health, London, UK

Kevin W. Southern PhD MRCP MBChB
Senior Lecturer and Honorary Consultant in Pediatric Respiratory Medicine, Institute of Child Health, University of Liverpool, and Royal Liverpool Children's Hospital, Liverpool, UK

Harm A. W. M. Tiddens MD PhD
Associated Professor in Pediatric Pulmonology, Chair CF-Team, Department of Pediatrics, ErasmusMC-Sophia Children's Hospital

Catherine E. Urch PhD MRCP
Honorary Senior Lecturer, UCL and Imperial College London; Consultant Palliative Medicine, Department Palliative Care, St Mary's and Royal Brompton Hospitals, London, UK

Colin Wallis MBChB DCH FCP MD MRCP FRCPCH
Respiratory Pediatrician, Great Ormond Street Hospital for Children, London, UK

Sarah Walters OBE MB FRCP FFPH
Senior Clinical Lecturer in Public Health and Epidemiology, Department of Public Health & Epidemiology, University of Birmingham, Birmingham, UK

David Westaby MA FRCP
Consultant Gastroenterologist and Hepatologist, Hammersmith Hospitals Trust, Honorary Senior Lecturer, Imperial College Medicine School, London, UK

Susan P. Wolfe BSc DipDiet RD
Chief Pediatric Dietitian, Regional Pediatric Cystic Fibrosis Unit, St James' University Hospital, Leeds, UK

Preface

Just as the face of cystic fibrosis has changed, from a respiratory and digestive disease of children to a multisystem disease predominantly of adults, so the 3rd edition of this book is radically different from the 2nd edition, published in 2000. The chapters have been reorganized into seven main sections, and all have been completely rewritten. Many of the authors from the previous edition have been retired, with great thanks, and some have taken on new tasks, and more than thirty new authors, and a third editor, have been recruited. We have tried to keep this edition the same length as its predecessor, by ensuring the old was excised to make way for the new.

Although this is, in effect, a completely new book, the opening chapter is rooted in the past, with an account of the great achievements of our forebears in describing and understanding the treatment and science of cystic fibrosis. This is followed by an epidemiological description of where we are now. Subsequent chapters describe basic science for the clinician, diagnostic aspects of the disease (including how to manage the screened patient), the clinical aspects, monitoring of the disease, and a complete section, that evolved from a single chapter, on multidisciplinary care. It ends with a chapter which looks to the future – which may be required reading in ten years time,

as an illustration of how wrong the most educated of guesses may be.

This is a book aimed primarily for clinicians with all degrees of experience, who we hope will learn from our authors – as we have done. It is predominantly a clinical book, but with scientific sections that are intended to be accessible to the interested clinician. We also hope that the scientist who wishes to find out more about cystic fibrosis will find the clinical sections informative.

We want to thank all the authors for their hard work and forbearance of our importuning; the publishers, in particular Heather Fyfe, for keeping us on track and ensuring the highest standards in production of the volume; and we ask the partners, family and friends of all concerned, authors, publishers and editors, to forgive us for the long hours consumed during the gestation of this volume. We hope the end-product in small measure repays their patience.

Finally, our chief thanks are due to our teachers – the patients and their families – from whom we have learned all we know about cystic fibrosis.

Margaret Hodson
Duncan Geddes
Andrew Bush

PART 1

INTRODUCTION: WHAT IS CYSTIC FIBROSIS?

1   History of cystic fibrosis   3
    James M. Littlewood
2   Epidemiology of cystic fibrosis   21
    Sarah Walters and Anil Mehta

History of cystic fibrosis

JAMES M. LITTLEWOOD

Cystic fibrosis (CF) is the most common life-shortening inherited disorder of Caucasian people. The incidence of around 1 in 2500 births is remarkably high as, until relatively recently, most affected children died in infancy or early childhood from pneumonia and malnutrition.

BEFORE THE NINETEEN THIRTIES

The first accurate description of the *swollen hardened gleaming white pancreas* likely to be due to CF was in an autopsy report on a supposedly 'bewitched' 11-year-old girl in 1595 by Pieter Pauw, Professor of Botany and Anatomy at Leiden (1564–1617). From the middle of the seventeenth century there were many reports of infants who almost certainly had CF described in detail by Busch [1,2,3] even earlier than the well-known quotation of Rochholz that 'The child will soon die whose brow tastes salty when kissed' in an almanac of children's songs and games from Switzerland [4]. Other versions of this prophecy include 'If it tastes salty when someone is kissed on the brow then this person is hexed [bewitched]' in a dictionary of the Swiss–German language [5]. In 1838, Rokitansky described the autopsy findings of ileal perforation and meconium peritonitis in a premature child likely to have had meconium ileus [6]. Landsteiner gave a clear description of the pancreatic lesions in an infant with meconium ileus [7].

In 1888, Samuel Gee described children with the appearances of severe intestinal malabsorption as having the 'celiac affection' with an arrest of growth, a distended abdomen, and attacks of diarrhea with large, pale, foul-smelling stools [8]. The cause was unknown but it became apparent that the syndrome was caused by a number of different conditions. The causative role of gluten in celiac disease, as we know it today, was not identified until 1950 [9]. There were infants reported with the clinical syndrome described by Gee who at autopsy had definite histological changes in the pancreas and lungs [10–14]. The pancreatic histology of all these patients was typical of the changes that Dorothy Andersen subsequently described using the term 'cystic fibrosis' [15].

THE NINETEEN THIRTIES

'CYSTIC FIBROSIS OF THE PANCREAS' RECOGNIZED AS A SPECIFIC ENTITY

Margaret Harper of Sydney, who earlier had reported two children with congenital pancreatic steatorrhea [16], described a further eight children with clinical features compatible with cystic fibrosis. At autopsy four had typical pancreatic changes [17]. Blackfan and Wolbach, reviewing the histological changes in eleven children with vitamin A deficiency, noted six had extensive pancreatic lesions characterized by 'dilatation of the acini and ducts, inspissated secretion, atrophy of the acini, lymphoid and leukocyte infiltration to some degree and fibrosis'; they noted the lesions were 'all identical and presumably representing a disease entity' [18]. In 1936, Fanconi described two children with 'celiac syndrome' where 'the changes in the lungs and pancreas, two vital organs, are so profound that their failure appears understandable' [19]. Blackfan and May reported a further 35 infants with characteristic pancreatic histology and chronic lung infection [20], and other similar reports appeared in 1938 [21,22].

However, it was Dorothy Andersen (Fig. 1.1), the pathologist at the Babies' and Children's Hospital at Columbia Presbyterian Medical Center in New York, whose 1938 publication resulted in CF being recognized as a specific entity [15]. Andersen's meticulous study was initiated to review the clinical, laboratory and autopsy findings of children with celiac disease to define the criteria for identifying those whose condition was caused by pancreatic disease. She collected cases in which the presence of a definite pancreatic histological abnormality had been identified, and she described in

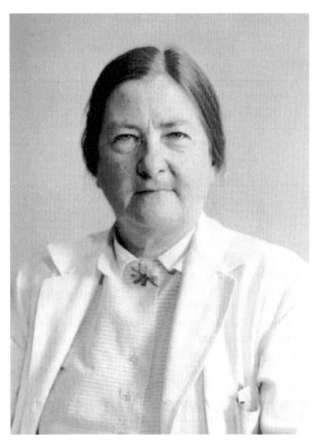

Figure 1.1 Dorothy Andersen 1901–1963.

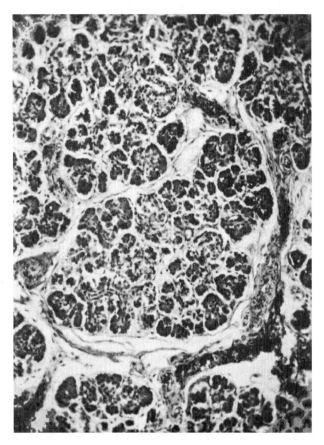

Figure 1.2 Normal pancreas in an infant at 3 days.

great detail the clinical and autopsy findings of 49 such children – 20 from her own hospital and others from colleagues and the literature. She described neonatal intestinal obstruction, later intestinal and respiratory complications and many other features, but particularly the striking characteristic pancreatic histology (Figs 1.2 and 1.3) [15]. The epithelial metaplasia characteristic of vitamin A deficiency was present in 14 of the 49 infants, and Andersen suggested that vitamin A deficiency, resulting from the severe intestinal malabsorption, predisposed to the respiratory infections and bronchiectasis [23,24].

THE NINETEEN FORTIES

A RECESSIVELY INHERITED MULTISYSTEM DISORDER

Despite Andersen's clear description of CF in 1938, 'knowledge and recognition of the disease were almost nil for several years' [25]. The few publications on CF came from North America; also Europe was heavily involved in the Second World War. Charles May, from the Babies' Hospital, New York, then a major in the US army, spoke on CF at a meeting of the Royal Society of Medicine in London and gave a succinct description of the 35 children with CF identified in Boston from 2800 pediatric autopsies over 15 years [26].

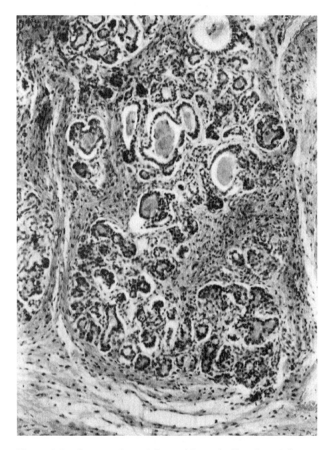

Figure 1.3 Pancreas in an infant with cystic fibrosis at 6 days [15], showing dilatation of the acini and ducts, inspissated secretions, atrophy of the acini, leukocyte infiltration and fibrosis.

The familial incidence of CF was soon noted and a Mendelian recessive mode of inheritance recognized [27,28]. Sydney Farber, pathologist at the Children's Hospital, Boston, recognized that CF was a generalized disorder affecting organs other than the pancreas and introduced the term 'mucoviscidosis'. He concluded: 'The inspissation of altered secretions in the pancreatic acini is only a part of a generalized disorder of secretory mechanisms involving many glandular structures but exerting its greatest effect on the pancreas' [29].

RECENTLY AVAILABLE ANTIBIOTICS HAD AN OBVIOUS BENEFICIAL EFFECT

Paul di Sant'Agnese, for a time a pediatric colleague of Andersen's in New York, attributed the improved prognosis, which had occurred during the decade, to 'an appropriate diet began promptly and continued consistently, use of sulphadiazine during the stage of chronic cough, and the use of [nebulized] penicillin' [30]. The use of sulphonamides, particularly in the early phases of the chest infection, and penicillin from 1944 and later other antibiotics (chlortetracycline from 1948, oxytetracycline from 1950, chloramphenicol from 1951 and erythromycin from 1951), soon became the mainstay of the treatment. Most children soon became infected with *Staphylococcus aureus*, which responded convincingly to small, frequent doses of penicillin aerosol (20 000 units seven times daily) alone or with intramuscular penicillin. Di Sant'Agnese observed: 'In most patients the results were dramatic. From death's door, slowly dying from chronic pulmonary disease while we watched helplessly, patients revived in a few days' [25].

NUTRITION A MAJOR PROBLEM

Nutritional treatment in the 1940s included a high-protein diet, relatively crude pancreatic extract with meals and large doses of intramuscular vitamin A, deficiency of which Andersen still considered to be the underlying cause of the respiratory problems [24]. Although not all pediatricians were convinced pancreatin was of benefit, Archie Norman and colleagues in London showed considerable improvement in both fat absorption (increased from 46% to 71% of intake) and nitrogen excretion (decreased from 23.1 g to 10.7 g per day) in children with CF treated with 15 g of pancreatin four times daily [31].

The availability of penicillin from 1944 had an obvious beneficial effect in prolonging the survival of affected infants. But throughout the decade few people, including most doctors, had even heard of CF and the outlook remained very poor; for example 64% of patients in one Mayo Clinic series failed to reach 7 years [32].

THE NINETEEN FIFTIES

THE SWEAT TEST: A NEW ERA IN DIAGNOSIS

The diagnosis of CF was not straightforward and still relied on a combination of symptoms and signs of intestinal malabsorption supported by laboratory evidence of fat malabsorption and pancreatic insufficiency – the latter confirmed by measurement of enzyme activity in duodenal fluid obtained by intubation. A less invasive test to demonstrate trypsin activity in the stool, by digesting gelatine from X-ray film, had been described and received considerable attention, but problems occurred with the effects of intestinal bacteria [33].

During a New York heat wave in 1948, five of ten infants admitted to hospital with marked dehydration, fever and signs of circulatory collapse were already known to have CF; in two the serum chloride values were low [34]. Noticing that in subsequent summers children with CF seemed to be particularly intolerant of the heat, in 1952 di Sant'Agnese investigated sweating function of two teenagers with CF and two controls. The patients with CF had considerably higher sweat chloride, sodium and to a lesser extent potassium levels than the controls. Although initially these findings were received with considerable scepticism by some authorities, this quite fundamental observation was soon confirmed in a larger series of patients [35]. Unfortunately attempts by others to obtain sufficient sweat for analysis occasionally led to problems and at least one fatality was reported when, to promote sweating, 'the patient was placed in a plastic bag up to the neck and covered with a blanket' [36]. Fortunately, in 1959, Gibson and Cooke described their pilocarpine iontophoresis method of sweat stimulation, which still remains the standard method [37]. Using the sweat test, patients with sufficient pancreatic function to maintain normal intestinal fat absorption could be confirmed as having CF, and the infants whose intestinal malabsorption syndrome was due to CF could be more easily identified. Unfortunately, with more widespread use of the sweat test there was considerable potential for mistakes when inexperienced people carried out the test [38].

TREATMENT AND OUTLOOK CONTINUE TO IMPROVE AT A FEW CENTERS

In the USA the names of Paul di Sant'Agnese and Harry Shwachman are closely linked with many of the advances in treatment. In London, from 1950, Winifred Young recommended postural drainage, the traditional treatment for bronchiectasis, for children with cystic fibrosis [39]. Jocelyn Reed was the first to recommend 'tipping the patient so that gravity will assist in drainage, clapping and pressure vibrations during expiration are the most effective forms of mechanical stimulus to eliminate secretions' [40]. These so-called 'English' methods of physiotherapy were introduced in North America. Details of breathing exercises and postural drainage were published when Barbara Doyle, an Irish physiotherapist, was working with Shwachman in Boston during 1956–58 [41]. Although physiotherapy was accepted as an important component of treatment, some pediatricians remained unconvinced of its value – 'the ritual of carefully positioning the patient to drain every pulmonary segment separately is usually an exercise in futility' [42].

ANTIBIOTICS BECOME THE MAINSTAY OF TREATMENT

The definite benefits of antibiotic therapy became increasingly apparent. In 1958, Shwachman and Kulczycki described an improving outlook for children with CF and noted that survival into adult life occurred with increasing frequency [43]. Antibiotics (chlortetracycline or oxytetracycline) were recommended for episodes of infection and continuously for those who were chronically infected; large oral doses combined with chloramphenicol or erythromycin were given for more severe infections. Aerosol antibiotics, penicillin and streptomycin or neomycin and polymyxin, were added for more severe infections [44]; subsequently the latter were abandoned because of ototoxicity. The numerous side-effects resulting from the unusually prolonged and repeated use of antibiotics, now becoming an established feature of CF treatment, were reviewed in detail at a later date; e.g. allergic reactions, renal, auditory, eye problems and many others including bacterial resistance [45]. Penicillin-resistant *Staphylococcus aureus* and the appearance of mucoid *Pseudomonas aeruginosa* were, even then, emerging problems [46].

NEW FEATURES WITH LONGER SURVIVAL

As survival improved, many additional features of CF were described. The first studies of lung function in six patients aged 12–14 years clearly identified most of the important features of impaired lung function [47], confirmed in later studies [48]. The beneficial effect of bronchodilators was recognized by the end of the decade [49], also that cor pulmonale developed [50]. Bronchial obstruction with the typical upper lobar atelectasis and emphysema was described [51], as was the early generalized emphysema, which is present even in the absence of infection reflecting the airway obstruction [52]. Nasal polyposis, unusual in non-CF children, was reported [53].

NEONATAL AND GASTROINTESTINAL ADVANCES

Although the first infants to survive with meconium ileus were reported in 1942 [54], the Bishop and Koop ileostomy significantly improved the outlook [55]. Intestinal obstruction in an older child was described in 1941 [56]; later Jensen coined the term 'meconium ileus equivalent' [57] for the condition now termed 'distal intestinal obstruction syndrome' – still a common problem.

Other new features reported were patients with preservation of sufficient pancreatic function to achieve normal fat absorption [58]. The 'pancreatic sufficient' patients had a fat absorption of over 90% without enzyme replacement therapy, yet two that died had typical pancreatic histological changes [59]. Rectal prolapse was recognized as a relatively common occurrence in untreated patients [60]. Two patients with appendicular abscesses were mentioned as occurring from among 700 patients [61].

LIVER INVOLVEMENT RECOGNIZED AS A MAJOR FEATURE

Small areas of biliary fibrosis had been recognized previously at autopsy [15,28,29], and massive steatosis had been described in 1950 [62]. The authors of a more detailed report of five patients with hepatic cirrhosis suggested that protein deficiency secondary to the pancreatic dysfunction was responsible for the liver damage [63] – analogous to the earlier belief that the bronchial changes were secondary to vitamin A deficiency. Di Sant'Agnese gave a detailed description of the multilobular biliary cirrhosis present in seven of their 325 patients and also of the associated portal hypertension and suggested that liver involvement should be added to the major manifestations of the condition [64,65].

THE CLEVELAND TREATMENT PROGRAM: A PARADIGM FOR MODERN CF CARE

In 1957 in Cleveland, a young pediatrician, Leroy Matthews, was appointed to plan and initiate a 'comprehensive and prophylactic [preventive] treatment program' for CF, initially suggested and funded by the parents of children with cystic fibrosis [66]. The treatment program which Matthews developed included accurate early diagnosis by sweat tests, and *from diagnosis* (a major feature of the program) included regular physiotherapy, frequent follow-up with monthly respiratory cultures to guide antibiotic therapy using special microbiology techniques for CF sputum, regular nebulized treatment using phenylephrine as decongestant and propylene glycol as a mucolytic, and nocturnal mist tents [67]. The method of management had a significant effect on survival, reducing the annual mortality rate there from over 10% to 2% by 1960. The details and impressive results of Matthew's comprehensive treatment program from 1957 onwards were published in 1964 and 1965 [67–69]. In commenting on the Cleveland program, di Sant'Agnese questioned the need to start the full prophylactic therapy at diagnosis, tending to favor the more usual practice of starting treatment when there is an indication of 'incipient pulmonary involvement' [70]. The obvious success of CF center care was influential in the development of the US CF Foundation's Care Teaching and Research Center Program, which started in 1961.

The nineteen fifties – science

THE BASIC PATHOPHYSIOLOGY WAS CONFUSING

As Paul Quinton later observed, it was obvious to the pathologist that the disease was caused by abnormal mucus or proteinaceous inspissations in the lumen of the pancreas, lung and intestine. On the other hand, the sweat gland with its abnormally salty secretion, that produced no mentionable amount of mucus and showed no structural defects, became the clearest criterion for diagnosis [71].

Andersen also observed that the abnormal salt loss could not be attributed to an abnormality of mucus, suggesting the basic defect did not lie in the molecular structure of mucoproteins [72]. Abnormalities of the hormonal or autonomic control of pancreatic secretion were suggested even as far as affecting the respiratory physiology [73]. Stimulation of various abdominal viscera could cause bronchospasm. This excited considerable interest and even prompted an unsuccessful trial of splanchnicectomies (interruption of the splanchnic nerves to the pancreas) in 24 patients with CF [74].

THE NINETEEN SIXTIES

THE START OF NATIONAL AND INTERNATIONAL CF ORGANIZATIONS

The 1960s saw the start of many national CF organizations, usually following pressure from parents and engendering a collaborative approach between the medical community and the CF families. In North America, the National Cystic Fibrosis Research Foundation (now the Cystic Fibrosis Foundation) had been founded in 1955 and the Canadian Cystic Fibrosis Foundation in 1959. In Europe, the UK Cystic Fibrosis Research Trust (now the Cystic Fibrosis Trust) was formed in 1964, and in the following year the French Association Française de lutte contre la Mucoviscidose (now Vaincre la Mucoviscidose). Other national CF organizations followed in Western Europe and then Australia and New Zealand, and from the 1970s in South America [75].

In 1965, the International Cystic Fibrosis (Mucoviscidosis) Association (ICFMA), the predecessor of CF Worldwide, was formed at a steering meeting in Paris in 1964 under the medical chairmanship of Paul di Sant'Agnese, who endeavored to involve those European physicians with an interest in cystic fibrosis. He had visited Europe in 1960, meeting several interested Europeans including Guido Fanconi and Ettori Rossi in Switzerland, Andre Heenequet and Jan Feigleson in France, Archie Norman and David Lawson in England, de Toni in Italy, and Weijers, Dicke and van de Kamer in Holland. The aims of the ICFMA were to improve the care of children and adults who had CF, to foster research and to disseminate information. In 1969, there was the first informal meeting of Europeans in Interlaken organized by Ettori Rossi and then the first meeting of the European Working Group for Cystic Fibrosis in Cambridge, England (in 1998 this became the European Cystic Fibrosis Society).

EARLY NEONATAL CF SCREENING

The increased protein content of CF meconium [76] resulted in the development the BM (Boehringer–Mannheim) meconium test for neonatal CF screening; this was later abandoned due to the high incidence of false positive and false negative results. Other possibilities suggested for neonatal CF screening were analysis of the electrolyte content of nail clippings [77] or of the parotid secretion [78], or of sweat using a chloride electrode [79], the chloride plate test [80] and the immunoreactive trypsin test using the blood spots obtained for Guthrie testing [81]; the last was subsequently adopted by a number of neonatal CF screening programs.

PANCREATIC FUNCTION TESTS AND OTHER GASTROENTEROLOGICAL ADVANCES

Beat Hadorn used pancreozymin–secretin stimulation tests of pancreatic function in children with CF, using a triple lumen tube and showed the pancreatic secretion to be of low volume with low enzyme and bicarbonate levels; he considered this to result in stagnation of pancreatic secretion and enzymes causing damage to the pancreatic ducts [82]. However, as the sweat test was now the main diagnostic test available in larger units, rather than the enzyme content of duodenal fluid, pancreatic insufficiency was more conveniently confirmed by the less invasive measurement of fecal trypsin and chymotrypsin activity [83]. The new technique of per-oral small intestinal biopsy to identify the characteristic duodenal subtotal villous atrophy of gluten-induced celiac disease allowed further clear separation of this condition from CF [84]. Celiac disease is slightly more common in CF than in the general population [85]. The characteristic histological appearance of the small intestine [86] and rectal mucosa [87] were described in detail. When the sweat test result was marginal and the diagnosis in doubt, the failure of oral 9α-fluorohydrocortisone to significantly decrease the sweat electrolyte levels in people with CF was helpful [88].

PSEUDOMONAS AERUGINOSA INFECTION AND OTHER RESPIRATORY DEVELOPMENTS

The mucoid form of *Pseudomonas aeruginosa* was described in 1964 but opinions still differed as to its importance as a pathogen [89]. Measures of respiratory function were becoming more common to show the day-to-day variability and the response to bronchodilators [90], and improvement in respiratory function of infants less than 9 months old after inhaled propylene glycol and bronchodilators [91]. The important association of allergic bronchopulmonary aspergillosis and CF was reported in 1965 [92]. There were a number of reports of pneumothorax following the initial recognition of this complication [93]. The side-effects resulting from the prolonged and repeated use of antibiotics – particularly staining of the teeth from tetracyclines [94] and optic atrophy from prolonged chloramphenicol therapy [95] – were an increasing cause for concern.

THE RISE AND FALL OF THE MIST TENT

The use of nocturnal mist tents to moisten the airway secretions became a major component of CF treatment in North America. Originally suggested by Robert Denton, the mist tent is the only major component of the Cleveland program not used today [96]. Some objective evidence of clinical improvement during mist tent therapy was published [97]; in fact, di Sant'Agnese commented: 'It is generally accepted by almost all clinicians who have had adequate experience with this disease that patients have considerable benefit from such a treatment program' [98]. However, further studies were deemed to show little or no lung deposition of fluid or improvement in pulmonary function and the treatment was eventually discontinued [99].

MAINTAINING A GOOD NUTRITIONAL STATE IN OLDER CHILDREN: A MAJOR PROBLEM

The growth and nutritional state of most children who survived was poor, with progressive deterioration through childhood as their condition worsened [100]. More invasive methods of nutritional support were not introduced until the 1980s. Hence the great interest in anabolic steroids, which were reported to achieve 'remarkable gains in weight' in some children with CF [101] and gained some popularity [102]. Acetyl cysteine was recommended for recurrent abdominal pain [103] and gastrografin enemas for meconium ileus [104]. An infant was described with both celiac disease and CF [105]. The association with diabetes mellitus was recognized [106], and there was considerable literature on the relationship with CF from many centers around Europe including reports of the glucose and insulin levels in children with cystic fibrosis [107].

A FEW ADULTS BUT A BLEAK OUTLOOK FOR MOST CHILDREN

Although there were reports of an improving outlook from a few centers, most affected children still died in early childhood and the nature of the basic defect remained unknown. Sir Robert Johnson, a CF parent and founder member of the UK Cystic Fibrosis Trust, recalls the situation facing most CF families in the UK in the 1960s: 'The general picture here was of ignorance and distress, unmitigated by hope or practical effective action' [108]. However, there were a few reports of older children and adults with CF, and the first clinic for adults was started in London by Sir John Batten [109]. Some adult patients had presented unusually late in childhood or adolescence; for example, 31 of Shwachman's 65 older patients were not diagnosed until after 10 years of age, and 65% were males – features noted in some subsequent reports of older patients [110]. This suggested that some were patients with milder disease, supported by the fact that their condition did not correlate with the age of diagnosis or length or adequacy of follow-up. Shwachman also mentioned other important factors that contributed to improved survival, including:

> our constant availability for guidance and harmonious relationship to the family physician or pediatrician and of highly skilled experts in our medical center, our

attempt to secure financial assistance and provide continuous long-term care by the same group of individuals regardless of the age of the patient coupled with efforts to instruct our parents and above all our positive approach undoubtedly contributes to the relative success of our programme and survival of some of these patients beyond adolescence.

Infertility of virtually all men with CF was reported [111] due to structural abnormalities of the vas deferens and epididymis [112]; also, the first pregnancy of a woman with CF was reported but the patient died 6 weeks after the birth [113].

The nineteen sixties – science

FEW PEOPLE WITH CF AND FEW SCIENTISTS INVOLVED IN CF RESEARCH

Diverse subjects investigated at the time included the composition of the airway secretions [114] and the characteristics of human epithelium [115]. Cultured fibroblasts from CF patients developed more metachromatically stained granules compared with those from unaffected subjects [116]. There was considerable interest in the finding that serum from people with CF induced marked dyskinesia in the action of the cilia in rabbit tracheal tissue when applied to the surface [117], a finding repeated with oyster cilia [118]. John Mangos and co-workers reported that when sweat or saliva from people with CF was applied to the surface of rat salivary gland ducts or human gland ducts, active sodium absorption was inhibited [119]. None of these observations significantly clarified the basic pathophysiology of the condition but did raise the possibility of a circulating 'CF factor'.

THE NINETEEN SEVENTIES

IMPROVED EXPECTATIONS, TREATMENT AND OUTCOME IN SELECTED CENTERS

There were few specialist CF centers in any country and many children were treated at their local hospital and most died in childhood. Even in some recognized CF centers, 'the care was relatively unsophisticated. Patients were seen in the clinic at intervals of several months, were admitted to the hospital only when they developed serious pulmonary disease and were generally expected to die early' [120].

Yet there were some encouraging reports. The results of Margaret Mearns and Winifred Young at the Queen Elizabeth Hospital in London, one of the few UK centers, were comparable with best centers in the USA with a 45% survival to age 20 years. From the mid-1950s their young patients had received prophylactic antistaphylococcal drugs, usually erythromycin, for the first year, early appropriate and prolonged antibiotic treatment for new respiratory symptoms, regular physiotherapy and frequent follow-up. Although there was still some question as to the pathogenicity of *Pseudomonas aeruginosa*, intravenous gentamicin and carbenicillin were used if the patient was generally ill [121,122]. David Lawson advocated the use of continuous prophylactic anti-staphylococcal antibiotics from diagnosis [123], a practice eventually supported to the age of 2 years by a relatively small trial in the UK [124], but the evidence is still not completely clear [125]. Intravenous antibiotics were used more frequently in some CF centers and regimens for their use in CF were established. In some CF centers in the United States, the 50% survival increased to well beyond age 18 years and was attributed to improvements in antimicrobial therapy, routes of delivery, and increased therapeutic aggressiveness [126]. The increasing prevalence of *Pseudomonas aeruginosa* respiratory infection and the use of gentamicin and tobramycin, and later carbenicillin and ticarcillin, all of which required systemic administration, resulted in the more general use of the intravenous rather than the intramuscular route.

CYSTIC FIBROSIS: 'A NOT SO FATAL DISEASE'

Douglas Crozier (who, in 1958, started the CF clinic at the Hospital for Sick Children, Toronto) reflected this improving outlook in his paper 'Cystic fibrosis – a not so fatal disease' [127]. As early as 1972, his patients were advised to take a high-saturated-fat diet of whole milk, butter, eggs and animal fats which did require them to take between 60 and 100 pancreatic enzyme capsules (Cotazym) each day, compared with the then conventional advice to have a low-fat diet to reduce unpleasant abdominal symptoms. Later, the better survival of these Toronto patients than others in Canada and in Boston was attributed to their superior nutritional state [128].

THE DANISH APPROACH IMPROVES THE PROGNOSIS

In some European clinics this lack of acceptance of the status-quo approach was also evident. For example, the Danish CF clinic in Copenhagen, where 80% of the country's 225 patients were treated, was established as a national CF center in 1968 by Erhard Flensborg [129]. In 1976, it was shown that the presence of chronic *Pseudomonas aeruginosa* infection was closely associated with a poor prognosis [130]. Therefore a policy of regular 3-monthly courses of intravenous anti-pseudomonal antibiotics for chronically infected patients was started and was associated with a fall in annual mortality from 10–20% in 1976 to only 1–2% in 1984–85 [131]. Also, from 1981, cohort isolation of patients in the clinic was introduced – separating those with chronic *Pseudomonas aeruginosa* from uninfected patients. Long-term inhaled colistin was introduced in 1987 for chronically infected patients [132], and from 1989 inhaled colistin and oral ciprofloxacin was used to eradicate early *Pseudomonas*

infection [133]. These treatment changes were eventually reflected by an impressive improvement in survival [134].

LONGER SURVIVAL WITH WORSENING CHRONIC INFECTION COMPROMISED NUTRITION

As survival improved there was an increasing interest in the chronic nutritional problems that developed in the adolescents. A number of important studies in the late 1970s and early 1980s reported that the daily energy intake of people with CF, most of whom were on a restricted fat intake, was frequently even less than that recommended for healthy children of their age [135]. There was considerable interest in a nutritional supplement consisting of beef serum protein hydrolysate, a glucose polymer and medium-chain triglycerides (the 'Allan diet') that was reported to improve weight gain [136], a finding supported by subsequent trials [137]. However, the more effective new acid-resistant pancreatic enzymes were soon to become available, permitting most patients a normal fat intake – a more palatable way of increasing their energy intake. Towards the end of the 1970s there was further evidence that a good nutritional state was shown to be associated with a better prognosis [138]. A new complication, recurrent acute pancreatitis, was reported in ten adolescents and young adults, all of whom were pancreatic sufficient [139].

Abnormalities of essential fatty acids had been noted by many authors from the 1960s [140] and subsequently [141] and were even suggested as the primary metabolic abnormality. Bob Elliott in New Zealand reported an unusually favorable clinical course in a child with CF treated with intravenous infusions of soya oil emulsion, which contains mainly linoleic acid, as well as in further treated children [142,143].

IMMUNOREACTIVE TRYPSIN: A RELIABLE TEST FOR NEONATAL CF SCREENING

The measurement of immunoreactive trypsin (IRT) in the blood spots collected from newborns for metabolic screening was the first reliable test for neonatal CF screening [81]. The test was soon used in a number of neonatal CF screening programs and eventually in most combined with DNA testing [144]. However, it was apparent from the West Midlands and Wales UK study during the 1980s that early diagnosis following neonatal screening must also be followed by effective treatment, of the type available at a CF center, to show a long-term advantage for the screened infants [145]. Now that more effective treatment is available, early diagnosis is an established advantage in terms of growth [146] and even cognitive development [147].

NATIONAL CF REGISTRIES: AN ESSENTIAL PROVISION TO MONITOR PROGRESS

Data collection was becoming increasingly important on both a national and local CF center basis. The CF

Foundation's patient registry, developed by Warren Warwick from 1964 onwards [148], had demonstrated a rise in median survival from 14 years in 1968 to 20 years in 1977. Also, Norman and colleagues published a series of papers between 1966 and 1975 recording the improving prognosis in the UK [149]. Between 1943 and 1964, 80% died by age 5 years and 90% by age 10 years; and 70% of infants with meconium ileus succumbed by age 3 months. Mary Corey had started data collection at the Toronto CF clinic during the 1970s [150]. In 1995, the UK CF Database (www.cystic-fibrosis.org.uk) replaced the original CF Survey started by the working party in 1982 [151]; the UK CF Database was replaced by CF Trust's CF Registry in 2007.

As a result of data from various registries, it became clear that, although there was a steady improvement in the condition and survival of many people with CF, there were significant differences in the treatment, condition and even survival of patients attending different CF centers. In a study reflecting care through the 1970s, the median survival ages at three recognized US centers were 9.5, 18.1 and 22.8 years, respectively; it was considered that the differences reflected the different degree of supervision (number of clinic visits) and intensity of treatment (days of intravenous antibiotics) the patients received [152]. The philosophy of a comprehensive treatment program recommended by Matthews and his colleagues, by Shwachman, and subsequently by Crozier and others, had a major influence on CF care in the 1970s but unfortunately remained confined to a few CF centers and available to only a minority of people with cystic fibrosis.

The nineteen seventies – science

INTERESTING BUT DISPARATE FINDINGS: A SEARCH FOR THE 'CF FACTOR'

Scientists continued to search in vain for a lead to the basic defect. As one experienced CF center director observed: 'Not professing to be a scientist or bench researcher, the unmet challenges that confront me every day as a clinician seem more distant and insolvable than they did thirty years ago' [153].

A unique protein band was described in CF serum electrophoresed through a pH gradient to its point of electric focus [154]. However, despite a great deal of research, neither isoelectric focusing nor using gels from isoelectric focusing to raise antibodies permitted accurate identification of the elusive 'CF factor' [155]. Lieberman described an elevated protein with lectin-like binding properties in the blood that was postulated to stimulate increased mucus production [156]. A variety of other metabolic abnormalities were described. Extensive research into bronchial mucus and its glycoproteins led to no definite conclusions, which had a bearing on the etiology [157]. However, Yeates's paper on mucociliary transport rates in humans did stimulate research into the epithelial transport of water and electrolytes [158].

In summary, although during the 1970s some clinical progress was made in a few centers in controlling the secondary effects of the CF defect, generally progress was limited. Neither the location of the CF gene nor the underlying mechanisms of its serious pathophysiological effects were known.

THE NINETEEN EIGHTIES

A DECADE OF EXCEPTIONAL CLINICAL AND SCIENTIFIC PROGRESS

At the start of the 1980s the basic defect was unknown and the chromosome on which the CF gene was located had not been identified but by the end of the decade the CF gene and its main function had been identified [159–161].

During the decade pre-natal diagnosis was pioneered by David Brock of Edinburgh [162], which improved in accuracy when new linked probes were described in 1985 [163] allowing families with an affected child to have reliable pre-natal diagnosis in subsequent pregnancies [164].

There were major advances in clinical care virtually all of which occurred at the increasing number of CF centers. Cystic fibrosis center care was already well established in a few, but by no means all, cities in the UK but still available to only a minority of families. Survival was reported to be better in Victoria, Australia, where all patients had specialist CF center care, than in England and Wales where the majority attended the pediatric clinic at their local hospital [165]. These results prompted the formation of the British Paediatric Association's UK Working Party on Cystic Fibrosis (WPCF) in 1982, whose main recommendation was that all people with CF should have some contact with a specialist CF center, as only half the UK patients had such contact at the time [166].

NEW TECHNIQUES OF PHYSIOTHERAPY

Various new devices and physiotherapy techniques were described during the decade [167–169] and exercise received more attention. An increasing proportion of people with CF received treatment from physiotherapists experienced in cystic fibrosis. In the USA, the mechanical therapy vest proved increasingly popular with many patients but, even now, it is rarely used in the UK [170].

MORE ANTIBIOTICS AND IMPROVED METHODS OF ADMINISTRATION

There was renewed interest in the use of nebulized anti-pseudomonal antibiotics after nebulized gentamicin and carbenicillin were shown to stabilize the condition of adults chronically infected with *Pseudomonas aeruginosa* [171]. This proved to be a major advance despite some initial reservations regarding the development of bacterial resistance. Also there was a short report of successful eradication of early infection with *P. aeruginosa* using nebulized colomycin, thus delaying or preventing chronic *P. aeruginosa* infection [172]. The feasibility and success of early eradication of *P. aeruginosa* was later confirmed in a controlled trial from Denmark using nebulized colomycin and oral ciprofloxacin [133]. Early eradication gradually became established practice in Europe [173] and resulted in a significant reduction in the number of patients with chronic *Pseudomonas* infection in centers where early treatment was used [174,175]. Early eradication of *P. aeruginosa* eventually became accepted practice in North America following a controlled trial of inhaled tobramycin [176].

During the decade there was earlier, more frequent and more effective use of intravenous antibiotics at all stages of infection [177]. Expert microbiological support, the use of two antibiotics, ensuring adequate blood levels, allowing for the altered pharmacokinetics in CF and also for the stage of the infection, gradually became routine practice in most CF centers. Intensive courses of intravenous antibiotics became routine treatment for exacerbations of chest infection, and in Denmark regular 3-monthly 2-week courses of intravenous antibiotics were given to most patients who were chronically infected with *P. aeruginosa* [178]. New anti-pseudomonal antibiotics became available permitting a wider choice of treatment as bacterial resistance became more common (azlocillin from 1980, piperacillin from 1982, netilmicin from 1982, ceftazidime from 1983, aztreonam from 1986 and oral ciprofloxacin from 1986). With more frequent use of antibiotics, however, side-effects were an increasing problem [45,94,95].

There were improved techniques for establishing and maintaining intravenous access with heparin locks [179], butterfly cannulas, percutaneous silastic catheters, long lines and central venous catheters. Constant intravenous infusion pumps permitted maintenance of intravenous lines for many days at very slow flow rates (particularly useful in small children), and totally implantable venous access devices greatly reduced the stress and trauma of repeated venous access [180,181]. From 1984, EMLA local anesthetic cream was routinely applied before venepunctures – a major advance for all children requiring repeated venepunctures [182] The increasing reliance on and more frequent use of intravenous antibiotics resulted in an increasing use of home intravenous antibiotics supervised by specialized CF staff – usually a CF Specialist Nurse [183,184].

There were hopes that regular oral corticosteroids would reduce the damaging effects of inflammation [185]; but although children receiving alternate-day prednisone had better pulmonary function and reduced morbidity compared to controls, the frequent side-effects precluded the more general use of oral steroids.

TREATMENT FOR CF-RELATED LIVER DISEASE

In 1989, Carla Colombo from Milan reported the beneficial effect of regular ursodeoxycholic acid treatment in improving liver function tests in CF-related liver disease [186]. Prior to this there had been no specific treatment for liver involvement. The suggestion by Kevin Gaskin that common bile duct stenosis was important in CF liver disease [187] was not supported by subsequent studies [188]. Liver transplantation has been used successfully in patients with CF and the results are surprisingly good. Lung function, far from deteriorating as a result of the long operation, improved in some patients [189]. Successful heart–lung–liver transplantations [190] and lung–liver transplantations have been performed [191].

ACID-RESISTANT PANCREATIC ENZYMES: A MAJOR NUTRITIONAL ADVANCE

The nutritional state of many patients continued to improve due the more widespread identification and correction of their inadequate energy intake [192]. The new acid-resistant enzymes were obviously more effective than the older unprotected preparations [193–195]. Undoubtedly these new enzymes were one of the major advances in treatment during the decade. They improved not only fat absorption and the nutritional state but also the symptoms and quality of life of the many patients, most of whom could now tolerate a normal fat intake [196].

MORE AGGRESSIVE NUTRITIONAL SUPPORT

Enteral feeding, first by the nasogastric route [197] and then by gastrostomy [198,199], allowed rehabilitation of those with severe malnutrition, allowing reasonable nutritional state to be maintained even in many of the most severely affected patients (e.g. those awaiting transplantation). The first of a number of studies reported increased energy expenditure to be a major factor contributing to malnutrition [200]. Fat-soluble vitamin deficiencies were identified and corrected by appropriate doses of suitable supplements with varying success [201–203]. Oral gastrografin was introduced as a treatment for meconium ileus equivalent – a treatment that is still widely used [204].

ORGAN TRANSPLANTATIONS

A major advance, for those who had reached the end stages of their disease, was the successful introduction of heart–lung transplantation in 1985 [205,206]. The possibility of successful treatment in the terminal stages of the condition had an obvious major influence not only on the prognosis but also on the treatment of severely affected individuals. The first results of heart–lung transplantations were quite remarkable and were related to surgical skills, to concentrated medical expertise in assessment and to aftercare, as well as to the availability of more effective immunosuppressive therapy to prevent organ rejection [207]. Later, double lung transplants became more popular [208]. Living-donor lung transplants have proved successful in some centers and will be chosen by some families [209].

INCREASING NEED FOR MORE CF CENTERS FOR ADULTS

As the population and age of people with CF increased, pediatric CF centers developed in most large cities in many countries. Towards the end of the 1980s, as a reflection of the improving survival, more CF centers for adults were required and gradually developed [210]. Arrangements for transition from pediatric to adult care received, and continues to receive, much attention [211].

The nineteen eighties – science

FROM EPITHELIAL TRANSPORT ABNORMALITY TO THE IDENTIFICATION OF THE GENE

In 1981, Michael Knowles and colleagues demonstrated an abnormal potential difference in the nasal mucosa of patients with CF thus providing direct evidence of primary epithelial dysfunction [212]. In 1983, Paul Quinton showed that the chloride impermeability he had demonstrated in sweat glands was the basis for the raised sweat electrolytes in patients with cystic fibrosis [213]. These were the most important advances to date in understanding the basic defect as a cell membrane transport problem and provided the first description of the basic cellular defect that has since been seen in all CF-affected cells. It was apparent that the problems with mucus were not due to abnormalities with its synthesis or composition, rather the fluid environment into which it was secreted.

SEARCH FOR AND IDENTIFICATION OF THE CF GENE

From the early 1980s, various groups attempted to identify the CF gene by using 'reverse genetics', as the protein was unknown. Families with more than one affected child were studied. In 1985, using this technique, Eiberg in Copenhagen demonstrated a linkage to the enzyme paraoxinase, which exists in two forms but was present in the same form in 90% of CF siblings [214]. In the same year, Lap-Chee Tsui in Toronto, in a series of mouse hybrid experiments, demonstrated a marker on chromosome 7 linked to both paraoxinase and cystic fibrosis [215]. Other markers, known to be on chromosome 7, were closely linked to CF, the *Met* oncogenes, *Met H* and *Met D* from Ray White in Salt Lake City [216] and the DNA probe pJ3.11 from Bob Williamson's laboratory in London [217]. In 1989, the CF gene was eventually identified by teams headed by Lap-Chee Tsui, Francis Collins and Jack Riordan and termed the 'cystic fibrosis transmembrane conductance regulator'. This was reported in three papers in a memorable issue of *Science* [159–161].

IMPLICATIONS OF IDENTIFICATION OF THE GENE

Since 1989, well over 1000 different CF gene mutations have been described (www.genet.sickkids.onca/cftr). There have been a number of practical benefits for the patients and their families. Carrier detection, accurate antenatal diagnosis and incorporation of DNA testing into the many IRT neonatal screening programs have been major advances. Attempts to correlate phenotype and genotype have proved less successful than at first expected but the major influence of environmental factors has been a confounding factor [218]. However, the definite correlation of so-called 'mild' mutations with preservation of sufficient pancreatic function to achieve normal fat absorption ('pancreatic sufficiency') and better clinical condition is now well established [219]. Also, certain mild mutations are associated with late-presenting disease often with normal pancreatic function and normal or near-normal sweat electrolytes [220]. An association of congenital bilateral absence of the vas deferens (CBAVD) in infertile males has been associated with a high incidence of CF mutations, some with two mutations, the most common being *DF508/R117H* – somewhat blurring the edges of the traditional CF diagnosis [221]. A significant proportion of people with idiopathic pancreatitis, but who do not have CF, have been found to be carriers of a CF mutation [222].

NOW AND THE FUTURE

The improvements in clinical care at the CF centers, which characterized the 1980s, continue to the present. The realization that cross-infection with both *Burkholderia cepacia* [223, 224] and *Pseudomonas aeruginosa* [225,226] was a major problem had a profound influence on both hospital practice and the social lives of people with cystic fibrosis. Neonatal screening, early diagnosis and treatment before any chronic pulmonary damage, early eradication treatment of *Pseudomonas* to prevent or delay chronic infection, the introduction of effective new drugs such as rhDNase [227], antibiotic formulations designed specifically for inhalation [228] and the widespread use of the macrolides [229] are likely to be reflected in a continuing improvement in health and survival of people with cystic fibrosis. However, the increasing number of adults with CF has resulted in more attention being given to problems of diabetes mellitus [230], osteoporosis [231], liver disease [232], pregnancy [233] and infertility [234].

In slightly less than 70 years CF has moved from a little known genetic condition, usually fatal in infancy and early childhood, to a complex multisystem disorder now affecting as many adults as children. The abnormality of cell membrane transport has been recognized and finally the CF gene identified. The increasingly successful control of the secondary effects of the basic defect is due largely to advances in treatment developed at CF centers which have resulted in clear treatment protocols [235,236] and efforts to ensure that these are available to all people with cystic fibrosis [237]. Treatment to correct or modify the basic defect by gene replacement or pharmacological means are showing considerable promise and likely to have a major influence on treatment regimens within a few years.

REFERENCES

1. Busch R. On the history of cystic mucoviscidosis. *Deutsche Gesundhs* 1978; **33**:316.

2. Busch R. The history of cystic fibrosis. *Acta Univ Carol Med* 1990; **36**:13–15.

3. Busch R. What do we know about the history of cystic fibrosis? *Quebec Adult CF Newsletter* 2005; 28–30.

4. Rochholz EL. 'The child will soon die whose brow tastes salty when kissed'. In the *Almanac of Children's Songs and Games from Switzerland*. Leipzig, JJ Weber, 1857.

5. Pfyffer JX. Zit bei 46: *Zitierend aus dem Wörterbuch der Schweizerdeutschen Sprache* 7, 1848, 899.

6. Rokitansky C von. *Sections-Protokoll und Gutachten*. Wien, 4. April 1838.

7. Landsteiner K. Darmverschluss durch eingedichtes Meconium. Pankreatitis. *Zentralbl f. Allg Path* 1905; **16**:903–907.

8. Gee S. On the coeliac affection. *St Bartholomew's Hospital Report* 1888; **24**:17–20.

9. Dicke WK, Weijers HA, van de Kamer JH. Coeliac disease: the presence in wheat of a factor having a deleterious effect in cases of coeliac disease. *Acta Paediatr Scand* 1953; **42**:344–399.

10. Passini F. Pankreaserkrangkung als Ursache des Nichtgedeihens von Kindern. *Deutsch Med Wchnschr* 1919; **45**:851–853.

11. Clarke CG, Hadfield G. Congenital pancreatic disease with infantilism. *Q J Med* 1924; **17**:358–364.

12. Burghard E. Diseases of the pancreas in infancy. *Klin Wchnschr* 1925; **4**:2305.

13. Gross F. Pancreatic atrophy in infancy and childhood. *Jahrb f Kinderh* 1926; **112**:251.

14. Hess JH, Saphire O. Celiac disease. Chronic intestinal indigestion: a report of three cases with autopsy findings. *J Pediatr* 1935; **6**:1–13.

15. Andersen DH. Cystic fibrosis of the pancreas and its relation to celiac disease: a clinical and pathological study. *Am J Dis Child* 1938; **56**:344-9-9.

16. Harper MH. Two cases of congenital pancreatic steatorrhoea with infantilism. *Med J Aust* 1930; **2**:663.

17. Harper MH. Congenital steatorrhoea due to pancreatic defect. *Arch Dis Child* 1938; **13**:45–56.

18. Blackfan KD, Wolbach SB. Vitamin A deficiency in infants: a clinical and pathological study. *J Pediatr* 1933; **3**:679–706.

19. Fanconi G, Uehlinger E, Knauer C. Das coeliakie syndrom bei angeborener zystischer pancreasfibromatose und bronchiektasien. *Wien Med Wchnschr* 1936; **86**:753–756.

20. Blackfan KD, May CD. Inspissation of secretion and dilatation of ducts and acini: atrophy and fibrosis of the pancreas in infants. A clinical note. *Pediatrics* 1938; **13**:624–637.

21. Thomas J, Schultz FW. Pancreatic steatorrhoea. *Am J Dis Child* 1938; **56**:336–343.

22. Rauch S, Litvak AM, Steiner M. Congenital familial steatorrhoea with fibromatosis of the pancreas and bronchiectasis. *J Pediatr* 1939; **14**:462–490.

23. Andersen DH. Cystic fibrosis of the pancreas, vitamin A deficiency and bronchiectasis. *J Pediatr* 1939; **15**:763–771.

24. Andersen DH. The present diagnosis and treatment of cystic fibrosis. *Proc R Soc Med* 1949; **42**:25–31.

25. di Sant'Agnese PA. Experiences of a pioneer researcher: discovery of the sweat electrolyte defect and the early medical history of cystic fibrosis. In: Doershuk CF (ed.) *Cystic Fibrosis in the 20th century*. Cleveland, AM Publishing, 2001, pp17–35.

26. May CD. Fibrosis of pancreas in infants and children. *Proc R Soc Med* 1943; **37**:311–313.

27. Andersen DH, Hodges RC. Celiac syndrome. V: Genetics of cystic fibrosis of the pancreas with a consideration of etiology. *Am J Dis Child* 1946; **72**:62–80.

28. Bodian ML (ed.) in collaboration with Norman AP, Carter CO. *Fibrocystic Disease of the Pancreas. A Congenital Disorder of Mucus Production (Mucosis)*. London, W Heinemann, 1952.

29. Farber S. Pancreatic insufficiency and the celiac syndrome. *N Engl J Med* 1943; **229**:653–657.

30. di Sant'Agnese PEA, Andersen DH. Chemotherapy in infections of the respiratory tract associated with cystic fibrosis of the pancreas; observations with penicillin and drugs of the sulphonamide group, with special reference to penicillin aerosol. *Am J Dis Child* 1946; **72**:17–61.

31. Harris R, Norman AP, Payne WW. The effect of pancreatin therapy on fat absorption and nitrogen retention in children with fibrocystic disease of the pancreas. *Arch Dis Child* 1955; **30**:424–427.

32. Kennedy RLJ. Cystic fibrosis of the pancreas. *Nebr Med J* 1946; **31**:493–496.

33. Shwachman H, Patterson PR, Laguna J. Studies in pancreatic fibrosis: Simple diagnostic gelatine film test for stool trypsin. *Pediatrics* 1949; **4**:222–230.

34. Kessler WR, Andersen DH. Heat prostration in fibrocystic disease of the pancreas and other conditions. *Pediatrics* 1951; **8**:648–656.

35. di Sant'Agnese PA, Darling MD, Perera G, Shea E. Abnormal electrolyte composition of sweat in cystic fibrosis of the pancreas: clinical significance and relationship to the disease. *Pediatrics* 1953; **12**:549–563.

36. Misch KA, Holden HM. Sweat test for diagnosis of fibrocystic disease of the pancreas: report of a fatality. *Arch Dis Child* 1958; **33**:179–180.

37. Gibson LE, Cooke RE. Test for concentration of electrolytes in sweat in cystic fibrosis of the pancreas utilizing pilocarpine by iontophoresis. *Pediatrics* 1959; **23**:545–549.

38. Smalley CA, Addy DP, Anderson CM. Does that child really have cystic fibrosis? *Lancet* 1978; **ii**:415–417.

39. Mearns MB. Cystic fibrosis: the first fifty years. In: Dodge JA, Brock DJH, Widdicombe JH (eds) *Cystic Fibrosis – Current Topics. Volume 1*. Chichester, John Wiley, 1993, pp217–250.

40. Reed JMW. Physiotherapy for chest diseases. In: Marshall G, Perry KMA (eds) *Diseases of the Chest, Volume 2*. St Louis, Butterworth, 1952, pp395–413.

41. Doyle B. Physical therapy in treatment of cystic fibrosis. *Phys Ther Rev* 1959; **39**:24–27.

42. Docter JM. Unmet challenges in cystic fibrosis. In: Warwick WJ (ed.) *1000 Years of Cystic Fibrosis*. Minnesota, University of Minnesota, 1981, pp1–4.

43. Shwachman H, Kulczycki LL. Long-term study of 105 cystic fibrosis patients. *Am J Dis Child* 1958; **96**:6–15.

44. Shwachman H. Therapy of cystic fibrosis. *Pediatrics* 1960; **25**:155–163.

45. Shwachman H. Cystic fibrosis: iatrogenic complications and related issues. In: Lloyd-Still JD (ed.) *Textbook of Cystic Fibrosis*. Boston, John Wright, 1983, pp409–448.

46. Doggett RG, Harrison GM, Stillwell RN *et al.* An atypical *Pseudomonas aeruginosa* associated with cystic fibrosis of the pancreas. *J Pediatr* 1966; **68**:215–221.

47. West JR, Levin MS, di Sant'Agnese PA. Studies of pulmonary function in cystic fibrosis of the pancreas. *Pediatrics* 1954; **13**:155–164.

48. Wessel HU. Lung function in cystic fibrosis. In: Lloyd-Still JD (ed.) *Textbook of Cystic Fibrosis*. Massachusetts, John Wright, 1983, pp199–216.

49. Gandevia B, Anderson CM. The effect of bronchodilator aerosol on ventilatory capacity in fibrocystic disease of the pancreas. *Arch Dis Child* 1959; **34**:511–515.

50. Royce SW. Cor pulmonale in infancy and early childhood: report on 34 patients, with special reference to the occurrence of pulmonary heart disease in cystic fibrosis of the pancreas. *Pediatrics* 1951; **8**:255–274.

51. di Sant'Agnese PA. Bronchial obstruction with lobar atelectasis and emphysema in cystic fibrosis of pancreas. *Pediatrics* 1953; **2**:178–190.

52. Keats TE. Generalized pulmonary emphysema as an isolated manifestation of early cystic fibrosis of the pancreas. *Radiology* 1955; **65**:223–226.

53. Lurie MH. Cystic fibrosis of the pancreas and the nasal mucosa. *Ann Otol Rhinol Laryngol* 1959; **68**:478–486.

54. Hiatt R, Wilson P. Celiac syndrome. VII: Therapy of meconium ileus, report of eight cases with review of the literature. *Surg Gynecol Obstet* 1948; **87**:317–327.

55. Bishop HC, Koop CE. Management of meconium ileus, resection, Roux-en-Y anastomosis and ileostomy irrigation with pancreatic enzymes. *Ann Surg* 1957; **50**:835–836.

56. Rasor R, Stevenson C. Cystic fibrosis of the pancreas, a case history. *Rocky Mt Med J* 1941; **38**:218–220.

57. Jensen KG. Meconium ileus equivalent in a fifteen-year-old patient with mucoviscidosis. *Acta Paediatr* 1962; **51**:344–348.

58. Gibbs GE, Gershbein LL. Incomplete pancreatic deficiency in cystic fibrosis of the pancreas. *Proc Soc Exp Biol Med* 1950; **37**:320–325.

59. Di Sant'Agnese PA. Fibrocystic disease of the pancreas with normal or partial pancreatic function: current views on pathogenesis and diagnosis. *Pediatrics* 1955; **15**:683–697.

60. Kulczycki LL, Shwachman H. Studies in cystic fibrosis of the pancreas: occurrence of rectal prolapse. *N Eng J Med* 1958; **259**:409–412.

61. di Sant'Agnese PA, Andersen DH. Cystic fibrosis of the pancreas in young adults. *Ann Intern Med* 1959; **50**:1321–1330.

62. Lelong M, Joseph R, Le Tan Vinh, Bouvattier P. Cystic fibrosis of the pancreas and massive hepatic steatosis. *Arch Franc Ped* 1950; **7**:234–240.

63. Webster R, Williams H. Hepatic cirrhosis associated with fibrocystic disease of the pancreas: clinical and pathological reports of 5 patients. *Arch Dis Child* 1953; **28**:343–350.

64. di Sant'Agnese PA. A distinctive type of biliary cirrhosis of the liver in patients with cystic fibrosis of the pancreas. *Pediatrics NY* 1956; **3**:387–409.

65. di Sant'Agnese PA. Cirrhosis of the liver with portal hypertension in cystic fibrosis of the pancreas. *Bull NY Acad Med* 1955; **31**:406–407.

66. Doershuk CF. The Matthews Comprehensive Treatment Programme: a ray of hope. In: Doershuk CF (ed.) *Cystic Fibrosis in the Twentieth Century*. Cleveland, AM Publishing, 2001, pp63–78.

67. Matthews LW, Doershuk CF, Wise M *et al.* A therapeutic regimen for patients with cystic fibrosis. *J Pediatr* 1964; **65**:558–575.

68. Doershuk CF, Matthews LW, Tucker AS *et al.* A 5-year clinical evaluation of a therapeutic program for patients with cystic fibrosis. *J Pediatr* 1964; **65**:677–693.

69. Doershuk CF, Matthews LW, Tucker A, Spector S. Evaluation of a prophylactic and therapeutic program for patients with cystic fibrosis. *Pediatrics* 1965; **36**:675–688.

70. di Sant'Agnese PA. In: Gellis SS (ed.) *Year Book of Pediatrics, 1966/1967*. Chicago, Year Book Publishers, 1967, pp257–259.

71. Quinton PM. Physiological basis of cystic fibrosis: a historical perspective. *Physiol Rev* 1999; **79**:3–22.

72. Andersen DH. Cystic fibrosis of the pancreas: a review. *J Chron Dis* 1958; **7**:58–90.

73. Baggenstoss AH, Power MH, Grindlay JH. The relationship of fibrocystic disease of the pancreas to deficiency of secretin. *Pediatrics* 1948; **2**:435.

74. Ayers WB, Stowens D, Ochsner A, Platou RV. Splanchnicectomy for cystic fibrosis of the pancreas: analysis of results in 24 patients. *Pediatrics* 1951; **8**:657–676.

75. Morrison C, Morrison R. National and International Cystic Fibrosis Associations. In: Dodge JA, Brock DJH, Widdicombe JH (eds) *Cystic Fibrosis – Current Topics*. Chichester, John Wiley, 1993, pp319–345.

76. Wiser WC, Beier FR. Albumin in the meconium of infants with cystic fibrosis: a preliminary report. *Pediatrics* 1964; **33**:115–119.

77. Kopito I, Mahmoodian A, Townley IT *et al.* Studies in cystic fibrosis: analysis of nail clippings for sodium and potassium. *N Eng J Med* 1965; **272**:504–509.

78. Lawson D, Westcombe P, Saggers B. Pilot trial of an infant screening programme for cystic fibrosis: measurement of parotid salivary sodium at 4 months. *Arch Dis Child* 1969; **44**:715–718.

79. Gurson CT, Sertel H, Gurkan M, Pala S. Newborn screening for cystic fibrosis with the chloride electrode and neutron activation analysis. *Helv Paediatr Acta* 1973; **28**:165–174.

80. Shwachman H, Mahmoodian A. Reappraisal of the chloride plate test as screening test for cystic fibrosis. *Arch Dis Child* 1981; **56**:137–139.

81. Crossley JR, Elliott RB, Smith PA. Dried blood spot screening for cystic fibrosis in the newborn. *Lancet* 1979; **i**:472–474.

82. Hadorn B, Johansen PG, Anderson CM. Pancreozymin secretin tests of exocrine pancreatic function in cystic fibrosis and the significance of the result for the pathogenesis of the disease. *Can Med J* 1968; **98**:377–384.

83. Barbero GJ, Siblinga MS, Marino JM, Seibel R. Stool trypsin and chymotrypsin: value in the diagnosis of pancreatic insufficiency in cystic fibrosis. *Am J Dis Child* 1966; **112**:536–540.

84. Anderson CM. Histologic changes in duodenal mucosa in coeliac disease: reversibility during treatment with wheat gluten free diet. *Arch Dis Child* 1960; **35**:419–427.

85. Valetta EA, Mastella G. Incidence of coeliac disease in a cystic fibrosis population. *Acta Paediatr Scand* 1989; **78**:784–785.

86. Freye HB, Kurtz SM, Spock A, Capp MP. Light and electron microscopic examination of the small bowel of children with cystic fibrosis. *J Pediatr* 1964; **64**:575–579.

87. Parkins RA, Eidleman S, Rubin CE, Dobbins WO. The diagnosis of cystic fibrosis by rectal suction biopsy. *Lancet* 1963; **38**:851–856.

88. Lobeck CC, McSherry NR. Response of sweat electrolyte concentrations to 9 alpha-fluorohydrocortisone in patients with cystic fibrosis and their families. *J Pediatr* 1963; **62**:393–398.

89. Doggett RG, Harrison GM, Wallis ES. Comparison of some properties of *Pseudomonas aeruginosa* isolated from infections in persons with and without cystic fibrosis. *J Bacteriol* 1964; **87**:427–443.

90. Mearns MB. Simple tests of ventilatory capacity in children with cystic fibrosis. I: Clinical and radiological findings in 85 patients. II: Three-year follow-up on 50 patients. *Arch Dis Child* 1968; **43**:528–539.

91. Phelan PD. Gracey M. Williams HE. Anderson CM. Ventilatory function in infants with cystic fibrosis: physiological assessment of inhalation therapy. *Arch Dis Child* 1969; **44**:393–400.

92. Mearns M, Young W, Batten J. Transient pulmonary infiltrations in cystic fibrosis due to allergic aspergillosis. *Thorax* 1965; **20**:385–392.

93. Bernard E, Israel L, Debris MM, Tip M. Mucoviscidosis and idiopathic spontaneous pneumothorax. *J Fr Med Chir Thor* 1962; **16**:105–109.

94. Zegarelli EV, Kutscher AH, Denning CR *et al.* Coloration of teeth in patients with cystic fibrosis of the pancreas: II. *Oral Surg Oral Med Oral Pathol* 1962; **15**:929–933.

95. Lietman PS, di Sant'Agnese PA, Wong V. Optic neuritis in cystic fibrosis of the pancreas: role of chloramphenicol therapy. *J Am Med Assoc* 1964; **189**:924–927.

96. Denton R. Clinical use of continuous nebulization in bronchopulmonary disease. *Dis Chest* 1955; **28**:123–140.

97. Matthews LW, Doershuk CF, Spector S. Mist tent therapy of obstructive pulmonary lesion of cystic fibrosis. *Pediatrics* 1967; **39**:176–185.

98. di Sant'Agnese. Comment in *Year Book of Pediatrics 1967/68.* Gellis SS (ed.). Chicago, Year Book Publishers, 1968, p197.

99. Chang N, Levison H, Cunningham K *et al.* An evaluation of nightly mist tent therapy for patients with cystic fibrosis. *Am Rev Resp Dis* 1973; **107**:672–675.

100. Sproul A, Huang N. Growth patterns in children with cystic fibrosis. *J Pediatr* 1964; **65**:664–676.

101. Kunstadter RH, Mendelsohn RS. Norethandrolone in children with and without cystic fibrosis of the pancreas. *Illinois Med J* 1961; **120**:156–161.

102. Dooley RR, Moss AJ, Wright PM, Hassakis PC. Norethandrolone in cystic fibrosis of the pancreas. *J Pediatr* 1969; **74**:95–102.

103. Gracey M, Burke V, Anderson CM. Treatment of abdominal pain in cystic fibrosis by oral administration of n-acetyl cysteine. *Arch Dis Child* 1969; **44**:404–405.

104. Noblett HR. Treatment of uncomplicated meconium ileus by gastrografin enema: a preliminary report. *J Pediatr Surg* 1969; **4**:190–197.

105. Hide DW, Burman D. An infant with both cystic fibrosis and coeliac disease. *Arch Dis Child* 1969; **44**:533–535.

106. Rosan RC, Shwachman H, Kulczycki LI. Diabetes mellitus and cystic fibrosis of the pancreas: laboratory and clinical observations. *Am J Dis Child* 1962; **104**:625–634.

107. Milner AD. Blood glucose and serum insulin levels in children with cystic fibrosis. *Arch Dis Child* 1969; **44**:351–355.

108. Johnson Sir R. *History of the Cystic Fibrosis Research Trust.* 20th Anniversary Meeting, Brighton, 1984, pp3–6.

109. Batten J. Cystic fibrosis: a review. *Br J Dis Chest* 1965; **59**:1–9.

110. Shwachman H, Kulczycki, Khaw Kon-Taik. Studies in cystic fibrosis: a report of sixty-five patients over 17 years of age. *Pediatrics* 1965; **36**:689–699.

111. Denning CR, Sommers SC, Quigley HJ. Infertility in male patients with cystic fibrosis. *Pediatrics NY* 1968; **41**:7–17.

112. Kaplan E, Shwachman H, Perlmutter AD *et al.* Reproductive failure in males with cystic fibrosis. *N Eng J Med* 1968; **279**:65–69.

113. Siegel B, Siegel S. Pregnancy and delivery in a patient with cystic fibrosis of the pancreas. *Obstet Gynecol* 1960; **16**:438–440.

114. Chernick WS, Barbero GJ. Composition of tracheobronchial secretions in cystic fibrosis of the pancreas and bronchiectasis. *Pediatrics* 1959; **24**:739–745.

115. Lev R, Spicer SS. An historical chemical comparison of human epithelial mucins in normal and in hypersecretory states including pancreatic cystic fibrosis. *Am J Path* 1965; **46**:23–47.

116. Danes BS, Bearn AG. A genetic cell marker for cystic fibrosis. *Lancet* 1968; **18**:1061–1063.

117. Spock A. Abnormal serum factor in patients with cystic fibrosis of the pancreas. *Pediatr Res* 1967; **1**:173–177.

118. Bowman BH, Lockhart LH, McCombs ML. Oyster ciliary inhibition by cystic fibrosis factor. *Science* 1969; **164**:325–326.

119. Mangos JA, McSherry N. Sodium transport: inhibitory factor in sweat of patients with cystic fibrosis. *Science* 1967; **158**:135–136.

120. Wood RE. Pediatric flexible bronchoscopy: the inside story. In: Doershuk CF (ed.) *Cystic Fibrosis in the 20th Century.* Cleveland, AM Publishing, 2001, 112–119.

121. Mearns MB. Treatment and prevention of pulmonary complications of cystic fibrosis in infancy and early childhood. *Arch Dis Child* 1972; **47**:5–11.

122. Mearns MB. Cystic fibrosis. *Br J Hosp Med* 1974; October: 497–506.

123. Lawson D. Panel discussion on microbiology and chemotherapy of the respiratory tract in cystic fibrosis. In: Lawson D (ed.) *Proceedings of the 5th International CF Conference, Cambridge, 1969*. London, Cystic Fibrosis Research Trust, 1969, p225.

124. Weaver LT, Green MG, Nicholson K *et al*. Prognosis in cystic fibrosis treated with continuous flucloxacillin for the neonatal period. *Arch Dis Child* 1994; **70**:84–89.

125. Stutman HR, Lieberman JM, Nussbaum E, Marks MI. Antibiotic prophylaxis in infants and young children with cystic fibrosis: a randomized controlled trial. *J Pediatr* 2002; **140**:299–305.

126. Wood RE, Boat TF, Doershuk CF. Cystic fibrosis: state of the art. *Am Rev Resp Dis* 1976; **113**:833–878.

127. Crozier DN. Cystic fibrosis: a not so fatal disease. *Pediatr Clin North Am* 1974; **21**:935–948.

128. Corey M, McLaughlin FJ, Williams M *et al*. A comparison of survival growth and pulmonary function in patients with cystic fibrosis in Boston and Toronto. *J Clin Epidemiol* 1988; **41**:588–591.

129. Nielsen OH, Schiotz PO. Cystic fibrosis in Denmark in the period 1945–1981: evaluation of centralized treatment. *Acta Paediatr Scand* 1982; Suppl 301:107–119.

130. Hoiby N. Antibodies against *Pseudomonas aeruginosa* in serum from normal persons and patients colonised with mucoid or non-mucoid *P. aeruginosa*: results obtained by crossed immunoelectrophoresis. *Acta Pathol Microbiol Immunol Scand* 1977; **85**:142–148.

131. Szaff M, Hoiby N, Flensborg EW. Frequent antibiotic therapy improves survival of cystic fibrosis patients with chronic *Pseudomonas aeruginosa* infection. *Acta Paediatr Scand* 1983; **72**:651–657.

132. Jensen T, Pedersen SS, Garne S, Heilmann C *et al*. Colistin inhalation therapy in cystic fibrosis patients with chronic *Pseudomonas aeruginosa* lung infection. *J Antimicrob Chemother* 1987; **19**:831–838.

133. Valerius NH, Koch C, Hoiby N. Prevention of chronic *Pseudomonas aeruginosa* infection in cystic fibrosis by early treatment. *Lancet* 1991; **338**:725–726.

134. Frederiksen B, Lanng S, Koch C, Hoiby N. Improved survival in the Danish Cystic Fibrosis Centre: results of aggressive treatment. *Pediatr Pulmonol* 1996; **21**:153–158.

135. Chase HP, Long MA, Lavin MH. Cystic fibrosis and malnutrition. *J Pediatr* 1979; **95**:337–347.

136. Allan JD, Mason A, Moss AD. Nutritional supplementation in treatment of cystic fibrosis of the pancreas. *Am J Dis Child* 1973; **26**:2–26.

137. Yassa JG, Prosser R, Dodge JA. Effects of an artificial diet on growth of patients with cystic fibrosis. *Arch Dis Child* 1978; **53**:777–783.

138. Kraemer R, Rudeberg A, Hadorn B *et al*. Relative underweight in cystic fibrosis and its prognostic value. *Acta Paediatr Scand* 1978; **67**:33–37.

139. Shwachman H, Lebenthal E, Khaw P-T. Recurrent acute pancreatitis in patients with cystic fibrosis with normal pancreatic enzymes. *Pediatrics* 1975; **55**:86–94.

140. Kuo PT, Huang NN. The effect of medium chain triglyceride upon fat absorption and plasma lipid and depot fat of children with cystic fibrosis of the pancreas. *J Clin Invest* 1962; **44**:1924–1933.

141. Strandvik B, Gronowitz E, Enlund F *et al*. Essential fatty acid deficiency in relation to genotype in patients with cystic fibrosis. *J Pediatr* 2001; **139**:650–655.

142. Elliott RB. A therapeutic trial of fatty acid supplementation in cystic fibrosis. *Pediatrics* 1976; **57**:474–479.

143. Chase HP, Cotton EK, Elliot RB. Intravenous linoleic acid supplementation in children with cystic fibrosis. *Pediatrics* 1979; **64**:207–213.

144. Southern KW, Littlewood JM. Newborn screening programmes for cystic fibrosis. *Paediatr Respir Rev* 2003; **4**:299–305.

145. Chatfield S, Owen G, Ryley HC *et al*. Neonatal screening for cystic fibrosis in Wales and the West Midlands: clinical assessments after 5 years of screening. *Arch Dis Child* 1991; **66**:29–33.

146. Farrell PM, Kosorok MR, Rock MJ *et al*. Early diagnosis of cystic fibrosis through neonatal screening prevents severe malnutrition and improves long-term growth. *Pediatrics* 2001; **107**:1–13.

147. Koscik RL, Farrell PM, Kosorok MR *et al*. Cognitive function of children with cystic fibrosis: deleterious effect of early malnutrition. *Pediatrics* 2004; **113**:1549–1558.

148. Warwick WJ, Pogue RE, Gerber HU, Nesbitt CJ. Survival patterns in cystic fibrosis. *J Chron Dis* 1975; **28**:609–622.

149. Robinson MJ, Norman AP. Life tables for cystic fibrosis. *Arch Dis Child* 1975; **50**:962–965.

150. Corey M, Levison H, Crozier D. Five- to seven-year course of pulmonary function in cystic fibrosis. *Am Rev Resp Dis* 1976; **114**:1085–1092.

151. Dodge JA, Morison S, Lewis PA *et al*. Incidence, population, and survival of cystic fibrosis in the UK, 1968–95. UK Cystic Fibrosis Survey Management Committee. *Arch Dis Child* 1997; **77**:493–496.

152. Wood RE, Piazza F. Survival in cystic fibrosis: correlation with treatment in three cystic fibrosis centres. Tenth International Cystic Fibrosis Congress, Sydney, 1988. *Excerpta Medica Asia Pacific Services* 74:79.

153. Docter JM. Unmet challenges in cystic fibrosis. In: Warwick WJ (ed.) *1000 Years of Cystic Fibrosis. Collected Papers*. University of Minnesota, Minnesota, 1981, pp1–3.

154. Wilson GB, Arnaud P, Monsher MT, Fudenberg HH. Detection of cystic fibrosis protein by electrofocusing. *Pediatr Res* 1976; **10**:1001–1002.

155. Manson JC, Brock DJH. Development of a quantitative immunoassay for the cystic fibrosis gene. *Lancet* 1980; i: 330.

156. Lieberman J, Costea N, Jakulis VJ, Kaneshiro W. Detection of a lectin in the blood of cystic fibrosis homozygotes and heterozygotes. *Trans Assoc Am Physicians* 1979; **92**:121–129.

157. Reid L. Bronchial mucus and its glycoproteins in cystic fibrosis. In: Warwick WJ (ed.) *1000 Years of Cystic Fibrosis*. Minnesota, University of Minnesota, 1981, pp79–84.

158. Yeates DB, Sturgess JM, Kahn SR *et al*. Mucociliary transport in trachea of patients with cystic fibrosis. *Arch Dis Child* 1976; **51**:28–33.

159. Rommens JM, Iannuzzi MC, Kerem B-S *et al*. Identification of the cystic fibrosis gene: chromosome walking and jumping. *Science* 1989; **245**:1059–1065.

160. Riordan JR, Rommens JM, Kerem B-S *et al*. Identification of the cystic fibrosis gene: cloning and characterization of the complementary DNA. *Science* 1989; **245**:1066–1073.

161. Kerem B-S, Rommens JM, Buchanan JA *et al*. Identification of the cystic fibrosis gene: genetic analysis. *Science* 1989; **245**:1073–1080.

162. Brock DJH, Befgood D, Barron L, Haward C. Prospective prenatal diagnosis of cystic fibrosis. *Lancet* 1985; i:1175–1178.

163. Farrall M, Law HY, Rodeck CH *et al*. First-trimester prenatal diagnosis of cystic fibrosis with linked DNA probes. *Lancet* 1986; i:1402–1405.

164. Lane B, Williamson P, Dodge JA *et al*. Confidential inquiry into families with two siblings with cystic fibrosis. *Arch Dis Child* 1997; **77**:501–503.

165. Phelan P, Hey E. Cystic fibrosis mortality in England & Wales and in Victoria, Australia. *Arch Dis Child* 1984; **59**:71–83.

166. British Paediatric Association Working Party on Cystic Fibrosis. Cystic fibrosis in the United Kingdom 1977–85: an improving picture. *Br Med J* 1988; **297**:1599–1602.

167. Pryor JA, Webber BA, Hodson ME, Batten JC. Evaluation of the forced expiration technique as an adjunct to postural drainage in treatment of cystic fibrosis. *Br Med J* 1979; **2**:417–418.

168. Webber BA, Hofmeyer JL, Morgan MDL *et al*. Effects of postural drainage, incorporating the forced expiration technique, on pulmonary function in cystic fibrosis. *Br J Dis Chest* 1986; **80**:353–359.

169. Falk M, Kelstrup M, Andersen JB *et al*. Improving the ketchup bottle method with positive expiratory pressure, PEP, in cystic fibrosis. *Eur J Resp Dis* 1984; **65**:423–432.

170. Hanson LG, Warwick WJ. High frequency chest compression system to aid in clearance of mucus from the lung. *Biomed Instrum Technol* 1990; **24**:289–294.

171. Hodson ME, Penketh ARL, Batten JC. Aerosol carbenicillin and gentamicin treatment of *Pseudomonas aeruginosa* in patients with cystic fibrosis. *Lancet* 1981; ii:1137–1139.

172. Littlewood JM, Miller MG, Ghoneim AT, Ramsden CH. Nebulised colomycin for early *Pseudomonas* colonisation in cystic fibrosis. *Lancet* 1985; i:865.

173. *Antibiotic Treatment for Cystic Fibrosis*. Bromley, London, Cystic Fibrosis Trust, 2001.

174. Frederiksen B, Koch C, Hoiby N. The changing epidemiology of *Pseudomonas aeruginosa* infection in Danish cystic fibrosis patients, 1974–1995. *Pediatr Pulmonol* 1999; **28**:159–166.

175. Lee TWR, Brownlee KG, Denton M *et al*. Reduction in prevalence of chronic *Pseudomonas aeruginosa* infection at a regional cystic fibrosis center. *Pediatr Pulmonol* 2004; **37**:104–110.

176. Gibson RL, Emerson J, McNamara S *et al*. Significant microbiological effect of inhaled tobramycin in young children with cystic fibrosis. *Am J Resp Crit Care Med* 2003; **167**:841–849.

177. Rabin HR, Harley FL, Bryan LE, Elfring GL. Evaluation of high dose tobramycin and ticarcillin treatment protocol in cystic fibrosis based on improved susceptibility criteria and antibiotic pharmacokinetics. In: Sturgess JM (ed.) *Perspectives in Cystic Fibrosis*. 8th International Cystic Fibrosis Congress, Toronto, Canada, 1980, pp370–375.

178. Jensen T, Pedersen SS, Hoiby N *et al*. Use of antibiotics in cystic fibrosis: the Danish approach. *Antibiot Chemother* 1989; **42**:237–246.

179. Stern RC, Doershuk CF, Matthews LW. Use of heparin lock to administer intermittent intravenous drugs. *Clin Pediatr* 1972; **11**:521–523.

180. Stead RJ, Davidson TI, Duncan FR *et al*. Use of a totally implantable system for venous access in cystic fibrosis. *Thorax* 1987; **42**:149–150.

181. Essex-Cater A, Gilbert J, Robinson T *et al*. Totally implantable venous access systems in paediatric practice. *Arch Dis Child* 1989; **64**:119–123.

182. Ehrenstrom Reiz GM, Reiz SL. EMLA: a eutectic mixture of local anaesthetics for topical anaesthesia. Controlled clinical trial. *Acta Anaesth Scand* 1982; **26**:596–598.

183. Winter RJD, George RJD, Deacock SJ *et al*. Self-administered home intravenous antibiotic therapy in bronchiectasis and adult cystic fibrosis. *Lancet* 1984; i:1338–1339.

184. Gilbert J, Robinson T, Littlewood JM. Home intravenous antibiotic treatment in cystic fibrosis. *Arch Dis Child* 1988; **63**:512–517.

185. Auerbach HS, Williams M, Kirkpatrick JA, Colten HR. Alternate-day prednisone reduces morbidity and improves pulmonary function in cystic fibrosis. *Lancet* 1985; ii:686–688.

186. Colombo C, Setchell KD, Podda M *et al*. Effects of ursodeoxycholic acid therapy for liver disease associated with cystic fibrosis. *J Paediatr* 1990; **117**:482–489.

187. Gaskin KJ, Waters DL, Howman-Giles R *et al*. Liver disease and common-bile-duct stenosis in cystic fibrosis. *N Engl J Med* 1988; **318**:340–346.

188. Nagel RA, Westaby D, Javaid A *et al*. Liver disease and bile duct abnormalities in adults with cystic fibrosis. *Lancet* 1989; ii:1422–1425.

189. Mieles LA, Orenstein D, Teperman L *et al*. Liver transplant in cystic fibrosis. *Lancet* 1989; i:1073.

190. Noble-Jamieson G, Barnes N, Jamieson N *et al*. Liver transplantation for hepatic cirrhosis in cystic fibrosis. *J R Soc Med* 1996; **89** (Suppl 27):31–37.

191. Couetil JP, Soubrane O, Houssin DP *et al*. Combined heart–lung–liver, double lung liver, and isolated liver transplantation for cystic fibrosis in children. *Transpl Int* 1997; **10**:33–39.

192. Littlewood JM, Kelleher J, Rawson I *et al*. Comprehensive assessment at a CF centre identifies suboptimal treatment

and improves management, symptoms and condition. 10th International Cystic Fibrosis Congress. Sydney, 1988. *Excerpta Medica Asia Pacific Services* **74**:89.

193. Holsclaw DS, Keith H. Long-term benefits of pH sensitive enteric coated enzymes in CF. In: *Perspectives in Cystic Fibrosis*. Proc. 8th International Cystic Fibrosis Congress, Toronto, 1980, p19a.

194. Mischler EH, Parrell S, Farrell PM, Odell GB. Comparison of effectiveness of pancreatic enzyme preparations in cystic fibrosis. *Am J Dis Child* 1982; **136**:1060–1063.

195. Beverley DW, Kelleher J, MacDonald A *et al.* Comparison of four pancreatic extracts in cystic fibrosis. *Arch Dis Child* 1987; **62**:564–568.

196. Littlewood JM, Wolfe SP, Conway SP. Diagnosis and treatment of intestinal malabsorption in cystic fibrosis. *Pediatr Pulmonol* 2006; **41**:35–49.

197. Bradley JA, Axon ATR, Hill GL. Nocturnal elemental diet for retarded growth in a patient with cystic fibrosis. *Br Med J* 1979; **1**(6157):167.

198. Shepherd R, Cooksley WGF, Cooke WD. Improved growth and clinical, nutritional and respiratory changes in response to nutritional therapy in cystic fibrosis. *J Pediatr* 1980; **7**:351–357.

199. Levy LD, Durie PR, Pencharz PB *et al.* Effects of long-term nutritional rehabilitation on body composition and clinical status in malnourished children and adolescents with cystic fibrosis. *J Pediatr* 1985; **107**:225–230.

200. Pencharz P, Hill R, Archibald E *et al.* Energy needs and nutritional rehabilitation in undernourished adolescents and young adult patients with cystic fibrosis. *J Pediatr Gastroenterol Nutr* 1984; **3**(Suppl 1):S147–153.

201. Congden PJ, Bruce G, Rothburn MM *et al.* Vitamin status in treated patients with cystic fibrosis. *Arch Dis Child* 1981; **56**:708–714.

202. Sitrin MD, Leiberman F, Jenson WE *et al.* Vitamin E deficiency and neurological disease in adults with cystic fibrosis. *Ann Int Med* 1987; **74**:314–318.

203. Rayner RJ, Tyrell JC, Hiller EJ *et al.* Night blindness and conjunctival xerosis caused by vitamin deficiency in patients with cystic fibrosis. *Arch Dis Child* 1989; **64**:1151–1156.

204. O'Halloran SM, Gilbert J, McKendrick OM *et al.* Gastrografin in acute meconium ileus equivalent. *Arch Dis Child* 1986; **61**:128–130.

205. Yacoub MH, Banner NR, Khaghani A *et al.* Heart–lung transplantation for cystic fibrosis and subsequent domino heart transplantation. *J Heart Transplant* 1990; **9**:459–466.

206. Scott J, Higgenbottam T, Hutter J *et al.* Heart–lung transplantation for cystic fibrosis. *Lancet* 1988; **ii**:192–194.

207. Hodson ME. Heart lung transplantation for cystic fibrosis. *Acta Univ Carol Med* 1990; **36**:207–209.

208. Pasque MK, Cooper JD, Kaiser LR *et al.* Improved technique for bilateral lung transplantation: rationale and initial clinical experience. *Ann Thorac Surg* 1990; **49**:785–791.

209. Cohen RG, Starnes VA. Living donor transplantation. *World J Surg* 2001; **25**:244–250.

210. Penketh AR, Wise A, Mearns MB *et al.* Cystic fibrosis in adolescents and adults. *Thorax* 1987; **42**:526–532.

211. Conway, SP. Transition programmes in cystic fibrosis centers. *Pediatr Pulmonol* 2004; **37**:1–3.

212. Knowles MR, Gatzy JT, Boucher RC. Increased bioelectric potential difference across respiratory epithelia in cystic fibrosis. *N Eng J Med* 1981; **305**:1489–1495.

213. Quinton PM. Chloride impermeability in cystic fibrosis. *Nature* 1983; **301**:421–422.

214. Eiberg H, Mohr J, Schmiegelow K *et al.* Linkage relationships of paraoxinase (PON) with other markers: evidence of PON-cystic fibrosis synteny? *Clin Genet* 1985; **28**:265–271.

215. Tsui L, Buchwald M, Barker D *et al.* Cystic fibrosis locus defined by a genetically linked polymorphic DNA marker. *Science* 1985; **230**:1054–1057.

216. White R, Woodward S, Leppert M *et al.* A closely linked genetic marker for cystic fibrosis. *Nature* 1985; **318**:382–384.

217. Wainwright BJ, Scambler PJ, Schmodtke J *et al.* Localization of cystic fibrosis locus to human chromosome 7cen-q22. *Nature* 1985; **318**:384–385.

218. McKone EF, Emerson SS, Edwards KL, Aitken ML. Effect of genotype on phenotype and mortality in cystic fibrosis: a retrospective cohort study. *Lancet* 2001; **361**:1671–1676.

219. Kristidis P, Bozon D, Corey M *et al.* Genetic determination of exocrine pancreatic function in cystic fibrosis. *Am J Hum Genet* 1992; **50**:1178–1184.

220. Mickle JE, Cutting GR. Genotype-phenotype relationships in cystic fibrosis. *Med Clin N Am* 2000; **84**:597–607.

221. Chillon M, Casals T, Mercier B *et al.* Mutations in the cystic fibrosis gene in patients with congenital absence of the vas deferens. *N Engl J Med* 1995; **332**:1475–1480.

222. Cohn JA, Friedman KJ, Noone PG *et al.* Relation between mutations of the cystic fibrosis gene and idiopathic pancreatitis. *N Engl J Med* 1998; **339**: 653–658.

223. LiPuma JJ, Dasen SE, Neilson DW *et al.* Person-to-person transmission of *Pseudomonas cepacia* between patients with cystic fibrosis. *Lancet* 1990; **336**:1094–1096.

224. Govan JR, Brown PH, Maddison J *et al.* Evidence for transmission of *Pseudomonas cepacia* by social contact in cystic fibrosis. *Lancet* 1993; **342**:15–19.

225. Cheng K, Smyth RL, Govan JRW *et al.* Spread of B-lactam-resistant *Pseudomonas aeruginosa* in a cystic fibrosis unit. *Lancet* 1996; **348**:639–642.

226. Jones AM, Govan JRW, Doherty CJ *et al.* Spread of a multiresistant strain of *Pseudomonas aeruginosa* in an adult cystic fibrosis clinic. *Lancet* 2001; **358**:557–558.

227. Fuchs HJ, Borowitz DS, Christiansen DH *et al.* Effect of aerosolized recombinant human DNase on exacerbations of respiratory symptoms and on pulmonary function in patients with cystic fibrosis. The Pulmozyme Study Group. *N Engl J Med* 1994; **331**:637–642.

228. Ramsey BW, Pepe MS, Quan JM *et al.* Intermittent administration of inhaled tobramycin in patients with cystic fibrosis. Cystic Fibrosis Inhaled Tobramycin Study Group. *N Engl J Med* 1999; **340**: 23–30.

229. Everard ML, Sly P, Brenan S, Ryan G. Macrolide antibiotics in diffuse panbronchiolitis and in cystic fibrosis. *Eur Resp J* 1997; **10**:2926.

230. Lanng S, Thorsteisson B, Nerup J *et al*. Influence of the development of diabetes mellitus on the clinical status in patients with cystic fibrosis. *Eur J Paediatr* 1992; **151**:684–687.

231. Gibbens DT, Gilsanz V, Boechat MI *et al*. Osteoporosis in cystic fibrosis. *J Pediatr* 1988; **113**:295–300.

232. Colombo C, Battezzati PM. Hepatobiliary manifestations of cystic fibrosis. *J Gastroenterol Hepatol* 1996; **8**:748–754.

233. Edenborough FP. Women with cystic fibrosis and their potential for reproduction. *Thorax* 2001; **56**:649–695.

234. Schlegel PN. Assisted reproductive technologies and sperm aspiration. *Pediatr Pulmonol* 1996; Suppl 13:119–120.

235. Clinical Standards and Accreditation Group. *Standards for the clinical care of children and adults with cystic fibrosis in the UK 2001*. Bromley: Cystic Fibrosis Trust.

236. Kerem E, Conway S, Elborn S *et al.*, for the Consensus Committee. Standards of care for patients with cystic fibrosis: a European consensus. *J Cystic Fibros* 2005; **4**:7–20.

237. Littlewood JM. European Cystic Fibrosis Society consensus on standards: a roadmap to 'best care'. *J Cyst Fibros* 2005; **4**:1–5.

Epidemiology of cystic fibrosis

SARAH WALTERS AND ANIL MEHTA

INTRODUCTION

Epidemiology may be defined as the study of the distribution and determinants of disease frequency in human populations [1]. *Clinical epidemiology* applies epidemiological principles to a clinical population; i.e. to a population already known to have a particular disease. An analogous definition might therefore be that clinical epidemiology is the study of the distribution of disease manifestations and determinants of disease outcome in a clinical population.

Clinical epidemiology is the basic science underpinning the practice of evidence-based medicine. Therefore a knowledge of the clinical epidemiology of cystic fibrosis (CF), and in particular a knowledge of risk factors for development of certain disease manifestations, and factors influencing overall prognosis, will be of value to all clinicians involved in the care of patients with CF.

This chapter examines and describes the epidemiology and clinical epidemiology of cystic fibrosis. It includes a description of clinical features and prognostic indicators, social and demographic features of the population, and finally some information about the application of clinical epidemiology to evidence-based practice in CF care.

This chapter could not have been written without the high-quality information that has been collected over the years by the US, Canadian and UK patient data registries. The main sources for this chapter are the US CF Foundation Patient Data Registry Reports of 1996 and 2004 [2,3], the Canadian CF Foundation Patient Data Registry Report of 2002 [4], and the UK CF Database Annual Report of 2003 [5]. Data from surveys of adults with CF in the UK in 1990, 1994 and 2000 are also used [6].

INCIDENCE AND PREVALENCE

Incidence (number of new cases per 100 000 population), birth prevalence (number of people with CF born per 10 000 live births) and population prevalence (number of people with CF per 100 000 population) vary according to the prevalence of CF genetic mutations in the underlying population. Calculation of incidence and prevalence also depends on access to a complete and accurate patient register.

Genotype distribution

The commonest mutation identified in the world is the *F508del* (formerly known as $\Delta F508$) mutation, which comprises 66% of global mutations, followed by *G451X* and *G551D* at 2.4% and 1.6% respectively [7]. However, its prevalence varies markedly among CF populations worldwide, and in some populations it is not the most common genotype. F508del comprises 70% of mutations detected in Northern Europe, and 74.6% in Australasians of European origin, but only 45% of mutations in Central and South America and 28.5% in the Middle East.

Even within individual countries, there are wide variations in gene frequency: in North America, frequency of F508del varies depending on ethnic origin of the population studied, varying from under 40% to over 80% of all mutations studied. This is of clinical importance for those providing medical services to such populations, because there is evidence that certain globally uncommon genotypes, which may be more common in particular populations such as ethnic minorities, are associated with a milder clinical phenotype, particularly class IV and class V mutations [8]. Such patients may not display classical CF symptoms from early childhood, may have a lower sweat chloride concentration, have improved survival, and in particular are more likely to be pancreatic sufficient.

Heterozygote prevalence, origins and effects

The commonest CF gene mutation, *F508del*, is at least 50 000 years old. Today the CF gene is found to be mutated

Table 2.1 CF case frequency and population incidence of specified CF genotypes.

Genotype	Gene frequency	Case frequency (per 100)	Live births per case (1000s)
ΔF508/ΔF508	0.67×0.67	45	6
ΔF508/single common	0.67×0.03	2.00	120
ΔF508/all common	0.67×0.18	12	21
ΔF508/single rare	0.67×0.0002	0.013	2×10^4
ΔF508/all rare	0.67×0.15	10	25
Single common/ single common	0.03×0.03	0.09	3×10^3
Single rare/single rare	0.0002×0.0002	4.0×10^{-6}	6×10^7
Single common/ single rare	0.03×0.0002	6.0×10^{-4}	4×10^5

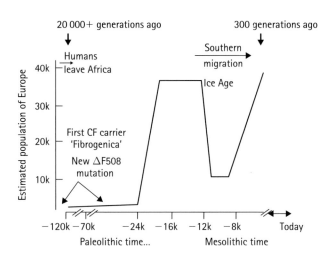

Figure 2.1 The ancient origin of the first CF mutation relative to changes in Northern European population numbers. The genetic record of haplotype mutation in nucleotide repeats suggests that the CF mutation *F508del* in the hypothetical progenitor Fibrogenica already existed when the population of the Indus Valley was only about 20 K and at a time when climate-driven mass movements of populations into Europe were occurring (ordinate in thousands, K). The fossil record shows that the last major volcanic super-eruption was at −70 000 years which left scattered shards of human population from which modern populations are derived. Thus CF mutation prevalence is a form of balanced natural selection whereby nature arrives at a steady state by offsetting a reproductive advantage gained against a (historical) lethal environmental factor(s) that kills a non-CF heterozygote peer group before they can reproduce.

in as many as 1 in 17 Irish citizens of Celtic descent, around 1 in 25 UK citizens of Anglo–Saxon descent, and 1 in 35 Continental Europeans of mixed descent (whether residing in Europe or North America). Table 2.1 summarizes the global frequency of CF genotypes.

There are considerable variations in the prevalence of genotypes in Caucasian populations [9], and the geographical distribution of these genotypes gives clues to potential origins. *F508del* occurs in almost 90% of Danish CF and only 20% of Turkish CF patients with a northwest to southeast gradient. *G542X* ranges in prevalence from 17% of Balearic Island CF chromosomes to less than 1% in Northern CF populations. A similar southern excess occurs for *N1303K* with 17% of Tunisian CF chromosomes being affected. The *G551D* mutation remains widespread in northwest and central Europe. *W1282X* is commonly found in Israel and its environs in about 1 in 3 CF chromosomes. In contrast, 17 other mutations have a combined prevalence of less than 1%.

The 7q31.2 chromosome region local to CFTR is in a genetically very stable region of DNA [9]. It has been suggested that *F508del*, *G542X* and *N1303K* have a common ancestry, albeit from different times in prehistory, but *G551D* and *W1282X* share a different, younger heritage. A reasonable working hypothesis is that *F508del* arose before *N1303K* and *G542X* approximately 35–50 thousand years ago (Fig. 2.1).

The high prevalence of F508del in Caucasian populations requires explanation, and there has been much debate about the nature of the selective pressure that generated the current pattern of CF carriage. *F508del* CFTR is prematurely degraded, and therefore fails to remain at the apical membrane compared to wild-type CFTR [10]. So, how could the remaining wild-type CFTR protect the heterozygote?

There are two possibilities. The first is that simply having 50% of normal wild-type CFTR in a heterozygote is sufficient to reduce the binding of *Salmonella enterica* serovar Typhi (or some other pathogen) and this afforded sufficient protection to prevent early death. Alternatively, it might be that a hitherto unknown positive function exists for *F508del* CFTR (and possibly other mutations) that interferes with the normal process by which the unknown environmental pressure kills infants and children before they have a chance to reproduce. The biological advantage for heterozygotes is discussed in greater depth in Appendix 2.1 to this chapter, and the reasons behind the variable frequency of CF mutations in different populations in Appendix 2.2.

CF heterozygotes may differ in phenotype from their peers. There is some evidence that they are shorter than their peers [11]. They may also have more upper airway inflammation than expected in the parents of affected children over and above the known clustering of rhinosinusitis in families [12]. This heightened inflammatory response might protect the host in single-gene dosage. Similarly, excess morbidity has been reported for nasal polyps, chronic pancreatitis, allergic bronchopulmonary aspergillosis and bronchiectasis. Heterozygosity for *CFTR* is also associated with chronic pancreatitis [13,14]. Up to half the cases of chronic pancreatitis may be associated with *CFTR* mutations

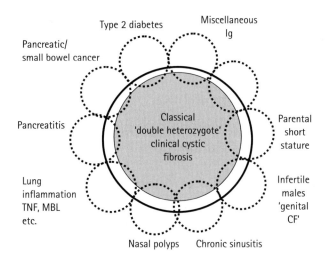

Figure 2.2 Definition problems in the epidemiology of CF. The central shaded circle represents CF patients located in disease registries; most having two classical *CFTR* mutations. The gap up to the outer circle defines patients that have partial, atypical or pre-clinical CF depending on the co-inherited tendencies shown in the dotted epicircles. CF can be considered as an inherited-disease inducing tendency whose severity depends on co-inheritance and acquired factors (or both). The boundaries of CF are fluid and will change further as the interactions of the CF gene/protein are understood. TNF, tumour necrosis factor; MBL, mannose-binding lectin. See text for references.

independently of other genetic forms. This is summarized in Fig. 2.2.

Birth prevalence

Birth prevalence of CF is higher in Caucasian populations than in those of other ethnic groups, and within the European population it generally increases upon moving westwards. Cystic fibrosis also occurs at a relatively high frequency in countries to which European populations have migrated, and at a much lower frequency in non-Caucasian populations. Among the Caucasian populations there are exceptional groups with very high birth prevalence due to relatively high CF gene frequency in small populations that are geographically or culturally isolated. It is quite difficult to estimate birth prevalence accurately because mild cases are diagnosed later in life. This means that a birth cohort must be followed for a long time so that all late diagnoses are included, in order to accurately estimate birth prevalence. Studies based only on neonatal screening are likely to be underestimates of birth prevalence.

Birth prevalence is traditionally cited as 1 in 2000 to 1 in 2500 live births in Caucasian populations. Evidence from more recent and detailed genetic studies and neonatal screening demonstrates that this is not always the case, and in some populations birth prevalence is either much higher

than expected (e.g. in Ohio Amish and Saguenay-Lac St Jean, Quebec) or lower than expected (e.g. in Norway and Finland). However, it should be noted that studies of birth prevalence in small populations are subject to a large level of random error, and some of these estimates may be very inaccurate.

Incidence estimates for countries should be based on large, long-term population studies that would negate the random variation seen in year-to-year birth prevalence [15]. A birth prevalence of 1 case in every 2500 births, giving a CF carrier frequency of 1 in 25 people and a CF gene frequency of 1 in 50, would seem to be the maximum reasonable estimate for any large Caucasian population. In communities showing unusually high birth prevalence, this has been attributed either to a founder effect (e.g. Ohio Amish) or unusually high prevalence of uncommon genetic mutations in a small, culturally or geographically isolated community.

Many Caucasian populations are reported as having a lower birth prevalence than 1 in 2500. In particular, in Finland the population has been reported as having a birth prevalence as low as 1 in 40 000 [16], and values for Sweden are quoted at 1 in 8000 [17–19]. Population subgroups having these antecedents might, therefore, have a substantially lower incidence than the maximum value suggested here.

For non-Caucasian countries, the problem of estimating birth prevalence of CF is even greater, and good estimates are lacking. In many countries, the diagnosis and treatment of CF is a low priority because in terms of its contribution to total infant mortality (IMR) there are other more substantial problems, many of which are more easily dealt with than CF. In these countries, birth prevalence will appear to be low due to a lack of detection as cases are not being actively sought. As developing nations improve their healthcare in childhood, birth prevalence of CF will appear to rise with active detection of cases, particularly in the Indian subcontinent [20].

Table 2.2 summarizes the reported birth prevalence of cystic fibrosis in Caucasian and non-Caucasian populations. In areas where either prenatal genetic screening or neonatal screening is offered, birth prevalence may be declining. This effect has been noted in Canada, Brittany (France), Scotland [21] and the Netherlands (see Table 2.2).

Population prevalence

Population prevalence of cystic fibrosis depends on both birth prevalence (incidence) and survival, which in turn depends on access to high-quality specialist treatment. Very few studies have reported population prevalence directly, but it can be calculated from population registers where sufficiently detailed information exists on both CF and the general population.

Only one population prevalence study has appeared in the peer-reviewed literature [22] – in Toronto, Canada, the population prevalence was reported by age group as being

Table 2.2 Birth prevalence (reported as number of live births per incident case) of CF as reported in different populations.

Country or group	Birth prevalence	Comments
Europe		
United Kingdom [103]	2415	Registry-based study
Northern Ireland [104]	1857	
Scotland [105]	1984	Estimate from carrier frequencies
Sweden [106]	2200–4500	Registry-based study
Sweden [107]	5600	
Norway [108]	6574	Screening study
Denmark [109]	4760	
Irish Republic 110]	1838	
Finland [111]	25 000	
Faroe Islands [112]	1775	
Italy [113]	4238	Registry-based study
Italy (Milan) [114]	3170	Screening study
West Brittany (France) [115]	2667	Calculated from figures in paper
Brittany (France) [116]	2838	
	1972 (if terminated pregnancies included)	
Netherlands [117]	3600 (from 1951 to 1965)	Registry study
	4750 (from 1974 to 1994)	
North America		
United States [118]	3419 (White)	
	12 163 (non-White)	
United States [119]	2500–3500 (White)	Review
	4000–10 000 (Hispanic)	
	15 000–20 000 (Black)	
United States [120]	3200 (White)	Review
	10 500 (Native American)	
	11 500 (Hispanic)	
	14 000–17 000 (Black)	
Canada (Ontario) [121]	2927	
Canada [122]	2500	Registry-based study
Canada [123]	2714 (1971 to 1987)	
	3608 (in 2000)	
Saguenay-Lac St Jean (Quebec) [124]	895	
Ohio Amish [125]	569	Founder effect
Zuni Native Americans [126]	333	
Middle East		
Ashkenazi Jews and Arabs [127]	1800–4000	
Bahrain [128]	5800	
Jordan [129]	2560	Neonatal screening study
Other		
New Zealand (non-Maori) [130]	3185	Not registry-based, likely to be underestimate
New Zealand (non-Maori) [131]	3179	Case-finding study
Australia [132]	2021 (British)	
	3625 (Italian)	
	3726 (Greek)	
Australia [133]	2874	
Japan [134]	355 000	From vital statistics
South Africa (Black) [135]	784–13924	Estimate from carrier frequencies
South Africa [136]	2000 (White)	Based on hospital referrals and diagnosis, likely
	12 000 (Colored)	to be underestimate

Table 2.3 Population prevalence of CF in the United Kingdom in 2003.

Age group	Population prevalence per 100 000
0–4	21.01
5–9	31.99
10–14	32.30
15–19	29.56
20–24	25.76
25–29	15.96
30–34	9.98
35 and over	1.79

1 in 6600 (15 per 100 000) in the white population aged 0 to 14 years, falling to 1 in 12 400 (8 per 100 000) in the white population aged over 25 years. For South Asians, the figures were 1 in 9200 (10.8 per 100 000) to 1 in 56 600 (1.8 per 100 000), respectively.

In the United Kingdom, 6861 patients were known to the patient registry in 2003 [5], with a UK population in the 2001 Census of 58.8 million, giving a crude UK population prevalence of 11.7 per 100 000. Table 2.3 shows UK prevalence by age group (2003 patients and 2004 population estimates). This represents prevalence in a country with high birth prevalence and also relatively high survival. The total number of patients was taken from the UK CF Database Annual Report 2003. Lower prevalence in the 0–9 age group than in the 10–14 group is likely to represent under-notification to the database because of late diagnosis; and overall prevalence is therefore likely to be higher than 11.7 per 100 000 when this under-ascertainment at younger ages is taken into account.

Prevalence for Canada can be calculated overall as 10.5 per 100 000 (based on 2002 patient registry data [4] and 2005 population estimates), and for the United States as 7.7 per 100 000 (based on 2004 patient registry data [3] and 2005 population estimates). Both figures are likely to be underestimates in younger age groups for the reasons given above. Prevalence within the states of the USA varies from 18.4 per 100 000 in Vermont, 14.3 in New Hampshire and 13.9 in Maine to 3.7 per 100 000 in the District of Colombia, 4.8 in New Mexico, 5.7 in Delaware and 6.0 in New Jersey. Prevalence varies according to a variety of factors, including ethnic mix of the states, as well as the proportion of patients accessing specialist healthcare for cystic fibrosis, the method by which they become known to the registry.

In the UK, the number of patients diagnosed exceeds deaths by about 100 patients per year, so prevalence is increasing by almost 0.2 per 100 000 per year. There is a similar increase in Canada and the United States. Decreases in birth prevalence are currently more than offset by increases in survival.

SURVIVAL

This section refers to population measures of survival, rather than prognosis and prognostic indicators in individual patients which are considered later in this chapter.

Survival at population level is a useful indicator of clinical outcome, and is likely to be influenced by a variety of factors, some of which are modifiable by health services (such as clinical care) and some of which are not (such as genotype and to some extent socioeconomic factors).

Mortality

Crude mortality is a measure of mortality, measured in deaths per 1000 population without adjustment for age and gender. Where adjustment for age and gender composition of the population is made, mortality is reported as directly standardized mortality rates.

As a cause of death in the general population, cystic fibrosis is uncommon. The crude death rate for CF in 2003 in the UK is only 0.17 per 100 000 general population. In the United States the crude death rate was reported as falling from 2.4 per million to 1 per million between 1979 and 1991 [23]. However, among younger age groups it is a significant cause of death, being responsible for 1–2% of all deaths in the UK between 5 and 24 years of age. In these age groups it is second only to pneumonia as a respiratory cause of death, exceeding asthma particularly in the 20–24 age group. Cystic fibrosis is therefore an important respiratory cause of death in young people at the population level.

Within the CF population, the crude mortality rates in the UK have varied between 13.5 and 15.0 per 1000 registered patients between 2001 and 2003 [5] (this is not calculated as person years at risk, because insufficient information was available). Between 1968 and 1995 the crude mortality in the UK was 21 per 1000 per year [15]. In the United States the crude mortality has been reported as 23.3 per 1000 between 1991 and 1999 [5], but in 2004 crude mortality rate was 15.6 per 1000 registered patients [3], and in 2002 the crude mortality rate in Canada was 14.8 per 1000 registered patients [4]. All these figures are consistent with falling mortality rates between 1968 and 2004, but it has been noted that mortality is falling more rapidly among young patients than among older patients [24].

Mortality-rate comparisons between different populations can be confounded by the different age structures of the populations. Thus while the overall all-causes population mortality rate for the UK in 1995 was 10.9 per 1000, for the CF population it was 21 per 1000, apparently only double the 'normal' rate. But the CF population is much younger than the non-CF population, and the 'standardized mortality ratio' (SMR) for the CF population, which adjusts for the age difference, has been calculated as 3300 – compared with a normal value of 100 [15].

In the United States, standardized mortality has been shown to vary significantly with genotype, being as low as

4.4 per 1000 person-years at risk for certain genotype combinations and as high as 25.0 per 1000 for others. Class IV mutations have lowest mortality at 7.8 per 1000 and class II mutations the highest at 21.2 per 1000 [8].

Median age at death

Median age at death is a convenient method of making a comparison of deaths between different populations (at national, regional or care-provider level). A low median age at death is taken to infer more premature deaths and therefore possibly suboptimal care. However, this can be a misleading inference. Median age at death will always be younger than survival measured by life-table methods, either using the current or cohort methods. This is because only those patients who have died are included in the measurement of median age at death, whereas all patients in a cohort or population are included in the latter methods.

This is important, because a population with otherwise excellent current or cohort survival, but which by chance has one or two deaths, some of which may not be CF-related, among relatively young patients, will appear to have relatively poor outcomes. However, in the population most of the patients are still alive, and *until they die they will not be included in median age at death statistics*. Thus a population of predominantly old, well and stable patients, but with a few deaths among young patients, may appear to have poor outcomes by chance. Median age at death is more likely to suffer from random error the smaller the population to which it is applied, and its use at clinic population level must be applied with great caution.

The UK CF Database reports the median age at death between 2001 and 2003 as being between 23 and 24.2 years [5]. An international comparison of median age at death has been made and has demonstrated a secular trend towards increased median age at death, but with significant international variations remaining [25]. During the period of study, the median age at death increased from 8 years to 21 years.

Current survival

Current survival curves are calculated using a statistical method that applies current age–sex specific mortality risks to a theoretical population to produce actuarial survival curves. The importance of this method is that is includes all the CF population, not just those who have died. However, it does not take into account cohort effects – for example the age-specific mortality risk for a patient aged 10 years may be different for current 10-year-olds than for those who will be 10 years old in 10 years' time. The difference is likely to become greater the older the age group being considered – it is difficult to predict what the age-specific mortality will be for children with CF being born this year in 30 or 40 years' time. Therefore, although it represents the

current actuarial situation for the current CF population, it *does not* represent the life expectancy of the current birth cohort. Calculation of accurate current survival curves depends on accurate and complete patient registers, as well as full ascertainment of deaths.

Historically, median survival was low. For the patients of one clinic for the period 1943–1964 life-table methods show that meconium ileus usually led to infant death, with about 15% surviving at 1 year. The non-meconium ileus median survival was about 9 months, with about 20% survival to 4 years [26].

More recent, and much improved, current median survival estimates have been reported for a number of populations. In 1994, the current UK survival for CF patients was 30 years [12], but this is likely to have improved since then, although no more recent reports exist. A very high median current survival age of 37.7 years was reported recently from Italy. Median survival ages have also been reported from the United States at 28 years in 1993 [27], but this had risen to 35.1 years by 2004 [3]. In Canada, median survival was reported in 1996 as 36.7 for males and 27.8 for females [28]. The Canadian CF Foundation Patient Data Registry Report in 2002 [4] showed improvements in current survival from 22.8 years in 1977 to 37.0 years in 2002, without the pronounced gender gap in the earlier published report.

It is important to remember that these survival curves apply only at the population level – an *individual* patient who has reached the median age of survival, for example 40 years, will have a probability of surviving another 10 years that is different from, and probably higher than, the average survival to 50 years, because they represent a special, survivor population who did not have what is now considered optimum healthcare from the time of birth or diagnosis. They are not, therefore, useful in estimating prognosis in individual cases.

Cohort survival

Cohort survival curves are similar to current survival curves, but calculated for individual birth cohorts in one-, two- or five-year groups. These are particularly valuable in showing how survival at various ages has changed over time. Although it is tempting to extrapolate a median survival from recent birth cohorts, a degree of caution has to be used, since it cannot be assumed that mortality risk at higher ages will be similar in recent birth cohorts to that in earlier birth cohorts, since members of the latter reaching advanced ages represent a survivor cohort who may have different clinical and survival characteristics.

Cohort survival has been reported from a number of countries including the UK, USA and Italy. Common to all studies are the findings that survival continues to improve with each successive birth cohort, and that the majority of the improvements in survival have come during the first few years of age. The 2004 US CF Foundation Patient Registry Annual Report [3] showed that the proportion surviving to age 12 years had increased from 93% in the 1980–84 birth cohort to 96.5% in the 1990–94 birth cohort. In the UK, the proportion surviving to age 15 years was approximately 49% and 54% for females and males, respectively, for the 1968–70 birth cohort, but had improved to 77% and 86%, respectively, for the 1980–82 birth cohort [15].

There is some evidence, however, that there has been a reduction in the rate at which median survival is improving in recent years [29]. The only country with published cohort survival curves for older birth cohorts is the UK. Survival at older ages has shown improvement with time, and there is no evidence that cohort survival curves are converging at older ages as might be expected if a substantial survivor effect was operating in the oldest birth cohorts. Over the age of 20 years mortality was 50 per 1000 per year for all birth cohorts (compared with an average over the same time period of 21 per 1000), suggesting that these older age groups are not experiencing the improvements in survival seen at younger ages [30].

Although caution must be used in extrapolating to the future because of the potential effect of unpredictable factors on mortality, if we assume that survival at older ages remains similar to current survival, median survival for the cohort born since 1990 is likely to exceed 50 years and may be as high as 60 years in the UK. It is predicted that 95% of those born in Sweden since 1991 will survive to their 25th birthday and the probability of surviving to 40 years was reported as 83% in Denmark [31]. A high proportion of current children with CF are therefore likely to reach middle-age or beyond, and planning of care and treatment needs to take into account this extended life span.

AGE DISTRIBUTION

The age distribution of patients in a population gives important information to planners of healthcare. It is a function in any population of birth rate, mortality rates and survival. In many countries the majority of patients are now adults (aged 16 or over). In the UK in 2003, 50.8% of patients were adults (aged 16 or over) [5]. In 2002, 47% of Canadian patients were aged 18 or over [4]. In the United States in 2004, 42% were aged 18 or over [3]. In Sweden, 45% were aged 18 or over in 1999.

The age distribution of UK patients in 2003 is shown in Fig. 2.3. Because births exceed deaths, and there are very few deaths in children, both number and proportion of adult patients is likely to continue to increase, even in areas where neonatal or prenatal carrier screening has reduced birth prevalence.

DIAGNOSIS

Although genotype analysis is readily available, diagnosis is usually made either on clinical grounds or on the basis of a screening program. Genetic analysis has made it possible

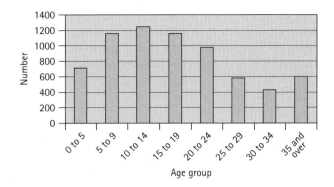

Figure 2.3 Age distribution of patients with CF in the United Kingdom in 2003. Data from UK Cystic Fibrosis Database Annual Report 2003 [5].

to identify homozygous CF in patients with few or no clinical manifestations, and for this reason the definition of cystic fibrosis has been modified by consensus statement. Patients with 'classic' CF must now have a coherent clinical syndrome, plus either evidence of CFTR dysfunction (abnormal sweat chloride or nasal potential difference) or confirmation of two abnormal CF-causing mutations [32]. Patients who do not meet these criteria, but with some CFTR abnormality, have CFTR-related disease but not cystic fibrosis.

In 1996, 6.2% of newly-diagnosed patients in the United States were diagnosed by neonatal screening [2]. The proportion diagnosed by screening in any population depends on the national or local screening policy, and in the UK the current proportion diagnosed by screening is likely to be 20% [33]. Regardless of whether the case presents clinically or through screening, diagnosis is confirmed by the sweat test. In the United States, 98% of patients had sweat sodium or chloride $\geqslant 61$ mEq/L, with a mean sweat chloride of 101.7 mEq/L (standard deviation 18.91 mEq/L). Of the 2% who were sweat test negative, 75% were diagnosed on the basis of two known mutations, 1% on transepithelial potential difference, and 24% on clinical manifestation [2].

Age at diagnosis

In the United States, 70% of all CF patients were diagnosed before their first birthday [2], and 90% before their eighth birthday. The proportion diagnosed before 1 year was similar, although slightly lower in series from New Zealand (61%) [34] and Ireland (55%) [35], although the latter patients were adolescents and adults. In the UK, the median age at diagnosis since 2001 has been 4–5 months; and of all newly-diagnosed children in 2003, 64% were diagnosed under the age of 1 year [5]. However, late diagnosis continues to be made, with occasional cases being diagnosed as late as the seventh decade of life (Fig. 2.4). In the UK, 12% of newly-diagnosed patients in 2003 were over 16 years of age [5].

Late diagnosis (after age 16) is associated with a milder clinical syndrome than seen in patients diagnosed as children [36]. This includes better lung function and nutritional status, and a lower prevalence of colonization by *Pseudomonas aeruginosa*. Late-diagnosed patients usually represent the mild end of the clinical spectrum presented by cystic fibrosis. This has very important implications when considering studies looking at the long-term benefits of neonatal screening for cystic fibrosis.

Neonatal screening

It seems reasonable to assume that early diagnosis of patients with cystic fibrosis before the onset of chronic bacterial colonization of the respiratory tract, and before the onset of clinical malnutrition, would lead to an improved clinical outcome. However, there is surprisingly little high-level evidence that long-term outcome is improved as a result of neonatal screening, the majority of evidence coming from observational studies.

The reasons for this include the lack of high-quality randomized studies, the majority employing either pseudo-randomization, or using historical or geographic controls, or no controls at all. In those studies where randomization has been employed, there is difficulty in interpretation of results because those diagnosed later in life have milder disease. This means that the screened cohort will include the majority of patients, including those with very mild disease, whereas the control cohort will include, at least initially, only those with more severe disease. Therefore reported differences in clinical outcome might be explained by this bias, unless this is accounted for in analysis. Also, some studies with randomized design have been let down by failure to analyze by intention-to-screen (i.e. analyze the groups as originally randomized); this usually means including those missed by screening (false negatives) in the group diagnosed

clinically. This would tend to enhance clinical differences between the groups.

In a pseudo-randomized study in the UK, which was not analyzed by intention-to-screen, there were few reported clinical benefits, the main one being reduced time in hospital in the screened cohort in the first year of life. However, this could be explained by the differential rates of inclusion of mild cases in the screened and unscreened cohorts under the age of 1 year [37]. The study with the most robust design and analysis comes from Wisconsin in the United States. This study has recently reported 10-year follow-up, demonstrating small but significant differences in favor of the screened cohort for nutritional parameters, especially in those with pancreatic insufficiency and homozygous for *F508del* [38]. A later report from the same study showed improved nutritional outcomes after 13 years' follow-up [39], but benefits do tend to converge over time. Effect of screening on pulmonary outcomes is less clear, and after 10 years screened children had worse chest X-ray scores, possibly due to early chronic *Pseudomonas aeruginosa* infection [40]. There are other less quantifiable benefits from running a screening program among neonates. This includes the ability to offer prenatal diagnosis to parents of infants detected by screening, the reduction of stress among parents seeking a diagnosis for their sick child, rapid determination of population prevalence in developing countries or areas where this is unknown, and the ability to research early development of respiratory and nutritional abnormalities in CF patients before clinical symptoms develop.

Limitations in design of published studies on neonatal screening have led to a cautious approach in implementing nationwide screening in several countries. In 2003, a Center for Disease Control and CF Foundation workshop considered that the benefits of neonatal screening outweighed the

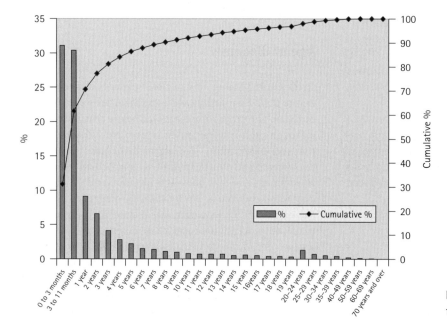

Figure 2.4   Age at diagnosis of cystic fibrosis. Data from [2].

potential risks and harms, and concluded that neonatal screening was justified, although implementation was left up to individual states [41]. Neonatal screening has also been recommended or implemented on a national basis in France, Scotland and England, and has been available in other countries and regions including Wales, Germany, Israel, Italy, Belgium, New Zealand and Australia, for varying periods of time.

Clinical presentation

The commonest clinical presentation of CF remains acute or persistent respiratory symptoms, appearing in 51% of all cases diagnosed in the United States [2]. Other common clinical features on presentation in this report were failure to thrive or malnutrition (43%), steatorrhea or abnormal stools (35%), and meconium ileus or intestinal obstruction (19.1%).

Clinical presentations of US patients in 1996 are summarized in Fig. 2.5. It is interesting to note that, although

overall only 3.5% were diagnosed by screening (prenatal or neonatal), this method of presentation comprised 9.1% of newly-diagnosed patients [2]. Genotype as a means presentation was 1.5% overall, but 5.8% of newly-diagnosed patients in 1996. This suggests that the number of patients with CF diagnosed before the onset of any clinical symptoms is increasing.

Congenital bilateral absence of the vas deferens (CBAVD) is a clinical syndrome recently described in which there is a relatively high prevalence of *CFTR* mutations, with 14.5% being homozygous for *CFTR* mutations, 48.1% being heterozygous, and 37.4% having no CFTR abnormalities [42]. A high proportion of patients with CBAVD homozygous for *CFTR* mutations have abnormal sweat chloride [43], and a few have some clinical symptoms suggestive of CF. This has led to a re-definition of cystic fibrosis, distinguishing it from CFTR-related disease that is not cystic fibrosis [20].

CLINICAL FEATURES

Lung function

In the UK in 2003, the median percentage predicted FEV_1 was 70–79% [5]. In Canada in 2002, the mean FEV_1 percentage predicted was 74.1% [4]. The distribution of percentage predicted FEV_1 percentiles for children and adults in the UK CF clinical population is summarized in Fig. 2.6.

FEV_1 by age in the US CF population is shown in Fig. 2.7. These data are difficult to interpret because of age-cohort effects. They represent all CF patients in the US Patient Data Registry, and therefore consist of several different birth cohorts, not all of which were exposed to current treatment practices throughout their life. In addition, there is a survivor effect – meaning that, in each cohort, lung function can be measured only in those remaining alive. As age increases, the proportion of each birth cohort that remains as

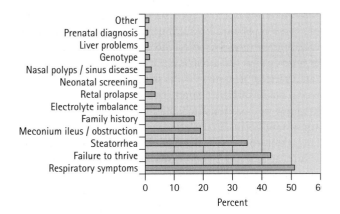

Figure 2.5 Clinical features suggesting the diagnosis of CF. These modes of clinical presentation are not mutually exclusive, and therefore the total is greater than 100%. Data from [2].

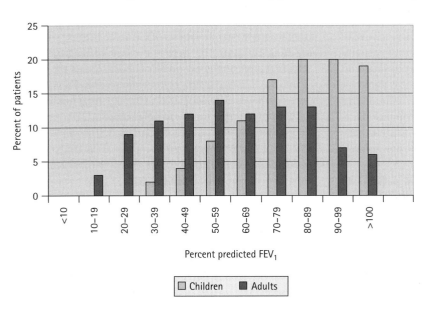

Figure 2.6 Lung function (percent predicted) in the UK CF clinical population. Number of patients with data = 4422. Data from [5].

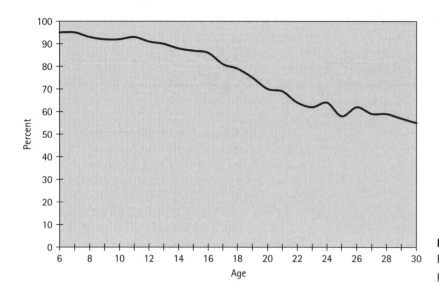

Figure 2.7 Median percentage predicted FEV$_1$ by age (years) in the US CF clinical population. Data from [3].

Table 2.4 Severity of lung function defect (FEV$_1$) by age.

Severity of FEV$_1$ defect	Children		Adults	
	n	%	*n*	%
Normal (>90% predicted)	780	38	317	13
Mild (70–89% predicted)	749	37	613	26
Moderate (40–69% predicted)	443	22	914	38
Severe (<40% predicted)	66	3	552	23

Data from *UK Cystic Fibrosis Database Annual Data Report 2003* [5].

survivors decreases. Those with worse lung function are usually the ones to die first. Those left therefore become the extreme survivors of that birth cohort, and therefore very atypical of the original group.

Difficulties with cohort and survivor effects mean that it is not possible to predict decline in lung function among a cohort of existing patients from these current lung function measurements. However, Fig. 2.5 demonstrates the pattern that might be expected in a population of patients who develop a progressive, predominantly obstructive respiratory function defect, followed by censoring of patients with a severe defect from the population either by death or transplantation. Increase in mean lung function parameters due to censoring are offset by decline among the remaining members of the cohort. There is evidence from the US CF Foundation Patient Registry that median percentage predicted FEV$_1$ has improved in all age groups since 1990 [3].

Fig. 2.6 demonstrates that the majority of patients at any point in time have good lung function, with only a few suffering from severe respiratory function defects, but this proportion is higher in the adult age group. Table 2.4 shows that the majority of those with moderate to severe lung disease are in the older age groups.

Average rates of decline of lung function with time have not been reported very frequently in the literature. Various

cohort studies of CF patients have demonstrated a lung function decline *in individual adult patients* of approximately 3–5% of predicted per annum in FEV$_1$ [44]. A recent study in the United States showed a mean decline of −3.89% predicted per annum (±4.11%). The range of variation was considerable, with some patients showing no or little decline (1.1% per annum) and others showing very rapid rates of decline (−8.1% per annum) [45]. The most recent data from the United States showed a rate of decline in those not participating in clinical trials of 1.52% per annum [46]. This is consistent with a recent study from the UK, which shows that the rate of FEV$_1$ decline per annum is low, and falling in successive birth cohorts. The mean annual decline in FEV$_1$ between the ages of 18 and 22 was 1.53%, but this fell from 2.49% to 0.65% with successive birth cohorts [47]. This suggests that earlier estimates of rate of decline are no longer valid for more recent groups of patients, and that the rate of lung function decline can be reduced to almost zero, even in adults.

Lung function is related to other aspects of clinical status in CF (Table 2.5). However, it is difficult to determine whether these manifestations of CF arose because of declining lung function, or were the cause of it, from cross-sectional data, and good-quality cohort studies are lacking.

In the UK in 2003, colonization with *Pseudomonas aeruginosa* was also associated with poor lung function [5]. Of those with *P. aeruginosa* colonization, 22% had poor lung function (FEV$_1$ under 40% predicted) compared with 6% of non-colonized patients. Only 11% of colonized patients had normal lung function (90% or more) compared with 35% of non-colonized patients.

Respiratory infection

The organism most frequently reported in sputum culture from cystic fibrosis patients is *Pseudomonas aeruginosa*. In the United States, 57% of patients had *P. aeruginosa* in their

Table 2.5 Association between lung function, microbial colonization and nutritional status in the US CF clinical population in 1996.

FEV$_1$ (% predicted)	n	%	% cultured Pseudomonas aeruginosa	% cultured Burkholderia cepacia	% under 5th centile for weight
Normal (90% or more)	4346	32	44.9	1.3	9.5
Mild (70–89%)	3884	24	64.1	3.0	14.4
Moderate (40–69%)	4182	28	80.9	5.6	31.3
Severe (<40%)	2295	16	87.3	8.4	61.2
Total	14707	100	67.2	4.2	25.1

Data from *US Patient Data Registry* [2].

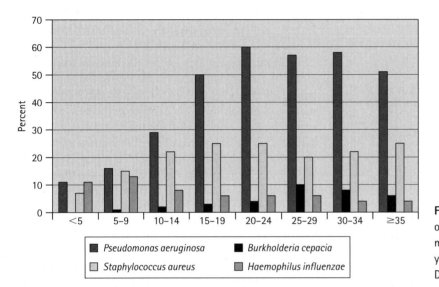

Figure 2.8 Age-related prevalence of microorganisms isolated from sputum on one or more occasion during the course of a single year. Number of patients with data = 5295. Data from [5].

sputum or other respiratory cultures in 2004 [3], but the proportion in the UK in 2003 was much lower at 38% [5].

The prevalence of *P. aeruginosa* infection varies between countries, and between treatment centers within countries. In Canada, for example, the isolation frequency for *P. aeruginosa* was 48% in 1995, but varied between treatment centers from 25% to 52% [48]. In UK pediatric centers in 2003, colonization rates ranged from 47% to 3%, and in UK adult centers from 84% to 47% [5]. The reported prevalence in New Zealand was 44% [22], and in *adults* in France was 62% [49] and Ireland 69% [23]. In Italy, prevalence was 49% [50].

Of the factors that affect infection rates with different micro-organisms, one of the most important is age. The prevalence of *Pseudomonas aeruginosa, Burkholderia cepacia, Aspergillus* spp and mycobacteria increase with age. The prevalence of *Haemophilus influenzae* falls with age. *Staphylococcus aureus* remains relatively common throughout life. These patterns are shown for the most frequently isolated organisms for the UK in 2003 in Fig. 2.8.

Recent recognition of highly-transmissible strains of *P. aeruginosa* has led to implementation of segregation and hygiene policies within clinics which may be responsible for

reduction in prevalence in sputum culture. In addition, chronic colonization can be prevented or delayed by early aggressive treatment upon first isolation, which has contributed to reduced prevalence of chronic colonization [51].

Other risk factors for colonization with *P. aeruginosa* that have been suggested include genotype (certain genotypes are associated with lower colonization rates), sex [52] (females may be colonized younger than males), pancreatic-insufficient phenotype, and nosocomial transmission within treatment centers where precautions were not taken to prevent cross-colonization [53]. *Pseudomonas aeruginosa* can appear in the respiratory tract of young infants with CF [54] prior to the onset of clinical respiratory disease, suggesting that this may be a primary infection, and prior lung damage by other micro-organisms is not necessary for infection to be established.

Likewise, although the overall prevalence of *Burkholderia cepacia* complex infection was only slightly higher in Canada than in the United States (9.2% in Canada, 3.6% in the USA), the prevalence varied from 2% to 21% in different treatment centers within Canada [48]. This is likely to represent both differences in the spread of risk factors for colonization for these organisms, and differences in policies to limit cross-infection operating in the different treatment centers. *Burkholderia cepacia* colonization has been clearly demonstrated to be associated with adverse clinical outcome, and as with *P. aeruginosa*, infection control measures implemented in treatment centers have led to a reduction in incidence of new cases of *B. cepacia* complex infection [55].

The frequency of all organisms isolated in UK patients in 2003 is shown in Fig. 2.9. Different countries, and different treatment centers within countries, show different patterns of respiratory infection. For example, the United States has a higher prevalence of *P. aeruginosa* infection in both children and adults than the UK (approximately 30% and 80%, respectively), and a high prevalence of *Stenotrophomonas maltophilia* infection at 12%, an organism seen less frequently in the UK. Knowledge of local bacteriology patterns in CF patients is of great importance not only to clinical care, but also in infection control.

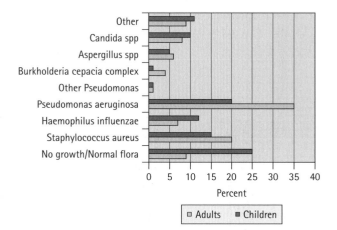

Figure 2.9 Percentage of patients colonized with common respiratory pathogens in cystic fibrosis. Number of patients with data = 5295. Data from [5].

Growth and nutritional status

The distribution of height and weight percentiles in the CF clinical population is bimodal, with one mode at 25th to 50th centile, and another mode at below 5th centile, representing a small group (10.5% of patients) with severe nutritional compromise. The distribution of height, weight and body mass index (BMI) centiles in the UK in 2003 are shown in Fig. 2.10. Adults tend to have a lower weight and body mass index centile than children, but similar height centile distributions, and a higher proportion of adult patients are severely underweight (22% as opposed to 13% of children). However, it should be noted that a proportion of patients maintain average nutrition or better (39% of adults and 46% of children are above 50th centile for BMI). In the UK, 12% of adults with CF meet the definition of overweight or obese (BMI over 25).

Again, the explanation of this distribution from cross-sectional data is difficult. Possible explanations include a cohort effect whereby adults did not benefit from current nutritional management when they were children, and hence now suffer from residual effects of malnutrition while young. There may also be a survivor effect operating, particularly in respect of the higher height centile, where the smaller and lighter children did not reach adult life, and the selective good prognosis of pancreatic sufficiency. There is another cohort effect that may be operating, namely the late maturation and growth of children with CF, meaning that full adult height is reached well after the age of 17 years. Finally, low weight among the adult group may be due to deteriorating clinical condition with age.

Average weight percentile is increasing at all ages up to 20 years in the United States, and is also increasing with successive birth cohorts [3]. The median weight centile at 5 years has increased from 30% in the 1980–84 birth cohort to 42% in the 2000 cohort. This is consistent with a report

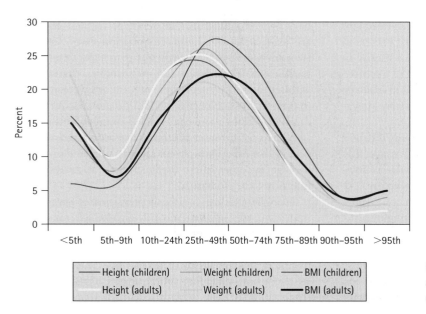

Figure 2.10 Distribution of height, weight and body mass index centiles in adults and children with CF. Data from [5].

from Australia showing the proportion of adults with BMI below 20 fell from 62% to 9% in the 17 years from 1983 to 2000 [56].

Complications

In addition to the classical clinical manifestations of CF – respiratory infection and malabsorption – there are a number of clinical complications affecting individuals with CF that are related to CF, but appear in only a minority of patients. The overall frequency of various complications in UK patients is shown in Fig. 2.11. The frequency of all complications rises with age, with the exception of allergic bronchopulmonary aspergillosis.

The most frequent major complications recorded in the CF clinical population are diabetes mellitus and abnormal liver function. In the UK in 2003, 14% of patients had diabetic glucose tolerance, and a further 3% impaired glucose tolerance [5]. The prevalence of diabetes rose from 1% in children under 10 years to a maximum of 43% in the

30–35 years age group, falling again to 33% over 35 years of age.

There have been varying reports of annual incidence and overall prevalence of diabetes mellitus in different CF clinical populations. This variation may in part be due to different ages of the clinical populations, in part to differences in the diagnostic tests and criteria applied to define diabetes in the CF population, and in part due to true differences in prevalence. The Danish cohort studies have been the most methodologically precise. In 1994, a prevalence of diabetes mellitus of 14.7% was reported in the Danish CF population [57]. Age was the only reported risk factor for development of diabetes; underlying severity of cystic fibrosis was not a risk factor. This study also reported that CF patients develop microvascular complications of diabetes at a similar rate to diabetics without CF. In a later report, the same authors recorded a mean age of diagnosis of diabetes at 21 years, and reported that impaired glucose tolerance (IGT) on a previous oral glucose tolerance test conferred a relative risk of 5.6 for development of diabetes, although some patients with IGT on one or more occasion did not go on to develop diabetes [58].

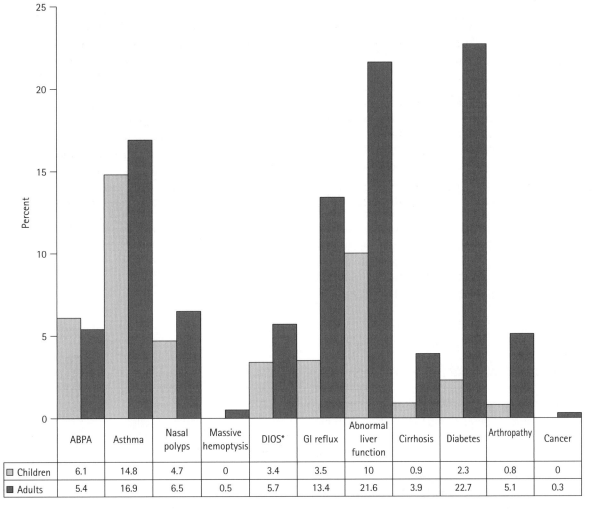

	ABPA	Asthma	Nasal polyps	Massive hemoptysis	DIOS*	GI reflux	Abnormal liver function	Cirrhosis	Diabetes	Arthropathy	Cancer
☐ Children	6.1	14.8	4.7	0	3.4	3.5	10	0.9	2.3	0.8	0
■ Adults	5.4	16.9	6.5	0.5	5.7	13.4	21.6	3.9	22.7	5.1	0.3

Figure 2.11   Proportion of patients with CF having different types of recorded complication. Rates are calculated as the proportion of patients with each complication. Number of patients with recorded data = 4897. Calculated from data in [5]. ABPI, allergic bronchopulmonary aspergillosis; DIOS, distal intestinal obstruction syndrome.

Liver disease is an important complication of CF because it is associated with an adverse prognosis and may require liver transplantation. In the UK, 15.4% of patients recorded abnormal liver function in 2003 [5], as did 8% of US patients in 2004 [3]. These data registry studies are probably an underestimate, and a cohort from Canada showed a prevalence of 41% at age 12 years, with 7.8% going on to develop cirrhosis [59]. Prevalence did not rise after the age of 12 in this cohort, but this does not mean that new cases cannot arise after that age.

The UK CF Database does not record the prevalence of bone disease. However, osteoporosis is a recently recognized important complication of CF, reported in 8% of the US CF population in 2004, and with a prevalence rising almost linearly with age to 20% of those aged 45 and over [3]. A high proportion of patients in one study had a bone mineral density below −1 Standard deviations (42.5%), and very low bone mineral density measurements are associated with low body mass index below 5th centile [60]. In adults and adolescents, prevalence was even higher at 61% for osteopenia or osteoporosis, and risk was highest in those with severe disease and taking corticosteroids [61]. The reasons for low bone mineral density in CF are not known. It is likely to arise due to a combination of a low rate of bone mineralization during childhood due to poor nutritional status, together with poorer preservation of bone mineralization due to poor nutrition and lack of weight-bearing exercise later in life. Indeed, in patients with normal levels of nutrition, bone mineral density appears to be normal in cystic fibrosis when compared with controls of similar height [62]. This suggests that low bone mineral density is not inevitable in CF, and that nutritional status is an important factor in etiology of CF-related bone disease.

Of recent interest is the question as to whether adults with CF are more susceptible to cancer. A large cohort study from the United States concluded that the risk of cancer among patients with CF overall was the same as that for the general population (RR 0.8; 95% CI 0.6 to 1.1). However, there was an increased risk of gastrointestinal cancer in both the US and European cohorts enrolled in the study, with a relative risk of 6.5 (3.5 to 11.1) and 6.4 (2.9 to 14.0), respectively [63].

SOCIAL AND DEMOGRAPHIC FEATURES IN ADULTS

Reported measurements of clinical outcome in CF have not been very sophisticated in reports of either clinical trials, or clinical case series. Measures tend to be confined to either survival, or measurements of lung function, nutritional status, clinical or x-ray scores, or biochemical parameters. While these are important indicators of clinical status, they do not necessarily reflect how the patient feels, and more importantly, whether his or her lifestyle matches that of peers without CF.

Demographic

In the US CF patient population in 1996, 33% of adult patients were married or cohabiting, with a further 5.2% separated, widowed or divorced [2], and this had risen to 36% and 5.2%, respectively, in 2004 [3]. Very similar figures were obtained from a survey of adults in the UK [6], where 30% were married or cohabiting with a further 2.6% divorced, separated or widowed in the year 2000. Similar proportions have been reported elsewhere [64]. The proportion married or cohabiting rises with age to over 60% in those over 30 years of age. Males are significantly less likely to be married or cohabiting than females, after adjustment for age and measures of clinical severity.

Male patients with CF were also significantly more likely to remain living with their parents than females, although as age increased, the differences between men and women decreased. (Fig. 2.12). This suggests that although it may be harder for young men with CF to achieve independence, it is delayed rather than prevented. A study from the Netherlands suggested that patients with CF were no more likely to be dependent on their parents than other young people [65]. In the UK in 2003, 56% of men and 37% of women aged 20–24 in the general population were still living with their parents [66], suggesting that young people with CF differ little from the general population, which also displays a gender difference. The figures for

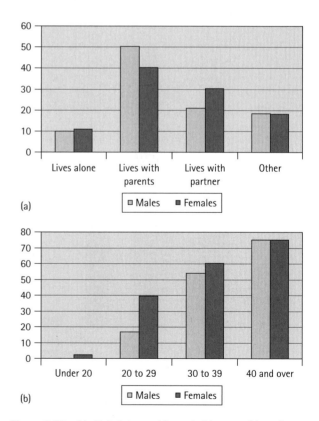

(a)

(b)

Figure 2.12 Marital status and household composition of adults with cystic fibrosis: **(a)** household composition; **(b)** proportion married or cohabiting by age and sex. Data from [6].

adults with CF in 2000 aged 20–29 were 54% and 33%, respectively.

Nine percent of adult patients in the year 2000 had parental responsibility for children of their own, and the proportion rose to 22% in those over 40 years of age. Two percent acted as carer for another adult, usually a parent or grandparent. As patients survive longer and get older, many will outlive their parents, and the proportion caring for elderly relatives is likely to increase. Those providing care for adults with CF need to recognize that many do not live with parents, and have their own responsibilities as carers of others.

Education

Despite the fact that CF patients from time to time miss periods of education due to episodes of illness, educational attainments of adults with CF are similar to those of the general population. In the United States, 27% of adult patients in 2004 had achieved a college degree or higher [3]. In the UK, the educational attainments of adults with CF were impressive, and were at least comparable to those of the general population of the same age, with 78% achieving GCSE or equivalent qualifications, 28% A-level or equivalent, 24% a degree qualification, and 4% a higher degree (Masters or Doctorate) [6]. Over 70% of patients take a further qualification after leaving school.

Any academic qualification is associated with an increased likelihood of employment (Fig. 2.13), even after adjustment for clinical status.

A study in the Netherlands suggested that educational attainments among adults with CF were higher than among the general population, with the CF population concentrating on traditional education, while the general population preferred vocational training [65].

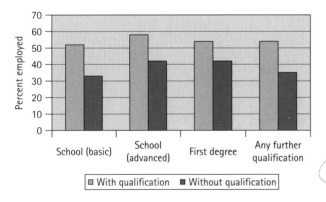

Figure 2.13 Association between educational attainments and employment status. School (basic) = GCSE, usually taken aged 16. School (advanced) = A-level, usually taken aged 18. Any further qualification includes professional and vocational qualifications as well as qualifications from higher education such as degrees and professional diplomas. Data from [6].

Employment

A high proportion of adult patients are able to work, either full or part-time. In the UK, adults achieved 80% of the employment rate of the general population of the same age and sex [67]. In both the United States and the UK, at least 50% of adults are in paid employment, with a further 24–25% students [3,6]. In the UK, 81% of adults with CF had ever been able to work, either full- or part-time, rising to over 98% by the age of 40 [6]. Half of those not currently employed in the UK were unable to work due to ill-health [6] (Fig. 2.14). In the UK, factors associated with *unemployment* were younger age, female gender, lower socioeconomic status, no basic or advanced school-leaving qualifications and more severe disease [6]. Older patients are more likely to give ill-health as a reason for not working. Some patients continue to work until normal age-related retirement.

Of particular interest is the fact that, although survival has been steadily increasing, the proportion of adults able to work has remained similar to studies reporting a decade ago, suggesting that continued survival increases have not been at the expense of quality of life. The majority of patients remain well for the majority of their lives.

Quality of life

Although there are CF-specific quality-of-life instruments, these do not permit comparison with other conditions, for which purpose a generic quality-of-life instrument is preferable. In 2000, the EuroQOL questionnaire [68] was included in a survey of adults with CF in the UK. Very few patients reported poor quality of life overall (6%). The proportion reporting problems in different domains of the EQ5D questionnaire are compared with the normal UK population in Fig. 2.15. The proportion of adults with CF reporting problems is higher than in the normal population, although the proportion reporting *severe* problems was under 3% in all domains, so the majority of these problems were not severe. However, the EQ5D score among adults with CF (0.77) does not differ greatly from reported scores in adults of similar ages with other chronic medical conditions, including asthma (0.73), chronic fatigue syndrome (0.76–0.86) and low back pain (0.69). The EQ5D and Visual Analogue Scale scores were both associated with markers of clinical severity [6].

PROGNOSIS

There have been many attempts to derive prognostic indicators for CF. This has been made more important by the advent of transplantation as a treatment for end-stage lung disease. It is therefore useful to have an index that will indicate when survival is expected to be poorer for the untreated patient than for a transplanted patient, and hence when referral for transplantation might be considered. Very few

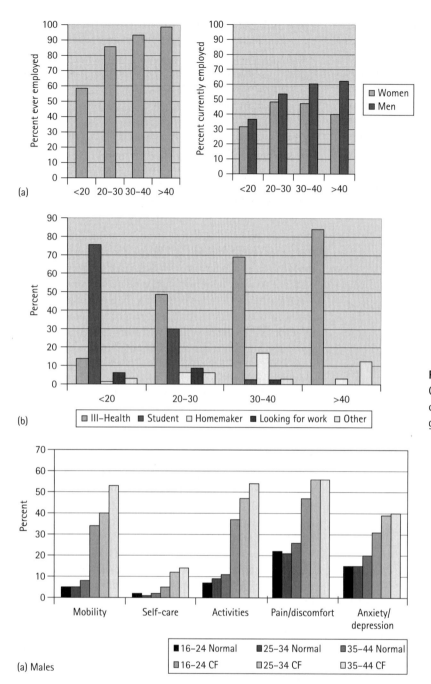

(a)

(b)

Figure 2.14 Employment status of adults with CF: **(a)** proportion ever employed and proportion currently employed by age group; **(b)** reasons given for not working, by age. Data from [6].

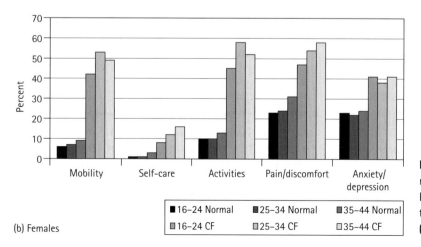

(a) Males

(b) Females

Figure 2.15 Proportion of adults with CF reporting any problems in each domain of the EuroQOL quality-of-life instrument compared with the UK population of the same age: **(a)** males; **(b)** females. Data from [5] and [102].

of these prognostic models have been validated by standard measures of sensitivity, specificity and predictive value to predict death over a pre-specified time period.

The problem with the studies reported in the literature is that they all start with different baseline populations: for example some consider children, others adults, and other all-age groups. They also use different survival times as an indicator, ranging from 2 to 10 years and over. They use different analytic methods that may produce different results in the same patient population. They also include slightly different subsets of clinical information in their multivariate models.

Genotype

Initial studies concentrated on the issue as to whether homozygosity for the *F508del* mutation conferred a particularly severe phenotype. However, the majority of these studies took place before a good classification of effects of different mutations on function of *CFTR* was produced. The majority of studies employing multivariate modeling that included genotype markers have concluded that homozygosity for *F508del* is *not* an adverse prognostic indicator, but different mutation classes may be. A cohort study has established that genotype not only affects phenotype, but also mortality. Significantly lower mortality rates were seen in patients carrying the *G551D, DeltaI507, R117H,* 3849 + 10 kb C → T, 2789 + 5 kb G → A alleles [8].

Pancreatic-sufficient phenotype

A pancreatic-sufficient phenotype is generally associated with milder clinical manifestations of cystic fibrosis. However, its association with survival is not as clear as for other risk factors, like pulmonary function. After accounting for major prognostic factors, pancreatic-sufficient phenotype has been a significant positive prognostic indicator in only a few studies [69,70].

Age

As for phenotype, once major prognostic factors are accounted for, age appears not to be a major determinant of survival, appearing as a determinant of survival in only one study [71].

Sex

It has been reported in some countries that average life expectancy is shorter for females than males with cystic fibrosis. However, it is not completely clear whether this is a gender-specific phenomenon *per se*, or whether it is related to increased prevalence of other poor prognostic indicators in women, such as poor lung function and nutritional

status. In the first year of life, survival is greater for girls, but after that, greater for boys, giving an overall survival advantage for males.

A study in a large US clinical cohort demonstrated that, after adjustment for a number of other prognostic factors, such as nutritional status, pulmonary function, pancreatic-sufficient phenotype, age at diagnosis, mode of presentation, race and airway microbiology, female sex conferred an additional risk of death before the age of 20 years (RR 1.6; 95% CI 1.4 to 1.8), but after the age of 20 years there was no significant difference [70]. A similar gender gap in survival in younger females (aged 2–20 years) was again reported in 2003 in the United States [72]. It has been suggested that this gender gap in survival may be due to very marked reduction in life expectancy among females with CF who also have diabetes [73]. Other possible explanations for the observation of shorter survival in females include poorer nutrition in females, which was felt to account for the reduced survival seen in Canadian females [29], and an earlier age at first colonization with *Pseudomonas aeruginosa*.

In some other studies, female sex emerged as an adverse prognostic indicator [74], but in other careful studies aimed at developing prognostic indices for CF, female sex was not an adverse prognostic indicator after other important markers for survival were accounted for [75]. In children in the UK, gender does not appear to be a prognostic indicator [76], nor does survival show a gender difference in Italy [77]. In general, studies demonstrating poorer survival among females have been from North America, and those showing no gender difference from the UK or Europe.

Pulmonary function

Almost every study employing multivariate modeling techniques identifies pulmonary function as a major determinant of survival. This includes several of the studies mentioned above [29,69,71,75]. In some studies, FEV_1 was the only lung function marker associated with survival, in others, FVC [75] or a marker of gas trapping (RV/TLC; residual volume/total lung capacity) were independently associated with survival [78]. In some studies, FEV_1 percentage predicted emerged as the only significant prognostic marker. Few have reported sensitivity and specificity of FEV_1 to predict mortality at various cut-off points using receiver–operator curves. One study reported that 54% of those below FEV_1 55% predicted died within 5 years and 96% of those above this value survived 5 years [79].

In a cohort study, we reported that FEV_1 was a better predictor of 2-year survival than the Shwachman clinical score [80]. With a cut-off of 47% predicted for FEV_1, sensitivity was 89% and specificity 80%, but positive predictive value was only 6% (i.e. 6% of those with an FEV_1 below 47% would die within 2 years) – too imprecise to be used for referral for transplantation. Another study reported a sensitivity of 42% and specificity of 95% for an FEV_1 below 30% predicted [81]. Rate of decline of lung function may be a better predictor of mortality in those with severe lung function limitation [82]. Predictors of mortality may differ in those who already have severely compromised lung function than in the general population, and this needs to be taken into account.

Exercise tolerance

A study from the United States suggested that exercise tolerance could be a more sensitive prognostic indicator than simple lung function tests. This study found that peak oxygen uptake ($V_{O2 \, peak}$) was a better predictor of 8-year survival in patients over 7 years of age than FEV_1 [83]. In this study, colonization with *Burkholderia cepacia* was the only other risk factor, age, sex, body mass index, FEV_1 and PCO_2 after exercise being unrelated to survival.

However, a more recent UK study in adults found that, although univariate analysis identified exercise performance as prognostic markers (including $VO_{2 \, peak}$, peak work rate, peak minute ventilation (VE) and VE/VO_2 ratio), multivariate analysis revealed only FEV_1 to predict 5-year survival [68]. FEV_1 over 55% predicted gave a 96% 5-year survival, but for an FEV_1 under 55% predicted 5-year survival was only 46%. In this study, colonization with *Burkholderia cepacia* was not a predictor of survival. As with several other studies, the predictive value was greater for survival than mortality.

Therefore it remains unclear as to whether exercise testing offers significantly improved prediction of survival when compared to simple pulmonary function tests alone. The populations in the two studies were of different ages, and it may be that exercise testing is more useful in children than adults.

Bacterial colonization

The majority of studies have considered the role of either *Pseudomonas aeruginosa*, *Burkholderia cepacia* or both in determining survival in cystic fibrosis patients. Most studies employing multivariate modeling techniques have failed to show colonization with either *P. aeruginosa* or more specifically with the mucoid subtype to be associated with survival, after accounting for other prognostic factors, particularly lung function [29,70,75]. However, mucoid *P. aeruginosa* was an adverse prognostic factor in one study which was also unusual in identifying age as an independent prognostic indicator [26]. In another study confined to infants diagnosed before the age of 2 years, with 10-year follow-up, *P. aeruginosa* was associated with poorer survival when *Staphylococcus aureus* had also been isolated before the age of 2 years [84].

The position with *Burkholderia cepacia* colonization is a little clearer in that, although it appears from some studies to selectively colonize those with poorer lung function and a poorer initial prognosis [85], it is also associated with a poorer prognosis after colonization, even after matching for initial lung function [29,70,82,86].

Nutritional status

Along with lung function, this appears to be one of the most important prognostic indicators in cystic fibrosis patients. Different studies use different indices of nutrition, but in a majority of studies, poor nutritional status appears to be independently associated with a poor prognosis [29,70,75,78].

Socioeconomic indicators

There have been very few studies looking at the effect of socioeconomic status on survival in cystic fibrosis, despite widespread knowledge that low socioeconomic status confers higher mortality rates from a wide variety of other common conditions. In the study by Britton [74], which examined mortality rates by region in the UK, there were only two significant predictors of premature death (death below the median age of survival): female sex (RR 1.47; CI 1.16 to 1.87) and manual social class (RR 2.75; CI 2.16 to 3.52).

In a recent study from the United States, patients who had health insurance, either privately or through Medicaid, had a median survival of 20.5 years, compared with just 6.1 years for those without insurance. Socioeconomic status and possession of insurance were both significantly and independently associated with survival in this study [87]. A more recent study using the US CF Foundation Patient Registry showed that Medicaid patients (used as a proxy for low socioeconomic status) had poorer clinical status and a relative risk of death of 3.65 compared with non-Medicaid patients. This was not related to frequency of visits to specialist clinics, and suggests that socioeconomic status may be a prognostic indicator independent of access to medical care [88]. Among adults with CF in the UK, access to specialist care is also not associated with socioeconomic status [6]. A further study based on the same data registry linked to US Census data showed a strong association between median household income, with a relative risk of death of 1.44 in the lowest income category [89].

Functional status

There has only been one published study showing that, although functional status appeared to be associated with survival, after adjustment for important clinical prognostic indicators, the association became non-significant [90].

Multivariate prognostic models

Several multivariate prognostic models have been published attempting to predict prognosis in cystic fibrosis based on cohort studies, and validated in subsequent cohorts. The first predictive system was proposed in 1992 [91]. This system was developed by retrospective analysis of data on a single cohort between 1977 and 1987. This system suggested that FEV_1 below 30% predicted was an indicator of poor prognosis over 2 years, as well as low PaO_2 and $PaCO_2$. Younger patients and female patients with a low FEV_1 had a poorer prognosis than older patients or males with the same FEV_1.

The modified Huang clinical score has also been evaluated as a predictor of survival at 6, 12, 18, 24 and 36 months. As well as showing reliability and internal consistency, the score provided a more accurate method than FEV_1 at predicting a poor prognosis, particularly at time intervals below 24 months [92].

Another model predicted survival for up to 6 years by retrospective analysis and was validated in a later cohort. The variables significantly associated with mortality and included in the final model were height (taller patients do better), hepatomegaly, FVC, FEV_1, and total white cell count [75].

A predictive model for 5-year survival was developed using the US patient register [93]. The model was developed from a randomly selected cohort and validated prospectively against a second randomly selected contemporaneous cohort. Their final model included age (older age implied worse survival), gender (male better), FEV_1 (percent predicted), weight for age z-score, pancreatic sufficiency (sufficient is better), diabetes mellitus (diabetes is worse), colonization with *Staphylococcus aureus* (better), *Burkholderia cepacia* (worse), number of acute exacerbations (more is worse) and an interaction term of *B. cepacia* and acute exacerbations.

Another model identified clinical predictors of 2-year survival was developed and sensitivity and specificity calculated at various cut-offs using receiver–operator curves. Their model included age (two terms, with a steeper slope under 21 than over 21), sputum bacteriology (*P. aeruginosa*, *B. cepacia*, both or neither), hospitalizations for acute exacerbation, courses of home intravenous antibiotics, height and FEV_1. Selecting a probability of dying >0.2 gave a sensitivity of only 52% but a specificity of 96%. Also, FEV_1 <30% gave a sensitivity of 42% and specificity of 95%. There was no difference between the two in terms of prognostic accuracy. Both FEV_1 and the new model were better at predicting survival than death [94].

Prognostic factors may differ for children. In children referred for transplant assessment (therefore already severely compromised), adverse prognostic factors included low FEV_1, low oxygen saturation during a 12-minute walk, high heart rate, young age, female gender, low albumin and low hemoglobin [95]. This model is likely to be applicable only to severely ill children.

PROVISION OF MEDICAL CARE

Although it seems reasonable to assume that care for patients with cystic fibrosis can best be provided by clinical teams specializing in treatment of this condition, it has proved difficult to subject this assumption to formal study and statistical analysis. There are theoretical risks of center-based care (such as increased risk of cross-infection with aggressive respiratory pathogens) as well as substantial theoretical advantages.

A randomized controlled trial of different models of is not possible, and non-randomized studies are made difficult because of the problem obtaining data about patients who do not attend specialist CF clinics. Patient data registries generally exclude patients who do not attend recognized CF clinics, making construction of cohort survival curves difficult, and ascertainment of deaths from cystic fibrosis may be incomplete. In addition, those who attend CF clinics may be a self-selected group with pre-existing good prognosis [74], although other studies have shown that there is no socioeconomic difference in access to specialist healthcare [6,88].

Early comparisons of care models were compromised by using historical controls (i.e. before and after establishment of a CF center) [96], or by relying on comparison of different median survival rates in countries with different methods of organizing healthcare. A study in the UK by the British Paediatric Association demonstrated that those patients attending centers where 40 or more patients were registered had better survival than those attending smaller treatment centers. Although the cut-off point was arbitrary, and it does not address the problem of self-selection of good prognosis patients, it provided the best evidence at that time that specialist center care improved outcome in cystic fibrosis [97].

Size of clinic is a crude measure of specialization, as is survival a crude measure of health status. We surveyed all known adults with CF in the UK in 1990, 1994 and 2000 [6]. One-third of the group surveyed in 1990 were not attending separate clinics for cystic fibrosis patients at any hospital, and were therefore deemed to be receiving non-specialist care. There were no social class differences between the groups. Patients attending the specialist clinics were more likely to have had simple but important clinical investigations performed recently, more likely to have had access to paramedical personnel (dietitians, physiotherapists, nurse specialists), more likely to have received home intravenous therapy, were taking higher doses of pancreatic enzymes with meals and snacks, had less severe symptom scores, and were more likely to be satisfied with professional aspects of their care [98]. These differences persisted in successive surveys, even when access to specialist care increased [6].

The proportion not receiving specialist care had fallen from one-third in 1990 to 23% in 1994 and just over 8% by 2000 [6]. Patients were also asked in 1994 and 2000 how they would prefer their care to be organized. This included the option of having care shared between a local hospital and a more distant specialist center. The results from 2000 are shown in Fig. 2.16. Only 2% of adult patients wanted care provided by a local general hospital. The rest would be prepared to travel at least 25 miles to a local specialist center,

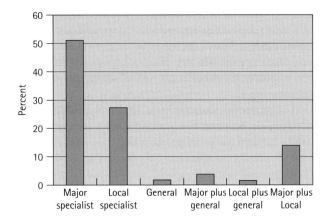

Figure 2.16   Preferences for organization of medical care expressed by adults with cystic fibrosis in the United Kingdom, 2000. Data from [6].

and many would be prepared to travel up to 100 miles to a major specialist center. These results were similar regardless of the type of care actually being received [6].

There is now wide consensus that specialist center care is of benefit to patients. The World Health Organization/ICF(M)A has recommended the establishment of such care centers as an appropriate model of care in countries where CF is thought to be more widespread than is appreciated by the medical profession [99]. In the UK, the Clinical Standards Advisory Group recommended that healthcare purchasers/commissioners ensure that all CF patients resident in their area should have access to specialist services [100]. The UK Cystic Fibrosis Trust has also published standards of care for patients with CF that recommend all patients should be cared for by centers specialising in the treatment of patients with CF [101] either directly or by shared-care arrangements.

TREATMENT OF CYSTIC FIBROSIS

This chapter on clinical epidemiology would not be complete without mentioning treatment of cystic fibrosis, but cannot possibly hope to cover the whole scope of management of this complex disease, nor to re-visit many areas already addressed in this book. Therefore this section addresses the way in which systematic reviews of the literature can assist the clinician in evidence-based practice in cystic fibrosis, and introduces the Cochrane Collaboration CF and Genetic Disorders Group.

Evidence-based medicine in CF

Evidence-based medicine is the process of applying published evidence regarding the epidemiology, diagnosis, investigation, treatment and prognosis of medical conditions to the individual patient. Although many doctors would contend this is what they do all the time, in practice

it is extremely difficult for practitioners to collect together, critically appraise and then put into practice the vast literature on a particular clinical area.

Traditional reviews, such as this chapter, of the medical literature have a number of problems, and are subject to the biased inclusion and exclusion of papers by the author, as well as the author's biased interpretation of the information contained in the selected papers. Therefore, although the primary research may be based on careful methodology and criteria, reviews of the research may be much less rigorous in their criteria for minimization of bias. In addition, traditional reviews may be out of date.

The systematic review of medical literature is an attempt to overcome some of the drawbacks of traditional reviews, while at the same time presenting the clinician with an overview that reduces the need to refer to the extensive primary literature. A systematic review will have a predetermined protocol, with explicit criteria for ensuring a thorough search of the literature, minimization of publication bias, selection of studies for inclusion in the review, pre-defined outcomes for consideration in the review, protocols for data extraction, and methods for undertaking statistical overviews, including methods for sensitivity analysis to check for bias.

The Cochrane Collaboration is an international collaboration that produces and maintains, in perpetuity, systematic reviews of randomized controlled trials of healthcare interventions. This covers the whole of medical practice. Cochrane reviews are produced according to a strict protocol, and updated each time new trials become available. A Cochrane CF and Genetic Disorders group has been established, and both protocols and reviews appear on the Cochrane Library, an electronic publication that is updated several times a year. The advantage of protocols appearing in the library is that criticism and feedback can be received before the review is performed. Input from patients and consumers of healthcare is encouraged to ensure that the outcomes considered in reviews are of relevance to consumers.

Access to abstracts of Cochrane Collaboration reviews is free online to all at http://www.thecochranelibrary.com. The CF and Genetic Disorders Group can be accessed at http://www.liv.ac.uk/cfgd/.

APPENDIX 2.1: BIOLOGICAL ADVANTAGE FOR CF HETEROZYGOTES

Carriage of the cystic fibrosis gene could be viewed as a potentially beneficial mutation. In this light, counselling for carrier status in clinical practice takes on a different hue because carriers do not carry a 'defective gene' as commonly stated; instead such endophenotypes could be viewed as the embodiment of Darwinian biological selection [137,138]. For example, CF heterozygotes might be protected against diarrheal diseases. Pier and co-workers showed that murine typhoid caused by *Salmonella enterica* (serovar Typhi) utilizes CFTR to enter epithelial cells in the gut of wild-type mice such that a survival advantage accrues for transgenic CF heterozygotes [139]. *F508del* heterozygote mice manifested 80% fewer invasive episodes of *Salmonella* infection [139,140]. Recently a typhoid protection hypothesis has been tested in humans in a case–controlled study in Indonesia with some evidence that naturally occurring variants of *CFTR* also protect against invasion of *Salmonella typhi* into the bloodstream in childhood [141]. This is a complex issue because this selective advantage ensues from wild-type non-coding (intronic) *CFTR* regions in the absence of the *F508del* mutation. Thus Indonesian populations that do not carry the common European variant to any significant penetrance (less than 1%) nevertheless accrue significant typhoid resistance dependent on an intronic inheritance pattern of *CFTR*. In this model, *CFTR* intron 4 carries two common variants bearing two different numbers of CA repeats that reduce the chances of finding typhoid bacteria in the bloodstream of those particular 'carriers'. These preliminary findings widen the concept of the heterozygote advantage for the mutant CF gene. Further supportive human data testing the typhoid hypothesis suggests that increments in *F508del* frequency occur after succeeding waves of typhoid. The cholera-protective hypothesis is more problematic in that *Vibrio cholerae* toxin has at least three different ways of entering the cell and it is unclear whether all (or some) of them are CFTR-dependent. Thus it is not unreasonable to presume that the elimination of carrier status might not be beneficial should catastrophic circumstances recur at some time in future generations.

APPENDIX 2.2: WHY IS THE FREQUENCY OF *CFTR* EXONIC MUTATION SO DIFFERENT IN DIFFERENT POPULATIONS?

The CFTR protein cycles from the epithelial cell interior to the apical cell surface facing the outside world and back again such that 50% of the resident CFTR molecules leave approximately every 15 hours [142]. Why this should be so is unknown. In contrast, *F508del CFTR* fails to traffic apically and may also exit more rapidly from the apical surface. The net result is a reduced residence time in the apical membrane. Current models invoke the idea that, when resident on the outer surface of the epithelial cell, the complexly glycosylated CFTR provides a docking site for one or more pathogens. This notion has important theoretical consequences for CF epidemiology.

Let us suppose that wild-type *CFTR* cycling was hijacked by a particularly lethal intra-epithelial pathogen and used to enter the cell from the apical membrane. Then, natural selection would eliminate surface-resident *CFTR* mutations because they enhanced pathogen entry. Random chance could also play a role in variability with the common mutation arising more than once but only surviving on one occasion. Alternatively, where CF is rare, it might be that there was no selective environmental pressure to maintain

a given mutant CF gene at high prevalence. Outside CF, such 'pressure-relief' decline is already happening in the USA where sickle cell homozygosity affects as many as 1 in 600 African–American neonates. Yet the sickle gene frequency is declining as the selective pressure from malaria wanes in African–Americans whereas no such decline has occurred in their parent populations in Africa. Thus for CF, as diarrheal disease becomes less prevalent in developed nations, the CF gene frequency might decline.

Acknowledgments

A lot of the data in this chapter has come from the UK CF Database, and we would particularly like to acknowledge the huge amount of work put in by Gita Mehta and her team at the University of Dundee. Their efforts in setting up and running the database have meant that good-quality information is available for this chapter. We would also like to thank all the clinicians who contribute data to the UK CF Database.

REFERENCES

1. McMahon B, Pugh TF. *Epidemiology: Principles and Methods.* Boston, Little, Brown, 1970.

2. Fitzsimmons SC. *Cystic Fibrosis Foundation Patient Data Registry Annual Data Report 1996.* Bethesda, Maryland, 1997.

3. Cystic Fibrosis Foundation. *Patient Registry 2004 Annual Report.* Bethesda, Maryland, 2005.

4. Canadian Cystic Fibrosis Foundation. *Report of the Canadian Patient Data Registry 2002.* Toronto, Ontario, 2002.

5. Cystic Fibrosis Trust. *UK CF Database Annual Data Report 2003.* Bromley, UK, 2005.

6. Walters S for the Cystic Fibrosis Trust. *Adults with Cystic Fibrosis: A Millennium Survey* (2001). Bromley, UK. Available at www.cfstudy.com/sarah/Report2000_2.pdf.

7. Cystic Fibrosis Mutation Database. Available at www.genet.sickkids.on.ca/cftr/ [accessed 16 January 2006].

8. McKone EF, Emerson SS, Edwards KL, Aitken M. Effect of genotype on phenotype and mortality in cystic fibrosis: a retrospective cohort study. *Lancet* 2003; **361**:1671–1676.

9. Mateau E, Calafell F, Ramos M *et al.* Can a place of origin of the main cystic fibrosis mutations be identified? *Am J Hum Genet* 2002; **70**:257–264.

10. Swiatecka-Urban A, Brown A, Moreau-Marquis S *et al.* The short apical membrane half-life of rescued F508-Cystic Fibrosis Transmembrane Conductance Regulator (CFTR): results from accelerated endocytosis of F508-CFTR in polarized human airway epithelial cells. *J Biol Chem* 2005; **280**:36762–36772.

11. Arrigo T, De Luca F, Sferlazzas C *et al.* Young adults with cystic fibrosis are shorter than healthy peers because their parents are also short. *Eur J Pediatr* 2005; **164**:781–782.

12. Wang X, Kim J, McWilliams R, Cutting G. Increased prevalence of chronic rhinosinusitis in carriers of a cystic

fibrosis mutation. *Arch Otolaryngol Head Neck Surg* 2005; **131**:237–240.

13. Teich N, Mossner J. Genetic aspects of chronic pancreatitis. *Med Sci Monitor* 2004; **10**(12):RA325–RA328.

14. Weiss FU, Simon P, Bogdanova N *et al.* Complete cystic fibrosis transmembrane conductance regulator gene sequencing in patients with idiopathic chronic pancreatitis and controls. *Gut* 2005: **54**:1456–1460.

15. Dodge JA, Morison S, Lewis PA *et al.* for the (UK Cystic Fibrosis Survey Management Committee). Incidence, population and survival of cystic fibrosis in the UK, 1968–95. *Arch Dis Child* 1997; **77**:493–496.

16. Nevanlinna HR. The finnish population structure, a genetic and genealogical study. *Hereditas* 1972; **71**:19.

17. Steinberg AG, Brown DC. On the incidence of cystic fibrosis of the pancreas. *Am J Hum Genet* 1960; **12**:416–424.

18. Kollnberg H. *Cystic Fibrosis in Sweden*. First Annual Meeting of the European Working Group for Cystic Fibrosis, Stockholm, 1970.

19. Isolair J, Witti J, Visakorpi JK. Screening of cystic fibrosis in the newborn. *Duodecium* 1979; **95**:1619 [in Finnish].

20. McCormick J, Green MW, Mehta G *et al.* Demographics of the UK cystic fibrosis population: implications for neonatal screening. *Eur J Hum Genet* 2002; **10**:583–590.

21. Cunningham S, Marshall T. Influence of five years of antenatal screening on the paediatric cystic fibrosis population in one region. *Arch Dis Child* 1998; **78**:345–348.

22. Mei-Zahav M, Durie P, Zielenski J *et al.* The prevalence of and clinical characteristics of cystic fibrosis in South Asian Canadian immigrants. *Arch Dis Child* 2005; **90**:675–679.

23. Halliburton CS, Mannino DM, Olney RS. Cystic fibrosis deaths in the United States from 1979 through 1991: an analysis using multiple-cause mortality data. *Arch Pediatr Adolesc Med* 1996; **150**:1181–1185.

24. Kulick M, Rosenfeld M, Goss CH, Wilmott R. Improved survival among young patients with cystic fibrosis. *J Pediatr* 2003; **142**:631–636.

25. Fogarty A, Hubbard R, Britton JD. International comparison of median age at death from cystic fibrosis. *Chest* 2000; **117**:1656–1660.

26. Mantle DJ, Norman AP. Life-table for cystic fibrosis. *Br Med J* 1966; **2**:1238–1241.

27. Fitzsimmons SC. The changing epidemiology of cystic fibrosis. *J Pediatr* 1993; **122**:1–9.

28. Corey M, Farewell V. Determinants of mortality from cystic fibrosis in Canada, 1970–1989. *Am J Epidemiol* 1996; **143**:1007–1017.

29. Corey M. Modelling survival in cystic fibrosis. *Thorax* 2001; **56**:743.

30. Lewis PA, Morison S, Dodge JA *et al.* (UK Cystic Fibrosis Survey Management Committee). Survival estimates for adults with cystic fibrosis born in the United Kingdom between 1947 and 1967. *Thorax* 1999; **54**:420–422.

31. Frederiksen B, Laang S, Koch C *et al.* Improved survival in the Danish Center-treated cystic fiboris patients: results of aggressive treatment. *Pedatr Pulmonol* 1996; **54**:420–422.

32. Rosenstein BJ, Cuttin GR for the Cystic Fibrosis Foundation Consensus Panel. The diagnosis of cystic fibrosis: a consensus statement. *J Pediatr* 1998; **132**:589–595.

33. Mehta G. Personal communication. January 2006.

34. Wesley A, Dawson K, Hewitt C, Kerr A. Clinical features of individuals with cystic fibrosis in New Zealand. *NZ Medical J* 1993; **106**:28–30.

35. Mulherin D, Ward K, Coffey M *et al.* Cystic fibrosis in adolescents and adults. *Ir Med J* 1991; **84**:48–51.

36. Gan KH, Geus WP, Bakker W *et al.* Genetic and clinical features of patients with cystic fibrosis diagnosed after the age of 16 years. *Thorax* 1995; **50**:1301–1304.

37. Chatfield S, Owen G, Ryley HC *et al.* Neonatal screening for cystic fibrosis in Wales and the West Midlands: clinical assessment after five years of screening. *Arch Dis Child* 1991; **66**:29–33.

38. Farrell PM, Kosorok MR, Laxova A *et al.* Nutritional benefits of neonatal screening for cystic fibrosis. *N Engl J Med* 1997; **337**:997–999.

39. Farrell PM, Kosorok MR, Rock MJ *et al.* for the Wisconsin Cystic Fibrosis Neonatal Screening Study Group. Early diagnosis of cystic fibrosis through neonatal screening prevents severe malnutrition and improves long-term growth. *Pediatrics* 2001; **107**:1–13.

40. Farrell PM, Li Z, Kosorok MR *et al.* Bronchopulmonary disease in children with cystic fibrosis after early or delayed diagnosis. *Am J Resp Crit Care Med* 2003; **168**:1100–1108.

41. Grosse SD, Boyle CA, Botkin JR *et al.* Newborn screening for cystic fibrosis: evaluation of the benefits and risks and recommendations for state newborn screening programs. *Morbid Mortal Wkly Rep* 2004; **53**(RR13):1–36. Available at www.cdc.gov/mmwr/preview/mmwrhtml/rr5313a1.htm. [accessed 16 January 2006].

42. De Brakeleer M, Ferec C. Mutations in the cystic fibrosis gene in men with congenital bilateral absence of the vas deferens. *Molec Hum Repro* 1996; **2**:669–677.

43. Colin AA, Sawyer SM, Mickle JE *et al.* Pulmonary function and clinical observations in men with congenital bilateral absence of the vas deferens. *Chest* 1996; **110**:440–445.

44. Rosenberg SM, Howatt WF, Grum CM. Spirometry and chest rontgenographic appearance in adults with cystic fibrosis. *Chest* 1992; **101**:961–964.

45. Rosenbluth DB, Wilson K, Ferkol T, Schuster DP. Lung function decline in cystic fibrosis patients and timing for lung transplantation referral. *Chest* 2004; **126**:412–419.

46. Goss CH, Rubenfeld GD, Ramsay BW, Aitken ML. Clinical trial participants compared with nonparticipants in cystic fibrosis. *Am J Resp Crit Care Med* 2006; **173**:98–104.

47. Cue C, Cullinan P, Geddes D. Improving rates of decline in FEV$_1$ in young adults with cystic fibrosis. *Thorax* (2005). Published Online First: 29 December 2005. thorax.bmj.com/cgi/content/abstract/thx.2005.043372v1.

48. Canadian Cystic Fibrosis Foundation. *Canadian Patient Data Registry National Report,* 1995.

49. Dureieu I, Bellon G, Vital Durand D *et al.* Cystic fibrosis in adults. *Presse Medicale* 1995; **24**:1882–1887 [review, in French].

50. Taccetti G, Campana S. Microbiologic data overview of Italian cystic fibrosis patients. *Eur J Epidemiol* 1997; **13**:323–327.

51. Cystic Fibrosis Trust. Pseudomonas aeruginosa *Infection in People with Cystic Fibrosis: Suggestions for Prevention and Infection Control*. London. November 2004.

52. Demko CA, Byard RJ, Davis PB. Gender differences in cystic fibrosis: *Pseudomonas aeruginosa* infection. *J Clin Epidemiol* 1995; **48**:1041–1049.

53. Tummler B, Bosshammer I, Breitenstein S *et al*. Infections with *Pseudomonas aeruginosa* in patients with cystic fibrosis. Behring Institute Mitteilungen 1997; **98**: 249–255 [in German].

54. Abman SH, Ogle JW, Harbeck RJ *et al*. Early bacteriologic, immunologic and clinical courses of young infants with cystic fibrosis identified by neonatal screening. *J Paediatrics* 1991; **119**:211–217.

55. Cystic Fibrosis Trust. Burkholderia cepacia *Complex: Suggestions for Prevention and Infection Control*. London. September 2004.

56. Richardson I, Nyulasi I, Cameron K *et al*. Nutritional status of an adult cystic fibrosis population. *Nutrition* 2000; **16**:255–259.

57. Lang S, Thorsteinsson B, Lund-Anderson C *et al*. Diabetes mellitus in Danish cystic fibrosis patients: prevalence and late diabetic complications *Acta Paediatr* 1994; **83**:72–77.

58. Lang S, Hansen A, Thorsteinsson B *et al*. Glucose tolerance in patients with CF: five-year prospective study. *Br Med J* 1995; **311**:655–659.

59. Lamireau T, Monnereau S, Martin S *et al*. Epidemiology of liver disease in cystic fibrosis: a longitudinal study. *J Hepatol* 2004; **41**:920–925.

60. Fok J, Brown NE, Zuberbuhler P *et al*. Low bone mineral density in cystic fibrosis patients. *Can J Dietetic Pract Res* 2002; **63**:192–197.

61. Conway SP, Morton AM, Oldroyd B *et al*. Osteoporosis and osteopenia in adults and adolescents with cystic fibrosis: prevalence and associated factors. *Thorax* 2000; **55**:798–804.

62. Hardin DS, Arumugam R, Seilheimer DK *et al*. Normal bone mineral density in cystic fibrosis. *Arch Dis Child* 2001; **84**:363–368.

63. Neglia JP, Fitzsimmons SC, Maisonneuve P *et al*. for the Cystic Fibrosis and Cancer Study Group. The risk of cancer among patients with cystic fibrosis. *N Engl J Med* 1995; **332**:494–499.

64. Penketh AR, Wise A, Mearns MB *et al*. Cystic fibrosis in adolescents and adults. *Thorax* 1987; **42**:526–532.

65. Sinnema G, Bonarius JC, Stoop JW, van der Laag J. Adolescents with cystic fibrosis in the Netherlands. *Acta Paed Scand* 1983; **72**:427–432.

66. STATBASE. Available at www.statistics.gov.uk/STATBASE/ ssdataset.asp? vlnk=7261 [accessed 20 January 2006].

67. Walters S, Britton J, Hodson ME. Social and demographic characteristics of adults with cystic fibrosis in the United Kingdom. *Br Med J* 1993; **306**: 549–552.

68. EuroQOL. Available at www.euroqol.org/web/ [accessed 23 January 2006].

69. Rosenfeld M, Davis R, Fitzsimmons S *et al*. Gender gap in cystic fibrosis mortality. *Am J Epidemiol* 1997; **145**:794–803.

70. Huang NN, Schidlow DV, Szatrowski TH *et al*. Clinical features, survival rate and prognostic factors in young adults with cystic fibrosis. *Am J Med* 1987; **82**:871–879.

71. Henry RL, Mellis CM, Petrovic K. Mucoid *Pseudomonas aeruginosa* is a marker of poor survival in cystic fibrosis. *Pediatr Pulmonol* 1992; **12**:158–161.

72. Kulich M, Rosenfeld M, Goss CH, Wilmott R. Improved survival among young patients with cystic fibrosis. *J Pediatr* 2003; **142**:631–636.

73. Milla CE, Billings J, Moran A. Diabetes is associated with dramatically decreased survival in female but not male subjects with cystic fibrosis. *Diabetes Care* 2005; **28**:2141–2144.

74. Britton JR. Effect of social class, sex, region of residence on age at death from cystic fibrosis. *Br Med J* 1989; **298**:483–487.

75. Hallyar KM, Williams SG, Wise AE *et al*. A prognostic model for the prediction of survival in cystic fibrosis *Thorax* 1997; **52**:313–317.

76. Verma N, Bush A, Buchdahl R. Is there still a gender gap in cystic fibrosis? *Chest* 2005; **128**:2824–2834.

77. Assael BM, Castellani B, Ocampo MB *et al*. Epidemiology and survival analysis of cystic fibrosis in an area of intense neonatal screening over 30 years. *Am J Epidemiol* 2002; **156**:397–401.

78. Grasemann H, Wiesemann HG, Ratjen F. The importance of lung function as a predictor of two year mortality in mucoviscidosis. *Pneumologie* 1995; **49**:466–469 [in German].

79. Moorcroft AJ, Dodge ME, Webb AK. Exercise testing and prognosis in adult cystic fibrosis. *Thorax* 1997; **52**:291–293.

80. Walters S, Mehta A, Mehta G, Tulley P. Prediction of 2-year mortality in CF: a comparison of Shwachman score and percent predicted FEV_1. *J Cyst Fibr* 2004; **3**:S112–S118.

81. Mayer-Hamblett N, Rosenfeld M, Emerson J *et al*. Developing cystic fibrosis lung transplant referral criteria using predictors of 2-year mortality. *Am J Respir Crit Care Med* 2002; **166**:1550–1555.

82. Milla CE, Warwick WJ. Risk of death in cystic fibrosis patients with severely compromised lung function. *Chest* 1998; **113**:1230–1234.

83. Nixon PA, Orenstein SM, Kelsey SF, Doershuk CF. The prognostic value of exercise testing in patients with cystic fibrosis. *N Engl J Med* 1992; **327**:1785–1788.

84. Hudson VL, Wielinski CL, Regelmann WE. Prognostic implications of initial oropharyngeal bacterial flora in patients with cystic fibrosis diagnosed before the age of two. *J Pediatr* 1993; **122**:854–860.

85. Lewin LO, Byard PJ, Davis PB. Effect of *Pseudomonas cepacia* colonisation on survival and lung function in cystic fibrosis patients. *J Clin Epidemiol* 1990; **43**:125–131.

86. Muhdi K, Edenborough RB, Gumery L *et al*. Outcome for patients colonised with *Burkholderia cepacia* in a Birmingham adult cystic fibrosis clinic and the end of an epidemic. *Thorax* 1996; **51**:374–377.

87. Curtis JR, Burke W, Kassner AW, Aitken ML. Absence of health insurance is associated with decreased life expectancy in cystic fibrosis. *Am J Resp Crit Care Med* 1997; **155**:1921–1924.

88. Schechter MS, Shelton BJ, Margolis PA, Fitzsimmons SC. The association of socio-economic status with outcomes in cystic fibrosis patients in the United States. *Am J Respir Crit Care Med* 2001; **163**:1331–1337.

89. O'Connor GT, Quinton HB, Kneeland T *et al*. Median household income and mortality rate in cystic fibrosis. *Pediatrics* 2003; **111**:e333–e339.

90. Shepherd SL, Hovell MF, Slymen DJ *et al*. Functional status as an overall measure of health in adults with cystic fibrosis: further validation of a generic health measure. *J Clin Epidemiol* 1992; **45**:117–125.

91. Kerem E, Reisman J, Corey M *et al*. Prediction of mortality in patients with cystic fibrosis. *N Engl J Med* 1992; **326**:1187–1191.

92. Matouk E, Ghezzo RH, Gruber R *et al*. Internal consistency reliability and predictive validity of a modified N. Huang clinical scoring system in adult cystic fibrosis patients. *Eur Resp J* 1997; **10**:2004–2013.

93. Liou TG, Adler FR, FitzSimmons SC *et al*. Predictive five-year survivorship model of cystic fibrosis. *Am J Epidemiol* 2001; **153**:345–352.

94. Mayer-Hamblett N, Rosenfeld M, Emerson J *et al*. Developing cystic fibrosis lung transplant referral criteria using predictors of 2-year mortality. *Am J Respir Crit Care Med* 2002; **166**:1550–1555.

95. Aurora P, Wade A, Whitmore P, Whitehead B. A model for predicting life expectancy of children with cystic fibrosis. *Eur Resp J* 2000; **16**:1056–1060.

96. Hill DJ, Martin AJ, Davidson GP, Smith GS. Survival of cystic fibrosis patients in South Australia: evidence that cystic fibrosis centre care leads to better survival. *Med J Australia* 1985; **143**:230–232.

97. Anonymous, for British Paediatric Association Working Party on Cystic Fibrosis. Cystic fibrosis in the United Kingdom 1977–85: an improving picture. *Br Med J* 1988; **297**:1599–1602.

98. Walters S, Britton J, Hodson ME. Hospital care for adults with cystic fibrosis: an overview and comparison between special cystic fibrosis clinic and general clinics using a patient questionnaire. *Thorax* 1994; **49**:300–306.

99. Anonymous. Implementation of cystic fibrosis services in developing countries: memorandum from a Joint WHO/ICF(M)A meeting. *Bull World Health Org* 1997; **75**:1–10.

100. Clinical Standards Advisory Group. *Access and Availability to Specialist Services: Cystic Fibrosis*. London, HMSO, 1993.

101. Cystic Fibrosis Trust. *Standards for the Clinical Care of Children and Adults with Cystic Fibrosis in the United Kingdom*. London, CF Trust, 2001.

102. Prescott-Clarke P, Primatesta P (eds). *Health Survey for England, 1996*. London, Stationery Office, 1996. Available at www.archive.official-documents.co.uk/document/doh/survey96/ehtitle.htm [accessed on 23 January 2006].

103. Dodge JA, Morison S, Lewis PA *et al*. for the UK Cystic Fibrosis Survey Management Committee. Incidence, population and survival of cystic fibrosis in the UK, 1968–95. *Arch Dis Child* 1997; **77**:493–496.

104. Nevin GB, Necin NC, Redmond AO. Cystic fibrosis in Northern Ireland. *J Med Genet* 1979; **16**:122–124.

105. Brock DJ, Gilfillan A, Holloway S. The incidence of cystic fibrosis in Scotland calculated from heterozygote frequencies. *Clin Genet* 1998; **53**:47–49.

106. Kollberg H. Incidence and survival curves of cystic fibrosis in Sweden. *Acta Paed Scand* 1982; **71**:197–202.

107. Lannefors L, Lindgren A. Demographic transition of the Swedish cystic fibrosis community: results of modern care. *Rest Med* 2002; **96**:681–685.

108. Edminson PD, Michalsen H, Aagenaes O, Lie SO. Screening for cystic fibrosis among newborns in Norway by measurement of serum/plasma trypsin-like immunoreactivity: results of a 2½ year pilot project. *Scand J Gastroenterol* 1988 (Suppl); **143**:13–18.

109. Nielsen OH, Thomsen BL, Green A *et al*. Cystic fibrosis in Denmark, 1945 to 1985: an analysis of incidence, mortality and influence of centralized treatment on survival. *Acta Paed Scand* 1988; **77**:836–841.

110. De Arce MA, Mulherin D, McWilliam P *et al*. Frequency of deletion 508 among Irish cystic fibrosis patients. *Hum Genet* 1990; **85**:403–404.

111. Kere J, Estivill X, Chillon M *et al*. Cystic fibrosis in a low-incidence population: two major mutations in Finland. *Hum Genet* 1994; **93**:162–164.

112. Schwartz M, Sorensen N, Brandt NJ *et al*. High incidence of cystic fibrosis in the Faroe Islands: a molecular and genealogical study. *Hum Genet* 1995; **95**:703–706.

113. Bossi A, Casazza G, Paddoan R for the Assemblea Dei Direttori Dei Centri. What is the incidence of cystic fibrosis in Italy? Data from the National Registry (1988–2001). *Hum Biol* 2004; **76**:455–467.

114. Corbetta C, Seia M, Bassotti A *et al*. Screening for cystic fibrosis in newborn infants: results of a pilot programme based on a two tier protocol (IRT/DNA/IRT) in the Italian population. *J Med Screening* 2002; **9**:60–63.

115. Scotet V, De Braekeleer M, Audrezet MP *et al*. Prevalence of CFTR mutations in hypertrypsinaemia detected through neonatal screening for cystic fibrosis. *Clin Genet* 2001; **59**:42–47.

116. Scotet V, Audrezet MP, Roussey M *et al*. Impact of public health strategies on the birth prevalence of cystic fibrosis in Brittany, France. *Hum Genet* 2003; **113**:280–285.

117. Slieker MG, Uiterwaal CS, Sinaasappel M *et al*. Birth prevalence and survival in cystic fibrosis: a national cohort study in the Netherlands. *Chest* 2005; **128**:2309–2315.

118. Kosorok MR, Wei WH, Farrell PM. The incidence of cystic fibrosis. *Statistics Med* 1996; **15**:449–462.

119. Grosse SD, Boyle CA, Botkin JR *et al*. Newborn screening for cystic fibrosis: evaluation of benefits and risks and recommendations for state newborn screening programs. *MMWR* 2004; **53**(RR13):1–36. Available at www.cdc.gov/mmwr/preview/mmwrhtml/rr5313a1.htm [accessed 16 January 2006].

120. American Lung Association. *Cystic Fibrosis Fact Sheet 2004*. Available at www.lungusa.org/site/pp.asp?c= dvLUK9OOE&b=35042 [accessed 16 January 2006.]

121. Sturgess JM, Czegledy-Nagy E, Corey M, Thompson MW. Cystic fibrosis in Ontario. *Am J Med Genet* 1985; **22**:383–393.

122. Corey M, Farewell V. Determinants of mortality from cystic fibrosis in Canada, 1970–1989. *Am J Epidemiol* 1996; **143**:1007–1017.

123. Dupuis A, Hamilton D, Cole DE, Corey M. Cystic fibrosis birth rates in Canada: a decreasing trend since the onset of genetic testing. *J Pediatr* 2005; **147**:312–315.

124. Rozen R, Schwartz RH, Hilman BC *et al.* Cystic fibrosis mutations in North American populations of French ancestry: analysis of Quebec French-Canadian and Louisiana Acadian families. *Am J Hum Genet* 1990; **47**:606–610.

125. Klinger KW. Cystic fibrosis in the Ohio Amish: gene frequency and founder effect. *Hum Genet* 1983; **65**:94–98.

126. Kessler D, Moehlenkamp C, Kaplan G. Determination of cystic fibrosis carrier frequency for Zuni native Americans of New Mexico. *Clin Genet* 1996; **49**:92–97.

127. Katznelson D, Ben-Yishay M. Cystic fibrosis in Israel: clinical and genetic aspects. *Israel J Med Sci* 1978; **14**:204–211.

128. Al-Mahroos F. Cystic fibrosis in Bahrain: incidence phenotype and outcome. *J Tropical Paed* 1998; **44**:35–39.

129. Nazer HM. Early diagnosis of cystic fibrosis in Jordanian children. *J Tropical Paed* 1992; **38**:113–115.

130. Robinson PG, Elliott RB, Fraxer J. Cystic fibrosis in New Zealand: incidence and mortality data. *NZ Med J* 1976; **83**:268–270.

131. Wesley AW, Stewart AW. Cystic fibrosis in New Zealand: incidence and mortality. *NZ Med J* 1985; **98**:321–323.

132. Allan JL, Phelan PD. Incidence of cystic fibrosis in ethnic Italians and Greeks and Australians of predominantly British origin. *Act Paed Scand* 1985; **74**:286–289.

133. Massie RJ, Olsen M, Glazner J *et al.* Newborn screening for cystic fibrosis in Victoria: 10 years' experience (1989–1999): *Med J Aus* 2000; **172**:584–587.

134. Imaizumi Y. Incidence and mortality rates of cystic fibrosis in Japan, 1969–1992. *Am J Med Genet* 1995; **58**:161–168.

135. Padoa C, Goldman A, Jenkins T, Ramsay M. Cystic fibrosis carrier frequencies in populations of African origin. *J Med Genet* 1999; **36**:41–44.

136. Hill ID, MacDonald WB, Bowie MD, Ireland JD. Cystic fibrosis in Cape Town. *SA Med J* 1988; **73**:147–149.

137. Harris EE, Malyango AA. Evolutionary explanations in medical and health profession courses: are you answering your students' 'why' questions? *BMC Med Edu* 2005; **5**(16):1–7.

138. Arrigo T, De Luca F, Sferlazzas C *et al.* Young adults with cystic fibrosis are shorter than healthy peers because their parents are also short. *Eur J Pediatr* 2005; **164**: 781–782.

139. Pier G, Grout M, Zaidi T *et al. Salmonella typhi* uses CFTR to enter intestinal epithelial cells. *Nature* 1998; **393**:79–82.

140. Lyczak J, Cannon C, Pier G. Lung infections associated with cystic fibrosis. *Clin Microbiol Rev* 2002; **15**:194–222.

141. Van de Vosse E, Ali S, De Visser A *et al.* Susceptibility to typhoid fever is associated with a polymorphism in the cystic fibrosis transmembrane conductance regulator (CFTR). *Hum Genet* 2005; **6**:123–142.

142. Swiatecka-Urban A, Brown A, Moreau-Marquis S *et al.* The short apical membrane half-life of rescued DF508-CFTR results from accelerated endocytosis of DF508-CFTR in polarized human airway epithelial cells. *Am Soc Biochem Mol Biol* 2005; **280**:36762–36772.

PART 2

BASIC SCIENCE FOR THE CLINICIAN

3 Molecular biology of cystic fibrosis: *CFTR* processing and functions, and classes of mutations 49
   Malka Nissim-Rafinia, Batsheva Kerem and Eitan Kerem

4 Pathophysiology: epithelial cell biology and ion channel function in the lung, sweat gland and pancreas 59
   Raymond D. Coakley and Richard C. Boucher

5 Immunology of cystic fibrosis 69
   Gerd Döring and Felix Ratjen

6a Genotype–phenotype correlations and modifier genes 81
   Jane C. Davies

6b Variability of clinical course in cystic fibrosis 87
   Michael Schechter

Molecular biology of cystic fibrosis: *CFTR* processing and functions, and classes of mutations

MALKA NISSIM-RAFINIA, BATSHEVA KEREM AND EITAN KEREM

THE *CFTR* PROCESSING AND FUNCTIONS

The *CFTR* gene was cloned in 1989 using positional cloning approach which included chromosome walking and jumping, linkage disequilibrium analysis and correlation of tissue expression pattern between CF and non-CF tissues [1,2,3]. The gene comprises 27 coding exons, spanning over 250 kb on chromosome 7q31.2, and the transcript is 6.5 kb (Fig. 3.1). The most common CF mutation is a 3bp deletion, causing a loss of phenylalanine at position 508 of the protein, *F508del* [1].

The protein encoded by the *CFTR* gene is a chloride (Cl$^-$) channel in the apical membrane of exocrine epithelial cells [3] (see Fig. 3.1). It comprises 1480 amino acids with a molecular weight of ~170 kDa. The protein comprised five domains: two membrane-spanning domains (MSD1 and MSD2), each composed of six transmembrane segments (TM1 to TM12) that form the channel, two nucleotide-binding domains (NBD1 and NBD2), capable of ATP hydrolysis, and a regulatory domain (R), which contains numerous phosphorylation sites [3,4] (Fig. 3.1). This protein structure indicates that the CFTR is part of the ATP-binding cassette (ABC) transporter proteins. Phosphorylation of sites in the R domain by protein kinase A (PKA), regulated by cyclic adenosine monophosphate (cAMP), and the hydrolysis of ATP by the NBDs, are essential for activating the chloride channel (reviewed in [4]). This complex multidomain assembly is thought to be responsible for the inefficient conformational maturation process of the CFTR (only 20–50%) in the endoplasmic reticulum (ER) (reviewed in [5]).

During its folding, the CFTR binds to molecular chaperones, such as the heat shock proteins Hsc70, Hsp40 and Hsp90, and calnexin, a calcium-binding transmembrane protein chaperone that assists newly synthesized proteins to fold into a normal structure in the ER (Fig. 3.2b). Complex formation with these chaperones is involved not only in facilitating folding but also in the degradation of non-native conformers; the latter are targeted for proteolysis by the ER-associated degradation (ERAD) to prevent the accumulation of toxic polypeptides in the cell (Fig. 3.2c) [6]. Folded CFTR is then transported out of the ER and into the Golgi to acquire cell type-specific carbohydrates in two alternative pathways, both regulated by coat protein complex II (COPII) (Fig. 3.2d). In the conventional pathway the CFTR is transferred via the *cis* and then the *trans* Golgi compartments. In the non-conventional pathway, the CFTR is trafficked to the *trans* Golgi prior to retrieval to the earlier compartment. The post-ER processing of the CFTR is modulated by several protein–protein interactions, through the C-terminal sequence of the CFTR protein, which forms a binding motif for interaction with PDZ-domain-containing proteins [7]. PDZ-mediated protein–protein interaction was detected between CFTR and CFTR-associated ligand (CAL), which is mainly localized at the *trans* Golgi compartment [8]. Mature CFTR level depends on CAL concentration, such that over-expression of CAL down-regulates CFTR expression. Another PDZ-domain-containing protein that was implicated in the regulation of CFTR trafficking is the Na$^+$/H$^+$ exchange regulatory factor (NHERF), localized at the apical surface (reviewed in [9]). Through NHERF, CFTR is tethered to the cytoskeleton actin filaments and couples with protein kinase A. Thus, NHERF is thought to contribute to CFTR apical expression and activation in cells. Deletion of CFTR C-terminal sequence led to CFTR protein accumulation at the membrane and caused almost complete loss of the PKA-activated CFTR function [10]. However, these results are inconsistent with the mild clinical phenotype in patients carrying the same C-terminal deletion [11]. In addition to the CFTR expression being regulated by NHERF, the CFTR seems to regulate the Na$^+$/H$^+$ exchanger (NHE3). Since both CFTR and NHE3 interact with the PDZ domain of NHERF and since CFTR is required for cAMP-mediated inhibition of NHE3, it is possible that a complex of these proteins is needed for NHE3 regulation [12]. Thus, the CFTR is not only regulated through its C-terminal interaction with PDZ-domain-containing proteins but also regulates such proteins. Another example for CFTR regulation of ion exchangers is the SLC26T family of Cl$^-$/HCO$_3^-$ exchangers. PDZ-mediated protein–protein interaction was detected between CFTR and these Cl$^-$/HCO$_3^-$ exchangers. Moreover, defective CFTR-dependent HCO$_3^-$ secretion was demonstrated in CF epithelia [13].

After the CFTR protein reaches the plasma membrane it undergoes a rapid endocytosis (Fig. 3.2f) and efficient recycling (Fig. 3.2g) back into the cell surface. This process is needed to maintain a long residence time of the CFTR at the cell surface. The PDZ binding motif was shown to play a role not only in the trafficking of the CFTR into the Golgi but also in its endocytic recycling. Deletion of the PDZ

binding motif reduced the half-life of CFTR in the apical membrane by decreasing CFTR endocytic recycling [14]. Two other motifs in the C-terminus of the CFTR, the tyrosine and the di-leucine based motifs, play a role in the CFTR clathrin-dependent endocytosis. CFTR forms a complex with clathrin, myosin VI, the myosin VI adaptor protein disabled-2 (Dab2), which facilitates CFTR endocytosis [15].

The pathophysiology of CF is complex and cannot be narrowed down to the loss of the CFTR function as a chloride channel. The CFTR appears to have an effect on a growing number of proteins (reviewed in [16]). In addition to the mentioned above effect of the CFTR on the Na$^+$/H$^+$ and Cl$^-$/HCO$_3^-$ exchangers, the CFTR modifies also the function and properties of ion transporters including chloride, sodium and potassium channels (Fig. 3.3). The CFTR has an inhibitory effect on the epithelial Na$^+$ channel ENaC. The loss of inhibition of ENaC by defective CFTR is regarded as an important cause for the enhanced epithelial Na$^+$ absorption found in the airways of CF patients. The CFTR has a similar effect on the cAMP regulated Cl$^-$ channel, the outward rectifying Cl$^-$ channel (ORCC). Therefore Cl$^-$ secretion, by the cAMP pathway,

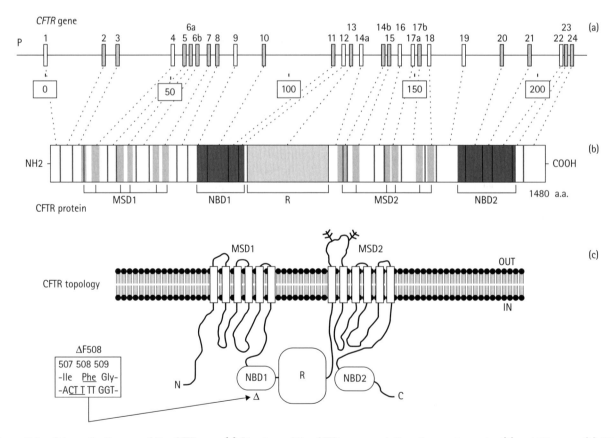

Figure 3.1 Schematic diagram of the *CFTR* gene. **(a)** Structure of the *CFTR* gene consisting of promoter region (P) and 27 exons. **(b)** CFTR polypeptide with predicted domains (highlighted). **(c)** Topology of the CFTR protein relative to the cytoplasmic membrane and position of the most common mutation, *F508del*. Box deletion of three nucleotides, CTT (underlined), and subsequent loss of phenylalanine 508 (underlined). Adapted from [42].

is markedly diminished in CF patients. However, in epithelial cells Cl$^-$ is secreted also through the Ca^{2+} regulated Cl$^-$ channel, the CaCC. Enhanced CaCC activity has been detected in human and murine CF airways [17]. Hence, high levels of CaCC expression in murine airways have been suggested to compensate for the lack of CFTR, thus

preventing the development of lung disease in CF mice [18]. The end result in human CF airways is reduced volume of airway surface fluid layer. This volume reduction is associated with reduced mucociliary clearance and impaired innate immunity leading to chronic infection and inflammation and lung damage.

CLASSIFICATION OF *CFTR* MUTATIONS

Over 1300 sequence variations (mutations, which are involved in disease expression and polymorphisms, which have no effect on the phenotype) have been identified so far along the entire *CFTR* gene [19]. *F508del* is found in ~70% of the CF chromosomes worldwide; however its frequency varies greatly among different ethnic groups, between 100% in the isolated Faroe Islands of Denmark to 18% in Tunisia. In Europe there is a clear decreasing gradient in the frequency of ΔF508 from northeast to southwest. All the other mutations are mostly rare and only 11 were found in more than 100 patients [20,21]. Several of the rare mutations however, appear with high incidence in isolated populations (Table 3.1).

As can be seen in Table 3.2, 48.7% of the mutations are missense, 19.5% are frameshifts caused by small insertions or deletions, 15.7% are splicing and 12.9% are nonsense mutations. The remaining (3.2%) affect other sequence variations, like in-frame insertions or deletions and mutations in the promoter [20]. Although hot spots for mutations along the *CFTR* gene were not found, several *CFTR* amino acids or even specific *CFTR* nucleotides show higher probability for mutations (e.g. amino acids R117, R347, I506, S549 and nucleotides 460 and 1058) [20]. Furthermore, the density of mutations is higher in the first half of the protein (particularly in MSD1 and NBD1), while very few occur in the R domain (Table 3.2), suggesting a different role for each domain. Recently it was shown that heterodimerization of the two *CFTR* NBDs exhibited 2- to 3-fold enhancement in ATPase activity relative to homodimerization of each NBD [22], which indicates a separate role for the two NBDs. Such a separate role was shown for another ABC protein, MRP1, in which ATP

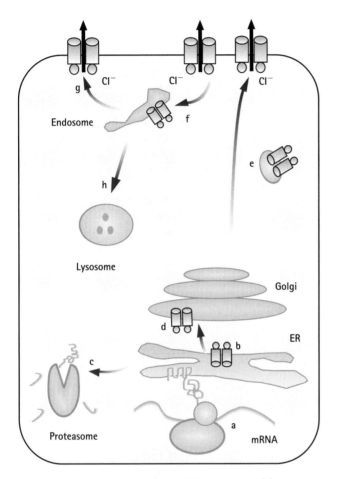

Figure 3.2 Schematic diagram of CFTR processing. **(a)** Translation. **(b)** Post-translational folding in the ER. **(c)** ER-associated degradation. **(d)** Acquirement of cell type-specific carbohydrates in the Golgi. **(e)** CFTR trafficking. **(f)** Endocytosis. **(g)** Recycling. **(h)** Degradation.

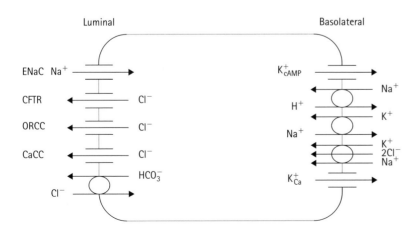

Figure 3.3 Schematic illustration of an epithelial cell. Ion transporters and channels modified by the CFTR are indicated.

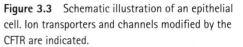

Table 3.1 *CFTR* mutations with high incidence in specific populations.

Mutation	Frequency (%) in specific populations[a]	Frequency (%) in the general population[b]	Ref.
Q359K/T360K	Georgian Jews (88)		[1]
M1101K	Hutterite Brethren (69)		[2]
S549K	United Arab Emirates (61.5)		[2]
W1282X	Ashkenazi Jews (48)	1.2	[1]
	Tunisian Jews (17)		
	Israeli Arabs (10.6)		
405 + 1G → A	Tunisian Jews (48)		[1]
	Libyan Jews (18)		
3120 + 1G → A	Bantu, Africa (46.4)		[2,3]
	South African (17.4)		
	African American, USA (13.9)		
	African American, Africa (12.2)		
	Saudi Arabia (10)		
N1303K	Egyptian Jews (33)	1.3	[1,2]
	Israeli Arabs (21)		
	Algeria (20)		
	Lebanon (10)		
G85E	Turkish Jews (30)		[1]
1898 + 5G → T	Taiwan (30)		[2]
394delTT	Finland (28.8)		[2]
	Estonia (13.3)		
621 + 1G → T	Saguenay Lac-Saint-Jean, Canada (24.3)	0.7	[2]
	Northern Greece (12.1)		
Y122X	Reunion Island (24)		[2]
3905insT	Amish, Mennonite (16.7)		[2]
	Switzerland (9.8)		
Y569D	UK, Pakistani (15.4)		[2]
T338I	Italy, Sardinia (15.1)		[4]
1548delG	Saudi Arabia (15)		[3]
R553X	Switzerland (14)	0.7	[2]
3120 + 1kb del8.6 kb	Israeli Arabs (13)		[5]
I1234V	Saudi Arabia (13)		[3]
R347P	Turkish population, Bulgaria (11.7)	0.2	[4]
Q98X	Pakistani, UK (11.5)		[2]
G542X	South Spain (11.4)	2.4	[4]
711 + 1G → T	Algeria (10)		[2]
4010del4	Lebanon (10)		[2]
R1162X	Northeast Italy (9.8)	0.3	[2]
1525 − 1G → A	Pakistani, UK (9.6)		[2]

[a] Mutations were included only if their frequency in a specific population was at least 10%, excluding ΔF508. The mutations are listed in a decreasing order of their frequency (in case of more than one population, the frequency was listed according to the highest).

[b] The frequency in the general population was listed only if it reached >0.1%, based on the CF mutation database [6].

binding affinity and hydrolysis differs between the two NBDs [23].

The cloning of the *CFTR* gene and the identification of its mutations has enabled extensive research into the association between genotype and phenotype, which has contributed to our understanding of the mechanisms responsible for the remarkable clinical heterogeneity of CF.

It is clear by now that most of the *CFTR* mutations are associated with the classical severe disease presentation. These patients carry two severe *CFTR* mutations and thus have the classical phenotype of early age of disease presentation and age at diagnosis (usually below 1 year), pancreatic insufficiency (PI), poor weight gain and nutritional status and elevated sweat chloride. It is important to

Table 3.2 Distribution of sequence variation (mutations and polymorphisms) along the *CFTR* gene.

(a) Mutation distribution											
	Pro	MSD1	ExLs1	InLs1	NBD1	R	MSD2	ExLs2	InLs2	NBD2	Other[a]	Total (%)
Missense		68	18	47	93	47	46	23	59	59	91	551 (48.7)
Frameshift (PTC)		20	5	18	27	33	15	6	22	26	49	221 (19.5)
Splicing		12	0	25	22	5	13	6	18	23	54	178 (15.7)
Nonsense (PTC)		13	4	7	17	26	12	2	10	15	40	146 (12.9)
In-frame in/del		2	1	4	4	2	1	0	5	2	7	28 (2.5)
Non-coding	8											8 (0.7)
Total mutations	8	115	28	101	163	113	87	37	114	125	241	1132

(b) Mutation density											
	Pro	MSD1	ExI1	InI1	NBD1	R	MSD2	ExI2	InI2	NBD2	Other[a]	Total
Total mutations	8	115	28	101	163	113	87	37	114	125	241	1132
Size (aa)		129	20	121	152	242	127	50	126	164	349	1480
Density[b]		0.89	1.4	0.83	1.07	0.47	0.69	0.74	0.9	0.176	0.69	0.76

(c) Variation distribution											
	Pro	MSD1	ExI1	InI1	NBD1	R	MSD2	ExI2	InI2	NBD2	Other[a]	Total
Total mutations	8	115	28	101	163	113	87	37	114	125	241	1132
Polymorphism	6	16	1	14	23	12	14	10	19	19	62	196
Total variations	14	131	29	115	186	125	101	47	133	144	303	1328

[a] Mutations in the intracellular domains.
[b] Number of mutations per domain size.
Pro, promoter; MSD, membrane-spanning domain; ExLs, extracellular loops within the MSD; InLs, intracellular loops within the MSD; NBD, nucleotide-binding domain; R, regulator; PTC, premature termination codon; in/del, insertion/deletion, aa, amino acid.
Data based on the CF mutation database [6].

emphasize that a small percentage of patients with pancreatic sufficiency (PS) will be found to carry two severe mutations, but the current data suggest that these patients will eventually develop PI. Only few mutations were found to be associated with the atypical phenotype. Patients carrying at least one atypical mutation (being dominant over the classical severe mutation) were diagnosed at a later age (usually after age 10 years), were older at the time of the study, had normal, borderline or mildly elevated sweat chloride levels, had better nutritional status, and most of them (60–70%) had PS. In some of these patients, CF diagnosis could be made only after genotype analysis was available. It is important to note that not all the patients who carry the atypical mutations have PS. There is a substantial variability in the extent of pulmonary involvement among patients carrying the same severe mutations and among patients carrying the same mild atypical mutations. In view of the current data, it appears that the variability in disease severity in patients with CF is not a consequence of relative preservation of pancreatic function but is a result of different CF gene mutants, together with additional factors, genetic and/or environmental.

So far, it has been shown that the location of a mutation along the *CFTR* gene has no direct effect on severity of CF disease. Likewise the type of mutation, either deletion, insertion, nonsense etc., is not directly affecting disease severity. Classical and atypical mutations were identified along the *CFTR* gene and in all types of mutation. The increased knowledge on the molecular mechanisms by which the mutations cause CF led to classify the different *CFTR* mutations into five major classes according to their effect on *CFTR* function (Fig. 3.4 and Tables 3.3 and 3.4).

Class I: defective protein synthesis

Class I includes mutations which lead to the disruption of the CFTR protein synthesis. The mutations in this class include nonsense and frameshifts, which lead to the creation of premature termination codons (PTCs) (>30%; Table 3.2). As can be seen in Table 3.1, PTCs (*W1282X*, *G542X*, etc.) are among the more frequent mutations in the population. PTCs were known to result in truncated proteins; however it is now apparent that they have additional

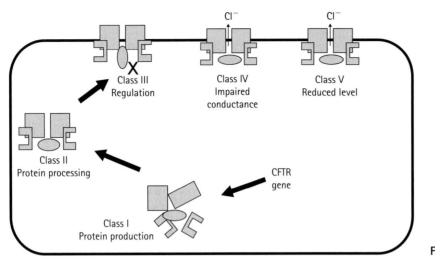

Figure 3.4   Classes of *CFTR* mutations.

Table 3.3   Classes of *CFTR* mutations: molecular mechanisms and potential therapies.

Class	Effect on CFTR	Functional CFTR	Presence of CFTR on cell membrane	Potential treatments[a]
I	Unstable RNA Production of truncated protein	No	No CFTR is degraded in the cytoplasm	Aminoglycosides PTC124
II	Impaired protein processing in the Golgi	No	No CFTR is degraded in the cytoplasm	Stabilizing chaperones – sodium-4-phenylbutyrate, ER Ca^{++} pump inhibitor – thapsigargin
III	Defective regulation	No	Yes	Alkylxanthines 8-cyclopentyl-1,3-dipropylxanthine (CPX), flavonoids – genistein
IV	Impaired function causing reduced chloride transport	Yes, but reduced	Yes	CFTR activators: Alkylxanthines 8-cyclopentyl-1,3-dipropylxanthine (CPX), *IBMX, DPCPX,* flavonoids – genistein, NS-004, milrinone, modulators of CFTR protein–protein interactions – with PDZ-binding proteins and syntaxins
V	Reduced synthesis of normal functioning CFTR	Depending on number of functional CFTR	Yes, depending on number of functional CFTR	Splicing factors that promote exon inclusion or factors that promote exon skipping depending on the molecular defect

[a] CFTR activators might be beneficial additives for all the classes of *CFTR* mutations.

effects on transcripts carrying these mutations. PTCs can dramatically decrease the half-lives of mutant mRNAs by the nonsense-mediated mRNA decay (NMD) pathway, as well as alter the pattern of pre-mRNA splicing. Therefore, such mutations are expected to produce little or no protein. Indeed, genotype–phenotype studies revealed that *CFTR* PTCs are associated with a severe form of the disease [24].

A specific therapy for PTCs has been suggested, aiming to read-through the nonsense codon, allowing synthesis of full-length proteins. Aminoglycoside antibiotics, in addition to their antimicrobial activity, can inefficiently interact with the A site of eukaryotic rRNA, leading to alteration in RNA conformation, which reduces the accuracy between

codon–anticodon pairing. This can lead to read-through of the PTCs by binding of any tRNA to the nonsense codon, thereby permitting protein translation to continue to the normal end of the transcript (reviewed in [25]). Since the normal termination of eukaryote genes consists of several termination codons, the aminoglycosides are not expected to affect the normal termination. In addition, in cases where even low levels of physiologically functional proteins are sufficient to restore the function, aminoglycosides might be suitable for treatment.

Several in-vitro studies demonstrated that aminoglycosides can read-through PTCs in the *CFTR* gene, and lead to functional full-length CFTR proteins [26]. Ex-vivo

Table 3.4 Classification of *CFTR* mutations.

Class	Mutations
I	Stop codons: W1282X, G542X, R1162X, R553X, E822X Splicing mutations that completely abolish protein synthesis: $1717 - 1G \rightarrow A$, $621 + 3A \rightarrow T$, $711 + 1G \rightarrow T$, $1525 - 1G \rightarrow A$, $2751 + 2T \rightarrow A$, $296 + 1G \rightarrow C$
II	F508del, D1507, S549R, S549I, S549N, S549R, S945D, S945L, H1054D, G1061R, L1065P, R1066C, R1066M, L1077P, H1085R, N1303K, G85E
III	G551D, S492F, V520F, R553G, R560T, R560S, Y569D
IV	R117H, R117C, R117P, R117L D1152H, L88S, G91R, E92K, Q98R, P205S, L206W, L227R, F311L, G314E, R334W, R334Q, I336K, T338I, L346P, R347C, R347H, R347L, R347P, L927P, R1070W, R1070Q
V	$3849 + 10\,kb\,C \rightarrow T$, $1811 + 1.6\,kb\,A \rightarrow G$, $3272 - 26A \rightarrow G$, IVS8-5T, D565G, G576A, c4006-1 $G \rightarrow A$, $2789 + 5G \rightarrow A$

Included in this table are mutations that have enough experimental data in the RNA/protein level to indicate their molecular mechanism.

exposure of airway cells from CF patients carrying nonsense mutations led to the identification of surface-localized CFTR in a dose-dependent fashion [27]. Clinical studies provided evidence that the aminoglycoside gentamicin can read-through PTCs *in vivo*. A pilot study in nine patients with CF carrying at least one nonsense mutation demonstrated a significant correction of the basic electrophysiological abnormalities characteristic of CF, using application of gentamicin drops to the nasal epithelium [28]. In most patients the main effect of gentamicin was activation of transmembrane chloride transport that approached the normal range. An additional clinical study in which systemic gentamicin was administrated also showed correction of the CFTR abnormalities [27]. Recently, in a double-blind placebo-controlled crossover study we have demonstrated expression of full-length CFTR proteins and restoration of CFTR function following topical application of gentamicin to the nasal epithelium of 19 CF patients carrying the *W1282X* mutation [29]. Complete normalization of the electrophysiological abnormalities was found in 21% of the patients and in 68% there was restoration of either chloride or sodium transport. Furthermore, a significant increase in peripheral and surface staining for full-length CFTR proteins was observed in the nasal epithelial cells of the patients following the treatment [29]. Together, these results suggest that gentamicin treatment can read-through PTCs. It is important to note that studies on other genetic diseases also showed that aminoglycoside have a potential to read-through PTCs, and restore the function of defective proteins encoded by nonsense alleles, both *ex vivo* and *in vivo* [25].

Class II: defective protein processing

Class II mutations are associated with defective protein processing. As discussed above, upon completion of the CFTR protein translation, the normal protein undergoes glycosilation and folding in the endoplasmic reticulum (ER) and the Golgi apparatus, which enable the protein trafficking to the apical membrane. Class II mutations cause impairment of this process, which leads to degradation of the abnormally processed protein. The major mutation, *F508del*, results in the synthesis of a CFTR protein that is unable to correctly fold into its appropriate tertiary conformation. Consequently, this protein is retained in the ER and abnormally degraded (>99% vs 75% in normal proteins). In addition, more recently it was found that Δ F508 CFTR proteins, on reaching the plasma membrane, undergo abnormal internalization and recycling into the membrane. However, most of the internalized *F508del* proteins will be marked for degradation and will not be recycled into the membrane [30]. This process further reduces the level of the defective protein in the membrane.

In-vitro studies of the *F508del*-CFTR protein demonstrated that this mutant polypeptide can function as a cAMP-dependent chloride channel once it reaches the cell membrane, suggesting that a therapy aimed at correcting protein folding and trafficking might partially correct the CFTR defect. A number of different chaperones within the lumen of the ER and in the cytosol can stabilize the misfolded structures and promote *F508del*-CFTR trafficking. Among the molecular chaperones are calnexin, Hsp70 and Hsc70, and sodium-4-phenylbutyrate, a histone deacetylase inhibitor that down-regulates Hsc70 and up-regulates Hsp70 [31]. The mutant CFTR undergoes a prolonged specific association with calnexin and with Hsp70.

Classes III and IV: defective protein regulation and altered conductance

Phosphorylation and dephosphorylation of the CFTR is considered the major pathway by which the chloride channel activity is physiologically regulated. In addition, the normal gating cycle of CFTR (both opening and closing) requires ATP binding and hydrolysis, at the two NBDs. Class III includes mutations that lead to the production of proteins (e.g. *G551D* and *Y569D*), which reach the plasma membrane; however their regulation is defective, so they cannot be activated by ATP or cAMP. Class IV mutations are associated with altered conductance (e.g. *R347P*, *R117H* and *D1152H*) such that the rate of chloride transport is reduced. Thus, mutations in both class III and IV lead to CFTR proteins that can be produced, processed, transported and inserted into the apical membrane, but display a defective conductance. Investigators have searched for exogenous compounds that are potential therapeutic activators of class III and IV mutant protein (including flavonoids, like genistein and NS-004, and xanthine derivatives, like CPX and IBMX). Genistein was shown to increase open probabilities of phosphorylated channels by binding directly to one or both of the NBDs without raising cAMP concentration and without affecting either protein kinases or protein phosphatases. IBMX seems, on the other hand, to affect CFTR through combined effects of raising cAMP levels and blocking protein phosphatases.

Class V: reduced CFTR level

Class V mutations lead to the production of normal proteins, but in reduced levels. This class includes promoter mutations that reduce transcription and amino acid substitutions that cause inefficient protein maturation. Yet, most of the mutations are splicing mutations, which affect the normal splicing of the pre-mRNA and thus reduce the levels of correctly spliced mRNA, by partial exon skipping or inclusion of intronic sequences. The alteration in the splicing pattern is caused by disrupting or generating intronic splicing motifs, required for exon recognition. These mutations account for >5% of *CFTR* mutations and include mutations that are relatively frequent in the general population (such as $3849 + 10\,kb\,C \rightarrow T$, the twelfth most common mutation) and/or in specific populations ($1898 + 5\,kb\,G \rightarrow T$, $3120 + 1\,kb\,del8.6\,kb$; see Table 3.1). In addition, there are mutations and polymorphisms that disrupt exonic splicing motifs, which also affect the splicing pattern. Class V splicing mutations (e.g. $3849 + 10\,kb\,C \rightarrow T$, $3272 - 26\,A \rightarrow G$, IVS8-5T, *D565G* and *G576A*) can lead to variable levels of correctly spliced transcripts among different patients and among different organs of the same patient (reviewed in [32] and [33]). These levels were found to inversely correlate with the variable disease expression, such that lower levels of correctly spliced transcripts are associated with a severe disease, while higher levels are associated with milder disease [34].

Splicing is regulated through the interaction of a complex repertoire of splicing factors with various splicing motifs (reviewed in [35]). Differences in the levels of functional splicing factors were found among different tissues, which have been suggested to regulate the level of alternatively spliced transcripts. Initially, the effect of over-expression of splicing factors on the level of correctly spliced *CFTR* transcripts were studied in minigenes carrying mutations, which lead to partial skipping of exons 9, 12, and the 5′ end of exon 13 and the $3849 + 10\,kb\,C \rightarrow T$ mutation, which results in partial inclusion of an 84-bp sequence from intron 19. Most (10/11) of the minigenes were modulated by splicing factors. Higher levels of correctly spliced transcripts were generated by several of these factors: Htra-α and E4-ORF3 promoted exon 13 and 9 inclusion, respectively, and hnRNP A1 and E4-0RF6 promoted skipping over the cryptic 84-bp exon (reviewed in [33]). Subsequently, we showed that Htra2-β1 and SC35 increased the level of correctly spliced mRNA transcribed from an endogenous *CFTR* allele carrying the $3849 + 10\,kb\,C \rightarrow T$

mutation [33]. Importantly, this increase activated the CFTR channel and restored its function. Over-expression of other splicing factors had no effect on the transcript level and did not restore the CFTR function.

Therapeutic approaches for this class aim to increase the level of correctly spliced transcripts and up-regulation of *CFTR* expression. One such approach is using antisense oligonucleotides designed to inhibit cryptic splicing. Antisense oligonucleotides for the 84-bp exon, cotransfected with CFTR cDNA carrying the $3849 + 10\,kb\,C \rightarrow T$ mutation, resulted in a decrease in the level of aberrant *CFTR* transcripts containing the 84-bp 'exon' [36]. Recently, a similar approach was taken for the *SMN2* (Survival Motor Neuron) and *BRCA1* (Breast Cancer) genes. Chimerical antisense oligonucleotides comprising two parts were designed, one complementary to the aberrantly spliced exon providing exon specificity, and the other containing binding motifs for recruitment of splicing factors to the mutation site [37]. An increase in the binding of splicing factors by such oligonucleotides resulted in an increased level of correctly spliced transcripts.

Another approach is the identification of small molecules that may lead to an increase in the level of correctly spliced transcripts. Recently it was shown that administration of sodium butyrate (NaBu), a histone deacetylase inhibitor that up-regulates the expression of splicing factors [38], led to a decrease in the level of aberrant *CFTR* transcripts containing the 84-bp 'exon'. Importantly, this decrease resulted in activation of the CFTR channel and restoration of the CFTR function [33]. Several other small molecules were shown to increase the level of correctly spliced mRNA transcribed from other genes, including aclarubicin, sodium vanadate and valproic acid in *SMN2* and *EGCG* ((−)-epigallocatechin gallate) and kinetin in IκAP (IκB kinase complex-associated protein) (reviewed in [33]). These molecules among others might be appropriate for CFTR therapy.

CFTR polymorphisms

As mentioned above, DNA sequence polymorphisms are defined as sequence variations that do not lead to disease expression. Yet, several polymorphisms in the *CFTR* gene were shown to modify disease severity. For example, the number of TG repeats in IVS8 correlates with the level of exon 9 skipping, and therefore with disease severity [39]. Similarly, *R668C* was shown to affect exon 12 skipping [40]. In addition, *M470V* was shown to have an effect on the CFTR channel activity and correlate with disease severity [39].

It should be mentioned that *CFTR* polymorphisms were also found in patients with CF-related diseases, with no other mutations in the *CFTR*. Thus, sequence variations that were defined as CF polymorphisms (not causing CF), can be defined as mutations causing CF-related diseases (listed in Table 3.5). The same CF-related diseases, atypical

Table 3.5 Phenotypes associated with increased incidence of *CFTR* mutations.

Obstructive azoospermia and congenital bilateral absence of the vas deferens
Chronic bronchitis
Chronic bronchiectasis
Pseudomonas bronchitis
Idiopathic disseminated bronchiectasis
Chronic sinusitis
Nasal polyposis
Allergic bronchopulmonary aspergillosis
Asthma
Neonatal hypertrypsinemia
Primary sclerosing cholangitis
Neonatal transitory hypertrypsinemia
Hypoelectrolytemia and alkalosis
Idiopathic chronic pancreatitis
Liver disease

cases of CF presenting in adolescence and manifested in only one or two organ systems, were also associated with carriers of *CFTR* mutations [41].

FUTURE PROSPECTS

Identifying all the mutations in the *CFTR* gene THAT are involved in the typical CF and CF-related diseases, and developing simple and inexpensive methods for screening a large number of mutations, will enable early genetic diagnosis of all the patients before the development of symptoms, at young individuals and even at neonates. Additional studies aiming to better understand the effect of different mutations along the *CFTR* gene on the CFTR function will broaden our understanding the different functions of the CFTR protein as well as the function of each CFTR domain. Further studies aiming to investigate the potential modulation of the CF phenotype by polymorphisms in the *CFTR* sequence and/or by other genes will enable us to learn more on the genetic complexity of the disease. Furthermore, development of mutation-specific therapies using high-throughput screening for small molecules will lead to pharmacotherapy targeting the basic *CFTR* defect.

REFERENCES

1. Kerem B, Rommens JM, Buchanan JA *et al.* Identification of the cystic fibrosis gene: genetic analysis. *Science* 1989; **245**:1073–1080.

2. Rommens JM, Iannuzzi MC, Kerem B *et al.* Identification of the cystic fibrosis gene: chromosome walking and jumping. *Science* 1989; **245**:1059–1065.

3. Riordan JR, Rommens JM, Kerem B *et al.* Identification of the cystic fibrosis gene: cloning and characterization of complementary DNA. *Science* 1989; **245**:1066–1073.

4. Sheppard DN, Welsh MJ. Structure and function of the CFTR chloride channel. *Physiol Rev* 1999; **79**:S23–45.

5. Riordan JR. Assembly of functional CFTR chloride channels. *Annu Rev Physiol* 2005; **67**:701–718.

6. Ellgaard L, Helenius A. Quality control in the endoplasmic reticulum. *Natl Rev Mol Cell Biol* 2003; **4**:181–191.

7. Short DB, Trotter KW, Reczek D. An apical PDZ protein anchors the cystic fibrosis transmembrane conductance regulator to the cytoskeleton. *J Biol Chem* 1998; **273**:19797–19801.

8. Cheng J, Moyer BD, Milewski M. A Golgi-associated PDZ domain protein modulates cystic fibrosis transmembrane regulator plasma membrane expression. *J Biol Chem* 2002: **277**:3520–3529.

9. Hung AY, Sheng M. PDZ domains: structural modules for protein complex assembly. *J Biol Chem* 2002; **277**:5699–5702.

10. Moyer BD, Duhaime M, Shaw C *et al.* The PDZ-interacting domain of cystic fibrosis transmembrane conductance regulator is required for functional expression in the apical plasma membrane. *J Biol Chem* 2000; **275**:27069–27074.

11. Mickle JE, Macek M, Fulmer-Smentek SB *et al.* A mutation in the cystic fibrosis transmembrane conductance regulator gene associated with elevated sweat chloride concentrations in the absence of cystic fibrosis. *Hum Mol Genet* 1998; **7**:729–735.

12. Weinman EJ, Minkoff C, Shenolikar S. Signal complex regulation of renal transport proteins: NHERF and regulation of NHE3 by PKA. *Am J Physiol Renal Physiol* 2000; **279**:F393–399.

13. Smith JJ, Welsh MJ. cAMP stimulates bicarbonate secretion across normal, but not cystic fibrosis airway epithelia. *J Clin Invest* 1992; **89**:1148–1153.

14. Swiatecka-Urban A, Duhaime M, Coutermarsh B. PDZ domain interaction controls the endocytic recycling of the cystic fibrosis transmembrane conductance regulator. *J Biol Chem* 2002; **277**:40099–40105.

15. Swiatecka-Urban A, Boyd C, Coutermarsh B. Myosin VI regulates endocytosis of the cystic fibrosis transmembrane conductance regulator. *J Biol Chem* 2004; **279**:38025–38031.

16. Kunzelmann K, Schreiber R, Nitschke R, Mall M. Control of epithelial Na$^+$ conductance by the cystic fibrosis transmembrane conductance regulator. *Pflugers Arch* 2000; **440**:193–201.

17. Knowles MR, Clarke LL, Boucher RC. Activation by extracellular nucleotides of chloride secretion in the airway epithelia of patients with cystic fibrosis. *N Engl J Med* 1991; **325**:533–538.

18. Clarke LL, Grubb BR, Yankaskas JR. Relationship of a non-cystic fibrosis transmembrane conductance regulator-mediated chloride conductance to organ-level disease in Cftr(-/-) mice. *Proc Natl Acad Sci USA* 1994; **91**:479–483.

19. Consortium of the Cystic Fibrosis Genetic Analysis Consortium. www.genet.sickkids.on.ca/cftr.

20. Consortium of the TCFGA. Population variation of common cystic fibrosis mutations. *Hum Mutat* 1994; **4**:167–177.

21. Zielenski J, Tsui LC. Cystic fibrosis: genotypic and phenotypic variations. *Annu Rev Genet* 1995; **29**:777–807.

22. Kidd JF, Ramjeesingh M, Stratford F *et al.* A heteromeric complex of the two nucleotide binding domains of cystic fibrosis transmembrane conductance regulator (CFTR) mediates ATPase activity. *J Biol Chem* 2004; **279**:41664–41669.

23. Hou YX, Riordan JR, Chang XB. ATP binding, not hydrolysis, at the first nucleotide-binding domain of multidrug resistance-associated protein MRP1 enhances ADP. Vi trapping at the second domain. *J Biol Chem* 2003; **278**:3599–3605.

24. Consortium of the TCFGP. Correlation between genotype and phenotype in patients with cystic fibrosis. *N Engl J Med* 1993; **329**:1308–1313.

25. Holbrook JA, Neu-Yilik G, Hentze MW, Kulozik AE. Nonsense-mediated decay approaches the clinic. *Nat Genet* 2004; **36**:801–808.

26. Bedwell DM, Kaenjak A, Benos DJ *et al.* Suppression of a CFTR premature stop mutation in a bronchial epithelial cell line. *Nat Med* 1997; **3**:1280–1284.

27. Clancy JP, Bebok Z, Ruiz F *et al.* Evidence that systemic gentamicin suppresses premature stop mutations in patients with cystic fibrosis. *Am J Respir Crit Care Med* 2001; **163**:1683–1692.

28. Wilschanski M, Famini C, Blau H *et al.* A pilot study of the effect of gentamicin on nasal potential difference measurements in cystic fibrosis patients carrying stop mutations. *Am J Respir Crit Care Med* 2000; **161**:860–865.

29. Wilschanski M, Yahav Y, Yaacov Y *et al.* Gentamicin-induced correction of CFTR function in patients with cystic fibrosis and CFTR stop mutations. *N Engl J Med* 2003; **349**:1433–1441.

30. Sharma M, Pampinella F, Nemes C *et al.* Misfolding diverts CFTR from recycling to degradation: quality control at early endosomes. *J Cell Biol* 2004; **164**:923–933.

31. Choo-Kang LR, Zeitlin PL. Induction of HSP70 promotes DeltaF508 CFTR trafficking. *Am J Physiol Lung Cell Mol Physiol* 2001; **281**:L58–68.

32. Nissim-Rafinia M, Kerem B. Splicing regulation as a potential genetic modifier. *Trends Genet* 2002; **18**:123–127.

33. Nissim-Rafinia M, Aviram M, Randell SH *et al.* Restoration of the cystic fibrosis transmembrane conductance regulator function by splicing modulation. *EMBO Rep* 2004; **5**: 1071–1077.

34. Kerem E, Rave-Harel N, Augarten A *et al.* A cystic fibrosis transmembrane conductance regulator splice variant with partial penetrance associated with variable cystic fibrosis presentations. *Am J Respir Crit Care Med* 1997; **155**:1914–1920.

35. Black DL. Mechanisms of alternative pre-messenger RNA splicing. *Annu Rev Biochem* 2003; **72**:291–336.

36. Friedman K, Kole J, Cohn JA *et al.* Correction of aberrant splicing of the cystic fibrosis transmembrane conductance regulator (CFTR) gene by antisense oligonucleotides. *J Biol Chem* 1999; **274**:36193–36199.

37. Cartegni L, Krainer AR. Correction of disease-associated exon skipping by synthetic by synthetic exon-specific activators. *Nat Struct Biol* 2003; **10**:120–125.

38. Chang JG, Hsieh-Li HM, Jong YJ *et al.* Treatment of spinal muscular atrophy by sodium butyrate. *Proc Natl Acad Sci USA* 2001; **98**:9808–9813.

39. Cuppens H, Lin W, Jaspers M *et al.* Polyvariant mutant cystic fibrosis transmembrane conductance regulator genes. The polymorphic (Tg)m locus explains the partial penetrance of the T5 polymorphism as disease mutation. *J Clin Invest* 1998; **101**:487–496.

40. Pagani F, Stuani C, Tzetis M *et al.* New type of disease causing mutations: the example of the composite exonic regulatory elements of splicing in CFTR exon 12. *Hum Mol Genet* 2003; **12**:1111–1120.

41. Boyle MP. Nonclassic cystic fibrosis and CFTR-related diseases. *Curr Opin Pulmon Med* 2003; **9**:498–503.

42. Zielenski J. Genotype and phenotype in cystic fibrosis. *Respiration* 2000; **67**:117–133.

4

Pathophysiology: epithelial cell biology and ion channel function in the lung, sweat gland and pancreas

RAYMOND D. COAKLEY AND RICHARD C. BOUCHER

INTRODUCTION

Cystic fibrosis (CF) is a lethal, autosomal recessive, multisystem disease, primarily affecting organs of epithelial origin. Although approximately 90% of the morbidity and mortality associated with CF is due to chronic suppurative lung disease, characteristic pathological findings are also evident in other organs, including the pancreas and intestinal, hepatobiliary and reproductive tracts. In addition, functional abnormalities in the sweat duct are well described and correlate with abnormally high sweat chloride content.

Despite its 'ancient' roots, CF was first described as a clinical syndrome in 1938 [1], and it was not until 1989 that mutations in the cystic fibrosis transmembrane conductance regulator (*CFTR*) gene were identified as its cause [2–4]. Since that time, links between aberrant *CFTR* expression and the diverse pathological manifestations of the condition have been vigorously (and largely successfully) sought.

Although not all aspects of CF pathogenesis have been fully elucidated, and some remain contentious, it is increasingly accepted that *CFTR* mutations promote disease by interfering with epithelial ion transport. Lack of functional *CFTR* expression has contrasting effects on ion transport in various organs, suggesting organ-specific mechanisms of disease pathogenesis. For instance, in the CF lung, isotonic liquid absorption dominates; in the gastrointestinal system, isotonic Cl^- and water secretion are impaired; in the CF pancreas, ductal $Na^+HCO_3^-$ and liquid secretion are abnormal; and in the sweat duct, hypertonic absorption of NaCl fails to occur. In this chapter, we will explore these concepts of CF pathogenesis and describe how our enhanced understanding of disease mechanism has advanced the goal of developing therapies that specifically address *primary defects* in CF, as opposed to merely tempering their consequences. We will focus most intensely on the lung, describing the accumulating evidence that abnormal ion transport causes inadequate hydration of luminal secretions and fosters the accumulation of viscous mucus in CF (of note, a condition formerly termed 'mucoviscidosis). This defect, in turn, compromises a key component of innate lung host defense, namely mucociliary clearance, leading to chronic infection, inflammation and, ultimately, parenchymal lung destruction.

GENETIC BASIS OF CF

CF is an autosomal recessive condition resulting from mutations in the cystic fibrosis transmembrane regulator (CFTR) gene, a ~250-kb gene located on the long arm of chromosome 7. Introns within the *CFTR* gene contain information that allows for alternative splicing. To date, more than 1000 candidate mutations in the CF gene have been identified and reported to the CF Gene Mutation Consortium in Toronto, Canada [5]. Targeting more common *CFTR* mutations has made population screening for CF feasible. However, even in patients in whom a diagnosis of CF has been made (based on positive sweat test and/or consistent nasal potential difference and an appropriate clinical context), it is not uncommon for *CFTR* mutations to evade detection (on one allele at least) and, occasionally, sequencing of the *CFTR* gene is undertaken where the diagnosis remains in doubt.

Mechanisms by which several classes of *CFTR* mutations disrupt protein function have been described and are dealt with in Chapter 3. The relationship between specific *CFTR* gene mutations and clinical manifestations of the disease are much more complex than was previously thought. In general, classes I, II and III are associated with the more severe phenotypic expression of the *CFTR* gene, while classes IV and V are associated with less severe clinical consequences. However, although the identification of *CFTR* mutations in a given individual has proven to be a reliable predictor of disease in the GI tract, pancreas and sweat duct, it is a less reliable as a predictor of lung disease severity. In fact, even in the presence of two mutations generally associated with a 'severe' extrapulmonary phenotype, there is a wide clinical spectrum of pulmonary disease. Some such adults may survive to adulthood with minimal lung disease. Clearly, both environmental and *CFTR*-independent genetic influences may be important in this regard. A variety of potential gene-modifiers have been suggested, including those that modulate innate lung defense [6–11]; also see Chapters 6a and 6b. However, the most rigorous and convincing evidence for a gene modifier of CF severity was provided in a comparative analysis of 808 *F508del* homozygous CF patients who manifested either mild or severe lung disease, in whom polymorphisms of the gene regulating TGFβ reproducibly predicted pulmonary severity [12]. The conjunction of such approaches in the future with proteomic analyses may lead to the generation of novel therapeutic targets.

MOLECULAR BASIS OF CF

Cystic fibrosis appears to reflect the relative absence of functional CFTR at an appropriate location in the apical cell membrane in epithelial organs. While a variety of *CFTR* mutation classes have been characterized, null mutations and those associated with CFTR non-function (in terms of ion transport) are rare. Most disease-causing mutations appear to result in misfolding of CFTR, with consequent failure of the mature protein to translocate to the plasma membrane. This mechanism was first suggested for the *ΔF508* mutation [13]. Since *ΔF508 CFTR* retains ion-transport function, the concept of manipulating protein trafficking to pharmacologically 'rescue' the protein and facilitate its passage to the apical membrane is an attractive one and is being actively explored [14]. However, it remains possible that even if some *F508del* CFTR protein reaches the apical membrane in the airway cell, it will be recycled too rapidly to function effectively, and excessive removal and degradation of CFTR could limit the therapeutic utility of such novel agents [15].

It is conceivable that accumulation of mutant CFTR within the cell may be deleterious, in a manner that is independent of absence of CFTR channel activity and analogous to functional derangements that occur in hepatocytes from patients with α_1-antitrypsin deficiency, due in accumulation of mutated 'z' α_1-antitrypsin protein in hepatocytes [16]. It has been suggested that such an 'unfolded protein response' would constitutively activate NFκB, thereby promoting dysregulation of inflammatory responses in affected subjects [17,18]. However, it has not been possible to show that inflammation is innately dysregulated in primary cell culture models of CF airway epithelia once environmental

influences are controlled for [19–21]. The severe phenotype in patients with null mutations also argues against this hypothesis [22].

PATHOPHYSIOLOGY OF LUNG DISEASE

Over the past five decades, a combination of clinical observations and experimental endeavors has led to a cogent and well-supported hypothesis to explain the pathophysiology of lung disease in CF, one that plausibly links the salty brow, viscid mucus and fibrocystic lung destruction that have been recognized for centuries.

Initially, divergent hypotheses were put forward to link altered Cl^- transport with lung disease in cystic fibrosis. In one, it was suggested that abnormally high *tonicity* of airway surface liquid (ASL), due to an inability of Cl^- to enter the cell via CFTR, might foster infection in CF airways by inactivation of endogenous salt-sensing antimicrobials including defensins [23–25]. However, more recent observations, in a variety of species (including human tissues and live subjects) and using a variety of investigative techniques, suggested instead that ASL is, in fact, isotonic in both CF and non-CF airways [26–29].

The weight of evidence now strongly favors an abnormal ASL *volume* hypothesis, to explain pathophysiological abnormalities in the CF lung. In this (now widely accepted) theory, lung disease in CF occurs due to ASL dehydration, which interferes with mucociliary clearance (MCC). Several innate mechanisms exist to meet the persistent challenge of inhaled bacteria. Although bacterial growth can also be suppressed by natural antibiotic substances secreted into the airway lumen (such as lacto-ferrin and lysozyme), the bactericidal capacity of these substances appears to be limited in magnitude and duration [30]. This observation emphasizes the primacy of physical clearance of bacteria to maintain sterility of the airways. This physical mode of bacterial clearance relies on their being trapped in airway mucus, which is in turn wafted in a cephalad direction by the coordinated beating of cilia. This activity requires not only the presence of normally beating cilia, but also sufficient periciliary liquid (PCL) to lubricate the transport of dense tangles of mucin molecules as well as to provide the necessary low-viscosity environment for efficient ciliary movement. Sufficient liquid must also be present to hydrate the 'mass' of mucin molecules in the mucus layer.

Failure of MCC (with consequent chronic suppurative lung disease) arises in patients with primary ciliary dyskinesia, due to abnormal ciliary motility [31]. It is believed that inappropriate dehydration of the periciliary and mucus layers underlies a similar but more severe phenomenon in CF. Several lines of evidence support this contention. First, using confocal immunofluorescence imaging studies of primary cultures of airway epithelium grown at an air–liquid interface, it has been possible to demonstrate that rotational mucus transport is maintained in normal cultures where the periciliary liquid layer is of the order of 7 μm (approximating the length of the outstretched cilium), but is impaired

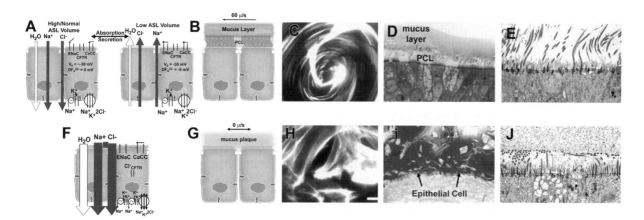

Figure 4.1 Ion and mucus transport in CF and non-CF airway epithelia. **(A)** Non-CF airway epithelia can exhibit both absorptive and secretory modes to regulate airway surface liquid (ASL) height. In the presence of an excess of liquid on airway surfaces, the dominant mode is Na$^+$-dependent volume absorption (active transcellular Na$^+$ transport with apical ingress via ENaC channels and passive paracellular Cl$^-$ transport). In contrast, when ASL is depleted, ENaC is inhibited and a more negative membrane potential favors apical secretion of Cl$^-$ via CFTR or the CaCC. **(B)** Schema illustrating optimal hydration of non-CF airway surfaces. Note that the adequate periciliary liquid (PCL) layer allows cilia to stretch upward and touch the underside of the mucus blanket, which floats above. **(C)** This optimal situation allows for rotational mucus transportation on primary cultures of non-CF airway epithelium (the image represents time lapse photography of fluorescent beads within an aggregation of rotating mucus upon the polarized culture surface). **(D)** Mucus layer in fixed specimen of a primary culture preparation of non-CF airway epithelia. **(E)** Electron microscopic imaging demonstrating normal PCL height and ciliary orientation in a primary cultured airway epithelial preparation grown at an air–liquid interface. **(F)** Schema illustrating ion-transport pathways in CF airway epithelial cells. Note that Na$^+$ absorption, via ENaC, is augmented and unopposed by Cl$^-$ secretion via CFTR, although the CaCC pathway remains intact. This results in adherence of mucus plaques to apical cell surfaces **(G)**, absent rotational mucus transport on cultured airway epithelial cells **(H)** and adherence and stagnation of mucus plaques on CF airway surfaces *in vitro* **(I)** and flattening and abnormal ciliary orientation in CF culture preparations **(J)**. Adapted from [124] and [125]. *See also Plate 4.1.*

in CF cultures, where PCL is notably depleted [32,33] (Fig. 4.1). This liquid depletion promotes direct apposition (and likely tethering) of mucus plaques and the apical membrane. Importantly, mucus transport can be restored in CF cultures by simply replacing depleted surface liquid [34]. Paralleling these in-vitro observations are key recent clinical trials which reveal benefits derived by CF patients from regular inhalation of 7% hypertonic saline, a measure designed to increase hydration of airway secretions [35,36].

The importance of airway surface hydration in MC and lung defense is reinforced by other lines of evidence. Mice genetically engineered to excessively hyperabsorb Na$^+$ and liquid from airway surfaces develop mucus accumulation and impaired host bacterial clearance [37]. In contrast to the *dehydration* of ASL in CF patients and β-ENaC over-expressing mice, humans with inherited *deficiencies* of airways Na$^+$ absorption, who exhibit *excessive* ASL hydration, actually manifest accelerated MCC [38]. This latter observation is interesting in that it is consistent with the notion that adding extra liquid to ASL may be an appropriate physiological response to inhaled toxins/infectious agents (see later).

REGULATION OF ASL VOLUME BY ACTIVE ION TRANSPORT

The volume of liquid on airway surfaces may be regulated by both passive and active forces. Passive regulation reflects

that capacity of the mucus layer to act as a liquid 'reservoir', adding water to, or extracting water from, the PCL, depending on its hydration state. However, active ion transport appears to represent a more dominant influence on ASL volume regulation [39]. Airway epithelium is relatively water-permeable [40]. Thus, ASL volume is adjusted by active transport of salt in either a mucosal or serosal direction.

- *Absorption* of liquid from the ASL occurs by active transport of Na$^+$ in a serosal direction, with the subsequent passive movement of (a) Cl$^-$ (paracellular route) to maintain electrochemical neutrality, and (b) water (transcellular route, via aquaporin water channels [41]) down an osmotic gradient. The driving force for Na$^+$ absorption is generated by a basolaterally located Na$^+$-K$^+$-ATPase, and the process is controlled at the apical membrane by tight regulation of apical Na$^+$ sodium channels (ENaC) (see Fig. 4.1A).
- *Secretion* of liquid into ASL occurs, in contrast, via active mucosal transport of Cl$^-$ in a mucosal direction, with passive movement of Na$^+$ and water following electrochemical and osmotic gradients, respectively (see Fig. 4.1A).

Normally, when ASL volume is excessive, Na$^+$ absorption dominates, but as ASL height approaches a level that appears to be physiologically optimal, Na$^+$ absorption is attenuated. In fact, under conditions where ASL is depleted or Na^+ transport is inhibited, Cl^- secretion can become dominant, facilitating repletion of ASL volume [39,42,43]. The surface 'factors' that transduce ASL volume regulatory signals, and control Na^+ absorption, are not fully characterized, though nucleotides, nucleosides and cell surface proteases appear to be important [44,45].

Egress of Cl^- via the apical membrane can occur via cAMP-regulated CFTR Cl^- channels, or by nucleotide-regulated Ca^{2+} activated Cl^- channels (CaCC) [42,43]. Under basal conditions, it appears that CFTR is the more active channel, whereas the function of both channels may be augmented in response to physiological or pathological stresses [42;43;46]. Of note, there appear to be regulatory interactions between components of the apical ion-transport apparatus. Most notably, CFTR and ENaC interact, via as yet unknown mechanisms, with resultant tonic inhibition of Na^+ absorption [47], a phenomenon that explains key in-vivo bioelectric findings (see later).

In CF airway epithelial cells, two derangements of ion transport contribute to abnormal regulation of ASL volume (see Fig. 4.1F). First, in-vitro approaches suggest that lack of functional CFTR in the apical membrane releases ENaC from tonic inhibition, thereby promoting hyperabsorption of Na^+ and depletion of surface liquid [32,34,42,43,48–52]. These observations are consistent with in-vivo studies that confirm (a) significantly more negative basal nasal potential difference (PD), and (b) markedly increased magnitude of its fractional amiloride-sensitive component [53]. In this regard, differences between CF and non-CF subjects are so striking that nasal PDs have been widely adopted as a secondary diagnostic investigation in clinical situations where CF is suspected but other diagnostic evaluations are equivocal. Further, CF epithelia also, as expected, exhibit defective Cl^- permeability [54,55]. This creates a doubly disadvantageous situation in CF; i.e. both hyperabsorption of Na^+ and an inability to compensate by secreting Cl^-. It is believed that the combination of defects promotes depletion of PCL and this ultimately results in adherence of mucus plaques in the airway and arrest of MCC.

Cl^- secretion in response to nucleotides (adenosine and uridine triphosphates; ATP, UTP) contained within ASL is not defective in CF. In fact, nasal PD studies in CF patients suggest that UTP responses are actually up-regulated when compared to non-CF controls [56]. However, likely because nucleotides are subject to rapid metabolism on airway surfaces, their elicited Cl^- secretory response is insufficient to compensate for the lack of CFTR. In this regard, less rapidly degraded nucleotides, administered by an inhalational route, may have therapeutic application in this patient population and, indeed, are currently undergoing clinical evaluation [57].

CFTR appears to act as a conduit for anions other than Cl^-, among which HCO_3^- is most physiologically relevant. In-vitro evidence suggests that pH on the surface of cultured CF airway epithelia is abnormally acidic [58,59]. Although CFTR channel conductivity for Cl^- exceeds that of HCO_3^-, it appears that the fraction of HCO_3^- versus Cl^- secreted may be actively regulated *in vitro*, with some conditions favoring

dominant HCO_3^- secretion [60]. While it has been known for decades that luminal pH in the CF pancreas, *in vivo*, is abnormally acidic [61,62], more recent evaluations extend similar phenomena to the male and female reproductive tracts [63,64]. The situation as it pertains to ASL pH is less well characterized, but recent reports indicate markedly acidic pH (~6.5) in diseased CF airway secretions [65] and abnormally low pH in liquid from freshly excised CF nasal submucosal glands compared to non-CF controls [66]. Taken together, there is a strong suggestion that surface airway pH is abnormally acidic in CF patients, though the pathological significance of these pH changes remains to be tested.

PATHOGENIC SEQUENCE OF BACTERIAL COLONIZATION/INFECTION

Despite accumulation of viscous, adherent mucus plaques in CF airways, it does not appear that a feedback mechanism exists to curtail mucin secretion. Indeed, mucin secretion is likely to be augmented in response to inflammation, bacterial proliferation, or viral infection in the CF airway. Normal host adaptations in ion transport, favoring liquid secretion, have been described [46,67]. These are likely to be important to hydrate the increased mass of mucus in airways following inflammatory provocation. However, since these compensatory responses involve up-regulation of CFTR function, they are likely to be defective in CF patients [46].

The concentrated mucus present in CF airways (up to 20% solids) (see Fig. 4.1) favors bacterial colonization and persistence for several reasons. Not only is MCC/cough clearance itself inhibited, but the mucus appears to be sufficiently thick to prevent penetration by host immune cells (dominantly neutrophils), while this is not the case for motile strains of *Pseudomonas* [68]. Moreover, the high epithelial O_2 consumption in CF airways (due to energy consumption required to drive the NA^+-K^+-ATPase that facilitates the high rates of basal Na^+ absorption) appears to render the plaques relatively hypoxic [69]. This environment appears to specifically select typical CF pathogens such as *Pseudomonas* [69]. This organism eventually established anaerobic biofilms, which are even more resistant to eradication by either host antimicrobial mechanisms or exogenously administered antibiotics. The result is a chronically infected and inflamed milieu with resultant gradual airway wall damage and, ultimately, lung parenchymal destruction.

Alternative hypotheses for selection of *Pseudomonas* in CF airways have been proposed. It has been suggested that CFTR itself is a receptor for *Pseudomonas* attachment, essentially immobilizing the organism, which would presumably be destroyed later by phagocytes [70,71]. However, this notion is inconsistent with the typical CF clinical disease and infection profile in patients with mutations that permit expression of CFTR in the apical membrane (in this case, mutants of CFTR whose channel function is disrupted, i.e. class IV). This hypothesis also fails to explain the observation that lung disease is established in CF patients prior to acquisition of *Pseudomonas*, though decline in FEV$_1$ does accelerate after chronic infection [72,73]. It has also been suggested that increased adhesivity of *Pseudomonas* to airway surfaces in CF may be the result of avid bacterial binding to defectively sialylated surface glycoconjugated proteins, a phenomenon postulated to occur secondary to abnormal acidification of intracellular vacuolar pH [74]. However, abnormal acidification of intracellular organelles in CF has not been easily reproduced in other studies [75], and morphological studies have identified virtually all bacteria in the luminal mucus and not on the cell surface [69].

PATHOPHYSIOLOGY OF PANCREATIC DISEASE IN CF

Many CF patients develop pancreatic exocrine and endocrine insufficiency. Exocrine insufficiency is more frequent and causes malabsorption, which ultimately leads to nutritional failure if appropriate compensatory therapeutic measures are not instituted. Fibrocystic damage with progressive fatty replacement of diseased pancreatic tissue occurs, and this abnormality parallels the rising prevalence of CF-related diabetes over time in pancreatic-insufficient patients. While most CF patients die of lung disease, the importance of pancreatic failure is borne out in the well-documented relationship between nutritional failure and rate of decline in lung function [76]. While the pathophysiology of pancreatic disease in CF is now better understood, no specific therapies to prevent or reverse pancreatic disease have been developed to date.

Ion-transport processes in the lung and pancreas differ, although disease in both ultimately reflects failure of apical membrane anion transport. In the pancreas, disease likely reflects a combination of both deficient liquid and HCO$_3^-$ secretion. In fact, among the earliest clinicopathological observations in CF was the deficient volume (resulting in inspissated mucus plugs), abnormally acidic pH, and increased concentration of digestive enzymes in CF pancreatic secretions [61,62,77]. These observations were later refined with the demonstration that the CF pancreas specifically lacks secretin-activated cAMP-dependent HCO$_3^-$ and liquid secretion.

Isotonic liquid is secreted in the pancreatic acinus, and its content (most notably HCO$_3^-$ content) is modified in the pancreatic duct (Fig. 4.2). Indeed, the pancreatic duct is capable of generating an exceptionally HCO$_3^-$-rich luminal liquid (up to 140 mEq/L) [78]. Though mechanisms of pancreatic HCO$_3^-$ secretion are not fully understood, it appears that basolateral HCO$_3^-$ uptake occurs via a Na$^+$/HCO$_3^-$ co-transporter, as well as the H$^+$/ATPase and Na$^+$/H$^+$ exchanger acting in concert with carbonic anhydrase [78]. There are several potential routes of HCO$_3^-$ exit from the apical membrane, and CFTR, which appears to be both expressed and functional in pancreatic ductal cells [79,80], may be implicated in several ways.

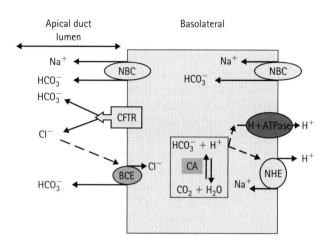

Figure 4.2 Ion transport properties of the pancreatic ductal epithelial cell. The pancreas secretes a liquid which is very rich in bicarbonate (up to 140 MEq/L). The pancreatic acinus produces isotonic fluid, and bicarbonate content and volume are modified in the pancreatic duct. Though mechanisms of pancreatic ductal HCO$_3^-$ secretion are not fully understood, it appears that basolateral HCO$_3^-$ uptake occurs via a Na$^+$/HCO$_3^-$ co-transporter (NBC), as well as H$^+$/ATPase and Na$^+$/H$^+$ exchanger (NHE) acting in concert with carbonic anhydrase (CA). Apical egress may occur (a) directly through CFTR (which also permits chloride secretion), (b) via (sometimes electrogenic) bicarbonate chloride exchangers (BCEs) such as SLCA3 and SLCA6, which may work in concert with CFTR (through which chloride is secreted), or (c) via an apically located NBC. In CF, absence of CFTR-dependent bicarbonate and chloride secretion results in abnormally acidic and hypovolemic secretions in response to stimuli such as secretin.

First, CFTR may itself act as the route of egress for HCO$_3^-$ ions. This activity might seem unlikely given the unfavorable concentration gradient in the pancreatic duct and generally low relative permeability of CFTR for HCO$_3^-$. However, it has been suggested that the ion selectivity of CFTR can be adjusted to favor HCO$_3^-$ either by intracellular events [60,81] or by low extracellular [Cl$^-$] [82]. Further, electrophysiological calculations suggest that a membrane potential of −60 mV would be sufficient to produce a luminal concentration of 190 mEq/L, even if the HCO$_3^-$ permeability of CFTR is modest (0.4 relative to Cl$^-$) [78].

Alternatively, it has been suggested that CFTR may play a role in HCO$_3^-$ secretion by interacting with the well-characterized DIDS(4,4-diisothiocyanostilbene 2,2-disulfonate)-sensitive apical HCO$_3^-$/Cl$^-$ exchange process; i.e. CFTR secretes Cl$^-$, which is exchanged for HCO$_3^-$ [83,84]. However, while this mechanism may facilitate secretion of moderate amounts of HCO$_3^-$, it is not likely that it could produce sufficient HCO$_3^-$ secretion to establish luminal concentration of the order of 140 mEq/L, since the exchange process would be reversed under these circumstances [85].

However, emerging evidence suggests that a class of (sometimes electrogenic) HCO$_3^-$/Cl$^-$ exchangers, the SLC26 class, whose properties include the potential to interact with CFTR, may be implicated in pancreatic HCO$_3^-$ secretion

[86,87]. Members thought to be important in the pancreas include SLCA3 (down-regulated in adenoma – DRA) and SLCA6 (putative anion transporter-1 – PAT-1), both of which are activated by CFTR [88–93].

Abnormally viscous and acidic ductal secretions likely lead to premature activation of proteolytic enzymes within the gland, with ensuing pancreatic inflammation and destruction. This notion is consistent with the emerging evidence that *CFTR* mutations are associated with pancreatitis in patients without CF [94].

Not all CF patients develop pancreatic insufficiency. Those who 'escape' this fate are now recognized to have characteristic *CFTR* genotypes (reviewed in Chapters 6a and 6b). Indeed, is has been suggested that some CFTR mutations result in a protein that retains the capacity to secrete Cl^-, but not HCO_3^-. However, in most cases, it appears that sparing of the pancreas reflects translocation of more functional but mutated CFTR protein to the apical membrane in patients with milder mutations than occurs with more 'severe' mutations.

PATHOPHYSIOLOGY OF DISORDERED SWEAT GLAND PHYSIOLOGY

Abnormal sweat chloride concentrations have been recognized in CF for more than 50 years, and the recognition of this defect constitutes one of the seminal observations in the field (95,96). Abnormal electric potential associated with sweating was first reported as early as the 1960s [97], hinting at subsequent findings from more comprehensive studies of CF sweat duct physiology.

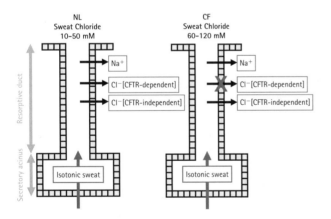

Figure 4.3   Ion transport in normal (NL) and CF sweat ducts. Isotonic sweat is produced in the secretory acinus. In the resorptive duct, both CFTR-dependent and CFTR-independent mechanisms of chloride resorption exist, reducing intraluminal chloride concentrations. Sodium absorption occurs in parallel and, as a result, hypotonic sweat (10–50 mmol/L) is normally secreted from the duct. However, in CF, the absence of CFTR in the apical membrane of resorptive duct cells results in defective chloride resorption and thus abnormally high sweat chloride concentrations (60–120 mmol/L).

It is now well established that abnormal physiology of the CF sweat reflects defective ductal resorption of Cl^- from isotonic liquid secreted in the gland acinus [98]. Relative ductal Cl^- impermeability results in an abnormal spontaneous transepithelial potential ($\sim$75 mV) in CF compared to non-CF ($\sim$7 mV) subjects [55] (Fig. 4.3). The observation that pilocarpine-stimulated sweat $[Cl^-]$ is less than 60 mM in non-CF subjects and above 80 mM in CF subjects (with virtually no overlap) forms the basis for the most widely adopted diagnostic test for CF [99,100]. In parallel with β-CFTR regulation in other organs, β-adrenergic-induced stimulation of acinar secretion was also found to be defective in CF patients [101], although no physiological significance of this observation has been identified.

PATHOGENESIS OF GASTROINTESTINAL AND HEPATOBILIARY DISEASE

Characteristic ion-transport defects are present in the gastrointestinal tract of CF patients and contribute to specific pathologies that are independent of pancreatic insufficiency. Most notable is the propensity for patients to exhibit delayed transit of GI contents, most classically manifesting as distal intestinal obstruction syndromes (DIOS). Accelerated glucose absorption, measured as increased nutrient-activated short-circuit current, was the first identified gut transport abnormality [102]. Subsequently, defective Cl^- secretion, consistent with that described in other organs (i.e. an inherent loss of Cl^- conductance), has been described in duodenum, jejunum, ileum, colon and rectum. Impaired anion secretion has been reported in response to a variety of agonists, including PGE2, dibutyl cAMP, acetylcholine, and the Ca^{++} ionophore A23187 [103–108].

As in the pancreas and gut, evidence also exists that HCO_3^- transport is also altered in CF intestine, though again, the pathophysiological significance has not been firmly established [109–112].

Paradoxically, impaired enteric anion secretory processes may have provided selective evolutionary pressure for the persistence of CFTR mutations, since it appears that they may confer a survival advantage in heterozygotes challenged with infectious diarrheal illnesses, such as those associated with cholera toxin or heat-stable *Escherichia coli* enterotoxin [113,114].

A spectrum of liver disease may also develop in CF patients, from transient biochemical abnormalities of cholestatic liver enzymes to cirrhosis and pulmonary hypertension [115], reviewed in more detail in Chapter 16b. The latter may be fatal. The underlying pathophysiological basis for CF liver disease is less well characterized than in other organs, but CFTR is known to be expressed in both biliary epithelial cells [116] and gallbladder epithelia [117], where it appears to play a role in normal bile formation. Defective biliary luminal anion secretion seems likely in CF, producing inspissated secretions within the biliary tree, which lead to obstruction, periductular inflammation, and eventually focal and then multilobular cirrhosis. Defective anion secretion in the gallbladder may increase the frequency of cholelithiasis. The restriction of severe liver disease to a small cohort of CF patients seemingly implicates modifier genes, which are the subject of current scrutiny [118].

PATHOGENESIS OF THE REPRODUCTIVE TRACT DISORDERS

Infertility in male CF patients is almost invariable and reflects congenital bilateral absence of the vas deferens (CBAVD). Seminal vesicles are also often hypoplastic. CFTR is expressed in the epididymis and vas deferens [119]. As in other affected epithelial organs, it is thought that CBAVD reflects obstruction of the developing vas with inspissated secretions, which may reflect defective Cl^- secretion, although it is worth also noting that abnormal pH of seminal secretions has been detected and defective HCO_3^- secretion may also play an important role [63]. Even in infertile males without a diagnosis of CF, mutations in CFTR are frequent and are thought to be pathophysiologically important [120].

Although many women with CF successfully conceive, fertility in CF females may be reduced [121]. CFTR is expressed in the uterus and cervix [119]. It has been suggested that dysregulation of intrauterine pH may be of pathophysiological relevance in female subfertility [64,122].

REFERENCES

1. Andersen DH. Cystic fibrosis of the pancreas and its relation to celiac disease: a clinical and pathologic study. *Am J Dis Child* 1938; **56**:344–399.
2. Kerem B, Rommens JM, Buchanan JA *et al.* Identification of the cystic fibrosis gene: genetic analysis. *Science* 1989; **245**:1073–1080.
3. Riordan JR, Rommens JM, Kerem B *et al.* Identification of the cystic fibrosis gene: cloning and characterization of complementary DNA. *Science* 1989; **245**:1066–1073.
4. Rommens JM, Iannuzzi MC, Kerem B *et al.* Identification of the cystic fibrosis gene: chromosome walking and jumping. *Science* 1989; **245**:1059–1065.
5. Cystic Fibrosis Gene Analysis Consortium. www.genet. cickkids.on.ca/cftr/.
6. Gabolde M, Guilloud-Bataille M, Feingold J, Besmond C. Association of variant alleles of mannose binding lectin with severity of pulmonary disease in cystic fibrosis: cohort study. *Br Med J* 1999; **319**:1166–1167.
7. Garred P, Pressler T, Madsen HO *et al.* Association of mannose-binding lectin gene heterogeneity with severity of lung disease and survival in cystic fibrosis. *J Clin Invest* 1999; **104**:431–437.
8. Hull J, Thomson AH. Contribution of genetic factors other than CFTR to disease severity in cystic fibrosis. *Thorax* 1998; **53**:1018–1021.
9. Mahadeva R, Stewart S, Bilton D, Lomas DA. Alpha-1 antitrypsin deficiency alleles and severe cystic fibrosis lung disease. *Thorax* 1998; **53**:1022–1024.
10. Arkwright PD, Laurie S, Super M *et al.* TGF-beta(1) genotype and accelerated decline in lung function of patients with cystic fibrosis. *Thorax* 2000; **55**:459–462.
11. Mahadeva R, Sharples L, Ross-Russell RI *et al.* Association of alpha(1)-antichymotrypsin deficiency with milder lung disease in patients with cystic fibrosis. *Thorax* 2001; **56**:53–58.
12. Drumm ML, Konstan MW, Schluchter MD *et al.* Genetic modifiers of lung disease in cystic fibrosis. *N Engl J Med* 2005; **353**:1443–1453.
13. Cheng SH, Gregory RJ, Marshall J *et al.* Defective intracellular transport and processing of CFTR is the molecular basis of most cystic fibrosis. *Cell* 1990; **63**:827–834.
14. Van Goor F, Straley KS, Cao D *et al.* Rescue of ΔF508 CFTR trafficking and gating in human cystic fibrosis airway primary cultures by small molecules. *Am J Physiol Lung Cell Mol Physiol* 2006; **290**(6): L117–130.
15. Swiatecka-Urban A, Brown A, Moreau-Marquis S *et al.* The short apical membrane half-life of rescued ΔF508-cystic fibrosis transmembrane conductance regulator (CFTR) results from accelerated endocytosis of ΔF508-CFTR in polarized human airway epithelial cells. *J Biol Chem* 2005; **280**:36762–36772.
16. Coakley RJ, Taggart C, O'Neill S, McElvaney NG. Alpha1-antitrypsin deficiency: biological answers to clinical questions. *Am J Med Sci* 2001; **321**:33–41.
17. Knorre A, Wagner M, Schaefer HE *et al.* DeltaF508-CFTR causes constitutive NF-kappaB activation through an ER-overload response in cystic fibrosis lungs. *Biol Chem* 2002; **383**:271–282.
18. Weber AJ, Soong G, Bryan R *et al.* Activation of NF-kappaB in airway epithelial cells is dependent on CFTR trafficking and Cl^- channel function. *Am J Physiol Lung Cell Mol Physiol* 2001; **281**:L71–L78.
19. Becker MN, Sauer MS, Muhlebach MS *et al.* Cytokine secretion by cystic fibrosis airway epithelial cells. *Am J Respir Crit Care Med* 2004; **169**:645–653.
20. Ribeiro CM, Paradiso AM, Schwab U *et al.* Chronic airway infection/inflammation induces a Ca^{2+}-dependent hyperinflammatory response in human cystic fibrosis airway epithelia. *J Biol Chem* 2005; **280**:17798–17806.
21. Ribeiro CM, Paradiso AM, Carew MA, Shears SB, Boucher RC. Cystic fibrosis airway epithelial Ca^{2+} i-signalling: the mechanism for the larger agonist-mediated Ca^{2+} i signals in human cystic fibrosis airway epithelia. *J Biol Chem* 2005; **280**:10202–10209.
22. Wong LJ, Wang J, Bowman CM. Two novel frame shift mutations of CFTR causing null alleles in a patient with a severe course of CF. *Am J Med Genet* 2001; **102**:389–390.
23. Smith JJ, Travis SM, Greenberg EP, Welsh MJ. Cystic fibrosis airway epithelia fail to kill bacteria because of abnormal airway surface fluid. *Cell* 1996; **85**:229–236.
24. Zabner J, Smith JJ, Karp PH *et al.* Loss of CFTR chloride channels alters salt absorption by cystic fibrosis airway epithelia *in vitro*. *Mol Cell* 1998; **2**:397–403.

25. Goldman MJ, Anderson GM, Stolzenberg ED *et al.* Human beta-defensin-1 is a salt-sensitive antibiotic in lung that is inactivated in cystic fibrosis. *Cell* 1997; **88**:553–560.

26. Caldwell RA, Grubb BR, Tarran R *et al.* In-vivo airway surface liquid Cl⁻ analysis with solid-state electrodes. *J Gen Physiol* 2002; **119**:3–14.

27. Jayaraman S, Song Y, Vetrivel L *et al.* Noninvasive in-vivo fluorescence measurement of airway-surface liquid depth, salt concentration, and pH. *J Clin Invest* 2001; **107**:317–324.

28. Knowles MR, Robinson JM, Wood RE *et al.* Ion composition of airway surface liquid of patients with cystic fibrosis as compared with normal and disease-control subjects. *J Clin Invest* 1997; **100**:2588–2595. Published erratum appears in *J Clin Invest* 1998; **101**:285.

29. Matsui H, Grubb BR, Tarran R *et al.* Evidence for periciliary liquid layer depletion, not abnormal ion composition, in the pathogenesis of cystic fibrosis airways disease. *Cell* 1998; **95**:1005–1015.

30. Cole AM, Dewan P, Ganz T. Innate antimicrobial activity of nasal secretions. *Infect Immun* 1999; **67**:3267–3275.

31. Regnis JA, Zeman KL, Noone PG *et al.* Prolonged airway retention of insoluble particles in cystic fibrosis versus primary ciliary dyskinesia. *Exp Lung Res* 2000; **26**:149–162.

32. Matsui H, Grubb BR, Tarran R *et al.* Evidence for periciliary liquid layer depletion, not abnormal ion composition, in the pathogenesis of cystic fibrosis airways disease. *Cell* 1998; **95**:1005–1015.

33. Matsui H, Randell SH, Peretti SW *et al.* Coordinated clearance of periciliary liquid and mucus from airway surfaces. *J Clin Invest* 1998; **102**:1125–1131.

34. Tarran R, Grubb BR, Parsons D *et al.* The CF salt controversy: in-vivo observations and therapeutic approaches. *Mol Cell* 2001; **8**:149–158.

35. Donaldson SH, Bennett WD, Zeman KL *et al.* Mucus clearance and lung function in cystic fibrosis with hypertonic saline. *N Engl J Med* 2006; **354**:241–250.

36. Elkins MR, Robinson M, Rose BR *et al.* A controlled trial of long-term inhaled hypertonic saline in patients with cystic fibrosis. *N Engl J Med* 2006; **354**:229–240.

37. Mall M, Grubb BR, Harkema JR *et al.* Increased airway epithelial Na⁺ absorption produces cystic fibrosis-like lung disease in mice. *Nat Med* 2004; **10**:487–493.

38. Kerem E, Bistritzer T, Hanukoglu A *et al.* Pulmonary epithelial sodium-channel dysfunction and excess airway liquid in pseudohypoaldosteronism. *N Engl J Med* 1999; **341**:156–162.

39. Tarran R, Grubb BR, Gatzy JT *et al.* The relative roles of passive surface forces and active ion transport in the modulation of airway surface liquid volume and composition. *J Gen Physiol* 2001; **118**:223–236.

40. Matsui H, Davis CW, Tarran R, Boucher RC. Osmotic water permeabilities of cultured, well-differentiated normal and cystic fibrosis airway epithelia. *J Clin Invest* 2000; **105**:1419–1427.

41. Kreda SM, Gynn MC, Fenstermacher DA *et al.* Expression and localization of epithelial aquaporins in the adult human lung. *Am J Respir Cell Mol Biol* 2001; **24**:224–234.

42. Boucher RC. Human airway ion transport: 2. *Am J Respir Crit Care Med* 1994; **150**:581–593.

43. Boucher RC. Human airway ion transport: 1. *Am J Respir Crit Care Med* 1994; **150**:271–281.

44. Donaldson SH, Hirsh A, Li DC *et al.* Regulation of the epithelial sodium channel by serine proteases in human airways. *J Biol Chem* 2002; **277**:8338–8345.

45. Caldwell RA, Boucher RC, Stutts MJ. Neutrophil elastase activates near-silent epithelial Na⁺ channels and increases airway epithelial Na⁺ transport. *Am J Physiol Lung Cell Mol Physiol* 2005; **288**:L813–L819.

46. Gray T, Coakley R, Hirsh A *et al.* Regulation of MUC5AC mucin secretion and airway surface liquid metabolism by IL-1beta in human bronchial epithelia. *Am J Physiol Lung Cell Mol Physiol* 2004; **286**:L320–L330.

47. Huang P, Gilmore E, Kultgen P *et al.* Local regulation of cystic fibrosis transmembrane regulator and epithelial sodium channel in airway epithelium. *Proc Am Thorac Soc* 2004; **1**:33–37.

48. Kunzelmann K, Schreiber R, Nitschke R, Mall M. Control of epithelial Na⁺ conductance by the cystic fibrosis transmembrane conductance regulator. *Pflugers Arch* 2000; **440**:193–201.

49. Chinet TC, Fullton JM, Yankaskas JR *et al.* Sodium-permeable channels in the apical membrane of human nasal epithelial cells. *Am J Physiol* 1993; **265**(4 Pt 1):C1050–C1060.

50. Chinet TC, Fullton JM, Yankaskas JR *et al.* Mechanism of sodium hyperabsorption in cultured cystic fibrosis nasal epithelium: a patch-clamp study. *Am J Physiol* 1994; **266** (4 Pt 1):C1061–C1068.

51. Boucher RC, Stutts MJ, Knowles MR *et al.* Na⁺ transport in cystic fibrosis respiratory epithelia: abnormal basal rate and response to adenylate cyclase activation. *J Clin Invest* 1986; **78**:1245–1252.

52. Jiang C, Finkbeiner WE, Widdicombe JH *et al.* Altered fluid transport across airway epithelium in cystic fibrosis. *Science* 1993; **262**:424–427.

53. Knowles M, Gatzy J, Boucher R. Increased bioelectric potential difference across respiratory epithelia in cystic fibrosis. *N Engl J Med* 1981; **305**:1489–1495.

54. Knowles MR, Stutts MJ, Spock A *et al.* Abnormal ion permeation through cystic fibrosis respiratory epithelium. *Science* 1983; **221**:1067–1070.

55. Quinton PM. Chloride impermeability in cystic fibrosis. *Nature* 1983; **301**:421–422.

56. Knowles MR, Clarke LL, Boucher RC. Activation by extracellular nucleotides of chloride secretion in the airway epithelia of patients with cystic fibrosis. *N Engl J Med* 1991; **325**:533–538.

57. Deterding R, Retsch-Bogart G, Milgram L *et al.* Safety and tolerability of denufosol tetrasodium inhalation solution, a novel P2Y2 receptor agonist: results of a phase 1/phase 2 multicenter study in mild to moderate cystic fibrosis. *Pediatr Pulmonol* 2005; **39**:339–348.

58. Coakley RD, Grubb BR, Paradiso AM *et al.* Abnormal surface liquid pH regulation by cultured cystic fibrosis bronchial epithelium. *Proc Natl Acad Sci USA* 2003; **100**:16083–16088.

59. Devor DC, Bridges RJ, Pilewski JM. Pharmacological modulation of ion transport across wild-type and DeltaF508 CFTR-expressing human bronchial epithelia. *Am J Physiol Cell Physiol* 2000; **279**:C461–C479.

60. Devor DC, Singh AK, Lambert LC *et al.* Bicarbonate and chloride secretion in Calu-3 human airway epithelial cells. *J Gen Physiol* 1999; **113**:743–760.

61. Johansen PG, Anderson CM, Hadorn B. Cystic fibrosis of the pancreas: a generalised disturbance of water and electrolyte movement in exocrine tissues. *Lancet* 1968; **1**:455–460.

62. Kopelman H, Durie P, Gaskin K *et al.* Pancreatic fluid secretion and protein hyperconcentration in cystic fibrosis. *N Engl J Med* 1985; **312**:329–334.

63. von Eckardstein S, Cooper TG, Rutscha K *et al.* Seminal plasma characteristics as indicators of cystic fibrosis transmembrane conductance regulator (CFTR) gene mutations in men with obstructive azoospermia. *Fertil Steril* 2000; **73**:1226–1231.

64. Wang XF, Zhou CX, Shi QX *et al.* Involvement of CFTR in uterine bicarbonate secretion and the fertilizing capacity of sperm. *Nat Cell Biol* 2003; **5**:902–906.

65. Yoon SS, Coakley R, Lau GW *et al.* Anaerobic killing of mucoid *Pseudomonas aeruginosa* by acidified nitrite derivatives under cystic fibrosis airway conditions. *J Clin Invest* 2006; **116**:436–446.

66. Song Y, Salinas D, Nielson DW, Verkman AS. Hyperacidity of secreted fluid from submucosal glands in early cystic fibrosis. *Am J Physiol Cell Physiol* 2006; **290**:C741–C749.

67. Galietta LJ, Pagesy P, Folli C *et al.* IL-4 is a potent modulator of ion transport in the human bronchial epithelium *in vitro*. *J Immunol* 2002; **168**:839–845.

68. Matsui H, Verghese MW, Kesimer M *et al.* Reduced three-dimensional motility in dehydrated airway mucus prevents neutrophil capture and killing bacteria on airway epithelial surfaces. *J Immunol* 2005; **175**:1090–1099.

69. Worlitzsch D, Tarran R, Ulrich M *et al.* Effects of reduced mucus oxygen concentration in airway *Pseudomonas* infections of cystic fibrosis patients. *J Clin Invest* 2002; **109**:317–325.

70. Armstrong DS, Grimwood K, Carlin JB *et al.* Lower airway inflammation in infants and young children with cystic fibrosis. *Am J Respir Crit Care Med* 1997; **156**(4 Pt 1): 1197–1204.

71. Schroeder TH, Reiniger N, Meluleni G *et al.* Transgenic cystic fibrosis mice exhibit reduced early clearance of *Pseudomonas aeruginosa* from the respiratory tract. *J Immunol* 2001; **166**:7410–7418.

72. Kosorok MR, Zeng L, West SE *et al.* Acceleration of lung disease in children with cystic fibrosis after *Pseudomonas aeruginosa* acquisition. *Pediatr Pulmonol* 2001; **32**:277–287.

73. Li Z, Kosorok MR, Farrell PM *et al.* Longitudinal development of mucoid *Pseudomonas aeruginosa* infection and lung disease progression in children with cystic fibrosis. *J Am Med Assoc* 2005; **293**:581–588.

74. Barasch J, Kiss B, Prince A *et al.* Defective acidification of intracellular organelles in cystic fibrosis [see comments]. *Nature* 1991; **352**:70–73.

75. Machen TE, Chandy G, Wu M *et al.* Cystic fibrosis transmembrane conductance regulator and H^+ permeability in regulation of Golgi pH. *JOP* 2001; **2**(4 Suppl):229–236.

76. Milla CE. Association of nutritional status and pulmonary function in children with cystic fibrosis. *Curr Opin Pulmon Med* 2004; **10**:505–509.

77. Hadorn B, Zoppi G, Shmerling DH *et al.* Quantitative assessment of exocrine pancreatic function in infants and children. *J Pediatr* 1968; **73**:39–50.

78. Steward MC, Ishiguro H, Case RM. Mechanisms of bicarbonate secretion in the pancreatic duct. *Annu Rev Physiol* 2005; **67**:377–409.

79. Marino CR, Matovcik LM, Gorelick FS, Cohn JA. Localization of the cystic fibrosis transmembrane conductance regulator in pancreas. *J Clin Invest* 1991; **88**:712–716.

80. Zeng W, Lee MG, Yan M *et al.* Immuno and functional characterization of CFTR in submandibular and pancreatic acinar and duct cells. *Am J Physiol* 1997; **273**(2 Pt 1):C442–C455.

81. Reddy MM, Quinton PM. Control of dynamic CFTR selectivity by glutamate and ATP in epithelial cells. *Nature* 2003; **423**:756–760.

82. Shcheynikov N, Kim KH, Kim KM *et al.* Dynamic control of cystic fibrosis transmembrane conductance regulator Cl^-/HCO_3^- selectivity by external Cl^-. *J Biol Chem* 2004; **279**:21857–21865.

83. Lee MG, Choi JY, Luo X *et al.* Cystic fibrosis transmembrane conductance regulator regulates luminal Cl^-. *J Biol Chem* 1999; **274**:14670–14677.

84. Namkung W, Lee JA, Ahn W *et al.* Ca^{2+} activates cystic fibrosis transmembrane conductance regulator- and Cl^--dependent HCO_3 transport in pancreatic duct cells. *J Biol Chem* 2003; **278**:200–207.

85. Sohma Y, Gray MA, Imai Y, Argent BE. A mathematical model of the pancreatic ductal epithelium. *J Membr Biol* 1996; **154**:53–67.

86. Mount DB, Romero MF. The SLC26 gene family of multifunctional anion exchangers. *Pflugers Arch* 2004; **447**:710–721.

87. Elgavish A, Meezan E. Altered sulfate transport via anion exchange in CFPAC is corrected by retrovirus-mediated CFTR gene transfer. *Am J Physiol* 1992; **263**(1 Pt 1):C176–C186.

88. Greeley T, Shumaker H, Wang Z *et al.* Downregulated-in-adenoma and putative anion transporter are regulated by CFTR in cultured pancreatic duct cells. *Am J Physiol Gastrointest Liver Physiol* 2001; **281**:G1301–G1308.

89. Jiang Z, Grichtchenko II, Boron WF, Aronson PS. Specificity of anion exchange mediated by mouse Slc26a6. *J Biol Chem* 2002; **277**:33963–33967.

90. Lohi H, Kujala M, Kerkela E *et al.* Mapping of five new putative anion transporter genes in human and characterization of SLC26A6, a candidate gene for pancreatic anion exchanger. *Genomics* 2000; **70**:102–112.

91. Lohi H, Lamprecht G, Markovich D *et al.* Isoforms of SLC26A6 mediate anion transport and have functional PDZ interaction domains. *Am J Physiol Cell Physiol* 2003; **284**:C769–C779.

92. Melvin JE, Park K, Richardson L *et al*. Mouse down-regulated in adenoma (DRA) is an intestinal Cl^-/HCO_3^- exchanger and is up-regulated in colon of mice lacking the NHE3 Na^+/H^+ exchanger. *J Biol Chem* 1999; **274**:22855–22861.

93. Xie Q, Welch R, Mercado A *et al*. Molecular characterization of the murine Slc26a6 anion exchanger: functional comparison with Slc26a1. *Am J Physiol Renal Physiol* 2002; **283**:F826–F838.

94. Cohn JA, Friedman KJ, Noone PG *et al*. Relation between mutations of the cystic fibrosis gene and idiopathic pancreatitis. *N Engl J Med* 1998; **339**:653–658.

95. Di Sant'Agnese PA, Darling RC, Perera GA, Shea E. Abnormal electrolyte composition of sweat in cystic fibrosis of the pancreas: clinical significance and relationship to the disease. *Pediatrics* 1953; **12**:549–563.

96. Di Sant'Agnese PA, Darling RC, Perera GA, Shea E. Sweat electrolyte disturbances associated with childhood pancreatic disease. *Am J Med* 1953; **15**:777–784.

97. Schulz IJ, Fromter E. Mikopunktionsuntersuchungen an schweibdrusen von mucoviscidosepatienten und gesunden versuchspersonen. In: Windorfer A, Stephan U (eds) *Mucoviscidose/Cystische Fibrose*. Stuttgart, Georg Thieme Verlag, 1968, pp21–25.

98. Quinton PM. Physiological basis of cystic fibrosis: a historical perspective. *Physiol Rev* 1999; **79**(1 Suppl):S3–S22.

99. Gibson LE, Gottlieb R, Di Sant'Agnese PA, Huang NN. Reliability of sweat tests in diagnosis of cystic fibrosis. *J Pediatr* 1972; **81**:193–197.

100. Wang L, Freedman SD. Laboratory tests for the diagnosis of cystic fibrosis. *Am J Clin Pathol* 2002; **117**(Suppl):S109–S115.

101. Sato K, Sato F. Defective beta adrenergic response of cystic fibrosis sweat glands *in vivo* and *in vitro*. *J Clin Invest* 1984; **73**:1763–1771.

102. Hardcastle J, Taylor CJ, Hardcastle PT *et al*. Intestinal transport in cystic fibrosis. *Acta Univ Carol [Med] (Praha)* 1990; **36**(1–4):157–158.

103. Teune TM, Timmers-Reker AJ, Bouquet J *et al*. In-vivo measurement of chloride and water secretion in the jejunum of cystic fibrosis patients. *Pediatr Res* 1996; **40**:522–527.

104. Taylor CJ, Baxter PS, Hardcastle J, Hardcastle PT. Absence of secretory response in jejunal biopsy samples from children with cystic fibrosis. *Lancet* 1987; **2**:107–108.

105. O'Loughlin EV, Hunt DM, Gaskin KJ *et al*. Abnormal epithelial transport in cystic fibrosis jejunum. *Am J Physiol* 1991; **260**(5 Pt 1):G758–G763.

106. Kunzelmann K, Mall M. Electrolyte transport in the mammalian colon: mechanisms and implications for disease. *Physiol Rev* 2002; **82**:245–289.

107. Bijman J, Veeze H, Kansen M *et al*. Chloride transport in the cystic fibrosis enterocyte. *Adv Exp Med Biol* 1991; **290**:287–294.

108. Berschneider HM, Knowles MR, Azizkhan RG *et al*. Altered intestinal chloride transport in cystic fibrosis. *FASEB J* 1988; **2**:2625–2629.

109. Pratha VS, Hogan DL, Martensson BA *et al*. Identification of transport abnormalities in duodenal mucosa and duodenal enterocytes from patients with cystic fibrosis. *Gastroenterology* 2000; **118**:1051–1060.

110. Hogan DL, Crombie DL, Isenberg JI *et al*. CFTR mediates cAMP- and Ca^{2+}-activated duodenal epithelial HCO_3^- secretion. *Am J Physiol* 1997; **272**(4 Pt 1):G872–G878.

111. Hogan DL, Crombie DL, Isenberg JI *et al*. Acid-stimulated duodenal bicarbonate secretion involves a CFTR-mediated transport pathway in mice. *Gastroenterology* 1997; **113**:533–541.

112. Clarke LL, Harline MC. Dual role of CFTR in cAMP-stimulated HCO_3^- secretion across murine duodenum. *Am J Physiol* 1998; **274**(4 Pt 1):G718–G726.

113. Goldstein JL, Sahi J, Bhuva M *et al*. *Escherichia coli* heat-stable enterotoxin-mediated colonic Cl^- secretion is absent in cystic fibrosis. *Gastroenterology* 1994; **107**:950–956.

114. Gabriel SE, Brigman KN, Koller BH *et al*. Cystic fibrosis heterozygote resistance to cholera toxin in the cystic fibrosis mouse model. *Science* 1994; **266**:107–109.

115. Flora KD, Benner KG. Liver disease in cystic fibrosis. *Clin Liver Dis* 1998; **2**:51–61.

116. Cohn JA, Strong TV, Picciotto MR *et al*. Localization of the cystic fibrosis transmembrane conductance regulator in human bile duct epithelial cells. *Gastroenterology* 1993; **105**:1857–1864.

117. Dray-Charier N, Paul A, Scoazec JY *et al*. Expression of delta F508 cystic fibrosis transmembrane conductance regulator protein and related chloride transport properties in the gallbladder epithelium from cystic fibrosis patients. *Hepatology* 1999; **29**:1624–1634.

118. Cutting GR. Modifier genetics: cystic fibrosis. *Annu Rev Genomics Hum Genet* 2005; **6**:237–260.

119. Tizzano EF, Silver MM, Chitayat D *et al*. Differential cellular expression of cystic fibrosis transmembrane regulator in human reproductive tissues: clues for the infertility in patients with cystic fibrosis. *Am J Pathol* 1994; **144**:906–914.

120. Cuppens H, Cassiman JJ. CFTR mutations and polymorphisms in male infertility. *Int J Androl* 2004; **27**:251–256.

121. Phillipson G. Cystic fibrosis and reproduction. *Reprod Fertil Dev* 1998; **10**:113–119.

122. Chan HC, Shi QX, Zhou CX *et al*. Critical role of CFTR in uterine bicarbonate secretion and the fertilizing capacity of sperm. *Mol Cell Endocrinol* 2006; **250**(1–2): 106–113.

5

Immunology of cystic fibrosis

GERD DÖRING AND FELIX RATJEN

INTRODUCTION

It is interesting how ideas on the role of inflammation in CF have come full circle. The apparent inability of the immune system to keep the airways free of bacterial pathogens led to early speculation that the then unknown genetic abnormality causes an immunological defect and that CF was, in fact, an immunological disorder (reviewed in [1]). With the knowledge that the CF gene codes for an epithelial ion-transport protein, and extensive data showing essentially normal systemic immune function in CF, immunology of CF was regarded to be similar to the immunology of any other chronic infection. However, recent data suggest again that CF respiratory epithelial cells differ from epithelial cells from normal individuals with regard to inflammation control. The consequences of these findings imply that, before onset of infection, inflammation is present in CF airways, triggering infection. Thereafter, the chronicity of the infection, and the chronic inflammatory response it induces, result in the production of potent inflammatory compounds which are present for prolonged periods in the airways. These have the potential for damaging not only airway cells but also cells of the inflammatory infiltrate. This in turn may contribute to the chronicity of bacterial infection, a situation that indeed deserves the description of a 'vicious cycle' [2].

A detailed knowledge of particular inflammatory products contributing to the disease pathology will allow more selective anti-inflammatory interventions, rather than risking the side-effects associated with potent but unselective drugs such as corticosteroids. The immunology of CF is, therefore, a particular example of the immunology of the host–parasite relationship, and the present review will focus on (1) host and bacterial factors leading to bacterial colonization, and subsequently to acute and chronic infection, (2) the humoral and cellular immune response against the major pathogens, particularly *Staphylococcus aureus* and

Pseudomonas aeruginosa, and, finally, on immunological strategies for prevention of infection.

HOST FACTORS IN BACTERIAL AIRWAY COLONIZATION

To maintain sterile lungs, the mucociliary clearance system as well as the mucosal and secretory immune system, act in concert with the constituents of the non-specific (or innate) immune system including secretory IgA, lymphocytes, sessile alveolar macrophages, mast cells, complement components, mobile neutrophils, antimicrobial peptides and proteins. The secretory immune system generally clears bacterial organisms such as *P. aeruginosa* rapidly, even when large doses are administered to normal airways [3]. This rapid clearance is mostly due to the influx of neutrophils which, as an immediate response to bacterial infection, reach the involved tissue site in high numbers within hours [4], eliminate the pathogens by phagocytosis and disappear by apoptosis [5]. Why does this not happen in CF airways? Although much has been learned, due to the complexity of the immune system and the relative lack of understanding concerning the physiological consequences of the basic defect, the answer to this question is still not clear. Several hypotheses have been proposed.

'Inflammation precedes bacterial lung infection'

Autopsy specimens from neonates with CF who have not yet developed lung disease show luminal dilation in submucosal glands [6]. This may indicate mucus accumulation. Indeed, elevated viscosity has been detected in CF submucosal glands, which was interpreted to promote bacterial colonization and airway disease in CF patients due to impaired mucociliary clearance and antimicrobial defense mechanisms [7]. Staining of immune cells revealed significant differences between CF and non-CF fetal airways concerning the numbers of mast cells and macrophages [8]. Already in the first months of life inflammatory infiltrates in bronchi and mucopurulent plugging of airways can be detected histologically [9]. Both the number of neutrophils and levels of a neutrophil-attracting IL-8 were increased in bronchoalveolar lavage (BAL) of CF infants as young as 4 weeks who had negative cultures for common bacterial CF-related pathogens [10,11]. Most probably, the neutrophils detected in BAL fluids are activated, since increased levels of the neutrophil lysosomal enzyme elastase have been also measured in plasma samples of uninfected CF infants [10] and in BAL fluids of young CF patients [12,13]. How is neutrophil activation related to infection? Lysosomal enzyme release and enhanced production of reactive oxygen species may facilitate bacterial infection. There is a large body of evidence that release of host proteases during acute and chronic inflammation may damage epithelial cells [14,15] thereby facilitating *P. aeruginosa* adhesion *in vitro* and *in vivo* [14,16,17].

The notion that inflammation precedes bacterial lung infection is also supported by cell culture studies, revealing increased toll-like receptor expression [18], increased NFκB activation [18,19] and increased baseline IL-8 production [20] in CF cells versus controls. Further support of this hypothesis stems from a study in germ-free raised CF mice which showed signs of inflammation [21] and sterile fetal CF airways, transplanted into severe combined immunodeficiency mice [22,23]. An increased IL-8 production and increased neutrophil infiltration was observed. Increased immune cell infiltration into the CF mucosa was also noticed in another study [24]. Furthermore, long-lived *C578L/6J CFTR−/−* mice develop CF-like disease [25,26]. Defective mucociliary transport alone can result in neutrophilic inflammation in the absence of infection as shown in mice over-expressing the beta subunit of the epithelial sodium channel [27].

CF BAL fluids contain low levels of IL-10, a cytokine that decreases pro-inflammatory responses [28,29]. In contrast, pro-inflammatory cytokines were highly elevated in BAL fluids from CF patients [28]. In *P. aeruginosa*-infected IL-10 knockout mice, more severe weight loss and lung inflammation were observed [30] and IL-10 treatment improved survival and reduced weight loss, neutrophil numbers and lung inflammation [31]. Also in the *CFTR−/−* mouse, challenged with lipopolysaccharide, increased inflammation was observed and contributed to low IL-10 expression [32]. Finally, *CFTR−/−* mouse strains are more susceptible to bacterial infection than normal mice [33–35].

However, others groups have not confirmed some of these findings. For instance, the inflammatory response in airway epithelial cells as well as IL-10 concentrations in BAL fluids isolated from CF patients did not differ from those of normal individuals [36–38]. Furthermore, since large regional variability of lung infection and inflammation is present in different lung lobes, sampling of BAL fluids in one lobe may yield inflammatory markers yet no bacterial organisms, whereas both can be found in another lobe [39]. Finally, in newly diagnosed CF infants under the age of 6 months [40], and in a group of CF patients up to 48 months of age [41], inflammatory BAL markers correlated with the presence of infection and decreased when pathogens were eradicated.

The debate is ongoing whether airway inflammation is a primary or secondary event, because it is unclear how *CFTR* mutations are mechanistically linked to the innate immune response and how inflammation triggers infection.

'Different membrane composition of CF epithelial airway cells'

Several observations argue for an increased binding of bacterial pathogens to membranes of CF epithelial cells. Increased or different sulfation of the glycocalix of CF epithelial cells has been demonstrated [42–45] which may facilitate binding of *S. aureus* [46,47]. Furthermore, it has been proposed that the apical membrane of CF bronchial epithelial cells is under-sialylated [48]. Both findings have been linked to the hypothesis that CFTR regulates endosomal acidification [48]. Defective acidification in CF cells would lead to increased levels of membrane-bound asialoganglioside-1 (aGM1) to which many pathogenic bacteria bind [49]. Increased binding of *S. aureus* and *P. aeruginosa* to CF bronchial epithelial cells has indeed been demonstrated [50,51]. However, in other studies this notion was not supported [52]. Rather, increased acidification was observed in CF cells which equally promoted adherence of *P. aeruginosa* [53]. Still other studies did not show significant differences in binding of *S. aureus* [54,55] or *P. aeruginosa* [56,57] to primary epithelial cells from CF patients and healthy individuals corroborating data showing absence of abnormal mucin O-glycosylation or sulfation in CF cells [58]. Regardless, whether the membranes of CF airway epithelial cells are structurally altered, it is unlikely that invading bacteria would directly interact with these membranes, since the ciliated respiratory epithelium is covered with airway surface liquid (ASL) containing mucins to which bacteria generally adhere.

'Impaired mucociliary clearance'

A number of studies demonstrated that *S. aureus* [55], *P. aeruginosa* [59], *Burkholderia cepacia* [60] or *Haemophilus influenzae* [61] bind to respiratory mucins. Significantly less binding is observed when mucus-producing cell balls of primary nasal epithelial cells from CF patients or healthy normal individuals are mucus depleted [55] (Figs 5.1 and 5.2). Further support for this notion comes from the same study in which *S. aureus* was located in CF airways by immunofluorescence [55]. Only a negligable amount of *S. aureus*

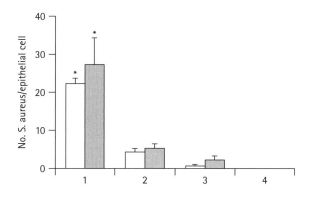

Figure 5.1 Adherence of *S. aureus* to primary nasal epithelial cell balls of five patients with cystic fibrosis (CF) (open columns) and five normal healthy individuals (N) (closed columns). Non-washed (with mucus) (1) and washed (without mucus) (2) cell balls were incubated with *S. aureus* for 2 h, non-adherent bacteria were removed using a cell strainer and centrifugation, and adherent bacteria quantified by scanning electron microscopy. 1: Unwashed cell balls; 2: washed, mucus-depleted cell balls; 3: cell balls, treated with 1 µg/mL neutrophil elastase prior to bacterial incubation; 4: cell balls, treated with 1 µg/mL neutrophil elastase after bacterial incubation. For quantification of adherent bacteria, about 500 cells from 10 cell balls were examined. Values represent means ± SD of five independent experiments for each of the individuals. *, CF 1–2, $p < 0.001$; N, CF 1–2, $p < 0.007$; Student's t-test. (Reproduced with permission from ref. 55.)

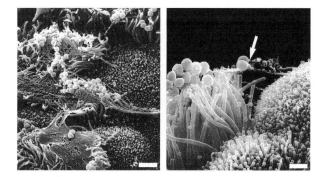

Figure 5.2 Scanning electron micrograph of primary nasal epithelial cells of a cystic fibrosis patient (a) and a healthy individual (b), grown as three-dimensional cell balls. Unwashed cell balls were inoculated with *S. aureus* for 2 hours. *S. aureus* can be seen adhering to mucus on cell balls. Note the *S. aureus*-free membranes. Magnifications: (a), ×5000; (b), ×8000. Bars: (a) 1.5 µm; (b) 1.3 µm. (Reproduced with permission from ref. 55.)

cells were adherent to the lung epithelium, whereas nearly all cells were found embedded in the mucus, distant from the epithelium. Similarly, *P. aeruginosa* was embedded in mucus rather than adhering to the epithelial membrane in lung tissue sections from CF patients [59].

The innate immune mechanism of mucociliary clearance is normally effective to eliminate bacterial pathogens which have bound to mucins in the airway surface liquid. However, defects in mucociliary clearance may allow bacterial multiplication and infection. The hypothesis of

defective mucociliary clearance in CF airways is based on the assumption that chloride secretion into the airway surface liquid is inhibited by mutated *CFTR*, leading to sodium hyperabsorption, leaving the luminal site hypotonic. To establish isotonic conditions, increased water absorption occurs from the luminal site which leads to a volume/height depletion of the airway surface liquid, resulting in mucus stasis [62,63]. The higher viscoelasticity of the CF mucus layer and submucosal gland secretions [6,7] may also influence innate immunity functions within these areas [64–66]. The failure to respond to the bacterial challenge 'in time' could increase the opportunity of the pathogens to change their phenotype and become resistant to a later phagocytic assault. Mucus stasis, seen in CF cell cultures may be less dramatic in CF airways, since young CF patients exhibit reduced but measurable rates of mucus clearance [67], which has been attributed to ATP release into the periciliary liquid during phasic motion of the lung *in vivo* [68]. Furthermore, and unexpected, administration of hypertonic saline to bronchial epithelial cells of CF patients increased ASL height for up to 6 hours *in vitro*, and also had a sustained effect on mucociliary clearance [69].

'Mutated *CFTR*'

A direct connection between mutations in *CFTR* and bacterial lung infections was suggested by the findings that normal CFTR functions as an epithelial cell receptor for *P. aeruginosa* [70–72] which endocytoses bound *P. aeruginosa*, followed by intracellular killing of the pathogen. Wild-type *CFTR* binds the outer core oligosaccharide of lipopolysaccharide of *P. aeruginosa* via amino acids 108–117 in the extracellular domain. Binding is followed by the accumulation of the CFTR–*P. aeruginosa* complex into lipid rafts [73] and clearance of the pathogen via internalization via larger ceramide-rich signaling platforms [74], accompanied by NF-κB activation [75] and cell apoptosis [74]. Thus, besides its role in ion transport, CFTR can be regarded as a component of innate immunity. Since mutant *CFTR* (*F508del*) does not bind *P. aeruginosa*, the organisms are thought to accumulate in the airway lumen, leading to infection [70–72]. However, *P. aeruginosa* has been shown to invade cells from CF patients which do not express CFTR [76] and transfection of cells not expressing CFTR with wild-type *CFTR* significantly reduced invasion of *P. aeruginosa* [77]. Furthermore, the question how other bacterial CF pathogens, which do not seem to bind to wild-type *CFTR*, cause chronic infections is open. In contrast to *P. aeruginosa*, *B. cepacia* may invade airway epithelial cells and resist killing [78].

'Abnormal sodium chloride concentrations in CF airway surface liquid'

This hypothesis links the basic CF defect to bacterial lung infection. It is based on the observation that cultured airway cells of normal individuals kill bacteria whereas cells from CF patients do not have this ability. Second, addition of salt to the bathing fluid on the apical membrane of normal cells prevented killing whereas dilution of this fluid from CF cells became bactericidal [79]. Indeed, increased extracellular chloride and sodium concentrations have been reported in the airway surface fluid of CF patients [80,81]. This led to the detection of salt-sensitive human antimicrobial peptides such as β-defensin-1 in human airways [82,83]. Although the in-vitro results were highly significant and the CF killing defect was mimicked in a human bronchial xenograft model [83], the major problem which prevents the unequivocal acceptance of this hypothesis is that the abnormal high salt concentrations in CF airways has been questioned [84]. Several reports demonstrate isotonic airway surface fluids in CF patients and CF mice, not significantly different from that of normal human individuals or normal mice [85–89].

'Impaired neutrophil functions'

Neutrophils are the predominant phagocytic cells in CF lung infections. Do neutrophils reach the airways in time? Neutrophils released from the marrow leave the circulation in response to chemoattractants which stimulate the cell via specific cell receptors. They adhere to the endothelial cells lining the blood vessels through integrins and then move through the space between the endothelial cells by a process known as diapedesis. They then move directly to the site of infection along a chemotactic gradient. In human newborns, decreased neutrophil chemotaxis until the age of 2 years [90,91] is caused by a reduced number of C3bi receptors (CD11b) on the neutrophil surface. Studies in infant animals show that pulmonary bacterial infections may be due to delayed recruitment of neutrophils into the airways [92,93]. Similarly, a delayed influx of neutrophils soon after birth in CF babies may faciliate bacterial lung infection. Neutrophil function may also be inhibited by the dehydration of ASL with regard to migration [68] or oxygen availability [59]. Furthermore, the ASL of CF patients may contain factors that negatively affect neutrophils [69]. Finally, chronic inflammation may have a negative impact on neutrophil function (see later).

Taken together, several mechanisms including lung inflammation, altered cell surface composition, impaired mucociliary clearance, mutated *CFTR*, inactivated defensins and immature neutrophil function may act together and cause the increased colonization and reduced clearance of micro-organisms in the CF lungs.

BACTERIAL PHENOTYPES IN CF AIRWAYS

Bacteria sense their environment and may change their phenotype accordingly. A pathogenic important phenotypic switch of *P. aeruginosa* during the course of chronic infection is the conversion from a non-mucoid strain to a mucoid one. Mucoidy is maintained *in vitro* under strict anaerobic growth conditions in the presence of nitrate [94] and triggered by an anaerobic environment [59] which could develop because bacteria, entrapped in the viscous, immotile mucus, consume all available oxygen. In addition, oxygen is consumed by respiratory epithelial cells from CF patients to a higher extent than by respective cells from normal individuals [95], contributing to microaerophilic growth conditions on the CF respiratory epithelium [59]. Impaired migration of neutrophils in the viscous mucus [68] may enlarge the time span for successful biofilm formation. There is evidence that the biofilm mode of growth protects bacterial cells from killing by phagocytic cells and that the matrix acts as a diffusion barrier to positively charged antibiotics and cationic antimicrobial peptides. Thus, biofilm formation is thought to be an important factor in the pathogenicity of lung disease in CF.

Similar to *P. aeruginosa*, *S. aureus* also adapts to the CF lung environment by forming biofilm-like aggregates [96,97] that differ genotypically and phenotypically significantly from environmental strains and strains from the nasal habitat [98]. Whether *Burkholderia cepacia* complex (BCC) strains form biofilms in CF airways is less clear.

THE HUMORAL IMMUNE RESPONSE: ANTIBODY PRODUCTION AND IMMUNE COMPLEXES

Pseudomonas aeruginosa infection provokes a rapid production of specific antibodies directed to a large number of *P. aeruginosa* antigens in CF patients [99–101]. Antibody titers may differ markedly from patient to patient. These differences most probably relate to regulatory immune response mechanisms, resulting in different ratios of Th1 to Th2 cells which determine antibody levels. Elevated antibody titers against *S. aureus* antigens in CF sera have not been described, suggesting that *S. aureus* has developed successful strategies for avoiding the immunological attack. Thus, until now, no certain correlation has been established between antistaphylococcal antibody titres and the severity of pulmonary disease. In many patients prolonged antibody production induces increased titers of immune complexes, detectable in patients' sputa, bronchial secretions or serum samples [102]. Immune complexes are thought to play an important role in the immunopathology of CF, since they can stimulate phagocytes directly or via bound complement components to release lysosomal enzymes, reactive oxygen species and antimicrobial substances which may lead to host tissue damage. In CF, therefore, high immune complex levels (and antibody titers) correlate with poor clinical status of the patients [102] as in other diseases characterized by type III hypersensitivity reactions.

NEUTROPHIL ACTIVATION

Neutrophil proteases and serine proteinase inhibitors

Even in CF patients with mild lung disease, there is ample evidence of ongoing inflammation reflecting local neutrophil activation [10–13]. Neutrophils are chemotactically attracted to the site of infection from the vascular space. Up to 10^8 neutrophils per milliliter of sputum or BAL fluid may be present in *P. aeruginosa* infected airways [103,104]. Once the neutrophil has reached the airways it will not return to the circulation and, during activation or cell death, lysosomal enzymes reach the extracellular space. Mainly the serine proteinase elastase has been detected in BAL or sputum samples of CF patients [105]. A mean value of $100\,\mu g$ of neutrophil elastase per milliliter of sputum supernatant fluid has been measured [105]. Other neutrophil-derived serine proteases such as cathepsin G [105] and proteinase 3 [106] are detectable and display enzymatic activities in CF airway. Due to the local cleavage of endogenous serine proteinase inhibitors, the major part of the immunologically detectable neutrophil elastase is also enzymatically active. However, neutrophil elastase is positively charged and thus may be bound to the DNA sputum matrix derived from decayed neutrophils resulting in its inhibition. The reason why such high levels of active neutrophil elastase are present in the inflamed CF airways is the local inactivation of about 90% of the endogenous α_1-proteinase inhibitor (α_1-PI) [105]. Immunoblots of sputum samples revealed that the majority of the inhibitor was present as low-molecular-mass degradation products [10], and addition

of radiolabeled neutrophil elastase to such samples showed no visible binding of α_1-PI with elastase (Fig. 5.3) [105]. On the other hand, α_1-PI is totally functional in the circulation [105]. Most probably, cleavage of α_1-PI is caused by high concentrations of released neutrophil elastase in the CF airways, although proteases of other yet unknown origin have been proposed in this context.

The other major serine proteinase inhibitor in the upper respiratory tract, secretory leukocyte proteinase inhibitor (SLPI), does not seem to compensate for the inactivation of α_1-PI *in vivo*. On the contrary, immunoblotting revealed that SLPI was also fragmented and inactive. Studies in healthy human individuals revealed that two-thirds of the SPLI recovered from the respiratory epithelium is nonfunctional, and the estimated ratio of functional SLPI to functional α_1-PI was 0.16. Thus, SLPI plays only a minor role in protecting the lower respiratory tract from neutrophil elastase. The same applies to the third important endogenous proteinase inhibitor, α_2-macroglobulin, which does not reach the inflamed airways in sufficient concentrations due to its high molecular mass of 725 000 Da.

Neutrophil elastase plays a major role in the pathophysiology of chronic inflammation in CF by cleaving a variety of substrates [107]. This notion is supported by the detection of elastin split products (desmosines) in CF sera and cleaved immunoglobulins, α_1-PI, cell surface receptors of neutrophil or lymphocyte origin in sputum or BAL fluids. Furthermore, elastase activity and desmosine concentrations correlated with the severity of CF lung disease. Additionally, many in-vitro experiments showed the broad biological effects of neutrophil elastase, including cleavage of fibronectin, transferrin, immune complexes, complement components, proteoglycans and surfactant proteins. Interestingly, there is a large overlap concerning the enzymatic activities of neutrophil and *P. aeruginosa* protease activities. Thus, *P. aeruginosa* may well take advantage of neutrophil proteases in the chronic infection state when its own proteases are neutralized by specific antibodies.

Successful opsonophagocytosis, mediated by alveolar macrophages, is dependent on intact opsonic immunoglobulins which bind to Fc cell receptors on the phagocytes through the Fc part of the immunoglobulin. Neutrophil-mediated phagocytosis is dependent on complement receptors such as CR1 and CR3, the receptors for deposited C3b and C3bi, respectively. Thus, intact antibodies, a functional complement system as well as sufficient receptor expression on the phagocytes are prerequisites for this process. Neutrophil elastase and cathepsin G cleave IgG, IgM and IgG or IgA immune complexes *in vitro*, leaving the antigen-binding site of the immunoglobulins intact. Cleavage occurs in the hinge region of the immunoglobulins and results in degradation of the Fc portion. This suggests that interaction of the truncated immune complex with a phagocytic cell is impaired. Consequently, neutrophil elastase-treated immune complexes were not able to stimulate the oxidative burst of neutrophils *in vitro*. When the Fc portions of immunoglobulins

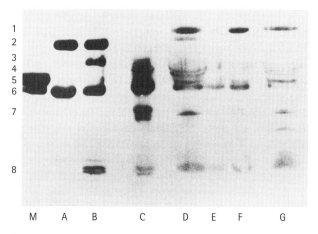

Figure 5.3 Immunoblot of cystic fibrosis sputa with specific antibodies against α_1-PI. M, α_1-PI marker; A, B, incubation of $\alpha_1$1-PI with PMN elastase for 30 min at 37°C; A, excess a1-PI; B, excess PMN elastase; C, sputum sample; D–G, ten-fold concentrated sputum; E, 1:2 diluted sample D. Molecular weights: 1, 90 000; 2, 78 000; 3, 70 000; 4, 66 000; 5, 54 000; 6, 50 000; 7, 42 000–45 000; 8, 25 000–30 000 Da. (Reproduced with permission from [105].)

are proteolytically degraded, also deposition of activated complement components on the CH2 domain is not any more possible. Complement deposition is furthermore directly impaired, since neutrophil elastase cleaves the central complement component of the classic and alternative pathway C3, as well as C5 and C3bi (but not C3b). Finally, the complement receptor for C3b (CR1) on human neutrophils (but not CR3) is cleaved by neutrophil elastase. Since C3b and CR3 are stable to neutrophil elastase and C3bi and CR1 are labile, the expression 'opsonin-receptor mismatch' was coined. Consequently opsonophagocytosis and killing of *P. aeruginosa*, as well as other CF-related pathogens such as *S. aureus*, *H. influenzae* and *S. pneumoniae*, has been shown to be markedly impaired. In summary, neutrophil elastase impairs opsonophagocytosis at the levels of opsonizing immunoglobulins, complement and the complement receptor CR1 on neutrophils.

An important consequence of this scenario is that free neutrophil elastase levels will decrease in the airway lumen, once the neutrophil cannot be stimulated further due to the damage to CR1, C3bi and Fc-Ig. Therefore, neutrophil elastase has been described as a regulatory enzyme in chronic inflammation [107]. It follows that as soon as neutrophil elastase levels are low, neutrophil stimulation will start again, thus creating fluctuating cycles of neutrophil elastase concentrations in chronic inflammatory states (Fig. 5.4). A longitudinal study of neutrophil elastase and immune complexes in CF sputa revealed such a course. Neutrophil serine proteases may have beneficial and deleterious consequences for the host: temporal down regulation of inflammation on the one hand, and allowance of bacterial survival on the other hand. Neutrophil elastase also cleaved receptors on lymphocytes in the CF airways such as CD4 and CD8 but not of CD2 [107].

Another trait of neutrophil elastase and cathepsin G is their ability to stimulate airway gland secretion [108,109]. Mucus hypersecretion may keep bacterial pathogens away from airway epithelial cells and shift them into the airway lumen. It had also been proposed that mucus layers lining the respiratory tract scavenge highly reactive oxygen-derived species [110], providing antioxidant protection to the underlying mucosal epithelial cells. Nevertheless, low levels of MUC5AC have been measured in CF sputum specimens [111], possibly related to non-functional CFTR [112,113].

The findings that neutrophil elastase-mediated airway inflammation is steroid-resistant has practical consequences for the treatment of CF patients with corticosteroids [114]. Induction of IL-8 expression by neutrophil elastase has been demonstrated to involve the toll-like receptor 4 (TLR4) [115]. Finally, neutrophil elastase activates epithelial Na^+ channels and thus increases airway epithelial Na^+ transport [116].

Other proteases

Besides neutrophil-derived serine proteases, other classes of proteases may act in a destructive way in CF lung

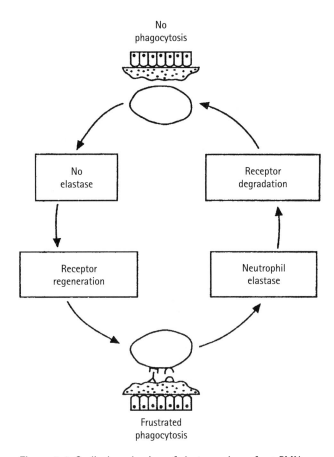

Figure 5.4 Cyclical mechanism of elastase release from PMN following frustrated phagocytosis.

inflammation and infection. However, since various inhibitors of metalloproteases are not able to reduce proteolytic effects in CF sputa or bronchial secretions, damage by at least this class of proteases (which includes both *P. aeruginosa* alkaline protease and elastase, interstitial collagenase, macrophage-derived metalloprotease and metalloproteases from neutrophils has been regarded as less important for the pathophysiology of CF airway disease than serine proteases. Nevertheless enzymatic activity due to neutrophil gelatinase (type IV collagenase) has been detected in CF sputa and lung damage, as assessed by increased type IV collagen degradation products in sputum, was significantly correlated to concentrations of a gelatinase. Cysteine proteases and the mast cell chymase which is also a potent secretagogue for airway gland serous cells have not been studied in CF airway samples.

Oxygen radicals

Neutrophils respond to stimulation with a burst of oxygen consumption – the respiratory burst – and the production of reactive oxygen species such as superoxide anion radical, H_2O_2, hydroxyl radical and possibly singlet oxygen. As with lysosomal proteases, these species are released not only into the phagolysosome but also outside the phagocyte where they may be toxic to the host. There is indirect evidence that toxic oxygen metabolites produced by stimulated neutrophils contribute to lung injury in CF: high sputum concentrations of extracellular myeloperoxidase (MPO), a neutrophil-derived enzyme which transforms H_2O_2 into highly reactive oxygen metabolites, have been detected in CF patients [105], and lung function has been inversely correlated with MPO levels. Glutathione deficiency may also contribute to an increased burden of reactive oxygen species in CF airways and there is evidence that mutated CFTR leads to reduced glutathione efflux. In addition, increased lipid peroxidation, reduced free-radical-trapping capacity, altered plasma antioxidant status, the oxidized DNA compound 8-hydroxydeoxy-guanosine and chloramines have been reported to occur in CF patients. Blood neutrophils from CF patients have been shown to release significantly higher amounts of MPO than healthy individuals, suggesting that these cells have been primed during the course of the infection. When H_2O_2 concentrations were measured in breath condensates of CF patients, no significant differences were noticed between CF patients and normal individuals.

This may be explained by a functional defect of neutrophils. As mentioned before, neutrophils generate much less superoxide anion radical in the presence of neutrophil elastase and activation of adherent neutrophils leads to a markedly attenuated release of superoxide anion per cell when neutrophils are activated at high density in comparison with cells activated at low cell density. Another explanation is the absence of oxygen in sputum plugs which would inhibit any oxidative burst of neutrophils and other inflammatory cells [59] and the presence of high concentrations of catalase (CAT), an enzyme which detoxifies H_2O_2 to oxygen and water, in CF sputum samples [117].

CYTOKINES

The inflammatory system in general communicates by a large repertoire of chemical messengers called cytokines. Elevated cytokine levels have been detected in CF patients. Many bacterial factors as well as host factors stimulate the release of ILs. The transcription factor NFκB plays a crucial role in the regulation of inflammation. NFκB is found in the cytoplasm where it is associated with an inhibitory protein known as IκB. Phosphorylation of IκB leads to accumulation of NFκB which activates gene transcription. Whereas some (but not all) studies show elevated cytokine concentrations in CF sera, BAL samples from CF patients infected with *P. aeruginosa* contain higher pro-inflammatory cytokine levels than healthy controls. These include tumor necrosis factor α (TNFα), IL-1, IL-6 and IL-8. Interestingly, sinus disease in CF patients differs with regard to inflammatory cell and cytokine profiles from that seen in other patients with chronic sinusitis. Particularly, higher numbers of neutrophils, macrophages and cells expressing messenger RNA for interferon γ and IL-8, as well as higher numbers of eosinophils and cells expressing messenger RNA for IL-4,

IL-5 and IL-10 were present in CF patients compared to other patients with chronic sinusitis or healthy controls.

If the inflammatory system is chronically activated, high cytokine levels may lead to deleterious consequences for the host. For example, TNFα may cause cachexia [118] and osteoporosis [119]. IL-8, the most important chemotactic attractant for neutrophils, may lead to a self-perpetuating inflammatory process.

NITRIC OXIDE

Nitric oxide (NO) originates from the biotransformation of L-arginine to L-citrulline by NO synthases (NOS). At least three isoforms of NOS exist of which the inducible NOS (NOS-2) is responsible for the large increase in NO production upon stimulation. The bronchial epithelilium expresses all three isoforms. NOS-2 appears to be responsible for the NO production measured in exhaled air. Also eosinophils and alveolar macrophages are sources of NO. Nitric oxide acts as a bronchodilator, affects immune responses and activates CFTR in cloned T cells by a cGMP-dependent mechanism. Other experiments have shown that cytokine-induced NO release in cell cultures is CFTR-dependent. Additionally, other chloride channels seem to be regulated by NO.

In CF patients, NO production is decreased, and low NO is found in exhaled air of CF patients. Also the airway epithelium from CF mice has been shown to have reduced expression of NOS-2. Low nitric oxide concentrations are thought to be a consequence of decreased NOS-2 expression in CF airways, which has been demonstrated in CF mice and human airways. Lowered NOS-2 expression has been found early in infancy, suggesting that low NOS-2 is related to the basic defect. Other explanations concern the availability of arginine, the substrate of NOS, in CF airways. High arginase activity has been detected in CF airways [120] which would impair NO production by NOS. Furthermore, NOS-2 expression is down-regulated by low arginine and downstream products of the arginase pathway such as spermine inhibit NOS expression and consequently NO production. Low NO in *P. aeruginosa*-infected airways of CF patients may allow bacterial proliferation since mucoid *P. aeruginosa* strains carrying the *MUC A* mutation have been shown to be sensitive to nitrite-dependent killing [121]. It may also compromise airways relaxation in CF, and may contribute to the bronchial obstruction. NO deficiency may serve as a therapeutic target and studies are currently under way to assess whether supplementation with L-arginine or NO donors can have a beneficial effect on CF lung disease.

IMMUNOLOGICAL STRATEGIES FOR PREVENTION OF INFECTION

Patients with CF may escape normal programs due to frequent hospital admissions and school absenteeism and may be more at risk to get 'vaccine-controlled' diseases at any age [122]. To avoid this situation, CF patients should follow national immunization programs without delay to obtain optimal vaccination coverage including viral vaccines against hepatitis A and B, varicella, influenza and pneumococci [122].

Furthermore, antibacterial vaccinations are necessary for prevention of lung infections. The historical development of vaccination against *P. aeruginosa* in CF and in other patients has been reviewed [123]. The first study of active immunization used an LPS vaccine and was carried out in patients already infected with *P. aeruginosa* [124]. Most patients in this study, therefore, already had high antibody titers to *P. aeruginosa* which were increased by the immunization. However, *P. aeruginosa* was not eliminated from the airways and the patients even deteriorated clinically. Two possible explanations are, first, that the increased antibody titers resulted in increased immune complex formation with the triggering of further inflammatory reactions; and second, that the known adverse reactions to the vaccine, which led to febrile responses in 20–40% of the patients, non-specifically worsened lung inflammation.

Improvements in the LPS vaccine preparation [125] led to a study in 28 CF patients who were not colonized with *P. aeruginosa* [126]. In this prospective study, the vaccine stimulated specific antibody production. However, neither the acquisition of *P. aeruginosa* nor the course of the disease differed from a non-vaccinated control group. Possibly, the vaccine did not protect against all different serotypes of *P. aeruginosa*. On the contrary, the clinical status of the vaccine group was lower than that of the control group for several years before both groups became indistinguishable. In several studies, a polysaccharide–exotoxin A conjugate vaccine was developed and revealed promising results in CF patients [127–132]. A phase III trial in approximately 500 CF patients in Europe is currently being carried out which will finally reveal whether this vaccine effectively prevents chronic *P. aeruginosa* lung infection in CF patients. Besides the polysaccharide–exotoxin A conjugate vaccine, a bivalent *P. aeruginosa* flagella vaccine has been tested in CF patients [133–136], but results from a phase III trial have not yet been published.

Experimental vaccines against *S. aureus* infections [137–139] have not been tested in CF patients. Although a very efficient *H. influenzae* type B vaccine has been developed [140], it will not be helpful in CF patients, since this pathogen does not produce a capsule in the airways.

SUMMARY

Much of the lung pathology in CF arises from an immune response chronically activated by micro-organisms which persist in the inherently abnormal CF airways. The reasons for initial bacterial infection of the lungs are complex and are thought to be consequences of an abnormal electrolyte transport in respiratory epithelial cells. Defective CFTR may affect various aspects of innate immunity, such as mucociliary clearance, oxygen levels in mucus layers, antimicrobial substances, the composition of epithelial cell membranes and phagocytic cell functions. There are only a few major bacterial pathogens infecting the lungs of many CF patients. Adaptation to the unique environment in the airways of CF patients leads to highly persisting phenotypes. Host inflammation is thought to be mainly responsible for the deterioration of lung function during chronic infection. Vaccines may be useful to reduce of prevent lung infections.

REFERENCES

1. Shapira E, Wilson GB (eds) *Immunological Aspects of Cystic Fibrosis.* Boca Raton, CRC Press, 1984.
2. Berger M. Inflammation in the lung in cystic fibrosis: a vicious cycle that does more harm than good? In: Moss RB (ed.) *Cystic Fibrosis: Infection, Immunopathology and Host Response.* New Jersey, Humana Press Clifton, 1990, pp119–142.
3. Döring G, Dauner H-M. Clearance of *Pseudomonas aeruginosa* in different rat lung infection models. *Am Rev Respir Dis* 1988; **138**:1249–1253.
4. Walker RI, Willemze R. Neutrophil kinetics and the regulation of granulopoiesis. *Rev Infect Dis* 1980; **2**:282–292.
5. Savill JS, Wyllie AH, Henson JE *et al.* Macrophage phagocytosis of aging neutrophils in inflammation: programmed cell death in the neutrophil leads to its recognition by macrophages. *J Clin Invest* 1989; **83**:865–875.
6. Boucher RC, Stutts MJ, Knowles MR *et al.* Na$^+$ transport in cystic fibrosis respiratory epithelia: abnormal basal rate and response to adenylate cyclase activation. *J Clin Invest* 1986; **78**:1245–1252.
7. Jayaraman S, Joo NS, Reitz B, Wine JJ, Verkman AS. Submucosal gland secretions in airways from cystic fibrosis patients have normal [Na$^+$] and pH but elevated viscosity. *Proc Natl Acad Sci USA* 2001; **98**:8119–8123.
8. Hubeau C, Puchelle E, Gaillard D. Distinct pattern of immune cell population in the lung of human fetuses with cystic fibrosis. *J Allergy Clin Immunol* 2001; **108**:524–549.
9. Lloyd-Still JD. Pulmonary manifestations, In: Lloyd-Still JD (ed.) *Textbook of Cystic Fibrosis.* Boston, John Wright, 1983, pp165–198.
10. Abman SH, Ogle JW, Harbeck RJ *et al.* Early bacteriologic, immunologic, and clinical courses of young infants with cystic fibrosis identified by neonatal screening. *J Pediatr* 1991; **119**:211–217.
11. Khan TZ, Wagener JS, Bost T *et al.* Early pulmonary inflammation in infants with cystic fibrosis. *Am J Respir Crit Care Med* 1995; 151:1075–1082.
12. Birrer P, McElvaney NG, Rudeberg A *et al.* Protease–antiprotease imbalance in the lungs of children with cystic fibrosis. *Am J Respir Crit Care Med* 1994; **150**:207–213.

13. Konstan MW, Hilliard KA, Norvel TM, Berger M. Bronchoalveolar lavage findings in cystic fibrosis patients with stable, clinically mild lung disease suggest ongoing infection and inflammation. *Am J Respir Crit Care Med* 1994; **150**:448–454.

14. Woods DE, Strauss DC, Johanson WGJr, Bass JA. The role of fibronectin in the prevention of adherence of *Pseudomonas aeruginosa* to buccal cells. *J Infect Dis* 1981; **143**:784–790.

15. Suter S, Schaad UB, Morgenthaler JJ *et al*. Fibronectin-cleaving activity in bronchial secretions of patients with cystic fibrosis. *J Infect Dis* 1988; **158**:89–100.

16. Niederman MS, Merrill WW, Polomski LM *et al*. Influence of sputum IgA and elastase on tracheal cell bacterial adherence. *Am Rev Respir Dis* 1986; **133**:255–260.

17. Plotkowski MC, Beck G, Tournier JM *et al*. Adherence of *Pseudomonas aeruginosa* to respiratory epithelium and the effect of leucocyte elastase. *J Med Microbiol* 1989; **30**:285–293.

18. Greene CM, Carroll TP, Smith SG *et al*. TLR-induced inflammation in cystic fibrosis and non-cystic fibrosis airway epithelial cells. *J Immunol* 2005; **174**:1638–1646.

19 Weber AJ, Soong G, Bryan R *et al*. Activation of NF-kappaB in airway epithelial cells is dependent on CFTR trafficking and Cl⁻ channel function. *Am J Physiol Lung Cell Mol Physiol* 2001; **281**:L71–L78.

20. Joseph T, Look D, Ferkol T. NF-kappaB activation and sustained IL-8 gene expression in primary cultures of cystic fibrosis airway epithelial cells stimulated with *Pseudomonas aeruginosa*. *Am J Physiol* 2005; **288**:L471–L479.

21. Zahm JM, Gaillard D, Dupuit F *et al*. Early alterations in airway mucociliary clearance and inflammation of the lamina propria in CF mice. *Am J Physiol* 1997; **272**:C853–C859.

22. Tirouvanziam R, de Bentzmann S, Hubeau C *et al*. Inflammation and infection in naive human cystic fibrosis airway grafts. *Am J Respir Cell Mol Biol* 2000; **23**:121–127.

23. Tirouvanziam R, Khazaal I, Peault B. Primary inflammation in human cystic fibrosis small airways. *Am J Physiol* 2002; **283**:L445–L451.

24. Hubeau C, Lorenzato M, Couetil JP *et al*. Quantitative analysis of inflammatory cells infiltrating the cystic fibrosis airway mucosa. *Clin Exp Immunol* 2001; **124**:69–76.

25. Du M, Jones JR, Lanier J *et al*. Aminoglycoside suppression of a premature stop mutation in a CFTR−/−mouse carrying a human CFTR-G542X transgene. *J Mol Med* 2002; **80**:595–604.

26. Durie PR, Kent G, Phillips MJ *et al*. Characteristic multiorgan pathology of cystic fibrosis in a long-living cystic fibrosis transmembrane regulator knockout murine model. *Am J Pathol* 2004; **164**:1481–1493.

27. Mall M, Grubb BR, Harkema JR *et al*. Increased airway epithelial Na⁺ absorption produces cystic fibrosis-like lung disease in mice. *Nat Med* 2004; **10**:487–493.

28. Bonfield TL, Panuska JR, Konstan MW *et al*. Inflammatory cytokines in cystic fibrosis lungs. *Am J Respir Crit Care Med* 1995; **152**:2111–2118.

29. Bonfield TL, Konstan MW, Burfeind P *et al*. Normal bronchial epithelial cells constitutively produce the anti–inflammatory cytokine interleukin-10, which is downregulated in cystic fibrosis. *Am J Respir Cell Mol Biol* 1995; **13**:257–261.

30. Chmiel JF, Konstan MW, Knesebeck JE *et al*. IL-10 attenuates excessive inflammation in chronic *Pseudomonas* infection in mice. *Am J Respir Crit Care Med* 1999; **160**:2040–2047.

31. Soltys J, Bonfield TL, Chmiel JF, Berger M. Functional IL-10 deficiency in the lung of cystic fibrosis (CFTR(−/−)) and IL-10 knockout mice causes increased expression and function of B7 costimulatory molecules on alveolar macrophages. *J Immunol* 2002; **168**:1903–1910.

32. Saadane A, Soltys J, Berger M. Role of IL-10 deficiency in excessive nuclear factor-kappaB activation and lung inflammation in cystic fibrosis transmembrane conductance regulator knockout mice. *J Allergy Clin Immunol* 2005; **115**:405–411.

33. Coleman FT, Mueschenborn S, Meluleni G *et al*. Hypersusceptibility of cystic fibrosis mice to chronic *Pseudomonas aeruginosa* oropharyngeal colonization and lung infection. *Proc Soc Natl Acad Sci USA* 2003; **100**:1949–1954.

34. Davidson DJ, Dorin JR, McLachlan G *et al*. Lung disease in the cystic fibrosis mouse exposed to bacterial pathogens. *Nat Genet* 1995; **9**:351–357.

35. Van Heeckeren AM, Tscheikuna J, Walenga RW *et al*. Effect of Pseudomonas infection on weight loss, lung mechanics, and cytokines in mice. *Am J Respir Crit Care Med* 2000; **161**:271–279.

36. Aldallal N, McNaughton EE, Manzel LJ *et al*. Inflammatory response in airway epithelial cells isolated from patients with cystic fibrosis. *Am J Respir Crit Care Med* 2002; **166**: 1248–1256.

37. Noah TL, Black HR, Cheng PW *et al*. Nasal and bronchoalveolar lavage fluid cytokines in early cystic fibrosis. *J Infect Dis* 1997; **175**: 638–647.

38. Muhlebach MS, Reed W, Noah TL. Quantitative cytokine gene expression in CF airway. *Pediatr Pulmonol* 2004; **37**:393–399.

39. Meyer KC, Sharma A, Rosenthal NS *et al*. Regional variability of lung inflammation in cystic fibrosis. *Am J Respir Crit Care Med* 1997; **156**:1536–1540.

40. Armstrong DS, Grimwood K, Carlin JB *et al*. Lower airway inflammation in infants and young children with cystic fibrosis. *Am J Respir Crit Care Med* 1997; **156**:1197–1204.

41. Armstrong DS, Hook SM, Jamsen KM *et al*. Lower airway inflammation in infants with cystic fibrosis detected by newborn screening. *Pediatr Pulmonol* 2005; **40**:500–510.

42. Frates RC, Kaizu TT, Last JA. Mucus glycoproteins secreted by respiratory epithelial tissue from cystic fibrosis patients. *Pediatr Res* 1983; **17**:30–34.

43. Cheng P-W, Boat TF, Cranfill K *et al*. Increased sulfatation of glycoconjugates by cultured nasal epithel cells from patients with cystic fibrosis. *J Clin Invest* 1989; **84**:68–72.

44. Lamblin G, Aubert JP, Perini JM *et al*. Human respiratory mucins. *Eur Respir J* 1992; **5**:247–256.

45. Zhang Y, Doranz B, Yankaskas JR, Engelhardt JF. Genotypic analysis of respiratory mucous sulfation defects in cystic fibrosis. *J Clin Invest* 1995; **96**:2997–3004.

46. Schwab UE, Thiel H-J, Steuhl K-P, Döring G. Binding of *Staphylococcus aureus* to fibronectin and glycolipids on corneal surfaces. *German J Ophthalmol* 1997; **5**:417–421.

47. Liang OD, Ascencio F, Franksson L-A, Wadström T. Binding of heparan sulfate to *Staphylococcus aureus*. *Infect Immun* 1992; **60**:899–906.

48. Barasch J, Kiss B, Prince A *et al.* Defective acidification of intracellular organelles in cystic fibrosis. *Nature* 1991; **352**:70–73.

49. Krivan HC, Roberts DD, Ginsburg V. Many pulmonary pathogenic bacteria bind specifically to the carbohydrate sequence Gal NAcβ1-4Gal found in some glycolipids. *Proc Natl Acad Sci USA* 1988; **85**:6157–6161.

50. Imundo L, Barasch J, Prince A, Al-Awqati Q. Cystic fibrosis epithelial cells have a receptor for pathogenic bacteria on their apical surface. *Proc Natl Acad Sci USA* 1995; **92**:3019–3023.

51. de Bentzmann S, Roger P, Dupuit F *et al.* Asialo GM1 is a receptor for *Pseudomonas aeruginosa* adherence to regenerating respiratory epithelial cells. *Infect Immun* 1996; **64**:1582–1588.

52. Seksek O, Biwersi J, Verkman AS. Evidence against defective trans-Golgi acidification in cystic fibrosis. *J Biol Chem* 1996; **271**:15542–15548.

53. Poschet JF, Boucher JC, Tatterson L *et al.* Molecular basis for defective glycosylation and Pseudomonas pathogenesis in cystic fibrosis lung. *Proc Natl Acad Sci USA* 2001; **98**:13972–13977.

54. Schwab UE, Wold AE, Carson JL *et al.* Increased adherence of *Staphylococcus aureus* from cystic fibrosis lungs to airway epithelial cells. *Am Rev Respir Dis* 1993; **148**:365–369.

55. Ulrich M, Herbert S, Berger J *et al.* Localization of *Staphylococcus aureus* in infected airways of patients with cystic fibrosis and in a cell culture model of *S. aureus* adherence. *Am J Respir Crit Care Med* 1998; **18**:1–9.

56. Plotkowski MC, Chevillard M, Pierrot D *et al.* Epithelial respiratory cells from cystic fibrosis patients do not possess specific *Pseudomonas aeruginosa*-adhesive properties. *J Med Microbiol* 1992; **36**:104–111.

57. Schroeder TH, Zaidi T, Pier GB. Lack of adherence of clinical isolates of *Pseudomonas aeruginosa* to asialo-GM(1) on epithelial cells. *Infect Immun* 2001; **69**:719–729.

58. Leir SH, Parry S, Palmai-Pallag T *et al.* Mucin glycosylation and sulphation in airway epithelial cells is not influenced by cystic fibrosis transmembrane conductance regulator expression. *Am J Respir Cell Mol Biol* 2005; **32**:453–461.

59. Worlitzsch D, Tarran R, Ulrich M *et al.* Effects of reduced mucus oxygen concentration in airway *Pseudomonas* infections of cystic fibrosis patients. *J Clin Invest* 2002; **109**:317–325.

60. Sajjan SU, Corey M, Karmali MA, Forstner JF. Binding of *Pseudomonas cepacia* to normal human intestinal mucin and respiratory mucin from patients with cystic fibrosis. *J Clin Invest* 1992; **89**:648–656.

61. Kubiet M, Ramphal R. Adhesion of nontypeable *Haemophilus influenzae* from blood and sputum to human tracheobronchial mucins and lactoferrin. *Infect Immun* 1995; **63**:899–902.

62. Boucher RC. New concepts of the pathogensis of cystic fibrosis lung disease. *Eur Respir J* 2004; **23**:146–158.

63. Matsui H, Grubb BR, Tarran R *et al.* Evidence for periciliary liquid layer depletion, not abnormal ion composition, in the pathogenesis of cystic fibrosis airways disease. *Cell* 1998; **95**:1005–1015.

64. Joo NS, Lee DJ, Winges KM *et al.* Regulation of antiprotease and antimicrobial protein secretion by airway submucosal gland serous cells. *J Biol Chem* 2004; **279**:38854–38860.

65. Matsui H, Verghese MW, Kesimer M *et al.* Reduced three-dimensional motility in dehydrated airway mucus prevents neutrophil capture and killing bacteria on airway epithelial surfaces. *J Immunol* 2005; **175**:1090–1099.

66. Moraes TJ, Plumb J, Martin R *et al.* Abnormalities in the pulmonary innate immune system in cystic fibrosis. *Am J Respir Cell Mol Biol* 2006; **34**:364–374.

67. Robinson M, Bye PT. Mucociliary clearance in cystic fibrosis. *Pediatr Pulmonol* 2002; **33**:293–306.

68. Tarran R, Button B, Picher M *et al.* Normal and cystic fibrosis airway surface liquid homeostasis. The effects of phasic shear stress and viral infections. *J Biol Chem* 2005; **280**:35751–35759.

69. Donaldson SH, Bennett WD, Zeman KL *et al.* Mucus clearance and lung function in cystic fibrosis with hypertonic saline. *N Engl J Med* 2006; **354**:241–250.

70. Pier GB, Grout M, Zaidi TS *et al.* Role of mutant CFTR in hypersusceptibility of cystic fibrosis patients to lung infections. *Science* 1996; **271**:64–67.

71. Pier GB. *CFTR* mutations and host susceptibility to *Pseudomonas aeruginosa* lung infection. *Curr Opin Microbiol* 2002; **5**:81–86.

72. Pier GB, Grout M, Zaidi TS. Cystic fibrosis transmembrane conductance regulator is an epithelial cell receptor for clearance of *Pseudomonas aeruginosa* from the lung. *Proc Natl Acad Sci USA* 1997; **94**:12088–12093.

73. Kowalski MP, Pier GB. Localization of cystic fibrosis transmembrane conductance regulator to lipid rafts of epithelial cells is required for *Pseudomonas aeruginosa*-induced cellular activation. *J Immunol* 2004; **172**:418–425.

74. Grassmé H, Jendrossek V, Riehle A *et al.* Host defense against *Pseudomonas aeruginosa* requires ceramide-rich membrane rafts. *Nat Med* 2003; **9**:322–330.

75. Schroeder TH, Lee MM, Yacono PW *et al.* CFTR is a pattern recognition molecule that extracts *Pseudomonas aeruginosa* LPS from the outer membrane into epithelial cells and activates NF-kappa B translocation. *Proc Natl Acad Sci USA* 2002; **99**:6907–6912.

76. Zaas DW, Duncan MJ, Li G *et al.* Pseudomonas invasion of type I pneumocytes is dependent on the expression and phosphorylation of caveolin-2. *J Biol Chem* 2005; **280**:4864–4872.

77. Darling KE, Dewar A, Evans TJ. Role of the cystic fibrosis transmembrane conductance regulator in internalization of *Pseudomonas aeruginosa* by polarized respiratory epithelial cells. *Cell Microbiol* 2004; **6**:521–533.

78. Burns JL, Jonas M, Chi EY *et al.* Invasion of respiratory epithelial cells by *Burkholderia* (*Pseudomonas*) *cepacia*. *Infect Immun* 1996; **64**:4054–4059.

79. Smith JJ, Travis SM, Greenberg EP, Welsh MJ. Cystic fibrosis airway epithelia fail to kill bacteria because of abnormal airway surface fluid. *Cell* 1996; **85**:229–236.

80. Joris L, Dab I, Quinton PM. Elemental composition of human airway surface fluid in healthy and diseased airways. *Am Rev Respir Dis* 1993; **148**:1633–1637.

81. Gilljam H, Ellin A, Strandvik B. Increased bronchial chloride concentration in cystic fibrosis. *Scand J Clin Lab Invest* 1993; **49**:121–124.

82. Cray PB, Bentley L. Human airway epithelia express a beta-defensin. *Am J Respir Cell Mol Biol* 1997; **16**:343–349.

83. Goldman MJ, Anderson GM, Stolzenberg ED *et al.* Human beta-defensin-1 is a salt-sensitive antibiotic in lung that is inactivated in cystic fibrosis. *Cell* 1997; **88**:553–560.

84. Smith JJ, Travis, SM, Greenberg EP, Welsh MJ. Erratum. *Cell* 1996; **87**:335.

85. Tarran R, Grubb BR, Parsons D *et al.* The CF salt controversy: in-vivo observations and therapeutic approaches. *Mol Cell* 2001; **8**:149–158.

86. Knowles MR, Robinson JM, Wood RE *et al.* Ion composition of airway surface liquid of patients with cystic fibrosis as compared to normal and disease-control subjects. *J Clin Invest* 1997; **100**:2588–2595.

87. Jayaraman S, Song Y, Vetrivel L *et al.* Noninvasive in-vivo fluorescence measurement of airway surface liquid depth, salt concentration, and pH. *J Clin Invest* 2001; **107**:317–324.

88. Hull J, Skinner W, Robertson C, Phelan P. Elemental content of airway surface liquid from infants with cystic fibrosis. *Am J Respir Crit Care Med* 1998; **157**:10–14.

89. Grubb BR, Chadburn JL, Boucher RC. In-vivo microdialysis for the determination of airway surface liquid ion composition. *Am J Physiol* 2002; **282**:C1423–C1431.

90. Berger M. Complement deficiency and neutrophil dysfunction as risk factors for bacterial infection in newborns and the role of granulocyte transfusion in therapy. *Rev Infect Dis* 1990; **12**:S401–S409.

91. Abughali N, Berger M, Tosi MF. Deficient total cell content of CR3 (CD11b) in neonatal neutrophils. *Blood* 1994; **83**:1086–1012.

92. Martin TR, Rubens CE, Wilson CB. Lung antibacterial defense mechanisms in infant and adult rats: implications for the pathogenesis of group B streptococcal infections in the neonatal lung. *J Infect Dis* 1998; **157**:91–100.

93. Sordelli DO, Djafari M, Garcia VE *et al.* Age-dependent pulmonary clearance of *Pseudomonas aeruginosa* in a mouse model: diminished migration of polymorphonuclear leukocytes to *N*-formyl-methionly-leucyl-phenylalanine. *Infect Immun* 1992; **60**:1724–1727.

94. Hassett DJ. Anaerobic production of alginate by *Pseudomonas aeruginosa*: alginate restricts diffusion of oxygen. *J Bacteriol* 1996; **178**:7322–7325.

95. Stutts MJ, Knowles MR, Gatzy JT, Boucher RC. Oxygen consumption and ouabain binding sites in cystic fibrosis nasal epithelium. *Pediatr Res* 1986; **20**:1316–1320.

96. McKenney D, Pouliot KL, Wang Y *et al.* Broadly protective vaccine for *Staphylococcus aureus* based on an in-vivo-expressed antigen. *Science* 1999; **284**:1523–1527.

97. Cramton SE, Ulrich M, Götz F, Döring G. Anaerobic conditions induce expression of the polysaccharide intercellular adhesin in *Staphylococcus aureus* and *Staphylococcus epidermidis*. *Infect Immun* 2001; **69**:4079–4085.

98. Goerke C, Wolz C. Regulatory and genomic plasticity of *Staphylococcus aureus* during persistent colonization and infection. *Int J Med Microbiol* 2004; **294**:195–202.

99. Döring G, Høiby N. Longitudinal study of immune response to *Pseudomonas aeruginosa* antigens in cystic fibrosis. *Infect Immun* 1983; **42**:197–201.

100. West SE, Zeng L, Lee BL *et al.* Respiratory infections with *Pseudomonas aeruginosa* in children with cystic fibrosis: early detection by serology and assessment of risk factors. *J Am Med Assoc* 2002; **287**:2958–2967.

101. Kappler M, Kraxner A, Reinhardt D *et al.* Diagnsotic and prognostic values of antibodies against *Pseudomonas aeruginosa* in cystic fibrosis. *Thorax* 2006; **61**:684–688.

102. Høiby N, Döring G, Schiøtz PO. The role of immune complexes in the pathogenesis of bacterial infections. *Ann Rev Microbiol* 1986; **40**:29–53.

103. Tournier JM, Jacquot J, Puchelle E, Bieth JG. Evidence that *Pseudomonas aeruginosa* elastase does not inactivate the bronchial inhibitor in the presence of leukocyte elastase. *Am Rev Respir Dis* 1985; **132**:524–528.

104. Bruce MC, Poncz L, Klinger JD *et al.* Biochemical and pathological evidence for proteolytic destruction of lung connective tissue in cystic fibrosis. *Am Rev Respir Dis* 1985; **132**:529–535.

105. Goldstein W, Döring G. Lysosomal enzymes and proteinase inhibitors in the sputum of patients with cystic fibrosis. *Am Rev Respir Dis* 1986; **134**:49–56.

106. Witko-Sarsat V, Halbwachs-Mecarelli L, Schuster A *et al.* Proteinase 3, a potent secretagogue in airways, is present in cystic fibrosis sputum. *Am J Respir Cell Mol Biol* 1999; **20**:729–736.

107. Döring G. The role of neutrophil elastase in chronic inflammation. *Am J Respir Crit Care Med* 1994; **150**:S114–S117.

108. Park JA, He F, Martin LD *et al.* Human neutrophil elastase induces hypersecretion of mucin from well-differentiated human bronchial epithelial cells *in vitro* via a protein kinase C{delta}-mediated mechanism. *Am J Pathol* 2005; **167**:651–661.

109. Voynow JA, Fischer BM, Malarkey DE *et al.* Neutrophil elastase induces mucus cell metaplasia in mouse lung. *Am J Physiol* 2004; **287**:L1293–L1302.

110. Cross CE, Halliwell B, Allen A. Antioxidant protection: a function of tracheobronchial and gastrointestinal mucus. *Lancet* 1984; **1**:1328–1330.

111. Henke MO, Renner A, Huber RM *et al.* MUC5AC and MUC5B mucins are decreased in cystic fibrosis airway secretions. *Am J Respir Cell Mol Biol* 2004; **31**:86–91.

112. Gray T, Coakley R, Hirsh A *et al.* Regulation of MUC5AC mucin secretion and airway surface liquid metabolism by IL-1beta in human bronchial epithelia. *Am J Physiol* 2004; **286**:L320–L330.

113. Montserrat C, Merten M, Figarella C. Defective ATP-dependent mucin secretion by cystic fibrosis pancreatic epithelial cells. *FEBS Lett* 1996; **393**:264–268.

114. Birrell MA, Wong S, Hele DJ *et al.* Steroid-resistant inflammation in a rat model of chronic obstructive pulmonary disease is associated with a lack of nuclear factor-kappaB pathway activation. *Am J Respir Crit Care Med* 2005; **172**:74–84.

115. Devaney JM, Greene CM, Taggart CC *et al.* Neutrophil elastase up-regulates interleukin-8 via toll-like receptor 4. *FEBS Lett* 2003; **544**:129–132.

116. Caldwell RA, Boucher RC, Stutts MJ. Neutrophil elastase activates near-silent epithelial Na$^+$ channels and increases airway epithelial Na$^+$ transport. *Am J Physiol* 2005; **288**:L813–L819.

117. Worlitzsch D, Herberth G, Ulrich M, Döring G. Catalase, myeloperoxidase and hydrogen peroxide in cystic fibrosis. *Eur Respir J* 1998; **11**: 377–383.

118. Moldawer LL, Lowry SF. Cachectin: its impact on metabolism and nutritional status. *Ann Rev Nutr* 1988; **8**: 585–609.

119. Teramoto S, Matsuse T, Ouchi Y. Increased production of TNF-alpha may play a role in osteoporosis in cystic fibrosis patients. *Chest* 1997; **112**:574.

120. Grasemann H, Schwiertz R, Matthiesen S *et al.* Increased arginase activity in cystic fibrosis airways. *Am J Respir Crit Care Med* 2005; **172**:1523–1528.

121. Yoon SS, Coakley R, Lau GW *et al.* Anaerobic killing of mucoid *Pseudomonas aeruginosa* by acidified nitrite derivatives under cystic fibrosis airway conditions. *J Clin Invest* 2006; **116**:436–446.

122. Malfroot A, Adam G, Ciofu O *et al.* Immunisation in the current management of cystic fibrosis patients. *J Cystic Fibrosis* 2005; **4**:77–87.

123. Cryz SJ. *Pseudomonas aeruginosa* vaccines. In: Cryz SJ (ed.) *Vaccines and Immunotherapy.* New York, Pergamon Press, 1991, pp156–165.

124. Pennington JE, Reynolds HY, Wood RE *et al.* Use of a *Pseudomonas aeruginosa* vaccine in patients with acute leukemia and cystic fibrosis. *Am J Med* 1975; **58**:629–636.

125. Miller JA, Spilsbury JF, Jones RJ *et al.* A new polyvalent *Pseudomonas aeruginosa* vaccine. *J Med Microbiol* 1977; **10**:19–27.

126. Langford DT, Hiller J. Prospective, controlled study of a polyvalent *Pseudomonas* vaccine in cystic fibrosis: three-year results. *Arch Dis Child* 1984; **59**:1131–1133.

127. Cryz SJ, Fürer E, Cross AS *et al.* Safety and immunogenicity of a *Pseudomonas aeruginosa* O-polysaccharide-toxin A conjugate vaccine in humans. *J Clin Invest* 1987; **80**:51–56.

128. Schaad UB, Lang AB, Wedgewood J *et al.* Safety and immunogenicity of *Pseudomonas aeruginosa* conjugate vaccine in cystic fibrosis. *Lancet* 1991; **338**:1236–1237.

129. Lang AB, Schaad UB, Rudeberg A *et al.* Effect of high-affinity anti-*Pseudomonas aeruginosa* lipopolysaccharide antibodies induced by immunization on the rate of *Pseudomonas aeruginosa* infection in patients with cystic fibrosis. *J Pediatr* 1995; **127**:711–717.

130. Lang AB, Horn MP, Imboden MA, Zuercher AW. Prophylaxis and therapy of *Pseudomonas aeruginosa* infection in cystic fibrosis and immunocompromised patients. *Vaccine* 2004; **22**(Suppl 1):S44–S48.

131. Lang AB, Rudeberg A, Schoni MH *et al.* Vaccination of cystic fibrosis patients against *Pseudomonas aeruginosa* reduces the proportion of patients infected and delays time to infection. *Pediatr Infect Dis J* 2004; **23**:504–510.

132. Zuercher AW, Imboden MA, Jampen S *et al.* Cellular immunity in healthy volunteers treated with an octavalent conjugate *Pseudomonas aeruginosa* vaccine. *Clin Exp Immunol* 2005; **142**:381–387.

133. Rotering H, Dorner F. Studies on a *Pseudomonas aeruginosa* flagella vaccine. *Antibiot Chemother* 1989; **42**:218–228.

134. Crowe BA, Enzensberger O, Schober-Bendixen S *et al.* The first clinical trial of Immuno's experimental *Pseudomonas aeruginosa* flagellar vaccines. *Antibiot Chemother* 1991; **44**:143–156.

135. Döring G, Pfeiffer C, Weber U *et al.* Parenteral application of a *Pseudomonas aeruginosa* flagella vaccine elicits specific anti-flagella antibodies in the airways of healthy individuals. *Am J Respir Crit Care Med* 1995; **151**:983–985.

136. Döring G, Dorner F. A multicenter vaccine trial using the *Pseudomonas aeruginosa* flagella vaccine IMMUNO in patients with cystic fibrosis. *Behring Inst Mitt* 1997; **98**:338–344.

137. Fournier J-M. *Staphyloccus aureus.* In: Cryz SJ (ed.) *Vaccines and Immunotherapy.* New York, Pergamon Press, 1991, 166–177.

138. Maira-Litran T, Kropec A, Goldmann DA, Pier GB. Comparative opsonic and protective activities of *Staphylococcus aureus* conjugate vaccines containing native or deacetylated staphylococcal poly-*N*-acetyl-beta-(1-6)-glucosamine. *Infect Immun* 2005; **73**:6752–6762.

139. Fattom A, Fuller S, Propst M *et al.* Safety and immunogenicity of a booster dose of *Staphylococcus aureus* types 5 and 8 capsular polysaccharide conjugate vaccine (StaphVAX) in hemodialysis patients. *Vaccine* 2004; **23**:656–663.

140. Sood SK, Daum RS. Haemophilus influenzae type B conjugate vaccine. In: Cryz SJ (ed.) *Vaccines and Immunotherapy.* New York, Pergamon Press, 1991, 36–58.

Genotype–phenotype correlations and modifier genes

JANE C. DAVIES

INTRODUCTION

The clinical spectrum of cystic fibrosis (CF) is highly variable, ranging from the classical 'severe' picture with pancreatic insufficiency and early lung involvement through to patients with much milder forms, some of whom appear to have single-organ disease or present much later in life. The correlation of *CFTR* gene mutation and phenotype in CF is relatively high in the pancreas and gastrointestinal tract but much lower in the lung, where other modifier genes and/or the environment are thought also to play a role. A small number of *CFTR* mutations have been identified which appear to confer a milder phenotype with pancreatic sufficiency (PS) and, in some cases, well-preserved lung function into later life. In general, these mild genes appear to dominate the more classical *CFTR* mutations, rendering patients who are compound heterozygotes for one mutation in each severity group, relatively mild. Additionally, increasing numbers of mutations outside the exons (coding region) are being described in association with partial disease phenotypes – for example, congenital bilateral absence of the vas deferens (CBAVD), a common cause of male infertility. Based in part on evidence from these studies, it is becoming clear that different organs may require different levels of CFTR function to achieve normal function; the vas deferens is exquisitely sensitive to partial loss of function, the lungs less so, and probably most resistant, is the pancreas.

CFTR MUTATIONS AND DISEASE SEVERITY

CFTR mutations, of which more than 1000 have now been described, fall into five classes based on their effect on protein structure and/or function [1]. Class I mutations are those from which, due to a premature stop mutation, no

full-length *CFTR* protein results. Class II mutations, of which by far the commonest is *F508del*, lead to protein misfolding and premature degradation with failure of the protein to reach the apical cell membrane. Classes III, IV and V mutations are those in which protein reaches the cell membrane, but fails to respond normally to stimulation or is present at abnormally low levels. In addition to the large number of mutations, around 130 genetic polymorphisms have been identified in the *CFTR* gene. These polymorphisms are variations in the gene sequence, which differ from mutations because they are also frequently (>1%) found in the general population. However, it has been well established that certain polymorphisms alter the amount of functional CF gene product. The best-studied example is the thymidine polymorphism in intron 8 of the CF gene [2]. This polymorphism exists as a 5-, 7- or 9-thymidine (T) variant. The 5T variant significantly reduces the amount of normal *CFTR* transcript, because intron 8 is incorrectly spliced, which leads to mRNA lacking exon 9.

Pancreatic function has been shown to correlate moderately well with *CFTR* mutation, classes I and II commonly being associated with pancreatic insufficiency, whereas classes IV and V are more likely to be found in patients with well-preserved pancreatic function [3]. However, correlations with lung disease are less clear. Patients with identical *CFTR* mutations, even siblings [4,5], can vary widely in severity of respiratory involvement. Individual, so-called 'mild' mutations have been described in small groups of patients, including *A455E* [6] and *R117H* [7], and these are thought often to be dominant to a more severe mutation in heterozygotes. However, in general, for an individual patient, it is difficult to predict respiratory prognosis on the basis of genotype. An extensive study based on the US database has recently reported lower lung function and decreased survival in patients possessing two class II mutations compared with those carrying at least one mutation of classes IV or V [8].

NON–CFTR GENES THAT MODIFY THE DISEASE PHENOTYPE (MODIFIER GENES)

The lack of correlation described above was, in part, responsible for the search for factors independent of CFTR which may influence disease severity, including both genetic and environmental influences (see Chapter 6b). Environmental influences are not further discussed here, although it must be remembered that there may be interactions between the environment (including therapies) and genetic makeup, as has been demonstrated in other diseases, for example the impact of polymorphisms in *glutathione S-transferase* on response to tobacco exposure [9].

THE BASIS OF GENETIC POLYMORPHISMS

The DNA sequence of any two unrelated individuals is approximately 99.9% identical. The remaining 0.1% contains variations (polymorphisms). If these affect either protein structure or function, they have the potential to influence the likelihood or severity of disease. The term 'polymorphism' refers either to single-base nucleotide substitutions (also known as single nucleotide polymorphisms or SNPs), deletion–insertion polymorphisms (DIPs), and repeat variations (short tandem repeats or STRs). In contrast to mutations, which occur at low frequencies (less than 1%) in the general population, polymorphisms are common genetic variants, occurring more frequently. Recently, SNPs have received most attention, mainly due to the development of high throughput analysis [10]. In 2002, the international HapMap project (www.HapMap.org) was founded, which aims to generate a SNP haplotype map of the human genome within 3 years. A similar project is being carried out in different strains of mice (www.jax.org).

SPECIFIC CF MODIFIER GENES

Evidence for CF modifier genes was first obtained in CF knockout mice, where the severity of intestinal disease depended on the presence of a particular genetic locus on mouse chromosome 7 [11]. More recently, an association between meconium ileus and a region of chromosome 19 has been demonstrated in humans [12]. However, in neither case has the exact gene(s) or protein product(s) been identified.

Genes involved in inflammation, antiproteases and antioxidants

Given the importance of inflammation in CF lung disease, this is a logical area of exploration. Tumour necrosis factor (TNF)-α, a cytokine found in high concentrations within the CF airway, is thought to be pivotal in the promotion of the neutrophil-dominated inflammatory response and has been inversely correlated with lung function [13]. In a small study, Hull and co-workers [14] found that a polymorphism in the promoter region of the TNF-α gene associated with high protein levels was linked to reduced FEV_1 and poor nutritional status. However, in a larger study including both adults and children, Arkwright and co-workers [15] found no such association, and in 269 adult patients we too found no link with any marker of severity [16]. In the CF airway, chronic inflammation results in an excess of destructive proteases such as neutrophil elastase. These overwhelm their inhibitors, the antiproteases, of which alpha$_1$-antitrypsin (α_1-AT) is one of the most abundant. Patients with inherited forms of α_1-AT deficiency are at risk of emphysema [17], and so it was postulated that CF patients with co-existing α_1-AT deficiency would demonstrate a more severe pulmonary phenotype. Studies examining effects on severity have reached conflicting conclusions: increased *Pseudomonas aeruginosa* infection without an adverse effect on pulmonary function [18]; a beneficial effect on lung function [19] (which was also observed for the related gene, α_1-antichymotrypsin [20]); and most recently, in the largest group, no effect on lung function, age at acquisition of *P. aeruginosa*, requirement for transplantation or death [21]. The glutathione S-transferase (GST) M1 allele, an enzyme involved in oxidative stress, has been reported to be linked to more severe chest radiograph and Schwachman score in homozygous children [14]. Polymorphisms leading to high levels of the profibrotic cytokine, tissue growth factor (TGF)-β, have previously been associated with increased pulmonary fibrosis after chemotherapy and radiotherapy and organ transplantation. Arkwright and co-workers [22] found that, in a cohort of 261 CF patients (children and adults), subjects with at least one high-expressing TGF-β haplotype had a significantly faster rate of decline in both FEV_1 and FVC than those with low-expressing variants. Subsequently, in one of the largest studies to date, Drumm and co-workers [23] studied 16 polymorphisms in over 800 patients; only TGF-β was found to be significant.

Host defense mechanisms and antigen presentation

The human leukocyte antigen (HLA) region is the most polymorphic in the human genome, encoding hundreds of genes including the major histocompatibility complexes (MHCs). MHC class II molecules are critical in antigen presentation and the ensuing inflammatory response. Two reports have linked certain polymorphisms with complications in CF: an association between DR7, high IgE levels and risk of *P. aeruginosa* infection [24] and between allergic bronchopulmonary aspergillosis (ABPA) and the DR2 allele [25]. Mannose-binding lectin (MBL), a liver-derived serum protein, exerts its innate defence effects both by direct opsonization of pathogens and by activation of complement [26]. Low levels of MBL have been shown to relate to a variety of infective processes including recurrent respiratory infections, and so the *MBL-2* gene was considered a likely candidate as a modifier in the CF lung. In the first study to examine such a link, Garred and co-workers [27] reported that both FEV$_1$ and FVC were significantly lower in subjects with either one or two structural *MBL-2* mutations, but only following chronic *P. aeruginosa* infection. Although numbers were small, the authors also reported an increased risk of infection with *Burkholderia cepacia*. In contrast, a second study found a significant reduction in lung function only in patients possessing two variant alleles [28]. In support of this, Buranawati and co-workers [29] have reported a significant survival disadvantage in American CF patients with two mutations. As part of a large study in almost 600 patients, we have recently found that adult patients possessing two structural mutations, but not heterozygotes, have significantly impaired lung function, oxygen saturations and raised inflammatory markers [30]. In contrast to the data from Garred *et al.* [27], this was not seen in our pediatric age group, in whom the majority had well-preserved lung function. This difference highlights an important point. Treatment regimens have evolved greatly over the last few years and, for example, a polymorphism that was significant in the era before the widespread use of anti-pseudomonal antibiotics may be less relevant now. Thus, in some cases comparisons with historical data might be flawed.

The antimicrobial effects of nitric oxide (NO) are being increasingly recognized. High numbers of the AAT trinucleotide repeat sequence in the *NOS-1* gene are associated with low levels of exhaled NO, and were found in CF patients to confer an increased risk of infection with both *P. aeruginosa* and *Aspergillus fumigatus*; interestingly, though, this did not lead to a more rapid decline in lung function [31]. This group has also recently related a polymorphism in the *NOS-3* gene with risk of infection [32]. This gene, expressed in vascular endothelium, respiratory epithelium and neutrophils, contains a functionally important polymorphism (894G/T), which affects the resistance of NOS-3 to proteolysis. Previous work has highlighted gender differences, by demonstrating that circulating estrogen increases the levels of NOS-3 in the vascular endothelium [33]. Grasemann and co-workers [34] reported higher exhaled NO levels and decreased frequency of *P. aeruginosa* infection in association with the 894T polymorphism in females only.

What is not clear from these two related studies is whether *NOS-1* and *NOS-3* are independent modifiers, or whether there is a confounding effect of one upon the other [35]. Further, in a letter on this subject, Mekus and Tummler [36] suggest that these genes may merely be 'hitch-hiking' with another gene of relevance, rather then being directly involved in disease modification themselves.

Airway function

Polymorphisms in the β-adrenergic receptor (β-AR) have been related to severity of asthma and response to treatment with β$_2$-agonist drugs [37]. Beta-AR are important regulators of cAMP in the airway, recent in-vitro data demonstrating that ion transport via protein kinase-regulated CFTR can be activated by β$_2$-agonists [38]. Buscher and co-workers [39] studied the effects of three polymorphisms in the β-AR in 87 young adults and children with CF. Subjects with either one or two copies of Gly16, an amino acid change leading to down-regulation of the receptor, had significantly reduced lung function and faster rates of decline than those patients homozygous for Arg16, an effect that was even more marked in the Δ*F508* homozygote patients. There were no differences in bronchodilator responsiveness, but in an in-vitro assay, lymphocytes from these subjects showed a blunted cAMP response to isoproterenol stimulation, suggesting that the clinical findings may relate to differences in level of CFTR function between the two groups. In contrast, Hart and co-workers [40] reported an effect of such polymorphisms on airway hyper-responsiveness, but this did not appear to relate to decline in lung function over a 5-year time period.

MODIFIER GENES FOR INTESTINAL AND LIVER DISEASE

Between 10% and 15% of CF patients are born with meconium ileus (MI). As mentioned above, a putative gene locus has been identified on human chromosome 19, and recently this locus has also been linked to liver disease [41]. Familial clustering of portal hypertension suggests that liver disease in CF may be under genetic influence, although few associations have been found with *CFTR* genotype. One of the major problems with studies of liver disease is that of phenotypic definition, which differs widely in clinical practice. Duthie and co-workers [42] performed a large multicenter study on 274 unrelated children and adults examining the effect of HLA status. Almost 30% of patients had evidence of chronic liver disease, a higher proportion than reported from most centers. DQ6 was found in 66% of patients with liver disease, but in only 33% of those without. Two other antigens in strong linkage disequilibrium with this locus, DR15 and B7, were also significant risk factors. When portal hypertension was used as a marker of chronicity, these markers were found to be significant for males only, but there was no association with age of onset. MBL deficiency was shown by one group to be a risk factor for the development of CF liver disease [43], although we could not replicate this in our study [44]. Arkwright and co-workers [45,46] have reported associations between liver disease and both high-expressing TGF-β haplotypes and ACE [46] (an enzyme involved in TGF-β activation) polymorphisms. Finally, Mekus and co-workers [47] identified loci in a partially imprinted region 3′ of *CFTR* as modifiers of both nutritional and pulmonary phenotype in 34 highly concordant or discordant sib pairs. This region includes both the leptin gene and a candidate for Russell-Silver dwarf syndrome, and is thus likely involved in growth, food intake and energy expenditure.

IMPORTANT ISSUES IN STUDY DESIGN

A large number of studies has been conducted to assess the contribution of selected candidate genes, although only a few highly significant modifiers have been described and in certain cases, subsequent studies in a second cohort reach conflicting conclusions. This may reflect several problems with study design [48]:

- heterogeneous patient populations studied or inadequately characterized phenotypes;
- small study size leading to underpowering;
- changes in clinical treatment over time precluding comparison of contemporary and historical cohorts;
- the likelihood that, rather than single modifier genes, combinations of genes may be important;
- the relative contributions of modifier genes being very small and variability in CF lung disease being mainly due to environmental factors, which are, in themselves difficult to quantify accurately.

Recent studies have begun to try and address at least some of these issues, with larger numbers and replication in a second, independent cohort.

We have progressed exponentially, within just over a decade, from no publications at all on the area, through to several hundred, many of which appear to contradict each other. With this experience comes, hopefully, recognition of the significant pitfalls, and methodological ways around them. Although it is hoped that such studies could broaden our understanding of disease pathogenesis in CF, and possibly lead to the rational design of novel therapeutic agents, there exists the very real possibility that other, non-genetic factors, such as the environment and treatments adhered to, have such a strong effect that the relatively modest effect of many modifier genes goes undetected.

REFERENCES

1. Lim M, Zeitlin PL. Therapeutic strategies to correct malfunction of CFTR. *Paediatr Respir Rev* 2001; **2**:159–164.

2. Noone PG, Pue CA, Zhou Z *et al*. Lung disease associated with the IVS8 5T allele of the CFTR gene. *Am J Respir Crit Care Med* 2000; **162**:1919–1924.

3. Kristidis P, Bozon D, Corey M *et al*. Genetic determination of exocrine pancreatic function in cystic fibrosis. *Am J Hum Genet* 1992; **50**:1178–1184.

4. Picard E, Aviram M, Yahav Y *et al*. Familial concordance of phenotype and microbial variation among siblings with CF. *Pediatr Pulmonol* 2004; **38**:292–297.

5. Castaldo G, Tomaiuolo R, Vanacore B *et al*. Phenotypic discordance in three siblings affected by atypical cystic fibrosis with the F508del/D614G genotype. *J Cyst Fibros* 2006; **5**(3):193–195.

6. Gan KH, Veeze HJ, van den Ouweland AM *et al*. A cystic fibrosis mutation associated with mild lung disease. *N Engl J Med* 1995; **333**:95–99.

7. Sheppard DN, Rich DP, Ostedgaard LS *et al*. Mutations in CFTR associated with mild-disease-form Cl⁻ channels with altered pore properties. *Nature* 1993; **362**(6416):160–164.

8. McKone EF, Emerson SS, Edwards KL, Aitken ML. Effect of genotype on phenotype and mortality in cystic fibrosis: a retrospective cohort study. *Lancet* 2003; **361**:1671–1676.

9. Gilliland FD, Li YF, Dubeau L *et al*. Effects of glutathione S-transferase M1, maternal smoking during pregnancy, and environmental tobacco smoke on asthma and wheezing in children. *Am J Respir Crit Care Med* 2002; **166**: 457–463.

10. Chen X, Sullivan PF. Single nucleotide polymorphism genotyping: biochemistry, protocol, cost and throughput. *Pharmacogenomics J* 2003; **3**(2):77–96.

11. Rozmahel R, Wilschanski M, Matin A *et al*. Modulation of disease severity in cystic fibrosis transmembrane conductance regulator deficient mice by a secondary genetic factor. *Nat Genet* 1996; **12**:280–287.

12. Zielenski J, Corey M, Rozmahel R *et al*. Detection of a cystic fibrosis modifier locus for meconium ileus on human chromosome 19q13. *Nat Genet* 1999; **22**:128–129.

13. Greally P, Hussein MJ, Cook AJ *et al*. Sputum tumour necrosis factor-alpha and leukotriene concentrations in cystic fibrosis. *Arch Dis Child* 1993; **68**:389–392.

14. Hull J, Thomson AH. Contribution of genetic factors other than CFTR to disease severity in cystic fibrosis. *Thorax* 1998; **53**:1018–1021.

15. Arkwright PD, Pravica V, Geraghty PJ *et al*. End-organ dysfunction in cystic fibrosis: association with angiotensin I converting enzyme and cytokine gene polymorphisms. *Am J Respir Crit Care Med* 2003; **167**:384–389.

16. Low T, Lympany PA, Davies JC *et al*. The effect of polymorphism in inflammatory mediators on clinical phenotype in CF. *Pediatr Pulmonol* 2003; Suppl **25**:219.

17. Mahadeva R, Stewart S, Bilton D, Lomas DA. Alpha-1 antitrypsin deficiency alleles and severe cystic fibrosis lung disease. *Thorax* 1998; **53**:1022–1024.

18. Doering G, Krogh-Johansen H, Weidinger S, Hoiby N. Allotypes of alpha 1-antitrypsin in patients with cystic fibrosis, homozygous and heterozygous for deltaF508. *Pediatr Pulmonol* 1994; **18**:3–7.

19. Mahadeva R, Westerbeek RC, Perry DJ *et al*. Alpha₁-antitrypsin deficiency alleles and the Taq-I G −>A allele in cystic fibrosis lung disease. *Eur Respir J* 1998; **11**:873–879.

20. Mahadeva R, Sharples L, Ross-Russell RI *et al*. Association of alpha(1)-antichymotrypsin deficiency with milder lung disease in patients with cystic fibrosis. *Thorax* 2001; **56**:53–58.

21. Frangolias DD, Ruan J, Wilcox PJ *et al*. Alpha 1-antitrypsin deficiency alleles in cystic fibrosis lung disease. *Am J Respir Cell Mol Biol* 2003; **29**(3 Pt 1):390–396.

22. Arkwright PD, Laurie S, Super M *et al.* TGF-beta(1) genotype and accelerated decline in lung function of patients with cystic fibrosis. *Thorax* 2000; **55**:459–462.

23. Drumm ML, Konstan MW, Schluchter MD *et al.* for the Gene Modifier Study Group. Genetic modifiers of lung disease in cystic fibrosis. *N Engl J Med* 2005; **353**:1443–1453.

24. Aron Y, Polla BS, Bienvenu T *et al.* HLA class II polymorphism in cystic fibrosis: a possible modifier of pulmonary phenotype. *Am J Respir Crit Care Med* 1999; **159**(5 Pt 1):1464–1468.

25. Aron Y, Bienvenu T, Hubert D *et al.* HLA-DR polymorphism in allergic bronchopulmonary aspergillosis. *J Allergy Clin Immunol* 1999; **104**(4 Pt 1):891–892.

26. Turner MW. The role of mannose-binding lectin in health and disease. *Mol Immunol* 2003; **40**:423–429.

27. Garred P, Pressler T, Madsen HO *et al.* Association of mannose-binding lectin gene heterogeneity with severity of lung disease and survival in cystic fibrosis. *J Clin Invest* 1999; **104**:431–437.

28. Gabolde M, Guilloud-Bataille M, Feingold J, Besmond C. Association of variant alleles of mannose binding lectin with severity of pulmonary disease in cystic fibrosis: cohort study. *Br Med J* 1999; **319**:1166–1167.

29. Buranawuti K, Boyle MP, Cheng S *et al.* Variants in mannose binding lectin and tumor-necrosis factor (alpha) affect survival in cystic fibrosis. *J Med Genet* 2006; Dec 11; [E-pub ahead of print].

30. Davies JC, Turner MW, Klein N for the London MBL CF Study Group. Impaired pulmonary status in cystic fibrosis adults with two mutated MBL-2 alleles. *Eur Respir J* 2004; **24**:798–804.

31. Grasemann H, Knauer N, Buscher R *et al.* Airway nitric oxide levels in cystic fibrosis patients are related to a polymorphism in the neuronal nitric oxide synthase gene. *Am J Respir Crit Care Med* 2000; **162**:2172–2176.

32. Grasemann H, van's Gravesande KS, Buscher R *et al.* Endothelial nitric oxide synthase variants in cystic fibrosis lung disease. *Am J Respir Crit Care Med* 2003; **167**:390–394.

33. Forstermann U, Boissel JP, Kleinert H. Expressional control of the 'constitutive' isoforms of nitric oxide synthase (NOS I and NOS III). *FASEB J* 1998; **12**:773–790.

34. Grasemann H, van's Gravesande KS, Buscher R *et al.* Endothelial nitric oxide synthase variants in cystic fibrosis lung disease. *Am J Respir Crit Care Med* 2003; **167**:390–394.

35. Accurso FJ, Sontag MK. Seeking modifier genes in cystic fibrosis. *Am J Respir Crit Care Med* 2003; **167**:289–290.

36. Mekus F, Tummler B. Cystic fibrosis and NOS3. *Am J Respir Crit Care Med* 2004; **169**:319–320.

37. Ramsay CE, Hayden CM, Tiller KJ *et al.* Polymorphisms in the beta2-adrenoreceptor gene are associated with decreased airway responsiveness. *Clin Exp Allergy* 1999; **29**:1195–1203.

38. Taouil K, Hinnrasky J, Hologne C *et al.* Stimulation of beta 2-adrenergic receptor increases cystic fibrosis transmembrane conductance regulator expression in human airway epithelial cells through a cAMP/protein kinase A-independent pathway. *J Biol Chem* 2003; **278**(19):17320–17327.

39. Buscher R, Eilmes KJ, Grasemann H *et al.* Beta2 adrenoceptor gene polymorphisms in cystic fibrosis lung disease. *Pharmacogenetics* 2002; **12**:347–353.

40. Hart MA, Konstan MW, Darrah RJ *et al.* Beta 2 adrenergic receptor polymorphisms in cystic fibrosis. *Pediatr Pulmonol* 2005; **39**:544–550.

41. Deering R, Algire M, McWilliams R *et al.* Meconium ileus and liver disease: an analysis of the CF twin and sibling study. *Pediatr Pulmonol* 2004; Suppl 27:224.

42. Duthie A, Doherty DG, Donaldson PT *et al.* The major histocompatibility complex influences the development of chronic liver disease in male children and young adults with cystic fibrosis. *J Hepatol* 1995; **23**:532–537.

43. Gabolde M, Hubert D, Guilloud-Bataille M *et al.* The mannose binding lectin gene influences the severity of chronic liver disease in cystic fibrosis. *J Med Genet* 2001; **38**:310–311.

44. Davies J, Johnson MM, Booth C *et al.* Age-specific effect of the cystic fibrosis modifier gene, MBL-2. *Pediatr Pulmonol* 2002; Suppl 23:223.

45. Arkwright PD, Laurie S, Super M *et al.* TGF-beta(1) genotype and accelerated decline in lung function of patients with cystic fibrosis. *Thorax* 2000; **55**:459–462.

46. Arkwright PD, Pravica V, Geraghty PJ *et al.* End-organ dysfunction in cystic fibrosis: association with angiotensin I converting enzyme and cytokine gene polymorphisms. *Am J Respir Crit Care Med* 2003; **167**:384–389.

47. Mekus F, Laabs U, Veeze H, Tummler B. Genes in the vicinity of CFTR modulate the cystic fibrosis phenotype in highly concordant or discordant F508del homozygous sib pairs. *Hum Genet* 2003; **112**:1–11.

48. Davies JC, Griesenbach U, Alton E. Modifier genes in cystic fibrosis. *Pediatr Pulmonol* 2005; **39**:383–391.

Variability of clinical course in cystic fibrosis

MICHAEL S. SCHECHTER

INTRODUCTION

Refinements in the treatment of cystic fibrosis (CF) have resulted in a dramatic preservation of lung function and prolongation of life in the current generation of people with CF compared to previous experience. At the same time it has also accentuated the degree of variability in the severity and progression of CF lung disease, as reflected in the distribution of age at diagnosis, age-related pulmonary function, and age at death [49] (Fig. 6.1).

A number of factors have been hypothesized or proven to influence disease severity and outcome, and these can be grouped into three major categories:

- genetic, which includes all biological factors intrinsic to the individual patient;
- environmental, which includes exposures that are secondary to socioeconomic and demographic factors;
- healthcare-related, which includes prescribed medical interventions and patient adherence to these recommendations (Fig. 6.2).

There are of course important interactions between these factors. Genetic explanations for variability in disease progression have been discussed in Chapter 6a, so here we will focus on non-genetic aspects.

ENVIRONMENTAL AND SOCIODEMOGRAPHIC CAUSES OF VARIABILITY OF CF OUTCOMES

Socioeconomic status as a marker of risk for adverse exposures

In the general population, health is worse and mortality is greater in groups with low socioeconomic status (SES) [50]. Pulmonary function is decreased in healthy Canadian schoolchildren with low SES scores compared to their higher SES peers [51]. Asthma, the most common cause of chronic respiratory illness in childhood, is more prevalent in low-SES groups, and indigent patients experience greater morbidity [52] and higher mortality [53].

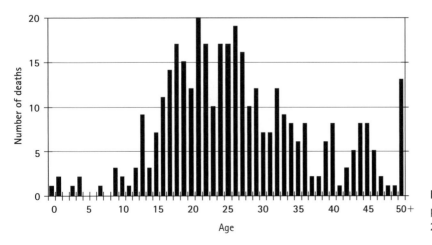

Figure 6.1 Age at death (years) of 364 CF patients reported to the US CF Registry in 2003.

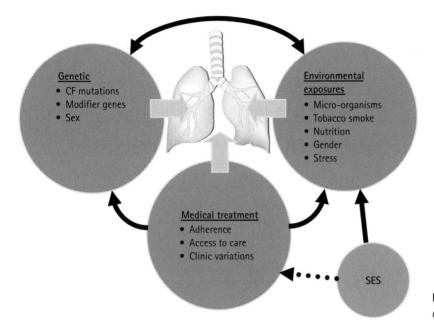

Figure 6.2   Influence/s on severity of CF lung disease. SES, socioeconomic status.

Several studies from the British Commonwealth were the first to document that sociodemographic factors influence CF prognosis. An analysis of all CF deaths over a 17-year period in England and Wales published in 1989 found that the odds of surviving beyond the median age of death varied by region of residence and were 2.75 times greater if the parental occupation was categorized as non-manual rather than manual [54]. A study of patients followed at the Belfast Hospital for Sick Children found that maternal age less than 19 years and single parenthood were associated with higher morbidity and greater likelihood of hospitalization. In South Africa, acquisition of *Pseudomonas aeruginosa* (PA) was reported to occur earlier in mixed-race children, and mortality in that group was higher than for European children [55].

Two publications by this author addressed the issue of SES and CF outcomes in the United States. An initial cross-sectional study at a single CF center using Medicaid* status as a proxy for low SES [56] was confirmed by a longitudinal analysis [57] of the US CF Foundation Patient Registry. Using registry data that spanned the years 1986 to 1994, we classified patients based on baseline Medicaid status, thereby establishing temporal sequence. By doing this and by including only pediatric patients we were able to reduce the likelihood that severity of illness was a cause rather than effect of poverty. The risk of Medicaid patients dying during the study period, adjusted for gender, race, pancreatic enzyme use and age, was 3.65 times higher than that of the non-Medicaid patients. Furthermore, the adjusted FEV_1 of surviving Medicaid patients was lower by 9.2% predicted compared to non-Medicaid patients. The difference between the groups was present at 6 years, the earliest age of recorded measurement, and was slightly age-dependent, increasing by 0.54% per year of age. In addition, Medicaid patients were 2.3 times more likely to be below the 5th percentile for height and weight. Similar results were found if SES was categorized as Medicaid status at diagnosis or by using median family income of the postal code of residence.

Two subsequent publications by O'Connor and co-workers confirmed and extended these findings. Linking US Census data with CF Registry data over the years 1982 to 1998, they found that patients living in postal codes with a median household income above US $50 000/year had a risk of death during that period that was 60% that of patients living in areas with a median household income below US $20 000/year [58]. Furthermore, they demonstrated a step-wise relationship between their five income categories and mortality, pulmonary function and nutrition, emphasizing that the relationship between outcomes and SES is an incremental rather than a dichotomous one that affects only the indigent [59].

The ideal measure of SES is unclear, as different aspects may impact upon health in different ways (e.g. family income impacts on financial resources; and maternal education affects disease self-management abilities [60]). The reason why low-SES patients suffer more severe consequences of CF is unclear, but a plausible starting point is to assume that poverty is associated with a clustering of detrimental environmental influences, health behaviors, and/or difficulties accessing optimal healthcare [61]. It follows that an understanding of the specific causes of SES-related disparities can provide important clues regarding the effects of adverse exposures for all patients with CF, independent of

---

*Medicaid is a US health insurance program for the indigent that is mandated by the Federal government but administered by individual states. Eligibility criteria vary by age and by state and may take healthcare-related spending into consideration. In 2004, 48% of children and 35% of adults with CF in the United States were eligible for Medicaid or state health insurance.

SES. The remainder of this discussion will draw upon general literature but point out where an association with SES is either proven or hypothesized to be present in CF.

Exposure to environmental tobacco smoke and other pollutants

It is clear from the general medical literature that environmental tobacco smoke (ETS) exposure exerts an effect on airway function prenatally as well as postnatally in children [62,63] and in adults [64]. The association of ETS exposure with poor lung function and growth in children with CF was initially reported in 1990 among attendees of a summer camp [65]. A dose-dependent relationship between reported ETS exposure and lung function, nutrition and rate of hospitalization was found, and those children who had been exposed to ETS at home gained significantly more weight during the two weeks of camp than did the children from smoke-free homes. The dose-dependent association of ETS exposure with lung function, nutritional status and number of hospitalizations has been confirmed in several subsequent publications [66–69], although the precise mechanism of this effect has not been investigated.

The importance of ETS exposure as an adverse influence on children with CF must be emphasized because of its pervasiveness. Thirty-five percent of children in the United States live in homes where residents or visitors smoke in the home on a regular basis [70]. While the prevalence of ETS exposure among children with CF is unknown, papers published in the last several years suggest rates comparable to this [65,69]. In 2003, 30% of the children attending 15 US CF centers participating in a quality improvement collaborative had at least one smoking parent (unpublished data). While comparable estimates of ETS exposure do not exist for CF patients in other countries, the overall prevalence of cigarette smoking among adults in the United States is equal to or lower than that for European and Latin American countries.

There is a strong association of smoking with lower SES in the general population [71], and a triangular association among ETS exposure, low SES, and worse lung function and nutrition has been reported from one US CF clinic [72]. ETS exposure is probably a significant contributor to health disparities among low-SES patients with CF.

Exposure to air pollution compromises lung growth in children [73] and leads to increased mortality in adults [74]. In a CF registry study investigating air pollution exposure by postal code of residence, exposure to ozone was associated with an increase in the number of pulmonary exacerbations, and exposure to particulates was associated with both an increased likelihood of pulmonary exacerbations and a decrease in FEV_1. This study adjusted for the possible confounding effect of SES, which is important because low-SES populations tend to live in areas with greater environmental pollution [75]. The authors of this study did not try to estimate to what extent air pollution

exposure might contribute to SES-related differences in disease outcome, but their study suggests that pollution is another contributor to SES-related disparities.

Exposure to and acquisition of infectious agents

There is an increasing consensus that acquisition of *Pseudomonas aeruginosa* (PA) in the CF airway leads to a more rapid deterioration in pulmonary function and nutrition [76], especially once the PA takes on mucoid characteristics [77]. The likelihood of acquisition is increased by a number of factors, including female sex [78], preceding use of anti-staphylococcal prophylaxis with cephalosporins [79,80], exposure to other CF patients with PA [81], nebulizer use [82], recent hospitalization and treatment with IV antibiotics [83], and (in infants) recent hospitalization for viral respiratory infection [84]. The impact of SES on acquisition of PA has not been well-investigated, but in a cohort of children diagnosed by newborn screening high maternal education was found to be protective [82].

The other important bacterial organism whose acquisition is associated with pulmonary deterioration and excessive mortality is *Burkholderia cepacia* (BC). Methodological issues related to surveillance and culture technique, and the recent recognition that the clinical consequence and relative contagiousness of the organisms comprising the BC complex vary by genovar [85], make it difficult to pinpoint the prognostic implication of acquisition of the organism. Nonetheless, BC acquisition has consistently been reported to lead to a more severe decline in pulmonary function [86]. It is also clear that the likelihood of acquisition is greatly increased by exposure to other patients with the organism; epidemic spread occurs but can be attenuated by infection control measures [86].

Respiratory viral infections may be associated with progression of CF airway disease, although this association is only well documented for the short term [87]. While respiratory syncytial virus gets significant attention due to the ease of its identification, it appears likely that all respiratory viruses are of equal virulence in this regard; what may be most important is the presence of lower versus upper tract involvement [87]. CF infants hospitalized with viral lower respiratory tract infections have decreased pulmonary function [87], increased inflammatory indices in BAL fluid, and are more likely to acquire PA over the ensuing 5 years [84].

A relationship of low SES to increased prevalence of respiratory viral infections is suggested but not well documented in the general medical literature, and postulated to be secondary to crowding [88]. A recent study reported lower SES scores in CF infants who sustained lower respiratory tract infections during the respiratory virus season; this difference was not statistically significant but the study was underpowered with regard to this relationship [87].

Stress

Stress appears to have a negative impact on the course of some diseases by impairing immune function [89]. Of greater potential importance for children with CF, however, is that parental experience of stress may lead to impaired personal and family functioning [90], which would have a direct and specific effect on adherence and other aspects of disease self-management.

Conceptual models of parental adjustment to having a child with chronic disease consider both the stress of caring for the child and the psychological and social mediators that affect how that stress is handled. A modified version of one schema [91] is shown in Fig. 6.3. Extrinsic stressors include the daily general irritants of life, and particularly those specific to parenting; those associated with major life events such as job loss or death of a loved one; and disease-specific stresses, which are due to living with the child's chronic illness and are experienced in proportion to the degree of the child's illness. Quittner and co-workers [92] reported that mothers of children with CF describe their most important source of stress as disease-specific, but their study did not consider SES, and others have shown a significant increase in the experience of all extrinsic stressors in low-SES parents [93]. The ability to process stress depends on psychological characteristics (temperament, coping skills, feelings of mastery and control, resilience) and social–ecological variables (family resources and social support) [94]. Most researchers on stress in CF have not specifically included SES in their theoretical models or in their investigations, but it is likely that poverty compromises the ability to process stress by decreasing the relative availability of financial and social resources [95].

Studies by Patterson and co-workers in the early 1990s suggested that stress and family dysfunction lead to decreased adherence and worse disease outcomes [90,96]. Excessive stress in caregivers can lead to depression, dysfunctional behaviors (including drug and alcohol abuse), and physical illness. A significant proportion of mothers of children with CF show depressive symptoms soon after diagnosis of their child, independent of the degree of the child's illness [92]. Many parents continue to report significant psychological distress years afterward [97]. There has been no investigation of a connection between parental stress and depression and the child's long-term outcome in CF, but it is likely that a reciprocal relationship exists; i.e. parental stress, depression, and/or anxiety leads to greater disease severity (due primarily to compromised disease self-management abilities), which in turn causes more disease-specific stress and also leads to a decrease in stress-processing resources in the parents.

Dietary and nutritional deficiencies

About 26% of CF patients in the United States are below the 10th percentile for weight [49]. Nutritional status is highly correlated with pulmonary function in patients with CF, and while the causal relationship is to some extent bidirectional [98], there is strong evidence that nutritional inadequacy is deleterious to long-term preservation of pulmonary function and survival [99]. The mechanism of this relationship is unclear, but it has been suggested that even subtle degrees of malnutrition may impair immunological defenses against infection [100] and that malnutrition may lead to respiratory muscle weakness [101].

Consensus guidelines suggest a high-energy and high-fat diet for patients with CF [102], but the recommended intake is not consumed by a significant proportion of patients [103,104]. In one study of 25 children with CF and mild lung disease, only 16% adhered to dietary recommendations, and dietary adherence was positively correlated with weight. Furthermore, maternal nutritional knowledge specific to CF significantly predicted children's dietary adherence score [104]. This is noteworthy because of the association between maternal nutritional knowledge and maternal educational attainment that was also linked to nutritional status in a report from North Carolina [72]. Aside from inadequate knowledge of and adherence to dietary guidelines, another possible reason for nutritional inadequacy in low-SES patients may be the inability to afford appropriate foods, nutritional supplements or even, in countries without a national health system, pancreatic enzymes (the latter being relevant only in healthcare systems where medication is not available free of charge). A relationship between SES and dietary quality has been shown for the general population [100], but there are no studies on food insecurity in patients with CF and its effect on intake. Another potential mechanism relating low SES and decreased nutritional status is the strong relationship

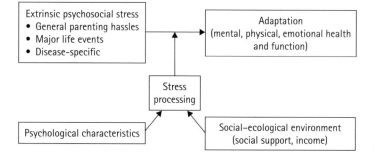

Figure 6.3 Schematic representation of stress processing.

between environmental tobacco smoke exposure and decreased weight that has been shown in CF patients [65].

Sex/gender

Several studies from the United States have shown that females with CF fare worse than males; they acquire PA infection at an earlier age [78], and have worse nutrition and pulmonary function and mortality [58,105]. Rosenfeld and co-workers evaluated US CF Registry data from 1988 to 1992 and demonstrated that the median age at death for women with CF was 3.1 years less than men, adjusted for nutritional status, pulmonary function, airway microbiology, and age at diagnosis [105]. The difference in survival was primarily seen in patients aged 1–20 years, and this gap had persisted despite global improvements in life expectancy for CF patients over 10 years (M. Rosenfeld, personal communication).

The mechanism of the disparity in outcomes between males and females is probably due to a mixture of biological and socioenvironmental effects, but there is little concrete information as to the relative importance of these. For the sake of this discussion, it is useful to distinguish *sex* as a biological category (which then may be considered to be a gene modifier) from *gender*, which is a cultural attribute that determines norms for a variety of attitudes and behaviors that may affect disease outcome. From the biological perspective, a study evaluating interleukin-10 (IL-10) knockout mice found that females were more susceptible to *Pseudomonas aeruginosa* infection than their male counterparts, and mounted a stronger inflammatory response; this is potentially relevant because IL-10 levels are relatively low in bronchoalveolar lavage fluid from CF patients [106]. It should be said that a strong inflammatory response could be beneficial (eliminating organisms) or detrimental (tissue damaging). A recent study reported that adjusted resting energy expenditure (REE) is higher in girls (111 ± 11% predicted) than boys (104 ± 8) with CF, and furthermore, girls with CF had a higher REE compared to control girls (103 ± 8), whereas there was no difference between boys with or without CF [107]. The significance of this finding is unclear [108]: while increased REE might make it harder to maintain an adequate nutritional status and thus predispose to worse overall outcome, the previously mentioned analysis [106] found increased mortality in girls even when controlling for their poorer nutritional status. It should be stated that the raised REE may be a marker that the disease is already worse, rather than a cause of the gender gap.

The concept of 'gendered embodiment' has been proposed to define how social contexts may alter and modify the material biological base [109]. For example, although participation in competitive sports might be beneficial for patients with CF [110], many young women might avoid team activities because they would be embarrassed if these cause them to cough and expectorate in public, an activity that is less deviant (and perhaps even normative) for young men.

Studies on American males and females with CF show systematic differences in attitudes towards the meaning of life, death, career, body image and regimen. Young men with CF are generally more activity oriented and less reflective and concerned about the impact of CF on their future, including career and life expectations [109]. There are also clear differences in body image: women with CF are generally more content with being thin, whereas the men want to be stronger and more muscular [111–113]. These gender-related differences in attitude towards body image are most notable in adolescents and adults, but can be found in younger children as well [114]. Furthermore, these attitudinal differences lead to behavior differences. Men are more aerobically fit [115] and are almost three times more likely than women to exercise regularly [109]. Furthermore, perception of self as underweight is associated with greater use of nutritional supplements [113], and men eat better and more frequently than women [109,113]. A possible explanation for the reported absence of a gender gap at a single CF center in London [116] might be that these cultural attitudes are less pronounced in the UK.

A provocative analysis of the CF Registry performed by investigators at the University of Wisconsin showed that American girls are diagnosed with CF at a significantly later age (12.7 months) than boys (8.7 months); this difference is even more striking when limited to children presenting with respiratory symptoms only (40.7 vs 22.3 months). This is not due to a tendency for boys to develop symptoms earlier than girls, which was verified by independently evaluating patients diagnosed from birth by the Wisconsin newborn screening program. Furthermore, boys in Wisconsin were more likely to be referred for sweat testing than girls. Thus, there appears to be a diagnostic bias against girls that could have significant implications [117].

Race

There is a large literature on the demography of race and the relative contribution of genetic versus cultural determinants of this category; it is debatable whether race should be discussed under a genetic or sociodemographic heading [118]. What literature exists on race in CF suggests that genetic determinants linked to race do not have an effect on CF disease severity. While some *CFTR* mutations (such as $3120 + 1\,G \rightarrow A$) are more common in the African–American population than in whites, a study evaluating racial differences found no difference in mortality or pulmonary dysfunction, but worse nutritional status, in *F508del* homozygotes when adjusted for age and sex [119]. However, this study was flawed by its failure to take SES into account. O'Connor and co-workers found a 48% increase in mortality associated with non-white race and a 85% increase in mortality associated with Hispanic ethnicity when they adjusted for SES as indicated by neighborhood median household income [59], but we found no difference in outcome by race when using Medicaid status as a proxy measure of SES [57]. These contradictory findings highlight the problem of measurement of SES and the difficulty of distinguishing the effect of SES and race often found in the general medical literature [120]. Medicaid status as a marker probably overestimates the effect of SES on disease because sicker patients are more likely to be eligible; neighborhood household income, which is an ecological (and thus imprecise) measure of SES, probably underestimates the effect of SES on disease and thus allows residual confounding to lead to an overestimation of the effect of race.

DIFFERENCES IN THE USE OF MEDICAL TREATMENT AS A CAUSE OF VARIABILITY IN CF OUTCOMES

Improvements in patient outcome over the last five decades demonstrate the overall effectiveness of medical interventions on the outcome of CF. While the relative contribution of individual therapies directed at nutritional rehabilitation airway clearance augmentation, reduction of airway infection and inflammation and detection and treatment of other complications is not clearly documented, it is likely that these are all synergistic. The CF Foundation in the United States the CF Trust in the UK, and their counterparts elsewhere have developed consensus guidelines and fostered a network of CF care centers with expertise in all of these treatment approaches [102,121,122]. The resulting CF international care system helps ensure the general availability and dissemination of medical expertise, promotes a focused research agenda, and maintains a registry of patient outcomes. While not all CF patients choose to attend designated CF care centers, the relative advantage of center-based care can be measured (even though this is made difficult by the presumed tendency for sicker patients to obtain care at accredited centers) [123].

Patient adherence to prescribed medical regimens

The high rate of non-adherence to CF treatment recommendations makes this an important consideration when examining reasons for variations in disease outcome [124]. However, significant difficulties in the accurate measurement of adherence exist, so any conclusions must be drawn with caution [125]. Studies have found that adherence correlates with optimism, disease knowledge [126], some measures of family functioning [90,96], and parental education [127]. Other factors associated with good adherence in CF include younger patient age and decreased parental stress [128]. The previously discussed relationship between stress, family function and disease outcome [90,96,128] is presumably mediated via a relationship to adherence.

Non-adherence may be more common in low-SES patients, although studies have not uniformly demonstrated this [124]. Many of the factors predicting adherence noted in the previous paragraph are seen more commonly in higher SES patients and families. Furthermore, given that a correlation between SES and health exists in parents as well as children, one would expect that lower SES parents are more likely to suffer physical and mental illness [129], which would negatively impact on adherence for the child with CF.

Knowledge of the treatment regimen and an understanding of its rationale is a prerequisite for adherence [130,131]. In one recent study of CF patients, non-adherence was specifically explained by the patient's misunderstanding of the prescribed regimen [132]. There is great variability in caregivers' knowledge of CF, and this has been shown to correlate with social class [133]. Families with less education or lower income might be intimidated or otherwise reluctant to ask questions, or may be stereotyped by caregivers as unable to understand and thus not offered information.

Differences in provision of evidence-based care

While CF treatment has improved dramatically, and the establishment of a care network using a standardized multidisciplinary approach makes CF care a model to be emulated, there is significant variance in disease outcomes such as mortality, pulmonary function and nutritional adequacy among credentialed CF care centers [49]. This variance persists even when comparisons are standardized to control for differences in the relative proportion of high-risk patients attending these centers [134]. The Epidemiological study of CF (ESCF) has demonstrated large variations in practice patterns regarding the use of various medications of proven efficacy [135] and outpatient monitoring [136], and has shown that these variations in care impact directly on outcome. Specifically, patients who are treated at care centers whose patients had better than average pulmonary function had more frequent monitoring of their clinical status (including lung function and airway cultures) and also received more interventions (particularly IV antibiotics) [137].

The between-center treatment differences do not appear to be associated with SES. Disparities in health and disease outcomes are often attributable to unequal access to quality care in countries such as the United States which lack an established national healthcare system [43,138]. However, SES-related barriers to care do not appear to be important for CF patients in the United States [105] and, as already mentioned, lower social class is also associated with worse outcomes in the UK where access to care is a government mandate [54]. A recent analysis from the US ESCF showed no SES-related differences in the use of chronic therapies or treatment of pulmonary exacerbations [139,140]. Nonetheless, it is possible that indigent CF patients receive qualitatively different medical care from that received by the middle class, as illustrated by apparent differences in teaching provided to low-SES CF patients [133,141] and the substandard care that inner-city asthma patients receive [138].

While some practice variations among CF care centers may reflect differences in scientific opinion among CF specialty physicians, variability in the implementation of consensus guidelines and evidence-based approaches to care is most likely to be due to inadvertently inconsistent application by the practice teams within a non-supportive system [142]. The care of patients with CF is complex. Certain aspects in the design of care involve decision-making processes that go beyond single clinical decisions to require interaction among many providers. A longitudinal perspective requires ongoing modifications of treatment in response to past and future considerations. On the other hand, many therapies and monitoring approaches are routine and need to be applied in a consistent and sometimes repetitive manner to almost all patients. This type of multifaceted care is best rendered within a system that is flexible and customizable but incorporates multicomponent strategies to limit reliance on isolated actions. The results obtained by a healthcare delivery system are a natural outcome of the design and operation of that system, and its ability to ensure that all steps in the process of care are supported and carried out correctly [143]. Thus, CF centers with the greatest successes regarding health outcomes appear to be those that have developed a system that supports the goal of allowing knowledgable practitioners to consistently provide the care they recognize to be appropriate to all of their patients [134].

The US CFF has recently begun to test methods of spreading beneficial organizational approaches to care via several quality improvement initiatives and also by reconfiguring its patient registry to make it a useful tool to track relevant patient- and center-based data. The underlying assumption is that a dramatic and relatively rapid improvement in life expectancy and quality of life for patients with CF would be obtained if all centers utilized systems that promote the efficient and consistent use of effective therapies [144]. This is discussed in more detail in Chapter 22.

CONCLUSION

While CF begins as a classic Mendelian autosomal recessive disease that is caused by alterations of the *CFTR* gene, its expression is influenced by a host of complex interactions with other genes, with the environment in which the patient lives, and by the efforts of healthcare providers. Just as we need to understand that the genetic milieu is an extraordinarily complex one with multiple opportunities ('gene modifiers') to affect disease expression, it is essential to appreciate that the human environment consists of specific biologic effectors (such as pollution and micro-organisms), and also a pervasive social and cultural setting which has

major implications for health. Furthermore, the disease course is modified in various degrees by the efforts of a healthcare delivery system that relies on the clinical expertise of knowledgable providers and on the success of a complex network that currently delivers appropriate interventions with uneven success. For any individual with CF, the course of the disease is impacted by the interaction of each of these three influences in varying ways (see Fig. 6.2), so it is of little wonder that, overall, there is a significant unpredictability regarding eventual outcome.

REFERENCES

49. Cystic Fibrosis Foundation Annual Data Report. *Patient Registry 2003*. Bethesda, MD, CFF, 2004.

50. Mackenbach JP, Kunst AE, Cavelaars AE *et al.* for the EU Working Group on Socioeconomic Inequalities in Health. Socioeconomic inequalities in morbidity and mortality in western Europe. *Lancet* 1997; **349**:1655–1659.

51. Dimissie K, Ernst P, Hanley JA *et al.* Socioeconomic status and lung function among primary school children in Canada. *Am J Respir Crit Care Med* 1996; **153**:719–723.

52. Ernst P, Demissie K, Joseph L *et al.* Socioeconomic status and indicators of asthma in children. *Am J Respir Crit Care Med* 1995; **152**:570–575.

53. Weiss KB, Gergen PJ, Crain EF. Inner-city asthma: the epidemiology of an emerging US public health concern. *Chest* 1992; **101**(Suppl 6):362S–367S.

54. Britton J. Effects of social class, sex, and region of residence on age at death from cystic fibrosis. *Br Med J* 1989; **298**:483–487.

55. Westwood AT. The prognosis of cystic fibrosis in the Western Cape region of South Africa. *J Paediatr Child Hlth* 1996; **32**:323–326.

56. Schechter MS, Margolis PA. Relationship between socioeconomic status and disease severity in cystic fibrosis. *J Pediatr* 1998; **132**:260–264.

57. Schechter MS, Shelton BJ, Margolis PA, FitzSimmons SC. The association of socioeconomic status with outcomes in cystic fibrosis patients in the United States. *Am J Respir Crit Care Med* 2001; **163**:1331–1337.

58. O'Connor GT, Quinton HB, Kahn R *et al.* Case-mix adjustment for evaluation of mortality in cystic fibrosis. *Pediatr Pulmonol* 2002; **33**:99–105.

59. O'Connor GT, Quinton HB, Kneeland T *et al.* Median household income and mortality rate in cystic fibrosis. *Pediatrics* 2003; **111**(4 Pt 1):e333–e339.

60. Krieger N, Williams DR, Moss NE. Measuring social class in US public health research: concepts, methodologies, and guidelines. *Annu Rev Pub Hlth* 1997; **18**:341–378.

61. Pincus T, Esther R, DeWalt DA, Callahan LF. Social conditions and self-management are more powerful determinants of health than access to care. *Ann Intern Med* 1998; **129**:406–411.

62. Stoddard JJ, Miller T. Impact of parental smoking on the prevalence of wheezing respiratory illness in children. *Am J Epidemiol* 1995; **141**:96–102.

63. Tager IB, Ngo L, Hanrahan JP. Maternal smoking during pregnancy. *Am J Respir Crit Care Med* 1995; **152**:977–983.

64. Eisner MD, Klein J, Hammond SK *et al.* Directly measured second hand smoke exposure and asthma health outcomes. *Thorax* 2005; **60**:814–821.

65. Rubin BK. Exposure of children with cystic fibrosis to environmental tobacco smoke. *N Engl J Med* 1990; **323**:782–788.

66. Smyth A, O'Hea U, Williams G *et al.* Passive smoking and impaired lung function in cystic fibrosis. *Arch Dis Child* 1994; **71**:353–354.

67. Kovesi T, Corey M, Levison H. Passive smoking and lung function in cystic fibrosis. *Am Rev Respir Dis* 1993; **148**:1266–1271.

68. Campbell PW, Parker RA, Roberts BT *et al.* Association of poor clinical status and heavy exposure to tobacco smoke in patients with cystic fibrosis who are homozygous for the F508 deletion. *J Pediatr* 1992; **120**(2 Pt 1):261–264.

69. Gilljam H, Stenlund C, Ericsson-Hollsing A, Strandvik B. Passive smoking in cystic fibrosis. *Respir Med* 1990; **84**:289–291.

70. Schuster MA, Franke T, Pham CB. Smoking patterns of household members and visitors in homes with children in the United States. *Arch Pediatr Adolesc Med* 2002; **156**:1094–1100.

71. Nelson DE, Emont SL, Brackbill RM *et al.* Cigarette smoking prevalence by occupation in the United States: a comparison between 1978 to 1980 and 1987 to 1990. *J Occup Med* 1994; **36**:516–525.

72. Schechter MS. Poverty and disease severity in CF: social and biological implications. *Pediatr Pulmonol* 1999; Suppl 19:156–157.

73. Gauderman WJ, Avol E, Gilliland F *et al.* The effect of air pollution on lung development from 10 to 18 years of age. *N Engl J Med* 2004; **351**:1057–1067.

74. Pope CA, Thun MJ, Namboodiri MM *et al.* Particulate air pollution as a predictor of mortality in a prospective study of U.S. adults. *Am J Respir Crit Care Med* 1995; **151**(3 Pt 1):669–674.

75. Wheeler BW, Ben-Shlomo Y. Environmental equity, air quality, socioeconomic status, and respiratory health: a linkage analysis of routine data from the Health Survey for England. *J Epidemiol Commun Hlth* 2005; **59**:948–954.

76. Emerson J, Rosenfeld M, McNamara S *et al. Pseudomonas aeruginosa* and other predictors of mortality and morbidity in young children with cystic fibrosis. *Pediatr Pulmonol* 2002; **34**:91–100.

77. Li Z, Kosorok MR, Farrell PM *et al.* Longitudinal development of mucoid *Pseudomonas aeruginosa* infection and lung disease progression in children with cystic fibrosis. *J Am Med Assoc* 2005; **293**:581–588.

78. Maselli JH, Sontag MK, Norris JM *et al.* Risk factors for initial acquisition of *Pseudomonas aeruginosa* in children with cystic fibrosis identified by newborn screening. *Pediatr Pulmonol* 2003; **35**:257–262.

79. Stutman HR, Lieberman JM, Nussbaum E, Marks MI. Antibiotic prophylaxis in infants and young children with cystic fibrosis: a randomized controlled trial. *J Pediatr* 2002; **140**:299–305.

80. Ratjen F, Comes G, Paul K *et al.* Effect of continuous antistaphylococcal therapy on the rate of *P. aeruginosa* acquisition in patients with cystic fibrosis. *Pediatr Pulmonol* 2001; **31**:13–16.

81. Jones AM, Dodd ME, Doherty CJ *et al.* Increased treatment requirements of patients with cystic fibrosis who harbour a highly transmissible strain of *Pseudomonas aeruginosa*. *Thorax* 2002; **57**:924–925.

82. Kosorok MR, Jalaluddin M, Farrell PM *et al.* Comprehensive analysis of risk factors for acquisition of *Pseudomonas aeruginosa* in young children with cystic fibrosis. *Pediatr Pulmonol* 1998; **26**:81–88.

83. Kerem E, Corey M, Stein R *et al.* Risk factors for *Pseudomonas aeruginosa* colonization in cystic fibrosis patients. *Pediatr Infect Dis J* 1990; **9**:494–498.

84. Armstrong D, Grimwood K, Carlin JB *et al.* Severe viral respiratory infections in infants with cystic fibrosis. *Pediatr Pulmonol* 1998; **26**:371–379.

85. LiPuma JJ. *Burkholderia cepacia*: management issues and new insights. *Clin Chest Med* 1998; **19**:473–486, vi.

86. Ledson MJ, Gallagher MJ, Jackson M *et al.* Outcome of *Burkholderia cepacia* colonisation in an adult cystic fibrosis centre. *Thorax* 2002; **57**:142–145.

87. Hiatt PW, Grace SC, Kozinetz CA *et al.* Effects of viral lower respiratory tract infection on lung function in infants with cystic fibrosis. *Pediatrics* 1999; **103**:619–626.

88. Gardner G, Frank AL, Taber LH. Effects of social and family factors on viral respiratory infection and illness in the first year of life. *J Epidemiol Commun Hlth* 1984; **38**:42–48.

89. Busse WW, Kiecolt-Glaser JK, Coe C *et al.* NHLBI Workshop summary. Stress and asthma. *Am J Respir Crit Care Med* 1995; **151**:249–252.

90. Patterson JM, Budd J, Goetz D, Warwick WJ. Family correlates of a 10-year pulmonary health trend in cystic fibrosis. *Pediatrics* 1993; **91**:383–389.

91. Wallander JL, Varni JW. Adjustment in children with chronic physical disorders: programmatic research on a disability-stress–coping model. In: LaGreca AM *et al.* (eds) *Stress and Coping in Child Health.* New York, Guilford Press, 1992, pp279–298.

92. Quittner AL, DiGirolamo AM, Michel M, Eigen H. Parental response to cystic fibrosis: a contextual analysis of the diagnosis phase. *J Pediatr Psychol* 1992; **17**:683–704.

93. Wright RJ, Rodriguez M, Cohen S. Review of psychosocial stress and asthma: an integrated biopsychosocial approach. *Thorax* 1998; **53**:1066–1074.

94. Quittner AL, DiGirolamo AM. Family adaptation to childhood disability and illness. In: Ammerman RT, Campo JV (eds) *Handbook of Pediatric Psychology and Psychiatry.* Boston, Allyn & Bacon, 1998, pp70–102.

95. Szanton SL, Gill JM, Allen JK. Allostatic load: a mechanism of socioeconomic health disparities? *Biol Res Nurs* 2005; **7**(1):7–15.

96. Patterson JM, McCubbin HI, Warwick WJ. The impact of family functioning on health changes in children with cystic fibrosis. *Social Sci Med* 1990; **31**(2):159–164.

97. Thompson RJ, Gustafson KE, Hamlett KW, Spock A. Psychological adjustment of children with cystic fibrosis: the role of child cognitive processes and maternal adjustment. *J Pediatr Psychol* 1992; **17**:741–755.

98. Borowitz D. The interrelationship of nutrition and pulmonary function in patients with cystic fibrosis. *Curr Opin Pulmon Med* 1996; **2**:457–461.

99. Konstan MW, Butler SM, Wohl ME *et al.* Growth and nutritional indexes in early life predict pulmonary function in cystic fibrosis. *J Pediatr* 2003; **142**:624–630.

100. James WP, Nelson M, Ralph A, Leather S. Socioeconomic determinants of health: the contribution of nutrition to inequalities in health. *Br Med J* 1997; **314**:1545–1549.

101. Schoni MH, Casaulta-Aebischer C. Nutrition and lung function in cystic fibrosis patients: review. *Clin Nutr* 2000; **19**(2):79–85.

102. Borowitz D, Baker RD, Stallings V. Consensus report on nutrition for pediatric patients with cystic fibrosis. *J Pediatr Gastroenterol Nutr* 2002; **35**:246–259.

103. Kawchak DA, Zhao H, Scanlin TF *et al.* Longitudinal, prospective analysis of dietary intake in children with cystic fibrosis. *J Pediatr* 1996; **129**:119–129.

104. Anthony H, Paxton S, Bines J, Phelan P. Psychosocial predictors of adherence to nutritional recommendations and growth outcomes in children with cystic fibrosis. *J Psychosom Res* 1999; **47**:623–634.

105. Rosenfeld M, Davis R, FitzSimmons S *et al.* Gender gap in cystic fibrosis mortality. *Am J Epidemiol* 1997; **145**:794–803.

106. Guilbault C, Stotland P, Lachance C *et al.* Influence of gender and interleukin-10 deficiency on the inflammatory response during lung infection with *Pseudomonas aeruginosa* in mice. *Immunology* 2002; **107**:297–305.

107. Allen JR, McCauley JC, Selby AM *et al.* Differences in resting energy expenditure between male and female children with cystic fibrosis. *J Pediatr* 2003; **142**:15–19.

108. Stallings VA. Gender, death and cystic fibrosis: is energy expenditure a component? *J Pediatr* 2003; **142**:4–6.

109. Willis E, Miller R, Wyn J. Gendered embodiment and survival for young people with cystic fibrosis. *Soc Sci Med* 2001; **53**:1163–1174.

110. Nixon PA, Orenstein DM, Kelsey SF, Doershuk CF. The prognostic value of exercise testing in patients with cystic fibrosis. *N Engl J Med* 1992; **327**:1785–1788.

111. Abbott J, Conway S, Etherington C *et al.* Perceived body image and eating behavior in young adults with cystic fibrosis and their healthy peers. *J Behav Med* 2000; **23**:501–517.

112. Anthony H, Paxton S, Catto-Smith A, Phelan P. Physiological and psychosocial contributors to malnutrition in children with cystic fibrosis: review. *Clin Nutr* 1999; **18**:327–335.

113. Walters S. Sex differences in weight perception and nutritional behaviour in adults with cystic fibrosis. *J Hum Nutr Diet* 2001; **14**(2):83–91.

114. Truby H, Paxton AS. Body image and dieting behavior in cystic fibrosis. *Pediatrics* 2001; **107**:E92.

115. Orenstein DM, Nixon PA. Exercise performance and breathing patterns in cystic fibrosis: male–female differences and influence of resting pulmonary function. *Pediatr Pulmonol* 1991; **10**:101–105.

116. Verma N, Bush A, Buchdahl R. Is there still a gender gap in cystic fibrosis? *Chest* 2005; **128**:2824–2834.

117. Lai HC, Kosorok MR, Laxova A *et al.* Delayed diagnosis of US females with cystic fibrosis. *Am J Epidemiol* 2002; **156**:165–173.

118. Braun L. Race, ethnicity, and health: can genetics explain disparities? *Perspect Biol Med* 2002; **45**:159–174.

119. Hamosh A, FitzSimmons SC, Macek M *et al.* Comparison of the clinical manifestation of cystic fibrosis in black and white patients. *J Pediatr* 1998; **132**:255–259.

120. Oliver MN, Muntaner C. Researching health inequities among African Americans: the imperative to understand social class. *Int J Health Serv* 2005; **35**:485–498.

121. Cystic Fibrosis Foundation. *Clinical Practice Guidelines for Cystic Fibrosis.* Bethesda, MD, CFF, 1997.

122. Yankaskas JR, Marshall BC, Sufian B *et al.* Cystic fibrosis adult care: consensus conference report. *Chest* 2004; **125**(Suppl 1):1S–39S.

123. Collins CE, MacDonald-Wicks L, Rowe S *et al.* Normal growth in cystic fibrosis associated with a specialised centre. *Arch Dis Child* 1999; **81**:241–246.

124. Quittner AL, Espelage DL, Ievers-Landis C, Drotar D. Measuring adherence to medical treatments in childhood chronic illness: considering multiple methods and sources of information. *J Clin Psychol Med Sett* 2000; **7**(1):41–54.

125. Greenberg RN. Overview of patient compliance with medication dosing: a literature review. *Clin Therap* 1984; **6**:592–599.

126. Gudas LJ, Koocher GP, Wypij D. Perceptions of medical compliance in children and adolescents with cystic fibrosis. *J Devel Behav Pediatr* 1991; **12**:236–242.

127. DiMatteo MR. Enhancing patient adherence to medical recommendations. *J Am Med Assoc* 1994; **271**:79–82.

128. Eddy ME, Carter BD, Kronenberger WG *et al.* Parent relationships and compliance in cystic fibrosis. *J Pediatr Health Care* 1998; **12**:196–202.

129. Hudson CG. Socioeconomic status and mental illness: tests of the social causation and selection hypotheses. *Am J Orthopsychiatry* 2005; **75**(1):3–18.

130. Ievers CE, Brown RT, Drotar D *et al.* Knowledge of physician prescriptions and adherence to treatment among children with cystic fibrosis and their mothers. *J Develop Behav Pediatr* 1999; **20**:335–343.

131. Lask B. Non-adherence to treatment in cystic fibrosis. *J R Soc Med* 1994; **87**(Suppl 21):25–27.

132. Quittner AL, Drotar D, Ievers-Landis C *et al.* Adherence to medical teatments in adolescents with cystic fibrosis: the development and evaluation of family-based interventions. In: Drotar D (ed.) *Promoting Adherence to Medical Treatment in Childhood Chronic Illness: Concepts, Methods and Interventions.* Mahwah, NJ, Erlbaum Associates, 2000.

133. Henley LD, Hill ID. Errors, gaps, and misconceptions in the disease-related knowledge of cystic fibrosis patients and their families. *Pediatrics* 1990; **85**:1008–1014.

134. Schechter MS. Demographic and center-related characteristics associated with low weight in pediatric CF patients. *Pediatr Pulmonol* 2002; Suppl **22**:156–157.

135. Konstan MW, Butler SM, Schidlow DV *et al.* Investigators and Coordinators of the Epidemiologic Study of Cystic Fibrosis. Patterns of medical practice in cystic fibrosis. II: Use of therapies. *Pediatr Pulmonol* 1999; **28**:248–254.

136. Konstan MW, Butler SM, Schidlow DV *et al.* Investigators and Coordinators of the Epidemiologic Study of Cystic Fibrosis. Patterns of medical practice in cystic fibrosis. I: Evaluation and monitoring of health status of patients. *Pediatr Pulmonol* 1999; **28**:242–247.

137. Johnson C, Butler SM, Konstan MW *et al.* Factors influencing outcomes in cystic fibrosis: a center-based analysis. *Chest* 2003; **123**:20–27.

138. Finkelstein JA, Brown RW, Schneider LC *et al.* Quality of care for pre-school children with asthma: the role of social factors and practice setting. *Pediatrics* 1995; **95**:389–394.

139. Schechter MS, Silva SJ, Morgan WJ, Rhoa M. Association of socioeconomic status with outpatient monitoring and the use of chronic cf therapies. *Pediatr Pulmonol* 2005; Suppl 28:330.

140. Schechter MS, Pasta D, Morgan WJ *et al.* Socioeconomic status and the likelihood of antibiotic treatment for pulmonary exacerbations. *Pediatr Pulmonol* 2005; Suppl 28:331.

141. Henley LD, Hill ID. Global and specific disease-related information needs of cystic fibrosis patients and their families. *Pediatrics* 1990; **85**:1015–1021.

142. Institute of Medicine Committee on Quality Health Care in America. *Crossing the Quality Chasm: A New Health System for the 21st Century*. Washington, DC, National Academy Press, 2001.

143. Berwick DM. Continuous improvement as an ideal in health care. *N Engl J Med* 1989; **320**:53–56.

144. Schechter MS, Margolis P. Improving subspecialty healthcare: lessons from cystic fibrosis. *J Pediatr* 2005; **147**:295–301.

PART 3

DIAGNOSTIC ASPECTS OF CYSTIC FIBROSIS

7 Diagnosis of cystic fibrosis   99
   Colin Wallis
8a The challenge of screening newborn infants for cystic fibrosis   109
   Kevin W. Southern
8b How to manage the screened patient   117
   Philip Robinson
9 Microbiology of cystic fibrosis: role of the clinical microbiology laboratory, susceptibility and
   synergy studies and infection control   123
   Samiya Razvi and Lisa Saiman

Diagnosis of cystic fibrosis

COLIN WALLIS

INTRODUCTION

Making the diagnosis of cystic fibrosis (CF) has lifelong implications and repercussions for the affected individual and their family. The diagnosis needs to be made accurately and as early as possible. A late diagnosis is often preceded by a history of hospital visits, family anguish, anger and guilt and a delay in the initiation or early treatment that may have an impact on long-term outcome. Equally disturbing is a small but increasing experience of the child or adult, diagnosed with CF, whom on review – often years later – is found to be normal [1].

In most cases, making the diagnosis is easy. A child has suggestive clinical symptoms or a family history and a positive sweat test confirms the suspicions of CF. A triad of clinical features based on recurrent chest infections, pancreatic insufficiency and failure to thrive were established in the 1960s and have been a useful phenotypic benchmark for a CF diagnosis for nearly 40 years [2]. The sweat test remains a very useful discriminator between those with and those without CF. But even before the identification of the CF gene, there were reported cases of 'sweat test negative CF' and the concept of a broader phenotypic range had been promulgated [3].

It was always hoped that the discovery of the gene for cystic fibrosis and its disease-causing mutations would provide diagnostic certainty. Two mutations within the *CFTR* gene would mean cystic fibrosis; normal genes would exclude the diagnosis. But it has not worked out that simply. Indeed, in the decade since the discovery of the CF gene, the situation is probably even more confusing and the number of 'atypical' or 'unusual' cases is growing. Over the last decade a number of developments have led to the question 'What makes a diagnosis of CF?'[4,5]. These include: (a) the recognition of an ever-widening phenotype for an individual with two *CFTR* mutations ranging from completely normal to a classical CF phenotype; (b) the development of screening programs whereby a newborn or fetus, on the basis of genetic information alone, could be given the CF label without necessarily developing clinical disease; (c) the recognition that a CF phenotype can emerge over time presenting *de novo* in adulthood; and (d) the development of sophisticated clinical investigations that allow detection of subtle changes in end organs that hitherto would have gone undetected – detailed CT scanning of pulmonary structure and the measurement of nasal epithelial potential difference being two examples.

Labels are important and the diagnosis of classical CF carries with it important implications. Failure to identify and label a patient with CF could lead to delays in effective therapies. But inappropriate categorization of a patient with an atypical form leads to an unnecessary burden of therapies and lifestyle restrictions. When considering the diagnosis of CF, clinicians must be aware of the expanding phenotype for this condition and the subclassification of CF into atypical or CFTR-related disorders.[6,7].

PRESENTING CLINICAL FEATURES

A Cystic Fibrosis Foundation Consensus Panel (USA) synthesized diagnostic criteria for CF, based on the presence of one or more characteristic clinical features or a history of CF in a sibling, or a positive newborn screening test, plus laboratory evidence of a CFTR abnormality [8]. The key features are summarized in Fig. 7.1. The basic premise of the consensus statement is that CF is a clinical and not a genetic diagnosis although it acknowledges that genetic testing may have a role in sorting out atypical clinical situations. Any such document must be considered a work in progress to accommodate new developments and acknowledge shortcomings [9].

The majority of children with CF present with a history of bulky offensive fatty stools, failure to thrive and recurrent chest infections [10]; 10–15% will present with meconium ileus shortly after birth. The range of clinical features

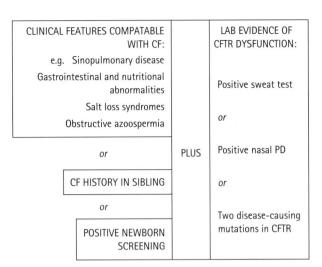

Figure 7.1 Diagnostic criteria for CF. PD, potential difference.

Table 7.1 Clinical features consistent with a CF diagnosis.

Sinopulmonary disease	Chronic cough or sputum production
	Wheeze
	Finger clubbing
	Nasal polyposis or chronic sinusitis
	Culture of characteristic CF organism eg *Pseudomonas aeruginosa* in sputum, 'staph' empyema
Gastrointestinal signs	
Intestinal	Meconium ileus, rectal prolapse, DIOS
Pancreatic	Pancreatic insufficiency, pancreatitis
Hepatic	Focal biliary cirrhosis, prolonged neonatal jaundice
Nutritional and salt-loss sequelae	Failure to thrive
	Acute salt loss
	Pseudo-Bartter syndrome, chronic metabolic alkalosis
	Hypoproteinemia–edema syndrome
	Kwashiorkor-like disease with skin changes
	Vitamin K deficiency
Obstructive azoospermia	Bilateral absence of the vas deferens

DIOS, distal intestinal obstruction syndrome.

suspicious of CF is listed in Table 7.1. The spectrum of presenting features is wide and vigilance is required to prevent missed diagnostic opportunities – especially in ethnic groups where CF is less common or in children who are considered 'too healthy'. The presenting features can vary with the age at time of clinical presentation as indicated in Table 7.2. In approximately 90% of children with access to modern healthcare, a CF diagnosis is established by the age of 1 year [11]. In atypical cases, however, the diagnosis is often delayed into adulthood. This latter group is often pancreatic sufficient with a milder (but not necessarily absent) pulmonary phenotype.

Table 7.2 Clinical features of CF at diagnosis in unscreened populations, grouped according to age and approximate order of frequency.

0–2 years
  Failure to thrive
  Steatorrhea
  Recurrent chest infections including bronchiolitis/bronchitis
  Meconium ileus
  Rectal prolapse
  Edema/hypoproteinemia/'kwashiorkor' dermatitis
  Severe pneumonia/empyema
  Salt depletion syndrome
  Prolonged neonatal jaundice
  Vitamin K deficiency with bleeding diathesis

3–16 years
  Recurrent chest infections or 'asthma'
  Clubbing and 'idiopathic' bronchiectasis
  Steatorrhea
  Nasal polyps and sinusitis
  Chronic intestinal obstruction, intussusception
  Heat exhaustion with hyponatremia
  CF diagnosis in a relative

Adulthood (often atypical CF)
  Azoospermia/congenital absence of the vas deferens
  Bronchiectasis
  Chronic sinusitis
  Acute or chronic pancreatitis
  Allergic bronchopulmonary aspergillosis
  Focal biliary cirrhosis
  Abnormal glucose tolerance
  Portal hypertension
  Cholestasis/gallstones

Reproduced with permission from [64]

In addition to suspicious clinical features, a clinician may need to confirm the diagnosis of CF in other settings: (a) postnatal confirmation may be required when an antenatal test has proven suspicious for CF; (b) a postnatal screening program may have identified a child as high risk for CF; or (c) an individual may be under investigation following the diagnosis of CF in a family member.

A clinical suspicion for the diagnosis of CF can be supported by a number of confirmatory tests and investigations.

CONFIRMATORY TESTS

The sweat test

The sweat test was first described in 1959 and remains the gold standard for the diagnosis of cystic fibrosis [12]. In the majority of CF patients with typical features and identified CFTR mutations, the sweat test is diagnostic. In atypical

Table 7.3 Examples of non-CF causes of a positive sweat test.

Adrenal insufficiency or stress
Anorexia nervosa
Autonomic dysfunction
Ectodermal dysplasia
Eczema
Fucosidosis
Glucose-6-phosphate dehydrogenase deficiency
Glycogen storage disease type 1
Hypoparathyroidism
Hypothyroidism
Malnutrition from various causes including HIV infection
Nephrogenic diabetes insipidus
Nephrosis
Pseudohypoaldosteronism

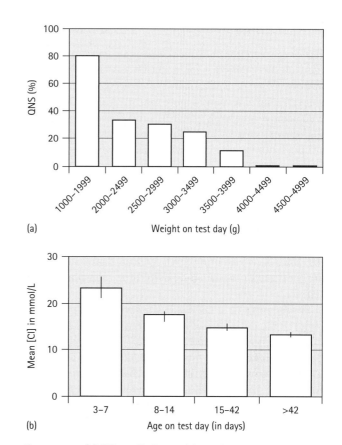

(a)

(b)

Figure 7.2 **(a)** Effect of infant weight at time of testing on likelihood of failure of collecting >75 mg of sweat (quantity not sufficient or QNS) on one arm as represented by a percentage failure rate on the y-axis. **(b)** Mean chloride concentration at different postnatal ages in infants without CF. Reproduced with permission from [18].

forms, the sweat chloride levels may fall into the intermediate range and there are rare examples of patients with CF, confirmed on genetic testing, who have a normal sweat test [13,14]. There are a number of other rare conditions (sometimes single case reports) that have been associated with a positive sweat test but these are usually clearly distinguishable by their clinical features. Examples are listed in Table 7.3.

The standard sweat test (Gibson and Cooke technique) requires skill and care and should be undertaken by accredited laboratories. Localized sweating is stimulated by the iontophoresis of pilocarpine into the skin. Sweat is collected on filter paper, gauze or in microduct tubing at a standardized rate. Guidelines for sweat testing procedures and precautions are published [15] and testing should be carried out by experienced personnel using standardized methodologies in facilities with a regular throughput.

PATIENT SELECTION

Sweat tests can be reliably performed after 2 weeks of age in infants greater than 3 kg who are normally hydrated and without significant systemic illness. During the first 24 hours after birth in full-term infants, sweat electrolyte values may be transiently elevated [16]. After the first week a decline in the levels occurs and an elevated value can be used to confirm a diagnosis of CF [17]. In a retrospective review of sweat tests in pre-term and full-term infants, collection of the requisite 75 mg of sweat could be obtained in infants over 36 weeks who weighed over 2 kg and were greater than 3 days postnatal age [18] (Fig. 7.2). Patients who are systemically unwell, edematous or on corticosteroids should have their testing delayed. Sweat tests can be performed in subjects on flucloxacillin [19]. Normal adolescents and adults tend to have higher sweat chloride levels (up to 60 mmol/L) and therefore borderline values in this age group may not reflect CF.

SWEAT COLLECTION

The flexor surface of the forearm is the preferred site for sweat collection although other sites may be considered if the arms are eczematous or otherwise unsuitable. Great care must be taken at all stages of the testing to avoid contamination. Electrodes should be of a suitable size and curvature to fit snugly on the patient's limb.

Sweat is collected on filter paper, gauze or in microduct tubing over a controlled period of time to ensure that the rate of sweating and the total sweat collected are sufficient and standardized. During the process of collection, the sweat must be protected from contamination and dehydration. Sweat should be collected for a period between 20 and 30 minutes. The National Committee for Clinical Laboratory Standards guidelines (Document C34-A2) state that iontophoresis should not be performed on a patient receiving oxygen by an open delivery system although no evidence is provided to support this statement. This would not apply to an infant in a headbox or a patient on nasal cannula oxygen.

SWEAT ANALYSIS

The sweat secretion rate, measured as an average rate over the collection period, should not be less than $1\,g/m^2$ per minute. Chloride is the analyte of choice [20,21]. A sweat chloride concentration of more than 60 mmol/L is considered positive and levels below 40 mmol/L are likely to be in the normal range – and CF is considered to be unlikely although not excluded. Intermediate levels between 40 and 60 mmol/L may be associated with atypical forms of CF and need to be interpreted with caution. Some normal adults can have values in the intermediate range. There is evidence from newborn screening that initial intermediate or high normal chloride readings may also occur in the affected premature infant or newborn and may need repeating [22]. Sweat chloride levels greater than 150 mmol/L are not physiological and should be questioned and repeated.

A false positive sweat test in the severely malnourished child, or the critically ill child in intensive care, needs cautious interpretation and follow-up. Case reports also describe a nonsense mutation in the *CFTR* gene associated with elevated sweat chloride in the absence of clinical features of CF [23]. The sweat sodium levels are less reliable and should never be used in isolation.

The osmolality of sweat records the total solute concentration in mmol/kg of sweat. The reference ranges for osmolality are wide: children with CF have sweat osmolality values greater than 200 mmol/kg with normal ranges falling between 50 and 150 mmol/kg. Positive and equivocal results (between 150 and 200 mmol/kg) should be followed up by a quantitative analysis of chloride concentration.

Research continues to explore the development of an easier sweat test. Collecting systems such as the nanoduct [24] are achieving credibility and the role of sweat conductivity as a diagnostic tool in CF is also gaining credence [25]. Conductivity represents a non-selective measurement of ions and good correlation between the results of sweat chloride concentrations and sweat conductivity have been shown. In one large trial the best conductivity cut-off value to diagnose CF was ≥90 mmol/L and the best conductivity cut-off value to exclude CF was <75 mmol/L [26] (Fig. 7.3) For conductivity, a provisional upper physiological limit of 170 mmol/L may be used pending further evidence. Currently, many clinicians and laboratories will chose to confirm a positive sweat conductivity result with a formal measurement of chloride concentration.

INDICATIONS FOR REPEAT SWEAT TESTING

The diagnosis of CF should never be based on a single positive sweat test result. If mutation analysis does not confirm the diagnosis then a repeat sweat test may be indicated. Similarly, patients with borderline results may require repeat testing especially if the basis of the testing was for failure to thrive or a positive family history. Sweat testing should be repeated in patients who are following an atypical course

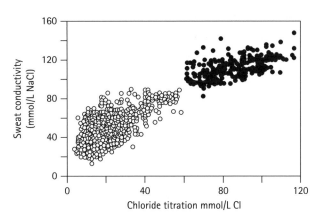

Figure 7.3   Comparison of conductivity method and chloride concentration in sweat of 3834 patients with CF (solid circles) and without CF (empty circles). Reproduced with permission from [26].

or where ancillary testing for end organ disease produces little supportive evidence for the diagnosis.

Mutation analysis

The identification of the CF gene in 1989 [27] and the characterization of its protein product (CFTR) held the promise that the diagnostic dilemmas for the condition were over. Two identifiable mutations meant you had the disease. Unfortunately, it has not worked out that simply. Although two disease-causing mutations are very supportive of the diagnosis of CF in the appropriate clinical setting there are a number of caveats.

First, there are over a thousand different CF gene mutations associated with CF disease. Examples of *CFTR* mutations are listed in Table 7.4. The dominance of the *F508del* mutation is highlighted – present in over 70% of CF alleles in Caucasian populations [10]. Confirming the diagnosis of CF based on the presence of two CF-producing mutations is highly specific but not very sensitive. Sensitivity is decreased due to the large number of CF alleles. Current techniques do not allow a full screen of the entire CF genome and most laboratories will search routinely for the commonest mutations only within their region. Customizing mutation panels to match the patient's ethnic background and clinical presentation can enhance the sensitivity of DNA testing in CF. For example, there are CF mutations which occur with increased frequency, in specific population groups such as the Ashkenazi Jewish (*W1282X*) or African ($3120 + 1\,kb\ G \rightarrow A$) patients and in patients with specific clinical features such as pancreatic sufficiency (*R117H* and *A445E*), male fertility ($3849 + 10\,kb\ C \rightarrow T$), or normal concentrations of sweat electrolytes ($3849 + 10\,kb\ C \rightarrow T$) [28,29].

Second, alterations in the *CFTR* gene designated as CF-causing mutations should fulfil at least one of the criteria as shown in Table 7.5 [30]. In addition to the 'disease-causing' mutations there are also recognizable polymorphisms that

Table 7.4 Common mutations that cause cystic fibrosis listed according to frequency[a].

Mutation	%
ΔF508	75.0
G551D	3.4
G542X	1.8
R117H	1.3
621 + 1 G → T	1.3
ΔI507	0.5
N1303K	0.5
R560T	0.4
Q493X	0.3
R1162X	0.3
R533X	0.3
W1282X	0.3
3659delC	0.3
1154insTC	0.3
E60X	0.2
G85E	0.2
P67L	0.2
R347P	0.2
V520F	0.2
1078delT	0.1
2184delA	0.1
A455E	0.1
R334W	0.1
S549N	0.1
2789 + 5 G → A	0.1
3849 + 10 kb C → T	0.1
711 + 1 G → T	0.1
1717 + 1 G → T	0.6
1898 + 1 G → T	0.6

[a]In Caucasian populations, variations in frequency can occur widely between different ethnic groups and geographic regions.
Reproduced with permission from [64].

Table 7.5 Features of a disease-producing mutation in the CFTR gene.

- A change in the amino-acid sequence that severely affects *CFTR* synthesis and/or function
- A deletion, insertion, or nonsense mutation which introduces a premature termination signal (stop mutation)
- Alteration to the first two or last two nucleotides of an intron splice site
- A novel amino-acid sequence that is not a 'normal' variant (found in at least 100 carriers within the subjects ethnic background)

do not necessarily result in a clinical phenotype but may influence the structure of the final protein product when associated with another mild mutation such as *R117H*. The thymidine run in intron 8 is a well-described example

Table 7.6 The range of clinical phenotypes associated with two mutations in the CF gene.

1. Classical CF
   Sinopulmonary disease with pancreatic insufficiency, gastrointestinal and nutritional consequences, high sweat chloride concentration and male infertility
2. Atypical CF (non-classical)
   Sinopulmonary disease, pancreatic sufficiency and positive sweat test
   Sinopulmonary disease and male fertility with a normal sweat test
   Severe sinusitis and congenital bilateral absence of the vas deferens
   Male infertility only
   Recurrent idiopathic pancreatitis
   Allergic bronchopulmonary aspergillosis
   Sclerosing cholangitis
   Positive sweat test only
3. No clinical features, including normal sweat chloride

where the 5T allele leads to a substantial reduction in functional protein compared with 9T; 7T is intermediate.

Failure to find two CF mutations from a selective or extended search does not exclude the diagnosis of CF. To exclude a patient with symptoms of CF and a positive sweat test from potentially beneficial treatment because the laboratory cannot detect two CF mutations would clearly be misguided. There are also rare reports of patients with classical CF symptoms and signs and a positive sweat test who do not appear to have any mutations in the CFTR gene – even when the entire gene has been sequenced – screening all 27 exons and the intron–exon boundaries [31]. These findings suggest that on these rare occasions CF may be caused by mutations within the promotor region of the *CFTR* gene, in one of the introns or even in a distant controlling gene from an unrelated locus [32].

Finally, although two mutations are very supportive of the diagnosis of CF in the appropriate clinical setting, two alterations in the gene for *CFTR* does not necessarily mean that you will develop classic CF disease. The clinical phenotype associated with two *CFTR* mutations is far broader than could ever have been anticipated [33]. Examples are listed in Table 7.6 and the importance of these atypical forms of cystic fibrosis are discussed further below.

CYSTIC FIBROSIS PHENOTYPES

There are four major contributing factors that influence the path from genotype to end-organ involvement and an individual's eventual phenotype.

SEVERITY OF THE INDIVIDUAL *CFTR* MUTATIONS

'Mild' mutations may cause milder phenotypic effects, but when there is a mixture of mild and severe mutations the final impact is unpredictable. Sometimes mild mutations may have a dominant effect on severe mutations with a 'corrective' effect. Similarly, co-existent polymorphisms hitchhiking within the *CFTR* gene may influence the final protein product. Pancreatic phenotype can sometimes be predicted by genotype, and pancreatic insufficiency is almost invariably associated with two 'severe' mutations. The correlation between genotype and phenotype for a pulmonary phenotype is not reliably predictive and the course of lung disease in CF is especially vulnerable to environmental and modifier genes [34].

MODIFYING GENES

Genes lying elsewhere in the genome have significant influence on the behavior of the CFTR protein [35]. These genes and their protein products can correct or exacerbate influencing pathological processes such as the biochemistry of the cell surface liquid, the innate and acquired immunity of the lungs and may even influence the predisposition to meconium ileus [36]. Each individual with CF is likely to have an immense and unique orchestra of modifying genes and proteins that are influential in his or her clinical outcome [37].

ENVIRONMENTAL FACTORS

The environment in which an individual with CF lives and grows has central bearing on the outcome of his or her disease [38]. Treatment and adherence to therapy, social circumstances and diet, exposure to infections such as *Pseudomonas* or viral infections in infancy can produce a sustained negative influence on the clinical course [39].

THE PASSAGE OF TIME

Cystic fibrosis is not necessarily an all-or-nothing disease. A clinical phenotype can emerge with time especially in some of the atypical forms. Effective therapies and adherence to treatment can help stall the disease progression. Patients with documented pancreatic sufficiency in childhood can become pancreatic insufficient in later life. Some but not all patients with CF will develop diabetes, liver disease and osteoporosis.

CLASSIFICATION OF CF PHENOTYPES

Classical cystic fibrosis

The diagnosis of classical CF needs to be made early and confidently. No racial group is exempt and children of ethnic minorities or mixed heritage are at greatest risk of a delayed or missed diagnosis. The clinical features of recurrent chest infections, malabsorption with pancreatic insufficiency in the majority (but not all) or an infant presenting with meconium ileus, rectal prolapse or unexplained

malnutrition requires investigation. Although pancreatic insufficiency is present in over 90% of classical CF patients, pancreatic-sufficient patients are not necessarily excluded from the classical CF category. A positive sweat test and/or two CFTR mutations is diagnostic. Appropriate therapy should be introduced without delay. Common causes for a delayed diagnosis include failure to consider the diagnosis because the patient looks 'too healthy'; inadequate sweat test methodology or misinterpretation of an inadequate sample of sweat; and the failure to repeat a previously borderline sweat test in the face of ongoing clinical concerns.

Atypical (non-classic) CF

There is an increasing group of children and adults who do not present with the full spectrum of clinical features associated with classical CF. The terms 'equivocal CF' or 'variant CF' have also been used to describe these atypical forms. There may only be single organ involvement. Sweat testing can be normal, equivocal or positive and *CFTR* analysis may reveal one, two or no mutations depending on the depth of analysis. In patients with atypical CF who have two identified *CFTR* mutations, one is usually a 'mild' mutation resulting in partial CFTR expression and function. Examples of such conditions are included in Table 7.6 and often represent the mildest end of the CF spectrum. Based on registry data, approximately 2% of individuals who fulfil the criteria for the diagnosis of CF fall in the atypical category. It is very probable, however, that this is an under-representation as it is likely that many of these atypical cases are undiagnosed or present in adult life [40,41].

Recent reviews have recognized that it is inappropriate to label individuals with these atypical forms as having classical CF [5,40]. Both the diagnostic labelling and medical management needs to be tailored to the patient's individual phenotype and requirements. The introduction of arduous therapies aimed at the patient with classical CF does not seem appropriate or beneficial. The negative connotations of a CF label can be avoided with a more considered approach to diagnostic categorization, embracing subcategorization and accepting the atypical forms of CF [42].

CFTR-related disorders

CFTR-related disease is a term coined to classify non-CF conditions that carry a higher incidence of *CFTR* mutations than could be expected by chance but have no other indicators of either classical or atypical CF. These conditions appear to be influenced by CFTR dysfunction but are under greatest influence from non-*CFTR* genes and environmental influences. The distinction from atypical CF (especially those with monosymptomatic disease and only one identified mutation) is not always clear-cut and in time this subgroup may require review. Examples of CFTR-related disorders include:

- allergic bronchopulmonary aspergillosis
- pancreatitis – acute or recurrent
- isolated obstructive azoospermia
- chronic rhinosinusitis
- disseminated bronchiectasis
- diffuse panbronchiolitis
- heat exhaustion.

Genetic predisposition for CF with no clinical sequalae

There is currently no satisfactory term to describe a very small but important group of individuals with the genetic potential to develop CF (i.e. two disease-causing mutations in the *CFTR* gene) but in whom, on careful and detailed clinical assessment, there is no evidence of end organ disease. Some authors have considered the term 'pre-CF' [7]: there is the potential that clinical features will emerge with time but there is insufficient clinical evidence to label the carrier of the gene mutations with a disease. Most clinicians would advise a program of surveillance in these cases and reserve therapy for a time when early changes occur. The role of prophylactic therapy in this situation (such as physiotherapy or antibiotics) is unclear.

ADDITIONAL SUPPORTIVE INVESTIGATIONS IN ATYPICAL PRESENTATIONS

Occasionally a clinician faces difficulties establishing the label of cystic fibrosis. The commonest situation is the patient with clinical features partially consistent with CF but a non-diagnostic sweat test and only one identified CF mutation. Further evaluation is required to determine whether the patient is a carrier for CF or has an atypical form. It is equally important to ensure that an alternative diagnosis has been excluded. Part of the differential diagnosis will include conditions such as immunodeficiency, Shwachman–Diamond syndrome, primary ciliary dyskinesia and allergic disease. It is also recognized that molecular abnormalities other than CFTR dysfunction can masquerade as atypical CF [43]. The following ancillary testing is suggested, tailoring these additional supportive investigations to the clinical picture.

Assessment of end organ effects

DETAILED STRUCTURAL IMAGING OF THE LUNG PARENCHYMA

Modern CT technology using high-resolution scans and 'combi' scans can demonstrate early structural changes to the small airways that are not readily visible on plain radiographic films [44]. In addition to assessing bronchial wall thickening and dilation in the smallest of bronchioles, the presence of air trapping representing early changes to the bronchioles may be visible on expiratory images.

EVALUATION OF THE PARANASAL SINUSES

The sinuses are highly sensitive to altered CFTR function. Plain X-rays, CT imaging and MRI views of the sinuses can show opacification and the presence of polyps. Normal sinuses on imaging are very unusual in CF.

PANCREATIC FUNCTION TESTING

Pancreatic insufficiency is usually clinically evident but further testing can be helpful in selected cases. Previously, pancreatic function testing required sophisticated technology with invasive sampling techniques and stimulation protocols. As an alternative, prolonged timed stool collections for fecal fat analysis have been suggested but remain unpopular with patients and laboratories. Recently, a simple test for quantification of fecal elastase 1 in a single small stool sample has shown considerable sensitivity and reliability and is not contaminated by exogenous enzyme administration [45,46]. It is likely that this test of pancreatic function will prove useful in the evaluation of borderline or equivocal cases. Caution is required in the interpretation of early stool samples especially in the premature infant or newborn within the first few days of life [47].

MICROBIOLOGICAL CULTURE

The culture of sputum, bronchoalveolar lavage fluid, oropharyngeal swabs or sinus aspirates for known CF pathogens can be important. If a child with 'idiopathic' bronchiectasis is found to be infected with typical CF pathogens such as *Staphylococcus aureus* or mucoid *Pseudomonas aeruginosa*, then re-evaluation of the possibility of a CF diagnosis is necessary. Infection with *P. aeruginosa* is highly associated with the presence of two deleterious CFTR mutations if the entire gene is sequenced, especially where there is elevation of sweat chloride [43].

SEMEN ANALYSIS

The seminal vesicles would appear to be acutely sensitive to lower levels of functioning CFTR and obstructive azoospermia is found in 98–99% of affected males [48,49]. In many atypical CF cases with minimal lung or pancreatic involvement, azoospermia may be the presenting feature [50,51]. Semen analysis should be considered in post-pubertal males. Ultrasound assessment for the bilateral absence of the vas deferens is possible in younger boys [52].

LUNG FUNCTION TESTING

Standard spirometry may be too insensitive to pick up the subtle alterations in lung function. Early changes would appear to affect the smallest airways first and lung function assessments should consider measurements that target these small airway changes. Newer technologies such as the multiple breath washout technique show promise [53,54].

Further assessment of CFTR dysfunction by potential difference testing

The transport of charged ions such as sodium and chloride across an epithelial surface such as that lining the entire respiratory tract (including the sinuses and the nose) generates a transepithelial potential difference (PD). This PD can be measured by placing an exploring electrode on the surface of the respiratory epithelium (most commonly on the floor of the nose or against the inferior turbinate) and

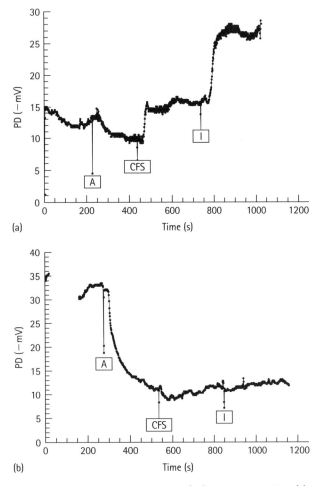

Figure 7.4   Nasal potential difference (PD) in a normal subject (a) and a CF patient (b) illustrating the response of the transepithelial PD to perfusion with amiloride (A), followed by the addition of a chloride-free solution (CFS) and the addition of isoproterenol (I). With acknowledgments to Dr A. Jaffe for the data.

a reference electrode into the subcutaneous tissue of the forearm or over an area of abraded skin [55]. The abnormalities of ion transport in CF produce a number of differences in PD measurements when compared to normal nasal mucosal measurements. Specifically, in CF: (a) there is a more negative basal PD in keeping with enhanced sodium ion transport; (b) a greater change in PD (less negative) occurs after the application of amiloride to the nasal epithelium; and (c) there is little or no response to perfusion of the mucosa with a chloride-free solution. A typical result for CF and normal nasal PD is shown in Fig. 7.4. A raised (more negative) PD is strong evidence for the diagnosis of CF and the presence of a large response to chloride-free perfusion is strong evidence against CF.

The technological considerations have been addressed in detail and require well-defined protocols and standardized procedures [56–58]. The test is technically difficult to perform and requires considerable cooperation from the subject and careful placement of the nasal electrode. Perfusion rate, the duration of the perfusion and the temperature of the solutions are all important variables. Results may be difficult to interpret in the presence of allergic or infectious rhinitis and nasal polyps. Adaptations of the technique have allowed measurements in newborns while asleep using an extremely low flow rate [59].

In general, for diagnostic dilemmas, nasal PDs are often also equivocal and indeterminate [60]. A relationship between PD and lung disease severity has been proposed [61]. Recently work has been published on the use of PD measurements in rectal biopsy specimens either *in vivo* or on biopsy specimens. This technology is not yet widely available [62,63].

REFERENCES

1. Shaw NJ, Littlewood JM. Misdiagnosis of cystic fibrosis. *Arch Dis Child* 1987; **62**:1271–1273.
2. Littlewood JM. The diagnosis of cystic fibrosis. *Practitioner* 1980; **224**:305–307.
3. Sarsfield JK, Davies JM. Negative sweat tests and cystic fibrosis. *Arch Dis Child* 1975; **50**:463–466.
4. Wilmott RW. Making the diagnosis of cystic fibrosis. *J Pediatr* 1998; **132**:563–565.
5. Dodge JA, Dequeker E. CF or not CF? That is the question. *J Cyst Fibros* 2002; **1**:3–4.
6. Knowles MR, Durie PR. What is cystic fibrosis? *N Engl J Med* 2002; **347**:439–442.
7. Bush A, Wallis C. Time to think again: cystic fibrosis is not an 'all or nothing' disease. *Pediatr Pulmonol* 2000; **30**:139–144.
8. Rosenstein BJ, Cutting G. The diagnosis of cystic fibrosis: a consensus statement. *J Pediatr* 1998; **132**:589–595.
9. Rosenstein BJ. Cystic fibrosis diagnosis: new dilemmas for an old disorder. *Pediatr Pulmonol* 2002; **33**:83–84.
10. McCormick J, Green MW, Mehta G *et al.* Demographics of the UK cystic fibrosis population: implications for neonatal screening. *Eur J Hum Genet* 2002; **10**:583–590.

11. Fitzsimmons SC. The changing epidemiology of cystic fibrosis. *J Pediatr* 1993; **122**:1–9.

12. Gibson LE, Cooke RE. A test for concentration of electrolytes in sweat in cystic fibrosis of the pancreas utilizing pilocarpine by iontophoresis. *Pediatrics* 1959; **23**:545–549.

13. LeGrys VA. Sweat testing for the diagnosis of cystic fibrosis: practical considerations. *J Pediatr* 1996; **129**:892–897.

14. Massie J, Robinson P. Cystic fibrosis: the twilight zone. *Pediatr Pulmonol* 1999; **28**:222–224.

15. Baumer JH. Evidence based guidelines for the performance of the sweat test for the investigation of cystic fibrosis in the UK. *Arch Dis Child* 2003; **88**:1126–1127.

16. Harpin VA, Rutter N. Sweating in pre-term babies. *J Pediatr* 1982; **100**:614–619.

17. Hardy JD, Davison SH, Higgins MU, Polycarpou PN. Sweat tests in the newborn period. *Arch Dis Child* 1973; **48**:316–318.

18. Eng W, LeGrys VA, Schechter MS *et al.* Sweat-testing in pre-term and full-term infants less than 6 weeks of age. *Pediatr Pulmonol* 2005; **40**:64–67.

19. Williams J, Griffiths PD, Green A, Weller PH. Sweat tests and flucloxacillin. *Arch Dis Child* 1988; **63**:847–848.

20. Gleeson M, Henry RL. Sweat sodium or chloride? *Clin Chem* 1991; **37**:112.

21. Green A, Dodds P, Pennock C. A study of sweat sodium and chloride; criteria for the diagnosis of cystic fibrosis. *Ann Clin Biochem* 1985; **22**(Pt 2):171–174.

22. Farrell PM, Koscik RE. Sweat chloride concentrations in infants homozygous or heterozygous for F508 cystic fibrosis. *Pediatrics* 1996; **97**:524–528.

23. Mickle JE, Macek MJ, Fulmer-Smentek SB *et al.* A mutation in the cystic fibrosis transmembrane conductance regulator gene associated with elevated sweat chloride concentrations in the absence of cystic fibrosis. *Hum Mol Genet* 1998; **7**:729–735.

24. Mastella G, Di Cesare G, Borruso A *et al.* Reliability of sweat-testing by the Macroduct collection method combined with conductivity analysis in comparison with the classic Gibson and Cooke technique. *Acta Paediatr* 2000; **89**:933–937.

25. Heeley ME, Woolf DA, Heeley AF. Indirect measurements of sweat electrolyte concentration in the laboratory diagnosis of cystic fibrosis. *Arch Dis Child* 2000; **82**:420–424.

26. Lezana JL, Vargas MH, Karam-Bechara J *et al.* Sweat conductivity and chloride titration for cystic fibrosis diagnosis in 3834 subjects. *J Cyst Fibros* 2003; **2**:1–7.

27. Kerem B, Rommens JM, Buchanan JA *et al.* Identification of the cystic fibrosis gene: genetic analysis. *Science* 1989; **245**:1073–1080.

28. Stewart B, Zabner J, Shuber AP *et al.* Normal sweat chloride values do not exclude the diagnosis of cystic fibrosis. *Am J Respir Crit Care Med* 1995; **151**(3 Pt 1):899–903.

29. Highsmith WE, Burch LH, Zhou Z *et al.* A novel mutation in the cystic fibrosis gene in patients with pulmonary disease but normal sweat chloride concentrations. *N Engl J Med* 1994; **331**:974–980.

30. Rosenstein BJ. Diagnosis. In: Hodson M, Geddes D (eds) *Cystic Fibrosis.* London, Arnold, 2000.

31. Mekus F, Ballmann M, Bronsveld I *et al.* Cystic-fibrosis-like disease unrelated to the cystic fibrosis transmembrane conductance regulator. *Hum Genet* 1998; **102**:582–586.

32. Groman JD, Meyer ME, Wilmott RW *et al.* Variant cystic fibrosis phenotypes in the absence of CFTR mutations. *N Engl J Med* 2002; **347**:401–407.

33. Wallis C. Atypical cystic fibrosis: diagnostic and management dilemmas. *J R Soc Med* 2003; **96**(Suppl 43):2–10.

34. Merlo CA, Boyle MP. Modifier genes in cystic fibrosis lung disease. *J Lab Clin Med* 2003; **141**:237–241.

35. Drumm ML, Konstan MW, Schluchter MD *et al.* Genetic modifiers of lung disease in cystic fibrosis. *N Engl J Med* 2005; **353**:1443–1453.

36. Zielenski J, Corey M, Rozmahel R *et al.* Detection of a cystic fibrosis modifier locus for meconium ileus on human chromosome 19q13. *Nat Genet* 1999; **22**:128–129.

37. Haston CK, Hudson TJ. Finding genetic modifiers of cystic fibrosis. *N Engl J Med* 2005; **353**:1509–1511.

38. Schechter MS. Non-genetic influences on cystic fibrosis lung disease: the role of sociodemographic characteristics, environmental exposures, and healthcare interventions. *Semin Respir Crit Care Med* 2003; **24**:639–652.

39. Kosorok M, Zeng L, West S *et al.* Acceleration of lung disease in children with cystic fibrosis after *Pseudomonas aeruginosa* acquisition. *Pediatr Pulmonol* 2001; **32**:277–287.

40. Boyle MP. Nonclassic cystic fibrosis and CFTR-related diseases. *Curr Opin Pulmon Med* 2003; **9**:498–503.

41. Boyle MP. Unique presentations and chronic complications in adult cystic fibrosis: do they teach us anything about CFTR? *Respir Res* 2000; **1**:133–135.

42. WHO/ICF(M)A/ECFTN. Classsification of cystic fibrosis and related disorders. *J Cyst Fibros* 2002; **1**:5–8.

43. Groman JD, Karczeski B, Sheridan M *et al.* Phenotypic and genetic characterization of patients with features of 'nonclassic' forms of cystic fibrosis. *J Pediatr* 2005; **146**:675–680.

44. Brody AS, Tiddens HA, Castile RG *et al.* Computed tomography in the evaluation of cystic fibrosis lung disease. *Am J Respir Crit Care Med* 2005; **172**:1246–1252.

45. Wallis C, Leung T, Cubitt D, Reynolds A. Stool elastase as a diagnostic test for pancreatic function in children with cystic fibrosis. *Lancet* 1997; **350**:1001–1002

46. Stein J, Jung M, Sziegoleit A *et al.* Immunoreactive elastase I: clinical evaluation of a new non-invasive test of pancreatic function. *Clin Chem* 1996; **42**:222–226.

47. Kori M, Maayan-Metzger A, Shamir R *et al.* Fecal elastase 1 levels in premature and full-term infants. *Arch Dis Child* 2003; **88**:F106–F108.

48. Denning CR, Sommers SC, Quigley HJ. Infertility in male patients with cystic fibrosis. *Pediatrics* 1968; **41**:7–17.

49. Kaplan E, Shwachman H, Perlmutter AD *et al.* Reproductive failure in males with cystic fibrosis. *N Engl J Med* 1968; **279**:65–69.

50. Noone PG, Pue CA, Zhou Z *et al.* Lung disease associated with the IVS8 5T allele of the CFTR gene. *Am J Respir Crit Care Med* 2000; **162**:1919–1924.

51. Kiesewetter S, Macek M, Davis C *et al.* A mutation in CFTR produces different phenotypes depending on chromosomal background. *Nat Genet* 1993; **5**:274–278.

52. Blau H, Freud E, Mussaffi H *et al.* Urogenital abnormalities in male children with cystic fibrosis. *Arch Dis Child* 2002; **87**:135–138.

53. Gustafsson PM, Aurora P, Lindblad A. Evaluation of ventilation maldistribution as an early indicator of lung disease in children with cystic fibrosis. *Eur Respir J* 2003; **22**:972–979.

54. Aurora P, Gustafsson P, Bush A *et al.* Multiple breath inert gas washout as a measure of ventilation distribution in children with cystic fibrosis. *Thorax* 2004; **59**:1068–1073.

55. Alton EW, Currie D, Logan-Sinclair R *et al.* Nasal potential difference: a clinical diagnostic test for cystic fibrosis. *Eur Respir J* 1990; **3**:922–926.

56. Knowles MR, Paradiso AM, Boucher RC. In-vivo nasal potential difference: techniques and protocols for assessing efficacy of gene transfer in cystic fibrosis. *Hum Gene Ther* 1995; **6**:445–455.

57. Middleton PG, Geddes DM, Alton EW. Protocols for in-vivo measurement of the ion transport defects in cystic fibrosis nasal epithelium. *Eur Respir J* 1994; **7**:2050–2056.

58. Standaert TA, Boitano L, Emerson J *et al.* Standardized procedure for measurement of nasal potential difference: an outcome measure in multicenter cystic fibrosis clinical trials. *Pediatr Pulmonol* 2004; **37**:385–392.

59. Southern KW, Noone PG, Bosworth DG *et al.* A modified technique for measurement of nasal transepithelial potential difference in infants. *J Pediatr* 2001; **139**:353–358.

60. Wilson DC, Ellis L, Zielenski J *et al.* Uncertainty in the diagnosis of cystic fibrosis: possible role of in-vivo nasal potential difference measurements. *J Pediatr* 1998; **132**:596–599.

61. Fajac I, Hubert D, Guillemot D *et al.* Nasal airway ion transport is linked to the cystic fibrosis phenotype in adult patients. *Thorax* 2004; **59**:971–976.

62. Greger R. Role of CFTR in the colon. *Annu Rev Physiol* 2000; **62**:467–491.

63. Mall M, Kreda SM, Mengos A *et al.* The deltaF508 mutation results in loss of CFTR function and mature protein in native human colon. *Gastroenterology* 2004; **126**:32–41.

64. Wallis C. Diagnosis and presentation of cystic fibrosis. In: Chernick V, Boat TF, Wilmott RW, Bush A (eds) *Kendig's Disorders of the Respiratory Tract in Children*. 7th edn. Saunders Elsevier, 2006.

The challenge of screening newborn infants for cystic fibrosis

KEVIN W. SOUTHERN

INTRODUCTION

Screening newborn infants for cystic fibrosis (CF) provides two opportunities: (a) to prevent the long and sometimes traumatic journey to a diagnosis [1–3], and (b) to provide information for parents to enable them to make informed choices about future pregnancies [4,5]. Whether screening improves the clinical outcome for a child with CF is less clear [6–9]. The pathogenesis of CF lung disease suggests this is an ideal condition to benefit from the introduction of early proactive treatment [10], but two randomized controlled trials of newborn screening (NBS) have not shown clear long-term benefit for clinical outcomes [6,11]. In fact one study reports worse chest radiograph appearances in screened infants associated with earlier acquisition of *Pseudomonas aeruginosa* [7]. In addition, the process of NBS can cause anxiety through recognition of carriers and distress from poor handling of the result [8,12,13]. It is imperative, therefore, that NBS programs for CF are run efficiently with a view to minimizing unnecessary negative outcomes. Strategies to reduce negative outcomes will be discussed in this chapter.

Expectations have changed with regard to long-term survival and quality of life for people with CF [14]. Factors, such as the relationship between early nutritional well-being and cognitive function, are increasingly pertinent [15,16]. The argument for NBS for CF must be examined with a view to the changing outlook for infants born with CF.

THE EVIDENCE BASE FOR NEWBORN SCREENING

Randomized controlled trials

In 1985, two randomized controlled trials were commenced to examine the impact of newborn screening on clinical outcomes in children with CF. The first study screened infants across a large region of the UK on an alternate week basis [6]. Fifty-eight children were diagnosed with CF following screening. At 4 years of age they did not demonstrate significant differences in clinical outcomes compared to 44 children diagnosed following a clinical presentation (including nine who were missed by screening). The number of non-screened children diagnosed with CF was significantly lower than those recognized by screening and raises the question of incomplete case recognition (i.e. cases of CF remain unrecognized). In addition, screened infants who were not recognized to have CF (false negatives) until they presented clinically were analyzed as part of the non-screened group, making this a study of early versus late diagnosis rather than the screening intervention (this type of analysis should, however, bias in favor of screening). Four children in the non-screened cohort died from complications of CF compared to none in the screened cohort [6]. Further analysis, after ten years, confirms this to be a statistically significant difference – although the authors express caution in interpreting this result given the small numbers involved, and the fact that two of these children were diagnosed before 8 weeks (the median age of diagnosis of the screened infants) suggesting that NBS may not have altered the course of their disease [17].

The second study was based in Wisconsin, USA, and involved screening infants on an alternate basis (with results from the control samples stored until the children were 4 years of age) [11]. Screened infants were diagnosed at a mean age of 12 weeks. This is later than most NBS programs report (possibly as responsibility for organizing the sweat test was with the parents), but significantly earlier than with non-screened infants (mean 72 weeks). Screened infants had significantly better nutritional parameters at diagnosis, which were maintained over the first 4 years [11]. This is considered the most compelling argument for NBS, particularly in view of the close relationship between

Table 8.1 Publications resulting from the Wisconsin newborn screening project.

Year	Journal	First author	Primary outcome	Result	Comment
1992	J Dev Behav Pediatr	Tluczek	Parental concern following false positive result	Most, but not all, relieved by negative sweat test	Not to contact by telephone and follow up results
1997	Pediatrics	Farrell	Acquisition of PA	NSD between Sc and non-Sc	Center affect with increased acquisition in urban area
1997 [11]	N Engl J Med	Farrell	Height, weight and head circumference	Higher at diagnosis in Sc	Screening significantly reduced the odds of being below 10th centile for weight or height
1998 [62]	Pediatrics	Mischler	Reproductive behavior	No impact from screening	Misconceptions about increased risks
2001	Pediatrics	Farrell	Nutritional status	Results remain significant in favor of screening	Unblinding and complete identification of non-Sc children
2003 [7]	Am J Respir Crit Care Med	Farrell	Chest radiograph appearances	Significantly better at diagnosis in Sc, but then worse in Sc children at 10 years	Associated with earlier acquisition of PA. No difference in RFTs
2004 [15]	Pediatrics	Koscik	Cognitive function	NSD between Sc and non-Sc	Children with lower vitamin E levels at diagnosis had poorer cognitive function
2005 [13]	Pediatrics	Tluczek	Psychosocial risk associated with sweat test	Significantly higher scores on depression scale during wait for ST	Linked with knowledge of CF and promptness of ST
2005 [16]	J Pediatr	Koscik	Cognitive function	NSD between Sc and non-Sc. Positive correlation between vitamin E level at diagnosis and cognitive function	Results maybe affected by increased number of pancreatic-sufficient patients in non-Sc group
2005	J Pediatr	Koscik	Quality of life (QoL) as assessed by Child Health Questionnaire	NSD in QoL between Sc and non-SC children	Child Health Questionnaire probably not appropriate tool

PA, *Pseudomonas aeruginosa*; NSD, no significant difference; Sc, screened; RFTs, respiratory function tests; ST, sweat test.

vitamin E level at diagnosis and subsequent cognitive function [16]. However, this study did not demonstrate advantage regarding cognitive function in the screened group [15].

A number of publications have resulted from the Wisconsin NBS project (Table 8.1) and these have provided much information on NBS as well as the natural history of CF in the early years of childhood. Of concern has been the increased incidence of *Pseudomonas aeruginosa* lung infection in the screened infants with a trend towards worsening chest radiograph appearances [7]. It has been suggested that this may relate to a relative lack of patient segregation in one of the Wisconsin CF centers. However, taken overall, the children in this study have good respiratory function and there is no difference in forced expiratory volume in one second (FEV_1) between the screened and non-screened children [7,18].

Evidence from other studies

A number of groups have compared clinical outcomes in children who were screened with historical controls prior to screening [19]. Researchers from New South Wales in Australia have presented sequential data on a cohort of screened and non-screened children [20,21]. In the most recent review (at 15 years of age), the screened children had significantly improved respiratory function and chest radiograph scores, although there was no difference in nutritional status [21]. Data from this type of study are helpful, but need to be assessed with caution as the outlook ____ ____ over time, and this will potentially

... comes ... ermin- ... ed the ... n [22]. ... impro- ... ates of ... natched ... e partic- ... [7]. This ... t burden ... tly fewer

... c Fibrosis ... lemiolog- ... sor), have ... al studies ... this work ... association ... term respi- ... t examina- ... ining early ... ethos of CF ... BS becomes ... e an impor- ... f these pro- ... nts have the ... tabase.

...OSIS

... identified that ... munoreactive ... st week of life ... ken on a blood spot card, which ... dovetail with established NBS programs for phenylketonuria and congenital hypothyroidism [30]. A raised IRT in the first week of life is a sensitive test for CF, but is not specific [31]. It would not be feasible to sweat test all infants identified at this point; the amount of anxiety generated would be disproportionate and the logistics impractical. A second IRT measurement at 4 weeks of age is more specific as there is a natural decline in IRT [32]. Consequently a two-tier (IRT/IRT) system was implemented by many screening centers across the world with varied success [6,33–35]. A number of NBS programs began to incorporate recognition of the commonest CF mutation (*F508del*) in the second tier of their NBS programs (in order to improve specificity and

reduce the time to diagnosis in those infants with two ΔF508 mutations) [36–38]. Other *CFTR* mutations occur at significant frequency in populations and have subsequently been included in most programs. A number of reports have suggested that incorporating gene analysis into the screening program has improved performance [39], but there are no randomized controlled trials comparing IRT/IRT versus IRT/DNA [40]. A consequence of employing DNA testing in the second tier is the recognition of carriers. Families in this position require counselling as to the implications for them and the child [41]. In addition, as there are over 1000 mutations of the *CFTR* gene, the possibility that the child has a second unrecognized mutation needs to be addressed and CF excluded. This is discussed in the next section on reducing harm.

Researchers in France have proposed measuring the concentration of pancreatitis-associated protein (PAP), which is raised in the blood of CF infants [42,43]. They measured PAP from samples obtained through the French NBS program in CF infants with raised IRT. They suggest cut-offs for IRT and PAP that would provide the necessary sensitivity and specificity to avoid DNA analysis (and subsequent carrier recognition); however, there are insufficient population data to draw these conclusions at present and certainly no data to suggest that PAP is a better initial screen than IRT. A number of other potential screening tests have been described (Table 8.2), but at present IRT measurement in the first week of life remains the first part of all screening programs around the world [44].

AVOIDING HARM FROM NEWBORN SCREENING

There is now an evidence base to support newborn screening for CF. Previously NBS programs have generally been established on a regional basis, relying on enthusiastic support from a team or individual. Pioneers of CF NBS are often passionate in their advocacy. However, there is potential for incurring significant harm from a CF NBS program. Four main areas of potential harm will be considered in this section. Table 8.3 summarizes strategies to reduce potential harm.

The sweat test

Sweat testing an infant identified through the NBS program is a time of acute and extreme anxiety for parents and other family members [13,45]. Two straightforward ways of reducing stress are to ensure that the test is performed promptly (preferably the day after the parents have received the preliminary screening result) and that the result is available the same day. Although straightforward on paper, in practical terms the logistics can be extremely challenging, particularly in geographically widespread regions. Sweat tests need to be undertaken in centers with adequate

Table 8.2 Screening tests for CF.

Test	Sensitivity[a]	Specificity[a]	Comments
Echogenic bowel on antenatal ultrasound	Not known	Poor	An increasing issue as ultrasonography improves technically
Immunoreactive trypsinogen (week 1 of life)	Excellent	Poor	The universal 'first step' in CF NBS programs
Immunoreactive trypsinogen (weeks 3–4)	Less good	Better	More specific but may miss some index cases
Pancreatitis-associated protein	Excellent	Not known	More information needed to assess potential
Stool meconium albumin (increased albumin in CF)	Reasonable	Poor	Not adequate for stand-alone testing
Stool meconium lactase (increased lactase in CF)	Reasonable	Good	Requires good-quality sample of meconium
DNA analysis (for four commonest *CFTR* mutations)	Good	Excellent	Recognition of carriers
DNA analysis (for 30 commonest *CFTR* mutations)	Good	Excellent	Increased carrier recognition with minimal improvement in sensitivity

[a] For the purposes of this table, sensitivity is considered the ability of the test to recognize cases of CF and specificity, the ability not to incorrectly identify non-CF cases. Positive predictive value varies between programs and populations and is not included. Excellent sensitivity and specificity are required to comply with the principles of the 1968 WHO screening criteria [65]. NBS, newborn screening.

Table 8.3 Strategies to reduce the negative impact of CF NBS.

Strategy	Rationale	Practicalities
Increase cut-off level set for initial IRT measurement	Reduces recognition of carriers and ST referrals	In some areas with a diverse population may reduce case recognition
Restrict number of *CFTR* mutations examined for on initial panel	Reduces recognition of carriers and ST referrals	May reduce efficiency of second-tier testing to recognize cases (unlikely)
Repeat IRT measurement at 21–28 days if only one mutation recognized on initial DNA analysis	Only high-risk cases taken forward to ST, therefore reduces anxiety associated with ST	Does not reduce carrier recognition and may result in an increase in unrecognized cases
Engage parents/carers in the process of CF NBS	Enables parents to make informed choices about the health welfare of their infant	Significant resource implications to primary care. Change in culture needed
Ensure a smooth interface between the screening result and the family	Reduce anxiety associated with ST. Possibly reduce long-term psychological distress	There is no 'painless' method of delivering a positive CF NBS result but there are ways of making the situation much worse

ST, sweat test; NBS, newborn screening.

experience and where the families can be counselled after the test [46–49].

It has been suggested that a sweat test is unnecessary in infants in whom two *CFTR* mutations are recognized, but there is a strong argument for physiological confirmation of this molecular result. In addition, undertaking the sweat test may have some benefit from a psychological perspective in providing the parents with confirmatory evidence of the diagnosis. In the UK National Programme (due to be implemented in 2006), it was agreed that the family would be approached by their community nurse (who should be familiar to them), supported by a CF Nurse Specialist if necessary. A sweat test will have already been arranged for the following day. An information sheet is given to the family that evening explaining the screening process and how the sweat test will be undertaken. The aim is not to overwhelm the family with information at this stage.

Approved websites are highlighted should they wish to search for further information.

Another strategy to reduce the number of infants who require sweat testing is to reduce the level of IRT that prompts second-level testing. For example, if infants with the top 5% of IRT levels are taken forward to the second tier of testing more will require a sweat test than if the cut-off is placed at the top 0.5%. Measuring immunoreactive trypsinogen from blood spot cards is not straightforward. A good-quality blood spot sample is required and, at present, no quality control product is available to verify the accuracy of the IRT assay [50]. It is important that regions review their IRT results regularly and adjust their cut-offs accordingly to avoid unnecessary referrals for sweat testing or a reduction in the sensitivity of the program. Generally, the level of referral to the second tier is set above the 99.5th centile for results in that laboratory.

A number of CF NBS programs adopt a fail-safe mechanism to avoid missing CF infants with no common *CFTR* mutation (which might be the case in a child from a non-Caucasian background). Infants with very high initial IRT (for example over the 99.9th centile) who do not have a recognized *CFTR* mutation are taken through to the second tier of testing (further DNA analysis and repeat IRT). However, recent data reported from Victoria, Australia, suggest that this strategy does not result in a significant increase in case recognition in their population, regardless of how high the IRT threshold is set [51].

Identification of carriers

Any NBS program that incorporates DNA analysis will recognize carriers. Advances in molecular genetics mean that DNA panels will become available to examine for increasing numbers of *CFTR* mutations. The temptation is to incorporate a panel with as many mutations as possible. However, data suggest that the benefits from case recognition are soon outweighed by the negative impact of increased carrier recognition [40,52]. For example, increasing the number of mutations from one to four may increase recognition of cases from 87% to 95% (numbers will vary depending on the population). A panel for 30 mutations may increase recognition of cases only to 96%, but would significantly increase the number of carriers recognized. Increasing the panel to 100 or even a 1000 would have negligible impact on case recognition but would again increase carrier recognition. That carriers probably have higher IRT levels in the first week of life will exacerbate the problem (more than expected are recognized by the NBS program) [36,53,54]. In the UK, the screening program center has moved to a four-mutation panel as the initial screen for infants with a raised IRT. Infants with one mutation recognized will have this result confirmed by a further panel that incorporates a larger number of mutations (29 or 30 depending on local population).

Although carrier recognition is generally considered something that should be avoided, the counter argument is that this information empowers couples to make informed reproductive decisions [55]. In a study in New York, parents of carriers were randomized to receive standard information or special counselling. Only a small number participated but significantly more in the 'special' group opted for further genetic testing [56]. In time the general population may be more inclined to know their carrier status, but at present the evidence does not suggest this is the case [57].

Infants in whom one mutation is recognized will require a further test to exclude CF. Generally this is a sweat test, but in the UK a second IRT is being undertaken at between 21 and 28 days of life. At this point the IRT is a more specific test and only those infants with a raised second IRT are referred for sweat testing and clinical assessment [58]. Parents of infants with a low second IRT require information regarding the carrier status of their infant, the

implications for them and their family, and the fact that CF has not been excluded in their infant. This information sheet is available at the NBS Programme Centre website (www.ich.ucl.ac.uk/newborn/). By adopting the policy of undertaking a second IRT on children with one recognized mutation, the number of sweat tests and accompanying anxiety needed is reduced. However, some monitoring of how successful this protocol is in reducing anxiety will be needed.

Identification of non-paternity

Newborn screening programs that incorporate DNA will result in the occasional recognition of a gene abnormality in the infant that does not belong to either putative parent. For this reason, it is important that parents be engaged in the whole process of screening and understand the implications [59,60]. It has been highlighted in the screening literature that simply signing a card does not mean that parents appreciate the complexities of the process [8]. In the UK, parents are offered the choice of opting out of the CF NBS program.

Long-term psychological morbidity from the result

There are a lack of data regarding the long-term psychological morbidity from newborn screening and this is an area that requires study. There is some evidence to suggest that parents of infants in whom a diagnosis is excluded may have long-term anxieties and misunderstanding regarding the result [41,45,61]. This may have a negative impact on their relationship with their child. Cascade screening (in which a family gains information on carrier status through an index case) may have a positive impact on reproductive decisions, but this can also be a cause of family tensions with blame and denial [55]. The services of clinical genetics in providing clear and empathetic counselling are imperative. Finally the impact of the screening process on the family of a child recognized to have CF needs to be considered [1,13,62]. Although the family may be grateful for the opportunity of early intervention, they are now faced with the realization that their child has a life-long and potentially life-shortening condition. CF teams and carers need to be aware of the needs of these families who will be faced with the psychological tension of waiting for things to happen. It is important that these families be provided with a clear pathway and support [63,64].

SUMMARY

There are good reasons to screen newborn infants for CF. In the current climate of improving outlook, it seems incongruous to delay a diagnosis with the negative impact on nutritional status and stress for families. However, there is no perfect screening test for CF; and although relatively straightforward, there are a number of inherent complexities in CF NBS. It is important that all possible measures be taken to avoid negative outcomes and that parents/carers be engaged in the process. A screening program for CF requires clear and efficient pathways between numerous disciplines. In addition there must be a smooth interface between the screening result and the family. The challenges are not insurmountable and the risk–benefit balance is now leaning well towards screening infants for cystic fibrosis.

ACKNOWLEDGMENTS

The author thanks Rodney Pollitt for assistance with difficult data and concepts, and David Heaf and Elinor Burrows for comments on the contents of the chapter.

REFERENCES

1. Merelle ME, Huisman J, Alderden-van der Vecht A *et al*. Early versus late diagnosis: psychological impact on parents of children with cystic fibrosis. *Pediatrics* 2003; **111**:346–350.

2. Campbell PW, White TB. Newborn screening for cystic fibrosis: an opportunity to improve care and outcomes. *J Pediatr* 2005; **147**(3 Suppl):S2–S5.

3. Kharrazi M, Kharrazi LD. Delayed diagnosis of cystic fibrosis and the family perspective. *J Pediatr* 2005; **147**(3 Suppl):S21–S25.

4. Scotet V, de Braekeleer M, Roussey M *et al*. Neonatal screening for cystic fibrosis in Brittany, France: assessment of 10 years' experience and impact on prenatal diagnosis. *Lancet* 2000; **356**:789–794.

5. Pollitt R. Neonatal screening for cystic fibrosis: early diagnosis is important to parents even if it makes little difference to outcome. *Br Med J* 1998; **317**:411–412.

6. Chatfield S, Owen G, Ryley HC *et al*. Neonatal screening for cystic fibrosis in Wales and the West Midlands: clinical assessment after five years of screening. *Arch Dis Child* 1991; **66**(1 Spec No.):29–33.

7. Farrell PM, Li Z, Kosorok MR *et al*. Bronchopulmonary disease in children with cystic fibrosis after early or delayed diagnosis. *Am J Respir Crit Care Med* 2003; **168**:1100–1108.

8. Wilfond BS, Parad RB, Fost N. Balancing benefits and risks for cystic fibrosis newborn screening: implications for policy decisions. *J Pediatr* 2005; **147**(3 Suppl):S109–S113.

9. Farrell PM, Lai HJ, Li Z *et al*. Evidence on improved outcomes with early diagnosis of cystic fibrosis through neonatal screening: enough is enough! *J Pediatr* 2005; **147**(3 Suppl):S30–S36.

10. Boucher RC. New concepts of the pathogenesis of cystic fibrosis lung disease. *Eur Respir J* 2004; **23**:146–158.

11. Farrell PM, Kosorok MR, Laxova A *et al*. for the Wisconsin Cystic Fibrosis Neonatal Screening Study Group. Nutritional benefits of neonatal screening for cystic fibrosis. *N Engl J Med* 1997; **337**:963–969.

12. Comeau AM, Parad R, Gerstle R *et al*. Challenges in implementing a successful newborn cystic fibrosis screening program. *J Pediatr* 2005; **147**(3 Suppl):S89–S93.

13. Tluczek A, Koscik RL, Farrell PM, Rock MJ. Psychosocial risk associated with newborn screening for cystic fibrosis: parents' experience while awaiting the sweat-test appointment. *Pediatrics* 2005; **115**:1692–1703.

14. Davis PB. Cystic fibrosis since 1938. *Am J Respir Crit Care Med* 2005; **173**:475–482.

15. Koscik RL, Farrell PM, Kosorok MR *et al*. Cognitive function of children with cystic fibrosis: deleterious effect of early malnutrition. *Pediatrics* 2004; **113**:1549–1558.

16. Koscik RL, Lai HJ, Laxova A *et al*. Preventing early, prolonged vitamin E deficiency: an opportunity for better cognitive outcomes via early diagnosis through neonatal screening. *J Pediatr* 2005; **147**(3 Suppl):S51–S56.

17. Doull IJ, Ryley HC, Weller P, Goodchild MC. Cystic fibrosis-related deaths in infancy and the effect of newborn screening. *Pediatr Pulmonol* 2001; **31**:363–366.

18. Farrell PM, Li Z, Kosorok MR *et al*. Longitudinal evaluation of bronchopulmonary disease in children with cystic fibrosis. *Pediatr Pulmonol* 2003; **36**:230–240.

19. Dankert-Roelse JE, Merelle ME. Review of outcomes of neonatal screening for cystic fibrosis versus non-screening in Europe. *J Pediatr* 2005; **147**(3 Suppl):S15–S20.

20. Waters DL, Wilcken B, Irwing L *et al*. Clinical outcomes of newborn screening for cystic fibrosis. *Arch Dis Child* 1999; **80**:F1–F7.

21. McKay KO, Waters DL, Gaskin KJ. The influence of newborn screening for cystic fibrosis on pulmonary outcomes in new South Wales. *J Pediatr* 2005; **147**(3 Suppl):S47–S50.

22. Sims EJ, McCormick J, Mehta G, Mehta A. Neonatal screening for cystic fibrosis is beneficial even in the context of modern treatment. *J Pediatr* 2005; **147**(3 Suppl):S42–S46.

23. Sims EJ, McCormick J, Mehta G, Mehta A. Newborn screening for cystic fibrosis is associated with reduced treatment intensity. *J Pediatr* 2005; **147**:306–311.

24. Zemel BS, Jawad AF, FitzSimmons S, Stallings VA. Longitudinal relationship among growth, nutritional status, and pulmonary function in children with cystic fibrosis: analysis of the Cystic Fibrosis Foundation National CF Patient Registry. *J Pediatr* 2000; **137**:374–380.

25. Emerson J, Rosenfeld M, McNamara S *et al*. *Pseudomonas aeruginosa* and other predictors of mortality and morbidity in young children with cystic fibrosis. *Pediatr Pulmonol* 2002; **34**:91–100.

26. Wang SS, O'Leary LA, Fitzsimmons SC, Khoury MJ. The impact of early cystic fibrosis diagnosis on pulmonary function in children. *J Pediatr* 2002; **141**:804–810.

27. Konstan MW, Butler SM, Wohl ME *et al*. Growth and nutritional indexes in early life predict pulmonary function in cystic fibrosis. *J Pediatr* 2003; **142**:624–630.

28. Rosenfeld M. Overview of published evidence on outcomes with early diagnosis from large US observational studies. *J Pediatr* 2005; **147**(Suppl):S11–S14.

29. Lai HJ, Cheng Y, Farrell PM. The survival advantage of patients with cystic fibrosis diagnosed through neonatal

screening: evidence from the United States Cystic Fibrosis Foundation registry data. *J Pediatr* 2005; **147**(3 Suppl):S57–S63.

30. Crossley JR, Elliott RB, Smith PA. Dried-blood spot screening for cystic fibrosis in the newborn. *Lancet* 1979; 1:472–474.

31. Wesley AW, Smith PA, Elliott RB. Experience with neonatal screening for cystic fibrosis in New Zealand using measurement of immunoreactive trypsinogen. *Aust Paediatr J* 1989; **25**(3):151–155.

32. Rock MJ, Mischler EH, Farrell PM *et al.* Newborn screening for cystic fibrosis is complicated by age-related decline in immunoreactive trypsinogen levels. *Pediatrics* 1990; **85**:1001–1007.

33. Henry RL, Boulton TJ, Roddick LG. False negative results on newborn screening for cystic fibrosis. *J Paediatr Child Health* 1990; **26**(3):150–151.

34. Massie RJ, Olsen M, Glazner J *et al.* Newborn screening for cystic fibrosis in Victoria: 10 years' experience (1989–1998). *Med J Aust* 2000; **172**:584–587.

35. Sontag MK, Hammond KB, Zielenski J *et al.* Two-tiered immunoreactive trypsinogen-based newborn screening for cystic fibrosis in Colorado: screening efficacy and diagnostic outcomes. *J Pediatr* 2005; **147**(3 Suppl):S83–S88.

36. Gregg RG, Wilfond BS, Farrell PM *et al.* Application of DNA analysis in a population-screening program for neonatal diagnosis of cystic fibrosis: comparison of screening protocols. *Am J Hum Genet* 1993; **52**:616–626.

37. Larsen J, Campbell S, Faragher EB *et al.* Cystic fibrosis screening in neonates: measurement of immunoreactive trypsin and direct genotype analysis for delta F508 mutation. *Eur J Pediatr* 1994; **153**:569–573.

38. Spence WC, Paulus-Thomas J, Orenstein DM, Naylor EW. Neonatal screening for cystic fibrosis: addition of molecular diagnostics to increase specificity. *Biochem Med Metab Biol* 1993; **49**:200–211.

39. Gregg RG, Simantel A, Farrell PM *et al.* Newborn screening for cystic fibrosis in Wisconsin: comparison of biochemical and molecular methods. *Pediatrics* 1997; **99**:819–824.

40. Pollitt RJ, Dalton A, Evans S *et al.* Neonatal screening for cystic fibrosis in the Trent region (UK): two-stage immunoreactive trypsin screening compared with a three-stage protocol with DNA analysis as an intermediate step. *J Med Screen* 1997; **4**(1):23–28.

41. Parsons EP, Clarke AJ, Bradley DM. Implications of carrier identification in newborn screening for cystic fibrosis. *Arch Dis Child* 2003; **88**:F467–F471.

42. Sarles J, Barthellemy S, Ferec C *et al.* Blood concentrations of pancreatitis associated protein in neonates: relevance to neonatal screening for cystic fibrosis. *Arch Dis Child* 1999; **80**:F118–F122.

43. Sarles J, Berthezene P, Le Louarn C *et al.* Combining immunoreactive trypsinogen and pancreatitis-associated protein assays, a method of newborn screening for cystic fibrosis that avoids DNA analysis. *J Pediatr* 2005; **147**:302–305.

44. Southern KW, Littlewood JM. Newborn screening programmes for cystic fibrosis. *Paediatr Respir Rev* 2003; **4**:299–305.

45. Parsons EP, Bradley DM. Psychosocial issues in newborn screening for cystic fibrosis. *Paediatr Respir Rev* 2003; 4:285–292.

46. Farrell PM, Koscik RE. Sweat chloride concentrations in infants homozygous or heterozygous for F508 cystic fibrosis. *Pediatrics* 1996; **97**:524–528.

47. Dillard JP, Carson CL, Bernard CJ *et al.* An analysis of communication following newborn screening for cystic fibrosis. *Health Commun* 2004; **16**:197–205.

48. Massie J, Clements B. Diagnosis of cystic fibrosis after newborn screening: the Australasian experience. Twenty years and five million babies later: a consensus statement from the Australasian Paediatric Respiratory Group. *Pediatr Pulmonol* 2005; **39**:440–446.

49. Parad RB, Comeau AM, Dorkin HL *et al.* Sweat testing infants detected by cystic fibrosis newborn screening. *J Pediatr* 2005; **147**(3 Suppl):S69–S72.

50. Heeley ME, Travert G, Ferre C, Lemonnier F. The international quality assurance program (IRTIQAS) for the assay of immunoreactive trypsin in dried blood spots. *Pediatr Pulmonol* 1991; **7**(Suppl):72–75.

51. Massie J, Curnow L, Tzanakos N *et al.* Markedly elevated neonatal immunoreactive trypsinogen levels in the absence of cystic fibrosis gene mutations is not an indication for further testing. *Arch Dis Child* 2006; **91**:222–225.

52. Comeau AM, Parad RB, Dorkin HL *et al.* Population-based newborn screening for genetic disorders when multiple mutation DNA testing is incorporated: a cystic fibrosis newborn screening model demonstrating increased sensitivity but more carrier detections. *Pediatrics* 2004; **113**:1573–1581.

53. Castellani C, Picci L, Scarpa M *et al.* Cystic fibrosis carriers have higher neonatal immunoreactive trypsinogen values than non-carriers. *Am J Med Genet A* 2005; **135**(2):142–144.

54. Scotet V, De Braekeleer M, Audrezet MP *et al.* Prevalence of CFTR mutations in hypertrypsinaemia detected through neonatal screening for cystic fibrosis. *Clin Genet* 2001; 59:42–47.

55. Super M. Cystic fibrosis newborn screening and detection of carriers. *Arch Dis Child* 2003; **88**:F448–F449.

56. Lagoe E, Labella S, Arnold G, Rowley PT. Cystic fibrosis newborn screening: a pilot study to maximize carrier screening. *Genet Test* 2005; **9**:255–260.

57. Clayton EW, Hannig VL, Pfotenhauer JP *et al.* Teaching about cystic fibrosis carrier screening by using written and video information. *Am J Hum Genet* 1995; **57**:171–181.

58. Pollitt RJ. Newborn screening for cystic fibrosis: science, legislation, and human values. *J Inherit Metab Dis* 2003; 26:725–727.

59. McCabe LL, McCabe ER. Genetic screening: carriers and affected individuals. *Annu Rev Genomics Hum Genet* 2004; 5:57–69.

60. Dhondt JL. Implementation of informed consent for a cystic fibrosis newborn screening program in France: low refusal rates for optional testing. *J Pediatr* 2005; **147**(3 Suppl):S106–S108.

61. Baroni MA, Anderson YE, Mischler E. Cystic fibrosis newborn screening: impact of early screening results on parenting stress. *Pediatr Nurs* 1997; **23**(2):143–151.

62. Mischler EH, Wilfond BS, Fost N *et al.* Cystic fibrosis newborn screening: impact on reproductive behavior and implications for genetic counseling. *Pediatrics* 1998; **102**(1 Pt 1):44–52.

63. Dillard JP, Tluczek A. Information flow after a positive newborn screening for cystic fibrosis. *J Pediatr* 2005; **147**(3 Suppl):S94–S97.

64. Comeau AM, Parad R, Gerstle R *et al.* Communications systems and their models: Massachusetts parent compliance with recommended specialty care after positive cystic fibrosis newborn screening result. *J Pediatr* 2005; **147**(3 Suppl):S98–S100.

65. Therrell BL, Lloyd-Puryear MA, Mann MY. Understanding newborn screening system issues with emphasis on cystic fibrosis screening. *J Pediatr* 2005; **147**(3 Suppl):S6–S10.

How to manage the screened patient

PHILIP ROBINSON

INTRODUCTION

Prior to the introduction of newborn screening for cystic fibrosis (CF) many families had spent considerable time and effort in accessing medical services seeking explanations for a myriad of symptoms which were often dismissed as infant colic, food allergies, wind, irritability, inexperienced parenting skills and other non-issues. The eventual diagnosis of CF in these families was often associated with feelings of great anger, and also justification on behalf of the parents that their concern over their infant's health had in fact been warranted.

In contrast, the diagnosis of CF by newborn screening may result in medical services contacting a family who have recently experienced the joy of welcoming a new child into their family with the news of the presence of a still often clinically silent, incurable and life-limiting condition. The method in which such a diagnosis is presented to the parents and family members in this setting is very important in determining how the family will cope over the sensitive next few months after diagnosis. In addition, as the family comes to terms with new treatments and aspects of their child's future that may well have been inconceivable or at least irrelevant prior to the diagnosis, the support from a well-trained and informed treatment team is vital.

All major pediatric CF treatment centers will spend considerable time planning not only how to introduce a diagnosis of CF to a new family but how to follow-up that diagnosis with education and support. At the Royal Children's Hospital in Melbourne, Australia, the CF unit supervises the care of approximately 340 children aged under 18 years with CF. A newly diagnosed education and support program was developed within the unit soon after the introduction of newborn screening for CF in the state of Victoria in April 1989. This program is outlined in general below. While other centers will have their own program, most will be similar in aiming to support and educate families with up-to-date and relevant material.

Inherent in this program is the understanding that the optimal treatment for a newly diagnosed infant with CF is provided by an experienced, multidisciplinary treatment team based at a major pediatric treatment center. This team, as a minimum, should involve a physician with experience in treating children with CF and with experience in at least both the gastroenterological and respiratory manifestations of CF. In addition, the team should include a trained pediatric physiotherapist, dietitian and clinic nurse, as well as a social worker or psychologist and genetic counsellor.

Life expectancy for children diagnosed by newborn screening is into the fifth decade. The way in which the diagnosis of CF is introduced to a family with an infant only several weeks old will set the scene for many years to come as to the acceptance of theories and suggestions from, and relationships between, the pediatric treatment team, the future adult treatment team, as well as between parents, siblings and infants. This education program therefore requires detailed planning to ensure a well-educated and empowered family.

DIAGNOSIS: INITIAL CONTACT

Once a newly diagnosed patient has been identified by the newborn screening laboratory, either as a result of an identified homozygous genotype or a positive sweat test in a compound heterozygote, a trained genetic counsellor will liaise with staff in the CF clinic about the new case. The decision is then made as to who will contact the family in the first instance, to raise the diagnosis and invite attendance at a meeting with the CF team, ideally for the following day. If, from the details provided with the newborn screening sample, an already involved medical officer such as a family doctor or consultant obstetrician is identified, the genetic counsellor may decide to approach those medical personnel to enquire whether they would be willing to pass on to the family the initial diagnosis. While this often means that the family is first approached by someone they are familiar with, and may trust, it is even more important that the first person to raise the diagnosis of CF made by newborn screening is well educated on current CF treatment and prognosis. The recent Victorian Government-initiated review of cystic fibrosis services in the state of Victoria (2001) highlighted that, in the state of Victoria (drainage population approximately 5 million persons, 65 000 live births per annum), one family doctor in ten would see one person with CF in his or her lifetime. These figures raise the possibility that a person, perhaps experienced with the family but inexperienced in the latest up-to-date information on CF, will be the first person to discuss CF with the family. For this reason preference is given for an experienced and well-trained genetic counsellor to first approach the family by phone and suggest follow-up with the CF treatment team the following day. If geographical issues permit a home visit from a hospital-based CF clinical nurse consultant in association with a local doctor the family is already familiar with, this may be an alternative way to introduce the diagnosis.

Once the diagnosis of cystic fibrosis has been presented to the family it is important to try to minimize the time before a face-to-face discussion occurs between members of the CF treatment team and the family. This will reduce the amount of disinformation that can be gained by families from out-of-date or misleading sources, such as medical information books in the local library, or the Internet. One of the most powerful tools that patients and families can access for education and support about CF is the Internet, but the many excellent and helpful websites providing this service are indistinguishable to the inexperienced from dangerous and misleading sites.

DIAGNOSIS: INITIAL DIAGNOSIS INTERVIEW

Experience would suggest that parents do not retain much of the information provided during this initial interview, as it is understandably a very stressful time [66]. Recognition of this stress means that staff involved in this initial interview should be prepared to go over information several times and should also provide only relevant basics at the first meeting. The treating physician and clinic coordinator or nurse are ideally the two staff members who should be involved in this first interview. It is important that parental education levels, prior parenting experience and cultural issues be taken into account by the CF team when planning how to initially explain the diagnosis of CF. The same factors must also be taken into account when constructing the time frame for any educational period that may follow. An explanation of the basics of genetic inheritance is important to include at this early stage, stressing that no 'blame'

should be directed at one parent compared to another. In addition, it is important to outline that CF does not occur as a result of any risk-taking behavior or other lifestyle issues. Smoking, alcohol intake or recreational drug usage during or before pregnancy is not related to the birth of a child with CF, but have all been used at times by families to try to blame the occurrence of CF on partners or themselves. The basic pathophysiology of CF with general details regarding respiratory and gastrointestinal involvement should also be provided at this first meeting.

At the initial diagnosis interview families should be invited to attend an educational period over several days to meet all members of the CF treatment team. During this period, members of the treatment team provide education to the family on current and planned therapies, as well as assess the individual child for the presence of any clinical manifestation of CF – including cough, wheeze, steattorhea, failure to thrive and salt depletion. The outline of one such education week plan is set out in Table 8.4.

While this education period serves mainly to educate and empower family members, it allows medical staff to recognize early clinical manifestation of CF and to initiate appropriate therapy. Many pediatric hospitals have residential facilities for families (so-called 'care-by-parent units'), which are ideal places for families to reside in during the education week. As the newly diagnosed infant is rarely acutely unwell, and is often clinically asymptomatic, it is unnecessary for the child to be admitted to an acute bed of the hospital. However, using a residential facility attached to the hospital means that, between consultations with members of the CF team, the parents and related siblings can have quiet time to allow the new infant to feed and rest in quiet surroundings. We have found this to be a valuable resource by removing the family from distractions at home such as work, enquiring friends, etc., and it allows the family to concentrate on learning about CF in general and the therapies required. In a recent review of our education program, the residential basis for the education week was appreciated even by families who were in close geographical proximity to the hospital [67]. Of the 15 families interviewed as part of this review, 89% reported that not having to travel was a significant advantage.

The usual time between the first diagnostic interview and the commencement of the education week should be as short as possible for reasons outlined above. It is certain, however, that no matter how short this time period most families will attempt to access additional information regarding CF. In an attempt to provide up-to-date and accurate information on CF, a kit of educational material should be provided to the family at the first interview when the diagnosis is raised. In our clinic, families are given an education kit consisting of a set of booklets developed both within our own unit and from international CF support agencies. They discuss the basics of cystic fibrosis and its treatment, with particular emphasis on issues surrounding diagnosis and infancy. In addition, a DVD/video developed by our unit discusses the basics of CF. We have found this education

Table 8.4 Outline of roles that various members of the CF care team play in the educational week for families of infants diagnosed by newborn screening, as used at the Royal Children's Hospital Melbourne, Australia.

Day 1	Physician	Answer questions from initial discussion. Query presence of any symptoms including diarrhea, abdominal discomfort, cough
	Counsellor	Provide program for week with appointment times and locations. Orient family to hospital
	Dietician	Assess nutritional status. Organize tests of pancreatic function (usually random stool or 3-day fecal fat analysis)
	Physiotherapist	Detailed respiratory assessment. Discuss role of physiotherapy and describe and demonstrate infant physiotherapy techniques. Teach the signs and symptoms of a respiratory exacerbation
Day 2	Counsellor	Discuss grief, coping and adjustment. Reinforce that the infant with CF is well, stress importance of normal parenting. Discuss marital and family dynamics including sibling relationships. Arrange CXR, blood tests
	Dietician	Review results of screening tests for fat absorption and commence pancreatic enzyme therapy if indicated. Educate on principles of pancreatic enzyme replacement dosing and administration
	Physiotherapist	Demonstrate and teach modified drainage and percussion techniques. Discuss physiotherapy in the home setting including timing with feeds, involvement of siblings and back care for carers
Day 3	Physician	Meet with family to answer questions. Discuss cross-infection issues. Offer meetings with grandparents and other family members. Contact local family doctor to discuss ongoing center-based care
	Counsellor	Discuss community-based resources. Contact maternal and child health nurse and send out information package
	Dietician	Discuss vitamin and salt replacement. Assess efficiency of supplement enzyme therapy clinically and with random stool test
	Physiotherapist	Review parents' techniques and discuss importance of exercise in future development
Day 4	Physician	If required meet with other family members including grandparents. Discuss genetic basis of disease and reassure that is not a lifestyle choice condition
	Counsellor	Introduce CF community team – nurse and physiotherapist
	Dietician	Review end of 3-day fecal fat results, if performed, and commence therapy if required or, if enzyme therapy commenced, assess weight gain and feeding pattern for evidence of improved absorption. Discuss basis for high-energy high-fat diet
	Physiotherapist	Review and refine parents' techniques
	Genetic counsellor	Revisit genetic basis of disease and arrange for blood testing of parents for genotype analysis. Discuss antenatal testing
	Community CF team	Introduce themselves to family and discuss role of community-based team. Set up first appointment for 1–2 weeks post-discharge
Day 5	Physician	Review outstanding issues. Discuss results of chest x-ray. Provide discharge medication. Reinforce concept of center-based care and encourage them to access team members at any time for information and advice. Contact local health providers including family doctor and primary pediatrician
	Counsellor	Arrange clinic appointment for 2–3 weeks. Advise importance of cohorting in clinics and attention to attending on correct outpatient day
	Other team members	As required, or requested by parents

pack to be invaluable in helping inform and educate other family members who did not attend the initial interview.

EDUCATION WEEK

There are two main aims to the education week. First, the family of the child needs to be educated about various aspects of the pathophysiology of CF, as well as the various therapies used. In addition, the medical team will need to spend time with the child and the family in assessing the specific CF phenotype that the child currently manifests. During the week, each member of the care team will introduce himself or herself and explain his/her role in CF treatments, and then spend time describing specifics of both pathophysiology and treatments in their relevant area of expertise. In addition, each member will assess the infant for the need for such therapies.

TEAM MEMBER ROLES

The physician

In discussing the diagnosis of CF with parents an important balance between over-supply of information and missing important facts is essential. In the first interview during the education week any questions that have arisen since the initial diagnosis interview can be answered. These questions may stem from information that was unclear from the educational material provided, or arise from questions raised by family members or other sources of information such as the Internet.

It is often necessary to set out early what is planned to be achieved in the education week. Parents will often, at this early stage, be keen to hear about research and discuss various 'cures' that they may have heard about or hope exist. By setting out that the education week is simply to inform parents about CF and its various therapies, the parents can be directed to make the best use of the time during the week.

An open approach is vitally important at this early stage and willingness to answer any queries raised helps develop trust and faith in the treating team. It is important to try to keep the parents focused on issues relevant to their own child and the recent diagnosis of CF – the relevant therapies and plans for follow-up. Subjects such as research that may have been conducted on the Internet should be recognized but not allowed to become the focus of the discussions. Subsequent meetings with parents during the week allow additional time to raise specific points such as cross-infection issues, and cohorting, if such practices are employed at the particular clinic. The offer to speak to other family members in a group is often welcomed by grandparents or family members who are also of reproductive age. To ensure that there is a common level of understanding through all family members, such discussions with extended family members are generally best done with the immediate family, particularly mother and father, present. At the end interview on day 5 the opportunity for the parents to ask questions is again raised and there is discussion regarding the importance of regular contact and follow-up.

While in many situations few or no respiratory symptoms or signs will be yet evident, respiratory assessment at this stage generally involves an assessment of lower airway pathogens and the commencement of anti-staphylococcal therapy – which is generally continued for the first 12 months of life. Our unit's previous work on lower respiratory infections and inflammation in the newly diagnosed screened group showed that there was a much higher level of lower airway bacterial infection than expected. In a group of 45 newly diagnosed infants (32 by newborn screening) who had a bronchoalveolar lavage at a mean age of 2.6 months, 15 bacterial infections were diagnosed, 14 of which involved *Staphylococcus aureus* [68].

The clinic coordinator or clinic nurse

Many centers have different roles for their clinical coordinator, who often have differing levels and types of training, ranging from trained nurse to social worker to academic psychologist. The role and extent of involvement in actual education about CF will depend on the specific training of the coordinator, but the major role will be one of support and advice for the family, as well as serving as the coordinator of the education week as a whole.

Counselling parents about the expected stresses and various emotions is an important role of the clinic coordinator. While possibly not having formal psychological or counselling training, an experienced CF coordinator should be able to discuss issues with parents and refer to more formal services if this is considered necessary.

The dietitian

While over 90% of adults and adolescents with CF have clinically apparent pancreatic insufficiency requiring supplemental pancreatic enzyme therapy, some infants diagnosed on newborn screening may have sufficient residual pancreatic exocrine function to have acceptable fat absorption at the time of diagnosis. Waters and co-workers [69], in their review of the New South Wales screening program, found that of 78 patients diagnosed over a 7-year period, 49 (63%) were clinically pancreatic-insufficient at diagnosis. Of the remaining 29 (37%), a further six (8%) developed pancreatic sufficiency over the following 4 years. Pancreatic insufficiency may already be clinically evident as diarrhea, abdominal cramping, irritability and failure to gain weight; if a screening test such a random fecal fat microscopy analysis confirms the presence of abnormal levels of fat globules, pancreatic enzyme therapy can be started immediately. In such cases, by the end of the education week, similar repeat tests can confirm the correction of steatorrhea and improvement of clinical symptoms of malabsorption. The dietitian will also spend time discussing the basics of the high-energy diet and educating parents about enzyme therapy dosing and administration.

Breast-feeding mothers may worry that the need to introduce enzyme therapy means that breast-feeding has to be discontinued. The dietitian can encourage and support the mother through the first few feedings to try to ensure that breast-feeding is continued. In situations where breast-feeding cannot be continued, parents should be assured that adequate nutrition for the CF infant is achievable using commercially available formulas with pancreatic enzyme supplementation if required.

Deficiencies of fat-soluble vitamins A, D, E and K have been demonstrated in pancreatic-insufficient individuals with CF, including infants diagnosed on newborn screening programs [70]. In a review of 127 infants diagnosed by the US CF newborn screening program in Colorado, deficiency of one or more fat-soluble vitamins was present in 44 of 96 patients (46%) at age 4–8 weeks. Vitamin A was deficient in 29% of cases, vitamin D in 23% and vitamin E in 23%. During the education week the dietitian should organize measurement of fat-soluble vitamins and commence therapy as necessary with an appropriate vitamin supplement.

The physiotherapist

Education, assessment and initiation of airway clearance and aerosol therapy are the main role of the physiotherapist during the education week. Discussion with the parents of the importance of regular airway clearance and how this can be achieved and adjusted with advancing childhood age is provided. Commencement of any required aerosol therapy during the education week allows for several sessions to familiarize both the infant and parents with this treatment. Information about cross-infection issues and care, and cleaning of equipment, can also be provided. The spectrum of future physiotherapy techniques – including the importance of regular exercise – is also raised at this early stage. Modified postural drainage techniques are introduced, and parents are encouraged to continue this for 20 minutes a day after discharge from the education week. This permits continued reinforcement of the technique to both the infant and parents. There is little evidence-based research available on the need for physiotherapy at this early stage.

The genetic counsellor

It is important for the genetic counsellor to be available in the education week to answer queries about the inherited basis for CF. Family members of child-bearing age may particularly wish to discuss the ramifications for, and options available for, themselves. In cases of compound heterozygotes diagnosed through follow-up sweat testing, the genetic counsellor can organize genotyping of parents to attempt to identify the second gene mutation. Siblings of newly diagnosed infants are generally recalled for a sweat test following the diagnosis; the genetic counsellor can explain why this is desirable, to ensure understanding of the inherited nature of cystic fibrosis.

The community CF team

Towards the end of the education week, introduction to the community-based CF team should be made. The team may include a nurse alone, or a nurse and physiotherapist will discuss with parents issues regarding CF treatment within the home and will organize a follow-up visit at home within 1–2 weeks of the end of the education week. It is important that the community team be introduced in the hospital setting, as this will reinforce to the family the concept of one CF treatment team across both hospital and community settings.

RESEARCH IN THE EDUCATION WEEK

Several centers initiate research projects in newly diagnosed patients from screening programs. It is important in this initial week to concentrate on educating and supporting the family rather than enrolling them in research programs. Many families will mistakenly believe that by enrolling in such research they may 'cure' their child, or at least be seen in a favorable light by the treatment team. Enrolment in research programs should not be raised until the family has a good understanding of CF and how it relates to their child. In addition, once a relationship has been established between the parents and the treatment team, a more informed and ethical acceptance, or decline, of involvement can be obtained.

While most centers obtain a standard anteroposterior chest X-ray of an infant during the educational week, some centers are increasingly utilizing high-resolution CT scans in young infants as a way of examining, in detail, any structural problems that may already be present. This procedure will usually involve a general anesthetic in order to ensure proper films are available during expiration where early air trapping may be evident. While some CT scans can be performed under sedation or even while the infant is asleep, these will not provide detailed information on air trapping and thus will be less helpful. Some centers will also perform infant lung function measurements on newly diagnosed babies; however, the information obtained from these studies, as well as from high-resolution CT scans, is yet to drive clinical therapy in any direction, and they are mostly seen as research tools. Some centers are keen to perform bronchoscopic alveolar lavage soon after the diagnosis of CF. Given that this procedure will require a general anesthetic, attempts to include it as part of the education week should be avoided if at all possible, to allow the parents to concentrate on learning about CF and how it clinically affects their child.

Enrolment in research projects should be raised at the earliest at the follow-up clinic appointment two weeks after the education week. While it is inappropriate to attempt to enroll families in research at this early stage, many families will be reassured to learn that the unit they are now attached to has an active research program, and a general discussion of current research, without any offer or inducement to enrol in such projects will be informative to many families.

REFERENCES

66. Jedlicka-Kohler I, Gotz M, Eichler I. Parents' recollection of the initial communication of the diagnosis of cystic fibrosis. *Pediatrics* 1996; **97**:204–209.

67. Sawyer S, Glazner J. What follows newborn screening? An evaluation of a residential education program for parents of infants with newly diagnosed cystic fibrosis. *Pediatrics* 2004; **114**:411–416.

68. Armstrong D, Grimwood K, Carzino R *et al.* Lower respiratory infection and inflammation in infants with newly diagnosed cystic fibrosis. *Br Med J* 1995; **310**:1571–1572.

69. Waters DL, Dorney SF, Gaskin KJ *et al.* Pancreatic function in infants identified as having cystic fibrosis in a neonatal screening program. *N Engl J Med* 1990; **322**:303–308.

70. Feranchak A, Sontag M, Wagener J *et al.* Prospective, long-term study of fat-soluble vitamin status in children with cystic fibrosis identified by newborn screening. *J Pediatr* 1999; **135**:601–610.

Microbiology of cystic fibrosis: role of the clinical microbiology laboratory, susceptibility and synergy studies and infection control

SAMIYA RAZVI AND LISA SAIMAN

The clinical microbiology laboratory plays an important role in CF care. Ongoing communication between the clinical laboratory and the CF care team is critical to provide effective care, institute appropriate infection control practices and further an understanding of the epidemiology of pathogens in CF patients. This chapter will review current recommendations for the processing of CF respiratory tract secretions by the clinical microbiology laboratory, the preferred methods of antimicrobial susceptibility testing, the potential role of synergy testing, infection control for CF, and strategies to strengthen interactions among the microbiology laboratory, the CF care team, and the infection control team.

CHANGING EPIDEMIOLOGY OF CF MICROBIOLOGY

An understanding of the changing epidemiology of CF microbiology is essential to justify appropriate, and often time-consuming and costly, laboratory processing. Traditional CF pathogens include *Haemophilus influenzae*, *Staphylococcus aureus* and *Pseudomonas aeruginosa*. Over the past two decades there has been an increasing understanding of the tremendous diversity of potentially emerging pathogens in CF. These emerging pathogens include intrinsically multidrug-resistant organisms such as the genomovars (phenotypically indistinguishable species) of *Burkholderia cepacia* complex, *Stenotrophomonas maltophilia*, *Achromobacter xylosoxidans*, methicillin-resistant *S. aureus* (MRSA), non-tuberculous mycobacteria (NTM), and moulds such as *Aspergillus* and *Scedosporium* spp. Additional potentially emerging pathogens include *Ralstonia* and *Pandoraea* spp [1].

LABORATORY PROCESSING OF CF RESPIRATORY TRACT SPECIMENS

Numerous steps are required to ensure appropriate processing of CF respiratory tract specimens. The CF care team should understand the advantages and disadvantages of various types of specimen, the types of selective media used and the need for prolonged incubation to ensure adequate detection of all potential pathogens. In many countries, quarterly cultures of the respiratory tract are the current standard of care for CF as more frequent cultures improve detection of potential pathogens.

Types and adequacy of respiratory tract specimens

The best respiratory specimen for diagnostic testing in CF patients has traditionally been expectorated sputum. In the 1980s, Thomassen and co-workers [2] showed 100% concordance between sputum cultures and thoracotomy specimens in 17 CF patients. Nearly two decades later, Jung and co-workers [3] performed genotyping of *P. aeruginosa* strains recovered from sputum versus bronchoalveolar lavage (BAL) from 38 CF patients and noted that the results of sputum specimens were concordant with those obtained from BAL. To optimize results from spontaneously expectorated sputum, at least 1 mL should be obtained in the early morning to ensure an adequate volume for plating on selective media as described below. Gram staining can be used to determine the adequacy of the specimen. If too many squamous epithelial cells are noted [>10 cells per high-powered field (100× magnification)], the sample most likely represents saliva and oropharyngeal organisms rather than sputum. The presence of polymorphonuclear (PMN) cells implies sputum and an inflammatory process.

In non-expectorating patients, an oropharyngeal (OP) culture can be obtained as either a deep throat culture or a cough swab. The technique for obtaining a deep throat culture is described as swabbing the posterior oropharyngeal wall and the tonsillar pillars with a cotton-tipped swab while avoiding contamination by contact with oral mucosa and saliva [4]. Obtaining a cough swab is described as placing a cotton-tipped swab stick in the posterior pharynx and asking the subject to cough while not touching the posterior pharynx [5,6]. Cough swabs have been found to detect CF pathogens in non-expectorating children, both asymptomatic (18/235 swabs, 8%) and symptomatic (22/87 swabs, 26%). Finally, investigators have also studied the potential utility of cough plates [7]. The technique for obtaining a cough plate is described as asking the patient to cough twice on to a blood agar plate. In a pilot study of 20 expectorating subjects, when compared with sputum, cough plates detected more potential pathogens than cough swabs (16 vs 7 patients, respectively). In addition, cough plates were more tolerable to patients than cough swabs. However, an important limitation of this study is that selective media were not used.

To assess the concordance of OP cultures with the lower airway, several studies have compared simultaneous BAL (considered the 'gold standard' for establishing the presence of lower respiratory tract pathogens) and OP cultures. Ramsey and co-workers [4] showed that the positive predictive value of positive OP cultures in non-expectorating patients was 83%, and 91% for *P. aeruginosa* and *S. aureus*, respectively. However, the negative predictive value of OP cultures was lower, 70% for *P. aeruginosa* and 80% for *S. aureus*. Rosenfeld and co-workers [8] pooled results from three studies performed in 141 children with CF younger than 5 years of age and showed lower positive (44%) and similar negative (95%) predictive values. These authors concluded that a negative OP culture could be used to 'rule out' lower tract colonization/infection, but that a positive OP culture did not predict lower tract findings. The different findings in these studies may reflect differences in the patient populations. Thus, while OP cultures do not always reliably predict the lower respiratory flora, upper airway cultures are currently used for surveillance and to guide treatment, including early eradication antimicrobial strategies for *P. aeruginosa*.

Despite the widespread use of BAL with documented safety in the CF population, this procedure is not without risk. BAL is usually reserved for CF patients who fail to improve despite empiric treatment, for research protocols, and for lung transplant recipients. Gutierrez and co-workers [9] compared sequential BAL samples from the right middle and lingular lobes and noted that, while inflammatory indices correlated well with bacterial cell counts in each lobe, the bacterial distribution varied. Therefore, multiple sites should be sampled by BAL. Cytology should be used to assess adequacy of a BAL sample; excessive numbers of ciliated or squamous epithelial cells (>5%) indicate contamination by bronchial or oropharyngeal material.

In efforts to develop a less invasive and more accurate method for sampling lower airway secretions, there has been much recent interest in obtaining sputum or oropharyngeal cultures following induction with hypertonic saline. Ordonez and co-workers [10] sought to demonstrate the reproducibility of bacterial burden and the inflammatory markers interleukin (IL)-8 and IL-6, myeloperoxidase and neutrophil elastase in induced sputum specimens from 15 stable patients, 6–13 years of age with mild lung disease. While the measures of inflammation varied from week to week, the concentrations of bacteria were relatively consistent, although only 7 of the 15 children had an adequate sample with which to assess potential pathogens. Ho and co-workers [6] induced sputum sampling in 41 children (mean age 7.2 years) and concordant results were only noted for 25 of them. In contrast, one or more additional pathogens were detected in the induced ($n = 12$) or pre-induced ($n = 3$) specimens and one subject had different pathogens detected in the two specimens. Overall, management was altered by induced specimens in 13 patients (30%). Aitken and co-workers [11] assessed whether the duration of induced sputum collection would alter the content of the sample; aliquots taken during 4-minute intervals were shown to be consistent in clinically stable CF patients; but after 20 minutes, alveolar sampling occurred. Thus, sputum induction appears promising, but may not fully reflect pathogens detected in other types of specimen. Furthermore, processing induced specimens is complex and requires extensive training to ensure reliable and reproducible results. Multicenter studies are ongoing to determine appropriate measures to assess the adequacy of an induced sputum specimen and to determine the frequency of successful induction.

Collection and transport

Respiratory tract specimens from CF patients, including those obtained after lung transplantation, should be clearly labeled 'CF specimens' to ensure appropriate processing by the clinical microbiology laboratory. The processing of CF respiratory tract specimens may be delayed; prolonged refrigeration and delayed transport can decrease the viability of micro-organisms. Ideally, specimens should be received by the laboratory within 3–4 hours of collection or stored at 4°C and processed within 24 hours.

Specimen processing

Due to the viscosity of CF sputum specimens, quantitative Gram-stain examination does not correlate with culture results. Liquefaction and homogenization of sputum samples have been recommended to ensure accurate detection of pathogens. Early studies evaluated the efficacy of dithio-threitol (DTT) as a mucolytic agent, but more recent work has suggested that an enzyme mixture comprised of deoxyribonuclease, hyaluronidase and galactosidase may provide more accurate culture results. Quantitative cultures of CF sputum are not generally recommended for routine clinical care, but are reserved for research studies.

Selective media

The respiratory tract of CF patients can harbor high concentrations of several pathogens. The predominant organism is usually *P. aeruginosa*, which is often present in large numbers (10^7–10^9 colony-forming units [CFU] per gram of sputum) and may be mucoid; such organisms can overgrow and obscure slower growing, more fastidious organisms such as *H. influenzae* or *B. cepacia* complex. In 1968, Kilbourn reported the first use of selective media for CF specimens to promote the growth of Gram-negative bacilli and staphylococci [12]. Processing of CF specimens was then further refined to include selective agars for *P. aeruginosa* (cetrimide), streptococci (blood agar with neomycin and gentamicin), *H. influenzae* (*N*-acetyl-D-glucosamine medium, with anaerobic incubation) and staphylococci (mannitol–salt agar), particularly for thymidine-deficient strains [13,14].

Perhaps the most dramatic example of the importance of selective media occurred during the 1980s when patient-to-patient spread of *B. cepacia* complex (then called *Pseudomonas cepacia*) was initially recognized [15–17]. Studies conducted by the Centers for Disease Control and Prevention demonstrated that only a minority (<10%) of laboratories were using selective media for *B. cepacia* and that the use of selective media greatly improved the yield of *B. cepacia* [15]. In these landmark studies, 14 of 15 laboratories using selective media correctly recovered and identified

B. cepacia complex compared with only 22 of 100 laboratories not using selective media. Selective media for *Burkholderia* include: oxidative fermentative bacitracin polymyxin B lactose (OFBPL) agar, *P. cepacia* media, and *Burkholderia cepacia* selective agar (BCSA) which has been reported in some studies to be superior to OFPBL [17]. Prolonged incubation of respiratory specimens from CF patients is recommended to allow slower-growing organisms, such as *B. cepacia* complex, to be detected.

There is a recent appreciation of the anaerobic milieu of the CF lung, particularly within the proposed biofilm that is thought to be characteristic of chronic *P. aeruginosa* infection, with mucoid alginate production and formation of microcolonies [18]. However, routine anaerobic cultures are not recommended as these generally have no yield, due in part to the technical challenges of growing anaerobic bacteria. Investigations of the potential role of molecular identification of anaerobes within CF respiratory tract secretions using nucleic acid amplification strategies are ongoing.

Current recommendations for the use of selective media for specific respiratory pathogens are shown in Table 9.1. All types of respiratory tract specimens from patients with CF should be plated on selective media. However, the use of selective culture media is costly and time-consuming. Studies have documented that the use of selective growth media for CF specimens varies among laboratories, but over the past two decades the use of selective media has become more widespread [15,19]. Most recently, Zhou and co-workers [20] have demonstrated that the majority of clinical microbiology laboratories affiliated with CF care centers in the United States use selective media; of the 150 sites surveyed, 99%, 89% and 82% used selective media for *B. cepacia* complex, *H. influenzae*, and *S. aureus*, respectively. Examples of the laboratory practices that are assessed during site visits conducted by the US CF Center directors' committee are described in Table 9.2.

Table 9.1 Recommended culture media and processing to enhance recovery of CF pathogens from respiratory tract specimens.

Micro-organism	Recommended culture media and/or procedures
Pseudomonas aeruginosa and other *Pseudomonas* spp	MacConkey agar
Burkholderia cepacia complex	OFPBL[a], BCSA[b]
Staphylococcus aureus (including methicillin-resistant strains)	Mannitol–salt agar
Haemophilus influenzae (typeable and non-typeable species)	Horse blood or chocolate agar (with bacitracin)
Stenotrophomonas maltophilia	MacConkey agar with DNase agar for identification
Alcaligenes xylosoxidans	MacConkey agar
Aspergillus spp	Sabouraud's dextrose agar (also grows well, although not selectively, on OFPBL agar)
Non-tuberculous mycobacteria species	NALC–NaOH decontamination step
	Lowenstein–Jensen medium
Other Gram-positive organisms	Sheep blood agar (with neomycin and gentamicin)
Other Gram-negative organisms	MacConkey agar

[a] Oxidative fermentative bacitracin polymyxin B lactose agar (OFPBL).
[b] *Burkholderia cepacia* selective agar (BCSA).
Adapted from [36].

Table 9.2   Sample questions from a survey for clinical microbiology laboratories affiliated with CF care centers.[a]

Does the lab have a specific protocol for culturing respiratory secretions from patients with CF?

Does the lab employ the same protocol for oropharyngeal, expectorated sputum and BAL specimens from patients with CF?

Does the lab report the mucoid phenotype for *P. aeruginosa*?

Are commercial systems used for the identification of glucose non-fermenting Gram-negative rods?

Does the lab send isolates identified as *Burkholderia* spp to a reference lab for confirmation of identification?

Does the lab use an automated susceptibility system?

If clinically indicated, does the lab use a unique protocol (to avoid overgrowth of *P. aeruginosa*) for the isolation of non-tuberculous mycobacteria (NTM)?

[a] This survey was developed by the US Cystic Fibrosis Foundation to be administered to the directors of the clinical microbiology laboratories serving accredited CF care centers.

Detection of other potential pathogens: non-tuberculous mycobacteria, moulds and viruses

If non-tuberculous mycobacteria (NTM) are suspected, CF sputum must be processed using an additional decontamination step to avoid overgrowth by *P. aeruginosa*. Decontamination of specimens with *N*-acetyl-L-cysteine-sodium hydroxide (NALC-NaOH), followed by 5% oxalic acid treatment has been shown to minimize the contamination of Lowenstein–Jensen slants with *P. aeruginosa* and increase the recovery of mycobacteria [21]. However, this decontamination procedure may reduce recovery of NTM from specimens with a low concentration of organisms, due to killing of NTM by oxalic acid [22]. Three specimens with acid-fast bacilli smears are recommended to distinguish transient colonization or contamination from true infection. Prolonged incubation for 8 weeks is needed to accommodate slow-growing NTM. The diagnosis of NTM infection is further discussed in Chapter 10.

Aspergillus species (mainly *A. fumigatus*) are isolated from the respiratory tract cultures of approximately a third of CF patients. However, most CF patients are merely colonized, and only a minority of patients have allergic bronchopulmonary aspergillosis. *Aspergillus* spp grow on blood agar as well as Mycosel agar.

Respiratory viruses have long been implicated as causing pulmonary exacerbations in CF and can contribute to decline in pulmonary function. Identification of a viral pathogen can alter clinical care and inform infection control strategies for hospitalized patients. Detection of respiratory viruses in CF patients by nucleic acid amplification strategies has been hindered by the difficulty in detecting viruses in viscous sputum specimens. Thus, if a viral pathogen is suspected, nasopharyngeal washings should be obtained for rapid respiratory viral antigen detection using direct fluoroscence assays (DFA) or enzyme-linked immunosorbent assays (ELISA).

Species identification

For decades, it has been recognized that the CF lung may contain diverse pathogens and that accurate and timely laboratory identification of species is critical for diagnostic, therapeutic and epidemiological purposes. As early as 1976, Otto and associates published an identification method for non-lactose fermenting Gram-negative bacilli based on a biochemical profile of substrate oxidation; the majority of strains were identified in 24 (94%) and 48 hours (99%), with 99% reproducibility [23]. In the 1980s, modified MacConkey agar was used to both detect and identify *P. aeruginosa* by enhancing pyocyanin pigment production while inhibiting the growth of Gram-positive organisms [24]. When compared to routine biochemical methods, modified MacConkey agar identified 97% of *P. aeruginosa* strains within 24 hours, although highly mucoid strains without detectable pigment were detected within 48 hours. Another reproducible method of species identification, although less frequently used, is the analysis of cellular fatty acid composition by gas–liquid chromatography supplemented with a limited number of biochemical tests [25].

While automated, commercial systems are widely available, *P. aeruginosa* and other Gram-negative bacilli can be difficult to identify due to their marked phenotypic diversity and the presence of other closely related species. Kiska and co-workers [26] showed that commercial systems performed relatively poorly; only 57–80% of non-lactose fermenting Gram-negative bacilli were accurately identified. Microscan® Walk-away has been shown to have unacceptably high rates of misidentification of *P. aeruginosa* as only 57% (108 of 189) of multidrug-resistant non-mucoid strains and 40% (24 of 60) of mucoid strains were definitively identified, the most common misidentifications being *P. fluorescens/putida* and *Alcaligenes* spp [27]. The relative accuracy of several commercial systems for identifying *B. cepacia* complex has also been studied; the positive predictive values ranged from 71% to 98% and the negative predictive values ranged from 50% to 82% [28]. The species most frequently misidentified as *B. cepacia* was *Burkholderia gladioli*. Similarly, commercial systems may misidentify *S. maltophilia* and *A. xylosoxidans*. In a study of *A. xylosoxidans*, 84% (89 of 106) of strains were correctly identified by referring laboratories, but 12 (11%) were misidentified as *P. aeruginosa* ($n = 10$), *S. maltophilia* ($n = 1$) or *B. cepacia* ($n = 1$) [27].

As a result of these observations, experts had previously recommended the addition of expanded biochemical testing to assist in species identification. However, biochemical testing can also be inaccurate or inconclusive and not always readily available. In 2000, McMenamin and co-workers [29] reported that only one-third of 115 CF centers in the United States used conventional biochemical tests to augment commercial test systems for species identification.

As a result of widespread acknowledgment of the limitations of commercial and biochemical identification strategies, molecular methods of identification have been developed. For *B. cepacia* complex genomovars, reference laboratories

Table 9.3 Genomovars of *Burkholderia cepacia* complex in the United States in 2005.

Genomovar	Species designation	Approximate percentage[a]
I	*B. cepacia*	3
II	*B. mulitivorans*	40
III	*B. cenocepacia*	45
IV	*B. stabilis*	<1
V	*B. vietnamensis*	6
VI	*B. dolosa*	3
VII	*B. ambifria*	1
VIII	*B. anthina*	<1
IX	*B. pyrrocinia*	<1
Indeterminate	Not applicable	1

[a] Approximate percentage of infection among more than 1200 CF patients infected with *B. cepacia* complex.
Adapted from [1] and [65].

use species-specific PCR for definitive identification of these species [30]. The currently identified genomovars and their relative distribution in patients with CF are shown in Table 9.3. At the *B. cepacia* Research Laboratory and Repository at the University of Michigan, investigators demonstrated that 36% of unspeciated isolates or isolates referred as another species were identified as *B. cepacia* complex and that 10% of isolates referred as *B. cepacia* complex were other species including *B. gladioli, Stenotrophomonas, Pseudomonas, Alcaligenes, Ralstonia, Flavobacterium* or *Chryseobacterium* [1]. Thus, these molecular methods can also detect previously unrecognized species whose role as emerging pathogens in CF is unknown. Such molecular strategies have also been used to investigate possible nosocomial or person-to-person transmission of *B. cepacia* complex and to assess the link between the natural environment and clinical strains. However, molecular strategies have thus far been confined to research and reference laboratories.

Molecular identification strategies have also been developed for *P. aeruginosa*. Real-time PCR assays have been shown to have similar costs compared with biochemical testing, but much shorter turn-around times. Qin and co-workers [31] demonstrated that real-time PCR using two target sequences optimized identification of *P. aeruginosa* and non-*P. aeruginosa* Gram-negative bacilli. Spilker and co-workers [32] reported PCR-based assays with 100% sensitivity and specificity. Similarly, da Silva Filho and co-workers [33] described a PCR primer pair for *P. aeruginosa* with 100% sensitivity and specificity. This latter PCR method also detected *P. aeruginosa* in sputum and throat swab samples. While rapid detection is obviously of great value, particularly for empirical therapy and infection control, growth of an organism is required for susceptibility testing and for molecular epidemiology.

ANTIMICROBIAL SUSCEPTIBILITY TESTING METHODS

Optimal antimicrobial susceptibility testing methods

In 1989, wide variability in susceptibility to seven commonly used antibiotics, particularly aminoglycoside agents, was demonstrated using different testing procedures for *P. aeruginosa* [34]. This variability prevented meaningful comparisons of susceptibility trends among laboratories and CF care centers and contributed to confusion and frustration among microbiologists and clinicians.

The optimal methodologies for antimicrobial susceptibility testing for both mucoid and non-mucoid strains of *P. aeruginosa* have been elucidated. Burns and co-workers [35] studied 500 multidrug-resistant strains of *P. aeruginosa* from CF patients, and found that the agar-based diffusion methods (Kirby Bauer disks and the E-test) were most accurate, while the commercial microbroth dilution assays, Vitek® and Microscan®, had unacceptably high rates of very major errors (i.e. false-susceptibility) and major errors (i.e. false-resistance). Thus, the Clinical and Laboratories Standards Institute (formerly the National Committee for Clinical Laboratory Standards or NCCLS) endorsed the use of agar-based diffusion assays rather than automated commercial microbroth dilution systems for susceptibility testing of *P. aeruginosa* isolated from patients with CF [36]. Studies to determine the optimal methods of susceptibility testing for other multidrug-resistant organisms, such as *B. cepacia* complex, *S. maltophilia*, or *A. xylosoxidans*, are under way.

Biofilm susceptibility testing

It has been suggested that *P. aeruginosa* can exist in a biofilm mode of growth within the relatively hypoxic milieu of the CF airways [18]. Thus, there has been increasing interest in developing laboratory techniques to better approximate these in-vivo growth conditions in the hope that antibiotic susceptibility testing performed on bacteria grown under anaerobic and biofilm-inducing conditions will generate more clinically relevant results when compared with conventional susceptibility testing performed on bacteria grown planktonically under aerobic conditions. Hill and co-workers [37] demonstrated that multidrug-resistant *P. aeruginosa* strains, grown under both anaerobic and biofilm conditions, were less susceptible to single and combination antibiotics than when grown under conventional testing conditions. Moskowitz and co-workers [38] demonstrated the clinical feasibility of biofilm susceptibility assays by developing a reproducible assay to determine the biofilm inhibitory concentrations (BICs) in a clinical microbiology laboratory. This assay found the BIC to be much higher than the corresponding minimum inhibitory concentrations (MICs) for β-lactam antibiotics, but the BICs and MICs were similar for meropenem, ciprofloxacin and the aminoglycosides. In contrast, the BIC for azithromycin (2 μg/mL) was substantially lower than the MIC (128 μg/mL).

SYNERGY TESTING

With the use of prolonged and frequent courses of oral, aerosolized and parenteral antibiotics, the emergence of multidrug-resistant CF pathogens is inevitable. Since pulmonary exacerbations are generally treated with two agents from different classes of antibiotics, clinicians are often left with few therapeutic options, particularly for older patients with more advanced lung disease. Thus, there has been interest in the use of synergy testing to provide clinicians with potential antibiotic combinations.

Currently, two methods of synergy testing have been described for CF patients. The first is a checkerboard assay pairing two agents in serial two-fold dilutions of clinically achievable concentrations and calculating the fractional inhibitory concentration (FIC). In this method, agents from different classes are tested together (e.g. an aminoglycoside is paired with a β-lactam agent) and the MIC of each agent when paired together is compared to each agent tested alone [27,39]. The in-vitro results of this assay have been published for *P. aeruginosa* as well as *B. cepacia*, *Stenotrophomonas* and *Alcaligenes* spp. Susceptibility to individual agents did not predict synergistic combinations of agents. Most multidrug-resistant strains, including pan-resistant strains, are found to be inhibited by one or more combinations of agents. However, the efficacy of this assay has not been validated in a clinical trial although anecdotal data support its use.

The second method is the multiple combination bactericidal testing (MCBT). In this assay, two or three drugs are combined at their peak serum concentration and cidal activity is determined. Aaron and co-workers [40] performed a randomized, double-blind, controlled clinical trial of MCBT among CF patients experiencing a pulmonary exacerbation in Canada and Australia. In this pivotal study, the primary outcome was the time to next pulmonary exacerbation. These investigators showed no significant difference in the time to next exacerbation among the 64 subjects randomized to treatment guided by MCBT versus the 68 subjects randomized to treatment guided by conventional susceptibility testing. Among the secondary outcomes, there was no difference in the bacterial density at the end of treatment, the proportion of treatment failures, or improvement in lung function in the two treatment groups. Potential explanations for the apparent lack of clinical efficacy of MCBT included the fact that in-vitro susceptibility testing may not predict clinical response and that MCBT combinations were based on specimens obtained within 3 months of the exacerbation that did not always reflect the resistance profile of the organisms associated with the exacerbation.

INFECTION CONTROL

Over the past two decades there has been an increasing recognition of the importance of infection control for CF patients [36]. The clinical microbiology laboratory plays an important role in infection control as appropriate identification and accurate susceptibility testing inform the use of transmission precautions and help to assess the effectiveness of infection control strategies. Furthermore, the laboratory may provide the first evidence that patient-to-patient transmission is occurring.

Transmission of CF pathogens

While the source of many pathogens in CF patients remains unknown, there is increasing evidence that CF patients may acquire potential pathogens from the contaminated healthcare environment or from other patients with CF. Modes of acquisition include direct contact between CF patients (e.g. kissing), indirect contact with objects contaminated with infectious secretions (e.g. sharing personal items or patient care equipment), and droplets (e.g. infectious particles generated by coughing that can be transmitted within 1 meter).

For years, studies demonstrated that siblings with CF frequently shared the same strain of *P. aeruginosa*, suggesting either a common environmental source or cross-infection [36]. However, with the increasing use of molecular typing, shared strains of several pathogens, particularly *P. aeruginosa* and *B. cepacia* complex, have been demonstrated among unrelated patients with CF hospitalized at the same time, attending the same CF clinic, or participating in the same recreational event such as CF summer camp or educational retreats [41,42]. Studies have provided evidence of spread of *P. aeruginosa* within adult CF clinics in the UK and Wales [43–45]. In Australia, molecular typing methods were utilized to demonstrate transmission of a clonal strain of *P. aeruginosa* in a CF clinic caring for older children and young infants newly diagnosed with CF by newborn screening [46]. Overall, 56 of 118 children (47%) infected with *P. aeruginosa* shared the same predominant strain and an increased risk was noted among children hospitalized within the preceding 12 months. This strain was not isolated from the healthcare environment. The impact of patient segregation in this clinic was assessed to determine if strict infection control measures and cohort segregation interrupted transmission [47]. The prevalence of the epidemic strain significantly decreased from 21% to 14% ($p = 0.03$) over 3 years, providing additional indirect evidence for person-to-person transmission within the clinic setting.

However, there is some disagreement about the frequency of patient-to-patient transmission of *P. aeruginosa*. Speert and co-workers [48] performed molecular typing of *P. aeruginosa* isolates from 174 patients followed in the CF center in Vancouver. Overall, 34 strain types were shared by 2–21 patient clusters, but there was no history of contact (except among siblings) detected among patient clusters in the hospital, clinic or non-healthcare settings. These investigators concluded that *P. aeruginosa* was most likely acquired from the natural environment, and thus, segregation was not recommended.

The complexities of these issues are further highlighted by a report by Van Daele and co-workers [49], wherein the epidemiology of *P. aeruginosa* among 76 CF patients attending a CF rehabilitation center in Belgium was studied. Overall, 44 of the 76 patients (56%) shared a strain with another patient, so-called 'cluster genotypes'. Most patients ($n = 38$) infected with a cluster genotype had these strains upon arrival to the rehabilitation center, suggesting previous acquisition from the center. Eight patients acquired a new cluster genotype, but only three were persistently infected with the new clone. Thus, the risk of persistent patient-to-patient transmission was 4% (3 of 76) during the study period.

Other investigators have assessed transmission of additional CF pathogens. Kahl and co-workers [50] examined the molecular epidemiology of *S. aureus* during a 6-year study period and identified six dominant clones suggesting the possibility of patient-to-patient transmission. Kanellopoulou and co-workers [51] described a common clone of *A. xylosoxidans* among five patients. Most recently, Kalish and co-workers [52] described an outbreak of *B. dolosa* (genomovar VI) in their CF population associated with increased morbidity and mortality.

However, many unanswered questions remain. The frequency of patient-to-patient transmission, the role of the contaminated environment, a potential point source of acquisition of a common strain, the frequency of multiple genotypes in individual patients, bacterial virulence factors responsible for transmission, or host factors that facilitate transmission are not well understood.

General strategies to reduce transmission

This chapter will highlight four important principles of infection control in CF: standard precautions, transmission precautions, hand hygiene, and care of respiratory therapy equipment.

STANDARD PRECAUTIONS

Standard precautions embrace the concept that all body fluids, including the respiratory tract secretions of all patients with CF can harbor potentially transmissible infectious agents that could infect other patients. To prevent patient-to-patient or healthcare worker-to-patient transmission of infectious agents when caring for a patient, healthcare workers must use an appropriate combination of practices (e.g. hand hygiene and disinfection) and barrier precautions (e.g. gloves, gown, mask) based on the anticipated exposure. Since patient care equipment (e.g. ventilator) or other items (e.g. bed rails) can become contaminated by infectious secretions, standard precautions extend to inanimate objects and surfaces in the patient's environment. The components of standard precautions are shown in Table 9.4.

TRANSMISSION PRECAUTIONS

Transmission precautions are used for patients with documented or suspected infections caused by highly transmissible (e.g. MRSA or influenza) or epidemiologically important (e.g. *B. cepacia* complex) infectious agents that require additional precautions to prevent transmission. Categories of transmission precautions relevant to CF include *contact* (e.g. multidrug-resistant organisms), *droplet* (e.g. influenza), and much less commonly *airborne infection isolation* (e.g. in tuberculosis), as detailed in Table 9.5.

HAND HYGEINE

Hand hygiene, if appropriately performed by staff, patients and families, is the single most important practice to prevent transmission of infectious agents. Hand hygiene must be done before and after all contact with patients and following contact with contaminated patient equipment. Alcohol-based hand-rubs have been shown to reduce bacterial contamination of hands better than traditional hand washing with water and plain soap or antimicrobial-containing soap (e.g. chlorhexidine or triclosan) [53,54]. Furthermore, alcohol is more convenient, less expensive and, due in part to emollients contained within the hand-rub, associated with better skin condition including decreased skin cracking, water loss and erythema.

Table 9.4 Components of standard precautions as recommended for all CF patients in inpatient and outpatient settings.

Recommended practice	Healthcare situation
Hand hygiene	Contact with blood, body fluids, secretions, excretions, contaminated items
	Immediately after removal of gloves
	Before and after all patient contacts
Gloves	Required for handling blood, body fluids, secretions, excretions
	Contact with mucus membranes and abraded skin
	Contact with contaminated equipment or patient care items
Gown, mask, eye protection, face shield	Required for procedures and patient care activities likely to generate splashes or sprays of blood, body fluids, secretions, or excretions

Adapted from [36] and [66].

Table 9.5 Transmission precautions for potential pathogens in CF patients.

Transmission precaution	Potential pathogens
Standard	Applicable to all CF patients including those with: – non-tuberculous mycobacteria – *P. aeruginosa* (excluding multidrug-resistant strains) – methicillin-susceptible *S. aureus*
Contact	Applicable to all CF patients with multidrug-resistant organisms: – methicillin-resistant *S. aureus* (MRSA) – *B. cepacia* complex – multidrug-resistant *P. aeruginosa* *S. maltophilia* Viruses (respiratory syncytial virus, influenza and parainfluenza)
Droplet	Viruses: – influenza virus – adenovirus
Airborne	*Mycobacterium tuberculosis*

Adapted from [36].

Table 9.6 Recommendations for disinfection of respiratory therapy equipment in the home.

Method for disinfection[a]	Duration recommended
Immerse in:[b] – 1:50 dilution of 5.25–6.15% sodium hypochlorite (household bleach) – 70–90% ethyl or isopropyl alcohol or – 3% hydrogen peroxide	3 minutes
OR	
Boiling in water	5 minutes
OR	
Use of a standard cycle dishwasher	30 minutes at a temperature greater than 158°F (70°C)
OR	
Use of a home microwave (2.45 GHz)	5 minutes

[a] Must be permissible by the manufacturer.
[b] These preparations will lose activity with time, but the optimal storage time is unknown.
Adapted from [36].

CARE OF RESPIRATORY THERAPY EQUIPMENT

Care of respiratory therapy equipment includes cleaning, disinfecting and drying reusable respiratory therapy equipment to prevent acquisition of potential pathogens from contaminated equipment. As evidence of the importance of nebulizer care, the use of aerosolized medications was associated with earlier acquisition of *P. aeruginosa* in a newborn screening study [55]. Sterile water is recommended to rinse nebulizers as tap water may harbor NTM, fungi or *P. aeruginosa*. Furthermore, flora colonizing the oropharynx could potentially contaminate a medication delivery device such as a valve-holding chamber or nebulizer, which could subsequently be aerosolized into the lower respiratory tract [56]. Bacterial contamination of the spacer devices used to deliver metered-dose inhaled medications has been reported to occur [57]. Contamination rates were significantly lower when parents cleaned and dried spacer devices after each use [58]. Similarly, cleaning and drying home respiratory therapy equipment between uses decreased the risk of acquiring *B. cepacia* complex [59]. Sharing respiratory therapy equipment was found to be a risk factor for acquisition of *B. cepacia* complex [60]. Finally, nebulizer equipment may be a source of *S. maltophilia* in CF [61].

Thus, appropriate care of respiratory therapy equipment includes cleaning the equipment to remove all debris prior to disinfection, as disinfection may be less effective if dried or baked debris remains on equipment [62]. Experimental studies have shown that hot water and soap

removed most bacteria from a nebulizer [63]. Disinfection (if permissible according to the manufacturer) can be accomplished using one of several methods as described in Table 9.6. Acetic acid (vinegar), while active against *P. aeruginosa*, should not be used as a disinfectant as vinegar is not active against some Gram-positive (e.g. *S. aureus*) and Gram-negative (e.g. *Escherichia coli*) bacteria [64].

Surveillance strategies for CF microbiology

It is critical that clinical laboratories maintain an efficient system for communicating with the clinicians caring for CF patients and for communicating with the infection control team. Surveillance strategies for CF microbiology should be developed in collaboration with the CF center's infection control team and target *S. aureus*, including MRSA, *P. aeruginosa*, particularly multidrug-resistant strains, and *B. cepacia* complex. Surveillance for other potential pathogens such as *S. maltophilia*, *A. xylosoxidans* and NTM should be considered if epidemiologically indicated, such as when patient-to-patient transmission or an outbreak is suspected. Microbiological surveillance includes calculation of incidence and prevalence rates and longitudinal review of antimicrobial susceptibility summaries with trend analysis. Surveillance reports should be shared between the infection control and CF care teams at least on an annual basis, to evaluate effectiveness of the center's infection control program. Selected *B. cepacia* complex isolates, and non-fermenting Gram-negative bacilli for which species identification cannot be established after routine analysis, should be submitted to the designated reference laboratory for further study.

REFERENCES

1. Lipuma JJ. Update on the *Burkholderia cepacia* complex. *Curr Opin Pulmon Med* 2005; **11**:528–533.

2. Thomassen MJ, Klinger JD, Badger SJ *et al.* Cultures of thoracotomy specimens confirm usefulness of sputum cultures in cystic fibrosis. *J Pediatr* 1984; **104**:352–356.

3. Jung A, Kleinau I, Schonian G *et al.* Sequential genotyping of *Pseudomonas aeruginosa* from upper and lower airways of cystic fibrosis patients. *Eur Respir J* 2002; **20**:1457–1463.

4. Ramsey BW, Wentz KR, Smith AL *et al.* Predictive value of oropharyngeal cultures for identifying lower airway bacteria in cystic fibrosis patients. *Am Rev Respir Dis* 1991; **144**:331–337.

5. Equi AC, Pike SE, Davies J, Bush A. Use of cough swabs in a cystic fibrosis clinic. *Arch Dis Child* 2001; **85**:438–439.

6. Ho SA, Ball R, Morrison LJ *et al.* Clinical value of obtaining sputum and cough swab samples following inhaled hypertonic saline in children with cystic fibrosis. *Pediatr Pulmonol* 2004; **38**:82–87.

7. Maiya S, Desai M, Baruah A *et al.* Cough plate versus cough swab in patients with cystic fibrosis: a pilot study. *Arch Dis Child* 2004; **89**:577–579.

8. Rosenfeld M, Emerson J, Accurso F *et al.* Diagnostic accuracy of oropharyngeal cultures in infants and young children with cystic fibrosis. *Pediatr Pulmonol* 1999; **28**:321–328.

9. Gutierrez JP, Grimwood K, Armstrong DS *et al.* Interlobar differences in bronchoalveolar lavage fluid from children with cystic fibrosis. *Eur Respir J* 2001; **17**:281–286.

10. Ordonez CL, Kartashov AI, Wohl ME. Variability of markers of inflammation and infection in induced sputum in children with cystic fibrosis. *J Pediatr* 2004; **145**:689–692.

11. Aitken ML, Greene KE, Tonelli MR *et al.* Analysis of sequential aliquots of hypertonic saline solution-induced sputum from clinically stable patients with cystic fibrosis. *Chest* 2003; **123**:792–799.

12. Kilbourn JP, Campbell RA, Grach JL, Willis MD. Quantitative bacteriology of sputum. *Am Rev Respir Dis* 1968; **98**:810–818.

13. Bauernfeind A, Rotter K, Weisslein-Pfister C. Selective procedure to isolate *Haemophilus influenzae* from sputa with large quantities of *Pseudomonas aeruginosa*. *Infection* 1987; **15**:278–280.

14. Wong K, Roberts MC, Owens L *et al.* Selective media for the quantitation of bacteria in cystic fibrosis sputum. *J Med Microbiol* 1984; **17**:113–119.

15. Tablan OC, Carson LA, Cusick LB *et al.* Laboratory proficiency test results on use of selective media for isolating *Pseudomonas cepacia* from simulated sputum specimens of patients with cystic fibrosis. *J Clin Microbiol* 1987; **25**:485–487.

16. Garner JS. Guideline for isolation precautions in hospitals. *Infect Control Hosp Epidemiol* 1996; **17**:53–80.

17. Henry D, Campbell M, Mcgimpsey C *et al.* Comparison of isolation media for recovery of *Burkholderia cepacia* complex from respiratory secretions of patients with cystic fibrosis. *J Clin Microbiol* 1999; **37**:1004–1007.

18. Hoiby N. Understanding bacterial biofilms in patients with cystic fibrosis: current and innovative approaches to potential therapies. *J Cyst Fibros* 2002; **1**:249–254.

19. Shreve MR, Butler S, Kaplowitz HJ *et al.* Impact of microbiology practice on cumulative prevalence of respiratory tract bacteria in patients with cystic fibrosis. *J Clin Microbiol* 1999; **37**:753–757.

20. Zhou J, Garber E, Desai M, Saiman L. Compliance of clinical microbiology laboratories in the United States with current recommendations for processing respiratory tract specimens from patients with cystic fibrosis. *J Clin Microbiol* 2006; **44(4)**:1547–1549.

21. Whittier S, Hopfer RL, Knowles MR, Gilligan PH. Improved recovery of mycobacteria from respiratory secretions of patients with cystic fibrosis. *J Clin Microbiol* 1993; **31**:861–864.

22. Bange FC, Bottger EC. Improved decontamination method for recovering mycobacteria from patients with cystic fibrosis. *Eur J Clin Microbiol Infect Dis* 2002; **21**:546–548.

23. Otto LA, Pickett MJ. Rapid method for identification of Gram-negative, nonfermentative bacilli. *J Clin Microbiol* 1976; **3**:566–575.

24. Daly JA, Boshard R, Matsen JM. Differential primary plating medium for enhancement of pigment production by *Pseudomonas aeruginosa*. *J Clin Microbiol* 1984; **19**:742–743.

25. Veys A, Callewaert W, Waelkens E, Van Den Abbeele K. Application of gas-liquid chromatography to the routine identification of nonfermenting gram-negative bacteria in clinical specimens. *J Clin Microbiol* 1989; **27**:1538–1542.

26. Kiska DL, Kerr A, Jones MC *et al.* Accuracy of four commercial systems for identification of *Burkholderia cepacia* and other Gram-negative nonfermenting bacilli recovered from patients with cystic fibrosis. *J Clin Microbiol* 1996; **34**:886–891.

27. Saiman L, Chen Y, Tabibi S *et al.* Identification and antimicrobial susceptibility of *Alcaligenes xylosoxidans* isolated from patients with cystic fibrosis. *J Clin Microbiol* 2001; **39**:3942–3945.

28. Shelly DB, Spilker T, Gracely EJ *et al.* Utility of commercial systems for identification of *Burkholderia cepacia* complex from cystic fibrosis sputum culture. *J Clin Microbiol* 2000; **38**:3112–3115.

29. McMenamin JD, Zaccone TM, Coenye T *et al.* Misidentification of *Burkholderia cepacia* in US cystic fibrosis treatment centers: an analysis of 1051 recent sputum isolates. *Chest* 2000; **117**:1661–1665.

30. Whitby PW, Pope LC, Carter KB *et al.* Species-specific PCR as a tool for the identification of *Burkholderia gladioli*. *J Clin Microbiol* 2000; **38**:282–285.

31. Qin X, Emerson J, Stapp J *et al.* Use of real-time PCR with multiple targets to identify *Pseudomonas aeruginosa* and other nonfermenting Gram-negative bacilli from patients with cystic fibrosis. *J Clin Microbiol* 2003; **41**:4312–4317.

32. Spilker T, Coenye T, Vandamme P, Lipuma JJ. PCR-based assay for differentiation of *Pseudomonas aeruginosa* from other *Pseudomonas* species recovered from cystic fibrosis patients. *J Clin Microbiol* 2004; **42**:2074–2079.

33. da Silva Filho LV, Levi JE, Oda Bento CN *et al.* PCR identification of *Pseudomonas aeruginosa* and direct detection in clinical samples from cystic fibrosis patients. *J Med Microbiol* 1999; **48**:357–361.

34. Staneck JL, Glenn S, Dipersio JR, Leist PA. Wide variability in *Pseudomonas aeruginosa* aminoglycoside results among seven susceptibility testing procedures. *J Clin Microbiol* 1989; **27**:2277–2285.

35. Saiman L, Burns JL, Larone D *et al.* Evaluation of MicroScan® Autoscan for identification of *Pseudomonas aeruginosa* isolates from cystic fibrosis patients. *J Clin Microbiol* 2003; **41**:492–494.

36. Saiman L, Siegel J. Infection control recommendations for patients with cystic fibrosis: microbiology, important pathogens, and infection control practices to prevent patient-to-patient transmission. *Infect Control Hosp Epidemiol* 2003; **24**:S6–S52.

37. Hill D, Rose B, Pajkos A *et al.* Antibiotic susceptibilities of *Pseudomonas aeruginosa* isolates derived from patients with cystic fibrosis under aerobic, anaerobic, and biofilm conditions. *J Clin Microbiol* 2005; **43**:5085–5090.

38. Moskowitz SM, Foster JM, Emerson J, Burns JL. Clinically feasible biofilm susceptibility assay for isolates of *Pseudomonas aeruginosa* from patients with cystic fibrosis. *J Clin Microbiol* 2004; **42**:1915–1922.

39. Saiman L, Mehar F, Niu WW *et al.* Antibiotic susceptibility of multiply resistant *Pseudomonas aeruginosa* isolated from patients with cystic fibrosis, including candidates for transplantation. *Clin Infect Dis* 1996; **23**:532–537.

40. Aaron SD, Vandemheen KL, Ferris W *et al.* Combination antibiotic susceptibility testing to treat exacerbations of cystic fibrosis associated with multiresistant bacteria: a randomised, double-blind, controlled clinical trial. *Lancet* 2005; **366**:463–471.

41. Wolz C, Kiosz G, Ogle JW *et al. Pseudomonas aeruginosa* cross-colonization and persistence in patients with cystic fibrosis: use of a DNA probe. *Epidemiol Infect* 1989; **102**:205–214.

42. Lipuma JJ, Marks-Austin KA, Holsclaw DS *et al.* Inapparent transmission of *Pseudomonas (Burkholderia) cepacia* among patients with cystic fibrosis. *Pediatr Infect Dis J* 1994; **13**:716–719.

43. Jones AM, Govan JR, Doherty CJ *et al.* Spread of a multi-resistant strain of *Pseudomonas aeruginosa* in an adult cystic fibrosis clinic. *Lancet* 2001; **358**:557–558.

44. da Silva Filho LV, Levi JE, Bento CN *et al.* Molecular epidemiology of *Pseudomonas aeruginosa* infections in a cystic fibrosis outpatient clinic. *J Med Microbiol* 2001; **50**:261–267.

45. Scott FW, Pitt TL. Identification and characterization of transmissible *Pseudomonas aeruginosa* strains in cystic fibrosis patients in England and Wales. *J Med Microbiol* 2004; **53**:609–615.

46. Armstrong DS, Nixon GM, Carzino R *et al.* Detection of a widespread clone of *Pseudomonas aeruginosa* in a pediatric cystic fibrosis clinic. *Am J Respir Crit Care Med* 2002; **166**:983–987.

47. Griffiths AL, Jamsen K, Carlin JB *et al.* Effects of segregation on an epidemic *Pseudomonas aeruginosa* strain in a cystic fibrosis clinic. *Am J Respir Crit Care Med* 2005; **171**:1020–1025.

48. Speert DP, Campbell ME, Henry DA *et al.* Epidemiology of *Pseudomonas aeruginosa* in cystic fibrosis in British Columbia, Canada. *Am J Respir Crit Care Med* 2002; **166**:988–993.

49. Van Daele SG, Franckx H, Verhelst R *et al.* Epidemiology of *Pseudomonas aeruginosa* in a cystic fibrosis rehabilitation centre. *Eur Respir J* 2005; **25**:474–481.

50. Kahl BC, Duebbers A, Lubritz G *et al.* Population dynamics of persistent *Staphylococcus aureus* isolated from the airways of cystic fibrosis patients during a 6-year prospective study. *J Clin Microbiol* 2003; **41**:4424–4427.

51. Kanellopoulou M, Pournaras S, Iglezos H *et al.* Persistent colonization of nine cystic fibrosis patients with an *Achromobacter (Alcaligenes) xylosoxidans* clone. *Eur J Clin Microbiol Infect Dis* 2004; **23**:336–339.

52. Kalish LA, Waltz DA, Dovey M *et al.* Impact of *Burkholderia dolosa* on lung function and survival in cystic fibrosis. *Am J Respir Crit Care Med* 2006; **173**(4):421–425.

53. Boyce JM, Pittet D. Guideline for hand hygiene in health-care settings. *Infect Control Hosp Epidemiol* 2002; **23**:S3–S40.

54. Pittet D, Boyce JM. Revolutionising hand hygiene in health-care settings: guidelines revisited. *Lancet: Infect Dis* 2003; **3**:269–270.

55. Kosorok MR, Jalaluddin M, Farrell PM *et al.* Comprehensive analysis of risk factors for acquisition of *Pseudomonas aeruginosa* in young children with cystic fibrosis. *Pediatr Pulmonol* 1998; **26**:81–88.

56. Hutchinson GR, Parker S, Pryor JA *et al.* Home-use nebulizers: a potential primary source of *Burkholderia cepacia* and other colistin-resistant, gram-negative bacteria in patients with cystic fibrosis. *J Clin Microbiol* 1996; **34**:584–587.

57. Cohen HA, Cohen Z, Kahan E. Bacterial contamination of spacer devices used by children with asthma. *J Am Med Assoc* 2003; **290**:195–196.

58. Cohen HA, Cohen Z, Pomeranz AS *et al.* Bacterial contamination of spacer devices used by asthmatic children. *J Asthma* 2005; **42**:169–172.

59. Walsh NM, Casano AA, Manangan LP *et al.* Risk factors for *Burkholderia cepacia* complex colonization and infection among patients with cystic fibrosis. *J Pediatr* 2002; **141**:512–517.

60. Tablan OC, Chorba TL, Schidlow DV *et al. Pseudomonas cepacia* colonization in patients with cystic fibrosis: risk factors and clinical outcome. *J Pediatr* 1985; **107**:382–387.

61. Denton M, Rajgopal A, Mooney L *et al. Stenotrophomonas maltophilia* contamination of nebulizers used to deliver aerosolized therapy to inpatients with cystic fibrosis. *J Hosp Infect* 2003; **55**:180–183.

62. Merritt K, Hitchins VM, Brown SA. Safety and cleaning of medical materials and devices. *J Biomed Mater Res* 2000; **53**:131–136.

63. Rosenfeld M, Joy P, Nguyen CD *et al.* Cleaning home nebulizers used by patients with cystic fibrosis: is rinsing with tap water enough? *J Hosp Infect* 2001; **49**:229–230.

64. Rutala WA, Barbee SL, Aguiar NC *et al.* Antimicrobial activity of home disinfectants and natural products against potential human pathogens. *Infect Control Hosp Epidemiol* 2000; **21**:33–38.

65. Reik R, Spilker T, Lipuma JJ. Distribution of *Burkholderia cepacia* complex species among isolates recovered from persons with or without cystic fibrosis. *J Clin Microbiol* 2005; **43**:2926–2928.

66. Welch DF, Muszynski MJ, Pai CH *et al.* Selective and differential medium for recovery of *Pseudomonas cepacia* from the respiratory tracts of patients with cystic fibrosis. *J Clin Microbiol* 1987; **25**:1730–1734.

PART 4

CLINICAL ASPECTS OF CYSTIC FIBROSIS

10	Respiratory disease: infection	137
	Ian M. Balfour-Lynn and J. Stuart Elborn	
11	Respiratory disease: non-infectious complications	159
	Margaret Hodson and Andrew Bush	
12	Sleep, lung mechanics and work of breathing, including NPPV	175
	Brigitte Fauroux and Annick Clément	
13	Delivery of therapy to the cystic fibrosis lung	185
	Harm A. W. M. Tiddens and Sunalene G. Devadason	
14	The upper airway in cystic fibrosis	199
	William E. Grant	
15a	Gastrointestinal disease in cystic fibrosis	209
	Ian Gooding and David Westaby	
15b	Liver, biliary and pancreatic disease	225
	Vicky Dondos and David Westaby	
16	Insulin deficiency and diabetes related to cystic fibrosis	241
	Christopher D. Sheldon and Lee Dobson	
17	Growth and puberty	253
	Nicola Bridges	
18	Cystic-fibrosis-related low bone mineral density	261
	Sarah L. Elkin and Charles S. Haworth	
19	Other system disorders in cystic fibrosis	269
	Khin Ma Gyi	
20	Sexual and reproductive health	279
	Susan M. Sawyer	
21	Transplantation	291
	Paul Aurora, Khin Gyi and Martin Carby	

Respiratory disease: infection

IAN M. BALFOUR-LYNN AND J. STUART ELBORN

INTRODUCTION

Most people with cystic fibrosis (CF) die from respiratory failure, which is a consequence of progressive lung damage resulting from chronic infection and inflammation. The airways of people with CF are susceptible to initial colonization and subsequent infection by organisms that are not adequately cleared. A host–bacteria relationship is established with airway epithelium and alveolar tissue becoming injured due to the effects of a large number of inflammatory mediators and bacterial products. These include cytokines, bacterial and host defense proteases, and oxygen-derived free radicals [1]. Early in life *Staphylococcus aureus* is the main organism that infects the airway, but by the end of the second decade *Pseudomonas aeruginosa* is the dominant infecting organism (Fig. 10.1) [2]. Aggressive treatment of pulmonary bacterial infection with antibiotics is the most important and effective intervention in the treatment of CF. Respiratory viral infections also play an important role in the early natural history of airway infection. Non-tuberculous mycobacteria are being recognized as increasingly important pathogens. Finally, various species of fungi may cause infection and allergy in the airways.

BACTERIAL INFECTIONS

NATURAL HISTORY

There have been a number of important CF studies, which have sampled airway secretions (during bronchoscopy) in the first few years of life. They have shown that infection occurs early, particularly with *S. aureus, Haemophilus influenzae* and *P. aeruginosa* [3–6]. It is unusual for CF airways to be truly sterile. Indeed the concept of chronic bacterial colonization should be abandoned, as it is clear that bacteria in the airways are always harmful since a host response can be demonstrated with neutrophilic inflammation and pro-inflammatory cytokines and chemokines. Whether inflammation can occur in the absence of infecting organisms is controversial [6], but inflammation is more intense when organisms are isolated [5,6]. Airway plugging is caused by viscous airway secretions which are due to dehydration of airway surface liquid, mucins and DNA from necrotic neutrophils and bacteria [1]. The airways become bronchiectatic as a consequence of inflammatory damage to the epithelium and matrix proteins [7,8]. In the airway, neutrophils are in excess with insufficient macrophages to remove the apoptotic cells, so neutrophil

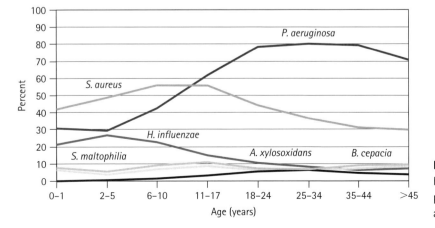

Figure 10.1 North American Cystic Fibrosis Foundation Registry data demonstrating the predominant infecting organisms according to age [2].

necrosis with release of toxic cellular compounds is prominent. In the case of *P. aeruginosa*, phagocytosis may be further frustrated by biofilm formation [9]. This sets the scene for further bacterial infection and a destructive cycle of infection, inflammation and lung injury.

PULMONARY EXACERBATIONS

Children and adults with CF have intermittent episodes of increased respiratory symptoms (Table 10.1), particularly cough and increased volume and purulence of sputum [10]. These are often accompanied by a reduction in pulmonary function and an acute-phase response with blood neutrophilia and elevation of acute-phase proteins such as C-reactive protein [10]. Such episodes are the most important cause of morbidity in CF. They are often used as an end-point in clinical trials, but this may be questionable, since the aim of antibiotic therapy is to institute treatment *before* a full-blown exacerbation is established.

Exacerbations can be precipitated by new infections, for example with *S. aureus* or *H. influenzae*, but can also occur in patients with chronic infection and no additional organisms isolated on sputum culture [11]. A recent study demonstrated that there is no clonal change in *P. aeruginosa* with these exacerbations, indicating that they are not necessarily due to infection with new strains [12]. It is also possible that exacerbations are part of a natural cycle of chronic infection with *P. aeruginosa*, as one study showed that adult patients seemed to regularly have three exacerbations per year [13]. Other microbes not isolated by routine methods, such as anaerobic bacteria, viruses and fungi, may also cause pulmonary exacerbations.

GENERAL PRINCIPLES FOR ANTIBIOTIC TREATMENT

The lower airways should be sterile, so the first aim of treatment is to render the lower airways as free from infection as is possible. Prophylactic use of antibiotics has some effect against *S. aureus*, but evidence is lacking for other organisms [14]. For new isolates, antibiotic treatment should be

Table 10.1 Typical symptoms of respiratory exacerbations [185].

Change in sputum color or volume
Increased cough
Increased dyspnea
New or increased hemoptysis
Malaise, fatigue and lethargy
Temperature above 38°C
Anorexia or weight loss
Sinus pain or tenderness
Change in sinus discharge
Change in physical examination of the chest (e.g. new crackles)
Decrease in pulmonary function by 10% or more
New radiographic changes indicative of pulmonary infection

appropriate for the organism, given at a sufficient dose and for a sufficient duration [15]. For some drugs, this is because of an increased volume of distribution in CF patients, but for others with normal pharmacokinetics it is necessary to deliver high doses to achieve adequate concentrations in sputum. It has been traditional to treat acute exacerbations for 14 days with intravenous antibiotics. but there are no studies demonstrating that a 14-day course is better than 7 days or less effective than 21 days.

A number of antibiotics are used as long-term therapy in CF. Antibiotic prophylaxis is frequently used in children to prevent infection with *S. aureus*. This strategy is effective in prevention of *S. aureus* infection but in some studies this has been at the cost of increasing the frequency of *P. aeruginosa* infection [14,16]. A recent Cochrane review suggested that there was still insufficient quality data to determine whether prophylactic antibiotic treatment was appropriate in CF [17]. In people with *P. aeruginosa* chronic infection, long-term treatment with nebulized Colomycin has been used for over 25 years in Europe. Although there is not a strong evidence base for efficacy, it has been demonstrated to reduce microbial burden assessed by colony counts of *P. aeruginosa* [18]. Nebulized tobramycin has also been used and the preservative-free formulation Tobi improves lung function and reduces the frequency of pulmonary exacerbations [19,20].

Most CF centers now offer the opportunity of having some intravenous antibiotic treatment for exacerbations delivered at home. This is driven by a number of factors, including patient preferences due to less social and school/work disruptions, as well as reducing the risk of cross-infection. It can be quite a burden for some families, with greater responsibility for treatment for a patient who is more unwell. Healthcare systems often encourage this because of lack of beds and the perceived lower costs of intravenous antibiotics. There are a few studies in the literature to support the use of home intravenous antibiotics; however, in the only randomized controlled trial, patients generally had a better quality of life and less sleep disruption at home, but there were some downsides – with better disease mastery (a domain in the Quality of Life score) and less fatigue with hospital-based intravenous antibiotics [21]. A recent non-randomized retrospective study also suggested that improvements in lung function and body weight are better in hospital compared to home intravenous treatment, perhaps due to the difficulties of delivering multidisciplinary care in the community [22] (the antibiotic itself is just one part of the package of care delivered in the hospital). In summary, home intravenous antibiotics are a good option, for carefully selected patients.

PHARMACOKINETICS OF INTRAVENOUS ANTIBIOTICS

An important feature of intravenous antibiotic treatment in CF is the need to deliver high doses. In children they are usually given at the high end of the dose range and in adults at two to three times the usual recommended dose [15].

This is because of the larger volume of distribution and more rapid clearance of most antibiotics in patients with CF [23,24]. Aminoglycosides represent a particular problem, as it is important to achieve appropriate peaks, in order to achieve bacterial killing and prolonged post-antibiotic effect [25]. Traditionally, aminoglycosides have been delivered three times daily, but a number of studies have shown similar efficacy between once and thrice daily [26,27]. In a recent randomized controlled trial, once-daily tobramycin had some limited short-term benefits, in terms of renal toxicity, particularly in children [27]. Repeated treatment with aminoglycosides can cause both vestibular nerve and renal toxicity so careful monitoring of hearing and renal function should be undertaken [25]. The long-term benefits/risks of once-daily dosing are unknown.

CHOICE OF ANTIBIOTICS

Treatment of pulmonary exacerbations is usually with two anti-pseudomonal antibiotics to reduce the development of resistance and provide an additive or synergistic effect on bacterial killing (Table 10.2) [2,15,28].

The choice of which antibiotic combination should be used is based on the antimicrobial sensitivities of recent sputum cultures. When the organism is resistant, an empirical choice is made [28]. Antimicrobial resistance is common and varies geographically; in the UK; ceftazidime is the most frequently prescribed antibiotic to which resistance has developed [29]. There are few clinical trials directly comparing antibiotic regimens and it is likely there are few differences between specific antibiotics [30]. Synergy testing has been advocated, but there is no convincing evidence that in-vitro determined synergistic antibiotics have any advantage over combinations decided empirically [28, 31,32]. Treatment of exacerbations in people with multi-resistant organisms resistant to all anti-pseudomonal antibiotics may still result in improvement in symptoms, lung function and systemic markers of inflammation, suggesting that there may be other effects in addition to bacterial killing [32,33]. The combination of antibiotics should avoid those likely to cause antagonism, such as a carbapenem and β-lactam. People with CF often know which combination works best for them and can often contribute to choosing the appropriate antibiotics.

Table 10.2 Antibiotics used for treatment of pulmonary exacerbations due to *Pseudomonas aeruginosa*. Usually a β-lactam-based compound is combined with an aminogylcoside and treatment is given for 14 days.

β-lactam	Aminoglycosides	Quinolone	Polymyxin
Ceftazidime	Tobramycin	Ciprofloxacin	Colistin
Aztreonam	Gentamicin		
Meropenem	Amikacin		
Tazobactam			

ALLERGY AND DESENSITIZATION

Allergic reactions to antibiotics are fairly common in people with CF. The mechanisms in CF are unclear, but most are not classic type-one anaphylactic reactions [34]. The most common form of reaction is an urticarial skin rash, though more serious reactions such as anaphylaxis have been described. Antibiotics based on the penicillin ring structure, such as piperacillin, have the highest reported frequency of reactions, in particular drug fever. Allergic reactions to aminoglycosides, macrolides and Colomycin are infrequent. With increasing survival and use of antibiotics, some patients become sensitive to multiple drugs and de-sensitization is required. This can be undertaken with incremental introduction of the antibiotic at low dose, usually with prior treatment with systemic corticosteroids and antihistamines. Once completed, a full course of intravenous treatment is then given [34].

MACROLIDE ANTIBIOTICS

Macrolides have been known for some time to improve the outcome of diffuse panbronchiolitis, a disease common in Japan and associated with chronic *P. aeruginosa* infection. Azithromycin is concentrated intracellularly, particularly in macrophages and may have important effects on biofilm formation and improve bacterial killing. It may also have anti-inflammatory effects [35]. Three studies have now reported a beneficial effect of regular azithromycin treatment in patients with CF [36–38]. All three studies demonstrated an improvement in lung function and quality-of-life measures, and reduction in CRP in one study. On the basis of these studies, many patients with CF with or without *P. aeruginosa* are now on regular macrolide therapy three times per week or every day. All of these studies lasted for 6 months, so it is unclear whether there are longer term benefits or adverse effects from this treatment.

I. *Pseudomonas aeruginosa*

Pseudomonas aeruginosa is the most common organism causing chronic lung disease in patients with CF. Chronic infection with *P. aeruginosa* is an important predictor of survival in CF and the most important cause of morbidity [39,40]. Infection usually occurs late in the first decade, or during the second decade of life [2]. By the third decade, over 80% of people with CF have chronic infection with *P. aeruginosa* (Fig. 10.1).

The factors leading to initial infection are increasingly understood and treatments that eradicate early infection are now available. However, once *P. aeruginosa* is established in CF airways, it is not possible to permanently eradicate it. At this point it has established a bacterium–host relationship which results in a sustained host inflammatory response. Prevention of chronic *P. aeruginosa* infection is one of the most important treatment goals in CF care. If correction of

CFTR function by gene therapy or biochemical means is to be achieved, an important outcome measure will be protection against chronic *P. aeruginosa* infection.

Pseudomonas species are complex bacteria that have adapted to various ecological niches. In the relatively hypoxic environment of CF airway mucus, they adapt by forming micro-colonies and developing a complex biofilm [39,41]. The biofilms are a key mechanism in protecting the organism from host defenses, and when organisms such as *P. aeruginosa* are in a biofilm, neutrophils are frustrated and become either apoptotic or necrotic, releasing damaging proteases and free radicals into the airway [9,42]. Biofilms are also associated with increased antibiotic resistance, protecting the organisms against drug penetration; the altered growth rates of biofilm organisms and other physiological changes may also be a factor [43,44]. Interfering with biofilm formation may be one of the mechanisms by which macrolide antibiotics have an effect in the long-term treatment of CF.

It has been known for some time that the conversion from non-mucoid to a mucoid phenotype is important in the development of chronic infection [2,39]. The mucoid phenotype is associated with acceleration in the decline in lung function and a poorer prognosis [40,45]. The mucoid phenotype over-produces the exopolysaccharide alginate [46], which occurs because of mutations in the suppressive regulatory genes *mec A, B, C* and *D*. These genes suppress the expression of *AlgT* gene and this allows expression of the genes important for alginate biosynthesis [47]. The cause of these mutations is not clear, though oxygen radical damage to DNA is a possible mechanism. Over-expression of alginate protects the bacteria from neutrophil phagocytosis [48]. Alginate may also inhibit important innate immune responses, thus protecting the organism from normal clearance from the airway [39]. It may also have a function in biofilm formation, though this has been recently challenged [49,50]. In addition, the *AlgT* gene negatively controls expression of the flagella gene [47]. This is important as loss of motility in mucoid CF isolates may help to further protect the organism from host antibody defenses.

Differences in the lipopolysaccharide (LPS) expressed by *P. aeruginosa* strains from CF airways may also be important in their virulence. *P. aeruginosa* from CF sputum frequently express LPS defective in O-side chains, making them less susceptible to complement-mediated killing [51,52]. These and other changes in P. *aeruginosa* may also impact the interaction of LPS with toll-like receptor 4 (TLR-4) [51]. The effect of this may be to amplify inflammatory responses.

SOURCES OF INFECTION AND PREVENTION

Pseudomonas aeruginosa is found in many warm and moist environments [53]. It has many natural habitats including organic matter and surface water and can be found associated with many plant species. It has been shown to contaminate hydrotherapy pools and jacuzzis/hot tubs, where it can cause pseudomonal folliculitis [54]. There are reports of people with CF being infected from such environments. *Pseudomonas* species have also been demonstrated in many habitats within the healthcare environment. Medical and dental equipment may be contaminated and are potential sources of infection. Sinks in hospital wards have been shown to be contaminated and strains from these were identical to those on the hands of staff, suggesting this may also be a mode of cross-infection [53]. Hospital environments should be maintained to a very strict standard to reduce the potential for nosocomial transmission.

Until recently, there has been little evidence of patient-to-patient spread of *P. aeruginosa*. A number of sibling studies in the 1980s, however, had demonstrated that sibling pairs usually, though not always, carried the same strains. Over the past 10 years or so evidence has emerged that patient-to-patient spread can occur, and a number of CF centers have reported that a proportion of their patients carried the same clone. This was first demonstrated in Liverpool, UK, during a study where sputum antibiograms (that were being analyzed as part of a clinical trial) suggested that there was a clonal variant resistant to ceftazidime [55]. Spread of clonal variants have now been demonstrated in other clinics in the UK and Australia [55–58]. It is not clear whether clonal strains affect survival, though in one study an increased mortality was seen in children [59,60]. *P. aeruginosa* cross-infection has also been demonstrated after camps [61]. These have now stopped in the CF community, because of concerns of some parents and patients about cross-infection.

A number of strategies are useful in reducing *Pseudomonas* infection [53,62]. Regular surveillance of sputum and/or cough swabs should be undertaken and new isolates typed using a molecular method such as pulsed field gel electrophoresis or random amplification of polymorphic DNA [58]. CF centers should practice good hygiene at all times and should have a detailed cross-infection policy. Many CF centers now segregate those patients who do not have *P. aeruginosa* from those who do. Taking this approach, a significant reduction in the incidence and prevalence of new infection with *P. aeruginosa* has been reported [63]. In some centers, clinics are organized to prevent patient-to-patient contact; this is more useful in pediatric centers where a patient's microbiological status is not always certain. This, however, increases social isolation.

TREATMENT

The approach to antimicrobial therapy in CF patients with chronic *P. aeruginosa* infection is radically different from the majority of other infectious diseases. The appropriate treatment for individual patients is dependent on the stage in the natural history of pseudomonal infection. The accurate identification of *P. aeruginosa* is therefore critically important. Specific media should be used for culture and identifications and sputum cultures checked at least 3-monthly [2,15]. Antibodies to *P. aeruginosa* can be detected and may be useful in confirming infections. Two recent studies, however, indicate that interpretation of such assays is most difficult in children in whom sputum samples are not available [64–68]. Antibody titers are usually elevated in patients with chronic infection and negative in those never infected. In intermittently infected people, the results are more difficult to interpret. There are three clinical situations where there is good evidence for useful effects of anti-pseudomonal antimicrobial treatment, which are outlined below.

i. First isolation

Aggressive treatment of early infection may be effective in delaying chronic infection, so regular monitoring of lower airway infection is essential to determine when treatment is appropriate [2]. This is difficult in newly diagnosed infants, and in some centers annual bronchoscopy samples are obtained until sputum is expectorated. It is not yet clear whether this approach is beneficial compared to more conventional methods such as regular cough swabs; a large study is currently under way in Australia to examine this approach.

In the early phase of pseudomonal infection of the CF airway, the organisms are usually motile, in low density, and have not yet become mucoid or developed into a biofilm [4]. So in these early stages of infection, it may be possible to clear *P. aeruginosa* with aggressive antibiotic use [15]. A common approach is to use nebulized colistin for 3 months and oral ciprofloxacin for 2–3 weeks [69]. Ciprofloxacin has a bitter taste and sometimes young children will not tolerate the liquid; for older children, tablets can be placed inside an empty enzyme capsule to make them more palatable. Sunblock must also be use as ciprofloxacin is photosensitizing, and this must be carried on for 4 weeks after a course has finished. If the repeat sputum culture is negative then some centers will not give further treatment. However, there may be some value in continuing the nebulized antibiotics for 3 months as this may increase the length of time before recurrence. If ciprofloxacin is contraindicated or cannot be tolerated, then a 2-week course of an intravenous anti-pseudomonal combination such as ceftazidime and tobramycin would be appropriate with continuation of nebulized colistin for a further 3 months [15]. Clearly if the patient is unwell at the time of first isolation, intravenous antibiotics are indicated.

A number of studies have also investigated the role of nebulized tobramycin for early eradication. One study was stopped because all eight patients who received tobramycin cleared *P. aeruginosa* from their airway after 28 days, compared to only 1 of 13 receiving placebo [70]. However, this effect did not persist after 1 year. A study of children following anti-pseudomonal treatment for their first infection demonstrated that the mean duration of eradication was around 8 months and that the majority subsequently became infected with a genetically distinct *P. aeruginosa* organism [71]. This suggests that long-term chronic suppressive therapy after eradication, with nebulized antibiotics, may be appropriate, though there are no studies to support this. Using nebulized antibiotics twice daily is very

challenging for patients and adherence to such regimens is generally poor [72]. The development of dry-powder inhalers or use of faster and quieter nebulizers to deliver antibiotics will be a very helpful addition to current treatment [73].

Aggressive early treatment of infection and careful infection control measures results in significant reductions in the prevalence of *P. aeruginosa* in CF centers [74].

ii. Acute exacerbations

People (especially adults) with CF have frequent episodes of acute pulmonary exacerbation, which in a clinical context are not difficult to define or diagnose. For the purposes of clinical trials, however, use of objective measures is more of a problem. A recent study observing the features in patients who had treatment for an exacerbation found pulmonary signs and symptoms associated with a reduction in lung function were the most helpful indicators [75,76]. In general, patients presenting with a significant exacerbation are treated for a period of 14 days on two anti-pseudomonal antibiotics [2,15]. This is usually a β-lactam-based antibiotic in combination with an aminoglycoside [16] (see Table 10.2). In addition to antibiotic treatment, airway clearance is intensified using a variety of techniques, and other aspects of lung symptoms such as bronchoconstriction are treated [2]. Pulmonary exacerbations are frequently associated with weight loss, so attention to nutrition is often required [77]. Treatment of pulmonary exacerbations in this way usually results in improvement of symptoms, lung function, exercise tolerance, and a reduction in sputum production and systemic markers of inflammation. Sometimes an empirical change of antibiotics is helpful if there is little response after 7–10 days.

Some centers advocate use of regular 3-monthly intravenous antibiotics regardless of symptoms [78]. This has been demonstrated to be more effective than historical controls treated for pulmonary exacerbations, but this type of comparison is less than ideal [79]. In a randomized controlled trial, no significant benefit was shown in regular therapy after 3 years [13]. However, the patients in the arm of the study where exacerbations were treated had three courses of antibiotics per year anyway, compared to four courses in those who were being treated with regular 3-monthly antibiotics. This suggests that the natural history of pseudomonal infection is for three or four exacerbations per year and that it is reasonable to treat pulmonary exacerbations rather than impose a regimen of regular therapy on patients. Routine intravenous antibiotics are very expensive, and also imposes 8 weeks in hospital per year, which must impact on quality of life. In patients where adherence to therapy is poor, regular hospital admissions for intensive physiotherapy and intravenous antibiotics have a useful role.

iii. Treatment of chronic infection

A number of antibiotics have been used in an attempt to suppress bacterial numbers, stabilize lung function and decrease morbidity [2]. This has now been most convincingly demonstrated in a large randomized controlled trial using high-dose tobramycin (Tobi® 300 mg twice daily) on alternate months [19]. The requirement for intravenous antibiotics was also reduced and there was no evidence of serious side-effects. The polymyxin colistin has also been used in this way for over 20 years, and been shown to reduce bacterial density and may have a similar effect on lung function; however, this has not been demonstrated in a randomized controlled trial although there is a wealth of experience in Europe [18,33]. All patients who have chronic infection with *P. aeruginosa* should be considered for long-term nebulized antibiotic therapy using colistin or tobramycin [15]. Use of long-term nebulized antibiotics for chronic infection is treatment rather than prophylaxis. It is not clear whether this form of treatment can be stopped in a patient (usually a child) who has not had *P. aeruginosa* isolated for a while (i.e. a number of years), with CF centers differing in their approaches.

II. *Burkholderia* species

Since the first report of infection with *Burkholderia cepacia* and its consequences in CF [80], it has become recognized that *Burkholderia* is a genus containing a number of species that can be distinguished by phenotypic tests [81–83]. Prior to this they were identified as genomovars [84] (Table 10.3).

All of the members of the *B. cepacia* complex group have been described as causing infection in CF. The majority of the infections are caused by *B. cenocepacia* (previously genomovar III) and *B. multivorans* (genomovar II). Of the other groups, *B. vietnamiensis* is the most common (genomovar V). A recent outbreak of *B. dolorosa* in Boston in the United States resulted in increased morbidity and mortality [85]. Other members of the *B. cepacia* complex are sporadically isolated from sputum and rarely cause chronic infection [86]. *B. cenocepacia* is particularly problematic because of its transmissibility and association with an acute, often fatal, cepacia syndrome [60,87–89]. There are a number of problematic issues, including identification, transmissibility, pathogenicity, management and infection control.

Table 10.3 *Burkholderia cepacia* complex species with previous genomovar typing.

Burkholderia multivorans	Genomovar I
Burkholderia cepacia	Genomovar II
Burkholderia cenocepacia	Genomovar III (a, b, etc)
Burkholderia stabilis	Genomovar IV
Burkholderia vietnamiensis	Genomovar V
Burkholderia dolosa	Genomovar VI
Burkholderia ambifaria	Genomovar VII
Burkholderia anthinia	Genomovar VIII
Burkholderia pyrrocinia	Genomovar IX

MICROBIOLOGICAL IDENTIFICATION

The accurate identification of *B. cepacia* complex organisms is critical. Because of the transmissibility of this organism, there are potentially serious consequences if it is misidentified [89]. It is important to use the appropriate selective medium for culture [90]; some commercial kits can report both false positive and false negative results. In particular, *Achromobacter (Alcaligenes) xylosoxidans* and *Stenotrophomonas maltophilia* can be misidentified as *B. cenocepacia* [91]. Around 10% of suspicious organisms sent to referral centers for confirmation of identification were false positives, while over 30% were reported as false negatives in the US referral center [91]. Further identification of species can be undertaken using biochemical tests, but the consensus is that molecular methods of identification – for example, specific polymerase chain reaction (PCR) based tests or sequencing methods – are more appropriate [82].

TRANSMISSIBILITY

Using a variety of such methods it is clear that *B. cenocepacia* is the most highly transmissible member of this complex [86–94]. There are some reports of patient-to-patient spread of *B. multivorans*, but in most published series from single centers this organism appears to be unique to individual patients, only showing clonal spread in siblings with CF [95]. In an outbreak of *B. multivorans* infections in Glasgow, Scotland, there did appear to be transmission of this organism but such outbreaks have not been confirmed elsewhere [96]. The clonal outbreak of *B. dolorosa* has occurred in Boston and was associated with a high level of transmissibility [85]. A number of outbreaks of *B. cenocepacia* related to electrophoresis type 12 (ET-12) have been described and it is clear that this organism is highly transmissible between patients [92,97]. Evidence of this comes from CF centers, summer camps and other forms of patient contact in social circumstances [98,99].

PATHOGENICITY AND CLINICAL CONSEQUENCES

Infection with *B. cepacia* complex is associated with increased morbidity and reduced survival in CF [92,97]. The individual response to this infection is very variable and is determined by the species involved and the host response to infection. With the clear designation of different species, there are now data available on clinical outcomes of *B. cenocepacia* and *B. multivorans* infection.

i. B. cenocepacia infection

The prognosis of CF patients infected with *B. cepacia* complex organisms is much worse than those infected with *P. aeruginosa*. *B. cenocepacia* is associated with a rapid deterioration and early death in up to one-third of patients who acquire the organism (cepacia syndrome); while others still have a more rapid deterioration in lung function than with *P. aeruginosa* [88,97]. However, there are also patients with *B. cenocepacia* complex who remain well and stable despite chronic infection with this organism [95]. The reasons for these differences are not clear, though may relate to the impact of modifier genes which determine responses to infection, or modulate inflammation.

ii. Cepacia syndrome

This term relates to patients who newly acquire, or have been chronically infected with, a *B. cepacia* complex organism and deteriorate rapidly [89]. Incidental events such as acute viral infections may occur, but a precipitating event is usually not apparent. In many, this syndrome rapidly leads to death over a few weeks to months. It is most commonly associated with *B. cenocepacia* subgroup A, and electrophoresis type 12 (ET-12). It occasionally occurs with *B. multivorans* infection [89,96]. It is usually associated with clinical signs of sepsis, weight loss and a sustained acute-phase response, and sometimes septicemia. The chest radiograph shows progressive infiltrates (Fig. 10.2).

All of this occurs despite aggressive antimicrobial treatment. Progression to early death can occur in a few weeks despite maximal therapy. Occasionally such patients stabilize for a time, and there is some anecdotal evidence that additional use of immunosuppressive agents such as ciclosporin may be of modest benefit in halting progression.

iii. Chronic infection with B. cepacia complex

For those patients who do not succumb to an acute cepacia syndrome, subsequent prognosis is still poor. This particularly applies to patients with *B. cenocepacia*. Most of the data available on such patients related to those infected with a common epidemic strain in Canada and the UK, the ET-12 strain [97,100]. This strain seems to be the most transmissible and also most virulent strain in the complex. Rather surprisingly, in studies examining airways inflammation in patients with CF, either when stable or during inflammatory exacerbations, markers of inflammation in patients with *B. cenocepacia* are similar to those with *P. aeruginosa*

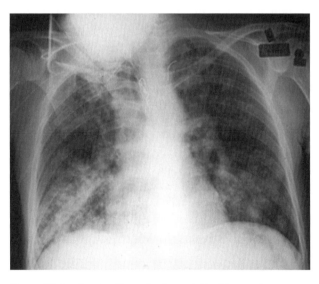

Figure 10.2 Chest radiograph of an adult with cepacia syndrome.

[9,100]. The outcomes from lung transplantation are significantly worse in people with *B. cenocepacia* infection compared to those with *P. aeruginosa* [101,102].

iv. B. multivorans infection

Infection with *B. multivorans* is generally less severe than with *B. cenocepacia* and a significant number of patients who isolate *B. multivorans* from sputum subsequently clear it [89]. This transient infection does not appear to be associated with significant morbidity. For those who do become chronically infected with *B. multivorans*, the natural history of the disease is comparable to patients with *P. aeruginosa* but worse than with *B. cenocepacia* [88,89]. It is currently not clear why this is the case, but it may relate to differences in the LPS from these species. Patients with *B. multivorans* infection also have a better prognosis following lung transplantation compared to those infected with *B. cenocepacia* [101].

MANAGEMENT OF RESPIRATORY EXACERBATIONS DUE TO *B. CEPACIA* COMPLEX

Burkholderia cepacia is almost always multiply-resistant and frequently pan-resistant to antibiotics [2]. This presents some problems in using in-vitro sensitivity to determine the selection of intravenous antibiotics. The choice is therefore often made empirically, based on the knowledge of the minimal inhibitory concentrations (MICs) of anti-pseudomonal antibiotics to this organism. Ceftazidime, meropenem, temocillin, tazobactam, co-trimoxazole, chloramphenicol and tetracyclines all show some activity [16]. The value of synergy testing has been recently evaluated in patients with *B. cepacia* complex infection. Response to treatment was not significantly different between empirically chosen combinations and those chosen after a checkerboard synergy test [103]. Nevertheless, the following combinations may be useful: meropenem or ceftazidime or temocillin in combination with an aminoglycoside [103]. Chloramphenicol, co-trimoxazole or tetracycline may be added as a third drug. There are no data on the effect of long-term antibiotic treatment in patients with *B. cepacia* complex infection. Nebulized aminoglycosides or oral macrolides have not been specifically tested. Because of the poor prognosis of these patients, they are generally excluded from antibiotic studies. However, it may be reasonable to extrapolate from *Pseudomonas* studies and use oral azithromycin three days per week. If there is co-infection with *P. aeruginosa*, nebulized antibiotic such as colistin or tobramycin is also appropriate [104].

INFECTION CONTROL

Burkholderia cepacia complex organisms are uncommon in the natural environment although they have been found around maize, onion fields and in soil associated with plants; they are also found in water, sinks and contaminated equipment [98,105]. It is likely that the majority of patients with *B. multivorans* infections acquire this organism from the environment whereas *B. cenocepacia* is more likely to be transmitted from patient to patient [105]. This can occur in hospital and in social environments. Close social contact such as attendance at a summer camp for people with CF, sharing a combined space such as a hotel room or car journey, sexual contact and sharing eating or drinking utensils, have all been implicated in patient-to-patient spread [99]. Contaminated respiratory equipment has also been shown to be associated with cross-infection. Air sampling studies demonstrate significant numbers of organisms for over an hour after coughing [99], but one study suggested that the air further than 3 feet (1 meter) from a patient is unlikely to contain aerosolized organisms [106].

There are important principles in infection control which particularly apply to *B. cepacia*, hence the importance of a precise diagnosis. Patients with different species should not be cohorted. Although patients with *B. multivorans* can probably attend the same outpatient clinic safely, if universal precautions are taken, patients with *B. multivorans* should under no circumstances mix with those with *B. cenocepacia* [62,98]. Although there is no definite evidence, patients with chronic infection with other members of the *B. cepacia* complex should be treated with universal precautions. Patients with *B. cenocepacia*, if they are all infected with the same clone, can reasonably be cohorted, though universal infection control precautions should be strictly adhered to. This means they may attend the same outpatient clinic and can be managed as inpatients in the same proximity but should have separate rooms and be discouraged from mixing with each other [62,98]. Infection control policies should be developed with an understanding of local epidemiology of this organism in the CF population.

III. *Staphylococcus aureus (MSSA)*

Methicillin-sensitive *Staphylococcus aureus* (MSSA) is the most common pathogen isolated in sputum of children with CF during the first decade [2,14]. It is an important pathogen throughout life and often occurs as a co-infecting organism in patients chronically infected with *P. aeruginosa*, *B. cepacia* complex and other Gram-negative organisms [107,108]. In children, it can be associated with an increase in respiratory symptoms but rarely causes a systemic inflammatory response [11]. There is still some debate as to its pathogenicity as it can be cultured in sputum without any change in symptoms [39]. Bronchoscopy studies indicate that up to 40% of infants aged under 3 years culture *S. aureus* from bronchoalveolar samples [109].

LONG-TERM PROPHYLAXIS/TREATMENT OF CHRONIC INFECTION

Some CF centers advocate the use of long-term prophylactic anti-staphylococcal treatment, while others treat on the basis of symptoms and positive sputum cultures [14,76,110]. It is a recommendation in the UK to treat all infants aged under 2

years with long-term flucloxacillin, but not in the USA [111]. However, it is only prophylaxis when the child has not yet had *S.aureus* cultured; more usually, the child is chronically infected and anti-staphylococcal antibiotics are used for treatment of chronic infection. Long-term flucloxacillin has been shown to result in a reduction in cough, antibiotic requirements, and number of hospital admissions [110]. However, no benefit in pulmonary function tests was described up to 2 years of age [112]. A further study compared cefalexin treatment to placebo and demonstrated no significant clinical benefits [17]. There was a reduction in the frequency of respiratory cultures positive for *S. aureus* but there was a significantly higher frequency of *P. aeruginosa* cultured; however cefalexin promotes biofilm formation, which may have contributed to this increase in *P. aeruginosa* infection. There is no strong evidence that anti-staphylococcal treatment is of benefit for patients over the age of 6 years, though many centers continue treatment into the second decade [113].

TREATMENT OF PULMONARY EXACERBATIONS

The alternative approach is to treat patients with *S. aureus* when they have symptoms of an exacerbation. This approach works best when there is frequent attendance for sputum or cough swab cultures (monthly) and treatment with antibiotics is started promptly. However, this approach has not been compared in a randomized controlled trial. A retrospective study from the Danish CF center reported eradication of *S. aureus* in 74% of patients with 14-day course of anti-staphylococcal antibiotics and in almost all after a 3-month treatment [114].

ANTIBIOTIC THERAPY

Oral flucloxacillin is usually sufficient to eradicate the organism when given for 2 weeks. For patients who are penicillin-allergic, azithromycin, clindamycin, rifampicin or sodium fusidate are suitable alternatives [16,115]. In a patient with deteriorating symptoms and lung function, treatment with intravenous flucloxacillin and an aminoglycoside can be effective [107]. Linezolid (an oxazolidinone), which is a new class of antibiotic with excellent bioavailability, has been used successfully in those with *S. aureus* who are deteriorating, but it is expensive and requires weekly blood tests. In patients receiving long-term anti-staphylococcal antibiotics, *S. aureus* may still be isolated from sputum. This should raise questions about adherence to treatment but, should it occur, and the patient is taking regular flucloxacillin, an alternative class of anti-staphylococcal antibiotic should be used.

IV. Methicillin-resistant *Staphylococus aureus (MRSA)*

Staphylococus aureus stains resistant to methicillin and other β-lactam antimicrobials have become an endemic problem in most healthcare facilities in the western world [116,117]. MRSA is usually acquired from the hospital environment but there is evidence that strains can be community-acquired. Patient-to-patient spread has also been well documented [119,120].

Not surprisingly the prevalence of MRSA in CF varies from center to center. It has been reported in up to 23% of centers in North America [118]. Infection with MRSA most frequently occurs in patients with poor lung function and may result in an increase in requirement for antibiotics [121]. However, other studies have not demonstrated any significant deterioration in CF patients infected with this organism [120].

This organism presents some problems when cultured from patients with CF. It is recommended that they should be isolated until they have had three clear sputum cultures over 6–12 months.

TREATMENT

Because of the potential of this organism to cause chronic infection, eradication should be attempted [107,122]. Patients should have sputum and appropriate swabs taken from flexor surfaces, perineum and anterior nares. Evidence of skin or nasal carriage should have treatment with tricosolan and mupirocin. For those who also isolate it from their sputum, treatment with appropriate oral antibiotics is recommended to eradicate the organism. A regimen of rifampicin and fusidic acid has been shown to be useful but treatment should be determined by in-vitro sensitivities [121]. Tetracycline and trimethoprim may also have activity against MRSA. Some centers now also use oral linezolid, though this drug needs to be used with care because of its expense and potential side-effect profile [123]. Intravenous vancomycin or teicoplanin are rarely required to treat MRSA in CF, particularly as vancomycin is thought to be less effective in lung infections.

V. *Haemophilus influenzae*

Haemophilus influenzae occurs reasonably frequently in patients with CF, but there is little evidence to indicate its significance [124,125]. This organism is pathogenic in non-CF bronchiectasis and chronic obstructive pulmonary disease, and there is no reason to suggest that is not the case in CF. It is often associated with increased symptoms and should be treated when isolated from sputum/cough swabs with an oral antibiotic such as co-amoxiclav [98]. It is more likely to cause symptoms in children under the age of 6 years due to their relatively immature IgG_2 immune response.

VI. *Stenotrophomonas maltophilia*

Stenotrophomonas maltophilia is an aerobic Gram-negative bacterium, previously called *Pseudomonas maltophilia* and *Xanthamonas maltophilia*. There are a number of other species in the *Stenotrophomonas* group but *S. maltophilia* is the only member to cause lung infection in CF. *S. maltophilia* is found in aquatic environments and in a wide range of environmental niches similarly to *P. aeruginosa* [126]. Biofilm formation has been described in *S. maltophilia*, although the clinical significance of this is unclear. The prevalence of *S. maltophilia* in patients with CF varies considerably from center to center [127,130]. Some European centers have reported prevalences of up to 30%. In a recent large study from North America using the CF Foundation Registry of 176 accredited centers (2755 patients aged over 6 years), the prevalence rate ranged from 3% to 7% [127]. The case rate varied from no cases in seven centers to 39% of patients in one center [127]. This was not significantly influenced by geographic region or center size. It has been generally accepted that *S. maltophilia* does not spread by cross-infection from patient to patient; using molecular typing techniques, studies have demonstrated that most patients have unique strains of the organism [128]. However, the North American data suggest that cross-infection may occur in some centers.

There are a number of risk factors described for acquisition of *S. maltophilia*, including high use of intravenous and nebulized antibiotics [126,129,130]. Oral quinolones have been specifically implicated. Carbapenems have been described as increasing the incidence of *S. maltophilia* particularly when used in intensive care, but this relationship is not apparent in CF. Other patient-associated characteristics include reduced body weight, steroid use, *Aspergillus fumigatus* and lung function [131].

CLINICAL IMPACT

A number of studies have demonstrated that *S. maltophilia* is not a cause of significant adverse morbidity or mortality in CF. A large study, using the CFF registry, demonstrated that 5-year mortality was no greater in people with CF infected with *S. maltophilia* compared to those with *P. aeruginosa* [127,130]. In addition, the rate of decline of lung function is less compared to patients infected with *P. aeruginosa*. The majority of patients with *S. maltophilia* have it transiently; in one study, only 11% of those who isolated *S. maltophilia* remained chronically infected [131]. However, some patients do become chronically infected, and have chronic symptoms as well as acute exacerbations in a similar way to those seen in *P. aeruginosa* infection. Some transplant centers consider *S. maltophilia* infection to be a relative contraindication to lung transplantation, because it is multiply-resistant to antibiotics.

TREATMENT

There are no clinical studies of antibiotic treatment in CF patients to indicate the most appropriate treatment regimen for a first or recurrent isolation of *S. maltophilia*. First isolates should probably be treated as a proportion may go on to develop chronic infection. In patients with chronic infection, pulmonary exacerbations may require treatment with intravenous antibiotics. *S. maltophilia* is constitutively multiply-resistant to antibiotics [126,132]; it is inherently resistant to carbapenems and high levels of resistance are usually seen to aztreonam, aminoglycosides, tazobactam and colistin [132]. Ceftazidime is probably the most active anti-pseudomonal antibiotic available [126]. *In vitro, S. maltophilia* is sensitive to a combination of co-amoxiclav and aztreonam despite being resistant to these antibiotics when tested alone. Intravenous tazobactam plus aztreonam or an aminoglycoside is a reasonable regimen. Patients with mild symptoms may respond to oral co-trimoxazole or doxycycline, as they also have useful activity against the organism [132,133].

VII. *Achromobacter (Alcaligenes) xylosoxidans*

Achromobacter xylosoxidans has a reported prevalence of around 15% in the North American CFF registry, though in a study of inhaled tobramycin the prevalence was 9% [134]. Not much is known about the environmental reservoirs of this organism or its potential for patient-to-patient spread; however, it is prudent to consider *A. xylosoxidans* as potentially transmissible and universal infection control measures should be utilized. It is usually multiply-resistant to antibiotics, but there are no studies to indicate that it has an adverse effect on prognosis in CF [134]. Treatment for pulmonary exacerbations in people who are chronically infected is usually empirical using two different classes of anti-pseudomonal antibiotics.

VIII. Non-tuberculous mycobacterial infection (NTM)

Mycobacterium avium complex (MAC) is the most common non-tuberculous mycobacterial infection in CF, accounting for around 70% of isolates, while *Mycobacterium abscessus* accounts for 16% [135]. In the largest series reported, the majority of those who cultured NTM had only one of three sputum cultures positive [135]. This suggests that either it causes transient infection or is present in low numbers. Patients with NTM infection compared to case controls do not show any acceleration in decline in lung function [136]. Patients acquiring NTM infection are older, tend to have better lung function, and have a low frequency of infection with *P. aeruginosa*. Cross-infection does not appear to be a problem, though there have only been a few studies using molecular typing of NTM. None of these have shown any clonal spread of organisms between patients [136]. *M. abscessus* seems to be more virulent than MAC or other types of NTM. This evidence comes mostly from case series, and it is only a proportion of people with CF who develop clinically relevant disease with this infection.

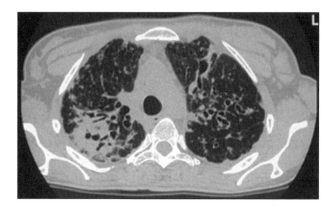

Figure 10.3 CT chest scan of an adult with non-tuberculous mycobacterial infection.

DIAGNOSIS

The diagnosis of clinically significant NTM infection is difficult [137]. The American Thoracic Society guidelines for diagnosis of NTM are of limited help and must be interpreted with an understanding of the overlap of symptoms and radiological changes with CF lung disease [138]. Systemic symptoms of mycobacterial infection, at least three sequential positive sputum cultures, a reduction in lung function, and new changes on high-resolution CT scanning of the chest are strongly suggestive of active infection (Fig. 10.3). However, all of these changes can occur with *P. aeruginosa* infection; and if this organism is co-infecting it is useful to treat it first. Only if symptoms and radiographic changes persist would treatment with an anti-mycobacterial regimen be considered.

TREATMENT

Non-tuberculous mycobacterial infection is usually resistant to standard anti-tuberculous antibiotics, but there are certain combinations that may be helpful [139,140]. Rifampicin, ethambutol, azithromycin and a fluoroquinolone (ciprofloxacin or moxifloxacin) have been shown to be of benefit in CF and non-CF populations. In difficult cases, particularly in *M. abscessus* infection, other regimens including cefoxatin, imipenem and amikacin (intravenously or by nebulizer) may also be of benefit [140]. Response to treatment should be monitored using symptoms, C-reactive protein, sputum cultures and serial high-resolution CT scans. The aim is to achieve 12 months with regular negative sputum cultures, before stopping treatment. This may be achieved in MAC infection but is much less likely with *M. abscessus*. Infection with NTM has been demonstrated to be associated with mutations of interferon-γ receptors and subsequent second messenger pathways. Patients with such defects may benefit from IFN-γ treatment [141].

RESPIRATORY VIRUSES

Respiratory viral infections have a significant impact on patients with CF, especially in the autumn (fall) and winter, and respiratory viruses may precipitate up to 40% of chest exacerbations [142–144]. Their effect has probably been under-estimated in the past, and this is likely due to difficulties in identifying them, especially from expectorated viscous sputum and thick mucoid airway secretions. Recently, however, it has been shown that combining a multiplex reverse transcriptase PCR with colorimetric amplicon detection can identify most respiratory viruses in the sputum of CF patients [145]. Viruses implicated in causing infections in CF are the same as those that may affect anyone, namely respiratory syncytial virus (RSV), adenovirus, parainfluenza virus types 1–3, influenza A and B, and rhinovirus [146]. There is no information yet on the relevance of human metapneumovirus in CF, but it is likely to be similar to that in previously healthy infants (less common than RSV but more common than parainfluenza) [147].

There is no evidence that infants, children or adults with CF are more susceptible to viral infections than healthy people, but the impact is greater, and the outcome worse as the lower respiratory tract is affected more often [142,146,148,149]. Viral infections may lead to increased frequency and duration of hospitalization for respiratory exacerbations [150], followed by deterioration in clinical status and lung function [142,144], which may persist for several months [149,150]. The viruses that have the greatest impact in CF are RSV and influenza. RSV predominates in infants although CF infants have the same number of RSV infections as non-CF infants in any season [151]. As well as causing acute pulmonary exacerbations and worsening of airway obstruction, RSV can sometimes cause more severe problems, including prolonged hospitalization, persistent hypoxemia and even a need for mechanical ventilation. Complications can last for several months after the acute infection; one study with a 2-year follow-up found increased respiratory symptoms and worse chest radiograph score in infants who had had RSV [143]. In older children and adults, influenza has the greatest effect, sometimes leading to a significant fall in lung function [152] and deterioration in clinical status [153]; primary influenza pneumonia can also occur.

Respiratory viral infections are also associated with onset of secondary bacterial infections, and the first isolation of a particular organism (particularly *P. aeruginosa*) often follows a viral infection [154,155]. One study, in which respiratory viral infections were confirmed on bronchoalveolar lavage (in 52% of infants hospitalized for respiratory disease), found at 12- to 60-month follow-up that first isolation of *P. aeruginosa* was more common in the infants who had been hospitalized for respiratory illness than those who were not (35% vs 6%) [156]. The pathophysiology is not well understood, but the association may be due to epithelial damage caused by the viruses with subsequent airway inflammation, as well as impairment of the cough reflex and mucociliary clearance. On the other hand, it may simply be that bacteria were already present in the lungs, but were isolated at the time of increased mucus production and expectoration only because of the viral

infection. This is more likely in children as sputum production is often minimal.

Antiviral strategies

The viruses have relatively short incubation periods (less than a week), and transmission occurs primarily via direct contact (skin or aerosol) with an infected person or something they have recently handled [38]. It is sensible to keep people with obvious upper respiratory tract infections away from CF infants if possible. Droplet infection via the nose and eyes can occur within 3 feet (1 meter) with influenza and adenovirus. In hospitalized infants, isolation in a cubicle or cohorting of infected patients is important, but success relies on rapid diagnosis, and a number of techniques are available. Staff must be meticulous with infection precautions, particularly hand-washing.

IMMUNIZATION

A Cochrane systematic review did not find any evidence that influenza immunization is beneficial to patients with CF [157]. However, the immunogenic effect in CF children is similar to normal children [158] and several studies have shown it to be safe [151]. Consequently, influenza immunization is recommended annually for CF patients aged over 6 months; immunization of immediate family members is also recommended [151]. There is no licensed vaccine for those aged under 6 months, and children aged 6–35 months require two half-doses 1 month apart. In addition, those aged 3–8 years who are receiving the vaccine for the first time also require two doses 1 month apart, but for succeeding years receive a single dose similarly to adults [151]. Currently there is no effective RSV vaccine available. Passive immunoprophylaxis with palivizumab (a monoclonal antibody to RSV) may have some benefit in expremature babies with chronic lung disease, but so far there are insufficient data to determine its effectiveness in CF infants. A number of studies investigating the efficacy of immunoprophylaxis are currently under way.

ANTIVIRAL DRUGS

There may be a role for the neuraminidase inhibitors oral oseltamivir or inhaled zanamivir when used early (ideally within a few hours of onset of symptoms, and at least within 48 hours) in influenza infection, as well as for prophylaxis of non-immunized patients exposed to influenza [159]. This is most likely to be valuable during an influenza epidemic. Evidence is lacking in CF, but one difficulty is recognizing a chest exacerbation as being due to influenza early enough in the illness for the drug to be effective. Amantadine is no longer recommended for treatment or prophylaxis of influenza [159].

Inhaled ribavirin (a nucleotide analogue) is licensed for use in RSV infection but has limited effectiveness and is rarely used in otherwise healthy infants; it is not indicated in CF. There is some evidence that the leukotriene receptor antagonist montelukast reduces respiratory symptoms (particularly cough) for a month post-RSV bronchiolitis, when given within 7 days of onset of symptoms [160]. Since it is free of adverse effects, it may be worthwhile trying in CF infants, although no study in this group has been undertaken.

Antibacterial prophylaxis

When patients have an upper respiratory tract infection (most commonly due to rhinovirus), unless symptoms are trivial, many clinicians advise antibiotic prophylaxis (principally against *H. influenzae*) – for example with co-amoxiclav for at least 2 weeks [15]. This is not based on trial evidence in CF patients, but is supported by clinical experience and a randomized controlled trial in non-CF patients with common colds. It was found that 5 days of co-amoxiclav benefited the 20% of patients whose nasopharyngeal secretions had also grown bacteria (*H. influenzae*, *Moraxella catarrhalis* or *Streptococcus pneumoniae*) [161]. Some centers advocate doubling the dose of the flucloxacillin the child is on for chronic *S. aureus* infection during colds, but that offers no additional benefit against *H. influenzae*.

FUNGAL INFECTIONS

Aspergillus is a widely-distributed spore-bearing fungus, and since it can grow at body temperature and the spores are respiratory particle-sized (2–4 μm) it can be associated with respiratory disease in humans. The presence of necrotic lung tissue and cavitating lung disease makes the CF lung an ideal environment for *Aspergillus* [162].

There are several species but *A. fumigatus* is most often implicated. *Aspergillus* lung disease may take the form of lung infection, aspergilloma, invasive aspergillosis or allergic bronchopulmonary aspergillosis (ABPA); it is the first and last that are most relevant to CF. An aspergilloma is a discrete fungal ball (mycetoma) found in an existing cavitatory lung lesion, which commonly causes hemoptysis. It is rare in children with CF but may be more common in adult patients, and is likely to be recognized more often with increased use of chest CT scanning [162]. Invasive aspergillosis occurs when the fungus invades the lung tissue; it is rare and more often associated with congenital or acquired immunodeficiency (including post-transplant); however, isolated cases in non-transplanted CF patients have been reported [163,164]. If immunosuppression becomes more widely used in CF then the frequency of this complication is likely to increase.

Aspergillus lung infection

Aspergillus is commonly found in the sputum in CF (variably reported as 1–60% [165]) and it is not always obvious

whether it is causing disease or just harmless colonization. *A. fumigatus* is commonest, but *A. clavatus*, *A. flavus*, *A. niger*, *A. terreus* and *A. nidulans* have also been isolated. If *Aspergillus* is repeatedly cultured, and especially if no bacteria are isolated, then in a patient who is symptomatic or chronically deteriorating, treatment with an antifungal agent is prudent. A typical regimen would be oral itraconazole for 1 month. *Aspergillus* has also been identified in a significant proportion of sinus cultures in a small series of patients with CF undergoing sinus surgery [166].

Allergic bronchopulmonary aspergillosis

PATHOPHYSIOLOGY

Allergic bronchopulmonary aspergillosis (ABPA) is a hypersensitivity disease of the lung due to an immune response to *A. fumigatus* antigens; it is seen most often in patients of all ages with CF and adults with asthma. Interestingly, heterozygosity for a CF gene mutation has been shown to predispose to ABPA in non-CF patients [167]. The inhaled spores are trapped in airway mucus, germinate and form mycelia which release allergens; the bronchus-associated lymphoid tissue (BALT) may be exposed to high levels of these allergens. This is followed by type I and type III immune responses with production of specific IgG and IgE antibodies. This is accompanied by an exaggerated T helper type-2 lymphocyte response leading to release of cytokines associated with allergy – interleukin (IL)-4, IL-5 and IL-13 [165]. Furthermore, the *Aspergillus* is bound to the surface epithelium and grows on and between the epithelial cells. It is not killed efficiently by monocytic and eosinophilic infiltrates, which results in chronic airway inflammation; this aids antigen transport across the epithelial cell layer and exposure of the antigens to further inflammatory cells. When the inflammation extends into the small airways and alveoli, it resembles eosinophilic pneumonia; the alveolar infiltrate is thought to cause the fleeting shadows seen on a chest radiograph.

EPIDEMIOLOGY AND RISK FACTORS

Prevalence data are hampered by poorly standardized diagnostic criteria and the difficulties of distinguishing symptoms of ABPA from other aspects of CF lung disease. Data from the European Epidemiologic Registry of CF (ERCF) on 12 447 patients in nine countries showed an overall prevalence of 7.8%, with a range of 2–14% (6% in the UK) [168]. ABPA seems to be less prevalent in North America, with the North American Epidemiologic Study of CF (ESCF) reporting on 14 210 patients as having a prevalence of 2% [169]. Differences may be partly due to the ESCF stricter diagnostic criteria (see both papers for different criteria used for these large databases) and this figure may be an under-estimate. It is also possibly due to less use of inhaled antibiotics in the United States in the past. An increased isolation of fungi

(*Aspergillus* and *Candida*) was detected in the active arm of the large North American inhaled TOBI study (although there was no reported increase in ABPA itself) [170], so use of inhaled tobramycin may now be a risk factor. Inhaled antipseudomonal antibiotics have been in use in Europe far longer than in the United States, although a small study did not show colistin (the principal one used before development of TOBI) to be associated with increased fungal colonization [171]. Both databases showed an increase with age and a low incidence in those under 6 years. ESCF data indicated increased prevalence in males, adolescents, those with poorer lung function and those with *P. aeruginosa* infection [169]. While they also reported an increased incidence in those with wheeze and asthma, that may simply have been symptoms of the ABPA itself. The ERCF found an association of ABPA with bacterial chronic infection, pneumothorax, massive hemoptysis, higher serum IgG levels and poor nutritional status [169]. Atopy is an important risk factor with ABPA occurring in 22% of atopic CF patients compared to 2% non-atopic patients [165]. In addition, HLA-DR2 and -DR5 may contribute to susceptibility while HLA-DQ2 may predispose to resistance [165]. Finally, a recent case–control study has found that sensitization to *A. fumigatus* (but not ABPA) was independently associated with higher cumulative doses of inhaled corticosteroids, although causation has not been proven [172].

CLINICAL PICTURE

This may vary but there are two classic scenarios of presentation. First, the patient may present relatively acutely with wheezing, dyspnea, chest pain and plugs of sputum with brown/black flecks. Sometimes there is fever, myalgia and malaise, an 'influenza-like' syndrome. Lung function is reduced with an obstructive pattern on the flow–volume curve and the chest radiograph shows new infiltrates (that tend to disappear with systemic corticosteroid therapy). The second scenario is more insidious with a chronic and generalized chest deterioration that does not respond to intravenous antibiotics. Bronchiectasis may be present, and when associated with ABPA tends to be found more centrally (inner two-thirds) on a chest CT scan. Diagnosis is not always obvious, however, as many features of ABPA are common to other aspects of CF lung disease. In addition, ABPA may be recurrent and episodic in nature.

DIAGNOSIS

Diagnosis relies on a combination of the clinical picture with evidence of *Aspergillus* exposure leading to a relevant immune response. A CF Foundation consensus conference has derived a set of criteria for diagnosing a 'classic case', as well as a set of minimal diagnostic criteria (Table 10.4) [165]; the UK CF Trust has also published guidelines (Table 10.5) [15].

However, the individual features are not enough for a diagnosis. For example, *Aspergillus* is frequently isolated in

Table 10.4 Diagnostic criteria for allergic bronchopulmonary aspergillosis (ABPA) proposed by the CF Foundation consensus conference [165].

Classic case

Acute or subacute deterioration (cough, wheeze, exercise intolerance, exercise-induced asthma, decline in lung function, increase in sputum) not attributable to another etiology

Serum total IgE >1000 IU/mL (unless receiving systemic corticosteroids)

Immediate cutaneous reactivity to *Aspergillus* or serum IgE antibody to *A. fumigatus*

Precipitating antibodies to *A. fumigatus* or serum IgG to *A. fumigatus*

New or recent abnormalities on chest radiography (infiltrates or mucus plugging) or chest CT (bronchiectasis) that have not cleared with antibiotics and standard physiotherapy

Minimal diagnostic criteria

Acute or subacute deterioration not attributable to another etiology

Serum total IgE >500 IU/mL; if total IgE level is 200–500 IU/mL, repeat test in 1–3 months

Immediate cutaneous reactivity to *Aspergillus* or serum IgE antibody to *A. fumigatus*

One of the following: (1) precipitins to *A. fumigatus* or IgG antibody to *A. fumigatus* or (2) new or recent abnormalities on chest radiography (infiltrates or mucus plugging) or chest CT (bronchiectasis) that have not cleared with antibiotics and standard physiotherapy

Table 10.5 Diagnostic criteria for allergic bronchopulmonary aspergillosis (ABPA) proposed by UK CF Trust [15].

The occurrence of asthma symptoms

New x-ray changes such as patchy atelectasis, consolidation, homogeneous bronchial shadowing or parallel 'tram-line' linear shadows

Increased IgE levels of >500 IU/mL or a 4-fold rise in IgE titers

Increased specific IgE radio-allergosorbent test (RAST) or positive skin prick tests

Eosinophilia >500/mm^3

Positive sputum culture or fungal hyphae identified on microscopy

the absence of ABPA; skin prick tests are commonly positive in CF patients (especially adults) with no ABPA [168]; precipitating antibodies are also found with no ABPA [165]; serum IgE may be raised due to atopy alone; eosinophilia may be associated with chronic *P. aeruginosa* infection; distal airways obstruction is non-specific; and radiographic infiltrates and bronchiectasis are common findings in CF patients. Some children have a chronically high serum IgE, and then an acute rise (2- to 4-fold) may be indicative of an ABPA exacerbation. Use of disease-specific recombinant *A. fumigatus* allergens may be helpful as non-secreted cytoplasmic allergens may be recognized by IgE only in patients with ABPA, whereas secreted allergens may be recognized by

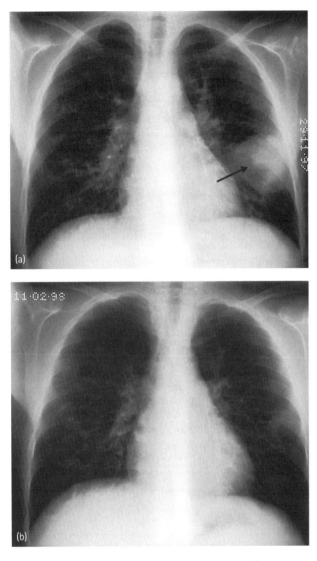

Figure 10.4 Chest radiographs of a child showing (a) infiltration due to ABPA (arrow) and (b) follow-up at 10 weeks later showing considerable improvement after oral corticosteroid therapy.

sensitized individuals whether or not they have ABPA [173]. An appropriate clinical response to corticosteroid therapy (with clearing of infiltrates on chest radiograph and reduction in IgE) will help confirm the diagnosis (Fig. 10.4).

The differential diagnosis includes bacterial chest exacerbation, CF asthma, atopy, severe small airways disease, gastroesophageal reflux with or without aspiration, and in the case of acute chest pain a pneumothorax.

SCREENING

The most important thing is for the clinician to have a high index of suspicion and consider the diagnosis. This is particularly so when there is a poor response to intravenous antibiotics, marked wheeze or pleuritic chest pain. Sputum cultures or cough swabs should be taken at every clinic visit. At annual review, ABPA serum markers should be measured; this baseline is then useful when markers are measured during chest exacerbations, since a rise in total and aspergillus-specific IgE can suggest the diagnosis. The CFF consensus recommends total IgE be measured annually in patients aged over 6 years, with further markers measured if >500 IU/mL and repeat IgE measurement if 200–500 IU/mL [165].

TREATMENT

When it is not obvious whether chest symptoms are due only to ABPA or whether bacterial infection is playing a part, intravenous antibiotics are usually started initially. There is surprisingly little evidence to inform clinicians how best to treat ABPA itself. Although there have been no randomized controlled trials in CF, the available data suggest that oral corticosteroids should be used to attenuate the inflammatory and immunological reaction [165]. Clinical experience has shown them to be effective in reducing symptoms (often within a few days), improve chest radiograph signs and reduce serum IgE and eosinophilia. While they are effective in suppressing acute exacerbations, it is unclear whether they affect progression of lung disease [174]. The starting dose of prednisolone is typically 2 mg/kg body weight (up to maximum of 60 mg) given for 2 weeks, reduced to 1 mg/kg for 2 weeks, 0.5 mg/kg for 2 weeks and then further gradual tapering of the dose depending on the clinical response, usually over 2–3 months. If there is no response to steroids the issue of non-adherence needs to be considered. It is also important not to prescribe enteric-coated preparations. There is little evidence for the role of inhaled corticosteroids [165], but they are sometimes used in adult patients. Relapse may occur during steroid tapering, in which case the dose is increased once more and tapered more slowly over several months. Recurrence is common within 2–3 years, in which case a full treatment course is required.

Oral antifungal agents are also used on the principle that it is beneficial to combat the airway fungal infection and thus reduce the antigenic burden. There have been no randomized controlled trials in CF [175], but evidence comes from trials in asthmatics with ABPA. Oral itraconazole led to a decrease in serum markers and eosinophilic inflammation, which was matched by a reduction in corticosteroid dose and clinical improvement [176,177]. In CF, there have been case series only, but they did demonstrate a small improvement [174]. Our practice is to prescribe oral itraconazole while the patient is taking corticosteroids, and usually for 1 month after the course is completed. CFF consensus recommends itraconazole for those with poor response to corticosteroids, those who are steroid-dependent, those with steroid toxicity and relapsed cases [165]. Unfortunately the drug is poorly absorbed but this is improved if taken with an acidic drink such as Coca Cola or orange juice (but grapefruit juice must be avoided because of its effect on gut CYP3A4 enzymes). Itraconazole has a number of drug interactions so concomitant medications must be checked before it is prescribed (e.g. clarithromycin, midazolam). In addition, it should not be taken at the same time as antacids such as ranitidine, omeprazole etc. The liquid preparation is better absorbed but fairly unpalatable. It is recommended that liver function be monitored when itraconazole is taken for a long time as transaminases can be transiently raised; our practice is to measure liver function at baseline and then 2–3 months later. Finally, there has been a report of adrenal suppression occurring when itraconazole was taken with inhaled corticosteroids (budesonide) in 11 of 25 people with CF; it is believed the itraconazole inhibited budesonide metabolism leading to suppressed adrenocorticotrophic hormone (ACTH) secretion, and recovery took many months after the itraconazole was stopped [178]. Resistance to itraconazole has now been noted in A. fumigatus but not other species [165].

Voriconazole is a newer antifungal agent and is a second-generation triazole (a derivative of fluconazole). The bioavailability is 96% so it is very well absorbed, even in patients with CF. It is licensed for use in invasive aspergillosis for those aged over 2 years. It has a number of recognized adverse effects including photosensitization, headaches, visual disturbances, skin rashes and hair loss. It is also rather expensive and liver function needs monitoring monthly. Nevertheless, we have used it in patients who do not respond to standard ABPA management or who cannot tolerate itraconazole; we have also tried it as monotherapy in patients who cannot (or will not) take corticosteroids, and have had a degree of success in some [179]. Voriconazole has also been used on occasions in patients with chronic Aspergillus infection (without evidence of ABPA) who have significantly deteriorating lung function.

Finally, there are circumstances where further therapy is needed. Some of these patients have recurrent relapses, and are steroid-dependent (often with significant adverse effects, particularly impaired glucose metabolism). Some do not respond to therapy in the first place and have a chronically elevated serum IgE (often in the thousands). Therapies that can be considered include long-term nebulized amphotericin, intravenous liposomal amphotericin (sometimes for several weeks), and monthly infusions of intravenous immunoglobulin [180]. For the future, it is tempting to speculate that anti-IgE monoclonal antibody (omalizumab) may have a role.

Avoidance of Aspergillus exposure is also important. Clearly damp housing conditions must be addressed as Aspergillus colonizes water-damaged walls and ceilings. Aspergillus is found in mouldy hay so is common in horse stables; if the patient insists on horse riding, a compromise is that he or she should only ride out in the open and not 'muck out' (clean) the stables. Aspergillus spores are commonly found in building sites so building work inside hospital grounds can also be quite a problem.

PROGNOSIS

The ERCF data have shown that ABPA had no effect on longitudinal decline in FEV_1 when divided into severity subgroups [168]. Nevertheless, some patients with chronic and recurrent ABPA are a difficult management problem, with constricted airways and sputum retention, and some become corticosteroid-dependent.

Other fungi

Candida albicans has been isolated in 75–90% of adult sputum samples [181,182] but does not seem to cause significant lung disease. Specific IgE antibodies to C. albicans have been detected in colonized CF patients although they were not associated with clinical disease [181]; rarely an allergic bronchopulmonary mycosis may be caused by Candida species [162]. Given the amount of antibiotics patients with CF receive, oral candidiasis is not uncommon, so it may often contaminate specimens; a positive sputum culture does not necessarily indicate pulmonary infection. A recent survey in over 100 adult patients revealed 70% had symptoms of oral and/or genital candidiasis, and Candida species was detected from mouth swabs in 35% [183]. Oral candidiasis should be treated with an agent such as oral fluconazole or topical treatment. Finally, Candida will sometimes infect an indwelling totally implantable venous access device leading to fungemia and possible seeding into distant organs such as the kidneys. Intravenous therapy (e.g. liposomal amphotericin or voriconazole) is required and the device is usually removed.

More recently, Scedosporium apiospermum has emerged as an isolate in children and adults with CF, reported in 9% sputum samples, with positive serology in 21% [184]. It was found from adolescence onwards and not in younger children, and was usually recovered from patients already colonized with A. fumigatus. The frequency of S. apiospermum is greater than expected from the prevalence of fungal spores in the environment (it is occasionally found in soil). Similarly to A. fumigatus, it can cause respiratory tract infection, sinusitis, lung mycetoma, necrotizing pneumonia and allergic bronchopulmonary mycosis [184]. However, its pathogenic role in CF is not well established, and it is usually considered as a simple colonizing agent. If treatment is warranted, oral itraconazole has been used effectively.

REFERENCES

1. Chimiel JF, Berger M, Konstan MW. The role of inflammation in the pathophysiology of CF lung disease. *Clin Rev Allergy Immunol* 2002; **23**:5–27.

2. Gibson RL, Burns J, Ramsey BW. Pathophysiology and management of pulmonary infections in cystic fibrosis. *Am J Resp Crit Care Med* 2003; **168**:918–951.

3. Dakin CJ, Numa AH, Wang H, Morton JR *et al.* Inflammation, infection and pulmonary function in infants and young children with cystic fibrosis. *Am J Respir Crit Care Med* 2002; **165**:904–910.

4. Rosenfeld M, Gibson RL, McNamara S et al. Early pulmonary infection, inflammation and clinical outcomes in infants with cystic fibrosis. *Pediatr Pulmonol* 2001; **32**:356–366.

5. Armstrong DS, Grimwood K, Carlin JB et al. Lower airway inflammation in infants and young children with cystic fibrosis. *Am J Respir Crit Care Med* 1997; **156**:1197–1204.

6. Balough K, McCubbin M, Weinberger M et al. The relationship between infection and inflammation in the early stages of lung disease from cystic fibrosis. *Pediatr Pulmonol* 1995; **20**:63–70.

7. McCauley, DF, Elborn JS. Cystic fibrosis: basic science. *Paediatr Respir* Rev 2000; **1**:93–100.

8. Knowles MR, Boucher RC. Mucus clearance as a primary innate defense mechanism for mammalian airways. *J Clin Invest* 2002; **109**:571–577.

9. Watt AP, Courtney J, Moore J et al. Neutrophil cell death, activation and bacterial infection in Cystic Fibrosis. *Thorax* 2005; **60**:659–64.

10. Bradley J, McAlister O, Elborn JS. Pulmonary function, inflammation, exercise capacity and quality of life in cystic fibrosis. *Eur Respir J* 2001; **17**:712–715.

11. Watkin SL, Elborn JS, Cordon SM et al. C-reactive protein is not a useful indicator of intermittent bacterial colonization in early lung disease of patients with cystic fibrosis. *Pediatr Pulmonol* 1994; **17**:6–10.

12. Aaron SD, Ramotar K, Ferris W et al. Adult cystic fibrosis excerbations and new strains of *Pseudomonas aeruginosa*. *Am J Respir Crit Care Med* 2004; **169**:811–815.

13. Elborn JS, Prescott RJ, Stack BH et al. Elective versus symptomatic antibiotic treatment in cystic fibrosis patients with chronic *Pseudomonas* infection of the lungs. *Thorax* 2000; **55**:355–358.

14. Elborn JS. Treatment of *Staphylococcus aureus* in cystic fibrosis. *Thorax* 1999; **54**:377–378.

15. Cystic Fibrosis Trust. *Antibiotic Treatment for Cystic Fibrosis*. Report of the UK CF Trust antibiotic group, 2nd edn. Bromley, Cystic Fibrosis Trust, 2002. Available at www.cftrust.org.uk.

16. Stutman HR, Lieberman JM, Nussbaum E, Marks MI. Antibiotic prophylaxis in infants and young children with cystic fibrosis: a randomized controlled trial. *J Pediatrics* 2002; **140**:299–305.

17. Smyth A, Walters S. Prophylactic anti-staphylococcal antibiotics for CF. *Cochrane Database of Systematic Reviews* 2003, Issue 3. Art. no. CD001912.

18. Littlewood JM, Koch C, Lambert PA et al. A ten year review of colomycin. *Respir Med* 2000; **94**:632–640.

19. Ramsey BW, Dorkin HL, Eisenberg JD et al. Efficacy of aerosolized tobramycin in patients with cystic fibrosis. *N Engl J Med* 1993; **328**:1740–1746.

20. Ramsey BW, Pepe MS, Quau JM et al. for Cystic Fibrosis Inhaled Tobramycin Study Group. Intermittant administration of inhaled tobramycin in patients with cystic fibrosis. *N Eng J Med* 1999; **340**:23–30.

21. Wolter JM, Bowler DS, Nolan PJ, McCormack JG. Home intravenous therapy in cystic fibrosis: a prospective randomised trial examining clinical, quality of life and cost aspects. *Eur Respir J* 1997; **10**:896–900.

22. Thornton J, Elliott R, Tully MP et al. Long-term clinical outcome of home and hospital intravenous antibiotic treatment in adults with cystic fibrosis. *Thorax* 2004; **59**:242–246.

23. de Groot R, Smith A. Antibiotic pharmacokinetics in cystic fibrosis: differences and clinical significance. *Clin Pharmacokinet* 1987; **13**:228–253.

24. Prandota J. Drug disposition in cystic fibrosis: progress in understanding pathophysiology and pharmacokinetics. *Pediatr Infect Dis J* 1987; **6**:1111–1126.

25. Tan KH, Mulheran M, Knox AJ, Smyth AR. Aminoglycoside prescribing and surveillance in cystic fibrosis. *Am J Respir Crit Care Med* 2003; **167**:819–823.

26. Bates RD, Nahata MC, Jones JW et al. Pharmacokinetics and safety of tobramycin after once-daily administration in patients with cystic fibrosis. *Chest* 1997; **112**:1208–1213.

27. Smyth A, Tan KH, Hyman-Taylor P et al. Once versus three times daily regimens of tobramycin treatment for pulmonary exacerbations of CF. The TOPIC study: A randomised controlled trial. *Lancet* 2005; **365**:573–578.

28. Chernish RN, Aaron SD. Approach to resistant Gram-negative bacterial pulmonary infections in patients with cystic fibrosis. *Curr Opin Pulm Med* 2003; **9**:509–515.

29. Pitt TL, Sparrow M, Warner M, Stefanidou M. Survey of resistance of *Pseudomonas aeruginosa* from UK patients with cystic fibrosis to six commonly prescribed antimicrobial agents. *Thorax* 2003; **58**:794–796.

30. Blumer JL, Saiman L, Konstan MW, Melnick D. The efficacy and safety of meropenem and tobramycin vs ceftazidime and tobramycin in the treatment of acute pulmonary exacerbations in patients with cystic fibrosis. *Chest* 2005; **128**:2336–2346.

31. Aaron SD, Vandemheen KL, Ferris W et al. Combination antibiotic susceptibility testing to treat excerbations of cystic fibrosis associated with multi-resistant bacteria: a randomised, double-blind, controlled clinical trial. *Lancet* 2005; **366**:463–471.

32. Foweraker JE, Laughton CR, Brown DF, Bilton D. Phenotypic variability of *Pseudomonas aeruginosa* in sputa from patients with acute infective exacerbation of cystic fibrosis and its impact on the validity of antimicrobial susceptibility testing. *Antimicrob Chemother* 2005; **55**:921–927.

33. Hodson ME, Gallagher CG, Govan JR. A randomised clinical trial of nebulised tobramycin or colistin in cystic fibrosis. *Eur Respir J* 2002; **20**:658–664.

34. Parmar JS, Nasser S. Antibiotic allergy in CF. *Thorax* 2005; **60**:517–520.

35. Saiman L. The use of macrolide antibiotics in patients with cystic fibrosis. *Curr Opin Pulm Med* 2004; **10**:515–523.

36. Wolter J, Seeney S, Bell S et al. Effect of long term treatment with azithromycin on disease parameters in cystic fibrosis: a randomised trial. *Thorax* 2002; **57**:212–216.

37. Equi A, Balfour-Lynn IM, Bush A, Rosenthal M. Long term azithromycin in children with cystic fibrosis: a randomised, placebo-controlled cross-over study. *Lancet* 2002; **360**:978–984.

38. Saiman L, Marshall BC, Mayer-Hamblett N *et al.* Azithromycin in patients with cystic fibrosis chronically infected with *Pseudomonas aeruginosa*: a randomized controlled trial. *J Am Med Assoc* 2003; **290**:1749–1756.

39. Lyczak JB, Cannon CL, Peir GM. Lung infections associated with cystic fibrosis. *Clin Microbiol Rev* 2002; **15**:194–222.

40. Demko CA, Byard PJ, Davis PB. Gender differences in cystic fibrosis: *Pseudomonas aeruginosa* infection. *J Clin Epidemiol* 1995; **48**:1041–1049.

41. Worlitzsch D, Tarran R, Ulrick M *et al.* Effects of reduced mucus oxygen concentration in airway *Pseudomonas* infections of cystic fibrosis patients. *J Clin Invest* 2002; **109**:317–325.

42. Courtney JM, Ennis M, Elborn JS. Cytokines and inflammatory mediators in cystic fibrosis. *J Cyst Fibros* 2004; **3**:223–231.

43. Drenkard E, Ausubel FM. *Pseudomonas* biofilm formation and antibiotic resistance are linked to phenotypic variation. *Nature* 2002; **416**:695–696.

44. Costerton JW, Stewart PS, Greenberg *et al.* Bacterial biofilms: a common cause of persistent infections. *Science* 1999; **284**:1318–1322.

45. Parad RB, Gerard CJ, Zurakowski D *et al.* Pulmonary outcome in cystic fibrosis is influenced primarily by mucoid *Pseudomonas aerugionsa* infection and immune status and only modestly by genotype. *Infect Immun* 1999; **67**:4744–4750.

46. Pedersen SS, Kharazmi A, Espersen F, Hoiby N. *Pseudomonas aeruginosa* alginate in cystic fibrosis sputum and the inflammatory response. *Infect Immun* 1990; **58**:3363–3368.

47. Garret ES, Perlegas D, Wozniak DJ. Negative control of flagellum synthesis in *Pseudomonas aeruginosa* is modulated by the alternative sigma factor AlgT (AlgU). *J Bacteriol* 1999; **181**:7401–7404.

48. Bayer AS, Speert DP, Park S *et al.* Functional role of mucoid exopolysaccharide (alginate) in antibiotic-induced polymorphonuclear leukocyte-mediated killing of *Pseudomonas aeruginosa. Infect Immun* 1991; **59**:302–308.

49. Nivens DE, Ohman DE, Williams J *et al.* Role of alginate and its O acetylation in formation of *Pseudomonas aeruginosa* microcolonies and biofilms. *J Bacteriol* 2001; **183**:1047–1057.

50. Hentzer M, Teitzel GM, Balzer *et al.* Alginate overproduction affects *Pseudomonas aeruginosa* biofilm structure and function. *J Bacteriol* 2001; **183**:5395–5401.

51. Hancock RE, Speert DP. Antibiotic resistance in *Pseudomonas aeruginosa*: mechanisms and impact on treatment. *Drug Resist Update* 2000; **3**:247–255.

52. Haijar AM, Ernst RK, Tsai JH *et al.* Human toll-like receptor 4 recognises host-specific LPS modifications. *Nature Immunol* 2002; **3**:354–359.

53. Cystic Fibrosis Trust. Pseudomonas aeruginosa *Infection in People with Cystic Fibrosis. Suggestions for Prevention and Infection Control.* Report of the Cystic Fibrosis Trust Infection Control Group. 2nd edn. Bromley, Cystic Fibrosis Trust, 2004. Available at www.cftrust.org.uk.

54. Moore JE, Heaney N, Millar BC *et al.* Incidence of *Pseudomonas aeruginosa* in recreational and hydrotherapy pools. *Comun Dis Public Health* 2002; **5**:23–26.

55. Cheng K, Smyth RL, Govan JR *et al.* Spread of a beta-lactam resistant *Pseudomonas aeruginosa* in a cystic fibrosis clinic. *Lancet* 1996; **348**:639–642.

56. Jones AM, Webb AK, Govan JR *et al. Pseudomonas aeruginosa* cross-infection in cystic fibrosis. *Lancet* 2002; **359**:527–528.

57. O'Carroll MR, Syrmis MW, Wainwright CE *et al.* Clonal strains of *Pseudomonas aeruginosa* in paediatric and adult cystic fibrosis units. *Eur Respir J* 2004; **24**:101–106.

58. Jones AM, Dodd ME, Govan JR *et al.* Prospective surveillance for *Pseudomonas aeruginosa* cross-infection at a cystic fibrosis center. *Am J Respir Crit Care Med* 2005; **171**:257–260.

59. Armstrong DS, Nixon GM, Carzino R *et al.* Detection of a widespread clone of *Pseudomonas aeruginosa* in a pediatric cystic fibrosis clinic. *Am J Respir Crit Care Med* 2002; **166**:983–987.

60. Elborn JS. Difficult bacteria, antibiotic resistance and transmissibility in cystic fibrosis. *Thorax* 2004; **59**:914–915.

61. Ojeniyi B, Frederiksen B, Hoiby N. *Pseudomonas aeruginosa* cross-infection among patients with cystic fibrosis during a winter camp. *Pediatr Pulmonol* 2000; **29**:177–181.

62. Saiman L, Siegel J. Infection control in cystic fibrosis. *Clin Microbiol Rev* 2004; **17**:57–71.

63. Griffiths AL, Jansen K, Carlin JB *et al.* Effects of segregation on an epidemic *Pseudomonas aeruginosa* strain in a CF clinic. *Am J Resp Crit Care Med* 2005; **171**:1020–1025.

64. Kappler M, Kraxner A, Reinhardt D. Diagnostic and prognostic value of serum antobides against *Pseudomonas aeruginosa* in cystic fibrosis. *Thorax* 2006; **61**:684–688.

65. Tramper-Stranders GA, van der Ent CK, Slieker MG *et al.* Diagnostic value of serological tests against *Pseudomonas aeruginosa* in a large cystic fibrosis population. *Thorax* 2006; **61**:689–693.

66. Farrell PM, Govan JW. Pseudomonas serology; confusion, controversy and challenges. *Thorax* 2006; **61**:645–647.

67. Burns JL, Gibson R, McNamara S *et al.* Longitudinal assessment of *Pseudomonas aeruginosa* in young children with cystic fibrosis. *J Infect Dis* 2001; **183**:444–452.

68. Nixon GM, Armstrong DS, Carzino R *et al.* Clinical outcome after early *Pseudomonas aeruginosa* infection in cystic fibrosis. *J Pediatr* 2001; **138**:699–704.

69. Frederiksen B, Koch C, Hoiby N. Antibiotic treatment of initial colonization with *Pseudomonas aeruginosa* postpones chronic infection and prevents deterioration of pulmonary function in cystic fibrosis. *Pediatr Pulmonol* 1997; **23**:330–335.

70. Marchetti F, Giglio L, Candusso M *et al.* Early antibiotic treatment of *Pseudomonas aeruginosa* colonisation in cystic fibrosis: a critical review of the literature. *Eur J Clin Pharmacol* 2004; **60**:67–74.

71. Munck A, Bonacorsi S, Mariani-Kurkdjian P *et al.* Genotypic characterization of *Pseudomonas aeruginosa* strains recovered from patients with cystic fibrosis after initial and

subsequent colonization. *Pediatr Pulmonol* 1998;
32:288–292.

72. Abbott J, Dodd M, Bilton D, Webb AK. Treatment compliance in adults with cystic fibrosis. *Thorax* 1994; **49**:115–120.

73. Westerman EM, Le Brun PP, Touw DJ *et al.* Effect of nebulised colistin sulphate and colistin sulphomethate on lung function in patients with cystic fibrosis: a pilot study. *J Cyst Fibros* 2004; **3**:23–28.

74. Lee TW, Brownlee KG, Conway SP *et al.* Evaluation of a new definition for chronic *Pseudomonas aeruginosa* infection in cystic fibrosis. *J Cyst Fibros* 2003; **2**:29–34.

75. Dakin C, Henry RL, Field P *et al.* Defining an exacerbation of pulmonary disease in cystic fibrosis. *Pediatr Pulmonol* 2001; **31**;436–442.

76. Marshall BC. Pulmonary exacerbations in cystic fibrosis: it's time to be explicit! *Am J Respir Crit Care Med* 2004; **169**:781–782.

77. Norman D, Elborn JS, Cordon SM *et al.* Plasma tumour necrosis factor alpha in cystic fibrosis. *Thorax* 1991; **46**:91–95.

78. Szaff M, Hoiby N, Flensborg EW. Frequent antibiotic therapy improves survival of cystic fibrosis patients with chronic *Pseudomonas aeruginosa* infection. *Acta Paediatr Scand* 1983; **72**:651–657.

79. Jensen T, Pederson SS, Hoiby N *et al.* Use of antibiotics in CF: the Danish approach. *Antibiot Chemother* 1985; **42**:237–246.

80. Isles A, Maclusky I, Corey M *et al. Pseudomonas cepacia* infection in cystic fibrosis: an emerging problem. *J Pediatr* 1984; **104**:206–210.

81. Kalish LA, Waltz DA, Dovey M *et al.* Impact of *Burkholderia dolosa* on lung function and survival in cystic fibrosis. *Am J Respir Crit Care Med* 2006; **173**:421–425.

82. Coenye T, LiPuma JJ. Molecular epidemiology of *Burkholderia* species. *Front Biosci* 2003; **8**:55–67.

83. Coenye T, Vandamme P, LiPuma JJ *et al.* Updated version of the *Burkholderia cepacia* complex experimental strain panel. *J Clin Microbiol* 2003; **41**:2797–2798.

84. Vandamme P, Holmes B, Vancanneyt M *et al.* Occurrence of multiple genomovars of *Burkholderia cepacia* in cystic fibrosis patients and proposal of *Burkholderia multivorans* sp. *Int J Syst Bacteriol* 1997; **47**:1188–1200.

85. LiPuma JJ, Spilker T, Gill LH *et al.* Disproportionate distribution of *Burkholderia cepacia* complex species and transmissibility markers in cystic fibrosis. *Am J Respir Crit Care Med* 2001; **164**:92–96.

86. McDowell A, Mahenthiralingam E, Dunbar KE *et al.* Epidemiology of *Burkholderia cepacia* complex species recovered from cystic fibrosis patients: issues related to patient segregation. *J Med Microbiol* 2004; **53**:663–668.

87. Manno G, Dalmastri C, Tabacchioni S *et al.* Epidemiology and clinical course of *Burkholderia cepacia* complex infections, particularly those caused by different *Burkholderia cenocepacia* strains, among patients attending an Italian Cystic Fibrosis Centre. *J Clin Microbiol* 2004; **42**:1491–1497.

88. Courtney JM, Dunbar KEA, McDowell A *et al.* Clinical outcome of *Burkholderia cepacia* complex infection in cystic fibrosis adults. *J Cys Fibros* 2004; **3**:93–98.

89. Jones AM, Dodd ME, Govan JRW *et al. Burkholderia cenocepacia* and *Burkholderia multivorans*: influence on survival in cystic fibrosis. *Thorax* 2004; **59**:948–951.

90. Henry DA, Campbell MR, LiPuma JJ, Speert DP. Identification of *Burkholderia cepacia* isolates from patients with cystic fibrosis and use of a simple new selective medium. *J Clin Microbiol* 1997; **35**:614–619.

91. McMenamin JD, Zaccone TM, Coenye T *et al.* Misidentification of *Burkholderia cepacia* in US cystic fibrosis treatment centers: an analysis of 1051 recent sputum isolates. *Chest* 2000; **117**:1661–1665.

92. Govan JR, Brown PH, Maddison J *et al.* Evidence for transmission of *Pseudomonas cepacia* by social contact in cystic fibrosis. *Lancet* 1993; **342**:15–19.

93. LiPuma JJ, Dasen SE, Nielson DW *et al.* Person-to-person transmission of *Pseudomonas cepacia* between patients with cystic fibrosis. *Lancet* 1990; **336**:1094–1096.

94. Mahenthiralingam E, Vandamme P, Campbell ME *et al.* Infection with *Burkholderia cepacia* complex genomovars in patients with cystic fibrosis: virulent transmissible strains of genomovar III can replace *Burkholderia multivorans*. *Clin Infect Dis* 2001; **33**:1469–1475.

95. Frangolias DD, Mahenthiralingam E, Rae S *et al. Burkholderia cepacia* in cystic fibrosis: variable disease course. *Am J Respir Crit Care Med* 1999; **160**:1572–1577.

96. Whiteford ML, Wilkinson JD, McColl JH *et al.* Outcome of *Burkholderia* (*Pseudomonas*) *cepacia* colonisation in children with cystic fibrosis following a hospital outbreak. *Thorax* 1995; **50**:1194–1198.

97. McCloskey M, McCaughern J, Redmond AOB, Elborn JS. Clinical outcome after acquisition of *Burkholderia cepacia* in patients with cystic fibrosis. *Irish J Med Sci* 2001; **170**:28–31.

98. Cystic Fibrosis Trust. Burkholderia cepacia *Complex: Suggestions for Prevention and Infection Control*. Report of the UK Cystic Fibrosis Trust Infection Control Group. 2nd edn. Bromley, Cystic Fibrosis Trust, 2004. Available at www.cftrust.org.

99. Jones AM, Dodd MR, Webb, AK. *Burkholderia cepacia*: current clinical issues, environmental controversies and ethical dilemmas. *Eur Respir J* 2001; **17**:295–301.

100. Jones AM, Martin L, Bright-Thomas RJ *et al.* Inflammatory markers in cystic fibrosis patients with transmissible *Pseudomonas aeruginosa*. *Eur Respir J* 2003; **22**:503–506.

101. DeSoyza A, McDowell A, Archer L *et al. Burkholderia cepacia* complex genomovars and pulmonary transplantation outcomes in patients with cystic fibrosis. *Lancet* 2001; **358**:1780–1781.

102. Aris RM, Routh JC, LiPuma JJ *et al.* Lung transplantation for cystic fibrosis patients with *Burkholderia cepacia* complex: survival linked to genomovar type. *Am J Respir Crit Care Med* 2001; **164**:2102–2106.

103. Aaron SD, Ferris W, Henry DA *et al.* Multiple combination bactericidal antibiotic testing for patients with cystic

fibrosis infected with *Burkholderia cepacia*. *Am J Respir Crit Care Med* 2000; **161**:1206–1212.

104. McManus TE, McDowell A, Moore JE, Elborn JS. Organisms isolated from adults with cystic fibrosis. *Ann Clin Microbiol Antimicrob* 2004; **3**:26.

105. Mahenthiralingam E, Baldwin A, Vandamme P. *Burkholderia cepacia* complex infection in patients with cystic fibrosis. *J Med Microbiol* 2002; **51**:533–538.

106. Saiman L, Siegel J for the Cystic Fibrosis Foundation. Infection control recommendations for patients with cystic fibrosis: microbiology, important pathogens, and infection control practices to prevent patient-to-patient transmission. *Infect Control Hosp Epidemiol* 2003; **24**(5 Suppl):S6–S52.

107. Conway S, Denton M. *Staphylococcus aureus* and MRSA. *Prog Respir Res* 2006; **34**:153–159.

108. McManus TE, Moore JE, Crowe M *et al.* A comparison of pulmonary exacerbations with single and multiple organisms in patients with cystic fibrosis and chronic *Burkholderia cepacia* infection. *J Infect* 2003; **46**:56–59.

109. Saiman L. Microbiology of early CF lung disease. *Paediatr Respir Rev* 2004; **5**(Suppl A):S367–S369.

110. Weaver LT, Green MR, Nicholson K *et al.* Prognosis in cystic fibrosis treated with continuous flucloxacillin from the neonatal period. *Arch Dis Child* 1994; **70**:84–89.

111. Smyth A. Prophylactic antibiotics in cystic fibrosis: a conviction without evidence. *Pediatr Pulmonol* 2006; **40**:471–476.

112. Beardsmore CS, Thompson JR, Williams A *et al.* Pulmonary function in infants with cystic fibrosis: the effect of antibiotic treatment. *Arch Dis Child* 1994; **71**:133–137.

113. Smyth A, Walters S. Prophylactic anti-staphylococcal antibiotics for cystic fibrosis. *The Cochrane Database of Systematic Reviews* 2003, Issue 3. Art. no. CD001912.

114. Koch C, Hoiby N. Diagnosis and treatment of cystic fibrosis. *Respiration* 2000; **67**:239–247.

115. Ratjen F, Doring G, Nikolaizik WH. Effect of inhaled tobramycin on early *Pseudomonas aeruginosa* colonisation in patients with cystic fibrosis. *Lancet* 2001; **358**:983–984.

116. Voss A. Preventing the spread of MRSA. *Br Med J* 2004; **329**:521.

117. Farr BM. Prevention and control of MRSA infections. *Eur Opin Infect Dis* 2004; **17**:317–322.

118. Palvecino E. Community acquired MRSA infections. *Clin Lab Med* 2004; **24**:403–418.

119. Miall LS, McKinley NT, Brownlee KG, Conway SP. Methicillin-resistant *Staphylococcus aureus* (MRSA) infection in cystic fibrosis. *Arch Dis Child* 2001; **84**:160–162.

120. Thomas SR, Gyi KM, Gaya H, Hodson ME. Methicillin-resistant *Staphylococcus aureus*: impact at a national cystic fibrosis centre. *J Hosp Infect* 1998; **40**:203–209.

121. Garske LA, Kidd TJ, Gan R *et al.* Rifampicin and sodium fusidate reduces the frequency of methicillin-resistant *Staphylococcus aureus* (MRSA) isolation in adults with cystic fibrosis and chronic MRSA infection. *J Hosp Infect* 2004; **56**:208–214.

122. Conway SP, Brownlee KG, Denton M, Peckham DG. Antibiotic treatment of multidrug resistant organisms in cystic fibrosis. *Am J Respir Med* 2003; **2**:321–332.

123. Saralaya D, Peckham DG, Hulme B *et al.* Serum and sputum concentrations following the oral administration of linezolid in adult patients with cystic fibrosis. *J Antimicrob Chemother* 2004; **52**:325–328.

124. Bilton D, Pye A, Johnson MM *et al.* The isolation and characterization of non-typeable *Haemophilus influenzae* in the sputum of adult cystic fibrosis patients. *Eur Respir J* 1995; **8**:948–953.

125. Rayner RJ, Hiller EJ, Isaphani P, Baker M. *Haemophilus* infection in cystic fibrosis. *Arch Dis Child* 1990; **65**:255–258.

126. Denton M, Kerr KG. Microbiological and clinical aspects of infection associated with *Stenotrophomonas maltophilia*. *Clin Microbiol Rev* 1998; **11**:57–80.

127. Goss CH, Otto K, Aitken ML *et al.* Detecting *Stenotrophomonas maltophilia* does not reduce survival of patients with cystic fibrosis. *Am J Respir Crit Care Med* 2002; **166**:356–361.

128. Goss CH, Mayer-Hamblett N, Aitken ML *et al.* Association between *Stenotrophomonas maltophilia* and lung function in cystic fibrosis. *Thorax* 2004; **59**:955–959.

129. Graff GR, Burns JL. Factors affecting the incidence of *Stenotrophomonas maltophilia* isolation in cystic fibrosis. *Chest* 2002; **121**:1754–1760.

130. Talmaciu I, Varlotta L, Mortensen J *et al.* Risk factors for emergence of *Stenotrophomonas maltophilia* in cystic fibrosis. *Pediatr Pulmonol* 2000; **30**:10–15.

131. Marchac V, Equi A, Le Bihan-Benjamin C *et al.* Case–control study of *Stenotrophomonas maltophilia* acquisition in cystic fibrosis patients. *Eur Respir J* 2004; **23**:98–102.

132. Krueger TS, Clark EA, Nix DE. In-vitro susceptibility of *Stenotrophomonas maltophilia* to antimicrobial combinations. *Diagn Microbiol Infect Dis* 2001; **41**:71–78.

133. Hutchinson ML, Bonell EC, Poxton IR, Govan JR. Endotoxic activity of lipopolysaccharides isolated from emergent potential cystic fibrosis pathogens. *FEMS Immunol Med Microbiol* 2000; **27**:73–77.

134. Hogardt M, Schmoldt S, Gotzfried M *et al.* Pitfalls of polymyxin antimicrobial susceptibility testing of *Pseudomonas aeruginosa* isolated from cystic fibrosis patients. *J Antimicrob Chemother* 2004; **54**:1057–1061.

135. Olivier KN, Weber DJ, Wallace RJ *et al.* Non-tuberculous mycobacteria. I: Multicenter prevalence study in cystic fibrosis. *Am J Respir Crit Care Med* 2003; **167**:828–834.

136. Olivier KN, Weber DJ, Lee JH *et al.* Non-tuberculous mycobacteria. II: Nested-cohort study of impact on cystic fibrosis lung disease. *Am J Respir Crit Care Med* 2003; **167**:835–840.

137. Olivier KN for the NTM in CF Study Group. The natural history of non-tuberculous mycobacteria in patients with cystic fibrosis. *Paediatr Respir Rev* 2004; **5**:S213–S216.

138. American Thoracic Society. Diagnosis and treatment of disease caused by non-tuberculous mycobacteria. [This official statement of the American thoracic Society was

approved by the Board of Directors, March 1997.] *Am J Respir Crit Care Med* 1997; **156**:S1–S25.

139. Leitritz L, Griese M, Roggenkamp A *et al.* Prospective study on non-tuberculous mycobacteria in patients with and without cystic fibrosis. *Med Microbiol Immunol* 2004; **139**: 209–217.

140. Forslow U, Geborek A, Hjelte L *et al.* Early chemotherapy for non-tuberculous mycobacterial infections in patients with cystic fibrosis. *Acta Paediatr* 2003; **92**:910–915.

141. Hallstrand TS, Ochs HD, Zhu O *et al.* Inhaled IFN-gamma for persistant non-tuberculous mycobacterial pulmonary disease due to functional IFN-gamma deficiency. *Eur Resp J* 2004; **24**:367–370.

142. Wang EE, Prober CG, Manson B *et al.* Association of respiratory viral infections with pulmonary deterioration in patients with cystic fibrosis. *N Engl J Med* 1984; **311**:1653–1658.

143. Abman SH, Ogle JW, Butler-Simon N *et al.* Role of respiratory syncytial virus in early hospitalizations for respiratory distress of young infants with cystic fibrosis. *J Pediatr* 1988; **113**:826–830.

144. Smyth AR, Smyth RL, Tong CY *et al.* Effect of respiratory virus infections including rhinovirus on clinical status in cystic fibrosis. *Arch Dis Child* 1995; **73**:117–120.

145. Punch G, Syrmis MW, Rose BR *et al.* Method for detection of respiratory viruses in the sputa of patients with cystic fibrosis. *Eur J Clin Microbiol Infect Dis* 2005; **24**:54–57.

146. Wat D, Doull I. Respiratory virus infections in cystic fibrosis. *Paediatr Respir Rev* 2003; **4**:172–177.

147. McIntosh K, McAdam AJ. Human metapneumovirus: an important new respiratory virus. *N Engl J Med* 2004; **350**:431–433.

148. Ramsey BW, Gore EJ, Smith AL *et al.* The effect of respiratory viral infections on patients with cystic fibrosis. *Am J Dis Child* 1989; **143**:662–668.

149. Hiatt PW, Grace SC, Kozinetz CA *et al.* Effects of viral lower respiratory tract infection on lung function in infants with cystic fibrosis. *Pediatrics* 1999; **103**:619–626.

150. Abman SH, Ogle JW, Harbeck RJ *et al.* Early bacteriologic, immunologic, and clinical courses of young infants with cystic fibrosis identified by neonatal screening. *J Pediatr* 1991; **119**:211–217.

151. Malfroot A, Adam G, Ciofu O *et al.* for the European Cystic Fibrosis Society (ECFS) Vaccination Group. Immunisation in the current management of cystic fibrosis patients. *J Cyst Fibros* 2005; **4**:77–87.

152. Pribble CG, Black PG, Bosso JA, Turner RB. Clinical manifestations of exacerbations of cystic fibrosis associated with nonbacterial infections. *Pediatrics* 1990; **117**:200–204.

153. Conway SP, Simmonds EJ, Littlewood JM. Acute severe deterioration in cystic fibrosis associated with influenza A virus infection. *Thorax* 1992; **47**:112–114.

154. Petersen NT, Høiby N, Mordhorst CH *et al.* Respiratory infections in cystic fibrosis patients caused by virus, *Chlamydia* and mycoplasma: possible synergism with *Pseudomonas aeruginosa*. *Acta Paediatr Scand* 1981; **70**:623–628.

155. Collinson J, Nicholson KG, Cancio E *et al.* Effects of upper respiratory tract infections in patients with cystic fibrosis. *Thorax* 1996; **51**:1115–1122.

156. Armstrong D, Grimwood K, Carlin JB *et al.* Severe viral respiratory infections in infants with cystic fibrosis. *Pediatr Pulmonol* 1998; **26**:371–379.

157. Bhalla P, Tan A, Smyth R. Vaccines for preventing influenza in people with cystic fibrosis. *The Cochrane Database of Systematic Reviews* 2000, Issue 1. Art. no. CD001753.

158. Gruber WC, Campbell PW, Thompson JM *et al.* Comparison of live attenuated and inactivated influenza vaccines in cystic fibrosis patients and their families: results of a 3-year study. *J Infect Dis* 1994; **169**:241–247.

159. National Institute for Clinical Excellence. Guidance on the use of zanamivir, oseltamivir and amantadine for the treatment of influenza. Technology Appraisal Guidance no. 58, 2003. Available at www.nice.org.uk.

160. Bisgaard H, for the Study Group on Montelukast and Respiratory Syncytial Virus. A randomized trial of montelukast in respiratory syncytial virus post-bronchiolitis. *Am J Respir Crit Care Med* 2003; **167**:379–383.

161. Kaiser L, Lew D, Hirschel B *et al.* Effects of antibiotic treatment in the subset of common-cold patients who have bacteria in nasopharyngeal secretions. *Lancet* 1996; **347**:1507–1510.

162. Que C, Geddes D. Respiratory fungal infections and allergic bronchopulmonary aspergillosis. *Progr Respir Res* 2006; **34**:166–172.

163. Brown K, Rosenthal M, Bush A. Fatal invasive aspergillosis in an adolescent with cystic fibrosis. *Pediatr Pulmonol* 1999; **27**:130–133.

164. Chow L, Brown NE, Kunimoto D. An unusual case of pulmonary invasive aspergillosis and aspergilloma cured with voriconazole in a patient with cystic fibrosis. *Clin Infect Dis* 2002; **35**:e106–e110.

165. Stevens DA, Moss RB, Kurup VP *et al.* Allergic bronchopulmonary aspergillosis in cystic fibrosis: state of the art: Cystic Fibrosis Foundation Consensus Conference. *Clin Infect Dis* 2003; **37**(Suppl 3):S225–S264.

166. Wise SK, Kingdom TT, McKean L *et al.* Presence of fungus in sinus cultures of cystic fibrosis patients. *Am J Rhinol* 2005; **19**:47–51.

167. Miller PW, Hamosh A, Macek M *et al.* Cystic fibrosis transmembrane conductance regulator (CFTR) gene mutations in allergic bronchopulmonary aspergillosis. *Am J Hum Genet* 1996; **59**:45–51.

168. Mastella G, Rainisio M, Harms HK *et al.* for the Epidemiologic Registry of Cystic Fibrosis. Allergic bronchopulmonary aspergillosis in cystic fibrosis: a European epidemiological study. *Eur Respir J* 2000; **16**:464–471.

169. Geller DE, Kaplowitz H, Light MJ, Colin AA for the Scientific Advisory Group, Investigators, and Coordinators of the Epidemiologic Study of Cystic Fibrosis. Allergic bronchopulmonary aspergillosis in cystic

fibrosis: reported prevalence, regional distribution, and patient characteristics. *Chest* 1999; **116**:639–646.

170. Burns JL, Van Dalfsen JM, Shawar RM *et al.* Effect of chronic intermittent administration of inhaled tobramycin on respiratory microbial flora in patients with cystic fibrosis. *J Infect Dis* 1999; **179**:1190–1196.

171. Jensen T, Pedersen SS, Garne S *et al.* Colistin inhalation therapy in cystic fibrosis patients with chronic *Pseudomonas aeruginosa* lung infection. *J Antimicrob Chemother* 1987; **19**:831–838.

172. Ritz N, Ammann RA, Casaulta Aebischer C *et al.* Risk factors for allergic bronchopulmonary aspergillosis and sensitisation to *Aspergillus fumigatus* in patients with cystic fibrosis. *Eur J Pediatr* 2005; **164**:577–582.

173. Crameri R. Recombinant *Aspergillus fumigatus* allergens: from the nucleotide sequences to clinical applications. *Int Arch Allergy Immunol* 1998; **115**:99–114.

174. Wark P. Pathogenesis of allergic bronchopulmonary aspergillosis and an evidence–based review of azoles in treatment. *Respir Med* 2004; **98**:915–923.

175. Elphick H, Southern K. Antifungal therapies for allergic bronchopulmonary aspergillosis in people with cystic fibrosis. *The Cochrane Database of Systematic Reviews* 2000, Issue 4. Art. no. CD002204.

176. Stevens DA, Schwartz HJ, Lee JY *et al.* A randomized trial of itraconazole in allergic bronchopulmonary aspergillosis. *N Engl J Med* 2000; **342**:756–762.

177. Wark PA, Hensley MJ, Saltos N *et al.* Anti-inflammatory effect of itraconazole in stable allergic bronchopulmonary aspergillosis: a randomized controlled trial. *J Allergy Clin Immunol* 2003; **111**:952–957.

178. Skov M, Main KM, Sillesen IB *et al.* Iatrogenic adrenal insufficiency as a side-effect of combined treatment of itraconazole and budesonide. *Eur Respir J* 2002; **20**:127–133.

179. Hilliard T, Edwards S, Buchdahl R *et al.* Voriconazole therapy in children with cystic fibrosis. *J Cyst Fibros* 2005; **4**:215–220.

180. Balfour-Lynn IM, Mohan U, Bush A, Rosenthal M. Intravenous immunoglobulin for cystic fibrosis lung disease: a case series of 16 children. *Arch Dis Child* 2004; **89**:315–319.

181. Máiz L, Cuevas M, Quirce S *et al.* Serologic IgE immune responses against *Aspergillus fumigatus* and *Candida albicans* in patients with cystic fibrosis. *Chest* 2002; **121**:782–788.

182. Bakare N, Rickerts V, Bargon J *et al.* Prevalence of *Aspergillus fumigatus* and other fungal species in the sputum of adult patients with cystic fibrosis. *Mycoses* 2003; **46**:19–23.

183. Woolnough E, Webb AK. *Candida albicans* infection in adults with cystic fibrosis. *J Roy Soc Med* 2006; **99**(Suppl 46):13–16.

184. Cimon B, Carrere J, Vinatier JF *et al.* Clinical significance of *Scedosporium apiospermum* in patients with cystic fibrosis. *Eur J Clin Microbiol Infect Dis* 2000; **19**:53–56.

185. Fuchs HJ, Borowitz DS, Christiansen DH *et al.* for the Pulmozyme Study Group. Effect of aerosolised recombinant human DNase on exacerbations of respiratory symptoms and on pulmonary function in patients with cystic fibrosis. *N Engl J Med* 1994; **331**:637–142.

Respiratory disease: non-infectious complications

MARGARET HODSON AND ANDREW BUSH

Rightly, much of the effort in pulmonary care is focused on prevention and treatment of chronic infection. However, there are a number of non-infective issues that are very important, and these are discussed in this chapter.

HEMOPTYSIS

Minor hemoptysis is common in cystic fibrosis (CF) and more so in older patients. The bleeding is usually from the bronchial arteries, two-thirds of which arise from the aorta and one-third from the mammary and intercostal vessels. Other vessels, which form collaterals with these, may also be a source of hemorrhage. Severe hemoptysis is usually associated with severe disease and is defined as 250 mL per 24 hours, or 100 mL per day in a 3–7 day period [1]. It occurs in about 7% of older patients. The CFF Patient Registry of 28 858 patients over a 10-year period showed that massive hemoptysis occurred with an annual incidence of 0.87% and overall 4.1% of patients experienced hemoptysis over a 2-year period. One in 100 patients will have a massive hemoptysis annually. The patients who had major hemoptysis were older (mean age 24 years) with more severe lung disease (60% had FEV_1 below 40% predicted). The major risk factors were *Staphylococcus aureus* in the sputum (OR 1.3) and diabetes (OR 1.1). There was an increased morbidity and mortality after massive hemoptysis (35% dying within 1 year, median survival after the first major hemoptysis being 5 years) [2].

Hemoptysis is due to chronic infection, leading to the formation of granulation tissue and small blood vessels, which rupture with coughing. There may also be damage to vessels by proteolytic enzymes released from leukocytes associated with the infection. Other factors include vitamin deficiency due to liver disease and malabsorption, and thrombocytopenia, the latter in patients with hypersplenism.

It is important for clinicians to distinguish between hemoptysis and hematemesis in this group of patients. Mild hemoptysis, namely blood streaking of the sputum, is usually of no great significance. Major bleeds are life-threatening due to asphyxiation, airflow obstruction, infection, hypotension, anemia, exacerbations of infection and respiratory failure.

History-taking should include what medications are being taken, and aspirin, non-steroidal anti-inflammatories and penicillin derivatives should be stopped. A chest radiograph should be performed to see if there is any new chest pathology. A full blood count, liver function tests, blood for cross-matching and arterial gases (at least in adults) should be performed. Coagulation should be checked including prothrombin time (PT), partial thromboplastin time (PTT) and platelet count. Sputum should be sent for culture. Clinicians used to bronchoscope patients before intervention such as embolization but recently this has been done less often as it has not been found to be particularly helpful.

For mild hemoptysis and blood streaking, reassurance is all that may be required. If the last sputum culture reveals any pathogen, this should be treated; coagulation should be checked and vitamin K given if appropriate. Moderate hemoptysis, which is more than streaking of the sputum but less than 250 mL/24 hours, should be treated by admission to hospital. Coagulation factors should be checked, drugs which may be exacerbating the situation stopped and physiotherapy and appropriate antibiotic therapy given. Oxygen saturation (SaO_2) should be monitored and oxygen given as required. Chest physiotherapy should be continued, but caution should be used, and an experienced physiotherapist is essential.

In severe hemoptysis, oxygen is essential and if it is known from which side the bleeding is coming the patient should be placed in the lateral position with the affected side down so that blood is not aspirated into the upper lung.

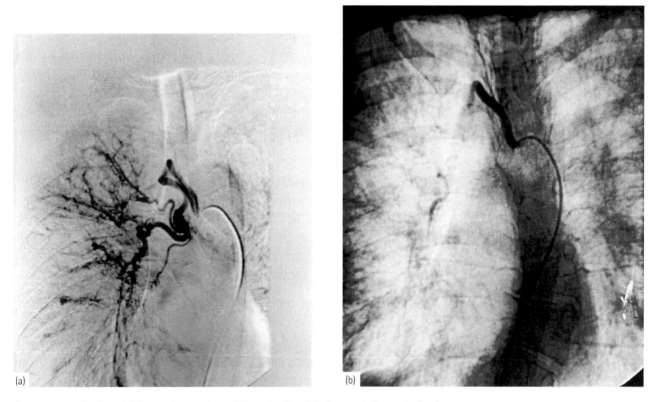

(a)
(b)

Figure 11.1   The bronchial artery in a patient with cystic fibrosis before and after embolization.

In this situation, pitressin derivatives have been found useful by some clinicians [3,4]. We have used vasopressin for a number a years, and more recently terlipressin with success. Two milligrams of terlipressin given intravenously are followed by 1–2 mg every 4–6 hours, up to 72 hours. A glycerine trinitrate patch and a diuretic should be given as fluid retention can occur. It is said that tranexamic acid can also be helpful [5] but this is not our experience. If severe hemoptysis continues, bronchial embolization (Fig. 11.1) can be extremely effective, at least in the short term [6–9]. A variety of substances can be used, such as gelatine pledgets, steel coils or polyvinyl alcohol. A group of 23 children (95%) stopped bleeding within 24 hours, but 55% of these needed re-embolization at between 5 days and 21 months [10]. Embolization also has the risk of paralysis if emboli are allowed to block the spinal arteries, and there are risks of other organ infarction or even death. However, in severe hemoptysis it can be life-saving. If embolization fails, the other options are intubation and endobronchial tamponade with balloon catheters or ligation of the bronchial artery or surgical resection of a lobe, which in a very sick patient has a very high mortality rate.

PNEUMOTHORAX

Pneumothorax occurs when there is air in the pleural space, usually due to rupture of a subpleural bleb in the visceral pleura; another cause is misplacement of a central line. Increase in intrapleural pressures due to inflammation and obstruction of the airways may cause check valve phenomena and sputum retention, increasing the risk of pneumothorax [11]. The incidence of pneumothorax increases in adolescence and adult life [12]; it is associated with a poor prognosis [13] and the median survival after pneumothorax is only 30 months. Pneumothoraces are often recurrent; indeed over 50% of patients may have more than one episode.

Pneumothorax in CF was studied [14] using the US National Cystic Fibrosis Patients Registry 1990–1999, which contains 28 588 patients with a follow-up of 10 years. Annual incidence of pneumothorax was 0.64% and occurred in 3.4% of patients. A pneumothorax occurs in 1 in 167 patients annually. Pneumothoraces were more common in older patients, mean age 22 years, and in those with severe lung disease (75% of patients had an FEV_1 of <40% predicted). Pneumothorax was increased in patients with: *Pseudomonas aeruginosa* (OR 2.3), *Burkholderia cepacia* (OR 1.8), *Aspergillus fumigatus* in the sputum (OR 1.3), FEV_1 <30% predicted (OR 1.5), enteral feeding (OR 1.7), pancreatic insufficiency (OR 1.4), allergic bronchopulmonary aspergillosis (OR 1.5) or a massive hemoptysis (OR 1.4). After a pneumothorax there was an increased rate and duration of hospital admissions and the 2-year mortality rate was increased: 49% vs 12% when compared to patients who had not had a pneumothorax ($p < 0.0001$).

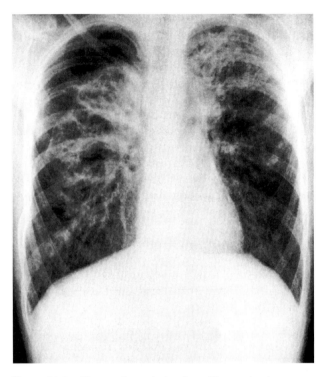

Figure 11.2   Chest radiograph showing widespread pulmonary disease and a right-sided pneumothorax.

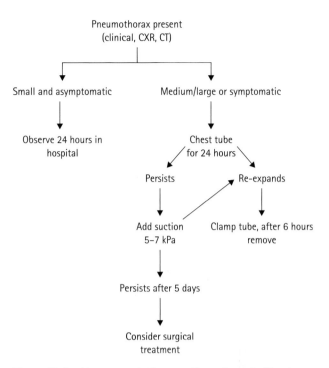

Figure 11.3   Management of pneumothorax in cystic fibrosis.

The patient may be asymptomatic or may have chest pain and/or breathlessness. Indeed any unexplained chest pain or breathlessness in a CF patient should prompt the clinician to exclude pneumothorax, particularly in older patients. A large pneumothorax, or tension pneumothorax, in patients with severe lung disease can be life-threatening and needs urgent treatment.

A small pneumothorax may be asymptomatic, but a patient with a larger pneumothorax may present with cyanosis, breathlessness, pallor, a raised respiration rate and be very distressed. On examination there will be reduced movement, increased resonance and decreased breath sounds over the affected side. If the mediastinum is displaced, as often happens with a tension pneumothorax, trachea and apex beat will be displaced away from the side of the pneumothorax. In tension pneumothorax there may be tachycardia and hypotension.

A PA chest radiograph will reveal the pneumothorax (Fig. 11.2) but often a lateral radiograph or CT scan is required to show the full extent and indicate the site for positioning an intercostal tube. Guidelines have suggested pneumothoraces of <2 cm from the chest wall are 'small' and large pneumothoraces are ⩾2 cm [15]. In the case of CF, in adults, we suggest small air rim ones <1 cm around the lung, moderate up to 2 cm, and large ⩾2 cm. Fortunately, pneumothorax is rare in young children with CF, but the recommendations above may be scaled down for children.

Management is summarized in Fig. 11.3 and reference [1]. Even a small and asymptomatic pneumothorax should be observed in hospital for 24 hours. Such a patient may require no treatment but the clinician must be satisfied the pneumothorax is not getting bigger and there is no associated hemothorax developing.

A moderate or large pneumothorax will require insertion of an intercostal tube connected to an underwater drainage system. The position is decided after studying the chest radiograph, but the usual position is at the 5th to 6th intercostal space in the mid-axillary line. The tube is directed to the apex and sufficient length is inserted. An alternative position is the 2nd intercostal space anteriorly. If the pneumothorax does not re-expand quickly, suction should be applied, at a pressure of 5–7 kPa. If it does not re-expand after 4–5 days, surgical advice should be obtained. The clinician should remember that it may take longer for a lung to re-expand if the patient has CF than in other idiopathic pneumothoraces as the CF lung is stiff.

If the lung does not re-expand the clinician has a dilemma. Extensive pleurectomy, or talc pleurodesis, may make the patient unsuitable for future transplantation. This is because dissection of the pleura would take a long time, causing a long ischemic time, and there is often extensive bleeding. The best treatment, in our view, is limited abrasion surgical pleurodesis. In patients not suitable for transplantation, chemical pleurodesis using bleomycin or talc has been used [16]. While the patient has a chest drain *in situ* physiotherapy should be continued with intravenous antibiotics as indicated. SaO$_2$ should be monitored and oxygen given to help reabsorb the air from the pneumothorax. High-dose oxygen, up to 10 L, may be helpful but the PaCO$_2$ must be carefully monitored. High-flow oxygen reduces the total pressure of gas in the capillaries, particularly nitrogen, and there is therefore a higher gradient between the pleural capillaries and the pleural cavity, and hence air is reabsorbed. High-flow oxygen can increase the rate of reabsorption of air by up to four times [17]. Appropriate analgesics should be given.

When a pneumothorax is diagnosed it should be treated quickly with an intercostal tube as re-expansion edema may occur when the lung is re-inflated after a period of time [18]. In the case of a tension pneumothorax, a 4-cm cannula can be inserted as an emergency procedure. Sometimes Heimlich valves can be used temporarily but, in our opinion, these are not as effective as an underwater drain seal.

Some patients in chronic respiratory failure are dependent on non-invasive positive pressure ventilation. There is a slightly increased incidence of pneumothorax in these patients but they can be managed using a ventilator at low pressure [19].

After non-surgical treatment of a pneumothorax patients should be provided with a letter stating they are CF patients who have had a pneumothorax. If they present to any hospital with breathlessness or chest pain, the clinician should request a chest radiograph to exclude a recurrent pneumothorax. Patients who have not had surgical procedures should not fly until a chest radiograph has confirmed that the lung is completely re-expanded, and probably should wait at least 6 weeks thereafter. Most regulatory authorities would prohibit scuba diving in anyone with airflow obstruction, and certainly after a pneumothorax.

LUNG OR LOBAR COLLAPSE

This is a relatively uncommon complication of CF in these days of effective antibiotics, airway clearance, and muco-active agents. Its occurrence should raise the possibility of a diagnosis of allergic bronchopulmonary aspergillosis (see Chapter 10), which should be excluded by standard tests. Anecdotally, a CT scan may help delineate optimal management. If the collapsed lobe is seen to contain a prominent

air bronchogram, it is likely that there is no proximal mucus plugging, and the changes represent chronic lobar destruction, which is irreversible.

Standard therapy includes the use of intensive physiotherapy, possibly augmented by positive airway pressure; either or both of rhDNase and hypertonic saline; and appropriate intravenous and nebulized antibiotics. If this fails, bronchoscopy should be performed, with the largest caliber flexible bronchoscope tolerated by the patient. There is evidence from case reports that directly instilling rhDNase endobronchially may be beneficial [20,21]. If there are really tenacious plugs of sputum that cannot be removed using the fiberoptic bronchoscope, rigid bronchoscopy may be considered.

Surgical removal of the collapsed lobe is occasionally contemplated in the patient with otherwise well-preserved lung architecture. However, in general a CT scan will reveal that the disease is not truly isolated, and there is widespread bronchiectasis elsewhere. The occasional patient may get short-term benefit from lobectomy [22], but only in the rare case of a destroyed non-functional lobe with well preserved lung elsewhere.

RESPIRATORY FAILURE, PULMONARY HYPERTENSION, AND SECONDARY CARDIAC COMPLICATIONS

Patients with end-stage CF become severely hypoxic (Fig. 11.4) and before that they develop significant desaturation during exercise and sleep [23]. Cor pulmonale is well recognized in patients with hypoxia and pulmonary hypertension. Right heart failure may be present before death in a small proportion of patients. The prognosis once heart failure occurs is grave [24].

The mechanism for pulmonary hypertension appears to be pulmonary vasoconstriction and subsequent vascular remodelling [25]. A study of 21 CF patients breathing air

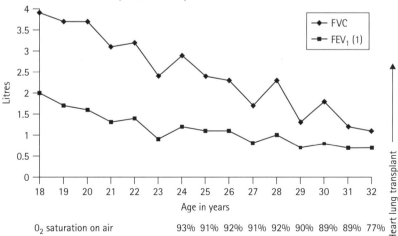

Deterioration in pulmonary function, over a 14-year period, in an adult with cystic fibrosis despite maximum medical treatment

O_2 saturation on air   93% 91% 92% 91% 92% 90% 89% 89% 77%

Figure 11.4 A cystic fibrosis patient developing progressive hypoxia despite maximal medical treatment as lung function deteriorates.

and oxygen mixtures showed the mean pulmonary artery pressure (PAP) to be abnormally high in 8 of 21, and the PAP correlated with the degree of hypoxia [25]. Patients with right heart failure may have ECG changes (Fig. 11.5) such as P pulmonale, and the chest radiograph may show cardiomegaly (Fig. 11.6).

Prolonged oxygen therapy has shown no survival advantage [26]. There is, however, no doubt that oxygen can provide symptomatic relief and should be given to hypoxic patients. When heart failure occurs it usually responds well to oxygen and diuretics. Some severely hypoxic patients continue to study or work using an oxygen concentrator at college or in the workplace.

More recently, echocardiography using Doppler techniques has been used to study the heart in CF patients. In some patients pulmonary hypertension was demonstrated,

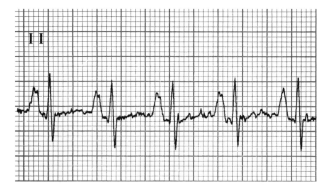

Figure 11.5   ECG of a CF patient with right heart failure showing tall P waves.

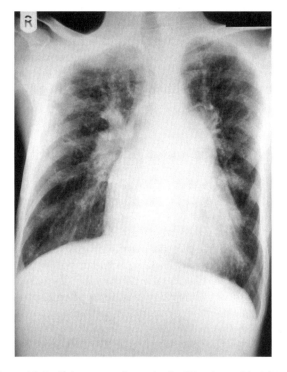

Figure 11.6   Pulmonary radiograph of a CF patient with right heart failure.

but in addition the presence of significant right ventricular systolic and diastolic dysfunction was demonstrated in patients with severe disease, in the absence of left ventricular abnormalities [27]. In 12 CF patients, circulating atrial natriuretic peptide (ANP) was higher in patients with pulmonary hypertension than in those without [28].

Patients with CF also develop mainly supraventricular arrhythmias [29]. This is probably caused by ventricular remodelling due to hypoxia, infection and/or sympathomimetic medication. Disease of the coronary arteries is rare, probably due to the low serum lipid levels found in CF. We have also seen a case of cardiomyopathy, and recently a number of patients with significant alterations in right and left ventricular filling with respiration demonstrated by Doppler echocardiography. On inspiration the right heart filling is increased and the left-heart filling is reduced. On expiration the right-ventricular filling is reduced (cardiac tamponade) and the left-ventricular filling increased. The authors suggest that the reduced filling of the left ventricle on inspiration may account for some of the unexplained neurological symptoms experienced by some CF patients [30].

PHARMACOLOGICAL ADJUNCTS TO MUCUS CLEARANCE

It must be stressed that these are only adjunctive to mechanical methods of airway clearance, which are reviewed in Chapter 29. The clearest evidence for mucolytic therapy is the use of rhDNase, followed by hypertonic saline. Other agents have been suggested, and are briefly reviewed, but there is little if any current evidence for efficacy in these other compounds.

Dornase alfa (rhDNase, Pulmozyme)

This must be the most studied medication in CF. Dornase alfa has been shown to decrease viscoelasticity in the sputum of patients with CF and this makes chest physiotherapy easier. Many studies have shown a clinical improvement in patients following treatment. Short-term studies showed an increase of FEV_1 [31,32]. A North American study of more than 900 patients showed that patients with moderate lung disease had an improvement of 5.8% in FEV_1 when treated with dornase alfa over a 6-month period ($p < 0.01$) [33]. Patients with mild pulmonary disease (i.e. $FEV_1 > 85\%$ predicted) and children aged 5–10 years have also shown a benefit [34]. A 2-year randomized placebo-controlled study showed benefit in young patients [35]. Patients with severe pulmonary disease also benefited [36,37]. An uncontrolled, open labeled study followed up patients for 2 years while they were taking dornase alfa and showed the FEV_1 stablized 6% above baseline [38]. A case–controlled study of dornase alfa which evaluated the impact on disease progression over a 4-year period also showed benefit [39].

The European Registry reported on patients treated with dornase alfa and showed that the treated patients benefited with an improved FEV_1 and reduced exacerbations of infection [40]. The possible anti-inflammatory effects of dornase alfa, which are less clear-cut than the physiological and clinical benefits, are discussed below.

Clinicians have been unsure whether to administer dornase alfa before or after physiotherapy. A recent study has shown that dornase alfa is equally effective when delivered before or after physiotherapy, but that patients who are chronically infected with *Pseudomonas aeruginosa* may derive more improvement in FEV_1 when dornase alfa is administered after physiotherapy [41].

A comparison of hypertonic saline with alternate-day or daily dornase alfa in children with CF showed hypertonic saline was not as effective as daily dornase alfa although there was no evidence of difference between daily and alternate day treatment with dornase alfa [42].

These studies with dornase alfa are encouraging, suggesting a reduction in the rate of pulmonary exacerbations and improved lung function. A recent evidence-based review has concluded that 'dornase alfa should be assessed in all patients over 6 years of age, particularly those with *Pseudomonas aeruginosa* infection' [43]. Therapeutic endpoints could include pulmonary function, weight, incidence of respiratory tract infection, breathlessness and patients' objective response. It should be noted that not all patients respond to rhDNase; between one-third and one-half get significant benefit in terms of lung function, although possibly a higher proportion may have a reduction in infective exacerbations with no change in lung function. It has been shown that lung function is a good predictor of response if the drug is administered for at least 6 weeks [44]. Clinicians should remember that adherence to treatment with dornase alfa may be variable [45]. It is hoped that the development of new nebulizers, shortening treatment time, may improve adherence to treatment regimens.

Hypertonic saline

Sputum induction with hypertonic saline (HS) is a well-established clinical and research procedure: a dose–response effect to increasing concentrations of HS, with a stepwise increase in mucociliary clearance (MCC) up to 6% HS, with no further increase going up to 12% [46]. Addition of amiloride to HS did not improve MCC [47]. These important studies underline the need for physiotherapists to try to increase the concentration of the saline solutions used up to 6–7%, and not be content with standard normal saline, provided the patient tolerates the escalation of the concentration without bronchospasm. It should be noted that HS may cause bronchoconstriction, but also subsequent bronchodilation, similar to the paradoxical bronchodilatation seen after exercise in some CF patients [48,49].

Efficacy studies of HS have focused on changes in lung function and changes in the weight of expectorated sputum.

Sputum induction and enhanced sputum clearance may not be the same procedure, however.

Short-term studies have demonstrated increases in pulmonary function with HS similar to those obtained with rhDNase in phase II studies [50, 51]. There have been two longer-term studies. A pediatric trial, in which children were randomly allocated in a cross-over design to either 7% HS, daily rhDNase or alternate-day rhDNase for 12 weeks showed that, for the group, there was no significant change in spirometry over baseline with HS [42]. Looking at individual patients, 35% did have an improvement in FEV_1 of at least 10% on HS, including some children who did not improve with rhDNase. The wide scatter emphasizes that there are important individual differences in response with this as with other treatments in CF. Patients already taking short-acting β_2 agonists were allowed to take them prior to nebulizing HS, and only three were unable to use HS. The study was not powered to show a difference in exacerbation rate. Benefit at 6 weeks was less than at 12 weeks, so this length trial was recommended on an individual basis.

By contrast, a much smaller short-term study concluded that efficacy for 5.85% HS and rhDNase was similar [1], but examination of the individual data reveals that there were marked individual differences in response.

In the second long-term study, normal saline and hypertonic (7%) given nebulized twice daily were compared over a 1-year period in 164 patients [52]. There was a statistically significant but clinically trivial (67 mL FEV_1) improvement in the hypertonic saline group, but a dramatic reduction in infective exacerbations (2.74 vs 1.30 per patient in favor of hypertonic saline) and improved work attendance. It should be noted that only 18% were using nebulized antibiotics, so it may be that the results are not applicable to patients using these. In an accompanying paper, it was suggested that 7% HS had a prolonged effect on MCC [53]. Curiously, this was abrogated by concurrent amiloride therapy.

Overall, this cheap treatment may be a useful adjunctive therapy in CF, and may possibly go some way towards correcting the effects of the basic defect by rehydrating the airway surface.

There have been concerns about the effects of HS on airway defences and its possible pro-inflammatory potential. Repetitive induction of sputum with HS has been reported to cause increased airway neutrophilia [54,55], which may be intrinsically undesirable in CF; however, in the large HS study reported above [42], HS had no pro-inflammatory effects and there were no correlations between changes in lung function and changes in inflammatory markers [56], suggesting that there is no clinically significant pro-inflammatory effect of HS over at least a 12-week period.

We conclude that the use of HS as an adjunct to physiotherapy should be evaluated on an individual basis. It is probable that patients who respond to both will prefer to use rhDNase because of the short nebulization time and less unpleasant taste. If there is no improvement in lung function or antibiotic usage with rhDNase, a trial of HS should be considered. The dose–response curve should be remembered [46] and 7% used if the patient can tolerate it. The trial duration should be longer than the standard rhDNase trial, and be of at least 12 weeks if lung function changes are to be detected [57], longer if an effect on antibiotic usage is to be documented. The major disadvantage is the requirement for two additional nebulized treatments, in a group of patients who are likely already using twice-daily nebulized antibiotics.

Sputum induction may also be used diagnostically. This has been routine in the context of HIV infection and tuberculosis, but we have been slower to introduce it in the context of CF. Compared with standard methods of collection of lower respiratory tract secretions, induced sputum was shown to lead to the isolation of more organisms [58]. It may even be that induced sputum is a better 'gold standard' than bronchoalveolar lavage (BAL), in which differences in culture results from different lobes in the same patient have been well documented [59]. The TB experience is that the technique can be used even in babies [60]. There are issues about cross-infection in CF as much as TB, and consideration must be given to ensuring that sputum induction does not lead to spread of infection. There is a need for comparisons between standard methods, such as cough swab and nasopharyngeal aspirates, with sputum induction, the use of cough plates, and BAL.

Other mucolytics

We can find no evidence in the published literature to support the use of any other agent as a mucolytic in CF or bronchiectasis. There have been three trials of N-acetyl-cysteine (NAC) as a mucolytic [60–62], none of which has shown any benefit. A recent systematic review confirmed the lack of benefit for either nebulized or oral acetyl–cysteine [64]. However, more recent work has suggested an immunomodulatory role for high-dose NAC, with reduction in sputum IL-8 levels [65], and a dose-finding study has established safety in high doses [66], so there may possibly be a role for NAC in CF in the future. However, it cannot be recommended generally as a treatment for CF lung disease.

Another agent that is currently being evaluated in CF is inhaled mannitol [67]. Mannitol has been used for airway challenges in the context of asthma in particular [68]. It has a number of actions that might make it potentially of interest in CF, including rehydration of airway secretions [67]. There may be secondary release of mediators, which could stimulate ciliary beat frequency [67]. It improved the tracheal mucus velocity of CF sputum placed on a bovine trachea [69]. In a pilot study, the effects of inhaled mannitol and 6% hypertonic saline were compared in 12 CF patients. The endpoint was mucus clearance using a radio-aerosol technique [67]. Both agents improved mucociliary clearance, and mannitol improved cough clearance. There was minor transient bronchoconstriction (mean falls in FEV_1 in the range 6–7%) despite bronchodilator premedication,

but this had improved by the end of the study. Mannitol has the advantage that it can be given as a dry powder, rather than nebulized. Worldwide, a number of trials are ongoing, and these will need to report before the place of mannitol in CF can be determined.

ANTI-INFLAMMATORY THERAPY

There is a widespread assumption that inflammation is a bad thing in CF, and must be suppressed [70]. This in part arose from the early prednisolone study (below), and in part from the study of the impressive catalog of toxic materials released from necrotic neutrophils, which are abundant in the airway. Furthermore, some, but not all, studies (reviewed in Chapter 5) have suggested that the CF airway is intrinsically pro-inflammatory, even in the absence of infection. However, it would be wrong to assume that all inflammation is bad and must be suppressed. Inflammation serves a beneficial function in very many circumstances. First, it is known that congenital immunodeficiencies characterized by absent or reduced lung defences result in devastating systemic infections, which, other than the dreaded cepacia syndrome, are unheard of in CF, at least in the untransplanted patient. Thus the neutrophil must have some protective function in CF. Second, early infection with *Pseudomonas aeruginosa* is frequently overcome, and it seems not unlikely that the host immune response is important in this. Third, a recent trial of an anti-inflammatory strategy, LTB_4 antagonism [71], had to be terminated prematurely because of increased serious adverse events, in particular infection, in the treated group. So the mantra 'inflammation bad, anti-inflammation good' should not be applied uncritically.

This section reviews potential anti-inflammatory medications currently available. More futuristic therapies are reviewed in Chapter 33b.

Oral steroids

An initial study was reported as showing that prednisone in a dose of 2 mg/kg on alternate days was beneficial in CF, with no side-effects [72]. This finding was tested in a multicenter double-blind randomized controlled trial of prednisone 2 mg/kg on alternate days versus 1 mg/kg on alternate days, and versus placebo [73]. Benefit was shown for both steroid treated groups, but only in patients chronically infected with *Pseudomonas aeruginosa*. However, the predictable side-effects led to the high-dose limb being halted after 2 years, and the lower dose after 4 years. We do not know whether a much lower dose of prednisolone might be beneficial (say 5–10 mg/day), nor is that trial likely ever to be done.

Currently, prednisolone as an anti-inflammatory can be recommended only in patients doing very badly on standard therapy. The new knowledge of the high prevalence of CF bone disease, and the potential role of prednisolone in pathogenesis, mandates extreme caution in the use of this medication unless there is clear likely benefit, for example in allergic bronchopulmonary aspergillosis.

Inhaled steroids

These medications are very widely prescribed in CF, often without much justification. Infants are sometimes prescribed them prior to diagnosis because their symptoms have been attributed to asthma. The word 'wheeze' is used very ambiguously, and another reason inhaled steroids are prescribed to known CF patients is the mistaken belief that the noise the patient or family is describing is related to bronchospasm, not airway secretions. Since CF is not known to be protective against asthma, one would expect by chance that 5–10% of the CF clinic will have coincident asthma and benefit from inhaled corticosteroids, but the diagnosis is very difficult to establish. Pointers in favor would be the presence of a personal or family history of atopy, acute reversibility to bronchodilator, and (when available) a raised rather than the more characteristically lower than normal exhaled nitric oxide, and sputum eosinophilia.

A recent large multicenter study of withdrawal of inhaled steroids showed no evidence of harm, in terms of time to next exacerbation [74]. The study had to be of withdrawal of therapy, not its institution, because insufficient inhaled steroid-naive CF patients could be recruited. This study has shed much needed light on the subject. Although a much longer-term benefit of inhaled steroids is theoretically possible, and might be suggested by results from the USCFF database [75] – only available as an abstract – most would believe that giving inhaled steroids to reduce CF-related inflammation is not a correct strategy. Therefore, the only indication for using them in CF is in the belief there is co-incident asthma, and they should therefore be used exactly as if the patient has asthma [76]. This means that every effort should be made to document one or more features of asthma (above); that if age appropriate, the response should be assessed using a period of home peak flow monitoring; and at each clinic visit an active decision should be taken as to whether the dose can be reduced. Furthermore, with new evidence that high-dose inhaled steroids may cause serious side-effects such as hypoglycemia [77], caution with their use is even more necessary. Fears have been expressed that inhaled steroids may actually increase the likelihood of infection with *Pseudomonas aeruginosa*, leading to premature termination of a trial; however, the result did not reach statistical significance, and has not been replicated.

Macrolides

There has been an explosion of interest in the immunomodulatory properties of macrolides, which have been reviewed in detail elsewhere (below). Diffuse panbronchiolitis is another neutrophilic disease, similar to CF, which afflicts almost exclusively middle-aged people in the Far East [78].

Presentation is with cough, chronic sputum production and breathlessness, with coarse crackles heard on auscultation. There is a mixed obstructive and restrictive pattern physiologically. High-resolution CT scanning reveals bronchiectasis. Sputum cultures are positive for *Hemophilus influenzae*, *Staphylococcus aureus* and, most strikingly, mucoid strains of *Pseudomonas aeruginosa*. As a result of chance observations, it became clear that long-term low-dose erythromycin dramatically improved prognosis, changing 10-year survival from less than 20% to more than 90% [79]. A series of elegant studies established that diffuse panbronchiolitis is characterized by a neutrophilic bronchoalveolar lavage, and that macrolide treatment therapy reduced lavage neutrophil chemoattractant activity and neutrophil counts [80]. The response did not depend on the patient being chronically infected with mucoid *Pseudomonas aeruginosa* [81]. Treatment with erythromycin or, if this fails, clarithromycin is essentially curative of a once fatal condition. This extraordinary result led to interest in the use of macrolides in CF, first in a series of case reports and a case study, and then in randomized controlled trials.

Three different double-blind randomized placebo-controlled trials have established a role for macrolides in some patients with CF, summarized in Table 11.1 [82]. These have established that macrolides improve lung function, reduce exacerbation rates, and possibly lead to increased weight gain [83–85]. As with many therapies in CF, there is individual variation in response to treatment, and not all will benefit. Any benefit is lost within 28 days of discontinuing therapy [85].

There are many potential anti-inflammatory and immunomodulatory mechanisms whereby macrolides could be beneficial in CF, which have been reviewed in detail elsewhere [86–88]. In patients with diffuse panbronchiolitis, it would appear that this is related to reduction of airway neutrophilia. However, there is no reason to suppose the mechanism is necessarily the same in CF, and in fact no group has been able to identify the actual mechanism. It is clearly not correction of the electrophysiological defect [89,90]. Challengingly, one group has even suggested that azithromycin may actually be pro-inflammatory [91], and that is the mechanism of benefit! There is a real practical need to find the mechanism; there are many hundreds of naturally occurring macrolides, with differing properties, and a designer macrolide, targeting a specific mechanism, could be highly beneficial.

In summary, these trials have confirmed that for many, but not all, individuals with CF, azithromycin therapy improves pulmonary function. No-one can predict which patients will benefit from treatment, nor is the mechanism of action known. Unlike in diffuse panbronchiolitis, there does not seem to be an effect on airway neutrophilia, but, as with diffuse panbronchiolitis, chronic *Pseudomonas aeruginosa* infection is not a prerequisite for benefit. The optimal dose and dosing frequency is not known. There are world-wide differences in how macrolides are used in CF. Some [92] use it as part of their routine treatment of chronic

Table 11.1 Summary of published clinical trials of azithromycin (AZM).

Centre [ref]	Trial design	AZM dose	n	Length of treatment (months)	FEV$_1$ drug vs placebo	Other clinical outcomes	Inflammatory markers	Adverse effects
Australia Two centers [83]	Parallel	250 mg daily	60 adults	3	Mean relative difference + 3.6%	↓ intravenous antibiotics ↑ quality of life	↓ CRP	Nil
UK Single center [84]	Cross-over	250 or 500 mg daily	41 children >8 years	6	Median relative difference +5.4%	↓ oral antibiotics	No difference sputum IL-8, neutrophil elastase	Nil
USA Multicenter [85]	Parallel	250 or 500 mg 3/week +adults	185 children >6 years	6	Mean relative difference +6.2%	↓ non-quinolone antibiotics ↓ exacerbation ↑ weight	Modest □ ↓ sputum elastase No difference in IL-8	Nausea, diarrhea, wheezing

Modified from [82] with permission from the authors.

infection with *Pseudomonas aeruginosa*. We are more cautious, having taken account of the lack of knowledge of possible long-term side-effects in children in particular; we carry out a 4- to 6-month therapeutic trial of daily azithromycin in those who are not doing well on conventional therapy, irrespective of their sputum bacteriology, and discontinue the medication if there is no benefit. This is clearly an area where more work is needed, but also an area in which clear-cut benefit for patients has been established.

Non-steroidal anti-inflammatory agents

A logical anti-inflammatory approach, given that oral steroids are too toxic and inhaled steroids ineffective, would be a non-steroidal anti-inflammatory medication such as ibuprofen. The first randomized controlled trial showed that ibuprofen slowed the rate of decline in lung function, in particular in the 5–13 age group [93]. The dose was carefully titrated, and it was impossible to predict blood levels, so these had to be measured. There are animal data that high-dose ibuprofen is anti-inflammatory, but low-dose ibuprofen may be pro-inflammatory [94], so if this therapy is to be used, regular venepuncture is necessary. Furthermore, ibuprofen may contribute to acute renal failure, especially with concurrent aminoglycoside treatment. Confirmation of a beneficial effect has been sought in a recent multicenter study, which has not yet been published.

Overall, the role of ibuprofen in CF is unclear [95]. More data are needed. There are clearly more risks, in particular of acute renal failure when combined with aminoglycosides [96,97], than were appreciated at first. The complications are probably rare, but devastating when they occur. The need to monitor blood levels, and the theoretical risk of doing harm if the dose is wrong, also indicates the need for caution. At the moment, ibuprofen cannot be recommended as a routine therapy; there may be scope for a related but safer agent to be used in the future in CF.

DNase

The strong physiological evidence for benefit of rhDNase therapy has been reviewed above. There have been suggestions in the literature of both pro- and anti-inflammatory effects. An initial in-vitro study suggested that addition of bovine rhDNase to CF sputum led to the release of IL-8 which had been bound to DNA by electrostatic forces [98]. However, a 3-month trial of rhDNase also looked at the change in sputum IL-8 and neutrophil elastase levels, and showed no change [56]. A recent study has suggested that there may be an additional, anti-inflammatory benefit of rhDNase [99]. There was no effect on inflammation in those who had no neutrophilia in the initial lavage. In those with an initial neutrophilia who were randomized to rhDNase there was no increase in lavage neutrophils; the placebo group showed increasing neutrophilia. It could be that the known effect of rhDNase in reducing exacerbations could have led to fewer neutrophils in the airway; unfortunately the group did not report data on exacerbations. Overall, the evidence is that rhDNase is not pro-inflammatory, may be neutral, but could have a bonus of anti-inflammatory effects which may give additional benefits in patients.

BRONCHODILATORS

Hypersensitivity of the airways in CF has long been recognized [100] and many patients with CF wheeze. This may be due to bronchospasm, mucosal edema or retained secretions in the airways. Once ABPA and gastroesophageal reflux have been excluded or treated one should think in terms of 'Is there any useful airway reversibility?' and treat accordingly.

Beta-adrenergic agonists enhance ciliary beat frequency and may affect mucus secretion. Terbutaline has been shown to stimulate chloride ion secretion in the lumen and may increase hydration of the airway [101]. All patients with CF should be tested to see if their spirometry improves after the use of a bronchodilator; e.g. salbutamol, terbutaline or ipratropium bromide given by aerosol or nebulizer [102–104]. Patients should have the bronchodilator stopped if no benefit is demonstrated. More than half the patients in the European database are taking regular bronchodilators [105]. During acute exacerbations patients may benefit from a regular bronchodilator and there is evidence, in some cases, intravenous administration may be more beneficial [106].

Long-acting β-agonists have also been shown to be beneficial in some patients [107,108] but long-term studies are required. Theophylline increases mucociliary clearance, diaphragmatic contractility and central nervous system drive to the respiratory centers [109], and may also be anti-inflammatory, at least in the context of asthma in the non-CF patient. However, if it is to be used, careful monitoring is required to avoid toxicity, especially nausea and vomiting. Some studies have shown theophylline to be beneficial [110,111]. Intravenous aminophylline can be helpful in acute exacerbations associated with carbon dioxide retention.

NOVEL THERAPIES

In this section we discuss briefly the anecdotal use of treatments that have been used more extensively in other contexts, and which may bring unexpected benefit to the patient who is not doing well. Treatments that have shown promise for the future, but not yet been studied in a controlled trial, and are not currently available as a clinical tool, are reviewed in Chapter 33b.

Potential current options

INTRAVENOUS IMMUNOGLOBULIN INFUSIONS

This therapy has been used in asthma with questionable benefit. The occasional CF patient may benefit from their use, as a steroid-sparing agent. An uncontrolled case series has shown that intravenous immunoglobulin in selected patients may allow reduction of steroid dosage, with no deterioration in lung function [112]. Our current practice in CF children is to use a 6-month trial in those with particularly distal airway disease and not much proximal bronchiectasis. Response is unpredictable.

CYTOTOXIC AGENTS

CF patients who have undergone orthotopic liver transplantation may show stabilization or even improvement in their lung function. One of several possible explanations is the post-transplant use of immunosuppressive agents. There are a few anecdotal reports of the use of immunosuppression with methotrexate [113] and ciclosporin A [114] in the pre-transplant stage. Clearly they all have side-effects, and the risks of a therapeutic trial must be balanced against benefit. In particular ciclosporin is nephrotoxic, and may therefore worsen aminoglycoside-induced renal impairment. The recently developed nebulized preparations of ciclosporin may offer a useful therapy for the future [115].

THE TRAVELLING CF PATIENT

Increasing numbers of adolescents and adults with CF wish to travel, often for long distances. This should be encouraged if their health permits. They should be advised to take out travel insurance and make sure it covers cystic fibrosis. They should take with them a letter documenting regular medications, lung function and sputum microbiology in case they need to see a doctor abroad. A letter for the customs officers should list any medications and air compressors, needles and/or syringes that they may be carrying. This can often save a lot of delay. Usually patients should have all appropriate immunizations advised for healthy travellers. However, immunosuppressed transplant patients should avoid live vaccines. A patient visiting hot countries should take salt supplements.

Some patients will require supplemental oxygen. Commercial aircraft cruise at 10 000–60 000 ft above sea level. The cabin pressure is approximately 5 000–6 000 ft above sea level, and the partial pressure of the oxygen is reduced to 80% of the sea-level values. So, for example, a patient who already has a PaO_2 of 9.6 kPa will drop to 6.3 kPa or less at an altitude of 8 000 ft after breathing air for 45 minutes [116]. The drop will be greater if the patient falls asleep [117]; and in non-commercial flights, the cabin may not be pressurized and an even lower FiO_2 may be encountered. Both the American Thoracic Society [118] and the British Thoracic Society [119] guidelines recommend a PaO_2 of above 6.6 kPa (50 mmHg) be maintained during flight. Patients with a sea-level PaO_2 of under 9.30 kPa or SaO_2 of 92% should be advised to have oxygen in flight. However, it has been pointed out that chronically hypoxic CF patients are often asymptomatic at these levels [120]. It has been recommended that CF patients with a baseline FEV_1 less than 60% and PaO_2 less than 10.5 kPa are most likely to need in-flight oxygen [121]. It is recommended that a hypoxic inhalation test be carried out on this group of patients using 15% oxygen and 85% nitrogen breathed for 15 minutes. If the saturation drops below 85% the CF patient should be recommended to receive oxygen in flight. It should be acknowledged that the risk of short periods of hypoxia in a CF patient is unknown, and that obtaining oxygen for flights on commercial airlines may be expensive; however, the cost of diverting a commercial jet because someone has become unwell may be as much as (US$40 000) £20 000, to say nothing of the inconvenience to other passengers, so flight assessments should not be undertaken lightly.

It has been reported that patients who went on skiing holidays at high altitude, without consulting their clinicians, developed right ventricular failure [122]. When discussing holiday arrangements with patients clinicians should take into account the altitude they wish to visit. Patients with any pneumothorax should not fly if at all possible. The pneumothorax will expand as the aircraft altitude rises, unless effectively drained. Patients attending a CF unit should be encouraged to discuss their holiday arrangements with their physician so that all the issues outlined above can be fully discussed.

MANAGEMENT OF THE CF PATIENT NEEDING SURGERY

Surgery may need to be performed as a result of CF-related complications (e.g. nasal polyps, insertion of percutaneous endoscopic gastrastomy, PEG) or for an unrelated condition. In all cases, the anesthetic and surgical team need to liaise closely with the CF center. Such close liaison may even preclude the need for surgery; for example, medical management of DIOS may obviate the need for a laparotomy.

The ideal is for procedures to be performed close to the CF unit, by surgeons and anesthetists who are familiar with CF and the treatment protocols. If this is not possible, the whole CF multidisciplinary team needs to liaise with their counterparts in the surgical service, to ensure airway clearance, nutritional and gastrointestinal issues are not neglected just because the patient is undergoing an orthopedic procedure for a fracture. As with much of CF care, recommendations are not evidence-based. It is also important that at all stages, routine care and detection of complications is not neglected because the team are preoccupied with non-CF-related issues.

Preoperative planning

If a CF patient is to have a general anesthetic, it is worth briefly considering whether other procedures should be performed opportunistically, particularly obtaining lower airway secretions from a patient who is unable to expectorate. This may be either by blind suction below the vocal cords performed by the anesthetist, or by fiberoptic bronchoscopy. If surgery is performed away from the CF center, it is essential that the lower airway secretions be cultured in the microbiology laboratory using appropriate media (Chapter 9).

Preoperative assessment of the patient

GENERAL

Ideally, the anesthetist and the CF physician should jointly see the patient. If this is not possible, at least a discussion of the current CF issues should take place. However, CF issues should not distract from the routine preoperative checks normally carried out by the anesthetist. In addition, there are a number of special CF-related issues that should be considered.

RESPIRATORY ISSUES

The anesthetist should arrange preoperative measurements of oxygen saturation in all CF patients, and spirometry in all those over aged 5 years, unless pain or another severe illness precludes an effective maneuver. All results should be compared with the patient's usual values at the CF center. For elective procedures, the patient's respiratory status should be optimized with intensive physiotherapy and antibiotics in particular. It is wise to obtain a sputum or cough swab culture prior to surgery, where this is practical. For all but minor procedures in well patients, a course of intravenous antibiotics should be considered, starting at least 48 hours prior to the procedure, and continuing until the patient is pain-free and has made a complete recovery. The anesthetist should enquire about current or past oral or high-dose inhaled corticosteroid therapy; the need for per- and postoperative steroid treatment should be judged on standard criteria. A preoperative chest x-ray should be obtained, in order to exclude a pneumothorax, or localized collapse, which might be treated with preoperative bronchoscopy. The possibility of bronchospasm should be considered although, in general, asthma complicating CF is over-diagnosed.

OTHER ISSUES

Nutritional status should be assessed, and postponement of all but emergency surgery considered if there is scope for optimizing this. Sodium and potassium depletion, with metabolic alkalosis, is not uncommon in hot weather [123], and urea and electrolytes need to be measured pre- and postoperatively, and any imbalance corrected. Any constipation should be treated vigorously, to avoid postoperative DIOS. Gastro-esophageal reflux is common in CF, and it should be noted whether this is present. CF patients on insulin should be managed using standard insulin-dependent diabetes protocols, but the anesthetist should be aware that the stress of surgery may precipitate hyperglycemia in the CF patient with borderline endocrine pancreatic function. Diabetic ketoacidosis is not a usual feature of CF-related diabetes.

Finally, the potential for drug interactions should be noted. The patient is usually already taking several other medications; there may be liver disease (which may also cause clotting factor deficiency, and thrombocytopenia if there is also hypersplenism); and renal insufficiency, particularly if multiple previous courses of aminoglycosides have been prescribed [124].

Peroperative management

Although gastroesophageal reflux is common, aspiration during anesthesia is rare, and there is no need routinely to use a rapid-sequence induction. Suxamethonium should probably be avoided, because this agent may cause postoperative pain which will impede the performance of efficient physiotherapy. Standard peroperative monitoring is performed as usual. The patient should be ventilated in such a way as to prevent as far as possible postoperative atelectasis. The anesthetist should be aware of the possibility of the build-up of secretions causing V:Q mismatch, or even blocking the endotracheal tube. In general, peroperative chest physiotherapy while the patient is anesthetized has not been shown to be useful [125]. Per- and postoperatively, oxygen and other inhaled gases should be humidified. Drugs that might cause postoperative suppression of cough, or constipation, should be avoided. Consideration should be given to inserting a regional blockade with, for example, marcaine, while the patient is still anesthetized.

Postoperative care

Adequate pain relief without cough suppression, to ensure efficient airway clearance, is essential. The continued close involvement of expert physiotherapists, ensuring adequate airway clearance and mobilization of the patient, is absolutely crucial. Opiates and dehydration may predispose to constipation, which should be treated aggressively to avoid progression to subacute bowel obstruction. If a prolonged period of ileus or other cause of failure of enteral nutrition is expected, then total parenteral nutrition should be instituted early.

REFERENCES

1. Schidlow DV, Taussig LM, Knowles MR. Cystic Fibrosis Foundation consensus conference report on pulmonary complications of cystic fibrosis. *Pediatr Pulmonol* 1993; **15**:187–198.
2. Flume PA, Yankaskas JR, Ebeling M *et al*. Massive hemoptysis in cystic fibrosis. *Chest* 2005; **128**:729–738.
3. Magee G, Williams MH. Treatment of massive hemoptysis with intravenous pitressin. *Lung* 1982; **160**:165–169.
4. Bilton D, Webb AK, Foster H *et al*. Life threatening haemoptysis in cystic fibrosis: an alternative therapeutic approach. *Thorax* 1990; **45**: 975–976.
5. Graff GR. Treatment of recurrent severe hemoptysis in cystic fibrosis with tranexamic acid. *Respiration* 2001; **68**:91–94.
6. Fairfax AJ, Ball J, Batten JC *et al*. A pathological study following bronchial artery embolization for haemoptysis in cystic fibrosis. *Br J Dis Chest* 1980; **74**:345–352.
7. Sweezey NB, Fellows KE. Bronchial artery embolization for severe hemoptysis in cystic fibrosis. *Chest* 1990; **97**:1322–1326.
8. Stern RC, Wood RE, Boat TF *et al*. Treatment and prognosis of massive hemoptysis in cystic fibrosis. *Am Rev Respir Dis* 1978; **117**:825–828.
9. Cohen AM. Haemoptysis: role of angiography and embolisation. *Pediatr Pulmonol* 1992; Suppl **8**:85–86.
10. Barben J, Robertson D, Olinsky A *et al*. Bronchial artery embolization for hemoptysis in young patients with cystic fibrosis. *Radiology* 2002; **224**:124–130.
11. Schramel FM, Postmus PE, Vanderschueren RG. Current aspects of spontaneous pneumothorax. *Eur Respir J* 1997; **10**:1372–1379.
12. Penketh AR, Knight RK, Hodson ME *et al*. Management of pneumothorax in adults with cystic fibrosis. *Thorax* 1982; **37**:850–853.
13. Spector ML, Stern RC. Pneumothorax in cystic fibrosis: a 26-year experience. *Ann Thorac Surg* 1989; **47**:204–207.
14. Flume PA, Strange C, Ye X *et al*. Pneumothorax in cystic fibrosis. *Chest* 2005; **128**:720–728.
15. Henry M, Arnold T, Harvey J. BTS guidelines for the management of spontaneous pneumothorax. *Thorax* 2003; **58**(Suppl. 2):ii39–ii52.
16. Egan TM. Treatment of pneumothorax in cystic fibrosis. *Pediatr Pulmonol* 1992; Suppl **8**:82–84.
17. Northfield TC. Oxygen therapy for spontaneous pneumothorax. *Br Med J* 1971; **4**(5779):86–88.
18. Miller WC, Toon R, Palat H *et al*. Experimental pulmonary edema following re-expansion of pneumothorax. *Am Rev Respir Dis* 1973; **108**:654–656.
19. Haworth CS, Dodd ME, Atkins M *et al*. Pneumothorax in adults with cystic fibrosis dependent on nasal intermittent positive pressure ventilation (NIPPV): a management dilemma. *Thorax* 2000; **55**:620–622.
20. Shah PL, Scott S, Hodson ME. Lobar atelectasis in cystic fibrosis and treatment with recombinant human Dnase 1. *Respir Med* 1994; **88**:313–315.
21. Slattery DM, Waltz DA, Denham B *et al*. Bronchoscopically administered human DNase for lobar atelectasis in cystic fibrosis. *Pediatr Pulmonol* 2001; **31**:383–388.
22. Lucas J, Connett GJ, Lea R *et al*. Lung resection in cystic fibrosis patients with localised pulmonary disease. *Arch Dis Child* 1996; **74**:449–451.
23. Coffey MJ, FitzGerald MX, McNicholas WT. Comparison of oxygen desaturation during sleep and exercise in patients with cystic fibrosis. *Chest* 1991; **100**:659–662.
24. Stern RC, Borkat G, Hirschfeld SS *et al*. Heart failure in cystic fibrosis: treatment and prognosis of cor pulmonale with failure of the right side of the heart. *Am J Dis Child* 1980; **134**:267–272.
25. Bright-Thomas RJ, Webb AK. The heart in cystic fibrosis. *J R Soc Med* 2002; **95**(Suppl 41):2–10.

26. Zinman R, Corey M, Coates AL *et al.* Nocturnal home oxygen in the treatment of hypoxemic cystic fibrosis patients. *J Pediatr* 1989; **114**: 368–377.

27. Florea VG, Florea ND, Sharma R *et al.* Right ventricular dysfunction in adult severe cystic fibrosis. *Chest* 2000; **118**:1063–1068.

28. Burghuber OC, Hartter E, Weissel M *et al.* Raised circulating plasma levels of atrial natriuretic peptide in adolescent and adult patients with cystic fibrosis and pulmonary artery hypertension. *Lung* 1991; **169**:291–300.

29. Sullivan MM, Moss RB, Hindi RD *et al.* Supraventricular tachycardia in patients with cystic fibrosis. *Chest* 1986; **90**:239–242.

30. Ketchell RL, Gyi KM, Badawi R *et al.* Cardiac compromise in end-stage cystic fibrosis. *Pediatr Pulmonol* 2004; **38**(Suppl 27):312.

31. Ranasinha C, Assoufi B, Shak S *et al.* Efficacy and safety of short-term administration of aerosolised recombinant human DNase I in adults with stable stage cystic fibrosis. *Lancet* 1993; **342**:199–202.

32. Ramsey BW, Astley SJ, Aitken ML *et al.* Efficacy and safety of short-term administration of aerosolized recombinant human deoxyribonuclease in patients with cystic fibrosis. *Am Rev Respir Dis* 1993; **148**:145–151.

33. Fuchs HJ, Borowitz DS, Christiansen DH *et al.* Effect of aerosolized recombinant human DNase on exacerbations of respiratory symptoms and on pulmonary function in patients with cystic fibrosis. The Pulmozyme Study Group. *N Engl J Med* 1994; **331**:637–642.

34. Accurso FJ. Aerosolised dornase alfa in cystic fibrosis patients with clinically mild lung disease. *Dornase alfa Clinical Series* 2006; **2**:1–6.

35. Quan JM, Tiddens HA, Sy JP *et al.* A two-year randomized, placebo-controlled trial of dornase alfa in young patients with cystic fibrosis with mild lung function abnormalities. *J Pediatr* 2001; **139**:813–820.

36. Shah PI, Bush A, Canny GJ *et al.* Recombinant human DNase I in cystic fibrosis patients with severe pulmonary disease: a short-term, double-blind study followed by six months open-label treatment. *Eur Respir J* 1995; **8**:954–958.

37. McCoy K, Hamilton S, Johnson C. Effects of 12-week administration of dornase alfa in patients with advanced cystic fibrosis lung disease. Pulmozyme Study Group. *Chest* 1996; **110**:889–895.

38. Shah PL, Scott SF, Geddes DM *et al.* Two years' experience with recombinant human DNase I in the treatment of pulmonary disease in cystic fibrosis. *Respir Med* 1995; **89**:499–502.

39. Shah PL, Conway S, Scott SF *et al.* A case-controlled study with dornase alfa to evaluate impact on disease progression over a 4-year period. *Respiration* 2001; **68**:160–164.

40. Hodson ME, McKenzie S, Harms HK *et al.* Dornase alfa in the treatment of cystic fibrosis in Europe: a report from the Epidemiologic Registry of Cystic Fibrosis. *Pediatr Pulmonol* 2003; **36**:427–432.

41. Fitzgerald DA, Hilton J, Jepson B *et al.* A crossover, randomized, controlled trial of dornase alfa before versus after physiotherapy in cystic fibrosis. *Pediatrics* 2005; **116**:e549–e554.

42. Suri R, Metcalfe C, Lees B *et al.* Comparison of hypertonic saline and alternate-day or daily recombinant human deoxyribonuclease in children with cystic fibrosis: a randomised trial. *Lancet* 2001; **358**:1316–1321.

43. Conway SP. Evidence-based medicine in cystic fibrosis: how should practice change? *Pediatr Pulmonol* 2002; **34**:242–247.

44. Suri R, Metcalfe C, Wallis C *et al.* Predicting response to rhDNase and hypertonic saline in children with cystic fibrosis. *Pediatr Pulmonol* 2004; **37**:305–310.

45. Burrows JA, Bunting JP, Masel PJ *et al.* Nebulised dornase alpha: adherence in adults with cystic fibrosis. *J Cyst Fibros* 2002; **1**:255–259.

46. Robinson M, Hemming AL, Regnis JA, *et al.* Effect of increasing doses of hypertonic saline on mucociliary clearance in patients with cystic fibrosis. *Thorax* 1997; **52**:900–903.

47. Robinson M, Regnis JA, Bailey DL *et al.* Effect of hypertonic saline, amiloride, and cough on mucociliary clearance in patients with cystic fibrosis. *Am J Respir Crit Care Med* 1996; **153**:1503–1509.

48. Rodwell LT, Anderson SD. Airway responsiveness to hyperosmolar saline challenge in cystic fibrosis: a pilot study. *Pediatr Pulmonol* 1990; **8**:4–11.

49. McFarlane PI, Heaf D. Changes in air flow obstruction and oxygen saturation in response to exercise and bronchodilators in cystic fibrosis. *Pediatr Pulmonol* 1990; **8**:4–11.

50. Eng PA, Morton J, Douglas JA *et al.* Short term efficacy of ultrasonically nebulised hypertonic saline in cystic fibrosis. *Pediatr Pulmonol* 1996; **21**:77–83.

51. Ballman M, von der Hardt H. Hypertonic saline and recombinant human DNase: a randomized cross-over pilot study in patients with cystic fibrosis. *J Cystic Fibrosis* 2002; **1**:35–37.

52. Elkins MR, Robinson M, Rose BR *et al.* National Hypertonic Saline in Cystic Fibrosis (NHSCF) Study Group: a controlled trial of long-term inhaled hypertonic saline in patients with cystic fibrosis. *N Engl J Med* 2006; **354**:229–240.

53. Donaldson SH, Bennett WD, Zeman KL, Knowles MR, Tarran R, Boucher RC. Mucus clearance and lung function in cystic fibrosis with hypertonic saline. *N Engl J Med* 2006; **354**:241–250.

54. Nightingale JA, Rogers DF, Barnes PJ. Effect of repeated sputum induction on cell counts in normal volunteers. *Thorax* 1998; **53**:87–90.

55. Holz O, Richter K, Jones RA, Speckin P, Mucke M, Magnussen H. Changes in sputum composition between two inductions performed on consecutive days. *Thorax* 1998; **53**:83–86.

56. Suri R, Marshall LJ, Wallis C *et al.* Effects of rhDNase and hypertonic saline on airway inflammation in children with cystic fibrosis. *Am J Respir Crit Care Med* 2002; **166**:352–355.

57. Suri R, Metcalfe C, Wallis C, Bush A. Predicting response to rhDNase and hypertonic saline in children with cystic fibrosis. *Pediatr Pulmonol* 2004; **37**:305–310.

58. Ho SA, Ball R, Morrison LJ *et al.* Clinical value of obtaining sputum and cough swab samples following inhaled hypertonic saline in children with cystic fibrosis. *Pediatr Pulmonol* 2004; **38**:82–87.

59. Guitierrez JP, Grimwood K, Armstrong DS *et al.* Interlobar differences in bronchoalveolar lavage fluid from children with cystic fibrosis. *Eur Respir J* 2001; **17**:281–286.

60. Zar H, Hanslo D, Apolles P *et al.* Induced sputum versus gastric lavage for microbiological confirmation of pulmonary tuberculosis in infants and young children: a prospective study. *Lancet* 2005; **365**:130–134.

61. Denton R, Kwart H, Litt M. *N*-acetylcysteine in cystic fibrosis. *Am Rev Respir Dis* 1967; **95**:643–651.

62. Howatt WF, DeMuth GR. A double-blind study of the use of acetylcysteine in patients with cystic fibrosis. *Univ Mich Med Centr J* 1966; **32**:82–85.

63. Ratjan F, Wonne R, Posselt HG et al. A double-bind placebo-controlled trial with oral ambroxol and *N*-acetylcysteine for mucolytic treatment in cystic florosis. *Eur J Pediatr* 1985; **144**: 374–378.

64. Duijvestijn YC, Brand PL. Systematic review of *N*-acetylcysteine in cystic fibrosis. *Acta Paediatrica* 1999; **88**:38–41.

65. Tirouvanziam R, Conrad CK, Bottiglieri T *et al.* High-dose oral *N*-acetylcysteine, a glutathione prodrug, modulates inflammation in cystic fibrosis. *Proc Natl Acad Sci USA* 2006; **103**:4628–4633.

66. App EM, Baran D, Dab I *et al.* Dose-finding and 24-h monitoring for efficacy and safety of aerosolized Nacystelyn in cystic fibrosis. *Eur Respir J* 2002; **19**:294–302.

67. Robinson M, Daviskas E, Eberl S *et al.* The effect of inhaled mannitol on bronchial mucus clearance in cystic fibrosis patients: a pilot study. *Eur Respir J* 1999; **14**:678–685.

68. Joos GF, O'Connor B on behalf of ERS Task Force. Indirect airway challenges. *Eur Respir J* 2003; **21**:1050–1068.

69. Wells PJ, Chan WM, Hall RL, Cole PJ. Ciliary transportability of sputum is governed by its osmolality. In: Baum GL *et al.* (eds) *Cilia, Mucus and Mucociliary Interactions.* Marcel Dekker, New York, 1998, pp281–284.

70. Geddes D, Inflammation: defense or offense. *Pediatr Pulmonol* 2005; Suppl **28**:122–123.

71. Konstan M, Doring G, Lands LC *et al.* Results of a Phase 11 clinical trial of B11L 284 BS (an LTB$_4$ receptor antagonist) for the treatment of CF lung disease. *Pediatr Pulmonol* 2005; Suppl **28**:125–126.

72. Auerbach HS, Williams M, Kirkpatrick JA, Colten HR. Alternate-day prednisone reduces morbidity and improves pulmonary function in cystic fibrosis. *Lancet* 1985; **2**:686–688.

73. Eigen H, Rosenstein B, Fitzsimmons S, Schidlow D. A multi-center study of alternate day prednisolone therapy in patients with cystic fibrosis. *J Pediatr* 1995; **126**:515–523.

74. Balfour-Lynn IM, Lees B, Hall P *et al.* Multicenter randomized controlled trial of withdrawal of inhaled corticosteroids in cystic fibrosis. *Am J Respir Crit Care Med* 2006; **173**:1356–1362.

75. Ren CL, Pasta DJ, Konstan MW *et al.* Inhaled corticosteroid (ICS) use is associated with a slower rate of decline in CF lung disease. *Pediatr Pulmonol* 2004; Suppl **25**:295.

76. Balfour-Lynn IM, Elborn JS 'CF asthma': what is it and what do we do about it? *Thorax* 2002; **57**:742–748.

77. Todd GR, Acerini CL, Ross-Russell R *et al.* Survey of adrenal crisis associated with inhaled corticosteroids in the United Kingdom. *Arch Dis Child* 2002; **87**:457–461.

78. Hoiby N. Diffuse panbronchiolitis and cystic fibrosis: East meets West. *Thorax* 1994; **49**:531–532.

79. Kudoh S, Azuma A, Yamamoto M *et al.* Improvement in survival of patients with diffuse panbronchiolitis treated with low dose erythromycin. *Am J Respir Crit Care Med* 1998; **157**:1829–1832.

80. Oda H, Kadota J, Kohno S, Hara K. Erythromycin inhibits neutrophil chemotaxis in bronchoalveolar lavage in diffuse panbronchiolitis. *Chest* 1994; **106**:1116–1123.

81. Nagai H, Shishido H, Yoneda R *et al.* Long-term, low-dose administration of erythromycin to patients with diffuse panbronchiolitis. *Respiration* 1991; **58**:145–149.

82. Hilliard TN, Balfour-Lynn IM. Anti-inflammatory agents: a clinical perspective. In: Bush A *et al.* (eds) *Progress in Respiratory Research. Cystic Fibrosis in the 21st Century.* Karger, Basel, 2005.

83. Wolter J, Seeney S, Bell S *et al.* Effect of long term treatment with azithromycin on disease parameters in cystic fibrosis: a randomised controlled trial. *Thorax* 2002; **57**:212–216.

84. Equi A, Balfour-Lynn I, Bush A, Rosenthal M. Long term azithromycin in children with cystic fibrosis: a randomized, placebo-controlled crossover trial. *Lancet* 2002; **360**:978–984.

85. Saiman L, Marshall BC, Meyer-Hamblett N *et al.* Azithromycin in patients with cystic fibrosis chronically infected with *Pseudomonas aeruginosa*: a randomized controlled trial. *J Am Med Assoc* 2003; **290**:1749–1756.

86. Jaffe A, Bush A. Anti-inflammatory effects of macrolides in lung disease. *Pediatr Pulmonol* 2001; **31**:464–473.

87. Bush A, Rubin BK. Macrolides as biologic response modifiers in cystic fibrosis and bronchiectasis. *Sem Resp Crit Care Med* 2003; **24**:737–747.

88. Jaffe A, Bush A. Macrolides in cystic fibrosis. In: Rubin BK, Tamaoki J (eds) *Progress in Inflammation Research. Antibiotics as Anti-inflammatory and Immunomodulatory Agents.* Birkhauser Verlag, Basel, 2005, pp167–191.

89. Barker PM, Gillie DJ, Schechter MS, Rubin BK. Effect of macrolides on in-vivo ion transport across cystic fibrosis nasal epithelium. *Am J Respir Crit Care Med* 2005; **171**:868–871.

90. Equi A, Davies JC, Painter H *et al.* Exploring the mechanisms of macrolides in cystic fibrosis. *Respir Med* 2006; **100**:687–697.

91. Ribeiro CP, O'Neal W, Wu Y *et al.* The macrolide azithromycin induces a pro-inflammatory response in human airway epithelia. *Pediatr Pulmonol* 2005; Suppl **28**:238–239.

92. Hansen CR, Pressler T, Koch C, Hoiby N. Long-term azithromycin treatment of cystic fibrosis patients with chronic *Pseudomonas aeruginosa* infection: an observational cohort study. *J Cyst Fib* 2005; **4**:35–40.

93. Konstan MW, Byard PJ, Hoppel CL, Davis PB. Effect of high dose ibuprofen in patients with cystic fibrosis. *N Engl J Med* 1995; **322**:848–854.

94. Rinaldo JE, Pennock B. Effects of ibuprofen on endotoxin-induced alveolitis: biphasic dose response and dissociation between inflammation and hypoxemia. *Am J Med Sci* 1986; **291**:29–38.

95. Dezateux C, Crighton A. Oral non-steroidal anti-inflammatory drug therapy for cystic fibrosis. *Cochrane Database Syst Rev* 2000; (2):CD001505.

96. Kovesi TA, Swartz R, MacDonald N. Transient renal failure due to simultaneous ibuprofen and aminoglycoside therapy in children with cystic fibrosis. *N Engl J Med* 1998; **338**:65–66.

97. Scott CS, Retsch-Bogart GZ, Henry MM. Renal failure and vestibular toxicity in an adolescent receiving gentamicin and standard-dose ibuprofen. *Pediatr Pulmonol* 2001; **31**:314–316.

98. Perks B, Shute JK. DNA and actin bind and inhibit interleukin-8 function in cystic fibrosis sputa: in vitro effects of mucolytics. *Am J Respir Crit Care Med* 2000; **162**:1767–1772.

99. Paul K, Rietschel E, Ballmann M *et al.* Effect of treatment with dornase alpha on airway inflammation in patients with cystic fibrosis. *Am J Respir Crit Care Med* 2004; **169**:719–725.

100. Eggleston PA, Rosenstein BJ, Stackhouse CM *et al.* Airway hyperreactivity in cystic fibrosis: clinical correlates and possible effects on the course of the disease. *Chest* 1988; **94**:360–365.

101. Davis B, Marin MG, Yee JW *et al.* Effect of terbutaline on movement of Cl⁻ and Na⁺ across the trachea of the dog *in vitro. Am Rev Respir Dis* 1979; **120**:547–552.

102. Ormerod LP, Thomson RA, Anderson CM *et al.* Reversible airway obstruction in cystic fibrosis. *Thorax* 1980; **35**:768–772.

103. Avital A, Sanchez I, Chernick V. Efficacy of salbutamol and ipratropium bromide in decreasing bronchial hyperreactivity in children with cystic fibrosis. *Pediatr Pulmonol* 1992; **13**:34–37.

104. van Haren EH, Lammers JW, Festen J *et al.* Bronchodilator response in adult patients with cystic fibrosis: effects on large and small airways. *Eur Respir J* 1991; **4**:301–307.

105. Koch C, McKenzie SG, Kaplowitz H *et al.* International practice patterns by age and severity of lung disease in cystic fibrosis: data from the Epidemiologic Registry of Cystic Fibrosis (ERCF). *Pediatr Pulmonol* 1997; **24**:147–154.

106. Finnegan MJ, Hughes DV, Hodson ME. Comparison of nebulized and intravenous terbutaline during exacerbations of pulmonary infection in patients with cystic fibrosis. *Eur Respir J* 1992; **5**:1089–1091.

107. Bargon J, Viel K, Dauletbaev N *et al.* Short-term effects of regular salmeterol treatment on adult cystic fibrosis patients. *Eur Respir J* 1997; **10**:2307–2311.

108. Hordvik NL, Sammut PH, Judy CG *et al.* Effects of standard and high doses of salmeterol on lung function of hospitalized patients with cystic fibrosis. *Pediatr Pulmonol* 1999; **27**:43–53.

109. Vaz Fragoso CA, Miller MA. Review of the clinical efficacy of theophylline in the treatment of chronic obstructive pulmonary disease. *Am Rev Respir Dis* 1993; **147**: S40–S47.

110. Pan SH, Canafax DM, Le CT *et al.* Bronchodilation from intravenous theophylline in patients with cystic fibrosis: results of a blinded placebo-controlled crossover clinical trial. *Pediatr Pulmonol* 1989; **6**:172–179.

111. Yankaskas JR, Marshall BC, Sufian B *et al.* Cystic fibrosis adult care: consensus conference report. *Chest* 2004; **125** (1 Suppl):1S–39S.

112. Balfour-Lynn I, Mohan U, Bush A, Rosenthal M. Intravenous immunoglobulin for cystic fibrosis lung disease: a case series of 16 children. *Arch Dis Child* 2004; **89**:315–319.

113. Ballmann M, Junge S, von de Hardt H. Low-dose methotrexate for advanced pulmonary disease for patients with advanced cystic fibrosis lung disease. *Respir Med* 2003; **97**:498–500.

114. Bhal GK, Maguire SA, Bowler IM. Use of cyclosporin A as a steroid sparing agent in cystic fibrosis. *Arch Dis Child* 2001; **84**:89.

115. Iacono AT, Johnson BA, Grgurich WF *et al.* A randomised trial of inhaled cyclosporine in lung-transplant recipients. *N Engl J Med* 2006; **354**:141–150.

116. Dillard TA, Berg BW, Rajagopal KR *et al.* Hypoxemia during air travel in patients with chronic obstructive pulmonary disease. *Ann Intern Med* 1989; **111**:362–367.

117. Buchdahl RM, Babiker A, Bush A, Cramer D. Predicting hypoxaemia during flights in children with cystic fibrosis. *Thorax* 2001; **56**:877–879.

118. Standards for the diagnosis and care of patients with chronic obstructive pulmonary disease (COPD) and asthma. *Am Rev Respir Dis* 1987; **136**:225–244.

119. Managing passengers with respiratory disease planning air travel: British Thoracic Society recommendations. *Thorax* 2002; **57**:289–304.

120. Fischer R, Lang SM, Bruckner K *et al.* Lung function in adults with cystic fibrosis at altitude: impact on air travel. *Eur Respir J* 2005; **25**:718–724.

121. Peckham D, Watson A, Pollard K *et al.* Predictors of desaturation during formal hypoxic challenge in adult patients with cystic fibrosis. *J Cyst Fibros* 2002; **1**:281–286.

122. Speechly-Dick ME, Rimmer SJ, Hodson ME. Exacerbations of cystic fibrosis after holidays at high altitude: a cautionary tale. *Respir Med* 1992; **86**:55–56.

123. Kennedy JD, Dinwiddie R, Daman-Willems C *et al.* Pseudo-Bartter's syndrome in cystic fibrosis. *Arch Dis Child* 1990; **65**:786–787.

124. Al-Aloul M, Miller H, Alapati S, *et al.* Renal impairment in cystic fibrosis patients due to repeated intravenous aminoglycoside use. *Pediatr Pulmonol* 2005; **39**:15–30.

125. Tannenbaum E, Prasad SA, Main E, Stocks J. The effect of chest physiotherapy on cystic fibrosis patients undergoing general anesthesia for an elective surgical procedure. *Pediatr Pulmonol* 2001; Suppl 22:315.

12

Sleep, lung mechanics and work of breathing, including NIPPV

BRIGITTE FAUROUX AND ANNICK CLÉMENT

INTRODUCTION

Most of the morbidity and mortality in cystic fibrosis (CF) is due to the involvement of the lung. Progressive airflow obstruction, due to mucus plugging and inflammation within the bronchial walls, and destruction of the lung parenchyma secondary to bronchiectasis, leads to progressive respiratory failure. This characteristic involvement of the airways and the lung parenchyma explains the details of the respiratory mechanics in CF. Although CF lung disease may be considered as a chronic obstructive pulmonary disease (COPD), the alterations observed in respiratory mechanics are not exactly similar to those of the 'classical' non-CF COPD. CF lung disease associates both an obstructive and a restrictive ventilatory defect, with an early decline in lung compliance, which constitutes the major determinant of the increase in respiratory muscle output [1]. Dynamic lung compliance represents the ratio of tidal volume to the esophageal pressure difference between the beginning and end of the inspiration, at an instant zero of flow in order to eliminate the load induced by the resistance, and thus the elastic properties of the lung. This decrease in lung compliance is the consequence both of hyperinflation (reaching the flat part of the compliance curve) and also of the inflammatory and infectious changes within the lung.

This chapter will focus on lung mechanics and work of breathing. The therapeutic strategies will be discussed, with a special emphasis on non-invasive positive pressure ventilation (NIPPV).

LUNG MECHANICS AND WORK OF BREATHING

The ability to sustain spontaneous ventilation can be viewed as a balance between neurological mechanisms controlling ventilation together with ventilatory muscle power on one side, and the respiratory load, determined by lung, thoracic and airway mechanics, on the other (Fig. 12.1). Significant dysfunction of any of these components of the respiratory system may impair the ability to spontaneously generate efficacious breaths. In normal individuals, central respiratory drive and ventilatory muscle power exceed the respiratory load, and they are thus able to sustain adequate spontaneous

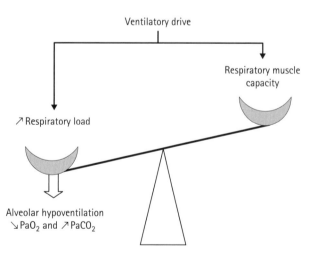

Figure 12.1 Spontaneous ventilation is the result of a balance between neurological mechanisms controlling ventilation together with ventilatory muscle power on one side, and the respiratory load, determined by lung, thoracic and airway mechanics, on the other. If the respiratory load is too high and/or ventilatory muscle power or central respiratory drive is too low, ventilation may be inadequate, resulting in alveolar hypoventilation with hypercapnia and hypoxemia. In patients with cystic fibrosis, the load imposed on the respiratory muscles is too high, which explains the occurrence of alveolar hypoventilation.

ventilation. However, if the respiratory load is too high and/or ventilatory muscle power or central respiratory drive is too low, ventilation may be inadequate, resulting in hypercapnia. Chronic ventilatory failure, then, is the result of an imbalance in the respiratory system, in which ventilatory muscle power and central respiratory drive are inadequate to overcome the respiratory load. If this imbalance cannot be corrected with medical treatment, the patient may benefit from long-term ventilatory support.

Respiratory load, ventilatory muscle power and the neurological mechanisms controlling ventilation have all been measured in patients with CF (see Fig. 12.1). The simplest way of estimating the patient's inspiratory effort is to measure the esophageal (PTP_{es}) and the diaphragmatic pressure–time product (PTP_{di}). The PTP_{es} is obtained by measuring the area under the esophageal pressure (P_{es}) signal between the time of onset of inspiratory effort and the end of inspiration, during one breath or during one minute. The PTP_{di} is obtained in a similar way, by measuring the area above the transdiaphragmatic pressure (P_{di}) signal during the same time periods as the P_{es}. Both pressure indexes reflect the respiratory muscle output, as they are significantly correlated with the oxygen consumption of the respiratory muscles themselves, of the global inspiratory muscles for PTP_{es}, and of the diaphragm for PTP_{di}. Thus, the greater these indexes, the greater the respiratory muscle output of the patient. PTP_{es} and PTP_{di} values measured in healthy adults are approximately $100 \, cmH_2O$-seconds per minute. In children and young adults with advanced pulmonary CF disease, as lung disease progresses, with a progressive fall in the forced expiratory volume in one second (FEV_1), there is an increase in the respiratory muscle load. Indeed, as FEV_1 falls, PTP_{es} and PTP_{di} and the elastic work of breathing increase [1]. Indeed, in a group of children with CF, having a FEV_1 between 30% and 50% of predicted value, PTP_{es} and PTP_{di} were increased 3- to 5-fold. As a result, the patients develop a compensatory mechanism of rapid shallow breathing pattern in an attempt to reduce the increase in load. Although this breathing strategy maintains the level of ventilation, partial arterial carbon dioxide pressure ($PaCO_2$) rises.

Ventilatory muscle power, or the capacity of the respiratory muscles, has also been evaluated in patients with CF (see Fig. 12.1). Previous studies provided inconsistent results with regard to the inspiratory muscle strength. These discrepancies could be explained by the different methods used, most being volitional tests, the results of which are dependent on motivation. More recently, diaphragmatic strength has been evaluated by a non-volitional test; i.e. the magnetic stimulation of the phrenic nerves [2]. In children with CF, this test showed that diaphragmatic strength was preserved in a group of young patients, aged 15 ± 3 years [3]. The diaphragm was weaker in those patients who were malnourished and in those who were hyperinflated, in the latter case presumably due to the muscle working at a mechanical disadvantage. Malnutrition, which is the consequence of poor caloric intake, malabsorption, increased

energy expenditure, less efficient pulmonary mechanics, and a catabolic intermediary metabolism, either as part of the primary defect or secondary to pulmonary infection and inflammation, seems to be the major determinant of diaphragmatic strength. Hyperinflation results in a shorter diaphragm length and imposes a mechanical disadvantage on the diaphragm, which causes a reduction in the generation of diaphragmatic pressure. In adults, magnetic stimulation of the phrenic nerves showed a decrease in diaphragmatic strength, but an increase in abdominal muscle strength [4]. Interestingly, the diaphragm and the abdominal muscle bulk were not affected by the general muscle wasting, which suggests that a training effect persists in patients with CF.

The third determinant of the ventilatory balance is central drive, which has also been evaluated in patients with CF (see Fig. 12.1). A classical test to evaluate central respiratory drive is the measure of the mouth pressure generated $100 \, ms$ after the onset of an occluded inspiratory effort ($P_{0.1}$). This measure reflects the central respiratory drive prior to any limitation from an abnormal respiratory mechanics. The results must be interpreted with caution in patients with chronic hyperinflation, such as CF. However, no study measuring $P_{0.1}$ in either adult or pediatric patients with chronic lung disease showed any alteration of central drive, except in those patients who were chronically hypercapnic.

Thus, in CF, an imbalance between the load imposed on the respiratory system and the capacity of the respiratory muscles explains the inability of the respiratory muscle pump to clear CO_2.

SLEEP

Sleep affects the three components of the respiratory balance. Physiological changes in respiratory and upper airway function, respiratory muscle power and ventilatory response lead to a degree of nocturnal hypoventilation even in normal subjects, causing a rise in $PaCO_2$ of up $3 \, mmHg$ ($0.4 \, kPa$) (Fig. 12.2). This explains why patients with chronic respiratory failure are more vulnerable during sleep. Sleep is associated with changes in respiratory mechanics, such as an increase in ventilation–perfusion mismatch, an increase in airflow resistance and a fall in functional residual capacity. Although the activity of the diaphragm is preserved, that of the intercostal and the upper airway muscles is decreased significantly. Finally, central drive and chemoreceptor sensitivity are less efficient during sleep than during wakefulness. All these abnormalities are most pronounced during rapid-eye-movement (REM) sleep.

Sleep disturbance seems to be common and occurs early in the course of CF. Sleep loss is known to have negative effects on mental and neurocognitive functions, and on multiple metabolic parameters including glucose metabolism. It has also been associated with alterations in the normal circadian cytokine network, the expression of adhesion

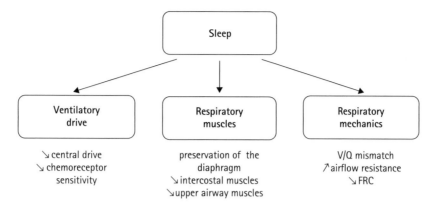

Figure 12.2 Sleep is associated with a degree of alveolar hypoventilation even in normal subjects, due to modifications in ventilatory drive, respiratory muscle function and respiratory mechanics. Central drive and chemoreceptor sensitivity are lower during sleep than during wakefulness. Although the activity of the diaphragm is preserved during sleep, those of the intercostal and the upper airway muscles decrease significantly. Changes in respiratory mechanics include an increase in ventilation–perfusion mismatch (V/Q), an increase in airflow resistance and a fall in functional residual capacity (FRC).

molecules, and the balance between cellular and humoral immune responses.

The Pittsburgh Sleep Quality Index (PSQI) is a validated questionnaire to assess subjective sleep quality in adults [5]. Sleep quality has been evaluated by means of this questionnaire in 37 patients with CF, having a mean FEV_1 of $36 \pm 12\%$ of predicted value. Their mean PSQI was 5.7 ± 4.0, a score higher than 5 reflecting poor self-perceived sleep quality. Better sleep efficiency ($p < 0.05$) and a greater percentage of REM sleep ($p < 0.05$) were found in those patients with a PSQI of $\geqslant 5$. Sleep efficiency has been evaluated by means of the actigraph, which is a miniature, wristwatch-like device that monitors activity levels for extended continuous periods. By means of this device, sleep quality has been evaluated in 44 children with CF, aged 8–18 years, having a large range of lung function, and 40 healthy control subjects [6]. CF patients had significantly lower sleep efficiency than control subjects. The FEV_1 of the patients correlated positively with sleep duration and efficiency, but even the patients with mild CF lung disease (as assessed by an FEV_1 between 70–89% of predicted) had a sleep efficiency of 93%, compared to 96% in patients with CF having a normal value of FEV_1 ($> 90\%$ predicted value). Sleep efficiency was only 82% in those with severe lung disease ($FEV_1 < 40\%$ predicted value). Sleep quality was assessed by the actigraph in 20 adult patients with CF and controls over a period of 14 days [7]. The patients had mild lung disease with a mean FEV_1 of $60 \pm 20\%$ predicted value and a normal mean body mass index of 23 ± 4. In this study, the CF patients had similar sleep duration, sleep latency and sleep efficiency, but a higher fragmentation index, and less immobile time than controls. The fragmentation index measures restlessness, and is calculated by summing the percentage of minutes spent moving, expressed as a percentage of the time spent in immobility; the immobile time is derived by dividing the number of minutes spent immobile by the assumed sleep time and multiplying by 100. Their mean PSQI score was also higher than controls. The underlying mechanisms are

unclear. Possibilities include nocturnal coughing, the need for nocturnal defecation, the use of β2 agonists before sleep, and an increased work of breathing.

As lung disease progresses, abnormal gas exchange and sleep-disordered breathing worsen. Compared to 10 healthy controls, 19 patients with CF and severe lung disease (mean FEV_1 $28 \pm 7\%$ of predicted value) tended to report more awakenings, and polysomnography revealed reduced sleep efficiency ($71 \pm 25\%$, vs $93 \pm 4\%$; $p = 0.004$), and a higher frequency of awakenings ($4.2 \pm 2.7 h^{-1}$ vs $2.4 \pm 1.4 h^{-1}$; $p = 0.06$) [8]. Mean SaO_2 was also significantly lower in the patients with CF ($84 \pm 7\%$ vs $94 \pm 2\%$; $p < 0.0001$) and was associated with reduced sleep efficiency. This sleep-disordered breathing translated into impairment of neurocognitive functions and daytime sleepiness.

A major issue is thus when to schedule a night-time sleep study in patients with CF. Daytime blood gases and parameters evaluating lung function and respiratory muscle performance correlated with nocturnal SaO_2 and transcutaneous CO_2 ($PtcCO_2$) in 32 patients with CF, in a stable condition, having FEV_1 below 65% predicted value [9]. Evening PaO_2 ($p < 0.0001$) and morning $PaCO_2$ ($p < 0.01$) were predictive of the average minimum SaO_2 per 30-second epoch of sleep ($p < 0.0001$). Evening PaO_2 was also predictive of the rise in $PtcCO_2$ seen from non-REM to REM sleep. In addition, there was some relationship between expiratory muscle strength, evaluated on the maximal expiratory pressure, and the REM respiratory disturbance index. Another study found only a weak relationship between FEV_1 and SaO_2 and nocturnal desaturation [10]. As might be expected, these sleep disturbances are enhanced during infective exacerbations [11].

Exercise and physiotherapy are also situations that can reveal or precipitate respiratory failure as minute ventilation (the load imposed on the respiratory muscles) increases [12,13]. As compared to sleep, alveolar hypoventilation is less important. Indeed, in a group of 14 patients with CF, hypoxemia was more severe during sleep (mean SaO_2

$82 \pm 2\%$) than during exercise ($89 \pm 5\%$), and $PtcCO_2$ was also higher during sleep (mean $PtcCO_2$ $48 \pm 7\%$), than during exercise ($43 \pm 6\%$) [12].

In conclusion, sleep disordered breathing, due to nocturnal alveolar hypoventilation, occurs early in the course of CF. Lung function parameters are poor predictors of nocturnal desaturation. Further studies are thus clearly needed to identify the symptoms and the lung function parameters that should lead to a request for polysomnography. The exact threshold of FEV_1 or daytime or nocturnal SaO_2 which should prompt a sleep sleep study is unknown (there is an ongoing study addressing this question). In practice, the presence of symptoms suggestive of nocturnal hypoventilation, such as frequent arousals, daytime fatigue or sleepiness, and morning headaches, as well as FEV_1 below 25–30% predicted, should lead to consideration of a sleep study. Because of the difficulty in obtaining full polysomnography in some centers, the monitoring of nocturnal SaO_2 could be used as a screening tool.

NON-INVASIVE POSITIVE PRESSURE VENTILATION

Although non-invasive positive pressure ventilation (NIPPV) is less commonly used in patients with CF than in other chronic lung diseases such as COPD, a definite physiological rationale has been demonstrated for its use in young CF patients with advanced lung disease. Short-term physiological studies, during awakefulness and sleep, have demonstrated that NIPPV reduces respiratory muscle load and work of breathing [14,15], increases minute ventilation [14,15], and thus improves alveolar ventilation and gas exchange. By definition, NIPPV is a non-invasive technique, that can be applied on demand, and preferably at night, because this is the time of greatest risk for hypoventilation, and also the period in which NIPPV can be applied with the least disruption to daily life. Despite these encouraging results, NIPPV is often not part of the routine management of severe lung disease in CF. Possible explanations include the lack of clearly validated criteria for when to propose this technique, controversies with regard to the optimal ventilatory modes and settings, scepticism with regard to long-term efficacy, and poor acceptance by patients who already spend a considerable amount of time on their treatment.

Benefits of NIPPV

In cystic fibrosis, NIPPV acts as an external respiratory muscle that unloads the respiratory muscles of the patient, and this has been confirmed by several short-term physiological studies, performed during wakefulness and sleep. This translates into an improvement in alveolar ventilation and gas exchange.

The efficacy of two ventilatory modes, a volume-targeted ventilation (AC/VT) and a pressure-targeted ventilation

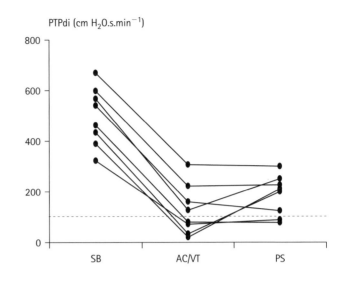

Figure 12.3 Individual variations of diaphragmatic pressure–time product per minute (PTP_{di}/min) in eight young patients with cystic fibrosis and chronic respiratory failure during non-invasive assist control/volume targeted (AC/VT) and pressure support (PS) ventilation, compared to spontaneous breathing (SB). The two ventilatory modes were associated with a significant reduction in PTP_{di}/min in all the patients [15]. The dotted line represents the normal value (100 cmH_2Os per minute).

(pressure support, PS) in reducing the work of breathing has been evaluated in children with stable, severe respiratory insufficiency (Fig. 12.3) [15]. Eight children (aged 11–17 years) were ventilated with PS and AC/VT ventilation in a random order. All indices of respiratory effort (PTP_{es}, PTP_{di}) decreased by about 60% during the two modes of NIPPV compared to spontaneous breathing. This unloading of the patient's respiratory muscles explained the significant improvement in tidal volume and minute ventilation, and consequently, in blood gas variables. Another short-term physiological study compared the unloading of the respiratory muscles in 12 adult patients with CF during PS and proportional assist ventilation [16]. The unloading of the respiratory muscles was evaluated on the change in surface diaphragmatic electromyography. On average, both PS and proportional assist ventilation reduced diaphragmatic activity (-30% with PS and -20% with proportional assist ventilation), improved ventilation ($+30\%$), tidal volume ($+30\%$) and $PtcCO_2$ (-7%).

The unloading of the respiratory muscles has also been demonstrated during sleep in several short-term studies. A study including seven adults with CF showed that, compared to a control night, continuous positive airway pressure (CPAP) ventilation resulted in a significant improvement in SaO_2 during both REM and non-REM sleep [17]. However, $PtcCO_2$ measurements were not significantly different between the control and the CPAP nights. Another interesting study compared the gas exchange and the quality of sleep in CF adults during three nights – a control night, a night with oxygen and a night with non-invasive bilevel positive

Table 12.1 Indications for non-invasive positive pressure ventilation (NIPPV).

Evidence based	Not-evidence based, but of probable benefit
Unloading of the respiratory muscles	Increase in survival
Improvement in alveolar ventilation and gas exchange during wakefulness, sleep, physiotherapy and exercise	Stabilization of the decline in lung function
	Accelerate the recovery during an acute respiratory exacerbation
	Improvement of respiratory muscle performance
	Improvement of quality of life
	Improvement of nutritional status

airway pressure (BiPAP) ventilation [18]. Similar significant improvements of SaO_2 and time spent in REM sleep were observed during the nights with oxygen and BiPAP ventilation. But, most importantly, the night with oxygen was associated with a significant increase in $PtcCO_2$, whereas BiPAP ventilation resulted in a significant decrease in $PtcCO_2$. A third study showed that non-invasive BiPAP ventilation was able to maintain a sufficient tidal volume and thus minute ventilation during sleep, whereas this was not observed during a control night, with or without oxygen [19]. A limitation of these sleep studies is their duration, comparing only two or three consecutive nights. Further studies, confirming these results on a long-term basis, are clearly needed.

This improvement of alveolar hypoventilation by NIPPV also leads to a persistent decrease of daytime hypercapnia within the first days of effective therapy [20]. Indeed, NIPPV may be responsible for a persistent decrease in the work of breathing during periods of spontaneous ventilation after the periods of NIPPV as a result of an increase in chest wall and lung compliance.

The more long-term benefits of NIPPV may also be explained by an increase in respiratory drive due to a reduction in cerebrospinal fluid bicarbonate concentration which resets the ventilatory response to CO_2, and to an improvement in sleep quality which influences the ventilatory response to CO_2 and respiratory muscle performance [21].

NIPPV has been associated with an improvement in respiratory muscle performance in patients with CF. Piper and co-workers [20] reported an increase in maximal expiratory and inspiratory pressures in four adults with CF after one month of NIPPV. However, improvement due to a learning effect or a better motivation cannot be excluded because of the volitional nature of these tests. We have observed a significant decrease in maximal expiratory and inspiratory pressures in 19 children with CF after a 20-minute physiotherapy session [13]. When the physiotherapy session was performed with PS ventilation administered by a nasal mask, a significant increase of these parameters was observed. The improvement of maximal inspiratory pressure after the PS session suggests that PS may 'rest' the inspiratory muscles during chest physiotherapy. The improvement of maximal expiratory pressure after the PS ventilation session could be explained by the increase in tidal volume during this ventilatory assistance. During PS, the tidal volume tends to the total lung capacity. Indeed, when the level of PS increases, the inspiration can be passive and tidal volume

can be assumed to be near the same as the inflation volume which is determined by the inspiratory pressure and the respiratory system compliance. In normal subjects, the respiratory system compliance is about $100 \, mL/cmH_2O$, so when PS is $10 \, cmH_2O$ the inflation volume is near 1 L. This allows a larger amount of energy passively to be stored, thereby facilitating expiration and a decrease in the expiratory muscles effort. These beneficial effects of NIPPV on respiratory muscle performance during chest physiotherapy have been validated in another study performed in 26 adult patients with CF [22]. Non-invasive BiPAP ventilation preserved maximal inspiratory pressure and was associated with a significant increase in maximal expiratory pressure compared to standard chest physiotherapy. These studies underline that NIPPV is able to improve respiratory muscle performance, at least in the short term, and during periods of increased respiratory effort such as chest physiotherapy.

Non-invasive CPAP ventilation has been associated with an improvement in exercise tolerance in 33 patients with CF [23]. Indeed, a 5-cmH_2O CPAP ventilation resulted in a decrease in oxygen consumption, respiratory effort, assessed by the transdiaphragmatic pressure (P_{di}), and dyspnea score. These beneficial effects during exercise were the most important in the patients with severe lung disease in whom the presence of intrinsic positive end-expiratory pressure (PEEP) may be favorably counteracted by CPAP.

Some studies have analyzed the benefits of NIPPV during acute exacerbations in patients with CF. Bilevel PAP ventilation has been used with success in nine adult patients with end-stage CF [24]. All the patients survived the intensive care unit stay and six underwent successful lung transplantation. The outcome of 76 patients with CF who had 136 intensive care unit admissions for a respiratory exacerbation was reported by Sood and co-workers [25]. Eighteen episodes occurring in 12 patients were managed with NIPPV. During these 18 episodes, four patients died and 14 survived, which represented a better outcome compared to those who required an endotracheal ventilation. However, it must be acknowledged that this difference in outcome may be confounded by the difference in severity between the two groups. The outcome and the efficacy of NIPPV has been recently evaluated in a large adult CF center in France [26]. NIPPV was used in 14 of 23 (63%) and 15 of 45 (33%) cases treated in the intensive care unit and pulmonary department, respectively. In the intensive care unit, the four patients who failed NIPPV and who required invasive mechanical ventilation died. In a multivariable analysis, independent factors influencing the risk of death were prior colonization with *Burkholderia cepacia*, hospitalization in the intensive care unit, and the severity of hypoxemia on admission. The ventilatory mode, either invasive or non-invasive, did not influence the 1-year outcome and mortality. The authors concluded that NIPPV represented a reasonable first therapeutic option in patients hospitalized for a severe respiratory exacerbation.

A major expectation of clinicians is that NIPPV could help to slow the ineluctable decline in lung function of patients with CF. The hypothesis is that the intermittent unloading of the respiratory muscles during periods of NIPPV could improve their performance during periods of spontaneous breathing, and thus contribute to preserving lung function. Indeed, the rate of decline in lung function, and in particular of FEV_1, has been proven to be a very strong predictive prognostic factor [26]. Unfortunately, such information is presently lacking but this hypothesis is worth evaluating, and if proven, may constitute a strong argument for a more widespread and earlier implementation of NIPPV in CF.

In a fatal disease such as CF, the impact of NIPPV on survival would constitute a major potential advantage. NIPPV is associated with an increase in survival in patients with neuromuscular diseases [27], but such data are not available for patients with CF. The benefit of pre-transplant NIPPV on post-transplant outcome remains controversial. Randomized studies will not be possible because of ethical issues. Data from national and international registers, with the restrictions and limitations due to real-life situations, will probably constitute the sole way to answer this very important question.

Few studies have evaluated the benefit of NIPPV on quality of life, especially in CF. Sleep-disordered breathing causes impairment in cognitive function and is associated with a poor quality of life. These adverse effects may impair the patient's daily life, and the school performances of a child, before the occurrence of daytime hypercapnia. The effect of an 'early' initiation of NIPPV should evaluate these outcomes, using age-appropriate techniques. For long-term studies, the benefits of NIPPV on quality of sleep, the ability to perform physiotherapy, daily activities, but also school attendance as well as work activities, clearly need to be evaluated. At the present time, an excellent theoretical basis for the use of NIPPV has been established; the acute use in severe exacerbations is common, and long-term use in chronic respiratory failure is increasingly offered, but there are no good-quality survival data to guide clinicians.

Criteria to initiate NIPPV

Several consensus conferences agree on the value of daytime hypercapnia as an indication for the initiation of NIPPV, because this is the hallmark of established ventilatory failure [28,29]. However, this classical criterion has been established

mainly for neuromuscular disorders. Daytime hypercapnia is preceded by a variable period of nocturnal hypoventilation during which treatable symptoms, such as frequent arousals, severe orthopnea, daytime fatigue and alterations in cognitive function, may impair the daily life of the patient. Also, criteria that apply for patients with neuromuscular disease are probably not applicable or may be less pertinent for patients with a lung disease such as CF [30].

There are no validated criteria to indicate the need to start NIPPV in CF. But, logically, a discussion of possible utilization should start the definite physiological and possible clinical benefits of NIPPV. The presence of a high respiratory effort and abnormal gas exchange, reflected by the presence of hypercapnia, constitutes a possible indication to offer NIPPV, especially if the patient experiences a downhill course with regard to his or her lung disease. Most groups systematically propose NIPPV to all their patients on a lung transplant list, but it is possible that the institution at an earlier stage may be accompanied by a greater benefit. Further data are needed to address this point.

A major issue is thus when is the best time to schedule a polysomnography [30]. A polysomnography should be performed without delay when the patient recognizes symptoms related to sleep-disordered breathing, but patients with CF may underestimate symptoms such as fatigue. Also, symptoms appear insidiously over long periods of time. The diagnosis of sleep-disordered breathing is difficult to establish in children because of reliance on parents and secondary caregivers who have a different perception of the child's disease. As discussed before, lung function parameters are poor indicators of nocturnal hypoventilation. A principal difficulty concerns the criteria that will be used for the definition of sleep-disordered breathing requiring NIPPV. Most often, the indication is based on a mean and/or cut-off level of SaO_2 and $PtcCO_2$, which is transgressed during a defined percentage of the sleep time or the study period. But other respiratory events during sleep, as those recently recommended for the diagnosis of sleep-related breathing disorders, such as sleep fragmentation, may be important to take into account.

NIPPV is also used during an acute exacerbation. An acute exacerbation does not represent an optimal physiological and psychological situation to start such a treatment; however, attempts to start earlier may be rejected by the patient if there is no perception of impaired well-being.

The respective indications for long-term oxygen therapy and NIPPV are not clearly known in CF. It seems logical to propose long-term oxygen therapy at an initial stage of respiratory failure, and/or when hypoxemia predominates; but even in this setting there is no evidence for improved mortality, and very little for an improvement in quality of life. However, when diurnal or significant nocturnal hypercapnia is documented, NIPPV is physiologically preferable. The consideration of practical and psychological aspects is very likely to be an important point is these decisions, particularly in the absence of any data on survival benefit. It is important to underline that NIPPV alone is not always able to correct hypoxemia. It is recommended to adjust supplemental oxygen therapy after the optimal setting of NIPPV.

Psychological considerations are of major importance in proposing NIPPV to patients with CF. It is essential that the patient, and the parents in child cases, should have the opportunity to discuss the NIPPV therapy in advance. Discussion should start long enough before the anticipated need to allow the patient and the family to evaluate options thoroughly and to discuss their feelings. NIPPV has here an essential first place as a non-invasive therapy but still represents an obvious escalation of treatment, reflecting a further step in the severity of lung disease. It is crucial to determine short-term and intermediate goals of NIPPV with the patient and the family, to explain the principles of NIPPV, to underline the fact that NIPPV will adapt to the patient and not the opposite. A wide range of ventilators and masks are available and great care must be taken to choose the most appropriate equipment and settings. The final objective is that NIPPV translates into well-being, a better quality of life, with a total acceptability to the patient and his or her family.

Ventilatory modes, setting and interfaces

Several different ventilatory modes have been used in patients with CF. Currently, the setting of the ventilator seems to be more important than the ventilatory mode.

Since the original publication by Sullivan and co-workers [31], nasal CPAP has become the treatment of choice for the management of obstructive events during sleep. Upper airway patency is maintained with nasal CPAP by a pneumatic splinting effect. In addition, it has been demonstrated that CPAP reduces the work of breathing in patients with flow limitation. If the main indication of CPAP is obstructive sleep apnea, it is also advocated in obstructive lung disease, when intrinsic positive end-expiratory pressure increases the work of breathing. In this way, this ventilatory mode has proved its efficacy in increasing exercise tolerance in patients with CF. Nasal CPAP used during exercise was associated with a decrease in oxygen consumption, heart rate, dyspnea score and respiratory effort, and a positive correlation was observed between the efficacy of the CPAP and the severity of the lung disease assessed by the percentage of decrease in FEV_1 [23]. However, because upper airway loading with complete or partial obstruction and intrinsic positive end-expiratory pressure are not the sole mechanisms of hypoventilation, CPAP may be insufficient in patients with significant respiratory function abnormalities.

Initial studies with long-term NIPPV in children with CF have used volume-targeted devices [32,33]. Volume-targeted ventilation is characterized by the delivery of a fixed, predetermined tidal volume. The main advantage of assisted-control/volume-targeted (AC/VT) ventilation is that a guaranteed minimal tidal volume is delivered, but

this can result in detrimentally high inspiratory airway pressures causing discomfort to the patient and poor tolerability. Another limitation of this mode is the absence of leak compensation. This mode has been developed mainly for patients with neuromuscular diseases where the ventilator acts as a substitute for the weakened respiratory muscles, which are unable to trigger the ventilator. The inspiratory triggers of these ventilators are not very sensitive, which necessitates a relatively high back-up rate. The recommendation of a high back-up rate is also supported by the fact that on most of the ventilators, the inspiratory/expiratory ratio is adjusted on the back-up rate of the ventilator and not on the patient's respiratory rate.

Pressure support is a more recent mode of ventilation. This ventilatory mode is pressure-targeted and each breath is triggered and terminated by the patient and supported by the ventilator; the patient can control the respiratory rate, inspiratory duration and tidal volume. This explains the relative ease in adapting to, and the greater comfort and synchrony of, this mode. In contrast to volume-targeted ventilation, tidal volume is not predetermined but depends on the level of PS, the inspiratory effort of the patient and the mechanical properties of the patient's respiratory system. During this mode, since there are no mandatory breaths present, an in-built low-frequency back-up rate is used to prevent episodes of apnea. Further, because the patient triggers the breaths, the sensitivity of the trigger is crucial. The sensitivities of the inspiratory triggers of the different ventilators designed for the home are variable but some are as sensitive as those of intensive care devices [34]. Because during PS, inspiratory muscle activity may influence respiratory frequency and tidal volume, this ventilatory mode is generally proposed in patients with lung disease, such as CF, who can breathe spontaneously for substantial periods of time and require mainly nocturnal ventilation [14,15].

Bi-level PPV is the combination of PS and PEEP, permitting an independent adjustment of the expiratory and the inspiratory positive airway pressures. In this mode, upper airway obstruction and/or work of breathing induced by intrinsic end-expiratory pressure are prevented by the expiratory positive airway pressure and thus PS can be triggered easily by the patient. This ventilatory mode has been used in patients with CF [24,35]

In conclusion, although all the different ventilatory modes have been tried in patients with CF, currently PS and bi-level positive pressure ventilation are used by the majority of the patients because of the better comfort and security with regard to the inspiratory pressure. Pressure support remains thus the preferred mode for domiciliary ventilation in patients with CF.

The ventilatory settings should be adjusted to relieve the symptoms associated with alveolar hypoventilation. In clinical practice, these settings are generally adapted according to non-invasive clinical parameters such as SaO_2, blood gases, tidal volume and respiratory rate, and sleep analysis. The analysis of more invasive parameters of respiratory effort, such as the PTP$_{es}$ and PTP$_{di}$, have rarely been used in children [14,15]. We demonstrated a correlation between the unloading of the respiratory muscles, assessed on the decreases in PTP$_{es}$ and PTP$_{di}$, and the subjective impression of comfort during NIPPV in children with CF receiving a PS or AC/VT ventilation by a nasal mask [15]. This observation led us to compare two methods of prescribing non-invasive PS ventilation: a clinical setting based on breathing pattern, gas exchange and comfort rate, and a physiological setting based on normalization of PTP$_{es}$ and PTP$_{di}$ [14]. Both methods improved breathing pattern and SaO$_2$ and reduced the respiratory effort. We found that patient–ventilator synchrony and patient comfort were better during the physiological setting. Thus, in patients with CF, PS ventilation is effective, independent of whether the ventilator settings are determined by the patient's breathing pattern and comfort or by an invasive evaluation of the patient's respiratory effort.

The nasal interface represents a crucial determinant of the success of NIPPV. The patient will be unable to tolerate and accept NIPPV if there is significant facial discomfort, skin injury, or significant air leaks. In children, nasal masks are preferred because they have less static dead-space, are less claustrophobic and allow communication and expectoration more easily than full-face masks. Some industrial masks are available for children. If there is intolerance of industrial masks, the manufacture of custom-made masks may improve the acceptance and the efficacy of NIPPV [36]. Because of the major importance of the interface, and the frequency of side-effects, a systematic maxillofacial evaluation, at the initiation of NIPPV, and during the follow-up, is strongly recommended.

Contraindications, side-effects and limits of NIPPV

In cystic fibrosis, NIPPV is contraindicated if there has been a recent pneumothorax. Also, in this population, nasal polyps are common and should be treated before the initiation of NIPPV. Abdominal distension is an uncommon problem, which can be lessened by switching to a PS ventilator or decreasing the tidal volume on a volume-targeted ventilator. A nasogastric tube can decrease the tolerance of a nasal mask, and also increase the risk of reflux. If NIPPV is to be used at night, nutritional support by means of a gastrostomy is preferable. Consideration should also be given to the performance of a fundoplication.

NIPPV is not always successful in adequately relieving hypoventilation. Air leaks have been shown to be an important cause of persistent hypercapnia in both invasively and non-invasively ventilated neuromuscular patients [37]. These observations in neuromuscular patients may also apply to patients with CF.

Side-effects caused by the interface and the delivery of a positive pressure are common in children receiving NIPPV. In our experience, skin injury, from transient erythema to

permanent skin necrosis, due to the nasal mask, has been observed in 53% of the 40 patients during their routine 6-month follow-up in our department [36]. These potential side-effects justify the systematic follow-up of children receiving NIPPV by a (pediatric) maxillofacial specialist.

Systematic humidification of the ventilator gas is not necessary for NIPPV because the upper airway, the physiological humidifier, is not bypassed. However, nasal intolerance due to excessive dryness can resolve after humidification of the ventilator gas.

CONCLUSIONS

There is a physiological rationale for NIPPV in cystic fibrosis. Clinical benefits have been demonstrated during acute exacerbations, nocturnal hypoventilation, exercise, and chest physiotherapy. Future studies should focus on determining the most pertinent criteria to propose NIPPV in these patients, and on evaluating whether there are long-term benefits in terms of survival, slowing the decline of lung function, and quality of life.

REFERENCES

1. Hart N, Polkey MI, Clément A et al. Changes in pulmonary mechanics with increasing disease severity in children and young adults with cystic fibrosis. Am J Respir Crit Care Med 2002; 166:61–66.

2. Mills GH, Kyroussis D, Hamnegard CH et al. Bilateral magnetic stimulation of the phrenic nerves from an anterolateral approach. Am J Respir Crit Care Med 1996; 154:1099–1105.

3. Hart N, Tounian P, Clement A et al. Nutritional status is an important predictor of diaphragm strength in young patients with cystic fibrosis. Am J Clin Nutr 2004; 80:1201–1206.

4. Pinet C, Cassart M, Scillia P et al. Function and bulk of respiratory and limb muscles in patients with cystic fibrosis. Am J Respir Crit Care Med 2003; 168:989–994.

5. Buysse DJ, Reynolds CI, Monk TII. The Pittsburgh sleep quality index: a new instrument for psychiatric practice and research. Psychiatr Res 1989; 28:193–213.

6. Amin R, Bean J, Burklow K, Jeffries J. The relationship between sleep disturbance and pulmonary function in stable pediatric cystic fibrosis patients. Chest 2005; 128:1357–1363.

7. Jankelowitz L, Reid KJ, Wolfe L et al. Cystic fibrosis patients have poor sleep quality despite normal sleep latency and efficiency. Chest 2005; 127:1593–1599.

8. Dancey DR, Tullis ED, Heslegrave R et al. Sleep quality and daytime function in adults with cystic fibrosis and severe lung disease. Eur Respir J 2002; 19:504–510.

9. Milross MA, Piper AJ, Norman M et al. Predicting sleep-disordered breathing in patients with cystic fibrosis. Chest 2001; 120:1239–1245.

10. Fragolias DD, Wilcox PG. Predictability of oxygen desaturation during sleep in patients with cystic fibrosis: clinical, spirometric and exercise parameters. *Chest* 2001; **119**:434–441.

11. Dobbin CJ, Bartlett D, Melehan K *et al.* The effect of infective exacerbations on sleep and neurobehavioral function in cystic fibrosis. *Am J Respir Crit Care Med* 2005; **172**:99–104.

12. Bradley S, Solin P, Wilson JW *et al.* Hypoxemia and hypercapnia during exercise and sleep in patients with cystic fibrosis. *Chest* 1999; **116**:647–654.

13. Fauroux B, Boulé M, Lofaso F *et al.* Chest physiotherapy in cystic fibrosis: improved tolerance with nasal pressure support ventilation. *Pediatrics* 1999; **103**:e32–e40.

14. Fauroux B, Nicot F, Essouri S *et al.* Setting of pressure support in young patients with cystic fibrosis. *Eur Resp J* 2004; **24**:624–630.

15. Fauroux B, Pigeot J, Isabey D *et al.* In-vivo physiological comparison of two ventilators used for domiciliary ventilation in children with cystic fibrosis. *Crit Care Med* 2001; **29**:2097–2105.

16. Serra A, Polese G, Braggion C, Rossi A. Noninvasive proportional assist and pressure support ventilation in patients with cystic fibrosis and chronic respiratory failure. *Thorax* 2002; **57**:50–54.

17. Regnis JA, Piper AJ, Henke KG *et al.* Benefits of nocturnal nasal CPAP in patients with cystic fibrosis. *Chest* 1994; **106**:1717–1724.

18. Gozal D. Nocturnal ventilatory support in patients with cystic fibrosis: comparison with supplemental oxygen. *Eur Resp J* 1997; **10**:1999–2003.

19. Milross MA, Piper AJ, Norman M *et al.* Low-flow oxygen and bilevel ventilatory support: effects on ventilation during sleep in cystic fibrosis. *Am J Respir Crit Care Med* 2001; **163**:129–134.

20. Piper AJ, Parker S, Torzillo PJ *et al.* Nocturnal nasal IPPV stabilizes patients with cystic fibrosis and hypercapnic respiratory failure. *Chest* 1992; **102**:846–850.

21. White D, Douglas N, Pickett C *et al.* Sleep deprivation and the control of ventilation. *Am Rev Respir Dis* 1983; **128**:984–986.

22. Holland AE, Denehy L, Ntoumenopoulos G *et al.* Noninvasive ventilation assists chest physiotherapy in adults with acute exacerbations of cystic fibrosis. *Thorax* 2003; **58**:880–884.

23. Henke KG, Regnis JA, Bye PTP. Benefits of continuous positive airway pressure during exercise in cystic fibrosis and relationship to disease severity. *Am Rev Resp Dis* 1993; **148**:1272–1276.

24. Caronia CG, Silver P, Nimkoff L *et al.* Use of bilevel positive airway pressure (BiPAP) in end-stage patients with cystic fibrosis awaiting lung transplantation. *Clin Pediatr* 1998; **37**:555–559.

25. Sood N, Paradowski LJ, Yankaskas JR. Outcomes of intensive care unit care in adults with cystic fibrosis. *Am J Respir Crit Care Med* 2001; **163**:335–338.

26. Ellafi M, Vinsonneau C, Coste J *et al.* One-year outcome after severe pulmonary exacerbation in adults with cystic fibrosis. *Am J Respir Crit Care Med* 2005; **171**:158–164.

27. Jeppesen J, Green A, Steffensen BF, Rahbek J. The Duchenne muscular dystrophy population in Denmark, 1977–2001: prevalence, incidence and survival in relation to the introduction of ventilator use. *Neuromuscular Dis* 2003; **13**:804–812.

28. Conference Report 1998. Management of pediatric patients requiring long-term ventilation. *Chest* 1998; **113**:322S–336S.

29. Conference Report 1999. Clinical indications for noninvasive positive pressure ventilation in chronic respiratory failure due to restrictive lung disease, COPD, and nocturnal hypoventilation. *Chest* 1999; **116**:521–534.

30. Fauroux B, Lofaso F. Noninvasive mechanical ventilation: when to start for what benefit ? *Thorax* 2005; **60**:979–980.

31. Sullivan CE, Issa FG, Berthon-Jones M, Eves L. Reversal of obstructive sleep apnea by continuous positive airway pressure applied through the nares. *Lancet* 1981; **1**:862–865.

32. Bellon G, Mounier M, Guidicelli J *et al.* Nasal intermittent positive ventilation in cystic fibrosis. *Eur Resp J* 1992; **2**:357–359.

33. Hodson ME, Madden BP, Steven MH *et al.* Noninvasive mechanical ventilation for cystic fibrosis patients: a potential bridge to transplantation. *Eur Resp J* 1991; **4**:524–527.

34. Lofaso F, Brochard L, Hang T *et al.* Home versus intensive care pressure support devices: experimental and clinical comparison. *Am J Respir Crit Care Med* 1996; **153**:1591–1599.

35. Padman R, Nadkarni VM, Von Nessen S, Goodill J. Noninvasive positive pressure ventilation in end-stage cystic fibrosis: a report of seven cases. *Respir Care* 1994; **39**:736–739.

36. Fauroux B, Lavis JF, Nicot F *et al.* Facial side-effects during noninvasive positive pressure ventilation in children. *Intens Care Med* 2005; **31**:965–969.

37. Gonzalez J, Sharshar T, Hart N *et al.* Air leaks during mechanical ventilation as a cause of persistent hypercapnia in neuromuscular disorders. *Intens Care Med* 2003; **29**:596–602.

13

Delivery of therapy to the cystic fibrosis lung

HARM A. W. M. TIDDENS AND SUNALENE G. DEVADASON

INTRODUCTION

In cystic fibrosis (CF), delivery of therapy directly to the lung encompasses many functions. Drugs are delivered to improve the qualities of the epithelial lining fluid, reduce the thickness of the sputum and treat infection or inflammation. In addition, oxygen can be administered to compensate for loss of lung tissue resulting in a reduced diffusion capacity of the lung. It is a technical challenge that aerosol therapy to the lung is required at all ages from infancy to adulthood and for the full range of early to end-stage disease. All these variables must be taken into account when considering therapeutic delivery options in cystic fibrosis. In this chapter the various therapeutic modalities will be addressed.

AEROSOL THERAPY

Aerosol therapy is an essential part of the treatment of CF lung disease. More than 75% of CF patients aged over 19 years are treated with some form of aerosol therapy [1]. Most have to inhale multiple drugs in various combinations, mainly delivered via nebulizer, on a daily basis. The value of nebulized drugs such as rhDNase or tobramycin for inhalation has been well established [2,3]. Although commonly prescribed to CF patients, the therapeutic value of other inhaled drugs, such as colistin, corticosteroids and bronchodilators, have not been fully investigated [4,5]. Furthermore, relatively little is known of the optimal method of aerosol delivery to the heavily obstructed regions of the CF-affected lung, which are more likely to require therapy. Aerosols are more likely to deposit in the better ventilated, healthier regions of the lung, where such treatment is needed less. A major disadvantage of currently used nebulizer therapy is that it is time-consuming, relatively inefficient, has a high risk of patient error, and infection control procedures are more difficult, resulting in contamination of nebulizers [6–8]. Fortunately, new delivery methods are in development. The choice of aerosol delivery device should consider the patient's requirements (ability to use the device, time constraints and severity of disease), the type of drug formulation (solution or suspension; stability issues), as well as the optimal site of action in the lung (peripheral or central). The burden of therapy to the patient should be minimized as far as possible.

Drugs that are available in quick and convenient delivery devices such as dry-powder inhalers (DPIs) or pressurized metered-dose inhalers (pMDIs) should be prescribed where possible. For patients with advanced lung disease, for young children, and for inhalation of drugs that are available only as fluids, a nebulizer system can be selected. Each drug available in nebulizer formulation should be used with the recommended delivery system as cited in the clinical data submitted to regulatory authorities. Alternative delivery methods should be used only after seeking regulatory approval based on sufficient laboratory and clinical data. Hence, the drug should be prescribed *with* an appropriate delivery device (as is the case for DPIs and pMDIs).

THE AEROSOL

An aerosol consists of fluid or solid particles distributed throughout a gas. The size of aerosol particles can vary between 0.01 and 100 μm and can be measured dynamically using cascade-impactors or laser diffraction techniques. An aerosol cloud measured with a cascade-impactor is characterized by the mass median aerodynamic diameter (MMAD). Half of the drug mass is present in particles smaller than the MMAD. The geometric standard deviation (GSD) is a measure of the size distribution of the aerosol particles. Aerosol particles between 2 and 5 μm are thought to have a high probability of deposition in bronchi and, therefore, are often referred to as respirable particles (Fig. 13.1). Larger particles have a higher probability of deposition in the upper airways. Very small particles have a higher probability

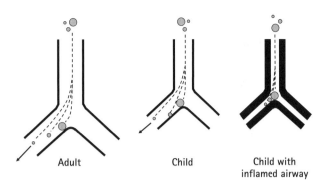

Figure 13.1 This figure explains the principle of deposition of aerosol particles in the lung. In the airways of an adult, particles with an aerodynamic diameter below 5 μm have a high probability of bypassing the upper airways and being deposited in the central and more peripheral airways. In this example, particles of 5, 3 and 1 μm are inhaled. The largest particle has the highest probability of being deposited against the airway wall due to inertial impaction. The small particle has the highest change of being deposited in more peripheral airways where the velocity of the airflow is low. In case of high inspiratory flows and/or secretions in the airway, a more turbulent flow pattern will result in increased central airway particle deposition. In children, the distance from the center of the airway to the airway wall is smaller and air velocity is higher. Therefore, even mid-sized particles have a high probability of being deposited against the airway wall. In a child with diseased airways due to airway wall thickening and mucus, even the smaller particles have a higher chance of being deposited in the central airways. Reproduced with permission from [9].

of entering the smaller airways and alveoli but may be exhaled, rather than sedimenting within the airways. It is important to realize that this 2–5 μm range is mostly derived from studies with healthy adult subjects. In case of severe airway obstruction in CF the deposition pattern is inhomogeneous, which favors deposition in the central airways [9]. The respirable fraction of an aerosol for a child with CF and severe lung pathology is largely unknown but is likely to be in the smaller particle range [10–13]. These particles are, therefore, important for the treatment of airway disease in CF since the major pathology is localized in the peripheral airways [14,15]. This is supported by a clinical study where treatment with rhDNase delivered as an aerosol with a MMAD of 2.1 μm was more effective than treatment with an aerosol with a MMAD of 4.9 μm [16]. The importance of particle size is likely to be highly relevant for all aerosol treatments including eradication therapy of *Pseudomonas* in young children.

DELIVERY SYSTEMS

Current delivery methods for medical aerosol can be classified into three different categories: nebulizer systems,

pressurized metered-dose inhaler (pMDI) systems and dry-powder inhalers (DPIs). It is important to keep in mind that most of these devices were primarily designed for use in adults and subsequently adapted for use in children. Relatively few data are available on the use of these devices in children. The advantages and disadvantages of the different devices are summarized in Table 13.1.

THE NEBULIZER

Principles

A nebulizer is a device that converts a liquid into aerosol droplets. There are three categories: jet, ultrasonic and the more recently developed mesh type. Traditionally, the jet nebulizer is the most important aerosol delivery system for therapy in CF patients. Nebulizers can be loaded with any liquid drug formulation. Hence, they are considered 'open' devices. The aerosol characteristics of a given nebulizer–compressor combination should be tested according to well-standardized procedures [17]. In the last decade it has been recognized by regulatory agencies that the output characteristics of any nebulizer–drug combination are unique and are important determinants of efficacy and toxicity. For this reason, specific nebulizer systems have been recommended for more recently developed drugs such as rhDNase and tobramycin for inhalation as part of the regulatory approval process. Hence, these drugs should be prescribed with these specific nebulizers. More modern nebulizer systems or disposable systems should be used only when these are included within the registration label [18]. This requires proper bioequivalence and/or clinical efficacy studies by the manufacturer of the drug. The effectiveness and risks of alternative nebulizer–drug combinations are difficult to predict and these should, therefore, be discouraged. Newer liquid drugs that are currently in development are often tested using more modern nebulizer systems.

The patient inhales the aerosol from the reservoir through a mouthpiece or face-mask. Young children usually use a face-mask since they are not able to breath through their mouth on demand. Optimal seal between face and face-mask is important to maximize efficiency [19]. A child old enough to inhale through a mouthpiece should do so since the efficiency of aerosol delivery can be twice as high relative to inhalation by face-mask [20]. The mouthpiece should be positioned in the center of the mouth between the teeth. The technique of inhalation should be regularly examined since many mistakes can be made. Some patients chew on their mouthpiece while inhaling (Fig. 13.2); others put their tongue in front of the opening, have the mouthpiece positioned eccentrically, or breath around the mouthpiece rather than through it. Clearly, poor inhalation technique results not only in adverse health outcome but also in a waste of scarce clinical resources and patient time.

Table 13.1   Aerosol delivery devices and CF.

Device	Advantages	Disadvantages
Jet nebulizer	All ages Tidal breathing Delivery of high doses over prolonged period Face-mask can be used Only for liquid drugs	Cumbersome Noisy Time-consuming Easily contaminated Poor reproducibility of dose and particle size Maintenance required Large inter-device variability
Breath-actuated nebulizer	Age at least 4 years Tidal breathing Improved dose reproducibility Improved particle size characteristics Only for liquid drugs	Time-consuming Easily contaminated Large size Maintenance required Large inter-device variability Cannot be used with face-mask Limited clinical data
Mesh nebulizer	Age at least 4 years Silent Small size Tidal breathing Improved dose reproducibility Improved efficiency Only for liquid drugs	Easily contaminated Maintenance required Cannot be used with face-mask Very limited clinical data
Pressurized metered-dose inhaler (pMDI)	Small, handy Quick Low dose-to-dose variability	Complicated hand–mouth coordination High oropharyngeal deposition Not suitable for children
Breath-actuated pMDI	Age at least 8 years Small, handy Quick Hand–mouth coordination not required Low inspiratory flow rate required Aerosol characteristics effort independent	High oropharyngeal deposition Deep inspiration required Only for bronchodilators and inhaled steroids
pMDI-spacer	All ages Tidal breathing possible Face-mask can be used Quick Reduction of oropharyngeal deposition Fewer local side-effects	Electrostatic charge of plastic spacers Large size Administration in ages 1–3 years is troublesome in 50% Many mistakes can be made
Dry-powder inhaler (DPI)	Age at least 6 years (for minimal inspiratory flow requirement of ≥30 L/min) Small, handy Quick Hand–mouth coordination not required Propellant free Microbiologically safe	Effort-dependent efficiency and particle size distribution Inspiratory flow critical Not suitable below 6–7 years High oropharyngeal deposition Currently only for bronchodilators and inhaled steroids Dry-powder inhaler for antibiotics in development

The breathing pattern required for inhalation from most nebulizers is tidal breathing. Aerosol produced during exhalation will be wasted (Fig. 13.3).

A more recent development are the adaptive aerosol delivery (AAD) devices. Aerosol delivery is triggered by the inspiratory flow of the patient and aerosol is produced only during a fixed fraction of the inspiration. Such a system clearly improves the efficiency of aerosol delivery. Some modern systems are, in addition, equipped with data logging options. With this logging system the time and duration of the aerosol treatment can be monitored. With other modern devices such as the AKITA Inhalation System®, nebulization can be restricted to any specific fraction of the inspiration. In addition, the inspiratory flow velocity with which the patient can inhale the aerosol is controlled for. With this device the volume and velocity for each inhalation can be preset to deliver maximum drug to the targeted airway site (central or peripheral) over a shorter time period. However, programmable inhalation devices such as these are more costly than conventional nebulizers, and tend to be used for more expensive medications (such as α_1-antitrypsin) or where the drug dose needs to be tightly controlled to minimize adverse effects (such as the delivery of insulin via inhalation).

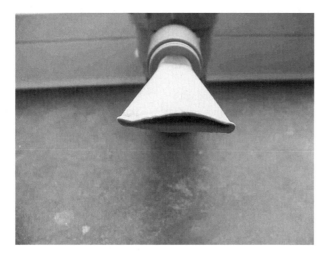

Figure 13.2   At the annual check-up the compressor–nebulizer combination used by a 14-year-old CF patient was inspected. It became clear that the patient was chewing on the mouthpiece while inhaling RhDNase and tobramycin for inhalation. This habit clearly reduced the efficacy of aerosol therapy substantially. Hence, time, health and resources were wasted and this could have been avoided by more frequent visual inspection of the technique and device used by the patient.

The jet nebulizer

FLOW AND PARTICLE SIZE

The traditional jet nebulizer consists of a compressor that is connected to the nebulizer by tubing. The compressor pushes ambient air at an increased pressure through the nebulizer bowl, which contains the drug formulation as a solution or suspension. Powerful compressors are able to generate a higher driving gas flow through the nebulizer which increases the rate of drug delivery, and reduces nebulization time. However, the maximal flow that a compressor can generate through a nebulizer is determined by the resistance of the nebulizer itself.

Jet nebulizers consist of a Venturi device where the flow of compressed air generates an area of low pressure within the nebulizer bowl. Droplets of liquid are drawn from the drug reservoir into the low-pressure region, forming droplets, or primary aerosol particles. The nebulizer baffle further disintegrates these droplets into smaller, secondary aerosol particles. Most of the primary and secondary aerosol particles fall back in the medication cup and will be re-nebulized. The particle size generated by a given nebulizer depends highly on the baffle design. During the nebulization process water evaporation can occur within the drug liquid reservoir. This process cools down the remaining fluid and can increase its osmolality [21,22]. Cold fluids with a high osmolality can induce bronchial obstruction due to bronchial smooth muscle contraction.

The design of the Venturi and the air flow through the system are important determinants of aerosol characteristics. In general, a high flow results in a low MMAD and a higher aerosol output of respirable particles [23]. The contrary is also true. A poorly functioning compressor, or low flow through the nebulizer, will result in a higher MMAD and lower output of respirable particles.

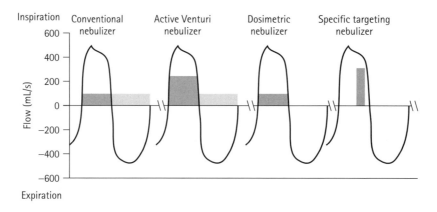

Figure 13.3   The effect of nebulization in relation to breathing pattern for four types of nebulizer system. Dark grey, aerosol delivered to the patient during inspiration; light grey, aerosol wasted during expiration. For conventional nebulizer systems, nebulization is continuous and independent of the breathing pattern. Aerosol produced during exhalation is lost. For active Venturi nebulizers, extra air entrains during inhalation which increases the amount of aerosol delivered to the patient during inhalation. For dosimetric nebulizers, aerosol is produced during a fraction of the inhalation time; no aerosol is produced during exhalation. For specific targeting nebulizers, aerosol is delivered only during a fraction of the inspiration and the inspiratory flow is controlled.

ENHANCEMENT AND VALVES

Approximately half the aerosolized drug generated by conventional nebulizers is wasted (see Fig. 13.3). This is because the rate of aerosol generation remains constant during both inspiratory and expiratory phases of the patient's tidal breathing pattern. Breath-enhanced nebulizers were developed to take advantage of the fact that, for most patients apart from infants and very young children, the tidal inspiratory flows are higher than the driving gas flow generated by portable compressors. This excess flow would normally be drawn from the surrounding ambient air [24]. However, using a system of one-way valves, the patient's inspiratory flow can be drawn through the nebulizer bowl, increasing aerosol delivery while the patient is inhaling. The inspiratory valve closes during exhalation, stopping expired air from entering the nebulizer bowl. An expiratory valve placed in the nebulizer mouthpiece enables the exhaled air to be vented directly from the mouthpiece to the environment, without passing back through the nebulizer. While drug wastage still occurs when using breath-enhanced nebulizers, due to the constant driving gas flow from the compressor, the proportion of drug inhaled by the patient is far greater than that wasted during exhalation. The higher the patient's tidal inspiratory flow, the greater the benefit of using the breath-enhanced system. Examples of such breath-enhanced nebulizers are the Pari LC Plus®, Pari LC Star®, Sidestream® and Ventstream®. The latter has valves to prevent exhaled air from passing through the nebulizer bowl.

REPEATED USE

In general, for daily maintenance therapy, a better quality, non-disposable nebulizer should be used. Long-life nebulizers need regular cleaning, undergo wear and tear and should be replaced at predetermined intervals that will vary between 3 months and 1 year. Due to the nebulization process the medication channels can increase slightly in diameter, which results in a slightly higher MMAD [6]. If the medication channels get partially obstructed, less drug will be nebulized and nebulization time will increase. It is not advisable to attempt to open up these channels with a sharp object. Even small scratches can have a major impact on aerosol output, MMAD and GSD. For some long-life nebulizers disposable equivalents are available. Clearly a 'disposable' nebulizer is designed for use only during a short period. In laboratory conditions it has been shown that some disposable nebulizers can resist repetitive cleaning quite well [18], but microbiological contamination was not evaluated. In addition, cleaning procedures for such disposable nebulizers are often not well defined. Hence it is not advisable to use a disposable nebulizer for maintenance therapy over longer periods of time.

The ultrasonic nebulizer

Ultrasonic (US) nebulizers use a piezoelectric crystal to generate vibrations in the medication fluid. On the air–liquid interface fountains of droplets are generated. As for jet nebulizers, large droplets drop back into the fluid. The smaller droplets can be inhaled by the patient inhaling air from the reservoir. Some US nebulizers have a small ventilator that can move the generated aerosol into the mouthpiece. An advantage of US nebulizers is that they are silent and can be small. In addition, depending on the energy released by the vibrating crystal, they can have a high aerosol output. A disadvantage is that they cannot nebulize suspensions or solutions of high viscosity very effectively. This can have the effect that the emitted particles contain relatively more water than drug, thus concentrating the liquid remaining in the nebulizer bowl. In addition, the vibrating crystal can heat up the liquid drug formulation, which can affect drug stability or function. Finally, the vibrations may effect the integrity of large molecules such as proteins, and so ultrasonic nebulizers cannot be used for drugs such as rhDNase. Currently, there are no drugs on the market for CF that should be nebulized by this system.

The vibrating mesh nebulizer

Recently vibrating mesh nebulizers have been launched on the market [25]. A key element of this technology is a membrane that contains a large number of holes in a mesh (Fig. 13.4a). This mesh is in contact with an annular piezo-element that is able to make the mesh vibrate at a very high frequency (Fig. 13.4b). As a result fluid is sucked up from the medication reservoir containing the liquid drug. On the side of the aerosol reservoir, aerosol particles are released by the mesh. The size of the particles is determined by the size and form of the holes in the mesh. The patient inhales the aerosol from the aerosol reservoir.

The mesh nebulizer has a number of important theoretical advantages over jet nebulizers. First, in contrast to jet nebulizers, the emitted aerosol particles have a low velocity, so only a small proportion of the aerosol particles should impact onto the walls of the aerosol reservoir. The aerosol leaves the reservoir as a standing cloud by inhalation of the patient. Hence, during exhalation time less aerosol is lost to the environment. Second, drug passes the mesh only once. Third, mesh nebulizers are silent. Fourth, the systems are substantially smaller compared to jet nebulizers. Cumbersome and noisy portable compressors are not required; only a small battery pack or AC adapter is required to generate the energy needed for aerosol production. Fifth, the volume of drug left in the medication chamber after the nebulization process is completed (dead volume) is substantially lower than with conventional nebulizers (0.1–0.3 mL). As a result, mesh nebulizer systems are more efficient than continuously operating jet nebulizers which have dead volumes up to 1.5 mL. Hence, the use of a mesh nebulizer should result in greater efficiency of drug use; a lower nominal or starting dose is required to obtain the same lung deposition.

Theoretically, most liquid drugs can be nebulized using this technology. With drug suspensions or highly viscous

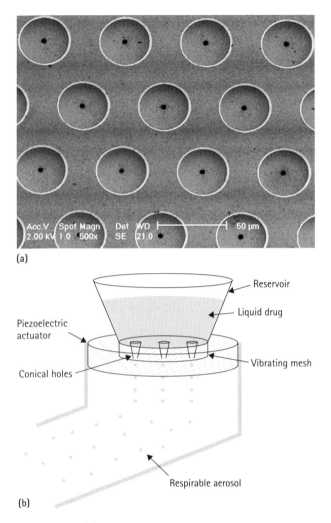

(a)

(b)

Figure 13.4 (a) A 500 × enlarged view of a mesh from a vibrating-mesh nebulizer. A key element of this technology is a membrane that contains a large number of holes. The size of the aerosol particles is determined by the size and form of the holes in the mesh. (b) Schematic view of a vibrating-mesh nebulizer. This mesh is in contact with an annular piezo-element that is able to make the mesh vibrate at a very high frequency. As a result, fluid is sucked up from the medication reservoir containing the liquid drug. On the side of the aerosol reservoir, aerosol particles are released by the mesh.

solutions there is a risk of occlusion of the holes. This will primarily increase the time needed by the patient to nebulize all drug from the medication reservoir. The aerosol output of mesh nebulizers ranges from 0.15 to 0.35 mL/min. Occlusion of the holes is thought not to affect particle size distribution but only the output rate.

Selection of nebulizer

Examples of nebulized drugs are tobramycin, rhDNase, acetylcysteine, colomycin and NaCl. Drugs such as rhDNase or tobramycin are registered to be delivered by a specific nebulizer–compressor combination. Hence, the drug comes with the aerosol delivery device. Alternative nebulizer–compressor systems or mesh nebulizers should be used only when

bio-equivalence and preferable clinical equivalence has been established. Nevertheless, for most drugs it is not possible to predict equivalence based on laboratory studies since such studies do not take patient-related factors into account. Examples of such factors are compliance, correct preparation of the device before each treatment, particle size characteristics in relation to breathing pattern, and dead volume. The use of alternative compressor–nebulizer systems requires that the prescribing physician is responsible for ensuring clinical equivalence in terms of both efficacy and side-effects. This can be difficult since one does not know the natural course of disease of that patient without the alternative intervention.

Mixing of drugs for nebulization is in general not recommended since interaction between drugs might occur and the aerosol characteristics may alter due to a change in the physicochemical properties of the mixture. Bronchodilators and inhaled steroids can be delivered more quickly and efficiently by pMDI-spacer, pMDI-autohaler or DPI.

Nebulizer maintenance

Adequate maintenance of the nebulizer–compressor is crucial. First, the nebulizer should be cleaned and dried after each use to prevent contamination. In case of inadequate cleaning there is a risk of bacterial contamination especially with *Pseudomonas* [26–28].

All nebulizer systems degenerate with time and regular use. In jet nebulizers the air filter on the compressor becomes polluted with dust particles, so it should be replaced at specified time intervals. Most long-life nebulizers need replacement once or twice a year. The compressor output of a jet nebulizer should be periodically tested according to manufacturer specifications. When pressure output is reduced nebulization time increases, and more importantly MMAD and GSD will increase, reducing the efficacy of the nebulized drug. As for jet nebulizers, mesh nebulizers require specific maintenance. The mesh should be replaced at regular intervals since the holes suffer from wear and tear and can get occluded, reducing aerosol output.

The importance of a comprehensive quality control program for aerosol therapy in CF cannot be sufficiently emphasized. The use of improperly functioning nebulizer–compressor systems results in a reduced treatment efficacy and wasted resources. Quality control of the compressor–nebulizer combination is therefore an obligatory part of nebulizer therapy in CF. A close visual examination of nebulizer and compressor and evaluation of the technique used by the patient to operate the device allows detection of issues that can affect the quality of aerosol therapy.

THE PRESSURIZED METERED-DOSE INHALER

In a pMDI, the drug is present as a solution or suspension in a propellant and/or surfactant mixture. In the case of a suspension formulation, the pMDI should be shaken vigorously before use to mix the drug as homogeneously as possible in the propellant carrier. When the pMDI is fired, an accurately metered dose is released at a high velocity. The mass of drug and its aerosol characteristics are largely independent on the inspiratory effort of the patient. This is of benefit for CF patients since a forced inspiratory maneuver is likely to be difficult for those with reduced pulmonary function due to exacerbations or lung infections. pMDIs are used primarily for treatment with bronchodilators and inhaled steroids.

The use of a spacer with a pMDI markedly improves the efficiency of aerosol delivery, by reducing unwanted oropharyngeal deposition and eliminating the need for coordinating the patient's inhalation with actuation of the pMDI. For children below the age of 4 years, a face-mask should be used. Great care should be taken to obtain an optimal seal between the child's face and the mask because a suboptimal seal will result in a substantial reduction of the aerosol output from the spacer [19,29]. A metal spacer is preferable to a plastic one as it avoids variation in drug delivery due to electrostatic charge on the wall of the spacer [11,30,31]. Washing a plastic spacer once a week in household detergent can reduce electrostatic charge effectively.

Another form of pMDI is the breath-actuated device (such as the Autohaler®), which is also ideal for most CF patients of 8 years and older. In these devices, aerosol emission is also propellant-driven. Hence, the particle size distribution of released aerosol particles is independent of the patient's effort. To prime the device, the patient has to load a spring by elevating a lever. Next, the patient exhales and then inhales through the device, with a slow and deep inspiratory maneuver. When the inspiratory flow reaches a minimum of 30 L/min, a valve opens, releasing the metered drug dose. The patient has to be trained to continue the inhalation up to total lung capacity level. Some patients are startled by the sudden sound or sensation as the drug is released, and may stop breathing without completing the inspiratory maneuver, resulting in increased drug impaction in the oropharynx, and little or no drug deposition in the lungs.

THE DRY-POWDER INHALER

In a dry-powder inhaler the drug is present in a single unit (e.g. Accuhaler®) or in a multi-dose chamber (e.g. Turbuhaler®). The drug can be present in a pure form or dispersed with lactose or other carrier substance. The mass of drug inhaled, and the MMAD and GSD of the resulting particles, depend on the inspiratory flow of the patient. For optimal DPI performance a CF patient should be able to inhale forcefully and deeply without coughing. In case of insufficient inspiratory flow through the DPI (<60 L/min for most inhaled steroids) the mass of drug that is released is reduced and the MMAD and GSD increased.

Sufficiently high and reproducible inspiratory flows through a DPI can be obtained in asthmatic children of 7 years and older but there are relatively few data for CF patients. Clearly many children and adults with CF have considerable structural lung damage that can affect their inspired volume and flow velocity [32]. In a controlled laboratory setting it was shown that 3 to 5-year-old CF patients could only inhale a lung dose of 6% from the Turbuhaler. Lung dose increased to 29% in the 13–16 years age range [33]. In a more recent study it was shown that from the age of 6 years most patients were able to generate an inspiratory flow of 30 L/min or higher and to inhale a volume of 1 L or more [34]. However, for patients who are not able to generate an inspired flow of 30 L/min or higher a DPI should not be used.

Routine lung function does not produce any reliable predictors for an inspiratory flow through a DPI. Ideally, peak inspiratory flow should be tested through a resistance that equals the resistance of the DPI that will be used by the patient. For high-resistance DPI devices testing of inspiratory flow should be considered for those below the age of 8 years or in patients with severe impairment of lung function [34]. Ideally, the inspiratory flow–volume curve through the appropriate resistor should be recorded to supply other relevant parameters such as the inhaled volume and time to peak inspiratory flow. In case of an insufficient inspired volume a second inhalation will be needed to mobilize all available drug from the capsule. When doing this the patient should not exhale through the DPI since humidity might affect the remaining drug.

Because the inspiratory flow profile for DPIs is rather critical it is recommended that a pMDI-spacer or breath-actuated pMDI should be used for the delivery of steroids or bronchodilators to CF-patients (see Table 13.1). Clearly, when antibiotics are prescribed to patients in DPI form, repetitive instructions and training should be given to the patient, and regular monitoring of his/her inhalation technique is advisable.

DRUGS INHALED FOR CYSTIC FIBROSIS

Antibiotics

Chronic bacterial infection of the lower airways is present in most CF patients early in life. It has become increasingly evident that early and aggressive antibiotic treatment reduces lung damage and improves life expectancy.

When antibiotics are nebulized, a filter on the expiration port is needed to prevent contamination of the environment by the exhaled antibiotic.

Intermittent maintenance therapy with inhaled tobramycin for patients with chronic *Pseudomonas* infection has been shown to be an efficacious strategy to improve lung function, reduce exacerbation rate, and improve quality of life [35–37]. Furthermore, nebulized tobramycin has been used for eradication of newly acquired *Pseudomonas* infection [38,39]. In most countries, tobramycin for nebulization is a registered antibiotic for nebulization. It should be nebulized using a Pari LC Plus nebulizer combined with a Pulmo-Aid or comparable compressor.

Colomycin is another nebulized antibiotic that is frequently prescribed for maintenance therapy against

Pseudomonas. The effectiveness of long-term maintenance therapy with Colomycin in relation to a specific aerosol delivery system has been less well documented [40,41]. Because of the lack of proper studies, Colomycin is not registered for nebulization in CF in many countries. Technically, Colomycin can be nebulized using a Pari LC® star or Hudson Updraft II® [42].

Other antibiotics for inhaled therapy are in development. Each of these has to be delivered with the system as specified in the registration studies. A wider choice of inhaled antibiotics will allow a more tailored treatment.

rhDNase

DNA levels in CF sputum are 3–5 times higher than in non-CF individuals and tend to be even higher in older CF patients. Recombinant human dornase (rhDNase) improves mucociliary clearance by hydrolyzing extracellular DNA present in elevated levels in lower airway secretions [43]. Large multicenter placebo-controlled trials have shown that maintenance treatment with nebulized rhDNase delivered by Portaneb compressor and Sidestream nebulizer improves lung function, and reduces the exacerbation rate in CF patients [2,44]. rhDNase should be delivered to the patient with a jet nebulizer as used in these studies. There are indications that administration of rhDNase by a compressor–nebulizer combination that delivers a high output rate and low MMAD is most effective [16]. However, this should be further investigated in well-designed clinical efficacy studies of sufficient size. rhDNase must not be mixed with other drugs for simultaneous nebulization.

In clinical use, rhDNase is commonly administered either before or after physiotherapy [1]. However, there are indications that nebulization of rhDNase should be done at a moment when the lungs are as clear as possible. For most patients this is towards the end of the day. Next, nebulization of rhDNase should be followed by physiotherapy within 30 minutes to maximally 4 hours to expectorate the liquefied sputum [45]. The optimal use of rhDNase with physiotherapy should be discussed with each individual patient, as the patient's preference is also important.

Bronchoscopic installation of rhDNase has been advocated for the treatment of lobar atelectasis that persists after intravenous antibiotics and physiotherapy [46,47]. Persistent atelectasis is associated with a poorer prognosis, so every attempt should be made to reverse the atelectasis. Direct installation of 2.5 mg rhDNase in 10 mL of normal saline has been effectively used to mobilize large quantities of mucopurulent secretions from the obstructed bronchus and to open up the atelectatic lobe.

Bronchodilators

Many older CF patients are treated with bronchodilators [1]. Some studies have shown that the lung function of CF patients improves after bronchodilator inhalation [48]. Furthermore, it has been suggested that the daily use of salbutamol reduces the number of exacerbations and the decline in lung function [49]; however the scope of this study is somewhat limited.

One should keep in mind that bronchodilators may have negative effects. In some patients, lung function worsens after inhalation of a bronchodilator [50,51]. This might be caused by a reduced stability of the central airways during a forced expiration [52]. Furthermore, the use of β_2-sympathomimetics increases the patient's metabolic rate. Based on the limited data on the effectiveness of bronchodilators on relevant end-points, it seems wise to restrict their use [53]. Bronchodilators can be used for those patients who show substantial reversibility of airflow obstruction after inhalation of bronchodilators and who report relief of symptoms after inhalation. In addition, bronchodilators should be used prior to the inhalation of drugs that may cause bronchial obstruction. This kind of obstruction can be the result of bronchial smooth muscle shortening but also of inflammatory changes to the airway wall.

For CF patients who need bronchodilators it makes sense to prescribe long-acting β_2-sympathomimetics [54]. The delivery device of first choice is a pMDI-spacer or a breath-actuated pMDI for reasons discussed earlier.

Corticosteroids

It has been shown by many authors that there is an exaggerated immune response in CF. This is probably the rationale for the massive use of inhaled steroids in CF patients [1]. Furthermore, inhaled corticosteroids are prescribed for patients who suffer from asthma-like symptoms or for the treatment of allergic bronchopulmonary aspergillosis. Unfortunately, as is the case for bronchodilator use, there are very limited data to support the current widespread use of inhaled corticosteroids [55]. Conclusive long-term studies on the dose–effect of inhaled corticosteroids at relevant end-points are lacking. Recently it has been shown that prescribed corticosteroid maintenance therapy could be withdrawn from most CF patients without significant changes in lung function or exacerbation rate [5].

When inhaled corticosteroids are indicated they can best be delivered by pMDI-spacer or with a breath-actuated pMDI. The minimum inspiratory flow recommended for DPI use in order to obtain a clinically effective dose is 60 L/min for most inhaled steroids. Flow dependency in deposition pattern between 30 and 90 L/min has been observed in pediatric CF patients using the Turbuhaler® [33], and with in-vitro drug delivery for both the Turbuhaler® and Accuhaler® [56].

Many CF-patients are not able to generate inspiratory flows of 60 L/min or higher [34]. Suboptimal flows can not only reduce the output of drug from the DPI but also increase particle size [56]. This is not desirable since larger particles are less likely to reach the peripheral airways where most pathology is localized in CF. When inhaled corticosteroids are prescribed they should be inhaled after physiotherapy to limit impaction in congested central airways and avoid immediate clearance from the lungs during physiotherapy. After inhalation, the patient should rinse the mouth to reduce the risk of *Candida* infection. Treatment with inhaled corticosteroids in CF should be restricted to patients with asthma-like symptoms.

Mucolytics

The effectiveness of specific delivery systems for administration of mucolytics other than rhDNase to CF patients has not been investigated in sufficiently large trials with relevant end-points [57]. In some countries mucolytics are still used on a large scale. The evidence supporting the use of mucolytics is thin [57]. Most sulfur-containing mucolytics should not be mixed with other drugs during nebulization. The optimal delivery system for mucolytics has not been defined.

Sodium chloride (NaCl)

Twice daily nebulization of 4 mL of hypertonic (7%) NaCl improves sputum expectoration, improves lung function, and reduces the number of exacerbations in CF patients [58–61]. The nebulizer system used in a large, double-blind, placebo-controlled clinical trial evaluating the use of hypertonic saline over a 12-month period was the Pari LC Plus® jet nebulizer and Pari Proneb® compressor [60]. Inhalation of hypertonic saline is known to induce bronchoconstriction in many patients. In the hypertonic saline trial mentioned above, 200 μg of albuterol was administered to patients via pMDI-spacer for bronchodilation prior to hypertonic saline inhalation. Importantly, all patients continued their routine medication regimen during this trial. Hence, the observed positive effect in the hypertonic saline treatment group was additional to the effect of normal rhDNase therapy. Fewer than 20% of patients in this study were using nebulized antibiotics.

Clearly, adding extra nebulization treatments to the daily treatment burden of CF patients would be unacceptable. Most CF patients would be required to undergo a minimum of two nebulization sessions twice daily, in addition to regular physiotherapy. An additional disadvantage is that, in most countries, 7% saline is not available in sterile ampoule form. In some countries 7% NaCl is obtained by mixing 10% NaCl from commercially available ampoules with sterile water. This clearly makes this therapy more inconvenient and increases the risk of contamination. The alternative is to use a lower strength NaCl preparation, which may be more readily available, although the efficacy of this option has not been tested.

Managing the aerosol package

It is clear that choices between therapies prescribed to CF patients have to be made. Unfortunately, there are few comparative data evaluating the efficacy of different combinations of drug therapy. An alternative is to mix two or more drugs for delivery during a single nebulization. However, the drug combinations would have to be stringently tested to rule out possible drug interactions, or that the activity or efficacy of individual drugs decreases. For example, rhDNase, being a protein, is highly likely to be denatured or deactivated by the addition of hypertonic saline for concurrent nebulization.

The more complicated aerosol therapy is for a CF patient the more likely it is that mistakes will be made and that adherence to the therapy will decrease. The aerosol therapy package prescribed for a CF patient should be critically evaluated on a yearly basis, if not more frequently. The number of drugs prescribed should be reduced to the absolute minimum. Many aerosolized drugs that are used in maintenance therapy for CF patients are not evidence-based and so can be deleted in the case of an overloaded therapeutic package for the patient [4].

The use of nebulizer–compressor systems for CF is cumbersome. The use of these systems should be restricted to drugs with proven efficacy and which are available only as nebulizer formulations. Regular maintenance of nebulizer–compressor systems and critical evaluation of the technical skills of the patients is crucial to optimize clinical efficacy, reduce adverse effects, and avoid wastage of both patient time and clinical resources. For each daily drug administration, the timing in relation to physiotherapy sessions should be discussed with the patient. This can prevent the suboptimal administration of inhaled medications such as antibiotics or steroids prior to physiotherapy [1].

ORAL AND INTRAVENOUS THERAPY

Many drugs can be administered to the lungs through the gastrointestinal route as an alternative for the inhaled route. A theoretical advantage is that the drug can target poorly ventilated but well-perfused areas of the lung. A second advantage of this route is its simplicity. Third, swallowing a pill or a liquid takes much less time than nebulization.

However, the oral route comes with some disadvantages. The most important disadvantage is adverse gastrointestinal effects. Second, drug absorption in CF patients can vary widely and the rate of absorption is often slower. Third, many oral drugs require exact timing before or after meals, increasing the complexity of CF therapy; it is likely that many mistakes are made in relation to adequate timing of oral drugs. Fourth, oral dosing involves systemic exposure to higher levels of the drug in question, rather than the relatively lower doses administered to the lungs via inhalation. Hence, oral dosing markedly increases the risk of adverse side-effects. Fifth, the unpleasant taste of many liquid drug formulations makes administration difficult, particularly to young children.

In this section we will discuss some specific issues related to orally administered antibiotics, and anti-inflammatory drugs, as well as the role of intravenous therapy in CF.

Bronchodilators will not be discussed, since it is evident from the multitude of studies carried out in asthmatic patients that the inhaled route of administration is superior to the oral route.

Antibiotics

For many antibiotics, the maximum dose that can be administered orally is much lower than can be administered intravenously, due to local oropharyngeal and gastrointestinal side-effects. High oral doses of antibiotics are often required to obtain sufficiently high therapeutic levels in CF sputum. This is particularly the case for drugs such as sulfamethoxazole in order to compensate for enhanced clearance of the drug [62,63]. Orally administered antibiotics can have a major impact on the microbiological environment of mouth and gut. Patients can develop symptoms such as diarrhea and *Candida* infection of the oral cavity. In addition, administration of doses that result in concentrations of the antibiotic at the site of action that are below the minimal inhibitory concentration may result in the development of antibiotic resistance. Very little is known about the doses of oral antibiotics needed to obtain sufficient concentrations above the minimal inhibitory concentration (MIC) in CF. Bioavailability of important oral antibiotics such as ciprofloxacin and azithromycin are thought not to be altered [64,65]. In contrast to the use of inhaled antibiotics, it has not been shown that micro-organisms in the lung can be eradicated solely by orally administered antibiotics [39].

Anti-inflammatory drugs

In trials that have investigated the effectiveness of anti-inflammatory agents, such as prednisone, ibuprofen and azithromycin, the drugs were administered orally [66–68]. It has not been shown that the use of inhaled corticosteroids is effective in CF [5].

The use of these oral anti-inflammatory medications has been shown to improve lung function in CF. However, oral treatment with prednisone is related to severe systemic side-effects. Oral treatment with ibuprofen is considered rather complicated since blood levels need to be controlled and precise timing is required [67,69]. Short-term studies with azithromycin showed improvement in lung function but it is associated with a substantial increase in resistance of *Staphylococcus aureus* and *Haemophilus influenzae* [70]. It is not clear whether the observed improvements are the direct result of a pulmonary effect or more of a systemic effect, or even of an antibiotic effect.

Intravenous therapy

Patients with CF frequently require intravenous (IV) antibiotics for treatment of pulmonary exacerbations. These courses are mostly given through a short peripheral catheter.

Unfortunately, the dwell time of peripheral catheters is short (days) and often complicated by phlebitis. For this reason alternatives such as the midline catheters and peripherally inserted central catheters (PICCs) are used for IV therapy in CF patients. These catheters are thought to allow longer courses of antibiotic treatment. Midline catheters are inserted in the antecubital region with the tip located in the axillary region. Catheters are made of biomaterial that softens and expands upon contact with body fluids. The dwell time is thought to be longer relative to short peripheral catheters and catheter phlebitis is thought to be less frequent. Complications that have been described are external breaks of the catheters, shoulder pain, phlebitis, catheter occlusion, accidental dislodgement, local irritation at the insertion site, and yeast infection at the insertion site. Another alternative for the short peripheral catheter is the placement of a peripherally inserted central catheter (PICC). PICCs are most often inserted in the antecubital veins. The PICC tip is located in the superior vena cava or right atrium. Complications associated with PICC insertion are infrequent, but include bleeding, tendon or nerve damage, cardiac arrhythmias, chest pain, catheter malpositioning, catheter embolism and difficult removal [71,72].

In general, the frequency of IV courses increases with disease severity. Following multiple peripheral IV placements more peripheral veins will become occluded. When venous access becomes troublesome and reduces therapeutic options, placement of a totally implantable venous access device (TIVAD) should be considered. A TIVAD might be positioned at the anterior chest wall at various locations (Fig. 13.5). For patients for whom the anterior thorax is not an attractive position, smaller devices are available that can be positioned on the upper arm. The life-span of these smaller devices placed on the arm is thought to be shorter relative to the larger ones placed on the thoracic wall. One-third of all adult CF patients has had a TIVAD at some time in their life. The average life-span of a TIVAD ranges from 440 to 1429

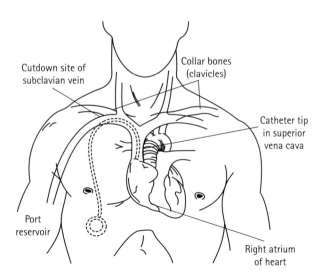

Figure 13.5 Possible locations for implantation of a totally implantable venous access device (TIVAD). From [85].

days [73–76]. Complications of a TIVAD can occur within one in 1065 to 2059 catheter days and have been described in up to a third of patients. The type of complication can vary from minor to severe (Table 13.2) [73]. The most common complication is thrombosis, either surrounding the catheter or adherent to the vein. This diagnosis can be made by using ultrasound or by injecting radiographic contrast into the TIVAD. Serious conditions like pulmonary embolism and superior vena cava syndrome can occur in these patients. It has been suggested that it might be helpful to do a hemostatic screening prior to TIVAD placement to identify patients with a thrombophilic state and in patients with a blocked TIVAD [77,78]. However, whether identification and treatment of patients with thrombophilia will help to prevent thrombotic events has not been investigated.

Oxygen delivery

Hypoxia during sleep and exercise may occur in CF patients with more advanced lung disease. These patients may develop pulmonary hypertension, reduced exercise tolerance, poor sleep quality, and deteriorating quality of life. It seems logical to treat these patients with oxygen therapy. Unfortunately, only few studies are available that evaluate the effectiveness of various forms of oxygen therapy [79,80]. Only one randomized controlled trial was published in 1989 where the effect of nocturnal oxygen therapy at a number of end-points was evaluated [81]. The authors concluded that nocturnal oxygen treatment in CF did not appear to affect mortality rates, frequency of hospitalizations, or the progression of disease. However, school and work attendance were maintained in the oxygen group but deteriorated in the placebo group. The authors stated that oxygen use should be instituted only after the development of symptoms to hypoxia.

There is no clear-cut definition for hypoxia in CF [79]. It is well recognized that patients with a resting SaO_2 below 93% have significant nocturnal desaturation. However, one-third of patients with SaO_2 above 93% became hypoxic at night. One of the definitions used to define sleep hypoxia is when a nocturnal SaO_2 of <93% is observed for more than 25% of the sleep study period. Other studies have selected a mean SaO_2 of <95%. Exercise-induced arterial hypoxia in children has been defined as a fall in SaO_2 during exercise of ≥4% from baseline. Hypoxia is reported to occur more frequently during sleep than on exercise, suggesting that for screening purposes a nightly SaO_2 profile might be appropriate. Due to this lack of randomized controlled trials the indication for oxygen therapy remains rather arbitrary.

In the American consensus guidelines it is recommended that night-time oxygen therapy is indicated for adults when SaO_2 is below 88–90% for at least 10% of the time, and oxygen during exercise is recommended if SaO_2 falls below 88–90% while exercising [82]. There is evidence of modest enhancement of exercise capacity and duration with oxygen supplementation especially in individuals with more advanced lung disease [80,83]. In a meta-analysis it was concluded by the authors that oxygen therapy should be reserved for those individuals with objective evidence of hypoxemia, when at rest while awake, or during either exercise or sleep [80]. Based on the levels of hypercapnia observed in the studies, there is no strong reason to suspect clinically important untoward side-effects in the short term. Attention to blood gas analysis is warranted in individuals with advanced lung disease.

OXYGEN DELIVERY SYSTEMS

Introduction of oxygen therapy is an emotional life event for a CF patient. First, it marks the poor pulmonary condition of the patient. Second, it adds substantially to the daily therapy burden. Introduction of oxygen should ideally be done when the patient is motivated and convinced of the potential benefit of such therapy. Clearly, introducing oxygen therapy in the home situation requires careful organization (Table 13.3).

When the initial flow to the patient is below 0.3 L/min oxygen can be delivered by cylinders. For higher flows an oxygen concentrator is preferred with back-up portable cylinders for breakdowns and for ambulatory use [84]. Many countries have guidelines for home oxygen programs. Flying and holidays spent at high altitudes can expose CF patients to a reduced inspired oxygen pressure. For a patient with severely impaired lung function this can result in a reduced oxygen saturation and increased work of breathing. From the

Table 13.2 Complications of totally implantable venous access devices (TIVAD).

Variables	Number of complications	Complications of catheter use (complications/days)
Thrombosis	0.185/1000 catheter days	1/5405
Infection	0.119/1000 catheter days	1/8403
Mechanical problem	0.079/1000 catheter days	1/12658
Superior vena cava syndrome	0.026/1000 catheter days	1/38461
Air embolism	0.013/1000 catheter days	1/76923
Pneumothorax	3.4% of catheter placements	–

Adapted from [73].

Table 13.3   Requirements for oxygen therapy in CF.

Instruction and support
Adequate training and written instructions on safe use of oxygen
   in home environment
24-hour technical and medical support in place

Equipment
Oxygen cylinders can be used for flow rates up to 0.3 L/min
Oxygen concentrator preferred for flow rates of above 0.3 L/min
Backup lightweight cylinders for breakdown and ambulatory use
Humidification system for flows at least 1 L/min for nasal
   comfort
Appropriately sized soft tin prong nasal cannulas
In cases of wheelchair use, consider cylinder fittings

literature it is not clear when in-flight oxygen is required or
when a holiday at high altitude should be discouraged. Some
authors suggest testing the patient with a 20-minute inhalation of a test-mixture of 15% oxygen and nitrogen. Others
suggest that pre-flight spirometric test may be better a predictor of desaturation during flight than a pre-flight hypoxic
challenge. To decide whether a patient requires in-flight oxygen, it is not only the desaturation which is of importance but
also the length of the flight. It is likely that a long flight will
have a higher risk of patient exhaustion due to the long duration with an increased work of breathing. If oxygen is
required, it is important that arrangements with the airline
be made well in advance.

REFERENCES

1. Borsje P, Tiddens HAWM, Mouton JW, de Jongste JC. Aerosol therapy in cystic fibrosis: a survey among 54 CF centers, *Pediatr Pulmonol* 2000; **30**:368–376.
2. Quan JM, Tiddens HAWM, Sy J *et al.* A two-year randomized, placebo controlled trial of dornase alfa in young cystic fibrosis patients with mild lung function abnormalities. *J Pediatr* 2001; **139**:813–820.
3. Ramsey BW, Pepe MS, Quan JM *et al.* for the Cystic Fibrosis Inhaled Tobramycin Study Group. Intermittent administration of inhaled tobramycin in patients with cystic fibrosis. *N Engl J Med* 1999; **340**:23–30.
4. Cheng K, Smyth RL, Motley J *et al.* Randomized controlled trials in cystic fibrosis (1966–1997) categorized by time, design, and intervention [in process citation]. *Pediatr Pulmonol* 2000; **29**:1–7.
5. Balfour-Lynn IM, Lees B, Hall P *et al.* Multicenter randomized controlled trial of withdrawal of inhaled corticosteroids in cystic fibrosis. *Am J Respir Crit Care Med* 2006; **173**(12):1356–1362.
6. Struycken VHJ, Tiddens HAWM, van den Broek ET *et al.* Problemen met gebruik, reiniging en onderhoud van vernevelapparatuur in de thuissituatie. *Neder Tijdsch voor Geneesk* 1996; **140**:654–658.
7. Rosenfeld M, Emerson J, Astley S *et al.* Home nebulizer use among patients with cystic fibrosis. *J Pediatr* 1998; **132**:125–131.
8. Vassal S, Taamma R, Marty N *et al.* Microbiologic contamination study of nebulizers after aerosol therapy in patients with cystic fibrosis. *Am J Infect Control* 2000; **28**:347–351.
9. Tiddens HAWM. Facts and fiction in inhalation therapy. *Ital J Pediatr* 2003; **29**:39–43.
10. Janssens HM, de Jongste JC, Hop WCJ, Tiddens HAWM. Extra-fine particles improve lung delivery of inhaled steroids in infants: a study in an upper airway model. *Chest* 2003; **123**:2083–2088.
11. Janssens HM, Heijnen EM, de Jong VM *et al.* Aerosol delivery from spacers in wheezy infants: a daily life study, *Eur Respir J* 2000; **16**:850–856.
12. Laube BL, Jashnani R, Dalby RN, Zeitlin PL. Targeting aerosol deposition in patients with cystic fibrosis: effects of alterations in particle size and inspiratory flow rate [in process citation]. *Chest* 2000; **118**:1069–1076.
13. Mallol J, Rattray S, Walker G *et al.* Aerosol deposition in infants with cystic fibrosis. *Pediatr Pulmonol* 1996; **21**:276–281.
14. Tiddens HAWM, Koopman LP, Lambert RK *et al.* Cartilaginous airway wall dimensions and airway resistance in cystic fibrosis lungs. *Eur Resp J* 2000; **15**:735–742.
15. Goris ML, Zhu HJ, Blankenberg F *et al.* An automated approach to quantitative air trapping measurements in mild cystic fibrosis. *Chest* 2003; **123**:1655–1663.
16. Geller DE, Eigen H, Fiel SB *et al.* for Group ftDAN. Effect of smaller droplet size of dornase alfa on lung function in mild cystic fibrosis. *Pediatr Pulmonol* 1998; **25**:83–87.
17. Boe J, Dennis JH, O'Driscoll BR *et al.* European Respiratory Society Guidelines on the use of nebulizers. *Eur Respir J* 2001; **18**:228–242.
18. Standaert TA, Morlin GL, Williams-Warren J *et al.* Effects of repetitive use and cleaning techniques of disposable jet nebulizers on aerosol generation. *Chest* 1998; **114**:577–586.
19. Esposito-Festen JE, Ates B, van Vliet FJM *et al.* Effect of a facemask leak on aerosol delivery from a pMDI-Spacer system. *J Aerosol Med* 2004; **17**:1–6.
20. Chua HL, Collis GG, Newbury AM *et al.* The influence of age on aerosol deposition in children with cystic fibrosis. *Eur Resp J* 1994; **7**:2185–2191.
21. Dahlback M. Behavior of nebulizing solutions and suspensions. *J Aerosol Med* 1994; **7**:S13–S18.
22. Schoni MH, Kraemer R. Osmolality changes in nebulizer solutions. *Eur Respir J* 1989; **2**:887–892.
23. Hess D, Fisher D, Williams P *et al.* Medication nebulizer performance: effects of diluent volume, nebulizer flow, and nebulizer brand [see comments]. *Chest* 1996; **110**:498–505.
24. Rau JL. The inhalation of drugs: advantages and problems. *Respir Care* 2005; **50**:367–382.
25. Vecellio L. The mesh nebulizer: a recent technical innovation for aerosol delivery. *Breathe* 2006; **2**:253–260.
26. Kosorok MR, Jalaluddin M, Farrell PM *et al.* Comprehensive analysis of risk factors for acquisition of *Pseudomonas*

aeruginosa in young children with cystic fibrosis [see comments]. *Pediatr Pulmonol* 1998; **26**:81–88.

27. Demko CA, Byard PJ, Davis PB. Gender differences in cystic fibrosis: *Pseudomonas aeruginosa* infection. *J Clin Epidemiol* 1995; **48**:1041–1049.

28. Nixon GM, Armstrong DS, Carzino R *et al*. Clinical outcome after early *Pseudomonas aeruginosa* infection in cystic fibrosis. *J Pediatr* 2001; **138**:699–704.

29. Esposito-Festen JE, Ates B, Vliet F *et al*. Aerosol delivery to young children by pMDI-spacer: is facemask design important? *Pediatr Allergy Immunol* 2005; **16**:348–353.

30. Wildhaber JH, Devadason SG, Eber E *et al*. Effect of electrostatic charge, flow, delay and multiple actuations on the in-vitro delivery of salbutamol from different small volume spacers for infants. *Thorax* 1996; **51**:985–988.

31. Wildhaber JH, Devadason SG, Hayden MJ *et al*. Electrostatic charge on a plastic spacer influences the delivery of salbutamol. *Eur Respir J* 1996; **9**:1943–1946.

32. de Jong PA, Lindblad A, Rubin L *et al*. Progression of lung disease on computed tomography and pulmonary function tests in children and adults with cystic fibrosis. *Thorax* 2006; **61**:80–85.

33. Devadason SG, Everard ML, MacEarlan C *et al*. Lung deposition from the Turbuhaler in children with cystic fibrosis. *Eur Respir J* 1997; **10**:2023–2028.

34. Tiddens HAWM, Standaert TE, Challoner P *et al*. Effect of dry powder inhaler resistance on the inspiratory flow rates and volumes of cystic fibrosis patients of six years and older. *J Aerosol Med* 2006; **19**(4):456–465.

35. Ramsey BW, Dorkin HL, Eisenberg JD *et al*. Efficacy of aerosolized tobramycin in patients with cystic fibrosis. *N Engl J Med* 1993; **328**:1740–1746.

36. Quittner AL, Buu A. Effects of tobramycin solution for inhalation on global ratings of quality of life in patients with cystic fibrosis and *Pseudomonas aeruginosa* infection. *Pediatr Pulmonol* 2002; **33**:269–276.

37. Moss RB. Long-term benefits of inhaled tobramycin in adolescent patients with cystic fibrosis. *Chest* 2002; **121**:55–63.

38. Ratjen F, Doring G, Nikolaizik WH. Effect of inhaled tobramycin on early *Pseudomonas aeruginosa* colonisation in patients with cystic fibrosis. *Lancet* 2001; **358**:983–984.

39. Gibson RL, Emerson J, McNamara S *et al*. Significant microbiological effect of inhaled tobramycin in young children with cystic fibrosis. *Am J Respir Crit Care Med* 2003; **167**:841–849.

40. Littlewood JM, Miller MG, Chonheim AT, Ramsden CH. Nebulised colomycin for early *Pseudomonas* colonisation in cystic fibrosis. *Lancet* 1985; **1**:865.

41. Jensen T, Pedersen SS, Garne S *et al*. Colistin inhalation therapy in cystic fibrosis patients with chronic *Pseudomonas aeruginosa* lung infection. *J Antimicrobial Chemother* 1987; **19**:831–838.

42. Katz SL, Ho SL, Coates AL. Nebulizer choice for inhaled colistin treatment in cystic fibrosis. *Chest* 2001; **119**:250–255.

43. Shak S, Capon DJ, Hellmiss R *et al*. Recombinant human DNase I reduces the viscosity of cystic fibrosis sputum. *Proc Natl Acad Sci USA* 1990; **87**:9188–9192.

44. Fuchs HJ, Borowitz DS, Christiansen DH *et al*. for the Pulmozyme Study Group. Effect of aerosolized recombinant human DNase on exacerbations of respiratory symptoms and on pulmonary function in patients with cystic fibrosis. *N Engl J Med* 1994; **331**:637–642.

45. van der Giessen LJ, De Jongste JC, Gosselink R, Hop WCJ, Tiddens HAWM. RhDNase before airway clearance therapy improves airway patency in children with CF.

46. Slattery DM, Waltz DA, Denham B *et al*. Bronchoscopically administered recombinant human DNase for lobar atelectasis in cystic fibrosis. *Pediatr Pulmonol* 2001; **31**:383–388.

47. Shah PL, Scott SF, Hodson ME. Lobar atelectasis in cystic fibrosis and treatment with recombinant human DNase I. *Respir Med* 1994; **88**:313–315.

48. Cropp GJ. Effectiveness of bronchodilators in cystic fibrosis. *Am J Med* 1996; **100**:1S–19S.

49. Konig P, Poehler J, Barbero GJ. A placebo-controlled, double-blind trial of the long-term effects of albuterol administration in patients with cystic fibrosis. *Pediatr Pulmonol* 1998; **25**:32–36.

50. Zach MS, Oberwaldner B, Forche G, Polgar G. Bronchodilators increase airway instability in cystic fibrosis. *Am Rev Respir Dis* 1985; **131**:537–543.

51. Hellinckx J, de Boeck K, Demedts M. No paradoxical bronchodilator response with forced oscillation technique in children with cystic fibrosis. *Chest* 1998; **113**:55–59.

52. Tiddens HAWM, Hofhuis W, Bogaard JM *et al*. Compliance, hysteresis, and collapsibility of human small airways. *Am J Respir Crit Care Med* 1999; **160**:1110–1118.

53. Halfhide C, Evans H, Couriel J, Halfhide C. Inhaled bronchodilators for cystic fibrosis. *Cochrane Database Syst Rev* 2005; CD003428

54. Bargon J, Viel K, Dauletbaev N *et al*. Short-term effects of regular salmeterol treatment on adult cystic fibrosis patients. *Eur Respir J* 1997; **10**:2307–2311.

55. Bisgaard H, Pedersen SS, Nielsen KG *et al*. Controlled trial of inhaled budesonide in patients with cystic fibrosis and chronic bronchopulmonary *Psuedomonas aeruginosa* infection. *Am J Respir Crit Care Med* 1997; **156**:1190–1196.

56. Broeders ME, Molema J, Burnell PK, Folgering HT. Ventolin Diskus and Inspyril Turbuhaler: an in-vitro comparison. *J Aerosol Med* 2005; **18**:74–82.

57. Duijvestijn YC, Brand PL. Systematic review of *N*-acetylcysteine in cystic fibrosis. *Acta Paediatr* 1999; **88**:38–41.

58. Robinson M, Hemming AL, Regnis JA *et al*. Effect of increasing doses of hypertonic saline on mucociliary clearance in patients with cystic fibrosis. *Thorax* 1997; **52**:900–903.

59. Wark PA, McDonald V, Jones AP. Nebulised hypertonic saline for cystic fibrosis. *Cochrane Database Syst Rev* 2005; CD001506.

60. Elkins MR, Robinson M, Rose BR *et al*. A controlled trial of long-term inhaled hypertonic saline in patients with cystic fibrosis. *N Engl J Med* 2006; **354**:229–240.

61. Donaldson SH, Bennett WD, Zeman KL *et al.* Mucus clearance and lung function in cystic fibrosis with hypertonic saline. *N Engl J Med* 2006; **354**:241–250.

62. Rey E, Treluyer JM, Pons G. Drug disposition in cystic fibrosis. *Clin Pharmacokinet* 1998; **35**:313–329.

63. Touw DJ. Clinical pharmacokinetics of antimicrobial drugs in cystic fibrosis. *Pharm World Sci* 1998; **20**:149–160.

64. Beringer P, Huynh KM, Kriengkauykiat J *et al.* Absolute bioavailability and intracellular pharmacokinetics of azithromycin in patients with cystic fibrosis. *Antimicrob Agents Chemother* 2005; **49**:5013–5017.

65. Christensson BA, Nilsson-Ehle I, Ljungberg B *et al.* Increased oral bioavailability of ciprofloxacin in cystic fibrosis patients. *Antimicrob Agents Chemother* 1992; **36**:2512–2517.

66. Eigen H, Rosenstein BJ, FitzSimmons S, Schidlow DV for Group CFFPT. A multicenter study of alternate-day prednisone therapy in patients with cystic fibrosis. *J Pediatr* 1995; **126**:515–523.

67. Konstan MW, Byard PJ, Hopel CL, Davis PB. Effect of high-dose ibuprofen in patients with cystic fibrosis. *N Engl J Med* 1995; **332**:848–854.

68. Saiman L, Marshall BC, Mayer-Hamblett N *et al.* Azithromycin in patients with cystic fibrosis chronically infected with *Pseudomonas aeruginosa*: a randomized controlled trial. *J Am Med Assoc* 2003; **290**:1749–1756.

69. Han EE, Beringer PM, Louie SG *et al.* Pharmacokinetics of ibuprofen in children with cystic fibrosis. *Clin Pharmacokinet* 2004; **43**:145–156.

70. Phaff SJ, Tiddens HAWM, Verbrugh HA, Ott A. Macrolide resistance of *Staphylococcus aureus* and *Haemophilus* species, associated with long-term azithromycin use in cystic fibrosis. *J Antimicrob Chemother* 2006; **57**:741–746.

71. Thiagarajan RR, Ramamoorthy C, Gettmann T, Bratton SL. Survey of the use of peripherally inserted central venous catheters in children. *Pediatrics* 1997; **99**:E4.

72. Miall LS, Das A, Brownlee KG, Conway SP. Peripherally inserted central catheters in children with cystic fibrosis: eight cases of difficult removal. *J Infus Nurs* 2001; **24**:297–300.

73. Aitken ML, Tonelli MR. Complications of indwelling catheters in cystic fibrosis: a 10-year review. *Chest* 2000; **118**:1598–1602.

74. Burdon J, Conway SP, Murchan P *et al.* Five years' experience of PAS Port intravenous access system in adult cystic fibrosis. *Eur Respir J* 1998; **12**:212–216.

75. Deerojanawong J, Sawyer SM, Fink AM *et al.* Totally implantable venous access devices in children with cystic fibrosis: incidence and type of complications. *Thorax* 1998; **53**:285–289.

76. Kariyawasam HH, Pepper JR, Hodson ME, Geddes DM. Experience of totally implantable venous access devices (TIVADs) in adults with cystic fibrosis over a 13-year period. *Respir Med* 2000; **94**:1161–1165.

77. Balfour-Lynn IM, Malbon K, Burman JF, Davidson SJ. Thrombophilia in children with cystic fibrosis. *Pediatr Pulmonol* 2005; **39**:306–310.

78. Barker M, Thoenes D, Dohmen H *et al.* Prevalence of thrombophilia and catheter-related thrombosis in cystic fibrosis. *Pediatr Pulmonol* 2005; **39**:156–161.

79. Urquhart DS, Montgomery H, Jaffe A. Assessment of hypoxia in children with cystic fibrosis. *Arch Dis Child* 2005; **90**:1138–1143.

80. Mallory G, Fullmer J, Vaughan D, Mallory G. Oxygen therapy for cystic fibrosis. *Cochrane Database Syst Rev* 2005; CD003884.

81. Zinman R, Corey M, Coates AL *et al.* Nocturnal home oxygen in the treatment of hypoxemic cystic fibrosis patients. *J Pediatr* 1989; **114**:368–377.

82. Yankaskas JR, Marshall BC, Sufian B *et al.* Cystic fibrosis adult care: consensus conference report. *Chest* 2004; **125**:1S–39S.

83. McKone EF, Barry SC, FitzGerald MX, Gallagher CG. The role of supplemental oxygen during submaximal exercise in patients with cystic fibrosis. *Eur Respir J* 2002; **20**:134–142.

84. Balfour-Lynn IM, Primhak RA, Shaw BN. Home oxygen for children: who, how and when? *Thorax* 2005; **60**:76–81.

85. www.mayoclinic.org.gi-jax/images/venous.gif/

14

The upper airway in cystic fibrosis

WILLIAM E. GRANT

INTRODUCTION

Cystic fibrosis (CF) is an autosomal recessive disease with multisystem involvement, but with particularly devastating respiratory impact. The respiratory tract can be considered to extend from the lips and nostrils to the alveoli, being divided into an upper and lower airway at the level of the larynx, and lined throughout with respiratory pseudostratified ciliated epithelium. From the point of view of the exocrine dysfunction of cystic fibrosis, the upper airway sites most significantly affected by the disease are the nose and paranasal sinuses.

Thickened viscid secretions overwhelm mucociliary clearance mechanisms and lead to mucus stasis and infection in the paranasal sinuses and lower segmental airways alike. Chronic inflammation in the nasal airways may lead to nasal polyposis, a condition rarely seen in childhood outside cystic fibrosis. Significant sinonasal symptoms arise in some 30–45% of sufferers, and these may be debilitating. Chronic catarrhal and cough symptoms with nasal obstruction, anosmia and headache are typical presenting features. The sinuses may become chronically infected by organisms such as *Pseudomonas aeruginosa* [1]. Interestingly, the incidence of primary otological disease, or of dysfunction secondary to Eustachian tube failure due chronic sinonasal disease, appears to be no higher than in the general population [2,3].

Physicians focusing on the life-threatening lower respiratory symptoms suffered by these patients may under-treat and under-appreciate the extent, impact and significance of sinonasal disease in this condition. The inflammatory burden of upper airway disease may contribute, by mechanisms as yet not fully understood, but involving sinobronchial reflex pathways, eosinophilia, and humoral mechanisms, to worsening of already profound lower respiratory tract dysfunction.

Improved medical and surgical management of sinonasal disease, both of which have seen dramatic developments in recent years, contribute to secondary improvement in control of pulmonary inflammatory and infective disease in non-CF patients [4–8]. As might be expected given the underlying pathophysiology of CF, studies in this population show varied, but less dramatic, response of the lower airway to improved upper airway disease management.

As CF patients are recognized to under-report upper airway symptoms, optimal treatment of upper airway disease will ideally involve input from rhinologically specialized ENT practitioners in a multidisciplinary setting. Improved management may thus result in benefit not only for the primary nasal symptoms, but may also improve lower respiratory function and general well-being.

PATHOPHYSIOLOGY

Mucus stasis inevitably leads to secondary infection, and in the nose it also results in sinus ostial obstruction with failure in ventilation and drainage, which are the major predisposing factors in the development of sinus disease in normal subjects [9]. Infective organisms isolated from the sinuses tend to be *Pseudomonas aeruginosa*, *Staphylococcus aureus* and *Haemophilus influenzae* and anaerobes [1]. Disease manifestations are likely to result from a combination of inflammation secondary to the failure to clear thickened secretions, sinus ostial obstruction, and superadded infection, rather than simply being primarily infective.

MUCOCILIARY FUNCTION

Cystic fibrosis patients are traditionally thought to have reduced mucociliary clearance [10,11]. More recently, a study aimed at differentiating primary (CFTR ion transport-related) from secondary (inflammatory) causes of delayed mucociliary clearance challenged the idea that CFTR dysfunction on its own caused delayed clearance from the nose [12]. Fifty children with cystic fibrosis, primary ciliary dyskinesia, and no respiratory disease were studied. Normal and CF children had normal mucociliary clearance times and pro-inflammatory cytokine levels. The finding that CF children actually had normal mucociliary function suggests that adults with cystic fibrosis had impaired ciliary clearance secondary to inflammatory airway changes. There is no doubt that chronic inflammation results in secondary changes including goblet cell hyperplasia, as well as squamous metaplasia and loss of ciliated cells. Bacterial toxins, such as the pyocyanin and 1-hydroxyphenazine produced by *Pseudomonas* spp [13,14], as well as inflammatory byproducts such as neutrophil elastase, can further impair ciliary motility [15]. This, coupled with the greatly increased mucus viscosity, results in severely disturbed mucociliary clearance.

Within the paranasal sinuses, alteration in the viscoelastic properties of the mucus in CF contributes to a mechanical obstruction of the sinus ostia. The secondary mucostasis, infection and inflammation that develops results in intrasinus hypoxia, hypercarbia, reduction in pH, leading to further mucosal inflammation, edema, and yet further mucociliary impairment and the opportunity for bacterial infection and colonization.

NASAL POLYPOSIS

Nasal polyposis in children is exceptionally rare outside the cystic fibrosis population, and once identified the diagnosis of CF must be pursued.

The incidence of nasal polyposis in CF was probably underestimated in earlier studies before the advent of endoscopic techniques, and more recent figures quoting a range 32–45% are probably more accurate [2,16]. Hadfield and co-workers [17] reported an incidence of 37% in a large series of 211 adults with cystic fibrosis from the Royal Brompton Hospital. Slieker and co-workers [18] reported half the children in a series of 140 children with CF had polyps, but that only 59% of these were symptomatic.

The pathophysiology of the development of nasal polyposis in CF is, however, unclear, as indeed it is in non-CF polyposis. Why some patients develop symptomatic sinusitis, some remain relatively asymptomatic, and why some, but by no means all, go on to develop nasal polyposis is not understood. The incidence of nasal polyposis is no higher in patients with allergic rhinitis than in the general population [19]. Tos and co-workers [20] have hypothesized that polyps result from nasal mucosal inflammation where epithelial damage allows prolapse of the lamina propria, and suggested a similar pathogenesis in inflammatory and non-CF polyps, based on histological appearance. Subsequent studies (more of which below) have, however, shown that the histological features of polyps in CF demonstrate specific differences to the polyps in chronic rhinosinusitis.

The presence of expansive polypoid disease in the ethmoids may result in widening of the nasal bridge and the appearance of hypertelorism (Fig. 14.1) [2]. The relatively elastic bones of younger children with massive polyposis in

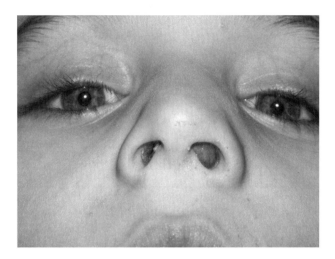

Figure 14.1 Photograph demonstrating nasal polyposis with complete occlusion of left nasal airway and broadening of nasal dorsum secondary to extensive anterior ethmoid polyposis. *See also Plate 14.1.*

the ethmoid labyrinth may be responsible for the broad nasal dorsum sometimes seen in pediatric cystic polyposis – a pseudohypertelorism or Woakes' syndrome. In CF the anterior ethmoid grows faster than the posterior compartment which may also relate to the broadening of the nasal dorsum seen with massive polyps. There is a higher frequency of chronic lower airway infection with *Pseudomonas aeruginosa* in CF patients with nasal polyps compared with patients with no polyps [21].

MICROBIOLOGY

While in the non-CF population *Haemophilus* and *streptococcal* organisms are responsible for chronic infective rhinosinusitis, in cystic fibrosis *Pseudomonas aeruginosa* and *Staphylococcus aureus* are more frequently cultured. The majority of the bacterial isolates recovered from the sinuses are also present in sputum cultures, as demonstrated by genotyping [22].

There has been little in the literature regarding fungal disease in CF in spite of debate in recent years regarding the role of fungi in chronic rhinosinusitis and nasal polyposis in the general population. One group found that fungal cultures were positive in 33.3% of cases [23]. *Candida albicans* was the commonest, with one each of *Aspergillus fumigatus*, *Penicillium* species, *Exserohilum* and *Bipolaris*. There appeared to be no correlation between presence of fungal isolates and requirement for revision surgery. Two patients were diagnosed as having allergic fungal sinusitis (AFS), according to the criteria of Bent and Kuhn [24]. The role of these fungi in the pathogenesis of sinonasal disease in CF is unclear at this time; while they may be incidental isolates, in some patients, in particular with *Aspergillus*, chronic low-grade presence may provoke IgE-mediated hypersensitivity and allergic fungal sinusitis, in a manner similar to allergic bronchopulmonary mycosis.

SINONASAL SYMPTOMS

There is a low self-reporting of symptoms by CF patients and poor correlation between symptoms and disease severity [25–27]. Patients may accept upper airway symptoms as normal because they may have been present from an early age [25]. Common symptoms include nasal obstruction, purulent rhinorrhea, headache, anosmia, facial pain, snoring and voice change [28,29]. Headache and periorbital pain are the commonest reported symptoms in those with chronic rhinosinusitis, and anosmia the commonest symptom in those with polyps [30]. Headache is difficult to quantify but tends to be reported more in adolescent and adult patients.

CLINICAL AND ENDOSCOPIC FINDINGS

Much can be gleaned from simple inspection of the child or adult in the clinic. Observation of mouth breathing tendencies may point to severity of nasal obstructive disease. Typical 'adenoidal' type facies, due to nasal obstruction may be evident. Broadening of the nasal bridge along with pseudohypertelorism is a further common clinical finding (see Fig. 14.1) [29].

Intranasal examination can be performed with a bright headlight or perhaps with an otoscope following the application of a topical decongestant. Rhinitic inferior turbinates are frequently misinterpreted as polyps and referral for examination by a collaborative rhinologist with an interest in this condition is the ideal. While gross polyps are easily seen, up to 25% of polyps can be missed by direct visualization alone [29]. Inspection is ideally carried out with either a rigid 2.7-mm Hopkins rod endoscope in adults and older children, or with a flexible endoscope in younger children (Fig. 14.2). This commonly reveals degrees of nasal polyposis, purulent secretions emanating from one or more of the recognized drainage pathways, or medial bulging of the lateral nasal wall. Appraisal of the postnasal space for obstructive adenoid enlargement may allow for a simple intervention that might improve the nasal airway and function. A work-up for coexisting allergy should be undertaken. A complete ENT examination should be considered on a regular basis in the interest of overall well-being of the CF patient [31].

ALLERGY

Most studies demonstrate increased atopy based on skin prick tests in patients with CF, and specifically increased hypersensitivity to *Aspergillus* fungal species has been noted. Atopy does not appear to influence the development of nasal polyps [17,32], but *Aspergillus* allergy is commoner in

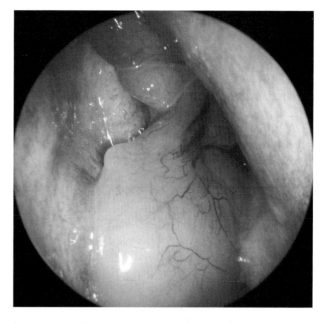

Figure 14.2   Endoscopic view of nasal polyposis, shrunken following application of vasonstricting agent. *See also Plate 14.2.*

CF patients with polyps than without [33]. A genetic link between CF and ABPA is suggested by the finding of a high frequency of homozygous and heterozygous CFTR gene mutations in patients with ABPA and normal sweat tests and without cystic fibrosis [34,35]. The term 'sinobronchial allergic mycosis' has been proposed for coexisting ABPA and allergic fungal sinusitis [36].

POST–TRANSPLANT LYMPHOPROLIFERATIVE DISORDER

Post-transplant lymphoproliferative disorder (PTLD) may be defined as uncontrolled lymphoproliferation in a setting of pharmacological immunosuppression. Sinonasal PTLD is rare [37] and early detection is prognostically critical. Clinician awareness that post-transplant immunosuppressed patients may not simply be suffering with a further recurrence of CF nasal polyposis is therefore of great importance.

IMAGING

Plain sinus radiographs have little if any role [38]. The imaging modality of choice in the evaluation of paranasal sinus disease is the CT scan. These scans play an important role in determining the extent and nature of disease, and are indispensable in guiding surgical intervention where that is required. Rapid-acquisition spiral CT techniques are satisfactorily tolerated and radiation exposure is relatively low. CT findings in cystic fibrosis patients almost invariably show extensive pan-sinus opacification, with certain findings specific to this population not seen in chronic sinusitis.

CT may not always clearly distinguish between polyp and fluid, whether pus or retained secretions. Varying signal return may indicate the presence of pus of varying degrees of inspissation, fluid and polyp. Normal CT scans are exceptionally rare in CF, most series reporting almost universal opacification [8,27,29].

Extensive paranasal sinus opacification (Fig. 14.3), sinus agenesis or hypoplasia (Fig. 14.4), and medial bulging of the lateral nasal wall with thinning or loss of bony landmarks (Fig. 14.5) are the hallmarks of the cystic fibrosis sinus CT series [2,16,39–41].

The common finding of medialization of the lateral nasal wall is particularly interesting and the pathogenesis is incompletely understood. This medial bulging of the lateral nasal wall has been defined as a soft tissue mass extending medially from the maxillary sinus in the area of the middle meatus to at least half the distance from the lamina papyracea (medial orbital bony plate) to the nasal septum [39] (see Fig. 14.5). However, the condition appears to be distinct from simple mucocele formation, as multiloculated collections of pus and thickened infected secretions are surrounded by gross thickening of the maxillary lining which is frequently polypoid – therefore the terms mucopyosinusitis or pseudomucocele have been proposed. Thinning of the bone of the medial wall and expansion of the natural maxillary sinus ostium from a few millimeters in healthy individuals to many times this is a common finding (see Fig. 14.5). The destruction of the bony walls of the antrum may be attributable to osteitis [42], pressure necrosis, demineralization [43] or osteolysis. Pseudomucocele of the antrum may be age-related, being present in all CF children under 5 years, more than 85% in age group 5–8, but in only 60% of CF adolescents [2]. When present it is usually bilateral.

The frontal sinuses classically remain hypoplastic as do the sphenoid sinuses. This is thought to reflect failure to develop due to inadequate ventilation which reduces pneumatization in a fashion analogous to the sclerotic mastoid bone system with reduced air cell development seen in chronic suppurative ear disease [44]. Primary ciliary dyskinesia is the only other disease with a clear association with frontal sinus hypoplasia. However, agenesis of one or both frontal sinuses can be seen in the absence of any sinonasal disease in 10% of healthy individuals [45].

In summary, CT imaging of the paranasal sinuses is recommended in symptomatic sinusitis and polyposis and where significant medial bulging of the lateral nasal wall is perceived.

MRI imaging tends to be very sensitive to inflammatory change, and can be used to monitor treatment, but it does not reveal bony detail, so is less used in sinus imaging. Gadolinium enhancement of T1-weighted images allows distinction between mucosal edema and fluid/secretions. Patients who have undergone FESS surgery (functional endoscopic sinus surgery) may be monitored postoperatively with STIR and T1-weighted MRI imaging to detect pus-filled loculations that can be eradicated with further

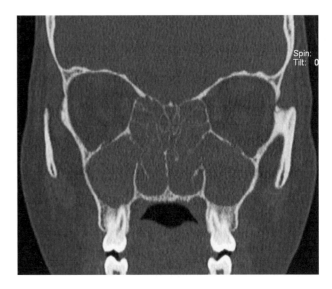

Figure 14.3 CT showing extensive pan-sinus opacification with no airway patency and middle meatal expansion.

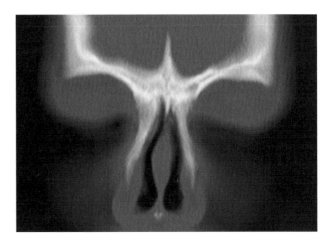

Figure 14.4 CT showing typical frontal sinus agenesis.

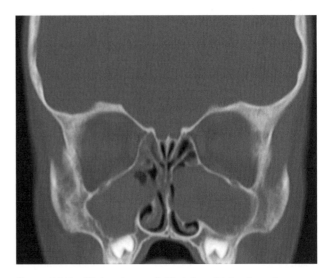

Figure 14.5 CT showing medial bulging of lateral nasal wall with complete opacification of the maxillary antra.

surgery, avoiding both unnecessary further irradiation, and unnecessary surgery for misdiagnosed simple mucosal disease [46].

HISTOPATHOLOGY

Nasal polyps in non-CF patients are benign mucosal swellings histologically characterized by edema, goblet cell hyperplasia of the epithelium, thickening of the basement membrane, and the presence of numerous leukocytes, predominantly eosinophils [47]. Many histological similarities exist between polyps in cystic fibrosis and non-CF patients [48].

Ultrastructurally, CF polyps differ significantly from non-CF polyps. Histological features specific to nasal polyposis in cystic fibrosis are a thin delicate basement membrane of surface epithelium, lack of extensive infiltration with eosinophils, and a preponderance of acid mucin in glands and cysts of the polyps (characteristically neutral in 'allergic polyps') – see Fig. 14.6 [49–52]. The CF nasal polyps show specific characteristics of (a) minimal damage to surface epithelium, (b) the presence of a mucus blanket lining the apical epithelium, (c) occasional intracytoplasmic lumina, (d) continuous and fenestrated type capillaries, (e) numerous degranulated mast cells, (f) many plasma cells often morphologically atypical and with intracisternal Russell bodies, and (g) a smaller number of eosinophils in comparison with non-CF polyps [53].

Further evidence in support of a different etiology for CF and non-CF nasal polyposis is becoming available from biochemical and molecular genetic studies. Nasal polyps from CF patients have different glycohistochemical properties to non-CF polyps, showing higher levels of lectin-reactive galactoside residues [54]. Studies of innate markers like human beta-defensins and toll-like receptors and inflammatory mediators such as myeloperoxidase, IgE and interleukins have shown significant differences between CF and non-CF nasal polyps [55].

Inflammatory cell and cytokine pathways have been well documented in the lower respiratory tract and in chronic rhinosinusitis, but relatively little has been reported regarding these mechanisms in chronic rhinosinusitis in patients with CF. Sinus mucosal specimens were found to have higher numbers of neutrophils, macrophages and cells expressing messenger RNA for interferon-γ and IL-8 in patients with cystic fibrosis than in patients with chronic rhinosinusitis or controls. Conversely the number of eosinophils and cells expressing RNA for IL-4, IL-5 and IL-10 was higher in patients with chronic sinusitis. These differing inflammatory mechanisms may in part explain differences in response to treatments in the CF group [56].

NITRIC OXIDE

Nitric oxide is synthesized in the nasal sinuses and may be low in the presence of normal synthetic activity if the sinus ostia are blocked, such as in nasal polyposis [57]. Children with cystic fibrosis have been shown to have lowered nasal levels of nitric oxide, but exhaled levels in the normal range [58,59]. Lowered nasal airway concentration of nitric oxide results from reduced NO synthase expression in the upper respiratory tract, and may be in part responsible for reduction in elimination of bacteria such as *Pseudomonas* [60].

MEDICAL MANAGEMENT

Medical management involves the use of anti-inflammatory and antimicrobial therapy coupled with attempts at promoting clearance of static secretions with irrigation techniques. Most medical treatment strategies derive from those used in non-CF polyposis and rhinosinusitis and have a limited evidence base for their use in either condition, and must be considered empirical. Combinations of oral and topical treatments are used depending on clinical symptom severity. The recognition that sinonasal disease in cystic fibrosis is incurable leads to efforts to control disease medically, reserving surgery for those with more severe symptoms. Topical decongestants aim to open sinus ostia occluded by mucosal edema and promote sinus ventilation and drainage in the acute infective exacerbation only; in the chronic situation there is little role for topical decongestant therapy. There is increasing enthusiasm for nasal saline irrigations, either isotonic or hypertonic, to aid in clearing thick secretions, and trials in non-CF patients have shown benefit in chronic rhinosinusitis in symptom reduction, endoscopic appearance and quality-of-life outcome measures [61]. Hypertonic solutions provide an osmotic gradient favoring fluid transport into the nose resulting in an 'osmotic decongestion' of sinus mucosa, and may be more effective than isotonic solutions.

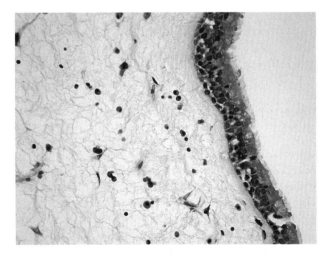

Figure 14.6 Area of polypoid mucosa showing sub-surface edema with chronic inflammatory cells (few eosinophils). H&E × 200. *See also Plate 14.6.*

Corticosteroids

There is good evidence for the use of systemic steroids to bring about reduction in polyps and symptoms in studies in non-CF patients with persistent rhinosinusitis with nasal polyposis. There also exists good evidence to support a role for use of postoperative steroids in reducing polyp recurrence [62]. Betamethasone drops may significantly reduce polyp size when compared to placebo [63]. Concerns regarding systemic adrenal suppression with long-term nasal steroid drop therapy lead to the recommendation that this form of treatment might alternate or rotate with periods of simple nasal steroid sprays in which systemic bioavailability is much lower.

Antibiotics

Infection secondary to thickened secretions and impaired ciliary function have led to the use of protracted courses of oral antibiotic treatment. The choice of antibiotic therapy is governed by likely infective organisms. The nasal sinuses, like the lungs, may become chronically infected by *Pseudomonas* and *Staphylococcus*, as well as non-typeable *Haemophilus influenzae* [1,22]. Empirical oral antibiotic treatment for sinusitis is recommended for a duration of 3–6 weeks for subjective increases in postnasal drainage, congestion and cough symptoms [64,65]. Complete eradication of *Pseudomonas* is unlikely [65]. Macrolides may be beneficial in chronic rhinosinusitis in non-CF children [66,67], but there have been no studies of macrolide therapy in CF sinonasal disease. Some authors have recommended regular nasal and postsinus surgical sinus cavity irrigation with tobramycin, particularly in lung transplant patients to reduce the risk of *Pseudomonas* pulmonary seeding and infection from infected sinuses [68,69].

Deoxyribonuclease

Recombinant human deoxyribonuclease-1 (dornase alfa) lyses extracellular DNA released by leukocytes involved in airway infection and inflammation, thereby reducing mucus viscosity. There is some evidence for benefit from nasal applications in patients undergoing sinus surgery [70,71].

SURGICAL MANAGEMENT

Surgical options range from simple nasal polypectomy where the polyps are simply amputated or avulsed, to meticulous clearance of all diseased mucosa with removal of the ethmoid labyrinth, usually with preservation of the turbinate structures and wide opening of the maxillary, and if present sphenoid and frontal sinuses (Fig. 14.7).

The time to recurrence to some extent appears to depend on the extent of surgical disease clearance. Simple

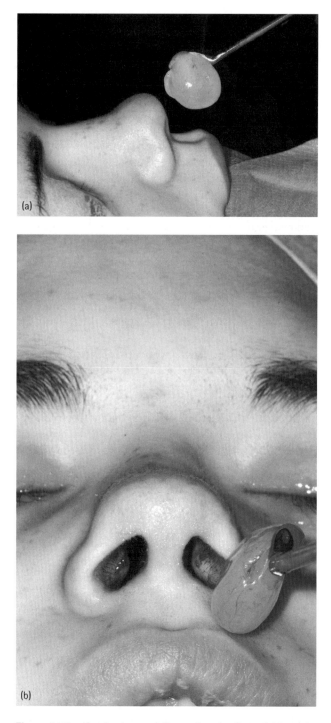

Figure 14.7 Nasal polyp on delivery. *See also Plates 14.7a and 14.7b.*

polypectomy surgery was associated with a tendency to earlier recurrence [72] than polypectomy with efforts to clear disease more thoroughly at intranasal ethmoidectomy [3,73]. The basic tenet of endoscopic sinus surgery in sinusitis is that restoration of ventilation and drainage of a sinus cavity allows restoration of normal function with return of chronically inflamed mucosa to normal. Endoscopic sinus surgical techniques have been hugely successful in the general population in restoring nasal function.

There was early enthusiasm that improved lung function might be brought about by sinus surgery in CF patients. As the lower respiratory tract suffers from the identical difficulties of greatly thickened mucus and secondary mucociliary failure, it is not surprising that problems persist in spite of adequate and maximal surgical and medical sinus treatment.

While nasal polyposis is frequently the obvious disease on inspection of the nasal cavities, the presence of trapped and infected pockets of mucopus within the obstructed ethmoid chambers and within the antrum is the usual finding at surgery (Fig. 14.8). It is often an over-simplification to consider polyposis and chronic rhinosinusitis as separate entities and polyps may be best considered as 'the extreme outcome of unchecked mucosal inflammation in the ethmoid sinuses' [74]. The degree of polyp formation, however, varies from extensive to little at all, for reasons which remain obscure, but which may be related to manifestations of different CFTR mutations. In turn such differing disease may indicate the likelihood of different response to surgery [75].

While accepting incurability of the sinonasal disease, this is not to say that considerable benefit may not be conferred by surgery. The aim of surgery is the relief of symptoms, the clearance of disease and its inflammatory burden, the elimination of reservoirs of infected mucus (especially in the severely affected population undergoing heart–lung transplant surgery), and minimization of likelihood of recurrence of disease. The excision of the ethmoid labyrinth of many small bony compartments, creating an open cavity, along with the creation of large drainage and ventilation antrostomies into the maxillary antra that might allow gravitational drainage, helped by irrigation with saline sprays and douches, would seem likely to help reduce mucus stasis and infection and allow ingress of medication and therefore decrease infection and inflammation.

In spite of almost universal disease presence on CT imaging, surgery has in the main been offered to patients with more severely diseased noses as these have been the ones associated with more severe symptoms. Some authors have recommended conservative surgery on the basis that the disease is highly likely to recur and that prolonged procedures and anesthetics should be avoided in this population with respiratory and occasional coagulation compromise [76]. Others advocate that if a procedure is to be undertaken, that as definitive a disease clearance as possible be achieved with optimization of anatomy for future management. This would include the addition of adenoidectomy in children and, for example, septoplasty where indicated.

SYMPTOM BENEFIT

Improvement following non-endoscopic [72,73] and subsequently endoscopic [2,76–80] sinus surgery of symptoms relating to nasal polyposis and chronic rhinosinusitis is universally reported. Recurrence of sinonasal disease is

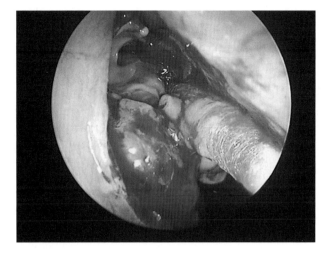

Figure 14.8 Endoscopic photograph showing both polyp and release of pocket of *Pseudomonas* pus from infected ethmoid air cell. *See also Plate 14.8.*

ultimately the rule, and persistence of radiological abnormality on CT imaging is inevitable [77,78,80]. Most studies are retrospective case series and duration of follow-up is frequently unclear.

In one prospective study of patients undergoing endoscopic sinus surgery with mean follow-up of 34 months, there were reported improvements in nasal obstructive symptoms, olfactory acuity, and reduction in purulent nasal discharge [28]. A mucopyocele-like disease process affecting the ethmoid and maxillary sinuses was frequent, but in spite of addressing this surgically, the nasal cavities remained abnormal.

In another study, patients became asymptomatic or improved in most cases [76]. They found on endoscopic appraisal of the nasal cavities that there was a 50% chance of returning to preoperative state by 18–24 months. They suggest that surgery was more effective at relieving infective processes than preventing recurrence of aggressive polyposis. Half of a subset who had had prior surgery in childhood had an average symptom-free period of 11.3 years before recurrence in adulthood.

Impact on pulmonary function

Although small studies have reported an improvement in lung function after sinus surgery, most have shown no change [65,81–83]. It must be borne in mind that this population is prone to wide variation in pulmonary function depending on infective exacerbations and intercurrent treatment, and this may render flawed small studies looking at pulmonary function at a given postoperative time-point.

Benefit to lung-transplant patients

Patients with advanced lung damage who are candidates for heart–lung transplantation have been recommended to undergo sinus surgery to reduce the likelihood of the sinuses acting as reservoirs for *Pseudomonas*. One pre-transplant protocol consists of FESS and wide antrostomy with postoperative saline and tobramycin irrigation to avoid pseudomonal and related pulmonary infection, with reports of only rare recurrent polyposis, and success in preventing pseudomonal pulmonary infection, although the time frame is not described [84]. Another group reported a significant decrease in the need for revision surgery with the use of postsinus surgical tobramycin irrigation in non-transplant CF patients [74]. *Pseudomonas* strain typing suggested that the sinuses were likely to be acting as a reservoir for bacterial spread, indicating that disease eradication or reduction in the sinuses might result in less secondary pulmonary infection [85].

Complications

Cystic fibrosis patients with significant respiratory compromise are not ideal candidates for protracted surgical procedures under general anesthetic [76]. The potential for disturbed clotting pathways secondary to vitamin K deficiency, malabsorption and thrombocytopenia secondary to hypersplenism is further cited as a risk factor for this surgery. Despite this, a retrospective review of surgical experience over a 42-year period found no complications from general anesthesia and no excessive bleeding or hypoxia postoperatively [86]. Complications are reported as similar in frequency and type to the non-CF population [87].

CONCLUSIONS

Cystic fibrosis is a complex multi-organ disease. The same pathophysiological processes affect the upper and lower airways alike. Chronic rhinosinusitis, with or without nasal polyposis, is manifest in a high proportion of sufferers. Developments in endoscopic and imaging techniques, and improved understanding of disease mechanisms, have led to improvements in diagnosis and treatment. Adequate management of sinonasal disease results in improved overall well-being and reduction in upper airway symptoms, and may have further impact in secondary benefit to lower respiratory function.

There is reasonable evidence to support the role of surgery to address symptomatic sinonasal disease in terms of improvement in symptom scores. The impact on lower respiratory function is less clear, but patients, in particular transplant patients, may benefit from the removal of a reservoir of infection in obstructed sinuses. However, the disease must be considered an incurable sinopathy and recurrence is inevitable. The time to recurrence appears to be related to the extent of disease clearance achieved at surgery. The extent of surgery undertaken should at least restore the airway and allow the disease to be controlled medically for prolonged periods.

REFERENCES

1. Shapiro ED, Milmoe GJ, Wald ER *et al*. Bacteriology of the maxillary sinuses in patients with cystic fibrosis. *J Infect Dis* 1982; **146**:589–593.
2. Brihaye P, Jorissen M, Clement PA. Chronic rhinosinusitis in cystic fibrosis (mucoviscidosis). *Acta Otorhinolaryngol Belg* 1997; **51**:323–337.
3. Cepero R, Smith RJ, Catlin FI *et al*. Cystic fibrosis: an otolaryngologic perspective. *Otolaryngol Head Neck Surg* 1987; **97**:356–360.
4. Adinoff AD, Cumming NP. Sinusitis and its relationship to asthma. *Pediatr Ann* 1989; **18**:785.
5. Rachelefsky GS, Katz RM, Siegel SC. Chronic sinus disease with associated reactive airway disease in children. *Pediatrics* 1984; **73**:526–529.
6. McFadden EA, Kany RJ, Fink JN, Toohill RJ. Surgery for sinusitis and aspirin triad. *Laryngoscope* 1990; **100**(10 Pt 1):1043–1046.
7. Nishioka GJ, Cook PR, Davis WE *et al*. Functional endoscopic sinus surgery in patients with chronic sinusitis and asthma. *Otolaryngol Head Neck Surg* 1994; **110**:494.
8. Parsons DS, Phillips SE. Functional endoscopic surgery in children: a retrospective analysis of results. *Laryngoscope* 1993; **103**:899–903.
9. Stammberger H, Posawetz W. Functional endoscopic sinus surgery: concept, indications and results of the Messerklinger technique. *Eur Arch Otorhinolaryngol* 1990; **247**(2):63–76.
10. Rutland J, Cole PJ. Nasal mucociliary clearance and ciliary beat frequency in cystic fibrosis compared with sinusitis and bronchiectasis. *Thorax* 1981; **36**:654–658.
11. Armengot M, Escribano A, Carda C *et al*. Nasal mucociliary transport and ciliary ultrastructure in cystic fibrosis: a comparative study with healthy volunteers. *Int J Pediatr Otorhinolaryngol* 1997; **40**(1):27–34.
12. McShane D, Davies JC, Wodehouse T *et al*. Normal nasal mucociliary clearance in CF children: evidence against a CFTR-related defect. *Eur Respir J* 2004; **24**:95–100.
13. Wilson R, Pitt T, Taylor G *et al*. Pyocyanin and 1-hydroxyphenazine produced by *Pseudomonas aeruginosa* inhibit the beating of human respiratory cilia *in vitro*. *J Clin Invest* 1987; **79**:221–229.
14. Munro NC, Barker A, Rutman A *et al*. Effect of pyocyanin and 1-hydroxyphenazine on in-vivo tracheal mucus velocity. *J Appl Physiol* 1989; **67**:316–323.
15. Amitani R, Wilson R, Rutman A *et al*. Effects of human neutrophil elastase and *Pseudomonas aeruginosa* proteinases on human respiratory epithelium. *Am J Respir Cell Mol Biol* 1991; **4**:26–32
16. Coste A, Gilain L, Roger G *et al*. Endoscopic and CT-scan evaluation of rhinosinusitis in cystic fibrosis. *Rhinology* 1995; **33**:152–156.
17. Hadfield PJ, Rowe-Jones JM, Mackay IS. The prevalence of nasal polyps in adults with cystic fibrosis. *Clin Otolaryngol Allied Sci* 2000; **25**:19–22.
18. Slieker MG, Schilder AG, Uiterwaal CS, van der Ent CK. Children with cystic fibrosis: who should visit the

otorhinolaryngologist? *Arch Otolaryngol Head Neck Surg* 2002; **128**:1245–1248.

19. Drake-Lee A. Nasal polyps. In: Mygind N, Naclerio RM (eds) *Allergic and Non-allergic Rhinitis.* Copenhagen, Munksgaard, 1993.

20. Tos M, Mogensen C, Thomsen J. Nasal polyps in cystic fibrosis. *J Laryngol Otol* 1977; **91**:827–835.

21. Henriksson G, Westrin KM, Karpati F *et al.* Nasal polyps in cystic fibrosis: clinical endoscopic study with nasal lavage fluid analysis. *Chest* 2002; **121**:40–47.

22. Taylor RF, Morgan DW, Nicholson PS *et al.* Extrapulmonary sites of *Pseudomonas aeruginosa* in adults with cystic fibrosis. *Thorax* 1992; **47**:426–428.

23. Wise SK, Kingdom TT, McKean L *et al.* Presence of fungus in sinus cultures of cystic fibrosis patients. *Am J Rhinol* 2005; **19**:47–51.

24. Bent JP, Kuhn FA. Diagnosis of allergic fungal sinusitis. *Otolaryngol Head Neck Surg* 1994; **111**:580–588.

25. King VV. Upper respiratory disease, sinusitis, and polyposis. *Clin Rev Allergy* 1991; **9**(1–2):143–157.

26. Kerrebijn JD, Poublon RM, Overbeek SE. Nasal and paranasal disease in adult cystic fibrosis patients. *Eur Respir J* 1992; **5**:1239–1242.

27. Cuyler JP, Monaghan AJ. Cystic fibrosis and sinusitis. *J Otolaryngol* 1989; **18**:173–175.

28. Nishioka GJ, Barbero GJ, Konig P *et al.* Symptom outcome after functional endoscopic sinus surgery in patients with cystic fibrosis: a prospective study. *Otolaryngol Head Neck Surg* 1995; **113**:440–445.

29. Brihaye P, Clement PA, Dab I, Desprechin B. Pathological changes of the lateral nasal wall in patients with cystic fibrosis (mucoviscidosis). *Int J Pediatr Otorhinolaryngol* 1994; **28**(2–3):141–147.

30. Gentile VG, Isaacson G. Patterns of sinusitis in cystic fibrosis. *Laryngoscope* 1996; **106**:1005–1009.

31. Nishioka GJ, Cook PR. Paranasal sinus disease in patients with cystic fibrosis. *Otolaryngol Clin N Am* 1996; **29**:193–205.

32. Raj P, Stableforth DE, Morgan DW. A prospective study of nasal disease in adult cystic fibrosis. *J Laryngol Otol* 2000; **114**:260–263.

33. Cimmino M, Cavaliere M, Nardone M *et al.* Clinical characteristics and genotype analysis of patients with cystic fibrosis and nasal polyposis. *Clin Otolaryngol Allied Sci* 2003; **28**:125–132.

34. Miller PW, Hamosh A, Macek M *et al.* Cystic fibrosis transmembrane conductance regulator (CFTR) gene mutations in allergic bronchopulmonary aspergillosis. *Am J Hum Genet* 1996; **59**:45–51.

35. Marchand E, Verellen-Dumoulin C, Mairesse M *et al.* Frequency of cystic fibrosis transmembrane conductance regulator gene mutations and 5T allele in patients with allergic bronchopulmonary aspergillosis. *Chest* 2001; **119**:762–767.

36. Venarske DL, deShazo RD. Sinobronchial allergic mycosis: the SAM syndrome. *Chest* 2002; **121**:1670–1676.

37. Pickhardt PJ, Siegel MJ, Hayashi RJ, Kelly M. Posttransplantation lymphoproliferative disorder in children:

clinical, histopathologic, and imaging features. *Radiology* 2000; **217**:16–25.

38. McAlister WH, Lusk R, Muntz HR. Comparison of plain radiographs and coronal CT scans in infants and children with recurrent sinusitis. *Am J Roentgenol* 1989; **153**:1259–1264.

39. Nishioka GJ, Cook PR, McKinsey JP, Rodriguez FJ. Paranasal sinus computed tomography scan findings in patients with cystic fibrosis. *Otolaryngol Head Neck Surg* 1996; **114**:394–399.

40. Kim HJ, Friedman EM, Sulek M *et al.* Paranasal sinus development in chronic sinusitis, cystic fibrosis, and normal comparison population: a computerized tomography correlation study. *Am J Rhinol* 1997; **11**:275–281.

41. Krzeski A, Kapiszewska-Dzedzej D, Jakubczyk I *et al.* Extent of pathological changes in the paranasal sinuses of patients with cystic fibrosis: CT analysis. *Am J Rhinol* 2001; **15**(3):207–210.

42. Mackay IS, Djazaeri B. Chronic sinusitis in cystic fibrosis. *J R Soc Med* 1994; **87**(Suppl 21):17–19.

43. Kim HJ, Friedman EM, Sulek M *et al.* Paranasal sinus development in chronic sinusitis, cystic fibrosis, and normal comparison population: a computerized tomography correlation study. *Am J Rhinol* 1997; **11**(4):275–281.

44. Davidson TM, Murphy C, Mitchell M *et al.* Management of chronic sinusitis in cystic fibrosis. *Laryngoscope* 1995; **105**(4 Pt 1):354–358.

45. Bolger WE, Woodruff WW, Morehead J, Parsons DS. Maxillary sinus hypoplasia: classification and description of associated uncinate process hypoplasia. *Otolaryngol Head Neck Surg* 1990; **103**(5 Pt 1):759–765.

46. Eggesbo HB, Dolvik S, Stiris M *et al.* Complementary role of MR imaging of ethmomaxillary sinus disease depicted at CT in cystic fibrosis. *Acta Radiol* 2001; **42**(2):144–150.

47. Hellquist HB. Nasal polyps update: histopathology. *Allergy Asthma Proc* 1996; **17**(5):237–242.

48. Tos M, Mogensen C, Thomsen J. Nasal polyps in cystic fibrosis. *J Laryngol Otol* 1977; **91**:827–835.

49. Oppenheimer EH, Rosenstein BJ. Differential pathology of nasal polyps in cystic fibrosis and atopy. *Lab Invest* 1979; **40**:445–449.

50. Sorensen H, Mygind N, Tygstrup I *et al.* Histology of nasal polyps of different etiology. *Rhinology* 1977; **15**(3):121–128.

51. Ramsey B, Richardson MA. Impact of sinusitis in cystic fibrosis. *J Allergy Clin Immunol* 1992; **90**(3 Pt 2):547–552.

52. Rowe-Jones JM, Shembekar M, Trendell-Smith N, Mackay IS. Polypoidal rhinosinusitis in cystic fibrosis: a clinical and histopathological study. *Clin Otolaryngol Allied Sci* 1997; **22**:167–171.

53. Beju D, Meek WD, Kramer JC. The ultrastructure of the nasal polyps in patients with and without cystic fibrosis. *J Submicrosc Cytol Pathol* 2004; **36**(2):155–165.

54. Hassid S, Choufani G, Decaestecker C *et al.* Glycohistochemical characteristics of nasal polyps from patients with and without cystic fibrosis. *Arch Otolaryngol Head Neck Surg* 2000; **126**:769–776.

55. Claeys S, Van Hoecke H, Holtappels G *et al.* Nasal polyps in patients with and without cystic fibrosis: a differentiation by innate markers and inflammatory mediators. *Clin Exp Allergy* 2005; **35**:467–472.

56. Sobol SE, Christodoulopoulos P, Manoukian JJ *et al.* Cytokine profile of chronic sinusitis in patients with cystic fibrosis. *Arch Otolaryngol Head Neck Surg* 2002; **128**:1295–1298.

57. Colantonio D, Brouillette L, Parikh A, Scadding GK. Paradoxical low nasal nitric oxide in nasal polyposis. *Clin Exp Allergy* 2002; **32**:698–701.

58. Balfour-Lynn IM, Laverty A, Dinwiddie R. Reduced upper airway nitric oxide in cystic fibrosis. *Arch Dis Child* 1996; **75**:319–322.

59. Lundberg JO, Nordvall SL, Weitzberg E *et al.* Exhaled nitric oxide in paediatric asthma and cystic fibrosis. *Arch Dis Child* 1996; **75**:323–326.

60. Dotsch J, Puls J, Klimek T, Rascher W. Reduction of neuronal and inducible nitric oxide synthase gene expression in patients with cystic fibrosis. *Eur Arch Otorhinolaryngol* 2002; **259**:222–226.

61. Rabago D, Pasic T, Zgierska A *et al.* The efficacy of hypertonic saline nasal irrigation for chronic sinonasal symptoms. *Otolaryngol Head Neck Surg* 2005; **133**:3–8.

62. Fokkens W, Lund V, Bachert C *et al.* EAACI position paper on rhinosinusitis and nasal polyps: executive summary. *Allergy* 2005; **60**:583–601.

63. Hadfield PJ, Rowe-Jones JM, Mackay IS. A prospective treatment trial of nasal polyps in adults with cystic fibrosis. *Rhinology* 2000; **38**(2):63–65.

64. Ramsey B, Richardson MA. Impact of sinusitis in cystic fibrosis. *J Allergy Clin Immunol* 1992; **90**(3 Pt 2):547–552.

65. Halvorson DJ, Dupree JR, Porubsky ES. Management of chronic sinusitis in the adult cystic fibrosis patient. *Ann Otol Rhinol Laryngol* 1998; **107**(11 Pt 1):946–952.

66. Iino Y, Sasaki Y, Miyazawa T, Kodera K. Nasopharyngeal flora and drug susceptibility in children with macrolide therapy. *Laryngoscope* 2003; **113**:1780–1785.

67. Hashiba M, Baba S. Efficacy of long-term administration of clarithromycin in the treatment of intractable chronic sinusitis. *Acta Otolaryngol Suppl* 1996; **525**:73–78.

68. Davidson TM, Murphy C, Mitchell M *et al.* Management of chronic sinusitis in cystic fibrosis. *Laryngoscope* 1995; **105**(4 Pt 1):354–358.

69. Lewiston N, King V, Umetsu D *et al.* Cystic fibrosis patients who have undergone heart–lung transplantation benefit from maxillary sinus antrostomy and repeated sinus lavage. *Transplant Proc* 1991; **23**(1 Pt 2):1207–1208.

70. Raynor EM, Butler A, Guill M, Bent JP. Nasally inhaled dornase alfa in the postoperative management of chronic sinusitis due to cystic fibrosis. *Arch Otolaryngol Head Neck Surg* 2000; **126**:581–583.

71. Cimmino M, Nardone M, Cavaliere M *et al.* Dornase alfa as postoperative therapy in cystic fibrosis sinonasal disease. *Arch Otolaryngol Head Neck Surg* 2005; **131**:1097–1101.

72. Drake-Lee AB, Morgan DW. Nasal polyps and sinusitis in children with cystic fibrosis. *J Laryngol Otol* 1989; **103**:753–755.

73. Crockett DM, McGill TJ, Healy GB *et al.* Nasal and paranasal sinus surgery in children with cystic fibrosis. *Ann Otol Rhinol Laryngol* 1987; **96**:367–372.

74. Moss RB, King VV. Management of sinusitis in cystic fibrosis by endoscopic surgery and serial antimicrobial lavage: reduction in recurrence requiring surgery. *Arch Otolaryngol Head Neck Surg* 1995; **121**:566–572.

75. Jarrett WA, Militsakh O, Anstad M, Manaligod J. Endoscopic sinus surgery in cystic fibrosis: effects on pulmonary function and ideal body weight. *Ear Nose Throat J* 2004; **83**:118–121.

76. Rowe-Jones JM, Mackay IS. Endoscopic sinus surgery in the treatment of cystic fibrosis with nasal polyposis. *Laryngoscope* 1996; **106**(12 Pt 1):1540–1544.

77. Duplechain JK, White JA, Miller RH. Pediatric sinusitis: the role of endoscopic sinus surgery in cystic fibrosis and other forms of sinonasal disease. *Arch Otolaryngol Head Neck Surg* 1991; **117**:422–426.

78. Cuyler JP. Follow-up of endoscopic sinus surgery on children with cystic fibrosis. *Arch Otolaryngol Head Neck Surg* 1992; **118**:505–506.

79. Jones JW, Parsons DS, Cuyler JP. The results of functional endoscopic sinus (FES) surgery on the symptoms of patients with cystic fibrosis. *Int J Pediatr Otorhinolaryngol* 1993; **28**(1):25–32.

80. Yung MW, Gould J, Upton GJ. Nasal polyposis in children with cystic fibrosis: a long-term follow-up study. *Ann Otol Rhinol Laryngol* 2002; **111**(12 Pt 1):1081–1086.

81. Madonna D, Isaacson G, Rosenfeld RM, Panitch H. Effect of sinus surgery on pulmonary function in patients with cystic fibrosis. *Laryngoscope* 1997; **107**:328–331.

82. Umetsu DT, Moss RB, King VV, Lewiston NJ. Sinus disease in patients with severe cystic fibrosis: relation to pulmonary exacerbation. *Lancet* 1990; **335**:1077–1078.

83. Rosbe KW, Jones DT, Rahbar R *et al.* Endoscopic sinus surgery in cystic fibrosis: do patients benefit from surgery? *Int J Pediatr Otorhinolaryngol* 2001; **61**(2):113–119.

84. Davidson TM, Murphy C, Mitchell M *et al.* Management of chronic sinusitis in cystic fibrosis. *Laryngoscope* 1995; **105**(4 Pt 1):354–358.

85. Holzmann D, Speich R, Kaufmann T *et al.* Effects of sinus surgery in patients with cystic fibrosis after lung transplantation: a 10-year experience. *Transplantation* 2004; **77**(1):134–136.

86. Schulte DL, Kasperbauer JL. Safety of paranasal sinus surgery in patients with cystic fibrosis. *Laryngoscope* 1998; **108**:1813–1815.

87. Albritton FD, Kingdom TT. Endoscopic sinus surgery in patients with cystic fibrosis: an analysis of complications. *Am J Rhinol* 2000; **14**:379–385.

Gastrointestinal disease in cystic fibrosis

IAN GOODING AND DAVID WESTABY

INTRODUCTION

The gastrointestinal tract is a major source of morbidity in cystic fibrosis (CF). Clinical entities such as distal intestinal obstruction syndrome (DIOS) and fibrosing colonopathy are essentially peculiar to CF, while other gastrointestinal conditions are encountered more frequently or behave differently in CF. In general, these conditions respond well to good medical management or prompt surgical intervention when indicated. The prevalence of various gastrointestinal entities relevant to CF is shown in Table 15.1.

MOLECULAR BIOLOGY

Cystic fibrosis transmembrane regulator (CFTR) is expressed on the luminal membrane of enterocytes. The pathophysiology of electrolyte and water movements across the intestinal

Table 15.1 Prevalence of gastrointestinal entities relevant to CF.

Condition	Prevalence
Malabsorption	85%
Gastro-esophageal reflux disease	26.5–80%
Rectal prolapse	20%
Distal intestinal obstruction syndrome	16%
Meconium ileus	6–20%
Appendicitis	1.5%
Intussusception	1%
Celiac disease	0.4%
Crohn's disease	0.22%
Volvulus	Case reports only
Peptic ulcer disease	Rare
Fibrosing colonopathy	Now rare

mucosa in CF is extensively discussed in a recent review [1]. Three separate mechanisms are affected. First, and probably most important, is the loss of Cl^- secretion via CFTR in response to stimulation (e.g. by acetylcholine and serotonin). Normally, this Cl^- flux creates a negative potential on the luminal side of the epithelium which causes a Na^+ flux into the lumen through tight junctions between the cells, with water following osmotically. Second, the inhibition of electroneutral NaCl absorption from the lumen into the enterocyte via a CFTR-independent mechanism is impaired. Third, the co-transport of Na^+ with nutrients such as glucose and alanine across the brush border is increased. All three mechanisms act to reduce the flow of water into the lumen (Fig. 15.1).

ABNORMAL FINDINGS IN CF

The following pathological and physiological abnormalities have been demonstrated in CF. What contribution these phenomena make to the clinical syndromes seen in CF is unclear and the evolution of most of the entities discussed in this chapter is poorly understood. This has to be seen in the context or our limited understanding of the control of gastrointestinal (GI) motility and secretion in normal physiology. However, there seems no doubt that the changes in the luminal milieu resulting from abnormalities of pancreatic and intestinal secretion is a dominant factor.

Histopathology

Farber described the presence of inspissated mucus and dilated mucosal glands in the duodenum and esophagus in 1944 [2]. Electron microscopy studies have shown abnormalities of goblet cells, tight junctions, mitochondria and Golgi apparatus in enterocytes [3]. Brush border morphology is normal.

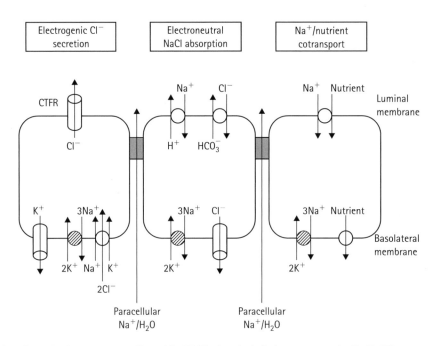

Figure 15.1 Electrolyte fluxes in the enterocyte affected in CF. The hatched circles represent the Na/K-ATPase pump. Flow of sodium, chloride and water into the lumen via all three mechanisms is reduced in CF. CFTR is only directly involved in electrogenic chloride secretion but may interact with other transport proteins to increase sodium influx into the cell via the other two mechanisms. Reproduced from [1] with permission from Karger AG, Basel.

Radiology

Contrast studies of the stomach and small intestine show thickened mucosal folds, nodular filling defects and variable dilatation in 80% [4]. Ultrasound studies have shown a marked increase in small and large intestinal wall thickness [5]. The histopathological changes behind these observed visceral wall changes (whether dilated glands and mucus in the crypts, fibrosis or edema) are not entirely clear. Pneumatosis intestinalis is also commonly seen, as in other chronic respiratory diseases, and is clinically silent.

pH studies

Some studies show an increased gastric acid output in CF, although whether this indicates genuine hypersecretion is unclear as acid secretion is usually expressed relative to body weight. In any case, gastric pH is normal. Duodenal pH, however, is reduced, especially post-prandially, and jejunal pH is probably low too [6]. This is undoubtedly a consequence of reduced pancreatic bicarbonate but duodenal bicarbonate secretion is also reduced [1]. This may inhibit both endogenous and exogenous pancreatic enzyme activity.

Motility

A number of parameters of gastrointestinal motility have been investigated, to a varying extent. There is conflicting

evidence regarding esophageal motility and gastric emptying (see later). Small bowel manometry has not been assessed. Lactulose/hydrogen breath testing showed a marked delay in oro–cecal transit in a number of studies [6], although this test depends on luminal bacterial populations, which may be disturbed in CF for a variety of reasons. There has been limited assessment of colonic transit and motility.

Intestinal permeability

There is a 4- to 10-fold increase in small intestinal paracellular permeability, with no change in transcellular permeability in CF. The paracellular pathway leaks large, water-soluble molecules through tight junctions, while the transcellular route transfers small or lipid-soluble molecules through membrane pores. This seems to be in keeping with the electron microscopy findings. Proton pump inhibitor therapy has been shown to partly correct abnormal intestinal permeability [7].

Inflammation

A number of lines of evidence point to chronic inflammation in the CF gastrointestinal tract. Chronic inflammation was demonstrated in duodenal biopsies [8]. High levels of calprotectin (a non-specific marker of GI inflammation) were found in fecal samples [8] and of cytokines in whole-gut lavage fluid [9].

Gastrointestinal hormone levels

Elevated motilin, neurotensin, enteroglucagon and peptide YY have been demonstrated in CF [6].

MALABSORPTION

The major factor causing malabsorption in CF is deficiency of pancreatic lipolytic and proteolytic enzymes. The pathological changes of the pancreas are described in Chapter 15b. Pancreatic insufficiency (PI) is present in 85% of CF patients, but 99% of ΔF508 homozygotes. PI is most often present from birth. In common with other causes of PI, steatorrhea and azotorrhea generally do not appear until lipase and trypsin levels are below 1–2% of normal. In approximately 15% of CF individuals, pancreatic changes are less severe and sufficient functional pancreatic exocrine tissue remains to allow normal fat and protein digestion. However, such pancreatic-sufficient (PS) individuals do not as a group have normal pancreatic exocrine function. Immunoreactive trypsinogen (IRT) levels tend to remain elevated in CF patients who are PS [10]. Deficiencies of pancreatic exocrine function can usually be demonstrated if more sensitive tests such as studies of fluid and bicarbonate secretion, total enzyme output or IRT response to pancreatic stimulation are performed [10–13]. The cholecystokinin (CCK)–secretin test is also usually abnormal in PS patients and this test can be helpful in making the diagnosis of CF when sweat tests and DNA analysis have not resolved the issue. Patients who are pancreatic-sufficient have been reported to have better nutrition and an improved prognosis with regard to the development of respiratory disease [12]. With increasing age, PS individuals may eventually become PI, particularly if they have 'severe' mutations, including *F508del* [14,15].

A number of luminal factors may also be relevant, especially to cases where pancreatic enzyme replacement alone does not lead to resolution of steatorrhea. Small intestinal acidity, secondary to reduced pancreatic bicarbonate production, may impair absorption in three ways. First, lipase activity is directly reduced in acidic conditions. Second, a low pH causes the precipitation of bile acids so that bile acid concentrations fall below the critical concentration for formation of micelles, inhibiting emulsification of fats which is essential for their digestion and absorption. Third, the enteric coatings used in modern pancreatic enzyme preparations are designed to release their contents as the pH rises on passage from the stomach to the small intestine. A low duodenal pH may impair this release and lead to treatment failure. Additionally, the cholestasis of CF liver disease impairs the delivery of bile acids to the duodenum, reducing small bowel bile acid concentrations and fat absorption. Intestinal uptake of fatty acids after enzymatic digestion may also be abnormal in some individuals [16].

Clinical presentation of pancreatic insufficiency

The clinical triad of ravenous appetite, steatorrhea and malnutrition or failure to thrive in an infant or young child is highly suggestive of CF with pancreatic insufficiency. A diagnostic sweat test is mandatory in such patients. Abdominal pain, bloating, foul flatus and rectal prolapse are also frequent and prominent symptoms. Additionally, PI can lead to edema, caused by hypoalbuminemia, and hemolytic anemia caused by vitamin E deficiency. Some CF infants with PI may avoid overt malnutrition or failure to thrive by means of pre-duodenal (lingual or gastric) lipase and lipases present in human breast milk [17]. These presymptomatic PI infants may nonetheless have significant nutritional deficiencies. In one study of such infants detected by IRT screening, deficiencies of fat-soluble vitamins such as D (35%), E (38%) and A (21%), were present by 3 months of age [18].

The first prerequisite of pancreatic enzyme replacement therapy in CF is to establish that such therapy is required. This is most accurately determined by measurement of 72-hour fecal fat excretion but more simply by measurement of human fecal elastase-1 on a small sample of stool. Specific pancreatic function tests such as the CCK–secretin test may be useful in this respect.

Therapy of pancreatic insufficiency

Therapy of pancreatic insufficiency in CF patients is based on the oral replacement of pancreatic enzymes. Numerous preparations are commercially available and important differences exist between them. All currently available preparations use enzymes of porcine origin. Enteric-coated microspheres, microtablets or granules are the modern preferred form of administration. The enteric coating protects the enzymes from denaturation by gastric acid. The coating disintegrates at higher pH to deliver greater duodenal enzyme concentrations than the older powder preparations. The differing chemical nature of the various enteric coatings may be of significance for the risk of fibrosing colonopathy (see later). Another variable is particle size which may influence the rate of passage through the pylorus [19,20]. The resulting separation of the enzyme dose from the meal may impair efficacy.

Once the requirement for pancreatic enzyme therapy is established, for patients over 1 year of age, a standard enteric-coated pancreatic enzyme preparation should be started at a dose of 500 units of lipase per kilogram body weight per meal, and half of this dose per snack. Enzymes are required with each fat- or protein-containing meal, snack or drink, but not for juices or fruit. It is often advised that enzymes be administered both at the beginning and during the meal to ensure thorough mixing of enzymes and meal throughout its small intestinal passage. A simpler alternative is to take enzymes at the start of the meal, as this is more readily remembered and convenient. There is also evidence that enteric-coated preparations are more effective when given at the start of a meal [21]. There is evidence of differential rates of gastric emptying for food and microspheres in some children, necessitating the giving of enzymes before and during the meal.

For young children who cannot yet swallow capsules, these may be opened and given in a teaspoon of apple sauce or similar medium. However, care must be taken to ensure that the child does not chew and break the microspheres. Enzyme-and-food mixtures should not be exposed to excessive heat and should not be stored for more than 1 hour.

Once enzymes have been started, the dosage is then gradually adjusted at 3- to 4-day intervals. The most practical tool for assessing adequacy of dose is the stool pattern. Dosages are adjusted upwards to achieve normal or near-normal stool pattern with formed, non-greasy stools of normal odor and absence of abdominal pain or excessive and malodorous flatus. Stool microscopy for fat globules may be helpful in some cases to monitor efficacy of therapy [22]. The maximum recommended dose is of 2500 units of lipase/kg per meal or 10 000 units of lipase/kg each day. These limits have been advised by the Committee on Safety of Medicines on account of the risk of fibrosing colonopathy. Higher dosages should only be considered after careful investigation into compliance, exclusion of other pathology and after trials of alternative enzyme preparations and adjuvants. Three-day fecal fat collections should be done to demonstrate that the increased dose is leading to an improved absorption and close supervision is required.

Management of enzyme therapy in the newly diagnosed CF infant requires special care. In this age group the number of feeds per day will change as the infant grows. Therefore enzyme intake will require frequent adjustment not only to cover increasing intake but also to accommodate changing meal patterns. Enteric-coated preparations should always be used – microspheres or microtablets should be emptied from the capsule, divided equally and given in a small amount of apple sauce immediately before each feed. The same regimen can be used for breast-fed infants, since the enteric coating protects the mother's nipple. When an infant's next feed occurs within 1–2 hours of the previous enzyme dose, it is generally not necessary to repeat the dose. A suitable initial dose for a full-term infant is 1000–2000 units of lipase per feed. This usually approximates to 250–500 units/kg body weight per feed. This initial dosage will require revision at 3- to 4-day intervals until the stooling pattern is normalized and normal growth is attained. As the infant grows, the number of feeds per day will naturally decrease. By one year of age, the infant is usually taking three meals and two snacks per day, and required enzyme dosage is usually in the range 500–2000 units of lipase/kg per meal and half that per snack.

CF patients receiving enteral tube feeding (via a nasogastric, gastrostomy or jejunostomy tube) present a problem as enteric-coated enzyme preparations can lead to tube blockage. A solution is 'Creon Micro', an enteric-coated formula that can go down nasogastric tubes. It is half the strength of Creon 10 000 (5000 lipase units per scoop, as opposed to 10 000), and needs significant volumes of flush if the granules are to clear the tube.

Inadequate therapeutic response and adjuvant therapies

Despite appropriate titration of enzyme dosage, 10% or more of CF patients continue to have significant fat malabsorption or poor growth [23]. This situation requires careful investigation.

The most common cause is non-compliance. Often this may be a sign that the patient or family has failed to come to terms with the implications of having CF. If careful explanation and discussion does not improve the situation, such patients and families may require psychological or psychiatric counselling.

The efficacy of the enzyme preparation should be considered and the way it is handled discussed with the patient and family. Substandard potency and inadequate dissolution characteristics have been reported with some generic or alternative-brand enzyme preparations [24]. Since pancreatic enzymes are biological products, faulty or prolonged storage may result in significant loss of activity. If there is any question about potency or dissolution characteristics of a product, these should either be assayed, or a new supply obtained and response to its use assessed before progressing to further investigation.

A stool sample should be taken for microscopy and culture. Giardiasis is a possible cause or treatment failure, which is reported to be more common in CF (see below for investigation and treatment).

If none of the above provides an explanation, the next step is to try an adjuvant therapy to increase gastric pH, such as antacids, H_2-histamine receptor antagonists or proton pump inhibitors. The administration of sodium bicarbonate or other antacids with the oral enzyme preparation (such as aluminium hydroxide) is effective, but magnesium- or calcium-based antacids should not be used as they have been reported to interact with glycine-conjugated bile salts. Proton pump inhibitors have been shown to decrease fecal fat loss and increase fat absorption [25] with improvements in weight, height, fat mass and bone mineral content [26].

Finally, it is appropriate to experiment with different enzyme preparations, as they have different characteristics as outlined above.

Adverse effects of enzyme therapy

A number of side-effects are associated with enzyme therapy. Perioral and perianal irritation are common in infants. Enteric-coated preparations and lower doses are less likely to cause problems. Protective barrier creams are also useful. Infants also have a propensity to develop watery diarrhea and crampy abdominal pain or colic when dosages are excessive. These may resemble the signs of PI and can be mistaken for the consequences of inadequate enzyme dose. Large doses have been associated with hyperuricemia and hyperuricosuria related to purine contamination or the enzyme preparations [24]. For a discussion of fibrosing colonopathy, see later.

MECONIUM ILEUS

Meconium ileus (MI) occurs in 6–20% of CF neonates. With early detection and appropriate therapy, it is now uncommon for infants to die of this complication and long-term outcome equals that of other CF patients [27].

Pathophysiology

Small intestinal obstruction is caused by an accumulation of abnormally viscid meconium, which becomes inspissated within the lumen. Meconium ileus is also found in normal neonates, in conditions unrelated to CF (including congenital pancreatic abnormalities) and in pancreatic-sufficient CF. Nevertheless, most neonates with meconium ileus have CF with pancreatic insufficiency and it appears to correlate with *F508del*, *G242X* and other mutations which are severe with respect to pancreatic phenotype [14]. Within the CF population, the tendency to express the MI phenotype may also be influenced by non-*CFTR* genes [1].

Clinical presentation and diagnosis

The usual clinical presentation is with bowel obstruction within 48 hours of birth. History may reveal polyhydramnios, fetal hyperechogenic bowel and failure to pass meconium, although small amounts may be passed. A perforation and meconium peritonitis may be diagnosed antenatally. There may be bile staining of vomit. Abdominal distension and dilated bowel loops are usually apparent on inspection and palpation, and there may be a right lower quadrant or pelvic mass. Rectal examination produces only a small amount of sticky meconium or a dry mucus plug. Abdominal radiograph may demonstrate calcification in about a quarter of cases of CF and MI [28]. The classic right lower quadrant speckled 'ground-glass' or 'soap-bubble' appearance on x-ray is seen in about one-third to one-half of patients. However, this appearance may also be seen in Hirschsprung's disease, small bowel atresia, meconium plug syndrome, small left colon syndrome, imperforate anus and obstruction due to a duplication cyst. Distended bowel loops are typical, usually with no air–fluid levels [29]. Contrast enema may show microcolon with meconium pellets in the distal ileum.

About 40% of cases present with complicated MI. This results when MI is accompanied by intestinal atresia, volvulus or antenatal perforation with meconium peritonitis. Small bowel ischemia due to volvulus or damage to the bowel wall may lead to jejunal atresia, which usually appears in the third trimester [30], and to calcification which is usually intramural. After an antenatal perforation, the bowel may seal over before birth. Liberated meconium may be contained as a pseudocyst or disseminated as meconium peritonitis. This chemical peritonitis may lead to the rapid development of serosal or scrotal calcification (although the most common cause of meconium peritonitis is small bowel atresia without CF) [29].

Meconium ileus in CF can often be detected *in utero* by ultrasound from early in the second trimester [29]. The finding of hyperechoic or dilated fetal bowel persisting after 20 weeks' gestation is suggestive of CF and MI, but is not specific and mandates a careful diagnostic evaluation for which a useful algorithm has been published [30].

Therapy

Therapy of uncomplicated MI involves decompression and relief of obstruction. This can often be accomplished by use of a gastrografin enema [31]. The gastrografin enema may need to be repeated for successful treatment. Neonates with MI which fails to respond to gastrografin enema require operative intervention. The surgical treatment of choice is laparotomy with gastrografin or *N*-acetylcysteine irrigation of the obstructed segment through the dilated ileum or appendiceal stump [32]. Temporary ileostomy to allow a microcolon time to enlarge may be useful measures in this regard [33].

There has been concern that the use of hypertonic contrast agents such as gastrografin may irritate the neonatal bowel mucosa, and deaths from necrotizing enterocolitis following use of gastrografin or renografin for MI have been reported [29]. Non-ionic, less hyperosmolar contrast agents or dilute ionic contrast agents mixed with *N*-acetylcysteine may be safer.

Complicated MI requires surgical management, consisting of bowel resection, irrigation anastomosis or creation of an enterostomy as appropriate [32]. Finally, since MI is not pathognomonic of CF with PI, the diagnosis and pancreatic status should always be confirmed with appropriate tests.

MECONIUM PLUG SYNDROME

Abnormal meconium occasionally produces colonic, rather than distal ileal, obstruction. The meconium plug syndrome may often be confused with MI, but is a separate and distinct entity. Affected infants have mild abdominal distension and fail to pass meconium at birth. Rectal examination reveals a tight anal canal. Contrast enema shows a normal colonic caliber with distal colonic obstruction by meconium [29]. The meconium plug is often expelled, with relief of symptoms, after rectal examination or enema. Twenty-five percent of infants with the meconium plug syndrome have underlying CF [34].

GASTROESOPHAGEAL REFLUX DISEASE

Since the first description of an association between gastroesophageal reflux (GER) and CF in 1975 [35], there has been an increased awareness of the importance of this association. GER is important for its effects on quality of life. However, it may also adversely impact on respiratory function and nutritional status.

Prevalence

A number of studies now point to a strong association between CF and gastroesophageal reflux. Heartburn was reported in 26.5% and regurgitation in 20.6% of patients (mean age 13 years), compared to 4.4% and 0%, respectively, in a control group composed of siblings without CF [36]. In adults, 80% admitted to heartburn and 52% to regurgitation in an uncontrolled study [37]. The most objective method of assessing gastroesophageal reflux is ambulatory esophageal pH monitoring. No controlled studies have been reported but the observational data paints a similar picture. Studies in young children (under 5 years) have demonstrated increased esophageal acid exposure in 76% [38] and 80% [39] of patients. Similarly, in older children abnormal results were found in 55% [40] and 66% [41]. Studies quoting the reflux index (percentage of time the esophageal pH is below 4) give values of 12.6% [36] and 7.9% [42] compared to a published normal value of 1.5%. Barrett's esophagus, a condition that is thought to develop as a consequence of extensive esophageal exposure to refluxate over many years, has been reported in two CF patients, aged 14 and 16 years, indicating the extent of acid exposure that can occur early in life [43].

Pathogenesis

The mechanisms behind gastroesophageal reflux in CF are not well understood. In general, GER has a multifactorial pathogenesis. The condition results from impaired function of the muscular barrier to reflux (the combination of the lower esophageal sphincter and the crural diaphragm) together with impaired esophageal clearance of refluxate and delayed gastric emptying. The lower esophageal sphincter is a 3- to 4-cm long segment of tonically contracted circular smooth muscle at the distal end of the esophagus. The majority of reflux episodes are caused by transient relaxations of the sphincter (TLOSRs) which are a vagally-mediated physiological reflex response to gastric distension, permitting belching. A minority of patients have a hypotensive lower esophageal sphincter (LOS). A hiatus hernia disrupts the anatomical relationship of the crural diaphragm to the LOS and may promote reflux during stress maneuvers such as coughing. In addition, hiatus hernia impairs esophageal clearance of refluxate.

It was initially postulated that GER in patients with CF was as a consequence of respiratory disease. An elevated prevalence of GER of comparable magnitude to that seen in CF has been demonstrated in asthma, recurrent pneumonia, chronic obstructive pulmonary disease and idiopathic pulmonary fibrosis. Whether a causal link is operative (in either direction) remains an unresolved question. A depressed diaphragm may affect the anatomy of the lower esophageal sphincter. Coughing and altered tidal volumes may lead to a transient pressure gradient between the abdomen and the thorax, which overcomes the LOS barrier. However, in CF, the finding of GER in young children together with evidence of declining prevalence with age (as the pulmonary disease usually progresses) argue against this.

A number of studies have looked at esophageal manometry to elucidate the basis of GER in CF. The most comprehensive of these used simultaneous ambulatory manometry and pH monitoring in fourteen children aged 5 months to 16 years, finding that 53.3% of reflux events in CF were attributable to TLOSRs with only 6.6% related to LOS hypotension [44]. Importantly this pattern was also seen in non-CF children with GER whereas those with respiratory complications of GER were more likely to have LOS hypotension. Other studies, using stationary manometry, have found normal LOS resting pressure in children [36,41], but LOS hypotension in six of ten adults [37]. These studies also looked for esophageal body dysmotility (which could impair esophageal clearance of refluxate); this was absent in children [41] but present in three of ten adults [37]. Malnutrition could theoretically contribute to GER by causing muscular atrophy and weakening LOS, diaphragmatic and esophageal body function. Only the single small adult study lends any objective weight to this hypothesis.

Gastric emptying has been assessed in CF in a number of studies but no consistent picture has emerged. Tests performed without administration of supplemental enzymes found emptying to be rapid. This is not surprising and is in keeping with results for patients with pancreatic insufficiency not due to CF. However, rapid gastric emptying of liquids has been found, even with administration of pancreatic enzymes. Studies of solid-phase emptying in CF have yielded conflicting results [45,46].

A controversial issue is whether postural drainage techniques contribute to GER. In infants, fewer episodes of reflux were found comparing techniques employing a 30-degree head-up tilt with conventional physiotherapy with a 30-degree head-down tilt. However, the reflux index, which is likely to be more important, was unchanged [47]. In older children, physiotherapy conducted during ambulatory pH studies did not cause reflux, but it is not clear which techniques were used [44].

LOS pressure is reduced by a number of drugs used by CF patients such as β-agonists (others include theophylline, calcium antagonists, opioids and benzodiazepines). Dietary fat causes both a post-prandial fall in LOS pressure and delayed gastric emptying, but is a necessary part of a high-calorie diet in many patients, especially those with diabetes. Alcohol also lowers LOS pressure.

In summary, physiological testing has failed to reveal a consistent abnormality in CF which might be responsible for GER. As with GER in the general population, most reflux events seem to coincide with TLOSRs, but it is not clear if TLOSRs are more common or if reflux is more likely during TLOSR in CF patients.

Clinical presentation

The most common symptoms of GER are heartburn and acid regurgitation (the effortless return of gastric or esophageal contents to the pharynx and mouth without nausea or retching). Odynophagia, chest pain, nausea and dysphagia are less frequent manifestations. Asymptomatic GER is common in CF [42].

GER may adversely affect respiratory function. Two theories have been advanced. The *reflux* theory proposes that this is mediated by aspiration of gastric contents into the lung. Animal studies have shown that tracheal infusion of miniscule amounts of acid is associated with profound bronchoconstriction. Tracheal acidification was demonstrated in 4 of 11 CF patients with GER symptoms, although PEFR was largely unaffected [48]. The *reflex* theory proposes that esophageal acidification causes bronchoconstriction via stimulation of esophageal vagal afferents.

Only one study has looked at whether the severity of GER correlates with the severity of respiratory disease in CF. In 12 CF patients (median age 14.4 years), there was a significant correlation between a score based on esophageal physiology testing and reduced first-second forced expired volume (FEV_1) and increased volume of trapped gas, although the correlation with a spirometry score fell short of statistical significance [41]. Obviously, the direction of causation is unclear in this correlation. Evidence that GER may exacerbate respiratory disease may be inferred from studies of treatment of GER in other respiratory conditions. Andze and co-workers [49] reported on 500 infants with a variety of respiratory problems (apnea, asthma, recurrent pneumonia, recurrent bronchiolitis, and chronic cough) who had had esophageal pH studies. They showed high prevalence of GER in all the categories of respiratory disease and high rates of response of the respiratory condition to medical or surgical treatment of the GER [49]. Treatment of GER results in symptomatic and objective improvement of asthma in a minority of adult patients.

GER may impair nutritional status by inducing nausea or by post-prandial worsening of GER leading to reduced intake. Occasionally, esophageal strictures may cause dysphagia which may be amenable to endoscopic treatment [50]. In Gustafsson's study, the esophageal physiology score showed a significant correlation with reduced body weight (the same qualifier about the direction of causation applies) [41].

Diagnosis

Generally speaking, it is reasonable to proceed to a trial of medical therapy for GER on clinical grounds alone and reserve invasive tests for those who fail to respond. Occult GER should be considered in the differential diagnosis of the patient with deteriorating pulmonary function, especially if the reasons are unclear.

Esophagogastroduodenoscopy (EGD) allows exclusion of peptic ulceration, other causes of esophagitis and also gastric outlet obstruction which may cause GER. If typical findings of reflux esophagitis are found the diagnosis of GER is confirmed (although EGD is commonly normal in GER). The presence of complications such as esophageal stricture and Barrett's esophagus can be assessed. Respiratory function permitting, EGD should be performed in patients with dysphagia, severe symptoms unresponsive to medical therapy and if there is a clinical suspicion of peptic ulceration. Barium swallow and meal is a less adequate alternative for those who cannot tolerate EGD.

In selected cases, 24-hour ambulatory esophageal pH monitoring, preceded by a stationary esophageal manometry study, may confirm the presence of GER and exclude forms of esophageal dysmotility such as achalasia. pH studies are useful in cases where there is doubt regarding whether GER is the cause of symptoms. An example would be a patient with symptoms that are typical for GER but which have failed to respond to PPI therapy. pH studies should also be conducted prior to surgery or endoscopic therapy. If episodes of pulmonary aspiration are suspected then esophageal physiological assessment may extend to impedance studies. This technique assesses liquid volume regurgitation which may occur in the absence of acid content [51].

Treatment

Standard non-pharmacological recommendations used include elevation of the head of the bed, avoidance of tight-fitting garments, restriction of alcohol intake and avoidance of lying down after meals. In infants thickened feeds can be used.

Drugs used fall into two groups, acid suppressants and prokinetics. Proton pump inhibitors (PPIs) are established as the highly efficacious agents for control of GER symptoms and healing of reflux esophagitis. Concerns about their long-term safety have lessened over the past ten years and certainly need not inhibit their use in CF. There have been a number of studies of PPIs in CF examining their effect on pancreatin efficacy, but none has assessed their effect on GER. However, whilst PPIs raise the pH of the refluxate, reflux (and the theoretical risk of aspiration) may continue. Prokinetic drugs that raise LOS tone and enhance gastric emptying have shown promise in GER. Cisapride has been used in two studies and produced improvements in pH recordings and endoscopic appearances [39,40]. In infants, cisapride also produced a growth spurt and disappearance of wheeze and cough [39]. Unfortunately, cisapride has been withdrawn due to an arrhythmogenic tendency. Domperidone and low-dose erythromycin are logical alternatives which have not been assessed in CF, but are likely to be less efficacious.

Surgical fundoplication is an option for patients who fail to respond to medical therapy. It has been reported in small numbers of CF patients [49,52,53]. However, chronic lung disease is the leading risk factor for failure of antireflux procedures in children [54]. There is concern that this applies to CF patients, perhaps with chronic cough causing failure of the wrap. A variety of endoscopic procedures to enhance the anatomical barrier to reflux has been introduced and would be attractive in these patients. However, none has yet shown sufficient efficacy to enter routine practice.

DISTAL INTESTINAL OBSTRUCTION SYNDROME

In 1962, Jensen first used the term 'meconium ileus equivalent' to describe intestinal obstruction due to inspissated intestinal contents after the neonatal period [55]. The term distal intestinal obstruction syndrome (DIOS) is now preferred, as the pathophysiology and treatment are distinct from meconium ileus, though related.

Pathophysiology

The pathophysiology of DIOS is not fully understood. The terminal ileum and/or right colon become obstructed by putty-like fecal material (Fig. 15.2). The following factors are likely to contribute:

- *Pancreatic exocrine deficiency.* Pancreatic insufficiency was once thought to be a prerequisite for DIOS, but the condition has been reported with normal pancreatic function [56]. Nonetheless the overwhelming majority of cases have pancreatic insufficiency [57]. It has been reported that DIOS is commoner in CF patients receiving suboptimal pancreatic enzyme therapy, but this finding is not uniform. However DIOS does not occur in other forms of pancreatic insufficiency, so other CF-related factors are necessary.
- *Abnormal electrolyte and fluid transport across the intestinal mucosa.* CF enterocytes display abnormalities of Cl^- secretion [6,58], reducing the water content of intestinal contents.
- *Abnormal intestinal motility.* A number of studies have shown prolonged oro–cecal transit times in CF [6], including one that demonstrated longer transit times in those with DIOS than in those without the syndrome

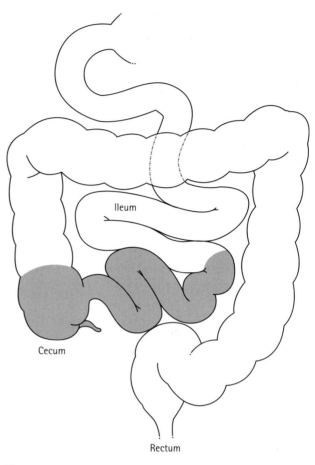

Figure 15.2   Diagram showing the pathophysiology of distal intestinal obstruction syndrome (DIOS), in which the distal small bowel and cecum become obstructed by putty-like fecal material (grey).

[59]. This may promote DIOS by increasing the time contents are in contact with intestinal mucosa and thus water absorption from the lumen and also indicate a defective ability of the intestinal smooth muscle to clear viscous material from the lumen.

Episodes of dehydration can precipitate DIOS. One study of dietary fiber found no evidence that deficient intake contributes to DIOS [60]. There is also no evidence that intestinal pH or bowel wall thickness affect the development of DIOS [5,59].

Prevalence

DIOS may occur at any time after the neonatal period and appears to be more common in adolescent and adult patients. Estimates range from less than 2% of CF patients aged under 5 years to 27% of those over 30 years [61]. The most recent study (a recall study in adults), gave an overall prevalence of 16%. In this study, 78% had a first episode after the age of 18, and 52% had recurrent episodes. DIOS was associated with pancreatic insufficiency, poor spirometry and more severe genotypes. There was no association with a history of meconium ileus, gastroesophageal reflux, malnutrition or

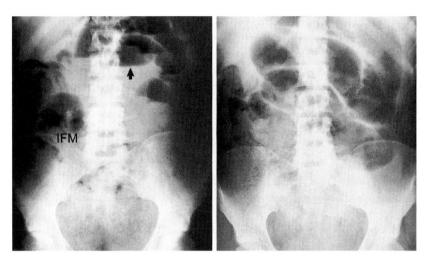

Figure 15.3 Plain abdominal radiographs of a patient with DIOS. Left radiograph shows an impacted fecal mass (IFM) and an air fluid level (arrow). Both radiographs show dilated small bowel.

increased mortality [57]. Acute DIOS has been reported in the postoperative period after lung transplantation [62,63] and may be precipitated by other systemic insults. Occasionally DIOS is the first presentation of CF [64].

CLINICAL FEATURES

A spectrum of clinical conditions results from partial or complete obstruction of the bowel. The two extremes of the spectrum are chronic recurring cramping abdominal pain and acute obstruction with vomiting, abdominal distension and pain.

One of the major clinical difficulties is distinguishing DIOS from a wide differential diagnosis: 'simple' constipation, appendicitis, intussusception, fibrosing colonopathy, volvulus, adhesions from previous abdominal surgery, inflammatory bowel disease, pancreatitis, biliary tract disease and pathology of the female reproductive tract. This distinction is critically important because DIOS can almost always be managed medically whereas some of the alternative diagnoses require prompt surgical intervention. In DIOS, a firm irregular mass or masses can often be palpated in the right iliac fossa. The mass is usually mobile and non-tender. This is a clinically useful sign, but one must also be aware that this sign may represent a distended appendix or intussusception [65].

No investigation will specifically confirm DIOS. A plain abdominal radiograph may show a granular, bubbly appearance extending from the terminal ileum with or without dilatation of proximal small bowel loops (Fig. 15.3) [32]. In the acute setting the main issue is to exclude a mechanical obstruction of the bowel before proceeding to specific therapy for DIOS. For this purpose contrast enema and abdominal CT are useful in selected cases [29].

THERAPY

The occurrence of DIOS may be reduced by attention to hydration in patients at risk. This is particularly the case in patients presenting with acute exacerbations of pulmonary infection during which fluid losses and relative dehydration

is common. Circulatory underfilling in the period after lung transplant has also been recognized as a risk factor and should be avoided.

Uncomplicated DIOS, once a surgical problem, now usually responds to medical management. In some cases, rehydration and adjustment of pancreatic enzyme dosage and dietary fiber may be sufficient. A stepwise approach is then employed:

- *Stool softeners* – such as lactulose (15–30 mL up to three times daily).
- *Oral* N-*acetylcysteine*. This is thought to work by reducing the viscosity of mucoprotein solutions by cleaving disulphide bonds. It can be given as 10 mL or more of a 20% solution three times daily in juice as the taste is unpleasant [66].
- *Gastrografin* (sodium meglumine diatrizoate). This is a hyperosmolar contrast medium that contains a small amount of detergent. Presumably the hypertonic fluid draws water into the lumen, softening the contents and may also stimulate peristalsis. It can be given orally as 100 mL in 400 mL of water or juice (for adults) or 50 mL in 200 mL (for children under 8 years). Gastrografin 100 mL enemas twice daily are also effective [67].
- *Intestinal lavage*. Balanced electrolyte solutions, such as Picolax or KleenPrep, are administered either orally or via nasogastric tube at a rate of 0.75–1.0 L/h to a total volume of 4–7 L [56,68].
- *Colonoscopy with instillation of gastrografin*. This has been described at our center for refractory DIOS in patients with significant cardiorespiratory comorbidity. The procedure was well tolerated with opiate and benzodiazepine sedation. Gastrografin 500 mL of 50% was instilled into the lumen at the limit of the examination. This was successful in 14 of 16 episodes [69].
- *Laparotomy*. With modern management this is required only occasionally. It is usually sufficient to milk the ileal contents distally. It should be noted that mortality from surgery is considerable [70].

Successful use of intravenous neostigmine has been reported in a single case [71]. There is the theoretical risk of perforation and more data are required before this can be recommended.

Management of more chronic presentations and prevention of recurrence of acute obstruction should start with avoidance of dehydration and reassessment of adequacy of pancreatic enzyme replacement (although the use of ever-increasing doses must nowadays be avoided). Oral NAC and/or lactulose should be used as maintenance therapy. Cisapride was also effective but has been withdrawn [72]. No other prokinetic has been trialled. In one case a modified anterograde continence enema procedure was performed with a good result [73]. This operation involves fashioning a stoma from the terminal ileum or appendix for the purpose of irrigation of the colon with saline or tap water and may be a useful treatment for difficult cases.

CONSTIPATION

Simple constipation, without obstruction or sufficient pain to warrant a diagnosis of DIOS, is also common in CF. The requirement for an energy-dense diet often leads to a low fiber intake [74]. Management involves attention to diet, fluid intake and enzyme dosage with use of laxatives as necessary. Constipation should not be confused with fat malabsorption, and treated with ever-increasing doses of pancreatic enzymes.

INTUSSUSCEPTION

Intussusception is an important complication of CF. In 1971, Holsclaw and co-workers [75] reported a series of 22 episodes in 19 individuals from a center with 2200 patients. The lifetime incidence is today likely to be higher than this survey indicated due to the increased CF life expectancy. The pathogenesis is different from idiopathic intussusception, which usually affects infants aged under 2 years. Thickened bowel contents tend to adhere to the bowel wall and serve as a lead point for the intussusception. A chronically distended appendix may also act as the lead point [76]. Asymptomatic intussusception is likely to be a common occurrence in CF patients, and indeed this was found in 5 of 90 patients in an ultrasound survey [5].

In the Holsclaw series, the mean age was 9.8 years. Compared to idiopathic intussusception, there was a tendency to a more chronic presentation (5 of 22) and hematochezia was seen in only 23%. Most intussusceptions were ileocolic or cecocolic [75]. A right iliac fossa mass may be palpable, but this sign is also present in DIOS, appendiceal disease and Crohn's disease. Plain abdominal radiography may demonstrate a soft tissue mass in 50–60%, and 25% have signs of small bowel obstruction. If the condition is suspected, a contrast enema should be performed and this may show an obstructing lobulated soft tissue mass with the coiled spring appearance of approximated mucosal folds. The intussusceptum may be reduced under fluoroscopic

guidance by performing a hydrostatic or pneumatic enema [29]. CT guidance may be helpful in difficult cases. Ultrasound can also be used to make the diagnosis. Most cases require operative intervention. Generally, manual reduction is relatively easy, but failing this a resection is carried out.

APPENDICEAL DISEASE

Characteristic changes of CF occur in the appendix. Increased numbers of goblet cells distended with mucus line dilated crypts. Eosinophilic casts of these crypts are extruded into the lumen of the appendix. The diagnosis of CF may be suspected on the basis of the histological appearance of the appendix.

However, acute appendicitis is apparently less common in patients with CF than in the general population, occurring in 1.5% of patients in one survey [76]. It has been suggested that the appendix may be protected to some degree from acute appendicitis by inspissated mucus. Most CF patients with acute appendicitis present in classical fashion, although they often do so late. Surveys suggest a higher rate of perforation [76] and of abscess formation [77], which is probably a consequence of delayed diagnosis and treatment. The only consistent radiological finding is an extrinsic compression of the cecum on contrast enema, the classic finding of a non-filling appendix being unreliable in CF patients [29]. CT and ultrasound have not proved reliable [32]. Acute appendicitis requires appendicectomy. If an abscess has developed, intravenous antibiotic treatment, with or without drainage, followed by an interval appendicectomy in one or two months may be appropriate management.

A second problem that can afflict the appendix in CF is mucoid distension, sometimes described as a 'sausage' appendix. This was found in 19 of 255 autopsies in one series [76], but not all autopsy series report this finding. The distended appendix can cause a syndrome of chronic intermittent pain and tenderness in the right lower quadrant which is relieved by appendicectomy. At histological examination, the appendix is distended with inspissated mucus but there are no features of appendicitis. Preoperative differentiation of this entity from DIOS is clearly difficult, but a contrast enema may show a cecal defect. Seven such patients (aged 10–24 years) were reported from a center with 1220 CF patients. A further four patients in this report had intussusception with a distended appendix acting as the lead point and three had a clinically silent distended appendix resected at cholecystectomy [76].

VOLVULUS

In the CF fetus or neonate, volvulus may complicate meconium ileus and lead to perforation and meconium peritonitis. This may be detectable *in utero* by ultrasound, or postnatally during investigation for neonatal bowel obstruction. Surgical relief is required.

In later life, small bowel volvulus – an uncommon condition in the general population – has been reported. However, no survey has assessed whether the condition is more common in CF. Large bowel volvulus (typically of sigmoid or cecum) can usually be detected on plain abdominal radiograph, and a contrast enema or CT will resolve doubt. For sigmoid volvulus, if there is no evidence of gangrenous bowel, decompression can be attempted with a flatus tube or colonoscope (although consideration will have to be given to fixation of the volvulus after the patient has recovered). Failures and other volvuli should then proceed to laparotomy.

FIBROSING COLONOPATHY

In 1994, Smyth and co-workers [78] published a series of four CF children who had been thought to have DIOS but had failed medical management and were found to have long segment strictures of the ascending colon at laparotomy. Resections were carried out and histology showed submucosal thickening by fibrous connective tissue, causing luminal narrowing without reduction in the external diameter of the colon. The epithelium was generally intact with very little inflammatory change.

A recent change from conventional-strength to high-strength pancreatic enzymes was the only common factor. High-strength preparations had been marketed in 1991. Further case reports appeared and two subsequent case–control studies confirmed a strong association between high-strength preparations (typically >24 000 units of lipase/kg body weight daily) and the new disease, named fibrosing colonopathy. It is unclear whether it is the pancreatic enzymes or the Eudragit L coating of some preparations (Nutrizym 22, Pancrease HL and Panzytrat 25 000) that are the injurious agent. Two case–control studies were conducted [79,80]. The UK study found no link with Creon 25 000, a high-strength preparation without Eudragit L. The US study found no significant difference between coatings, but Creon 25 000 was used by relatively few patients (just 4% of fibrosing colonopathy cases). Most cases occurred 7–15 months after commencing high-strength preparations. The great majority of cases have been children (mean age 5 years [80]), but adult cases have been described [81]. An adult patient without CF, but on high-dose Nutrizym 22, has been reported [82]. The picture is slightly clouded by two neonatal cases with no history of pancreatic enzyme supplementation [83,84]. The Committee on the Safety of Medicines recommended restrictions on dose to 10 000 units of lipase/kg daily and avoidance of Eudragit L coatings [85]; it was stated in 2001 that no cases in children associated with high-strength pancreatic enzymes had been reported since 1995.

Most patients have presented with abdominal pain, distension, vomiting and constipation, either acutely or insidiously. There have been cases of a colitic presentation with diarrhea and also ascites, occasionally chylous. Investigation is with contrast enema. Typical findings are mucosal irregularity and spiculation with loss of haustral folds, shortening of the colon and long-segment narrowing from mild stenosis to complete occlusion [29]. In most cases, involvement is limited to the right colon but the whole colon can be affected. Alternatively, an abdominal radiograph plus ultrasound can be obtained and contrast enema reserved for patients with a bowel wall thickness of more than 2 mm, reduced peristalsis or free fluid. Patients who are symptomatic should undergo laparotomy with resection of the strictured bowel. In most cases a right hemicolectomy is indicated. Those with total colonic disease require subtotal colectomy and ileostomy with a later procedure to restore continuity [32].

RECTAL PROLAPSE

Rectal prolapse occurs in as many as 20% of untreated CF patients under 5 years of age [86]. Approximately 11% of all pediatric patients with rectal prolapse have CF and sweat testing should be performed in any patient presenting with this complaint [87]. In most cases, prolapse resolves after initiation of adequate pancreatic enzyme therapy, high-fiber diet and improved nutrition.

ENTERIC INFECTIONS

It has long been speculated that the frequency of the CF gene in Caucasians reflects a heterozygote advantage due to resistance to certain enteric infections or enterotoxins. Jejunal mucosa from CF patients has been shown to be unresponsive to various enterotoxins *in vitro* [88]. This may well be a manifestation of *CFTR*-related abnormalities of electrolyte transport across the intestinal epithelium. This is not to say that enteric infections are unimportant in CF homozygotes. *Clostridium difficile* and *Giardia duodenalis*, in particular, are worthy of particular attention.

Clostridium difficile

Clostridium difficile is the cause of almost all pseudomembranous colitis and some cases of non-pseudomembranous antibiotic-associated diarrhea. It causes disease via elaboration of two toxins (A and B) and bacterial invasion of the mucosa does not occur. The disease is occasionally fulminant, with development of toxic megacolon and a high mortality rate.

A number of studies have shown carriage rates of *C. difficile* in feces from CF patients in the range 22–32% [89]. This is undoubtedly due to the high exposure of these individuals to antibiotics and hospitals. However, the great majority of patients carrying *C. difficile* are asymptomatic

[90] with negative toxin assays of cultures [89]. It is possible that CF confers some protection against *C. difficile*, either by exposure early in life promoting immunity or due to CFTR-related unresponsiveness [91]. However, reports of fulminant and fatal cases [92] counsel against complacency and a patient developing diarrhea with a recent inpatient stay and exposure to antibiotics should be tested. The initial test should be an assay for toxin in stool but this is falsely negative in approximately 21% [93]. Flexible sigmoidoscopy shows the very characteristic appearances of pseudomembranous colitis and this should be carried out in all patients with a negative toxin assay as *C. difficile* culture involves a delay and is not offered by many microbiology laboratories. Treatment involves discontinuation of antibiotics if possible, plus a 10-day course of oral metronidazole (400 mg three times daily) or oral vancomycin (125 mg four times daily). Relapse occurs in about 30% and a further course of the above antibiotics is given in the first instance.

Giardia duodenalis

A single study in Louisiana in 1988 found an increased carriage rate of *G. duodenalis* in CF patients versus controls from the same household (28% vs 6.3%) [94]. This was true especially for the older age groups. It is possible that altered bile composition in CF promotes *G. duodenalis* infection. There have been no further surveys and carriage rates show a marked geographical variability. Symptomatic giardiasis is likely to be missed in CF as the typical symptoms are diarrhea, steatorrhea, cramping abdominal pains and malabsorption. Stool microscopy for cysts has a sensitivity of only 50% although counter-immunoelectrophoresis for *G. duodenalis* antigens raises this to 95%. It is common gastroenterological practice to prescribe tinidazole 2 g as a single dose on clinical suspicion alone (a 2-day course of metronidazole is an alternative).

COMMON GASTROENTEROLOGICAL CONDITIONS IN CF

Peptic ulceration

Gastric and duodenal ulceration are reported to be frequent in CF autopsy series [95,96]. However, general clinical experience is that this condition is rare. The autopsy series may be misleading in so far as 'stress' ulceration is common in terminal disease. In addition the frequent use of protein pump inhibitor medication for GER and pancreatic enzyme therapy will provide protection.

In patients with persistent epigastric pain it is prudent to carry out a C^{13} urea breath test for *Helicobacter pylori* infection, as this is the dominant agent in causing peptic ulceration. Endoscopic examination can be reserved for those who are *H. pylori* negative or whose symptoms persist after *H. pylori* eradication.

Inflammatory bowel disease

Crohn's disease is associated with CF. A survey of 11 321 CF patients found a prevalence of 0.22%, which is 17-fold higher than published prevalence figures for comparable age groups [97]. The same survey found no evidence of an association with ulcerative colitis, which argues against this being an ascertainment bias.

Symptoms such as diarrhea, pain, weight loss or failure to thrive, and features of obstruction are again difficult to differentiate from manifestations of CF. A diagnosis of Crohn's disease should be sought in three groups of CF patients: (a) those with features suggestive of Crohn's such as perianal disease (abscess, fistula or skin tags), fistulation elsewhere or oral aphthous ulcers, (b) those with extraintestinal features suggestive of Crohn's (anterior uveitis, arthritis, erythema nodosum, pyoderma gangrenosum) and appropriate GI symptoms, and (c) after therapeutic failure of CF management. Contrast studies of the colon and small bowel are useful diagnostic tools. Endoscopy has the advantage of obtaining histological specimens which are essential for a firm diagnosis. This is not the place for a discussion of the management of this complex and difficult condition, in which a gastroenterologist should be involved. Attention to nutritional aspects of management is a high priority.

Celiac disease

Celiac disease is a lifelong disorder due to sensitivity to dietary gluten that can cause a wide spectrum of clinical manifestations, not all confined to the gastrointestinal tract, and many indistinguishable from CF. This is hardly surprising, since celiac disease and CF both emerged from the now archaic 'celiac syndrome'. Whereas CF was separated from the celiac syndrome in 1938 through the work of Dorothy Andersen, the true cause of celiac disease was not elucidated until the 1950s.

Velletta and co-workers [98] found celiac disease in five patients from a CF population of 1100 in the 1980s. These were overt cases and one would expect the rate to be somewhat higher if a CF population were to be screened with serology. The possibility of celiac disease should be considered in any CF patient with diarrhea or persistent loose stools, weight loss or failure to thrive despite enzyme replacement. A family history of the condition should also raise suspicion. Serum testing for anti-endomysial antibodies or tissue transglutaminase (tTG) has a sensitivity of 86–98%. EGD with distal duodenal biopsy is required to confirm diagnosis.

Treatment involves strict and lifelong adherence to a gluten-free diet. This involves avoidance of all wheat, barley and rye; the status of oats remains unclear. It is important that the high nutrient needs of the CF patient be recognized in dietary planning for the patient with both CF and celiac disease.

Lactose intolerance

Early studies suggested a link between hypolactasia and CF. A large study found no hypolactasia under age 5 years and a normal prevalence of hypolactasia in CF children older than 5 years [99]. Intestinal lactase levels normally fall dramatically after weaning but lactase persists throughout life, at lower levels in non-Caucasians. Hypolactasia can also be secondary to a range of small bowel diseases. If symptoms of diarrhea, bloating and pain are suspected to be related to lactose intake, a 2-week trial of a lactose-free diet, looking for symptomatic improvement, is the most practical measure. Lactose/hydrogen breath testing is an alternative, but would seem to offer few advantages.

GASTROINTESTINAL MALIGNANCY

A prospective study of the 28 858 patients registered by the US Cystic Fibrosis Foundation from 1990 to 1999 has established that the overall risk of malignancy in CF is similar to that in the non-CF population. However, there is an increased risk for cancers of the digestive tract [100]. The standardized incidence ratio (SIR) for digestive cancers overall is 5.1, among which cancers of the small bowel (SIR = 24.8), colon (7.4) and gallbladder and bile duct (39.0) are significantly more common. However, bearing in mind the young age of the population these are still rare tumors, the absolute excess risk (AER) attributable to CF for all digestive cancers being 9.1 per 100 000 patients per year. There is no association between digestive cancer and prior gastrointestinal conditions such as acute bleeding, cirrhosis or other liver disease, DIOS, fibrosing colonopathy, gallbladder surgery, pancreatitis, peptic ulcer or rectal prolapse.

Various possibilities have been advanced as explanations for the observed increase in malignancy of the digestive tract in CF. Cancer of the small bowel is also seen in other conditions which cause chronic malabsorption or intestinal stasis (e.g. celiac disease). Colonic cancer is associated with conditions that cause chronic inflammation (e.g. inflammatory bowel disease) for which there is also evidence in CF [9]. Cystic fibrosis patients ingest less dietary fiber and this has been shown to be a risk for colon carcinoma [74]. There may be a linkage between the CFTR gene and an oncogene. As the longevity of CF patients increases, malignant disease may assume a greater significance.

REFERENCES

1. Taylor CJ, Hardcastle J. Gut disease: clinical manifestations, pathophysiology, current and new treatments. *Prog Respir Res* 2006; **34**:232–241.
2. Farber S. Pancreatic function and disease in early life. V: Pathologic changes associated with pancreatic insufficiency in early life. *Arch Pathol* 1944; **37**:238–250.
3. Freye HB, Kurtz SM, Spock A *et al.* Light and electron microscopic examination of the small bowel of children with cystic fibrosis. *J Pediatr* 1964; **64**:575–579.
4. Taussig L, Saldino R, di Sant'Agnese P. Radiographic abnormalities of the duodenum and small bowel in cystic fibrosis of the pancreas (mucoviscidosis). *Radiology* 1973; **106**:369.
5. Haber HP, Benda N, Fitzke G *et al.* Colonic wall thickness measured by ultrasound: striking differences in patients with cystic fibrosis versus healthy controls. *Gut* 1997; **40**:406–411.
6. Gregory PC. Gastrointestinal pH, motility/transit and permeability in cystic fibrosis. *J Pediatr Gastroenterol Nutr* 1996; **23**:513–523.
7. Hendriks JH, van Kreel B, Forget PP. Effects of therapy with lansoprazole on intestinal permeability and inflammation in young cystic fibrosis patients. *J Pediatr Gastroenterol Nutr* 2001; **33**:260–265.
8. Bruzzese E, Raia V, Gaudiello G *et al.* Intestinal inflammation is a frequent feature of cystic fibrosis and is reduced by probiotic administration. *Aliment Pharmacol Ther* 2004; **20**:813–819.
9. Smyth RL, Croft NM, O'Hea U *et al.* Intestinal inflammation in cystic fibrosis. *Arch Dis Child* 2000; **82**:394–399.
10. Davidson AGF, Wong LTK, Kirby LT *et al.* Immunoreactive trypsin in cystic fibrosis. *J Pediatr Gastroenterol Nutr* 1984; **3**(Suppl 1):79–87.
11. Wong LTK, Turtle S, Davidson AGF. Secretin pancreozymin stimulation test and confirmation of the diagnosis of cystic fibrosis. *Gut* 1982; **23**:744–750.
12. Gaskin KJ, Durie P, Corey M *et al.* Evidence of a primary defect of bicarbonate secretion in cystic fibrosis. *Pediatr Res* 1982; **16**:554–557.
13. Davidson AGF, Wong LTK, Applegarth DA *et al.* Plasma immunoreactive trypsin levels after secretin pancreozymin stimulation. In: Warwick WJ (eds) *1000 Years of Cystic Fibrosis.* University of Minnesota Press, pp292–293.
14. Tsui L, Durie P. Genotype and phenotype in cystic fibrosis. *Hosp Pract* 1997; June:115–142.
15. Guy-Crotte O, Carrere J, Figarella C. Exocrine pancreatic function in cystic fibrosis. *Europ J Gastroenterol Hepatol* 1996; **8**:755–759.
16. Kalivianakis M, Minich DM, Bijleveld CM *et al.* Fat malabsorption in cystic fibrosis patients receiving enzyme replacement therapy is due to impaired intestinal uptake of long-chain fatty acids. *Am J Clin Nutr* 1999; **69**:127–134.
17. Manson W, Weaver L. Fat digestion in the neonate. *Arch Dis Child* 1997; **76**:F206–F211.
18. Sokol RJ, Reardon MC, Accurso FJ *et al.* Fat-soluble-vitamin status during the first year of life in infants with cystic fibrosis identified by screening of newborns. *Am J Clin Nutr* 1989; **50**:1064–1071.
19. Meyer JH, Lake R. Mismatch of duodenal deliveries of dietary fat and pancreatin from enterically coated microspheres. *Pancreas* 1997; **15**:226–235.
20. Taylor CJ, Hillel PG, Ghosal S *et al.* Gastric emptying and intestinal transit of pancreatic enzyme supplements in cystic fibrosis. *Arch Dis Child* 1999; **80**:149–152.

21. Brady MS, Rickard K, Yu PL *et al.* Effectiveness of enteric coated pancreatic enzymes given before meals in reducing steatorrhea in children with cystic fibrosis. *J Am Diet Assoc* 1992; **92**:813–817.

22. Walters MP, Kelleher J, Gilbert J *et al.* Clinical monitoring of steatorrhea in cystic fibrosis. *Arch Dis Child* 1990; **65**:99–102.

23. Littlewood JM. Implications of the committee on safety of medicines 10 000 IU lipase/kg/day recommendation for use of pancreatic enzymes in cystic fibrosis. *Arch Dis Child* 1996; **74**:466–468.

24. Kraisinger M, Hochhaus G, Stecenko A *et al.* Clinical pharmacology of pancreatic enzymes in patients with cystic fibrosis and in-vitro performance of microencapsulated formulations. *J Clin Pharmacol* 1994; **34**:158–166.

25. Proesmans M, De Boeck K. Omeprazole, a proton pump inhibitor, improves residual steatorrhoea in cystic fibrosis patients treated with high dose pancreatic enzymes. *Eur J Pediatr* 2003; **162**:760–763.

26. Tran TM, Van den Neucker A, Hendriks JJ *et al.* Effects of a proton-pump inhibitor in cystic fibrosis. *Acta Paediatr* 1998; **87**:553–558.

27. Coutts JA, Docherty JG, Carachi R *et al.* Clinical course of patients with cystic fibrosis presenting with meconium ileus. *Br J Surg* 1997; **84**:555.

28. Lang I, Daneman A, Cutz E *et al.* Abdominal calcification in cystic fibrosis with meconium ileus: radiologic–pathologic correlation. *Pediatr Radiol* 1997; **27**:523–527.

29. Agrons GA, Corse WR, Markowitz RI *et al.* Gastrointestinal manifestations of cystic fibrosis: radiologic–pathologic correlation. *Radiographics* 1996; **16**:871–893.

30. Gaillard D, Bouvier R, Scheiner C *et al.* Meconium ileus and intestinal atresia in fetuses and neonates. *Pediatr Pathol Lab Med* 1996; **16**:25–40.

31. Noblett H. Treatment of uncomplicated meconium ileus by gastrografin enema: a preliminary report. *J Pediatr Surg* 1969; **4**:190–197.

32. Beierle EA, Vinocur CD. Gastrointestinal surgery in cystic fibrosis. *Curr Op Pulm Med* 1998; **4**:319–325.

33. Waggett H, Bishop HC, Keep CE. Experience with gastrografin enema in the treatment of meconium ileus. *J Pediatr Surg* 1970; **5**:649–654.

34. Ellis DG, Clatworthy HW. The meconium plug syndrome revisited. *J Pediatr Surg* 1966; **1**:54–61.

35. Feigelsen J, Sauvegrain J. Reflux gastroesophagien dans la mucoviscidose. *N Press Med* 1975; **4**:2729–2730.

36. Scott RB, O'Loughlin EV, Gall DG. Gastroesophageal reflux in patients with cystic fibrosis. *J Pediatr* 1985; **106**:223–227.

37. Ledson MJ, Tran J, Walshaw MJ. Prevalence and mechanisms of gastro-oesophageal reflux in adult cystic fibrosis patients. *J R Soc Med* 1998; **91**:7–9.

38. Vic P, Tassin E, Turck D *et al.* Frequency of gastro-oesophageal reflux in infants and in young children with cystic fibrosis. *Arch Pediatr* 1995; **2**:742–746 [in French].

39. Malfroot A, Dab I. New insights on gastro-oesophageal reflux in cystic fibrosis by longitudinal follow up. *Arch Dis Child* 1991; **66**:1339–1345.

40. Brodzicki J, Trawinska-Bartnicka M, Korzon M. Frequency, consequences and pharmacological treatment of gastroesophageal reflux in children with cystic fibrosis. *Med Sci Monit* 2002; **8**:CR529–537.

41. Gustafsson PM, Fransson SG, Kjellman NI *et al.* Gastro-oesophageal reflux and severity of pulmonary disease in cystic fibrosis. *Scand J Gastroenterol* 1991; **26**:449–456.

42. Button BM, Toberts S, Kotsimbos TC *et al.* Gastroesophageal reflux (symptomatic and silent): a potentially significant problem in patients with cystic fibrosis before and after lung transplantation. *J Heart Lung Transplant* 2005; **24**:1522–1529.

43. Hassall E, Israel DM, Davidson AG *et al.* Barrett's esophagus in children with cystic fibrosis: not a coincidental association. *Am J Gastroenterol* 1993; **88**:1934–1938.

44. Cucchiara S, Santamaria F, Andreotti MR *et al.* Mechanisms of gastro-oesophageal reflux and severity of pulmonary disease in cystic fibrosis. *Scand J Gastroenterol* 1991; **66**:617–622.

45. Collins C, Francis J, Thomas P *et al.* Gastric emptying time is faster in cystic fibrosis. *J Pediatr Gastroenterol Nutr* 1997; **25**:492–498.

46. Cucchiara S, Raia V, Minella R *et al.* Ultrasound measurement of gastric emptying time in patients with cystic fibrosis and effect of ranitidine on delayed gastric emptying. *J Pediatr* 1996; **128**:485–488.

47. Button BM, Heine RG, Catto-Smith AG *et al.* Postural drainage and gastro-oesophageal reflux in infants with cystic fibrosis. *Arch Dis Child* 1997; **76**:148–150.

48. Ledson MJ, Wilson GE, Tran J. Tracheal microaspiration in adult cystic fibrosis. *J R Soc Med* 1998; **91**:10–12.

49. Andze GO, Brandt ML, Dickens St Vil *et al.* Diagnosis and treatment of gastroesophageal reflux in 500 children with respiratory symptoms: the value of pH monitoring. *J Pediatr Surg* 1991; **26**:295–300.

50. Bendig DW, Seilheimer DK, Wagner ML *et al.* Complications of gastroesophageal reflux in patients with cystic fibrosis. *J Pediatr* 1982; **100**:536–540.

51. Bredenoord AJ, Weusten BL, Timmer R *et al.* Reproducibility of multichannel intraluminal electrical impedance monitoring of gastroesophageal reflux. *Am J Gastroenterol* 2005; **100**:265–269.

52. Vinocur CD, Marmon L, Schidlow DV *et al.* Gastroesophageal reflux in the infant with cystic fibrosis. *Am J Surg* 1985; **149**:182–186.

53. Olsen MM, Gauderer MW, Girz MK *et al.* Surgery in patients with cystic fibrosis. *J Pediatr Surg* 1987; **22**:613–618.

54. Taylor CJ, Threlfall D. Postural drainage techniques and gastro-oesophageal reflux in cystic fibrosis. *Lancet* 1997; **349**:1567–1568.

55. Jensen K. Meconium ileus equivalent in a fifteen year old patient with mucoviscidosis. *Acta Paediatr Scand* 1962; **51**:433–438.

56. Davidson AC, Harrison K, Steinfort CL, Geddes EM. Distal intestinal obstruction syndrome in cystic fibrosis treated by oral intestinal lavage and a case of recurrent obstruction

despite normal pancreatic function. *Thorax* 1987; **42**:538–541.

57. Dray X, Bienvenu T, Desmazes-Dufeu N *et al.* Distal intestinal obstruction syndrome in adults with cystic fibrosis. *Clin Gastroenterol Hepatol* 2004; **2**:498–503.

58. O'Loughlin EV, Hunt DM, Gaskin KJ *et al.* Abnormal epithelial transport in cystic fibrosis jejunum. *Am J Physiol* 1991; **260**:G758–G763.

59. Dalzell AM, Heaf DP. Oro-caecal transit time and intra-luminal pH in cystic fibrosis patients with distal intestinal obstruction syndrome. *Acta Univ Carol [Med] (Praha)* 1990; **36**:159–160.

60. Proesmans M, De Boeck K. Evaluation of dietary fiber intake in Belgian children with cystic fibrosis: is there a link with gastrointestinal complaints? *J Pediatr Gastroenterol Nutr* 2002; **35**:610–614.

61. Rubinstein S, Moss R, Lewiston N. Constipation and meconium ileus equivalent in patients with cystic fibrosis. *Pediatrics* 1986; **78**:473–479.

62. Minkes RK, Langer JC, Skinner MA *et al.* Intestinal obstruction after lung transplantation in children with cystic fibrosis. *J Pediatr Surg* 1999; **34**:1489–1493.

63. Gilljam M, Chaparro C, Tullis E *et al.* GI complications after lung transplantation in patients with cystic fibrosis. *Chest* 2003; **123**:37–41.

64. Gardiner KR, Cranley B. Acute presentation of cystic fibrosis in an adult. *Postgrad Med J* 1989; **65**:471–472.

65. Martens M, De Boeck K, Van der Steen K *et al.* A right lower quadrant mass in cystic fibrosis: a diagnostic challenge. *Eur J Pediatr* 1992; **151**:329–331.

66. Gracey M, Burke V, Anderson CM. Treatment of abdominal pain in cystic fibrosis by oral administration of *N*-acetylcysteine. *Arch Dis Child* 1969; **44**:404–405.

67. O'Halloran SM, Gilbert J, McKendrick *et al.* Gastrografin in acute meconium ileus equivalent. *Arch Dis Child* 1986; **61**:1128–1130.

68. Koletzko S, Stringer DA, Cleghorn GJ *et al.* Lavage treatment of distal intestinal obstruction syndrome in children with cystic fibrosis. *Pediatrics* 1989; **83**:727–733.

69. Shidrawi RG, Murugan N, Westaby D *et al.* Emergency colonoscopy for distal intestinal obstruction syndrome in cystic fibrosis patients. *Gut* 2002; **51**:285–286.

70. Hodson ME, Mearns MB, Batten JC. Meconium ileus equivalent in adults with cystic fibrosis of pancreas: a report of six cases. *Br Med J* 1976; **2**:790–791.

71. Kurtzman TL, Borowitz SM. Successful use of neostigmine in a patient with refractory distal intestinal obstruction syndrome. *J Pediatr Gastroenterol Nutr* 2002; **35**:700–703.

72. Koletzko S, Corey M, Ellis L *et al.* Effects of cisapride in patients with cystic fibrosis and distal intestinal obstruction syndrome. *J Pediatr* 1990; **117**:815–822.

73. Clifton IJ, Morton AM, Ambrose NS. Treatment of resistant distal intestinal obstruction syndrome with a modified antegrade continence enema procedure. *J Cyst Fibros* 2004; **3**:273–275.

74. Gavin J, Ellis J, Dewar AL *et al.* Dietary fibre and the occurrence of gut symptoms in cystic fibrosis. *Arch Dis Child* 1997; **76**:35–37.

75. Holsclaw DS, Rocmans C, Shwachman H. Intussusception in patients with cystic fibrosis. *Pediatrics* 1971; **48**:51–58.

76. Coughlin JP, Gauderer MW, Stern RC *et al.* The spectrum of appendiceal disease in cystic fibrosis. *J Pediatr Surg* 1990; **25**:835–839.

77. Shields MD, Levison H, Reisman JJ *et al.* Appendicitis in cystic fibrosis. *Arch Dis Child* 1991; **66**:307–310.

78. Smyth RL, van Velzen D, Smyth AR *et al.* Strictures of ascending colon in cystic fibrosis and high-strength pancreatic enzymes. *Lancet* 1994; **343**:85–86.

79. Smyth RL, Ashby D, O'Hea U *et al.* Fibrosing colonopathy in cystic fibrosis: results of a case-control study. *Lancet* 1995; **346**:1247–1251.

80. Fitzsimmons SC, Burkhart GA, Borowitz D *et al.* High-dose pancreatic-enzyme supplements and fibrosing colonopathy in children with cystic fibrosis. *N Engl J Med* 1997; **336**:1283–1289.

81. Mack EH, Brett AS, Brown D. Fibrosing colonopathy in an adult cystic fibrosis patient after discontinuing pancreatic enzyme therapy. *South Med J* 2004; **97**:901–904.

82. Bansi DS, Price A, Russell C *et al.* Fibrosing colonopathy in an adult owing to over use of pancreatic enzyme supplements. *Gut* 2000; **46**:283–285.

83. Waters BL. Cystic fibrosis with fibrosing colonopathy in the absence of pancreatic enzymes. *Pediatr Dev Pathol* 1998; **1**:74–78.

84. Serban DE, Florescu P, Miu N. Fibrosing colonopathy revealing cystic fibrosis in a neonate before any pancreatic enzyme supplementation. *J Pediatr Gastroenterol Nutr* 2002; **35**:356–359.

85. Breckenridge A, Raine J. Concern about records of fibrosing colonopathy study. *Lancet* 2001; **357**:1527.

86. Stern RC, Izant RJ, Boat TF *et al.* Treatment and prognosis of rectal prolapse in cystic fibrosis. *Gastroenterology* 1982; **82**:707–710.

87. Zempsky WT, Rosenstein BJ. The cause of rectal prolapse in children. *Am J Dis Child* 1988; **142**:338–339.

88. Baxter PS, Goldhill, Hardcastle J *et al.* Accounting for cystic fibrosis. *Nature* 1988; **335**:211.

89. Peach SL, Borriello SP, Gaya H *et al.* Asymptomatic carriage of *Clostridium difficile* in patients with cystic fibrosis. *J Clin Pathol* 1986; **39**:1013–1018.

90. Pokorny CS, Bye PT, MacLeod C *et al.* Antibiotic-associated colitis and cystic fibrosis. *Dig Dis Sci* 1992; **37**:1464–1468.

91. Lloyd-Still JD. Co-existing gastrointestinal disorders in cystic fibrosis. *Pediatr Pulmonol Suppl* 1991; **2**:95–96.

92. Rivlin J, Lerner A, Augarten A *et al.* Severe *Clostridium difficile*-associated colitis in young patients with cystic fibrosis. *J Pediatr* 1998; **132**:177–179.

93. Johal SS, Hammond J, Solomon K *et al.* *Clostridium difficile* associated diarrhoea in hospitalised patients: onset in the community and hospital and role of flexible sigmoidoscopy. *Gut* 2004; **53**:673–677.

94. Roberts DM, Craft JC, Mather FJ *et al.* Prevalence of giardiasis in patients with cystic fibrosis. *J Pediatr* 1988; **122**:555–559.

95. Vawter GF, Shwachman H. Cystic fibrosis in adults: an autopsy study. *Pathol Annu* 1979; **14**:357–382.

96. Oppenheimer EH, Esterley JR. Pathology of cystic fibrosis: review of the literature and comparison with 146 autopsied cases. *Perspect Pediatr Pathol* 1975; **2**:241–278.

97. Lloyd-Still JD. Crohn's disease and cystic fibrosis. *Dig Dis Sci* 1994; **39**:880–885.

98. Valletta EA, Mastella G. Incidence of celiac disease in a cystic fibrosis population. *Acta Paediatr Scand* 1989; **78**:784–785.

99. Antonowicz I, Lebenthal E, Shwachman H. Disaccharidase activities in small intestinal mucosa in patients with cystic fibrosis. *J Pediatr* 1978; **92**:214–219.

100. Maisonneuve P, Fitzsimmons SC, Neglia JP *et al.* Cancer risk in nontransplanted and transplanted cystic fibrosis patients: a 10-year study. *J Nat Can Inst* 2003; **95**:381–387.

Liver, biliary and pancreatic disease

VICKY DONDOS AND DAVID WESTABY

INTRODUCTION

Liver involvement is well recognized in cystic fibrosis (CF) and may occasionally be a dominant manifestation. The reported prevalence and risk factors of CF-associated liver disease (CFALD) vary widely. There is a scarcity of long-term longitudinal studies; until recently populations studied have been small, and the lack of distinct sensitive and specific markers for diagnosis hinders comparison of studies, which have often used different diagnostic criteria. While early estimates from postmortems suggested that in excess of 70% of adults in the third decade of life had some evidence of focal biliary cirrhosis (the pathognomonic lesion of CF liver disease) [101], recent prospective studies report that approximately 20–25% of patients with CF will develop liver disease; 6–8% will have evidence of cirrhosis; and 2–3% will progress to liver decompensation.

Liver disease is a relatively early complication: the majority of patients will present in childhood or their early teens [102,103]. In the vast majority, liver disease appears to have a very limited impact on the clinical manifestations of CF until the most advanced stages. However, the rate of progression is extremely variable and occasionally rapid. Patient characteristics that may predict a higher risk of decompensation (as well as the initial development of liver disease) are as yet inadequately defined. The vast majority of cases are detected on routine clinical screening, but there is a very small group of patients who present with clinically overt liver disease, that progresses to decompensation.

There has been speculation that as a more elderly adult population of patients with CF evolved, an increasing proportion would develop liver disease. However, this has not been substantiated. Despite progressive improvements in life expectancy, great advances in the care of pulmonary complications of CF, as well as the availability of lung transplantation, prevalence of CFALD appears to decline in the third decade [104,105]. The possibility of premature mortality due to an occult adverse influence of liver disease remains a controversial issue (discussed further in the section on clinical features).

PATHOGENESIS OF CHRONIC LIVER DISEASE

See Fig. 15.4. The characteristic hepatic lesion in cystic fibrosis is a focal biliary cirrhosis consistent with that seen in partial biliary obstruction (Fig. 15.5).

Bile duct plugging

The plugging of intrahepatic bile ducts due to the enhanced viscosity of bile has been compared to that seen in the pancreatic ducts of CF patients [106]; i.e. it is a direct expression of the basic underlying gene defect [107]. The transmembrane conductance regulator (CFTR) has been localized to the apical membrane of the intrahepatic bile ducts [108]. Enhanced bile viscosity is likely to be due to the abnormalities of chloride transport inhibiting the hydration and alkalinization of the canalicular-produced

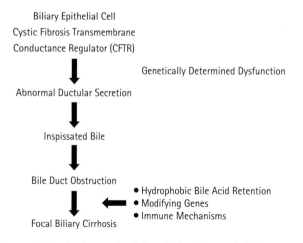

Figure 15.4 Pathogenesis of chronic liver disease in CF.

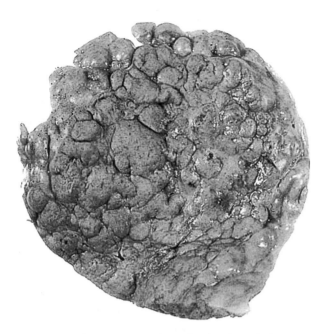

Figure 15.5   Postmortem specimen showing the typical multifocal nodularity of CF-related cirrhosis.

bile as well as the excessive production by intrahepatic biliary epithelial cells of mucus composed of proteoglycans [109]. Patchy plugging of the intrahepatic ducts with this high-viscosity bile results in an initial focal distribution of cirrhotic changes. With increasing ductular involvement over a variable time span the process becomes much more diffuse, producing a fully established biliary cirrhosis with extensive liver involvement.

Bile acid–related toxicity

Whether biliary duct obstruction alone is sufficient to account for this process remains controversial. A light and electron microscopic study of CF liver disease demonstrated features more in-keeping with a destructive bile duct lesion than a purely obstructive phenomenon [110]. Similar findings have been reported from a murine model of CF [111]. A bile-related toxin has been suggested as the most likely explanation for these findings. Initial analyses showed no significant difference in the serum bile acid profile between those with and without evidence of liver disease. However, given the significantly lower volume and thus higher concentration of bile produced in the presence of the CFTR gene defect [112,113], it could be speculated that bile reflux and retention caused by the partial or complete obstruction of ducts seen in CFALD dramatically increases the exposure of hepatocytes to potentially hepatotoxic lipophilic bile acids. A recent study has revisited the relationship between the bile acid profile and the presence of CFALD in children [114]. These authors identified an inverse correlation between the level of endogenous serum ursodeoxycholic acid (UDCA) and CFALD and suggested that this might represent a protective factor against liver injury. Why higher levels of endogenous UDCA levels are found in some patients has not been explained.

Risk factors

Although the above provides a possible etiological basis for chronic CFALD, it does not account for the absence of liver involvement in such a large proportion of patients and the wide spectrum of severity in those in whom liver disease does occur. A number of possible contributing or associated factors have been reported.

GENETIC INFLUENCES

Attempts to match a specific CF genotype with expression of liver disease have failed to show any significant correlation [115]. However, there is evidence that the presence of a severe genotype (class I, II and III mutations), associated with complete loss of CFTR function, has an independent association with the development of CFALD [105,116,117]. A relationship between HLA status has been reported with a significant increased prevalence of DQ6 in those with CFALD [118]. There is now accumulating evidence that other genetic factors may be extremely important in the pathogenesis of liver disease. Modifier genes are inherited independently of the CFTR mutation but may attenuate or exacerbate the CF phenotype by their influence on such factors as host defense and the inflammatory response. Polymorphisms in the α_1-antitrypsin and mannose-binding lectin genes have been identified as independent risk factors for CF liver disease [119]. There is also recent evidence that liver disease is associated with glutathione S-transferase P1 polymorphism [119,120].

MECONIUM ILEUS (MI)

A history of MI has been identified as a risk factor for CFALD in a number of reports [103,105]. A study reporting autopsy findings suggested that viscous mucus might accumulate simultaneously in the intestine, gallbladder and biliary tree leading to chronic damage [121]. Other studies have failed to confirm an association with MI [116,122], and as only a small proportion of patients who develop CFALD have a history of MI this should only be considered a possible contributory factor.

MALE GENDER

A male preponderance among CFALD patients has been reported in several studies [104,105]. There is further evidence that in female patients liver disease occurred only before puberty, while male patients presented up to the age of 18 years [105]. This male predominance may in part reflect the possible survival benefit of males in CF [123].

However, a role for estrogens and their receptors in modulating the development of CFALD should be considered.

COMMON BILE DUCT OBSTRUCTION

Distal common bile duct compression by pancreatic fibrosis is a well recognized cause of obstructive biliary injury in patients with chronic pancreatitis and has been postulated as a factor in the development of liver disease in CF [124]. However, imaging of the extrahepatic biliary tree in CFALD has shown this to be an unusual phenomenon and at best a contributory factor in a small proportion of cases [125].

ADDITIONAL CONTRIBUTING FACTORS

The presence of a sub population of lymphocytes, cytotoxic to hepatocytes and directed towards the liver-specific lipoprotcin, suggests that immune mechanisms might also be involved in the pathogenesis of CF liver disease [126]. Factors that may exacerbate existing liver injury include poor nutritional status (total parenteral nutrition may accelerate disease progression), drug toxicity, sepsis, medical treatment or compliance and recent abdominal surgery [102,107].

CLINICAL FEATURES OF LIVER DISEASE

Deep cholestasis secondary to common bile duct obstruction with inspissated bile may be the earliest manifestation of CF [127,128]. This condition rarely results in clinically significant liver disease, typically resolving spontaneously during the first months of life.

Fatty infiltration of the liver may sometimes produce massive hepatomegaly and abdominal distension, complicated by hypoglycemia [129,130]. It is the most frequent hepatic lesion associated with CF but does not seem to be caused directly by the CF secretory defect, being rather a consequence of the disease process outside the liver (e.g. conditions associated with insulin resistance [131]) and the effect of circulating cytokines resulting from chronic infection by respiratory pathogens [132]. Malnutrition has also been implicated in its pathogenesis; deficiencies in carnitine, fatty acids, trace elements and minerals may be associated [130]. A risk of progression to cirrhosis has not been specifically identified in CF but is recognized in children with other etiological causes of fatty liver [133].

Evidence of underlying cirrhosis may occur at any time, but new diagnoses are most frequently made during the first two decades of life (see above) and usually as part of routine follow-up in patients with an established diagnosis of CF. Clinical hepatosplenomegaly is perhaps the commonest presentation. Abnormal liver function tests are common in CF but may be of no significance. Many large centers have established routine surveillance including sequential ultrasound scanning (see later). This approach has identified a small proportion of patients with no other clinical or laboratory evidence of liver disease. Variceal bleeding

may be the presenting feature of established portal hypertension and may occur in the absence of any other signs of decompensation. As in other types of biliary cirrhosis, portal hypertension may occur in a pre-cirrhotic phase because of the pre-sinusoidal component to portal vascular resistance. Decompensated biliary cirrhosis – including jaundice, ascites or encephalopathy – are very unusual presenting features.

Overall, the clinical picture is one of a very slowly progressive liver disease, the natural history of which is usually interrupted by premature mortality related to pulmonary disease. The long natural history of cirrhosis in CF is not dissimilar to that seen in other biliary cirrhotic disease such as primary biliary cirrhosis or primary sclerosing cholangitis [134,135].

Controversy remains as to whether the adverse effect of liver disease in CF is restricted to the 2–3% of patients who have overt liver decompensation and a further 1–2% who experience variceal bleeding. There is some evidence that liver disease may have an adverse effect on the prognosis in CF independent of specific complications. A large time-dependent multiple regression analysis of survival risk factors in cystic fibrosis reported liver disease as an independent predictor of premature mortality, in addition to pulmonary function and nutrition [136]. As is typical in liver diseases characterized by initial involvement of bile ducts and later impairment of hepatocyte function, the systemic and pulmonary hemodynamic abnormalities of cirrhosis are often earlier and more prominent manifestations than features of liver failure per se [137,138]. Low peripheral vascular resistance, high cardiac output and increased pulmonary shunting might be expected to adversely affect patients with advanced pulmonary disease. However, recent studies provide evidence that impact on clinical course (with regard to pulmonary and nutritional complications) is not significant until the most advanced stages of liver disease are reached [105,139].

INVESTIGATIONS FOR LIVER DISEASE

LIVER FUNCTION TESTS

Standard laboratory liver-related tests have reasonable sensitivity but poor specificity as predictive factors for CF liver disease. This is not surprising as many potential factors might influence these tests (especially serum aminotransferase), including infection, hypoxemia and medications. Markers of a biliary component such as the alkaline phosphatase and gamma glutamine transpeptidase may be more helpful particularly when levels are elevated by a factor of 3–4 and this is sustained over a period of months [140]. A small proportion of patients with established cirrhosis will have entirely normal liver function tests [104,140]. The most important role for these standard liver function tests is to initiate a search for possible underlying liver disease through imaging.

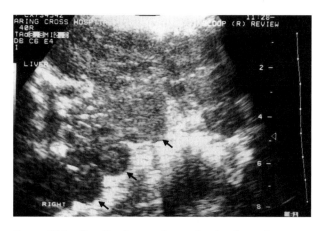

Figure 15.6 Hepatic ultrasound scan showing the surface nodularity of established cirrhosis (arrowed).

Table 15.2 The ultrasound scoring system.

	Score		
	1	2	3
Hepatic parenchyma	Normal	Coarse	Irregular
Liver edge	Smooth	–	Nodular
Periportal fibrosis	None	Moderate	Severe

IMAGING

The availability of high-quality transabdominal ultrasound scanning has provided a cheap and widely available means of detecting underlying chronic liver disease. In experienced hands ultrasound imaging provides diagnostic information with respect to a diffuse cirrhotic process as well as detecting earlier focal abnormalities [141]. Splenomegaly, a dilated portal vein and the presence of collateral vessels are all important markers of portal hypertension [141].

Parenchymal irregularity, periportal fibrosis and irregularity of the liver edge (Fig. 15.6) are factors incorporated in an ultrasound scoring system deemed effective in documenting established cirrhosis in adults (Table 15.2) [138].

The use of Doppler studies allows the detection of portal or splenic vein thrombosis with increased prevalence in CF, usually as a consequence of associated chronic pancreatitis. Transabdominal ultrasound has been widely adopted for the routine screening of CF populations [140].

Radionuclide imaging using derivatives of iminodiacetic acid (IDA) labeled with technetium-99m provides an alternative means of assessing the biliary tree [142]. IDA when injected systemically is taken up by hepatocytes and then cleared rapidly into bile. In established cirrhosis there is documented delay in hepatocyte uptake. Delay of excretion at the level of both the intra- and extrahepatic biliary tree has also been identified and may be one of the earliest abnormalities seen in those susceptible to the development of biliary

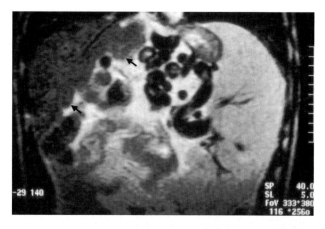

Figure 15.7 Abdominal MRI scan showing the surface nodularity of cirrhosis. There is splenomegaly and portal venous collateral vessels.

cirrhosis [143]. The introduction of quantitative IDA imaging raises the possibility of an objective means of monitoring the degree of both hepatocyte and biliary impairment as well as monitoring response to therapy [144].

Magnetic resonance imaging (MRI) and in particular magnetic resonance cholangiopancreatography (MRCP) techniques [145] produce excellent definition of the cirrhotic liver and the collateral circulation associated with portal hypertension. (Fig. 15.7) The MRCP technique is extremely effective in the detection and management of common bile duct stones and with improving resolution it may also define the intrahepatic biliary tree and the caliber abnormalities characteristic of CF-related liver disease [146].

ENDOSCOPIC RETROGRADE CHOLANGIOGRAPHY (ERCP)

The characteristic intraductular caliber irregularities associated with established CF cirrhosis (Fig. 15.8) are similar to the pattern of stricturing and dilatation described in primary sclerosing cholangitis [125]. This appearance was first visualized by trans-gallbladder and endoscopic contrast cholangiography [125,143] and found to be highly specific for established chronic liver disease, only being seen in patients with evidence of cirrhosis on ultrasound [125]. While endoscopic retrograde cholangiography still has a role in the management of common bile duct stones and in the small proportion of patients in whom there is evidence of common bile duct obstruction at the level of the head of pancreas (see above), it is no longer considered an appropriate investigation technique for evaluating CFALD. With the increasing resolution of MRI/MRCP there is every expectation that intrahepatic ductular changes will be adequately delineated by this non-invasive technique.

HISTOLOGY

Histological assessment forms a fundamental basis for most aspects of hepatology. Studies of CFALD and in particular

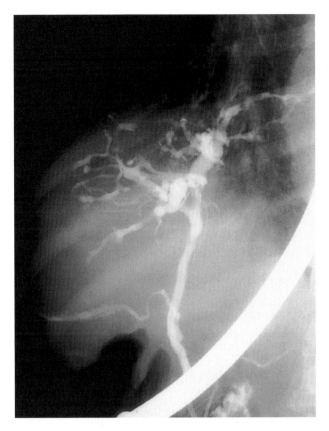

Figure 15.8 Endoscopic retrograde cholangiogram showing the irregularity of caliber of the intrahepatic ducts.

the response to therapy (see later) have been limited by an absence of a histological 'gold standard'. However, in CF liver disease the initial focal nature of the changes may result in considerable sampling error, even with the use of ultrasound guidance. Furthermore, the potential severity of a pneumothorax in CF (a well-recognized procedural risk) has rendered liver biopsy acceptable only as part of controlled studies of therapy or in a very small proportion of patients in whom other causes of liver damage need to be excluded. Liver biopsy is not useful in the routine clinic management of CFALD.

MANAGEMENT OF LIVER DISEASE

Bile acid therapy

Ursodeoxycholic acid (UDCA) is a hydrophilic bile acid that has been used extensively in cholestatic disorders [147]. It is normally present in human bile, albeit representing just 3% of the total bile acid pool. Proposed mechanisms of action are multifactorial and include the following.

- Protection of cholangiocytes against the cytotoxic influence of hydrophobic bile acid. In a mouse model of suppurative cholangitis, oral intake of UDCA reduced

cholangiocellular injury, portal inflammation and ductular proliferation [148]. Reduced inflammatory reaction around the intrahepatic ducts has been demonstrated in patients with primary biliary cirrhosis and primary sclerosing cholangitis managed with oral UCDA [149,150].
- Stimulation of biliary secretion through increasing the number and activity of carrier proteins in the apical membrane [151].
- Protection of hepatocytes against hydrophobic bile-acid induced apoptosis [152].
- An immunoregulatory effect in particular with respect to reversal of aberrant expression of HLA class-1 molecules on hepatocytes [153].

The optimum dose of UDCA appears to be between 15 and 20 mg/kg [154,155]. Attention has also been paid to the need for taurine supplementation as part of UDCA therapy; it has shown no additional effect upon liver function, but there may be a nutritional benefit [156]. Despite extensive use of UCDA in patients with CFALD, data from objective studies are sparse.

- Early uncontrolled data suggested both biochemical and clinical improvement with the use of UDCA in CF liver disease [156,157].
- A small unblinded controlled trial was the first to report both benefits in liver biochemistry as well as improvement in biliary excretion of IDA derivatives in those taking UDCA [143]. A further placebo-based controlled trial has also confirmed improvement in liver biochemistry as well as benefits with respect to a general illness score [158]. However, neither of these two trials has been of sufficient power or duration to comment on important end-points such as the development of decompensated liver disease, need for liver transplantation or associated mortality.
- A small study has evaluated the response of liver histology to UDCA therapy [139]. Liver biopsy was performed before and after one or two years of therapy. A scoring system reflecting bile duct proliferation, fibrosis and inspissation of bile as well as inflammatory changes was used. A significant histological benefit was confirmed [139].

The accumulated evidence with UDCA is insufficient to lay down clear guidelines for management [159]. It is highly unlikely that this drug is capable of reversing advanced liver disease, so there is considerable justification for focusing further studies on the introduction of this drug in patients with *early* imaging evidence of liver disease [140]. More objective therapy may evolve as risk factors predicting the development liver disease are identified (see above). In the meantime it is likely that this less than objective use of UDCA in patients with CF liver disease will continue based on the evidence that is available and in the setting of a drug that is well tolerated and has very few associated adverse effects.

Liver transplantation

Liver transplantation in advanced chronic liver disease has yielded survival rates in excess of 80% at 1 year and as high as 60% at 10 years. Criteria for inclusion of patients with CFALD are gradually expanding [160,161].

Fears that underlying pulmonary disease precluded isolated liver transplants in the large majority of patients with CF should be greatly allayed by the beneficial results reported in several small series of patients who have undergone this procedure. In appropriately selected patients, survival rates in the short and medium term (i.e. up to 5 years) appear to be similar as in other types of cirrhosis [162,163]. Perhaps more strikingly, despite the predicted increased risk of overwhelming pulmonary sepsis due to the immunosuppression required, there has been an observed improvement in pulmonary function after liver-only transplant. Potential explanations for this include the following:

- resolution of portal hypertension and the associated splenomegaly which may itself impair diaphragmatic function (resolution of chronic ascites may have a similar effect);
- improvement in intrapulmonary shunting secondary to the cirrhosis;
- a potential direct benefit of immunosuppression itself on CF lung disease.

Contraindications to liver transplantation remain:

- severely compromised lung function or frequent exacerbations of pulmonary infection;
- chronic infection with organisms such as some members of the *Burkholderia cepacia* family, or other multi-resistant organisms;
- a persistently raised arterial PCO_2 indicating underlying ventilatory failure as well as severe pulmonary hypertension.

The importance of portal hypertension and variceal bleeding as an indicator for liver transplantation is controversial. There are a number of liver transplant groups who have used the presence of portal hypertension and the history of variceal bleeding as specific risk factors incorporated in a scoring system identifying those suitable for isolated liver transplantation [160]. However, in our own published experience we observed long-term survival following presentation with variceal bleeding which was comparable to the general CF population (Fig. 15.9) [164].

This outcome appears to reflect the success of the new endoscopic techniques for managing variceal bleeding (see later) and the failure of the underlying liver disease to manifest other serious complications such as persistent ascites and encephalopathy. In the absence of such features of liver decompensation we would not consider portal hypertension

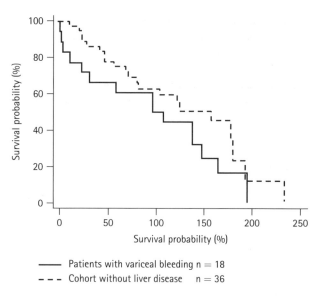

Figure 15.9 A Kaplan–Meier survival analysis for patients from the time of first variceal bleed compared to a cohort without evidence of liver disease [165].

and variceal bleeding to be an indication for isolated liver transplantation.

There remains a small but important group of patients in whom there is evidence of advanced liver disease as well as pulmonary disease of such severity that liver transplantation alone would not be feasible. There are a number of reports of heart, lung, liver or lung–liver transplantation in such cases [162,165,166]. With a shortage of donated organs there has been considerable reluctance to use those available in such a high-risk undertaking. However, there are small series reporting as high as a 70% 1-year survival in such cases although medium- and long-term data are not available [165].

INFLUENCE OF LIVER DISEASE ON ORGAN TRANSPLANTATION

For those patients in whom there is evidence of liver disease but not fully established cirrhosis, there should be no contraindication to lung transplantation. There is now evidence from small series that patients with well-compensated cirrhosis tolerate lung transplantation without difficulty and have not presented problems with decompensation. Furthermore there is no evidence that variceal bleeding has been precipitated [167]. In our own series, five patients with established cirrhosis and portal hypertension have undergone heart–lung or lung-only transplantation without specific liver-related complications.

Molecular biological therapy

Most emphasis on gene therapy has been directed towards pulmonary disease (see Chapter 33a). However, recombinant adenoviruses expressing the human CFTR gene have been infused into the biliary tree of a rat model [168]. Recombinant gene expression was achieved in virtually all the cholangiocytes and expression persisted for the duration of the 21 days over which the study was carried out. It remains to be seen whether this will offer a viable therapy for CF-related liver disease.

MANAGEMENT OF COMPLICATIONS OF LIVER DISEASE

The majority of patients with CFALD never develop specific complications associated with chronic liver disease. With the exception of UDCA no other liver-related therapy needs to be considered. However, some care should be taken with respect to nutritional requirements as there is evidence that patients with established cirrhosis have an increased resting energy expenditure [137]. There may also be established deficiencies of specific macronutrients, fat-soluble vitamins and clotting factors [169]. Such nutritional deficiencies may become much more prominent in patients with liver decompensation, particularly in the presence of persisting jaundice, ascites and following major variceal bleeding. Difficulties in maintaining nutrition are compounded by the contraindication to placing gastrostomy tubes in patients with established portal hypertension and particularly in the presence of ascites. It is essential that specific individualized attention be directed towards the nutritional management of CF patients with decompensated cirrhosis.

Jaundice

Outside the context of infantile bile duct obstruction (that typically resolves spontaneously), jaundice in established cirrhosis is an unusual event that must be considered a poor prognostic feature. In one published series only 20% of patients with CFALD had a history of jaundice [125]. Documentation of jaundice or a rising bilirubin level requires detailed investigation to exclude other possible treatable causes. Transabdominal ultrasound scanning is an essential to exclude bile duct obstruction, due either to bile duct stones or less frequently a distal common bile duct stricture (see above). Other possible etiological factors for jaundice in the absence of advanced cirrhosis include sepsis, drug toxicity or hemolysis. UDCA has been shown to improve liver function and may lead to at least transient resolution of the jaundice (see above).

Variceal bleeding

Variceal bleeding is the most common serious complication of CF liver disease, with a prevalence of less than 2% of the total CF population (20% of those with established cirrhosis). This compares to a 30% risk of variceal bleeding consistently reported for cirrhotic populations of other etiologies. This lower risk of a first variceal bleed is likely to reflect the well-maintained liver function seen in most cases of CFALD throughout life. Premature mortality secondary to pulmonary complications may also limit the timescale over which the risk of variceal bleeding may occur.

Management follows the same principles as in any other group of cirrhotic patients [169], initial priorities being basic resuscitation, replacement of blood loss, correction of any coagulopathy, prevention of sepsis with prophylactic antibiotics and attention to airway clearance [170].

Fiberoptic endoscopy is the basis of diagnosis and the optimal interventional technique for control of active bleeding. Success rates of 85–90% have been reported, with very low complication rates in experienced hands [171].

- Banding ligation has now replaced injecting sclerotherapy as the most effective therapeutic technique (Fig. 15.10) [171,172]. Anesthetic expertise should always be available but intubation and general anesthesia is not a prerequisite. There is an approximate 30% risk of early rebleeding; obliteration of the varices with repeated sessions of banding ligation between 1 and 3 weekly intervals (a total of three sessions are usually required) reducing this risk. In addition, the use of proton pump inhibitors [173] and sucralfate suspension – to prevent the mucosal ulceration associated with endoscopic therapy [174] – are of proven benefit in averting early recurrence.
- There is accumulating evidence of the benefit of banding ligation to prevent the first bleed in high-risk patients [175]. However, given the lower incidence of variceal hemorrhage in CF liver disease versus other cirrhotic conditions, the potential complications may well outweigh the benefits of such intervention.

Pharmacological agents are also widely used in the management of variceal bleeding.

- Vasopressin and somatostatin (and their respective analogues glypressin and octreotide) modulate portal blood flow and pressure by reducing splanchnic inflow and in the case of somatostatin by a direct effect on the portal circulation itself. These agents have been widely used for the management of an episode of variceal bleeding. The emphasis is on temporary reduction or control of bleeding prior to the early introduction of endoscopic therapy. Comparative studies suggest that glypressin has a greater a survival benefit in active bleeding than somatostatin or octreotide [176]; it is easy to administer as an intravenous bolus and has fewer cardiovascular side-effects than its predecessor vasopressin. There is also some evidence that continuing these agents for 4–5 days after endoscopic therapy reduces the risk of early rebleeding [177].

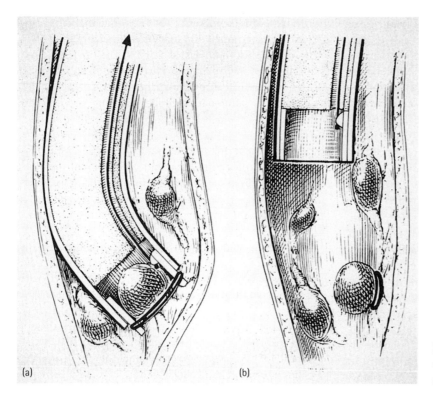

(a)   (b)

Figure 15.10 Diagrammatic representation of the technique of banding ligation of esophageal varices.

- While non-selective beta-adrenoreceptor blockers have been shown to be effective in both reducing the risk of first bleed and preventing an early rebleed in patients with esophageal varices, the risk of precipitating bronchoconstriction in the presence of pulmonary complications in CF precludes their use.

RESCUE TECHNIQUES FOR VARICEAL BLEEDING

Endoscopic management will arrest bleeding in 85–90% of cases. However, it is essential to establish a strategy for those who continue to bleed or have early recurrence. A further endoscopic procedure is justified but should be carried out by the most experienced operator and with alternative rescue techniques available if this further attempt should fail.

In the presence of life-threatening large-volume variceal bleeding, balloon tamponade using one of the commercially available balloon tubes has been shown to be effective at obtaining temporary hemostasis and allowing a short time window to carry out either endoscopic therapy or other rescue techniques [178]. Balloon tamponade is at best a very uncomfortable and unpleasant experience for the patient but in the presence of significant pulmonary disease may be poorly tolerated and associated with a high risk of complications (particularly pulmonary aspiration).

Historically the most commonly used rescue procedure was to create a portal systemic shunt. Initial experience dating back to the 1960s involved the surgical creation of such shunts. These were highly effective for the control of variceal bleeding and preventing recurrence but at the expense of a marked reduction in liver blood flow. A high

morbidity and mortality rate ensued from associated liver failure. Despite this, portal systemic shunt surgery was quite commonly used in CF [179]. Over the last decade it has been possible to create a portal systemic shunt by a radiological technique termed a 'transjugular intrahepatic portosystemic shunt' (TIPS). Because this is a much less invasive procedure operative morbidity and mortality is small and the benefits with respect to arresting bleeding and preventing re-bleeding have been maintained [180]. However, hopes that this intrahepatic shunt might maintain a higher level of blood flow to the liver as compared to shunt surgery have not been realized. Post-procedural liver decompensation, specifically encephalopathy, is a major drawback to this approach. There is, however, a small but important rescue role for this approach in patients in whom there has been a failure to control bleeding following the endoscopic technique, and this has been successfully applied in CF patients [181].

Ascites

The accumulation of a transudate within the peritoneal cavity is a well-recognized complication of cirrhosis and associated portal hypertension. The development of ascites in chronic liver disease is a poor prognostic factor, being a feature of advanced disease and decompensation (which may not be the case for variceal bleeding). Occasionally transient small-volume ascites may develop following a significant variceal hemorrhage or when there has been intravenous overload with sodium and water. If this resolves promptly without recurrence the prognostic implications may not be so profound. Management is that applied in any case of underlying cirrhosis [182].

Encephalopathy

Hepatic encephalopathy is an extremely infrequent complication in patients with very advanced CFALD. Where there is a clearly defined precipitating factor (such as ventilatory failure, sepsis, gastrointestinal hemorrhage or persistent constipation), the disturbed cerebration may revert promptly with resolution of the acute event. Prolonged encephalopathy in the absence of a specific precipitant is an extremely poor prognostic factor. Again, management is not different from that used more widely in the hepatological field [183].

Splenomegaly and hypersplenism

Splenomegaly is a very common observation in patients with CFALD. In most circumstances the degree of splenomegaly has no clinical significance. There are, however, a small proportion of patients who have associated morbidity which raises the question as to whether splenectomy is indicated. In patients with CF any abdominal surgery is a major undertaking and indications and risks need to be carefully assessed.

Pain alone is a very unusual indication for splenectomy. Occasionally splenomegaly may be gross with intractable pain particularly if accompanied by splenic infarction.

Significant impairment of diaphragmatic function may be considered an indication for splenectomy. In patients with decompensated liver disease, liver transplantation has led to a resolution of such ventilatory impairment and improvement in pulmonary function (see above).

Splenectomy (or partial splenectomy) may also be considered in the rare event of spontaneous bleeding in the context of low platelet counts due to hypersplenism [184,185]. An alternative approach is splenic artery embolization to reduce splenic size. TIPS has also been used as a means of reducing portal hypertension in this setting.

EXTRAHEPATIC BILIARY DISEASE

Pathology and pathophysiology

Structural abnormalities of the extrahepatic biliary system are commonly observed in cystic fibrosis. The failure to identify the gallbladder is a common finding in fetuses with documented CF [186]. Imaging studies of patients with CF have shown a wide spectrum of biliary abnormalities [141,145,167,187]. An undetectable or micro-gallbladder has been documented in up to 30% of cases. Stenosis or atresia of the cystic duct is also a common finding. These abnormalities account for the high proportion of patients

Table 15.3 Complications of gallstone disease.

Biliary colic(cystic duct or bile duct stone)
Acute cholecystitis
Empyema of the gall bladder
Bile duct obstruction
Cholangitis(obstruction with infection)
Gallstone pancreatitis

in whom the gallbladder is not functioning. Gallstones have been identified in 20–25% of cases, the prevalence increasing with age and representing a 4- to 5-fold elevation over aged-matched non-CF controls. Most stones are radiotranslucent and were believed to be of cholesterol composition. The bile salt deficiency identified in some cases of CF would represent a risk factor for such stones. However, this concept has been challenged by a study analyzing bile and gallstone composition in CF which showed calcium bilirubinate to be the major component [167]. Furthermore, there was no evidence of cholesterol saturation of bile. Calcium bilirubinate (pigment) stones are seen in conditions associated with hyperbilirubinbilia such as the hemolytic anemias. In CF there is experimental evidence that chronic bile salt loss from the small intestine might predispose to reabsorption of unconjugated bilirubin from the colon [188]. The resulting enterohepatic cycling of bilirubin increases the secretion of conjugated bilirubin into bile and enhances the risk of precipitation with calcium. There is recent evidence that in CF the co-inheritance of at least one Gilbert syndrome allele (UGT1A1) further enhances the risk of hyperbilirubinbilia and pigment stone formation [189]. It is likely that the development of gallstone disease is a multifactorial process encompassing the chemical compositon of bile, anatomical abnormalities as well as the impairment of bile flow.

Management of gallstone disease

Complications of gallstones have been reported in approximately 4% of CF patients [190] and encompass the full spectrum of pathologies (Table 15.3).

Management strategies do not differ from those applied to non-CF patients. Laparoscopic cholecystectomy is well tolerated even in patients with advanced pulmonary disease. It is not an unusual scenario to be managing patients with symptomatic gallstone disease in the period while they are waiting for lung transplantation. Stone-related bile duct obstruction is managed by standard endoscopic techniques. A small proportion of patients develop intrahepatic stones and may require repeated endoscopic intervention to clear them (Fig. 15.11). Management of stone disease requires close cooperation between CF and hepatobiliary (HPB) units. UDCA has proved ineffective as a pharmacological therapy for gallstones in CF (almost certainly reflecting the unfavorable chemical composition of the stones [191].

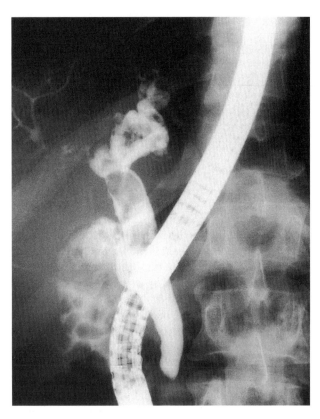

Figure 15.11 Endoscopic retrograde cholangiogram showing multiple gallstones in the gallbladder (GB), common hepatic duct (CHD) and left intrahepatic duct (IHD).

PANCREATIC DISEASE

The investigation and management of malabsorption is discussed in Chapter 15a.

Pathophysiology of pancreatic disease

In the majority of patients with CF, pancreatic insufficiency (PI) is evident from the neonatal period. Indeed, pancreatic insufficiency was an integral part of the early descriptions of CF. Only when sweat electrolytes were established as a diagnostic tool did it become apparent that approximately 10–15% of CF patients remained pancreatic-sufficient (PS). High concentrations of CFTR are present on pancreatic duct epithelium and produce a high-volume bicarbonate-rich secretion responsible for maintaining the solubility of acinar-derived enzymes and flushing these into the duodenum. In the presence of impaired CFTR function the volume of fluid and bicarbonate secreted is reduced, resulting in the increased viscosity of the secretion. There is considerable evidence from postmortem studies [192] and a murine model of CF [111] to suggest that the injury to the pancreas is secondary to ductular plugging by this viscous secretion. In most cases of PI it is likely that pancreatic injury commences *in utero* [192]. The initial ductular obstruction

results in progressive acinar replacement with fat and fibrosis. Endocrine tissue is almost always preserved into infancy and islets of Langerhans can be identified embedded into the areas replaced by the fat and fibrotic stroma.

There is debate as to the possible importance of other factors that might influence the evolution of pancreatic injury in CF. The role of an inflammatory response has been investigated in animal models of CF [193]. There is evidence that the failure of duodenal bicarbonate secretion initiates a pancreatic acinar stress response which is associated with activation of cellular inflammatory pathways. Such an inflammatory component to pancreatic damage might explain late progression from PS to PI in some cases.

Genotype–phenotype relationships

The pancreatic phenotype in CF has the closest correlation of all clinical manifestations with the underlying genotype. Early reports confirmed the very close relationship between PI and homozygosity for *F508del* [194]. These studies also identified certain compound heterozygotes (such as *R117H/F508*) in which PS was commonly identified. An increased understanding of the functional capacity of CFTR in relationship to specific mutant alleles has allowed a more accurate prediction of PI/PS.

Mutations belonging to classes I–III are predicted to have a severe effect upon CFTR function whereas those of classes 1V and V are associated with some residual function. Homozygosity or compound heterozygosity for class I, II or III mutations strongly correlates with PI whereas compound heterozygosity for class IV and V mutation is predictive of PS status [195]. The combination of a mild (class IV, V) and severe (class I, II, III) mutation is usually associated with PS status.

Symptomatic pancreatitis in CF

Symptomatic (pain associated) pancreatitis is a rare but well-recognized complication of CF [196]. In a recent multicenter study, episodes of symptomatic pancreatitis were reported in 125 (1.24%) of 10 071 patients [197]. This may underestimate the true incidence of symptoms associated with pancreatitis, as the study required significant elevations of serum amylase levels to define an episode. It is our experience that the majority of patients with pancreatitis-related pain have established chronic pancreatitis and episodes of pain may occur without such elevation. Most patients who experience symptomatic pancreatitis are PS at presentation and are compound heterozygous for class IV and V mutations (see above). However, a small subgroup experience episodes of pancreatitis despite having established PI [197,198]. The mean age of presentation is in the late teens and for almost 30% of those with symptomatic pancreatitis this is the presenting feature leading to the diagnosis of CF [197,198].

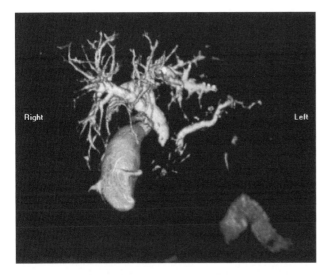

Figure 15.12 A workstation-constructed 3-D MRCP scan showing stricturing of both the distal pancreatic duct and common bile duct in a patient with established symptomatic chronic pancreatitis. Both strictures were managed by endoscopic stenting. *See also Plate 15.12.*

In the majority of cases of symptomatic pancreatitis the process is one of chronicity with recurrent episodes of pain. Possible trigger mechanisms such as alcohol excess and gallstone disease are rarely identified. Specific complications such as pseudocyst formation and common bile duct obstruction appear to be uncommon, and few cases of associated mortality are reported. Progression from PS to PI is well documented as part of the process of symptomatic pancreatitis and may be associated with resolution of pain [197].

In most cases a diagnosis of symptomatic pancreatitis is readily established based on typical pain, elevated amylase (or lipase) levels supplemented by imaging confirming an inflammatory process. This may be less apparent in cases with atypical pain or in whom the amylase levels do not rise (see above). High-quality transabdominal ultrasound and cross-sectional imaging are an essential aid to diagnosis in such cases. A high index of suspicion of this diagnosis should be attached to CF patients who are PS. Possible etiological factors such as common bile duct stones should be sought.

Management is usually restricted to pain control for individual episodes. For long-term management, acid suppression using proton pump inhibitors may be of benefit by reducing pancreatic stimulation. Pancreatic supplements have also been used to reduce pancreatic stimulation in other etiological types of pancreatitis and a trial of therapy is justified.

Endoscopic intervention for the management of pain in chronic pancreatitis is well established for other etiologies particularly in the presence of pancreatic stricture (and duct dilatation), pancreatic stones and pseudocyst formation [199]. We have intervened successfully in three cases of CF in whom poorly controlled pain was associated with a pancreatic stricture and intraductal stones. Endoscopic pancreatic sphincterotomy and temporary stenting was combined with shockwave lithotripsy to re-establish duct drainage (personal communication). Endoscopic biliary stenting is the first-line approach in the rare cases of common bile duct obstruction secondary to chronic pancreatitis (Fig. 15.12). Surgical management for symptomatic pancreatitis in CF is rarely indicated but should be considered for those with intractable pain who have failed endoscopic intervention. The optimum care of these rare complications of CF requires very close cooperation between CF and HPB centers.

CFTR mutations and idiopathic pancreatitis

It has been recognized for some time that there is an increased frequency of gene mutations encoding for *CFTR* in patients with recurrent acute and idiopathic chronic pancreatitis [108,200]. The most recent studies which have screened for the entire coding sequence for *CFTR* have suggested a frequency as high as 25% [201,202]. In most cases a single *CFTR* mutation could be identified (heterozygous) but a small proportion of patients were compound heterozygous (i.e. had CF with the presence of two different *CFTR* mutations). In this latter group are the patients in whom pancreatitis is the presenting feature of CF subsequently confirmed by sweat chloride. The same studies also identified cases of chronic pancreatitis who were transheterozygous for *CFTR* mutations and a mutation in the *SPINK-1* (serine protease inhibitor, Kazal type 1) or *PRSS1* (cationic trypsinogen) genes, both the latter being associated with inherited pancreatitis. *CFTR* mutations have also been identified with increased frequency in cases of pancreatitis seen in patients with alcohol abuse [100] and the congenital ductular abnormality pancreas divisum [203].

These data form the basis of an evolving theory of a multi-hit pathogenesis of recurrent acute and chronic pancreatitis, a theory in which *CFTR* mutations have a major role.

HEPATOBILIARY AND PANCREATIC MALIGNANCY

It is now well recognized that patients with CF have an increased risk of gut-related cancer [204], including malignancies of hepatobiliary and pancreatic origin. While reports of such malignancies are rare in the CF population, their occurrence in young adults is markedly increased as compared to age-matched cohorts. There have recently been two case reports of hepatocellular carcinoma in patients with CF-related cirrhosis [205,206].

Despite this documented increased risk of hepatobiliary and pancreatic malignancy, the overall risk of these occurring is low and does not justify the instigation of routine screening programs.

REFERENCES

101. Vawter GF, Shwachman H. Cystic fibrosis in adults: an autopsy study. *Pathol Annu* 1979; **14**(Pt 2):357–382.

102. Corbett K, Kelleher S, Rowland M *et al*. Cystic fibrosis-associated liver disease: a population-based study. *J Pediatr* 2004; **145**:327–332.

103. Lamireau T, Monnereau S, Martin S *et al*. Epidemiology of liver disease in cystic fibrosis: a longitudinal study. *J Hepatol* 2004; **41**:920–925.

104 Scott-Jupp R, Lama M, Tanner MS. Prevalence of liver disease in cystic fibrosis. *Arch Dis Child* 1991; **66**:698–701.

105. Colombo C, Battezzati PM, Crosignani A *et al*. Liver disease in cystic fibrosis: a prospective study on incidence, risk factors, and outcome. *Hepatology* 2002; **36**:1374–1382.

106. Marino CR, Gorelick FS. Scientific advances in cystic fibrosis. *Gastroenterology* 1992; **103**:681–963.

107. Colombo C, Battezzati PM. Liver involvement in cystic fibrosis: primary organ damage or innocent bystander? *J Hepatol* 2004; **41**:1041–1044.

108. Cohn JA, Friedman KJ, Noone PG *et al*. Relation between mutations of the cystic fibrosis gene and idiopathic pancreatitis. *N Engl J Med* 1998; **339**:653–658.

109. Bhaskar KR, Turner BS, Grubman SA *et al*. Dysregulation of proteoglycan production by intrahepatic biliary epithelial cells bearing defective (delta-f508) cystic fibrosis transmembrane conductance regulator. *Hepatology* 1998; **27**:7–14.

110. Lindblad A, Hultcrantz R, Strandvik B. Bile-duct destruction and collagen deposition: a prominent ultrastructural feature of the liver in cystic fibrosis. *Hepatology* 1992; **16**:372–381.

111. Durie PR, Kent G, Phillips MJ, Ackerley CA. Characteristic multiorgan pathology of cystic fibrosis in a long-living cystic fibrosis transmembrane regulator knockout murine model. *Am J Pathol* 2004; **164**:1481–1493.

112. Robb TA, Davidson GP, Kirubakaran C. Conjugated bile acids in serum and secretions in response to cholecystokinin/secretin stimulation in children with cystic fibrosis. *Gut* 1985; **26**:1246–1256.

113. Weizman Z, Durie PR, Kopelman HR *et al*. Bile acid secretion in cystic fibrosis: evidence for a defect unrelated to fat malabsorption. *Gut* 1986; **27**:1043–1048.

114. Smith JL, Lewindon PJ, Hoskins AC *et al*. Endogenous ursodeoxycholic acid and cholic acid in liver disease due to cystic fibrosis. *Hepatology* 2004; **39**:1673–1682.

115. Duthie A, Doherty DG, Williams C *et al*. Genotype analysis for delta F508, G551D and R553X mutations in children and young adults with cystic fibrosis with and without chronic liver disease. *Hepatology* 1992; **15**:660–664.

116. Lindblad A, Glaumann H, Strandvik B. Natural history of liver disease in cystic fibrosis. *Hepatology* 1999; **30**:1151–1158.

117. Efrati O, Barak A, Modan-Moses D *et al*. Liver cirrhosis and portal hypertension in cystic fibrosis. *Eur J Gastroenterol Hepatol* 2003; **15**:1073–1078.

118. Duthie A, Doherty DG, Donaldson PT *et al*. The major histocompatibility complex influences the development of chronic liver disease in male children and young adults with cystic fibrosis. *J Hepatol* 1995; **23**:532–537.

119. Salvatore F, Scudiero O, Castaldo G. Genotype–phenotype correlation in cystic fibrosis: the role of modifier genes. *Am J Med Genet* 2002; **111**:88–95.

120. Henrion-Caude A, Flamant C, Roussey M *et al*. Liver disease in pediatric patients with cystic fibrosis is associated with glutathione S-transferase P1 polymorphism. *Hepatology* 2002; **36**(4 Pt 1):913–917.

121. Maurage C, Lenaerts C, Weber A *et al*. Meconium ileus and its equivalent as a risk factor for the development of cirrhosis: an autopsy study in cystic fibrosis. *J Pediatr Gastroenterol Nutr* 1989; **9**:17–20.

122. Wilschanski M, Rivlin J, Cohen S *et al*. Clinical and genetic risk factors for cystic fibrosis-related liver disease. *Pediatrics* 1999; **103**:52–57.

123. Lai HJ, Cheng Y, Cho H *et al*. Association between initial disease presentation, lung disease outcomes, and survival in patients with cystic fibrosis. *Am J Epidemiol* 2004; **159**:537–546.

124. Gaskin KJ, Waters DL, Howman-Giles R *et al*. Liver disease and common-bile-duct stenosis in cystic fibrosis. *N Engl J Med* 1988; **318**:340–346.

125. Nagel RA, Westaby D, Javaid A *et al*. Liver disease and bile duct abnormalities in adults with cystic fibrosis. *Lancet* 1989; **2**:1422–1425.

126. Mieli-Vergani G, Psacharopoulos HT, Nicholson AM *et al*. Immune responses to liver membrane antigens in patients with cystic fibrosis and liver disease. *Arch Dis Child* 1980; **55**:696–701.

127. Vlaman HB, France NE, Wallis PG. Prolonged neonatal jaundice in cystic fibrosis. *Arch Dis Child* 1971; **46**:805–809.

128. Furuya KN, Roberts EA, Canny GJ, Phillips MJ. Neonatal hepatitis syndrome with paucity of interlobular bile ducts in cystic fibrosis. *J Pediatr Gastroenterol Nutr* 1991; **12**:127–130.

129. Roy CC, Weber AM, Morin CL *et al*. Hepatobiliary disease in cystic fibrosis: a survey of current issues and concepts. *J Pediatr Gastroenterol Nutr* 1982; **1**:469–478.

130. Treem WR, Stanley CA. Massive hepatomegaly, steatosis, and secondary plasma carnitine deficiency in an infant with cystic fibrosis. *Pediatrics* 1989; **83**:993–997.

131. Chitturi S, Farrell GC. Etiopathogenesis of nonalcoholic steatohepatitis. *Semin Liver Dis* 2001; **21**:27–41.

132. Feranchak AP, Sokol RJ. Cholangiocyte biology and cystic fibrosis liver disease. *Semin Liver Dis* 2001; **21**:471–488.

133. Roberts EA. Non-alcoholic fatty liver disease (NAFLD) in children. *Front Biosci* 2005; **10**:2306–2318.

134. Pares A, Rodes J. Natural history of primary biliary cirrhosis. *Clin Liver Dis* 2003; **7**:779–794.

135. Farrant JM, Hayllar KM, Wilkinson ML *et al*. Natural history and prognostic variables in primary sclerosing cholangitis. *Gastroenterology* 1991; **100**:1710–1717.

136. Hayllar KM, Williams SG, Wise AE *et al.* A prognostic model for the prediction of survival in cystic fibrosis. *Thorax* 1997; **52**:313–317.

137. Sokol RJ, Durie PR for the Cystic Fibrosis Foundation Hepatobiliary Disease Consensus Group. Recommendations for management of liver and biliary tract disease in cystic fibrosis. *J Pediatr Gastroenterol Nutr* 1999; **28**(Suppl 1): S1–S13.

138. Williams SG, Samways J, Innes JA *et al.* Systemic haemodynamic changes in patients with cystic fibrosis with and without chronic liver disease. *J Hepatol* 1996; **25**:900–908.

139. Lindblad A, Glaumann H, Strandvik B. A two-year prospective study of the effect of ursodeoxycholic acid on urinary bile acid excretion and liver morphology in cystic fibrosis-associated liver disease. *Hepatology* 1998; **27**:166–174.

140. Lenaerts C, Lapierre C, Patriquin H *et al.* Surveillance for cystic fibrosis-associated hepatobiliary disease: early ultrasound changes and predisposing factors. *J Pediatr* 2003; **143**:343–350.

141. McHugo JM, McKeown C, Brown MT *et al.* Ultrasound findings in children with cystic fibrosis. *Br J Radiol* 1987; **60**:137–141.

142. Krishnamurthy S, Krishnamurthy GT. Technetium-99m-iminodiacetic acid organic anions: review of biokinetics and clinical application in hepatology. *Hepatology* 1989; **9**:139–153.

143. O'Brien S, Keogan M, Casey M *et al.* Biliary complications of cystic fibrosis. *Gut* 1992; **33**:387–391.

144. Colombo C, Castellani MR, Balistreri WF *et al.* Scintigraphic documentation of an improvement in hepatobiliary excretory function after treatment with ursodeoxycholic acid in patients with cystic fibrosis and associated liver disease. *Hepatology* 1992; **15**:677–684.

145. King LJ, Scurr ED, Murugan N *et al.* Hepatobiliary and pancreatic manifestations of cystic fibrosis: MR imaging appearances. *Radiographics* 2000; **20**:767–777.

146. Durieu I, Pellet O, Simonot L *et al.* Sclerosing cholangitis in adults with cystic fibrosis: a magnetic resonance cholangiographic prospective study. *J Hepatol* 1999; **30**:1052–1056.

147. Paumgartner G, Beuers U. Ursodeoxycholic acid in cholestatic liver disease: mechanisms of action and therapeutic use revisited. *Hepatology* 2002; **36**:525–531.

148. Van Nieuwkerk CM, Elferink RP, Groen AK *et al.* Effects of ursodeoxycholate and cholate feeding on liver disease in FVB mice with a disrupted mdr2 P-glycoprotein gene. *Gastroenterology* 1996; **111**:165–171.

149. Poupon RE, Balkau B, Eschwege E, Poupon R for the UDCA-PBC Study Group. A multicenter, controlled trial of ursodiol for the treatment of primary biliary cirrhosis. *N Engl J Med* 1991; **324**:1548–1554.

150. Beuers U, Spengler U, Kruis W *et al.* Ursodeoxycholic acid for treatment of primary sclerosing cholangitis: a placebo-controlled trial. *Hepatology* 1992; **16**:707–714.

151. Fickert P, Zollner G, Fuchsbichler A *et al.* Effects of ursodeoxycholic and cholic acid feeding on hepatocellular transporter expression in mouse liver. *Gastroenterology* 2001; **121**:170–183.

152. Qiao L, Yacoub A, Studer E *et al.* Inhibition of the MAPK and PI3K pathways enhances UDCA-induced apoptosis in primary rodent hepatocytes. *Hepatology* 2002; **35**:779–789.

153. Calmus Y, Gane P, Rouger P, Poupon R. Hepatic expression of class I and class II major histocompatibility complex molecules in primary biliary cirrhosis: effect of ursodeoxycholic acid. *Hepatology* 1990; **11**:12–15.

154. Colombo C, Apostolo MG, Assaisso M *et al.* Liver disease in cystic fibrosis. *Neth J Med* 1992; **41**:119–122.

155. van de Meeberg PC, Houwen RH, Sinaasappel M *et al.* Low-dose versus high-dose ursodeoxycholic acid in cystic fibrosis-related cholestatic liver disease: results of a randomized study with 1-year follow-up. *Scand J Gastroenterol* 1997; **32**:369–373.

156. Cotting J, Lentze MJ, Reichen J. Effects of ursodeoxycholic acid treatment on nutrition and liver function in patients with cystic fibrosis and longstanding cholestasis. *Gut* 1990; **31**:918–921.

157. Colombo C, Setchell KD, Podda M *et al.* Effects of ursodeoxycholic acid therapy for liver disease associated with cystic fibrosis. *J Pediatr* 1990; **117**:482–489.

158. Colombo C, Battezzati PM, Podda M *et al.* for the Italian Group for the Study of Ursodeoxycholic Acid in Cystic Fibrosis. Ursodeoxycholic acid for liver disease associated with cystic fibrosis: a double-blind multicenter trial. *Hepatology* 1996; **23**:1484–1490.

159. Cheng K, Ashby D, Smyth R. Ursodeoxycholic acid for cystic fibrosis-related liver disease. *Cochrane Database Syst Rev* 2000; CD000222.

160. Noble-Jamieson G, Barnes N, Jamieson N *et al.* Liver transplantation for hepatic cirrhosis in cystic fibrosis. *J R Soc Med* 1996; **89**(Suppl 27):31–37.

161. Mack DR, Traystman MD, Colombo JL *et al.* Clinical denouement and mutation analysis of patients with cystic fibrosis undergoing liver transplantation for biliary cirrhosis. *J Pediatr* 1995; **127**:881–887.

162. Milkiewicz P, Skiba G, Kelly D *et al.* Transplantation for cystic fibrosis: outcome following early liver transplantation. *J Gastroenterol Hepatol* 2002; **17**:208–213.

163. Fridell JA, Bond GJ, Mazariegos GV *et al.* Liver transplantation in children with cystic fibrosis: a long-term longitudinal review of a single center's experience. *J Pediatr Surg* 2003; **38**:1152–1156.

164. Gooding I, Dondos V, Gyi KM *et al.* Variceal hemorrhage and cystic fibrosis: outcomes and implications for liver transplantation. *Liver Transpl* 2005; **11**:1522–1526.

165. Couetil JP, Soubrane O, Houssin DP *et al.* Combined heart–lung–liver, double lung–liver, and isolated liver transplantation for cystic fibrosis in children. *Transpl Int* 1997; **10**(1):33–39.

166. Dennis CM, McNeil KD, Dunning J *et al.* Heart–lung–liver transplantation. *J Heart Lung Transplant* 1996; **15**:536–538.

167. Angelico M, Gandin C, Canuzzi P et al. Gallstones in cystic fibrosis: a critical reappraisal. *Hepatology* 1991; **14**:768–775.

168. Yang Y, Raper SE, Cohn JA et al. An approach for treating the hepatobiliary disease of cystic fibrosis by somatic gene transfer. *Proc Natl Acad Sci USA* 1993; **90**:4601–4605.

169. Jalan R, Hayes PC for British Society of Gastroenterology. UK guidelines on the management of variceal haemorrhage in cirrhotic patients. *Gut* 2000; **46**(Suppl 3–4):III1–III15.

170. Garcia-Tsao G. Bacterial infections in cirrhosis. *Can J Gastroenterol* 2004; **18**:405–406.

171. Vlavianos P, Westaby D. Management of acute variceal haemorrhage. *Eur J Gastroenterol Hepatol* 2001; **13**:335–342.

172. Gross M, Schiemann U, Muhlhofer A, Zoller WG. Meta-analysis: efficacy of therapeutic regimens in ongoing variceal bleeding. *Endoscopy* 2001; **33**:737–746.

173. Gimson A, Polson R, Westaby D, Williams R. Omeprazole in the management of intractable esophageal ulceration following injection sclerotherapy. *Gastroenterology* 1990; **99**:1829–1831.

174. Polson RJ, Westaby D, Gimson AE et al. Sucralfate for the prevention of early rebleeding following injection sclerotherapy for esophageal varices. *Hepatology* 1989; **10**:279–282.

175. Schepke M, Kleber G, Nurnberg D et al. for the German Study Group for the Primary Prophylaxis of Variceal Bleeding. Ligation versus propranolol for the primary prophylaxis of variceal bleeding in cirrhosis. *Hepatology* 2004; **40**:65–72.

176. Nevens F. Review article: a critical comparison of drug therapies in currently used therapeutic strategies for variceal haemorrhage. *Aliment Pharmacol Ther* 2004; **20**(Suppl 3): 18–22; discussion 23.

177. de Franchis R. Somatostatin, somatostatin analogues and other vasoactive drugs in the treatment of bleeding oesophageal varices. *Dig Liver Dis* 2004; **36**(Suppl 1): S93–S100.

178. Vlavianos P, Gimson AE, Westaby D, Williams R. Balloon tamponade in variceal bleeding: use and misuse. *Br Med J* 1989; **298**:1158.

179. Stern RC, Stevens DP, Boat TF et al. Symptomatic hepatic disease in cystic fibrosis: incidence, course, and outcome of portal systemic hunting. *Gastroenterology* 1976; **70**(5 Pt 1): 645–649.

180. Luketic VA, Sanyal AJ. Esophageal varices. II: TIPS (transjugular intrahepatic portosystemic shunt) and surgical therapy. *Gastroenterol Clin N Am.* 2000; **29**: vi,387–421.

181. Pozler O, Krajina A, Vanicek H et al. Transjugular intrahepatic portosystemic shunt in five children with cystic fibrosis: long-term results. *Hepatogastroenterology* 2003; **50**:1111–1114.

182. Garcia-Tsao G. Portal hypertension. *Curr Opin Gastroenterol* 2003; **19**:250–258.

183. Shawcross D, Jalan R. Dispelling myths in the treatment of hepatic encephalopathy. *Lancet* 2005; **365**:431–433.

184. Zach MS, Thalhammer GH, Eber E. Partial splenectomy in CF patients with hypersplenism. *Arch Dis Child* 2003; **88**:649.

185. Westwood AT, Millar AJ, Ireland JD, Swart A. Splenectomy in cystic fibrosis patients. *Arch Dis Child* 2004; **89**:1078.

186. Duchatel F, Muller F, Oury JF et al. Prenatal diagnosis of cystic fibrosis: ultrasonography of the gallbladder at 17–19 weeks of gestation. *Fetal Diagn Ther* 1993; **8**:28–36.

187. Chaudry G, Navarro OM, Levine DS, Oudjhane K. Abdominal manifestations of cystic fibrosis in children. *Pediatr Radiol* 2006; **36**:233–240.

188. Vitek L. Intestinal metabolism of bilirubin in the pathogenesis of neonatal jaundice. *J Pediatr* 2003; **143**:810.

189. Wasmuth HE, Keppeler H, Herrmann U et al. Coinheritance of Gilbert syndrome-associated UGT1A1 mutation increases gallstone risk in cystic fibrosis. *Hepatology* 2006; **43**:738–741.

190. Stern RC, Rothstein FC, Doershuk CF. Treatment and prognosis of symptomatic gallbladder disease in patients with cystic fibrosis. *J Pediatr Gastroenterol Nutr* 1986; **5**:35–40.

191. Colombo C, Bertolini E, Assaisso ML et al. Failure of ursodeoxycholic acid to dissolve radiolucent gallstones in patients with cystic fibrosis. *Acta Paediatr* 1993; **82**:562–565.

192. Imrie JR, Fagan DG, Sturgess JM. Quantitative evaluation of the development of the exocrine pancreas in cystic fibrosis and control infants. *Am J Pathol* 1979; **95**:697–707.

193. De Lisle RC, Isom KS, Ziemer D, Cotton CU. Changes in the exocrine pancreas secondary to altered small intestinal function in the CF mouse. *Am J Physiol Gastrointest Liver Physiol* 2001; **281**:G899–G906.

194. The Cystic Fibrosis Genotype-Phenotype Consortium. Correlation between genotype and phenotype in patients with cystic fibrosis. *N Engl J Med* 1993; **329**:1308–1313.

195. Ahmed N, Corey M, Forstner G et al. Molecular consequences of cystic fibrosis transmembrane regulator (CFTR) gene mutations in the exocrine pancreas. *Gut* 2003; **52**:1159–1164.

196. Shwachman H, Lebenthal E, Khaw KT. Recurrent acute pancreatitis in patients with cystic fibrosis with normal pancreatic enzymes. *Pediatrics* 1975; **55**:86–95.

197. De Boeck K, Wilschanski M, Castellani C et al. Cystic fibrosis: terminology and diagnostic algorithms. *Thorax* 2006; **61**:627–635.

198. Durno C, Corey M, Zielenski J et al. Genotype and phenotype correlations in patients with cystic fibrosis and pancreatitis. *Gastroenterology* 2002; **123**:1857–1864.

199. Westaby D, Lombard M. *Therapeutic Gastrointestinal Endoscopy*. London, Martin Dunitz Publishers, 2002.

200. Sharer N, Schwarz M, Malone G et al. Mutations of the cystic fibrosis gene in patients with chronic pancreatitis. *N Engl J Med* 1998; **339**:645–652.

201. Noone PG, Zhou Z, Silverman LM et al. Cystic fibrosis gene mutations and pancreatitis risk: relation to epithelial ion transport and trypsin inhibitor gene mutations. *Gastroenterology* 2001; **121**:1310–1319.

202. Audrezet MP, Chen JM, Le Marechal C et al. Determination of the relative contribution of three genes – the cystic

fibrosis transmembrane conductance regulator gene, the cationic trypsinogen gene, and the pancreatic secretory trypsin inhibitor gene – to the etiology of idiopathic chronic pancreatitis. *Eur J Hum Genet* 2002; **10**:100–106.

203. Gelrud A, Sheth S, Banerjee S *et al.* Analysis of cystic fibrosis gene product (CFTR) function in patients with pancreas divisum and recurrent acute pancreatitis. *Am J Gastroenterol* 2004; **99**:1557–1562.

204. Maisonneuve P, FitzSimmons SC, Neglia JP *et al.* Cancer risk in nontransplanted and transplanted cystic fibrosis patients: a 10-year study. *J Natl Cancer Inst* 2003; **95**:381–387.

205. McKeon D, Day A, Parmar J *et al.* Hepatocellular carcinoma in association with cirrhosis in a patient with cystic fibrosis. *J Cyst Fibros* 2004; **3**(3):193–195.

206. Kelleher T, Staunton M, O'Mahony S, McCormick PA. Advanced hepatocellular carcinoma associated with cystic fibrosis. *Eur J Gastroenterol Hepatol* 2005; **17**:1123–1124.

Insulin deficiency and diabetes related to cystic fibrosis

CHRISTOPHER D. SHELDON AND LEE DOBSON

INTRODUCTION

The improved survival of cystic fibrosis (CF) patients has resulted in the emergence of cystic-fibrosis-related diabetes (CFRD) as a significant complication. Substantial evidence now confirms the negative clinical impact of CFRD. Loss of pancreatic function is usually first related to exocrine function followed by deteriorating endocrine function some years later. Acute-on-chronic infection contributes to variable resistance to the effects of insulin. The combination of gradual onset of insulin deficiency combined with variable insulin resistance is characteristic of CFRD. The deteriorating clinical status seen before the diagnosis of CFRD has directed attention away from the direct effects of blood glucose towards the potentially more important and widespread effects of insulin deficiency, the fundamental pathophysiological process underlying CFRD.

The recognition that clinical decline precedes frank diabetes has prompted a re-evaluation of diagnostic methods and the timing or choice of therapeutic interventions. In CFRD there appears to be a spectrum of impaired glucose metabolism varying from entirely normal to fasting hyperglycemia and persistently elevated blood glucose (Fig. 16.1). Due to increased survival patients are now developing the microvascular complications of chronic hyperglycemia previously seen only in the non-CF population.

INCIDENCE AND PREVALENCE

The reported prevalence of CFRD has been increasing since the first case report of its association in 1955 (Table 16.1) [1]. Though this is most likely a result of improvements in life expectancy, the increasing awareness of CFRD, the associated rise in screening for CFRD and the variation in patient populations or diagnostic criteria may also be contributing to this increase.

Lanng and co-workers [2] reported that a national cohort of 210 Danish patients, median age 14 years, had a prevalence of glucose intolerance of 26% (11% with CFRD, 15% with impaired glucose tolerance) and confirmed that this prevalence increased with age. Studies from the UK have reported similar results. Yung and co-workers [3] reported a diagnosis of CFRD in 74 (14.3%) out of the 518 CF subjects attending the Royal Brompton Hospital.

The most recent studies have come from large epidemiological surveys both in Europe [4] and the United States [5]. The European study reported levels of diabetes of 5% and

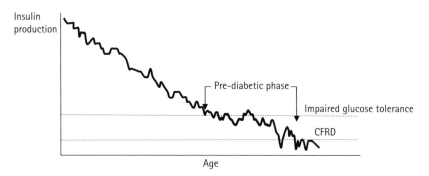

Figure 16.1 Visual representation of the progressively deteriorating beta-cell function (insulin deficiency) that precedes the diagnosis of CF-related diabetes (CFRD).

Table 16.1 Incidence and prevalence of CF-related diabetes.

Authors	*n*	Criteria	Prevalence/incidence
Prevalence			
Rosan (1962)	1300	–	<1%
Lanng (1991)	210	OGTT	11%
CFF (1996)	18 627	Use of insulin or OHA	5.1%
Moran (1998)	408	OGTT	11% (5–9 years: 9%; >30 years: 43%)
Koch (2001)		–	5% (10–14 years); 12.6% (15–19 years)
Marshall (2005)	8247	Use of insulin or OHA	14.3% (>35 years: 21.7%)
Incidence			
Lanng (1995)	191	OGTT	Annual incidence 3.8% (>10 years: 5.0%; >20 years: 9.3%)

OGTT, oral glucose tolerance test; CFF, Cystic Fibrosis Foundation (USA); OHA, oral hypoglycemic agent.

12.6% in the respective age groups 10–14 and 15–19 years. The US study reported data on 8247 patients. They confirmed that CFRD was associated with increased age (14.3% of patients aged over 13 years, 21.7% of those over 35 years) but also with female gender (17% females, 12% males).

The only estimate of incidence comes from a 5-year prospective study in 191 Danish CF patients with annual oral glucose tolerance testing (OGTT) from the age of 2 years showing an average annual incidence of 3.8% [6]. Incidence rates increased with age, with patients aged over 10 years and over 20 years having annual rates of 5.0% and 9.3%, respectively.

Importantly these studies underline the presence of a spectrum of glucose tolerance within the CF population, with a gradual transition from normal glucose tolerance to impaired glucose tolerance progressing finally to diabetes mellitus.

ETIOLOGY

The etiology of CFRD is complex and incompletely understood. The gradual development of insulinopenia is believed to be the result of functioning beta cell loss. However, the imbalance in the prevalence of CFRD compared to that of exocrine pancreatic insufficiency (which is present in the majority of CF patients) would suggest that another process is occurring in the pathogenesis of the disease.

Genetic susceptibility

The two most recent large epidemiological studies have provided some insight into this area. The Epidemiologic

Survey of Cystic Fibrosis reported that *F508del* homozygotes had a higher prevalence of CFRD when compared with the compound heterozygotes and other genotype groups [5]. They also noted that the prevalence of CFRD in the *F508del* homozygotes increased in each successive age group. This would be compatible with our current understanding that the genotype in CF is highly predictive of pancreatic status and the homozygous *F508del* genotype is known to be associated with pancreatic insufficiency in nearly all patients.

Cystic fibrosis transmembrane regulator mutations occur in six main classes and CFRD mainly occurs in people with severe class I–III mutations with background exocrine pancreatic deficiency [7]. The European Epidemiologic Registry of CF (ERCF) reported that 20% of patients carrying class I, II or III gene mutations developed CFRD in contrast to only 1.5% of patients carrying class IV and V mutations [4].

No link has been found with HLA alleles DR3, DR4, DR3/4, HDR2 which are associated with type 1 diabetes in the general population [8].

Autoimmune process

Autoantibodies to pancreatic islet cells and glutamic acid decarboxylase are present in people with type 1 diabetes and reflect the cell-mediated immune destruction that occurs. Researchers have looked for these markers in CFRD but they have rarely been found and their contribution to cellular injury remains unclear [9].

PATHOPHYSIOLOGY

CFRD results directly from mutations in the *CFTR* gene, so it is not just coincidental that type 1 or type 2 diabetes have a very different pathophysiology from CFRD (Table 16.2). A number of processes are believed to be involved in the pathophysiology of CFRD, including impaired beta-cell function, impaired alpha/pancreatic polypeptide cell function, reduced insulin sensitivity and altered insulin clearance.

Impaired beta-cell function

CFRD is primarily an insulinopenic condition characterized by impaired and delayed insulin secretion, as a consequence of beta-cell failure [10,11,12]. There is still decreased insulin secretion compared to normal subjects in CF patients with normal glucose tolerance [11]. Studies have also shown that this impairment worsens with deteriorating glucose tolerance [11,13,14]. This would suggest that there is a progressive deterioration in beta-cell function that precedes the diagnosis of diabetes and continues after diagnosis. Other factors are likely to be contributing

Table 16.2   Comparison of CF-related diabetes with type 2 diabetes.

	Type 2 diabetes	Type 1 diabetes	CF-related diabetes
Age of onset (years)	>40	<20	18–21
Prevalence (%)	5–7	1	5–10
Body habitus	Obese	Normal	Thin
Symptoms	Common	Common	Uncommon
Insulin secretion	↓	↓↓↓	↓↓
Insulin resistance	+++	+	+
Autoimmune etiology	No	Yes	No
Microvascular complications	Yes	Yes	Yes
Macrovascular complications	Yes	Yes	No
Diet	Calorie restrictive	Variable	Calorie high
Treatment	OHAs, insulin	Insulin	Insulin

OHA, oral hypoglycemic agent.

to the abnormal glycemic status seen in CFRD and support the concept of a clinically important pre-diabetic period.

Impaired function of alpha cells and pancreatic polypeptide cells

Alpha-cell function can be assessed either by measuring the suppressibility of glucagon production following a glucose load, or by the expected stimulation in glucagon production associated with the infusion of arginine. Studies implementing the latter method have shown the response to be normal [15] or decreased [10] in CF subjects with normal glucose tolerance, and decreased in subjects with CFRD [10]. The suppressibility of glucagon production after a glucose load has been shown to be normal [15] or impaired [11] in CF subjects with impaired glucose tolerance. Further studies are needed to clarify this finding as it would suggest the presence of a signaling defect rather than islet destruction leading to alpha-cell failure.

Both basal and stimulated pancreatic polypeptide levels have been shown to be reduced in CF subjects independent of the presence of diabetes [11,16].

In conjunction with the reduction in insulin secretion, these findings suggest the destruction of entire islets rather than a beta-cell specific defect. Postmortem studies have supported this by documenting fibrosis and fatty infiltration of the pancreas with a reduction in the absolute number of pancreatic islets [17,18]. However, there is a poor correlation between the number of islets lost and the degree of pancreatic fibrosis [19,20], implying that CFRD is not explained simply by the degree of islet obliteration [21]. As glucagon elevates blood glucose the reduced glucagon

response may also explain why in the setting of quite marked insulinopenia CF patients may not be diabetic.

Insulin resistance

In the general population the commonest cause of resistance to the peripheral actions of insulin is obesity, which is a major risk factor for type 2 diabetes. In CF, obesity is very uncommon but infections and corticosteroid administration can both result in insulin resistance (reduced insulin sensitivity). The contribution of insulin resistance to the etiology of CFRD is unclear. Results of studies have been conflicting with reports of increased [15], normal [22,23] and reduced insulin sensitivity [24,25]. Its reduction in some studies may simply be a reflection of chronic hyperglycemia as seen in type 1 diabetes, but predominantly the discrepancies are due to differences in the methodologies employed and the lack of uniformity between the cohorts of subjects studied.

It is unlikely that reduced insulin sensitivity is an important cause of CFRD, although the decreased insulin sensitivity probably contributes to the worsening glucose tolerance in acute infections.

Hepatic glucose production (HGP) is an important regulator of glycemic control. Insulin is a potent inhibitor of this pathway but the suppression of HGP by insulin has been shown to be reduced in non-CF diabetes. This condition has been termed 'hepatic insulin resistance' (HIR). HGP has been shown to be raised in CF subjects [24–26], and HIR has also been noted [27]. However, the exact contribution of hepatic insulin resistance is unclear and deserves further investigation.

Insulin clearance rate

Studies of insulin kinetics have shown that the insulin clearance rate is increased by 30–40% in CF patients whether or not they have CFRD [23,28]. Increased clearance combined with reduced insulin secretion could contribute to the observed insulinopenia. The relative contribution of increased insulin clearance to the pathophysiology of CFRD remains unclear.

Increased glucose uptake from the gut

Two studies have studied glucose absorption and both have reported an increased glucose uptake in CF when compared to non-CF controls [29,30]. Unfortunately the studies were small, and it is likely that the contribution to the pathophysiology of CFRD is small.

Summary

The abnormal pattern of glycemia in CFRD has many contributory factors. It is principally characterized by delayed and impaired insulin secretion but with some contribution from reduced insulin sensitivity and reduced glucagon response.

CLINICAL FEATURES

Due to the insidious nature of this condition the classic features of diabetes are present in only about one-third of patients at diagnosis, and many of the symptoms that are recognized may be due solely to the CF condition alone [6]. Ketoacidosis, a common presentation in type 1 diabetes, is unlikely to occur and there has only been one case reported in the literature [31].

The average age of onset of CFRD is 18–21 years [4,32,33], and there appears to be growing data to support a female to male preponderance (17.1% vs 12%; [5]), with its onset at a younger age [6].

Mortality and CFRD

The impact of diabetes mellitus on the prognosis of patients with CF has been the subject of much debate. This has been due to difficulties in interpreting survival data in epidemiological studies. Often there are variations between centers with respect to the age ranges of the cohorts studied, and the criteria used for diagnosis. In addition studies that have looked at survival from birth have introduced an element of bias due to the inclusion of patients in the non-CFRD group who died young but may have gone on to develop CFRD had they lived long enough.

Despite this, and in contradiction to original studies that reported that survival was unaffected [34], there now appears to be substantial evidence that there is excess mortality associated with CFRD [4,35].

Finkelstein and co-workers [32] reported that there was only a 25% survival in patients with CFRD by the age of 30 years, whereas survival was 60% in the non-CFRD group. The CF Patient Registry in the United States revealed that the mortality rate was 6-fold greater in patients with CFRD [36]. Recent prospective data found that patients with CFRD have a median survival of 24 years as compared with 34 years in non-diabetic controls [4]. There also appears to be a difference between the sexes, with median survival for females being over 15 years shorter than for males [35].

Morbidity and CFRD

The impact of improved longevity in CF patients has not only been an increased prevalence of CFRD, but also an increased duration with the condition and potentially a greater clinical impact. Consequently there are two aspects that need to be considered. First, can patients with CFRD develop the late diabetic complications recognized in the non-CF population? Second, does CFRD lead to a

Table 16.3 Microvascular complications of CF-related diabetes.

Authors	CFRD patients studied	Results
Chazan (1970)	62	36% abnormal retinal vessels
Rodman (1986)	24	8% retinopathy
Sullivan (1989)	19	16% retinopathy, 16% nephropathy, 21% neuropathy
Lanng (1994)	40	5% retinopathy, 5% nephropathy, 5% neuropathy
Rosenecker (2001)	28	11% retinopathy, 7% nephropathy, 7% neuropathy

decline in clinical status independent of diabetes-related complications?

Despite the lack of clarity in a few studies regarding whether universally accepted definitions of retinopathy, nephropathy and neuropathy have been applied, there is growing evidence that diabetes mellitus in the CF population can produce the recognized late complications of microvascular disease [37–44] (Table 16.3). Patients with CFRD should be screened routinely for complications but with some caution when deciding which screening measures to adopt from the non-CF population as few studies have been carried out to assess their application to CF patients. One such measure is microalbuminuria. This simple urine test is well established as a sensitive indicator of progression to diabetic nephropathy in non-CF diabetes, but confounding factors, such as increased urinary albumin excretion due to chronic sepsis and reduced urinary creatinine excretion due to a low muscle mass, may reduce its specificity in CF subjects [45].

Macrovascular disease, a common finding in the non-CF population, does not at present appear to be a complication of CFRD but this probably reflects the reduced life expectancy. There has been only one report of a CF patient with longstanding diabetes who at postmortem was noted to have diffuse atherosclerosis; however, the cause of death was respiratory in origin [46]. With the advent of improved treatments macrovascular disease may become more of a problem.

Initial studies reported no clinical decline with the onset of CFRD [34,41]. Consensus opinion, however, now seems more strongly to suggest the association of CFRD with deterioration in health status [4,5,13,44].

Milla and co-workers [13] followed 152 patients with CF for 4 years after a baseline OGTT was performed. They showed that the rates of decline in FEV_1 and FVC correlated with the degree of glucose intolerance. Rosenecker and co-workers [44], in a prospective multicenter study, followed 56 CF patients (28 with CFRD and 28 without CFRD) for 5 years; FEV_1 and FVC declined significantly over the study period in the group with diabetes, whereas patients without diabetes did not show a significant decline. The ESCF reported that patients with CFRD had more severe pulmonary disease, more frequent pulmonary exacerbations and poorer nutritional status compared to those without diabetes [5]. As with mortality there is some data to suggest that gender differences may again be present, with females having a 20% lower percentage predicted FEV_1 compared with control subjects [47].

Impact of pre-diabetes

The overall clinical status of CF patients gradually declines with age regardless of the presence or absence of diabetes. However, it is now becoming clearer that the pre-diabetic period accentuates this decline with CF subjects showing evidence of deteriorating health status years prior to a diagnosis of CFRD [32,48]. Finkelstein and co-workers [32], in their report on 448 CF patients, described clinical deterioration in National Institutes of Health scores for up to 2 years prior to the diagnosis of CFRD. Lanng and colleagues [48] reported decreases in weight, BMI, FEV_1 and FVC up to 4.5 years prior to the diagnosis of CFRD. Further support has come from trials assessing the impact of insulin therapy, reporting clinical decline prior to the introduction of insulin [49–52].

Analysis of this pre-diabetic phase has revealed declining insulin levels prior to the OGTT becoming diagnostic for diabetes [11,13]. Previous studies have shown that patients with CF have chronically elevated rates of protein catabolism [53]. Insulin is a key factor in fat and protein synthesis and storage as well as carbohydrate metabolism. It is therefore logical to assume that insulin deficiency is partly responsible for this catabolic state. Traditionally the OGTT has been used as the reference point for the introduction of insulin therapy, but it is possible that the anabolic roles in protein and lipid metabolism that are deficient with declining insulin levels may be more clinically relevant than glycemic control.

DIAGNOSIS AND SCREENING

Diagnostic criteria

The reversible and/or preventable clinical decline in the pre-diabetic and subsequent diabetic period reinforces the importance of accurate screening and diagnostic tools for CFRD. In the non-CF population the diagnosis is based on the widely accepted World Health Organization criteria (Table 16.4). The glycemic thresholds in a 75-g oral glucose tolerance test, that define diabetes, were derived from the glucose concentrations associated with glucose-specific complications (such as diabetic retinopathy) in epidemiological studies. Despite the lack of equivalent studies in CF, the same glycemic thresholds have been adopted as the standard for the diagnosis of CFRD. Whether these glycemic thresholds should apply is unclear and still the matter of some debate. The increased recognition of the clinically

Table 16.4   World Health Organization (WHO) diagnostic criteria for diabetes mellitus (1999).

In the presence of diabetes symptoms
Random venous plasma glucose >11.1 mmol/L
OR
Fasting plasma glucose >7.0 mmol/L
OR
2-hour glucose >11.1 mmol/L following an OGTT
No symptoms
At least one elevated glucose test greater than the concentrations above, with a second elevated glucose on another day

OGTT, oral glucose tolerance test (oral load of 75 g of anhydrous glucose in patients over 43 kg and a dose of 1.75 g/kg below this value).

relevant consequences of insulin deficiency other than the effects on glucose metabolism has cast further doubt. In the future, methods of defining insulin deficiency other than the degree of hyperglycemia may be more appropriate.

Strategies for testing for CFRD

Features unique to CF may make the diagnosis of CFRD difficult in that clinical status or treatment may alter the glycemic status of an individual. This may mean that glycemic status may be abnormal on one occasion (e.g. during an infective exacerbation) and normal on another [54].

Centers have adopted different strategies for testing patients for CFRD. These have included: random and fasting plasma glucose, post-prandial glucose testing, urine glucose testing, glycosylated hemoglobin (HbA_{1c}), and the oral glucose tolerance test (OGTT). A survey of physicians in the United States found that the two most popular methods were the measurement of HbA_{1c} and random plasma glucose [55]. The UK CF Trust currently suggests an oral OGTT annually after the age of 12 years [56]. Many UK centers use a series of post-prandial blood sugar measurements to detect hyperglycemia in the diabetic range (>11.1 mmol/L) . Clinical observations suggest that many CF patients may have their most significant hyperglycemia following their evening meal, and 1- to 2-hour post-prandial evening blood glucose estimations can be diagnostic.

Glycosylated hemoglobin (HbA_{1c})

HbA_{1c} levels provide a retrospective measure of glycemia and are not recommended by the WHO as a diagnostic tool for non-CF diabetes mellitus. Early reports had supported its use in detecting CFRD [57]; however, subsequent studies have revealed its poor sensitivity when compared to the OGTT [3,6,12,14,58]. It has been suggested that this is due to the red blood cell turnover time being shorter than 3 months in CF subjects resulting in low HbA_{1c} levels for the same degree of glycemia [59]. An alternative reason may be that early in the development of CFRD transient excursions of blood glucose into the diabetic range are insufficiently prolonged to cause a rise in HbA$_{1c}$.

The role of HbA$_{1c}$ in monitoring glycemic control once CFRD is diagnosed requires further validation. Theoretically the effects on red-cell turnover might lead to an underestimation of glycemic control and hence the requirement for lower targets than in non-CF subjects; however, recent work would suggest that it still retains good predictive value [60].

Random blood glucose

Random blood glucose (RBG) testing has been reported as being insufficiently sensitive in the diagnosis of CFRD [3], although a value greater than 7.0 mmol/L (126 mg/dL) has been adopted as a starting point for the investigation of CFRD in the American Consensus Conference screening protocol [36]. One criticism of previous studies that have analyzed the value of RBGs is the reliance on single measurements, when in fact the development of an RBG profile over a period of time may be more informative [49].

Urine glucose testing

The accuracy of urine glucose testing has not been fully evaluated in CF subjects. However, any benefit is unlikely as it is not sensitive in the diagnosis of type 2 diabetes in non-CF subjects.

Fasting blood glucose

Within the non-CF population, fasting blood glucose (FBG) is one of the accepted diagnostic approaches for diabetes mellitus [61], and a recent North American Consensus Statement has included its use in the diagnosis of CFRD [36]. There are, however, a number of drawbacks with its use. A genuine fasting status cannot always be guaranteed and the potential for false positive results is recognized within the non-CF population [62]. More importantly there are likely to be a considerable number of false negative results in a screening strategy based on fasting values. In studies in which CF subjects have been classified on the basis of the 2-hour glucose (in an OGTT), FBG will miss a significant proportion of subjects with CFRD [6,57]. More recently a further review of this method in light of the recent changes in the American Diabetes Association (ADA) criteria for impaired fasting glucose has revealed that it remains an unsuitable test for the early identification of patients with CFRD [63].

Oral glucose tolerance test

The OGTT remains the accepted gold standard and its use is widely advocated [3,36]. The test is laborious and time-consuming for both staff and patients and recent evidence suggests that it may be missing clinically relevant episodes of hyperglycemia in some subjects [64]. In addition, results may vary within an individual depending on the clinical status or treatment [54]. Various attempts to rationalize the use of OGTTs by combining the presence of symptoms with a variety of conventional measures have been described with some success [3]. It is important to remember that screening for non-CF diabetes, unlike in CFRD, is commonly guided by the presence of clinical features of hyperglycemia such as polyuria, polydipsia and weight loss. A reliance on these symptoms in the CF population would miss many cases of CFRD, as documented in a Danish study where diabetes mellitus was suspected on clinical grounds in only 33% of patients at the time of diagnosis [6].

Continuous glucose monitoring

The recent introduction of devices that provide a continuous glucose profile has revealed clinically relevant excursions in glycemia previously missed by conventional measures. These devices have been shown to be reliable and accurate and are widely used in the non-CF population [65,66]. We have shown that the correlations of a subcutaneous continuous glucose monitoring system (CGMS) with plasma glucose are similar to those in the non-diabetic population. This device has been shown to be well tolerated and able to provide a reliable glucose profile within CF subjects [64,67,68]. It may therefore be useful in assessing glucose tolerance in CF although its precise role in diagnosis remains unclear.

Summary

In conclusion, the use of urine glucose testing, HbA$_{1c}$ and FBG are not reliable in detecting CFRD. The consensus of opinion would suggest that the OGTT still remains the gold standard, but its limitations should be recognized. Random evening post-prandial blood glucose estimations may alert clinicians to significant episodes of hyperglycemia. Further studies are required to evaluate the current diagnostic criteria and methods and to determine whether new techniques, such as glucose profiles and continuous glucose monitors, will be of increased value.

TREATMENT OF CFRD

Although the etiology of CFRD is complex, the principal problem is absolute or relative insulin deficiency associated with varying insulin resistance. The logical treatment is additional insulin although there is debate regarding the initial use of oral hypoglycemic agents, especially in children. Regrettably there are few trial data available on which to decide best treatment for CFRD. Patients with CF have complex regimens of diet and medical treatment so a pragmatic treatment schedule which maintains quality of life by the relief of symptoms, minimizes the metabolic effects of insulin deficiency, reduces the risk of long-term vascular complications and does not jeopardize other components of treatment is essential. Detailed guidance on the management of CFRD has recently been published by the UK Cystic Fibrosis Trust [56].

Diet

Nutrition is usually impaired more by CF than by diabetes, so the nutritional strategy is to concentrate on good CF nutrition rather than dietary regulation for diabetic control. Dietary restriction to maintain euglycemia is not appropriate in cystic fibrosis. Appropriate nutrition is critical in those with CF to maintain body mass and lung function. Blood glucose should be controlled by adjusting insulin doses to the requirements of adequate food intake and not by calorie restriction. Cystic fibrosis patients generally require 120–150% of the estimated average requirement for energy, requirements rising with deteriorating clinical condition [69,70]. The aim is to encourage a diet providing 35–40% as fat, 20% as protein and 40–45% as carbohydrates, but this is often difficult to achieve [71]. To achieve this intake and reduce post-prandial blood glucose peaks, three main meals and at least three snacks are recommended, together with appropriate pancreatic enzyme supplements. Dietetic advice from a dietician experienced in the particular problems of CF and diabetes is essential. It is usually unnecessary to alter dramatically the eating patterns of patients already on good, established CF diets, but smaller meals taken more often may help limit hypo- or hyperglycemia and special diabetic foods are seldom appropriate.

Alcohol reduces gluconeogenesis so may cause hypoglycemia. In patients taking insulin, alcohol may cause severe hypoglycemia resulting in death or brain damage; coexisting liver disease in CF may exacerbate this. Patients should understand the effect of alcohol on their diabetes as there may be an initial rise in blood sugar due to the carbohydrate content of the drink or mixer followed by a rapid fall.

Oral agents

Sulphonylureas enhance insulin secretion by acting on a specific islet beta-cell receptor. Early in the course of CFRD some patients may have euglycemia with oral agents alone. A number of small studies have found some success using sulphonylureas [72], tolbutamide [73] or glipizide [74]. Repaglinide is a member of a class of oral hypoglycemic agents, the glitinides, which increase insulin secretion but have a more rapid onset and shorter duration of action than sulphonylureas. A study of repaglinide in North American

CF patients is currently under way after an initial study showed some benefit [75]. It is unknown whether sulphonylureas or early insulin therapy are preferable in the early treatment of CFRD, but sulphonylureas may provide a short period of sufficient insulin secretion before starting insulin therapy.

The thiazolidinediones (glitazones) antagonize the peroxisome proliferator-activated receptor (PPAR antagonists) and improve insulin sensitivity by acting on adipose tissue, liver and skeletal muscle. They are generally recommended for second- or third-line use in type 2 diabetes and there are no studies in CFRD. They are not currently recommended in CFRD.

Metformin improves hepatic insulin sensitivity. There are no studies of its use in CFRD but it is contraindicated where tissue hypoxia is likely due to a risk of lactic acidosis or with coexisting liver disease. Metformin is not recommended for use in CFRD.

Insulin

Insulin replacement is the recommended and most widely used method of treatment. Once frank diabetes is established with fasting hyperglycemia, post-prandial hyperglycemia or elevated HbA_{1c} then insulin is essential. There are no double-blind placebo-controlled trials of insulin regimens in cystic fibrosis [76]. Initially, small doses of insulin may can be surprisingly effective in improving lung function and weight [49]. A small study with relatively low doses of glargine have been effective in improving lung function and reducing the frequency of exacerbations [77]. Continuous insulin infusions have been used in small uncontrolled studies and may have some value when compliance is poor [78,79].

Transient diabetes during infections is common as insulin production declines and although this is often treated with insulin during an admission it is unknown whether continuing low-dose insulin in these patients in the absence of fasting hyperglycemia or elevated HbA_{1c} is beneficial. Given the underlying pancreatic pathology and declining production of insulin, a low threshold for introducing insulin seems logical but the optimum time to start long-term insulin treatment is unknown. In considering whether to start insulin it may be helpful to review recent trends in lung function, weight or frequency of hospital admissions, as decline in any of these features may indicate clinically significant insulin deficiency.

Tailoring the timing and dosage of insulin to individual patients is essential, and ideally this would match the normal pattern of insulin secretion with a basal level of insulin supplemented by short-acting insulin after meals. Optimal control is often not achievable due to poor compliance and complex treatment regimens. In patients with a normal fasting blood glucose and CFRD short-acting insulin with meals shown to cause hyperglycemia on home testing is probably sufficient, titrated to keep the post-meal reading under 7.0 mmol/L or the post-meal reading 0–2 mmol/L higher than the pre-meal reading. Those patients with CFRD and raised fasting glucose require both basal insulin and extra mealtime insulin. The dosage of insulin will frequently need to be significantly increased during infections or treatment with steroids.

Advice on appropriate insulin regimens is best sought from an experienced diabetologist. A joint clinic with close working together with a diabetic team interested in the special problems of CFRD is ideal for managing patients with CFRD, particularly to avoid conflicting advice from team members, ensure appropriate dietetic advice, detect complications and improve compliance.

Annual review

The annual review has become an established feature of CF care and an opportunity to review diabetic care at least annually is essential. The ever-increasing number of parameters to be checked and the desirability of a joint CF/diabetes team approach may mean that a separate annual diabetic review is more appropriate. The annual checklist should include the following, based on the NICE guidelines for the management of type 1 diabetes in adults [80]:

CF diabetic annual review

- *History* – clinical course including admissions, alcohol, smoking, infections, sexual dysfunction, exercise, episodes of distal intestinal obstruction syndrome (DIOS)
- *Dietetic review*
- *Weight* – a vital assessment of CF progress
- *Review of current control* – recording of hypoglycemia
- *Treatment and understanding of regimen*
- HbA_{1c} – aiming for under 7%
- *Kidney function* – the value of urine testing for albumin creatinine ratio to assess microalbuminuria is unclear as urinary albumin secretion is increased in CF (probably due to infection) and there is reduced creatinine due to low muscle mass
- *Blood pressure* – aiming for 140/80 mmHg or less
- *Lipids* – a total cholesterol of 5.0 mmol/L or less and fasting triglycerides of under 2.0 mmol are accepted as national targets
- *Legs and feet* – to assess skin, circulation and presence of any neuropathy
- *Fundoscopy* – each patient should be part of the local retinal screening program
- *Injection sites.*

Transplantation

The presence of insulin-dependent diabetes is not a contraindication to transplantation in adults. Diabetes does not appear to be associated with a poorer survival following lung transplantation [81,82]. Postoperative diabetes may develop due to sepsis or steroid use and should be treated with insulin. In one study, 22 of 77 patients (29%) were diabetic before transplantation and 49% of this cohort were diabetic after a median follow-up of 3.3 years from transplant [83]. Two patients have been reported whose preoperative diabetes was corrected after a simultaneous liver and pancreatic transplant for pre-existing cirrhosis, malabsorption and diabetes [84].

Diabetes and pregnancy

In non-CF individuals, pregnancy has a major impact on glucose tolerance. Insulin requirements are stable or reduced in the first trimester, rise in the second trimester and peak in the third trimester. Insulin requirements at the end of the third trimester may be 200–300% of preconception levels. Raised blood glucose levels in the first trimester are associated with an increased risk of teratogenesis and raised levels in the second and third trimester are associated with increased risks to both mother and fetus.

As survival improves, more CF patients will wish to become pregnant but many of these will be people with established CFRD or impending insulin deficiency. Close liaison between the CF team, specialist diabetes team and obstetric team is essential for all patients with CFRD or even transiently raised post-prandial blood glucose levels, ideally 3 months prior to a planned pregnancy. Complications are more common in women with CFRD or gestational diabetes. In one study of 33 successful pregnancies in 23 Scandinavia women, 43% were found to have established or gestational diabetes [85]. Preterm delivery was the commonest complication, and these women were more likely to have other CF complications including diabetes, asthma or liver disease.

Exercise

Exercise is a valuable form of therapy in CF for numerous reasons including airway clearance, muscular development, prevention of osteoporosis and general well-being. Patients should not be discouraged from taking appropriate exercise due to diabetes, but a reduction in insulin or increase in carbohydrate intake may be required for those increasing their exercise patterns above normal for them. Easily absorbed carbohydrate snacks should be available during and after exercise. Delayed hypoglycemia can occur 24–36 hours after exercise. Injection sites should be away from areas used during exercise when possible. Hydration and foot care are especially important.

Driving

The same rules apply to patients with CFRD as all other diabetics. In the UK all diabetics receiving treatment with insulin or tablets should inform the Driver and Vehicle Licensing Agency (DVLA). Regulations concerning all diabetics in the UK are updated on the DVLA website.

Patients should not drive if they do not recognize the symptoms of hypoglycemia or fail to reach required visual standards. Patients on insulin are barred from driving HGVs or passenger carrying vehicles (PCVs).

CONCLUSION

Cystic fibrosis related to diabetes is a complex disorder characterized by progressive insulin deficiency and varying insulin resistance. At times patients may clearly fulfil the conventional accepted diagnostic criteria for diabetes mellitus only to revert to apparently normal glucose metabolism at a later date when they are free of infection or in better health. Rather than attempt to fit CF patients into diagnostic categories designed for the non-CF population, a more helpful approach may be to consider whether the CF patient has sufficient insulin for his or her current metabolic requirements. Factors suggesting insulin deficiency include a decline in lung function, body weight and, at a later stage in some patients, transient and then persistently disordered glucose metabolism. The ideal treatment of early insulin deficiency in CF is unknown and current interventions are largely based on the benefits of insulin therapy in the non-CF diabetic population rather than randomized controlled trials in CF patients.

REFERENCES

1. Shwachman H, Leubner H, Catzel. Mucoviscidosis. *Adv Pediatr* 1955; **7**:249–323.
2. Lanng S, Thorsteinsson B, Erichsen G *et al.* Glucose tolerance in cystic fibrosis. *Arch Dis Child* 1991; **66**:612–616.
3. Yung B, Kemp M, Hooper J, Hodson ME. Diagnosis of cystic fibrosis related diabetes: a selective approach in performing the oral glucose tolerance test based on a combination of clinical and biochemical criteria. *Thorax* 1999; **54**:40–43.
4. Koch C, Cuppens H, Rainisio M *et al.* European Epidemiologic Registry of Cystic Fibrosis (ERCF): comparison of major disease manifestations between patients with different classes of mutations. *Pediatr Pulmonol* 2001; **31**:1–12.
5. Marshall BC, Butler SM, Stoddard M *et al.* Epidemiology of cystic fibrosis-related diabetes. *J Pediatr* 2005; **146**:681–687.
6. Lanng S, Hansen A, Thorsteinsson B *et al.* Glucose tolerance in patients with cystic fibrosis: five year prospective study. *Br Med J* 1995; **311**:655–659.
7. Vankeerberghen A, Cuppens H, Cassiman JJ. The cystic fibrosis transmembrane conductance regulator: an intriguing protein with pleiotropic functions. *J Cyst Fibros* 2002; **1**:13–29.
8. Lanng S, Thorsteinsson B, Pociot F *et al.* Diabetes mellitus in cystic fibrosis: genetic and immunological markers. *Acta Paediatr* 1993; **82**:150–154.
9. Nousia-Arvanitakis S, Galli-Tsinopoulou A, Dracoulacos D *et al.* Islet autoantibodies and insulin dependent diabetes mellitus in cystic fibrosis. *J Pediatr Endocrinol Metab* 2000; **13**:319–324.
10. Moran A, Diem P, Klein DJ *et al.* Pancreatic endocrine function in cystic fibrosis. *J Pediatr* 1991; **118**:715–723.
11. Lanng S, Thorsteinsson B, Roder ME *et al.* Pancreas and gut hormone responses to oral glucose and intravenous glucagon in cystic fibrosis patients with normal, impaired, and diabetic glucose tolerance. *Acta Endocrinol (Copenh)* 1993; **128**:207–214.
12. Garagorri JM, Rodriguez G, Ros L, Sanchez A. Early detection of impaired glucose tolerance in patients with cystic fibrosis and predisposition factors. *J Pediatr Endocrinol Metab* 2001; **14**:53–60.
13. Milla CE, Warwick WJ, Moran A. Trends in pulmonary function in patients with cystic fibrosis correlate with the degree of glucose intolerance at baseline. *Am J Respir Crit Care Med* 2000; **162**:891–895.
14. Yung B, Noormohamed FH, Kemp M *et al.* Cystic fibrosis-related diabetes: the role of peripheral insulin resistance and beta-cell dysfunction. *Diabet Med* 2002; **19**:221–226.
15. Lippe BM, Sperling MA, Dooley RR. Pancreatic alpha and beta cell functions in cystic fibrosis. *J Pediatr* 1977; **90**:751–755.
16. Nousia-Arvanitakis S, Tomita T, Desai N, Kimmel JR. Pancreatic polypeptide in cystic fibrosis. *Arch Pathol Lab Med* 1985; **109**:722–726.
17. Kopito LE, Shwachman H. The pancreas in cystic fibrosis: chemical composition and comparative morphology. *Pediatr Res* 1976; **10**:742–749.
18. Lohr M, Goertchen P, Nizze H *et al.* Cystic fibrosis associated islet changes may provide a basis for diabetes: an immunocytochemical and morphometrical study. *Virchows Arch A: Pathol Anat Histopathol* 1989; **414**:179–185.
19. Abdul-Karim FW, Dahms BB, Velasco ME, Rodman HM. Islets of Langerhans in adolescents and adults with cystic fibrosis: a quantitative study. *Arch Pathol Lab Med* 1986; **110**:602–606.
20. Soejima K, Landing BH. Pancreatic islets in older patients with cystic fibrosis with and without diabetes mellitus: morphometric and immunocytologic studies. *Pediatr Pathol* 1986; **6**:25–46.
21. Couce M, O'Brien TD, Moran A *et al.* Diabetes mellitus in cystic fibrosis is characterized by islet amyloidosis. *J Clin Endocrinol Metab* 1996; **81**:1267–1272.
22. Cucinotta D, De Luca F, Arrigo T *et al.* First-phase insulin response to intravenous glucose in cystic fibrosis patients with different degrees of glucose tolerance. *J Pediatr Endocrinol* 1994; **7**:13–17.
23. Lanng S, Thorsteinsson B, Roder ME *et al.* Insulin sensitivity and insulin clearance in cystic fibrosis patients with normal and diabetic glucose tolerance. *Clin Endocrinol(Oxf)* 1994; **41**:217–223.
24. Austin A, Kalhan SC, Orenstein D *et al.* Roles of insulin resistance and beta-cell dysfunction in the pathogenesis of glucose intolerance in cystic fibrosis. *J Clin Endocrinol Metab* 1994; **79**:80–85.

25. Moran A, Pyzdrowski KL, Weinreb J et al. Insulin sensitivity in cystic fibrosis. Diabetes 1994; 43:1020–1026.

26. Kien CL, Horswill CA, Zipf WB et al. Elevated hepatic glucose production in children with cystic fibrosis. Pediatr Res 1995; 37:600–605.

27. Hardin DS, Leblanc A, Para L, Seilheimer DK. Hepatic insulin resistance and defects in substrate utilization in cystic fibrosis. Diabetes 1999; 48:1082–1087.

28. Ahmad T, Nelson R, Taylor R. Insulin sensitivity and metabolic clearance rate of insulin in cystic fibrosis. Metabolism 1994; 43:163–167.

29. Frase LL, Strickland AD, Kachel GW, Krejs GJ. Enhanced glucose absorption in the jejunum of patients with cystic fibrosis. Gastroenterology 1985; 88:478–484.

30. Taylor CJ, Baxter PS, Hardcastle J et al. Glucose intolerance in cystic fibrosis. Arch Dis Child 1989; 64:759.

31. Atlas AB, Finegold DN, Becker D et al. Diabetic ketoacidosis in cystic fibrosis. Am J Dis Child 1992; 146:1457–1458.

32. Finkelstein SM, Wielinski CL, Elliott GR et al. Diabetes mellitus associated with cystic fibrosis. J Pediatr 1988; 112:373–377.

33. Rosenecker J, Eichler I, Kuhn L et al. Genetic determination of diabetes mellitus in patients with cystic fibrosis. Multicenter Cystic Fibrosis Study Group. J Pediatr 1995; 127:441–443.

34. Reisman J, Corey M, Canny G, Levison H. Diabetes mellitus in Patients with cystic fibrosis: effect on survival. Pediatrics 1990; 86:374–377.

35. Milla CE, Billings J, Moran A. Diabetes is associated with dramatically decreased survival in female but not male subjects with cystic fibrosis. Diabetes Care 2005; 28:2141–2144.

36. Moran A, Hardin D, Rodman D et al. Diagnosis, screening and management of cystic fibrosis related diabetes mellitus: a consensus conference report. Diabetes Res Clin Pract 1999; 45:61–73.

37. Rosan RC, Shwachman H, Kulczvcki LI. Diabetes mellitus and cystic fibrosis of the pancreas: laboratory and clinical observations. Am J Dis Child 1962; 104:625–634.

38. Chazan BI, Balodimos MC, Holsclaw DS, Shwachman H. Microcirculation in young adults with cystic fibrosis: retinal and conjunctival vascular changes in relation to diabetes. J Pediatr 1970; 77:86–92.

39. Allen JL. Progressive nephropathy in a patient with cystic fibrosis and diabetes. N Engl J Med 1986; 315:764.

40. Dolan TF. Microangiopathy in a young adult with cystic fibrosis and diabetes mellitus. N Engl J Med 1986; 314:991–992.

41. Rodman HM, Doershuk CF, Roland JM. The interaction of two diseases: diabetes mellitus and cystic fibrosis. Medicine (Baltimore) 1986; 65:389–397.

42. Sullivan MM, Denning CR. Diabetic microangiopathy in patients with cystic fibrosis. Pediatrics 1989; 84:642–647.

43. Lanng S, Thorsteinsson B, Lund-Andersen C et al. Diabetes mellitus in Danish cystic fibrosis patients: prevalence and late diabetic complications. Acta Paediatr 1994; 83:72–77.

44. Rosenecker J, Hofler R, Steinkamp G et al. Diabetes mellitus in patients with cystic fibrosis: the impact of diabetes mellitus on pulmonary function and clinical outcome. Eur J Med Res 2001; 6:345–350.

45. Dobson L, Stride A, Bingham C et al. Microalbuminuria as a screening tool in cystic fibrosis-related diabetes. Pediatr Pulmonol 2005; 39:103–107.

46. Schlesinger DM, Holsclaw DS, Fyfe B. Generalised atherosclerosis in an adult with CF and diabetes mellitus. 1997; Pediatr Pulmonol 16:365a.

47. Sims EJ, Green MW, Mehta A. Decreased lung function in female but not male subjects with established cystic fibrosis-related diabetes. Diabetes Care 2005; 28:1581–1587.

48. Lanng S, Thorsteinsson B, Nerup J, Koch C. Influence of the development of diabetes mellitus on clinical status in patients with cystic fibrosis. Eur J Pediatr 1992; 151:684–687.

49. Dobson L, Hattersley AT, Tiley S et al. Clinical improvement in cystic fibrosis with early insulin treatment. Arch Dis Child 2002; 87:430–431.

50. Lanng S, Thorsteinsson B, Nerup J, Koch C. Diabetes mellitus in cystic fibrosis: effect of insulin therapy on lung function and infections. Acta Paediatr 1994; 83:849–853.

51. Nousia-Arvanitakis S, Galli-Tsinopoulou A, Karamouzis M. Insulin improves clinical status of patients with cystic-fibrosis-related diabetes mellitus. Acta Paediatr 2001; 90:515–519.

52. Rolon MA, Benali K, Munck A et al. Cystic fibrosis-related diabetes mellitus: clinical impact of prediabetes and effects of insulin therapy. Acta Paediatr 2001; 90:860–867.

53. Moran A, Milla C, Ducret R, Nair KS. Protein metabolism in clinically stable adult cystic fibrosis patients with abnormal glucose tolerance. Diabetes 2001; 50:1336–1343.

54. Hardin DS, Leblanc A, Lukenbough S, Seilheimer DK. Insulin resistance is associated with decreased clinical status in cystic fibrosis. J Pediatr 1997; 130:948–956.

55. Allen HF, Gay EC, Klingensmith GJ, Hamman RF. Identification and treatment of cystic fibrosis-related diabetes: a survey of current medical practice in the US. Diabetes Care 1998; 21:943–948.

56. Stutchfield PR, O'Halloran S, Teale JD et al. Glycosylated haemoglobin and glucose intolerance in cystic fibrosis. Arch Dis Child 1987; 62:805–810.

57. Solomon MP, Wilson DC, Corey M et al. Glucose intolerance in children with cystic fibrosis. J Pediatr 2003; 142:128–132.

58. Hardin DS, Moran A. Diabetes mellitus in cystic fibrosis. Endocrinol Metab Clin N Am 1999; 28:787–800, ix.

59. Brennan AL, Gyi KM, Wood DM et al. Relationship between glycosylated haemoglobin and mean plasma glucose concentration in cystic fibrosis. J Cyst Fibros 2006; 1:27–31.

60. World Health Organization (1999) Part 1: Diagnosis and Classification of Diabetes. Definition, Diagnosis and Classification of Diabetes Mellitus and its Complications. 1999. Available at www.staff.ncl.ac.uk/phlip.home/ who_dmc.htm/who.dmg.pdf/

61. WHO Study Group on Diabetes Mellitus. Diabetes mellitus. WHO Technical Report Series 1985; 727:1–113.

62. Mueller-Brandes C, Holl RW, Nastoll M, Ballmann M. New criteria for impaired fasting glucose and screening for diabetes in cystic fibrosis. Eur Respir J 2005; 25:715–717.

63. Dobson L, Sheldon CD, Hattersley AT. Conventional measures underestimate glycaemia in cystic fibrosis patients. *Diabet Med* 2004; **21**:691–696.

64. Gross TM, Mastrototaro JJ. Efficacy and reliability of the continuous glucose monitoring system. *Diabetes Technol Ther* 2000; **2** (Suppl 1):S19–26.

65. Mastrototaro J. The MiniMed Continuous Glucose Monitoring System (CGMS). *J Pediatr Endocrinol Metab* 1999; **12** (Suppl 3):751–758.

66. Dobson L, Sheldon CD, Hattersley AT. Validation of interstitial fluid continuous glucose monitoring in cystic fibrosis. *Diabetes Care* 2003; **26**:1940–1941.

67. Jefferies C, Solomon M, Perlman K *et al.* Continuous glucose monitoring in adolescents with cystic fibrosis. *J Pediatr* 2005; **147**:396–398.

68. Cystic Fibrosis Trust. *Management of Cystic Fibrosis Related Diabetes Mellitus.* Bromley, Kent, CF Trust, 2004.

69. Pencharz PB, Durie PR. Pathogenesis of malnutrition in cystic fibrosis, and its treatment. *Clin Nutr* 2000; **19**:387–394.

70. Sinaasappel M, Stern M, Littlewood J *et al.* Nutrition in patients with cystic fibrosis: a European consensus. *J Cyst Fibros* 2002; **1**:51–75.

71. White H, Morton AM, Peckham DG, Conway SP. Dietary intakes in adult patients with cystic fibrosis: do they achieve guidelines? *J Cyst Fibros* 2004; **3**:1–7.

72. Rosenecker J, Eichler I, Barmeier H, von der Hardt H. Diabetes mellitus and cystic fibrosis: comparison of clinical parameters in patients treated with insulin versus oral glucose-lowering agents. *Pediatr Pulmonol* 2001; **32**:351–355.

73. Zipf WB, Kien CL, Horswill CA *et al.* Effects of tolbutamide on growth and body composition of nondiabetic children with cystic fibrosis. *Pediatr Res* 1991; **30**:309–314.

74. Culler FL, McKean LP, Buchanan CN *et al.* Glipizide treatment of patients with cystic fibrosis and impaired glucose tolerance. *J Pediatr Gastroenterol Nutr* 1994; **18**:375–378.

75. Moran A, Phillips J, Milla C. Insulin and glucose excursion following premeal insulin lispro or repaglinide in cystic fibrosis-related diabetes. *Diabetes Care* 2001; **24**:1706–1710.

76. Onady GM, Stolfi A. Insulin and oral agents for managing cystic fibrosis-related diabetes. *Cochrane Database Syst Rev* 2005; CD004730.

77. Franzese A, Spagnuolo MI, Sepe A *et al.* Can glargine reduce the number of lung infections in patients with cystic fibrosis-related diabetes? *Diabetes Care* 2005; **28**:23–33.

78. Reali MF, Festini F, Neri AS *et al.* Use of continuous subcutaneous insulin infusion in cystic fibrosis patients with cystic fibrosis-related diabetes awaiting transplantation. *J Cyst Fibros* 2006; **6**:67–68.

79. Sulli N, Shashaj B. Continuous subcutaneous insulin infusion in children and adolescents with diabetes mellitus: decreased HbA1c with low risk of hypoglycemia. *J Pediatr Endocrinol Metab* 2003; **16**:393–399.

80. National Institute for Health and Clinical Excellence. *Diagnosis and management of type 1 diabetes in adults.* July 2004. Available at www.nice.org.uk.

81. De SA, Archer L, Wardle J *et al.* Pulmonary transplantation for cystic fibrosis: pre-transplant recipient characteristics in patients dying of peri-operative sepsis. *J Heart Lung Transplant* 2003; **22**:764–769.

82. Doershuk CF, Stern RC. Timing of referral for lung transplantation for cystic fibrosis: overemphasis on FEV_1 may adversely affect overall survival. *Chest* 1999; **115**:782–787.

83. Hadjiliadis D, Madill J, Chaparro C *et al.* Incidence and prevalence of diabetes mellitus in patients with cystic fibrosis undergoing lung transplantation before and after lung transplantation. *Clin Transplant* 2005; **19**:773–778.

84. Fridell JA, Vianna R, Kwo PY *et al.* Simultaneous liver and pancreas transplantation in patients with cystic fibrosis. *Transplant Proc* 2005; **37**:3567–3569.

85. Odegaard I, Stray-Pedersen B, Hallberg K *et al.* Maternal and fetal morbidity in pregnancies of Norwegian and Swedish women with cystic fibrosis. *Acta Obstet Gynecol Scand* 2002; **81**:689–692.

17

Growth and puberty

NICOLA BRIDGES

INTRODUCTION

The improvements that have occurred in the management of cystic fibrosis (CF) over the last few decades, as well as reducing morbidity and increasing long-term survival, have reduced the impact the disease has on growth and pubertal development. However, longer survival makes problems with growth and puberty more significant. Cystic fibrosis may be originally diagnosed because of poor growth in infancy or early childhood, and then later have an adverse impact on prepubertal growth, cause delay in the onset of puberty and can reduce the amount of pubertal growth. Most individuals with CF have some loss of their adult height potential.

PREPUBERTAL GROWTH IN CF

Birth weight and length are reduced in CF [1]. There is a deficit in height for infants known to have a diagnosis of CF in the first year of life, probably related to poor nutrition and increased infection rates. The deficit seen in infancy is greater than that later in childhood. This suggests there is catching up in growth after diagnosis, at least until adolescence, when nutritional status may fall off again, as the disease progresses. Although most children with CF are diagnosed before 12 months of age, those with milder CF are more likely to be diagnosed after that age and may contribute to the relative increase in height compared to the normal population [2]. Height and weight for prepubertal children with CF are reduced by about 0.2–0.5 standard deviations compared with standards for healthy children, and this difference increases with age [2,3]. The increased height deficit in later childhood is partly explained by the delay in puberty in CF compared to the normal population [4]. Height, weight and lung function are closely linked [5]; poor lung function in early childhood is correlated with reduced height later on [6,7]. The assessment of changes of growth patterns in CF with time is complicated by the fact that the population being observed has changed, as more patients survive. An Australian study showed that the relative height position compared with the normal population for children with CF in one center deteriorated between 1986 and 1996. The difference was explained by an increase in the survival of children with very poor lung function in the more recently studied cohort. Those with the worst FEV_1 were shortest and because more children with poorer lung function survived they contributed to apparent worsening of average height position [8].

PUBERTAL TIMING AND GROWTH IN CF

Pubertal development is delayed in CF as is the case in most other chronic diseases. The mechanism for pubertal delay in chronic disease is poorly understood. In the general population, changes in nutritional status and reduction in childhood diseases are the most likely cause for the reduction in the age at onset of puberty which has occurred over time. In CF there is no evidence that the CF mutation of itself is responsible for changes in pubertal timing, and delay is likely to be related to nutritional defects and increased infections. This is supported by the fact that those with the most severe lung disease have the most marked pubertal delay, although delay is seen even in individuals with milder CF [9].

Age at peak height velocity in puberty is delayed for both sexes, with age at menarche for girls more significantly delayed than age at peak height velocity, suggesting that the speed of pubertal development is also slowed [4]. Pubertal delay is seen even in well-nourished girls with CF [9]. Once again, the fact that the population being studied has changed must be taken into account in interpreting trends in pubertal growth. Laursen examined pubertal growth from the 1950s to the 1990s in Danish CF patients, and found that average peak height velocity during puberty was greater in 1950 than in 1970, but increased again after this. The age at peak height velocity was delayed compared with the unaffected population and did not change over time. Individuals who survived to puberty in the 1950s mostly had milder CF mutations, and the later cohorts contained more severely affected individuals [10].

The fact that puberty in individuals with CF is delayed compared to the normal population is a factor when comparisons of growth are made during this phase. Cystic fibrosis individuals become relatively shorter after 10 years of age compared to the unaffected population, because fewer of them will have had their pubertal growth spurt. At this stage CF individuals will also have delayed bone maturation compared to the normal population. Their relative position will improve when they have their delayed pubertal growth spurt. In normal growth, peak height velocity in puberty is lower if the pubertal spurt is later, and this partly explains the fact that peak height velocity in puberty is reduced in CF compared with unaffected individuals [4,10]. Adult height is for most individuals within the normal range and within parental target heights [11], but the mean height of adults with CF is reduced compared with the unaffected population [2]. In females with CF there is an increased incidence of menstrual irregularity after menarche [12]. Males usually reach a normal adult testicular volume although most have obstructive azoospermia.

FACTORS AFFECTING GROWTH AND PUBERTY IN CF

There is no evidence of a defect in the hypothalamo–pituitary axis in CF and the control of growth hormone (GH) secretion is normal [13]. The growth and anabolic actions of GH are mediated by insulin-like growth factor 1 (IGF-1). GH binding to GH receptors on the cell membrane stimulates the secretion of IGF-1, and IGF-1 then acts through the IGF-1 receptor on the cell membrane. GH is the main regulator of IGF-1 levels but there are other factors, for example nutrition [14]. IGF-1 is secreted and acts as a paracrine (local) hormone (for example at the epiphyseal growth plate) and also acts in an endocrine fashion with circulating levels mainly generated in the liver. The action of IGF-1 is modulated by at least six IGF binding proteins (IGFBPs). IGFBP-3 is the most significant of these and is positively correlated with GH levels. IGFBP-1 is negatively correlated with insulin concentrations. Studies have shown that IGF-1 and IGFBP-3 concentrations correlate with height velocity in the pediatric population, but this complex system of regulation means that circulating levels have limited value as a measure of GH bioactivity in individuals.

In CF there is evidence of a relative resistance to GH, with IGF-1 and IGFBP-3 levels reduced despite normal GH secretion. Poor nutrition, insulin deficiency, infection and inflammation, steroid treatment and liver impairment are all potential factors influencing the secretion and action of IGF-1. IGF-1 and IGFBP-3 concentrations in CF correlate with height [3], but IGF-1 and IGFBP-3 concentrations, and IGF-1 bioactivity, are all reduced compared to controls [15].

Intensive nutritional input increases IGF-1 and IGFBP-3 [16]. Insulin concentrations may be one of the routes by which nutrition influences IGF-1 action. Insulin regulates hepatic GH receptors [17], as well as influencing IGFBP-1 concentrations. Individuals with type 1 diabetes develop GH resistance, with elevated circulating GH but reduced IGF-1 [17,18], probably because of reduced insulin levels in the hepatic circulation. Insulin levels decline with age in CF – abnormalities are detected in many children before 10 years, and by adolescence approximately 50% of individuals have abnormal glucose tolerance [19]. Insulin secretion is often reduced in CF even if glucose tolerance is normal on oral glucose tolerance test (OGTT) [20]. In adolescents with CF, there is a relationship between reduced fasting insulin levels, and reduced IGF-1 and IGFBP-3 levels, and IGF-1 bioactivity [15]. Insulin secretion in adolescents with CF, measured as area under the curve after OGTT, correlates with height velocity [21].

The negative effect of developing CF-related diabetes (CFRD) on body mass index (BMI) and lung function has been demonstrated in adults [22]. The decline starts years before the development of overt diabetes and improves with insulin treatment [22]. In adolescence, the decline in insulin secretion with age could have a negative impact on growth before the development of overt diabetes, but there are currently no studies demonstrating this. The trend towards better and earlier management of CFRD in adolescence is suggested as a factor in improved growth over time [13]. Insulin deficiency and diabetes are discussed in more detail in Chapter 16.

Studies in adolescents with disorders characterized by chronic inflammation such as inflammatory bowel disease (and also studies in animals with experimental inflammation or overexpression of cytokines) have demonstrated an interaction of inflammatory cytokines with growth factors. Adolescents with Crohn's disease and rats with induced colitis have normal stimulated GH secretion, but reduced IGF-1 concentrations [23]. Reduced sensitivity to GH in inflammation appears to be mediated by inflammatory cytokines like interleukin 6 (IL-6), interleukin 1β (IL-1β), and tumor necrosis factor α (TNFα), all of which are overexpressed in CF lung disease. In humans with inflammatory bowel disease, IL-6 and IL-1β correlated with reduced IGF-1 levels [24]. Transgenic mice which over-express IL-6 have growth retardation with reduced IGF-1 [25], and elevated levels of IL-6 in rats with experimental colitis correlate with growth failure and reduced IGF-1 levels [23]. IL-1β and TNFα inhibit the GH-stimulated secretion of IGF-1 from cultured rat liver cells [26]. There are no data relating cytokines and growth factors in CF, but TNFα and IL-6 concentrations are increased in CF [27,28] and it is likely that inflammation acts in the same manner to produce GH resistance and reduced IGF-1 levels. TNFα may also have an adverse effect on growth by increasing insulin resistance in CF. A trial of GH treatment in children with CF, which demonstrated in an increase in growth velocity and IGF-1 concentrations with treatment, found that GH reduced TNFα concentrations [29].

Many children and adolescents with CF receive short- or long-term courses of corticosteroids, or are on inhaled steroids. Steroid treatment acts by a number of different mechanisms to suppress linear growth. At the level of the hypothalamus and pituitary, steroids increase somatostatin tone (somatostatin suppresses GH secretion) and decrease responsiveness to GH-releasing hormone [30]. In Cushing's disease in adolescence, elevated circulating glucocorticoids result in reduced GH secretion and impaired growth [31]. Glucocorticoids still inhibit growth when used on alternate days [32]. Inhaled steroids can have significant bioavailability due to swallowing and lung absorption, and can act in the same way to inhibit growth [33]. Bone maturity, measured as bone age, is retarded in children treated with glucocorticoids [34].

INTERVENTIONS TO IMPROVE GROWTH IN CF

Poor growth velocity and reduced adult height seen in CF is related to a complex combination of factors. For an individual with CF there is rarely a single cause for poor growth, and the different influences can change with time. Changes in therapy and clinical condition (e.g. glucocorticoid therapy) can result in a pattern of growth showing fluctuations in growth velocity. In some individuals growth can stop entirely during severe illnesses or high-dose steroid treatment.

Obviously, the most important intervention for growth for children and adolescents with CF is the optimization of their treatment – managing infections, keeping steroid doses to a minimum and assessing whether insulin treatment is needed. Increasing insulin deficiency with the development of abnormal glucose tolerance is likely to contribute to the poor pubertal growth seen in CF and evidence in the adult population suggests that early intervention [35] improves nutritional status. Most clinicians avoid systemic steroid treatment if possible because of the effect on growth, but the short-term adverse effect may be balanced if the overall clinical state of the individual is improved (reduced inflammation or improved nutrition).

A number of agents have been examined as growth-promoting agents in CF.

Growth hormone

As discussed, the endocrinology of growth failure in CF is complex and not simply related to a reduction in GH secretion. GH has been used since the 1960s as a replacement therapy in children with GH deficiency, but the availability of recombinant GH has led to trials of its use in growth disorders where there is no GH deficiency. Children with true GH deficiency get the greatest benefit in terms of final height for the smallest doses. Where trials in non-GH-deficient short stature have demonstrated benefit, increments in adult height have been considerably smaller and the doses required larger than those needed for

'replacement' therapy. Studies to final height have demonstrated final height increments of 6–8 cm in girls with Turner syndrome, 4–6 cm in children who were small for gestational age, and slightly less in children with idiopathic short stature. GH is a potent anabolic agent and treatment results in increases in muscle bulk and reduced lean body mass. The anabolic effects of GH treatment have been studied in disorders characterized by wasting, such as HIV.

There have been a number of small trials of GH treatment in CF, which have looked at potential benefits in terms of height, and the value of GH as an anabolic agent. The results are summarized in Table 17.1. Short-term use of GH increases height velocity in CF. The study of GH in a wide range of potential clinical indications has confirmed that almost all children get an increase in height velocity with short-term GH treatment, but this does not necessarily correlate with increase in adult height. The anabolic effects of GH may be of value in CF independent of the effect on height. There appears to be a positive effect on weight gain, lean body mass and bone mineral density during treatment, but the effect on lung function is less clear.

Some children and adolescents with CF grow poorly because of long-term glucocorticoid treatment. There have been no studies in CF but the role of GH in reversing steroid-induced growth suppression has been examined in other disorders. GH can increase height velocity in glucocorticoid-treated children but there are no data as to final height. Response is negatively correlated with the steroid dose [36].

The value of GH simply as an agent to increase final height in CF is uncertain. Most individuals with CF attain an adult height in the normal range, and those who have a significantly reduced height potential are also most likely to have medical conditions, which will reduce the potential effect of treatment. GH treatment increases insulin resistance, and there must be concerns about the impact of treatment on glucose metabolism in CF children and adolescents with reduced insulin secretion. There have not been any reports of diabetes developing during GH treatment in CF. In one study fasting glucose was monitored during treatment and was unchanged [37]. GH treatment is delivered by daily subcutaneous injections, adding to the burden of treatment for children with CF, and the financial cost of treatment at the doses currently studied is approximately US$20 000–30 000 (£10–15 000) per year. There have been no studies comparing its use to other anabolic agents such as sex steroids.

Sex steroids to induce puberty

In normal children, mean growth velocity declines during childhood and continues to decline until the onset of puberty, whenever that occurs. A child with delay of puberty will continue to grow at a slowing height velocity until the onset of puberty. The more delayed the onset of pubertal growth, the smaller the pubertal height increment [38]. This means that although individuals with pubertal delay grow until they are older, there is no adult height gain from

Table 17.1 Studies of growth hormone treatment in CF.

Reference	Number treated	Age range (years)	Duration of treatment	Effect on height, weight and body composition	Effect on lung function	Other measurements
Hardin *et al.* [28]	10 (9 controls)	7–12	12 months	Increased height and weight velocity Increased lean body mass	Increased FVC	Reduced hospitalizations Reduced protein catabolism
Hutler *et al.* [49]	10	9–14	6 months	Increased height and weight velocity Increased lean body mass	No significant change	Increased exercise capacity
Schibler *et al.* [50]	10 (9 controls)	10–23	12 months	No significant change in weight	No significant change	Increased exercise capacity
Darmaun *et al.* [51]	9	7–13	4 weeks	Increased lean body mass	Not measured	Given in combination with glutamine
Hardin *et al.* [52]	25	13–16	12 months ($n = 12$) 24 months ($n = 13$)	Increased height and weight	Increased FVC and FEV_1	Increased bone mineral density Reduced hospital admissions
Hardin *et al.* [53]	18	Mean age 11.6 years	12 months ($n = 9$) 24 months ($n = 9$)	Increased height and weight velocity	No significant change	Increased bone mineral density Reduced hospital admissions

delayed puberty [39]. The difference in the size of the pubertal growth increment compensates for the age of onset of puberty over a very wide range [40]. Puberty is delayed in males and females with CF. The psychological impact of delay of puberty in healthy individuals is well recognized, and there is evidence of the positive effects of treatment [41,42]. Adolescents with CF have difficulties in self-esteem and body image related to their chronic disease, and pubertal delay plays a significant part in this [43,44]. Pubertal levels of sex steroids are important in achieving normal peak bone density. Normal individuals with delay of puberty achieve adult bone density in the normal range at the end of their development [45]. There is an increased incidence of reduced bone density in adults with CF (discussed in more detail in Chapter 18), and sex steroid deficiency may be a factor in this as well as nutritional deficiencies, and treatments such as corticosteroids [46]. The need to optimize bone density may be a reason to treat delay of puberty, in addition to psychological factors.

PRACTICAL ISSUES IN GROWTH AND PUBERTY

The growth of children with CF is much more carefully followed than in the general population, and all children should be regularly plotted on a centile chart. Ensuring consistent and accurate measurement is important in monitoring growth. The Harpenden stadiometer is a robust wall-mounted height measure that can maintain accuracy with constant use in an outpatient clinic. There are simpler

alternatives such as the Minimeter, Magnameter and the Leicester height measure (which can be folded into a case), which are accurate but slightly less robust. With care, accurate measurements can be made on very basic equipment – careful positioning of the child, proper installation, checking regularly to make sure the measure remains accurate, and ensuring consistency among the members of staff doing the measurement are the most important factors. The child's head should be supported by gently holding under the mastoid processes, and brought to the correct position with the lower margin of the eye socket on the same level as the external auditory meatus (called the Frankfurt plane). The child should be asked to relax the shoulders and the measuring arm brought firmly on to the head.

Parental 'target height' is a way of assessing the genetic contribution to height, calculated as:

$$(\text{father's height} + \text{mother's height})/2,$$

adding 7 cm for boys and subtracting 7 cm for girls.

There are limitations to the values of target height calculations – obviously the effect of CF on growth but also erratic estimates of parental height, and factors that may have affected parental height attainment. Assessment and recording puberty using Tanner pubertal stages is important in monitoring pubertal delay. Centiles for pubertal development are available and included in UK growth charts. When assessing male puberty, a Prader orchidometer (Fig. 17.1) should be used to measure testicular volumes.

In girls the first sign of puberty is usually breast development. The female pubertal growth spurt starts early in

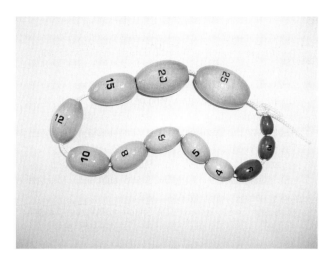

Figure 17.1   Prader orchidometer. The numbers are volume in milliliters, with a testicular volume of 4 mL or over marking the onset of puberty. Assessment of testicular volume is helpful in monitoring pubertal progress in boys. *See also Plate 17.1.*

puberty (at Tanner breast stage 2 to 3) and menarche does not occur until late in puberty (Tanner breast stage 4 to 5). Approximately 4–5 cm of growth normally occurs after menarche. In boys the first sign of puberty is testicular enlargement (4 mL volume) and the pubertal growth spurt does not start until mid puberty (10–12 mL testicular volume), with growth slowing at the end of puberty (15–20 mL testicular volume). The pace of development in puberty varies, with most children completing growth and development in 18–24 months from the onset of puberty.

Bone age is an estimate of growth potential from the development of the bones in the hand and wrist. Two methods are in use in the UK, Tanner Whitehouse 2 and Greulich and Pyle; both are operator-dependent. Bone age remains in the prepubertal range until the start of puberty whenever this occurs, and during puberty the bone age will often advance at more than 1 bone-age 'year' per chronological year [47]. Children with chronic diseases like CF usually have bone age delay [46]; periods of poor growth related to illness or steroid treatment may increase this. Bone age delay indicates that there is some potential for catch-up growth at a later stage, usually during puberty. Both bone age techniques allow for prediction of adult height. The prediction methods are based on the growth patterns of normal children, and become much less accurate for those with growth disorders or abnormal patterns of growth. The calculations assume normal pubertal growth and are therefore likely to be over-optimistic in children with CF who may have impaired growth at this stage. The reasons for poor growth in a child with CF are often obvious, and as discussed above there are usually several factors. It may be helpful to exclude other causes, such as thyroid disease, celiac disease, or Turner syndrome in girls. Growth hormone deficiency should be considered if growth velocity is consistently poor.

TREATMENT OF PUBERTAL DELAY

In the general population, children referred with pubertal delay are almost always male. Puberty is delayed in both sexes in CF but there is still a predominance of males who seek treatment. Height centile charts are an average for the population including early and late developers, so an adolescent with pubertal delay will fall in their position on the centiles over time, although their pattern of growth may be normal for their prepubertal state. Adolescents with pubertal delay usually complain of feeling relatively shorter compared to their peers. Lack of physical maturity is often a concern but adolescents may be reluctant to discuss this. Some adolescents will not raise the issue of their pubertal delay unless treatment options are offered, and some will deny there is any concern but then take the option of treatment enthusiastically. Sex steroid treatment to induce puberty has been widely used in adolescents with 'constitutional' delay of puberty and there have been a number of reports of treatment in CF [48].

The option for treatment should be discussed with anyone who is significantly delayed. Ninety-eight percent of normal girls have started pubertal development (reached Tanner breast stage 2) by 13.7 years, and 98% of boys have started development (increased testicular volume) by 14.2 years. It is sometimes appropriate to offer treatment to individuals slightly younger than this, and given in conventional doses (Table 17.2) this will not have an adverse effect on adult height. The decision to have treatment for those with moderate delay is largely on psychological grounds – how left behind the individual feels in terms of height and physical development. Individuals who are very delayed should probably be encouraged to have treatment even if they are not particularly concerned. If growth and development in puberty takes about 2 years to complete, someone who does not find their delay a problem at 16 is likely to experience difficulties if they still look very young at 18 or 19 years.

To induce puberty, sex steroids are given in low dose and gradually increased in an attempt to mimic the gradual increase in sex steroids seen in spontaneous puberty (see Table 17.2). Treatment can sometimes stimulate the onset of endogenous puberty; and it may become clear that the development exceeds what is expected for the dose being given. Liver function should be regularly monitored if there is liver impairment, and starting doses should be lower with slower increases, although liver impairment has not been reported with sex steroids at the doses used for pubertal induction. If endogenous puberty does not start, treatment is usually continued until nearly adult height is attained. Development should be monitored after stopping treatment, to check that endogenous puberty starts. If not, the patient may need further investigations and maintenance sex steroids. For boys who are already in early puberty, but have not yet had their pubertal growth spurt, oxandrolone is an alternative treatment option. This is an anabolic steroid given orally, 2.5 mg daily for 3 months. This will give acceleration in growth rate but will not have much effect on physical development.

Table 17.2 Steroid treatment for induction of puberty.[a]

Females

Increasing doses of oral ethinylestradiol:

– 2 or 2.5 μg daily for 6 months[b]
– 5 μg daily for 6 months
– 10 μg daily for 6 months
– 15 μg daily for 6 months
– 20 μg daily for 6 months

Add in progesterone when 15 μg ethinylestradiol is given, or before this if there is spotting:

– levonorgestrel 30 μg daily or norethisterone 5 mg daily for 7 days out of every 28 days

Males

Increasing doses of intramuscular depot testosterone esters as Sustanon 100 (100 mg in 1 mL)

– 50 mg i.m. every 4–6 weeks for 6 months
– 100 mg every 4 weeks for 6 months
– 100 mg every 3 weeks for 6 months
– 100 mg every 2 weeks for 6 months

[a] There are currently no reliable data to guide pubertal induction with topical sex steroids in males or females.
[b] Either 2-μg tablets or one quarter of a 10-μg tablet can be given.

CONCLUSIONS

Short stature in childhood, delay of puberty and reduced adult height are features of CF, which have assumed increasing importance as long-term survival has improved. Nutrition, chronic inflammation, insulin deficiency and the use of steroids are factors in poor growth, and management strategies that improve lung function and clinical condition will also improve growth and improve final height. The early use of insulin to manage CF-related diabetes and impaired glucose tolerance may be of benefit. Exogenous growth hormone has been studied as a growth and anabolic agent in CF but the value of this treatment is unclear. There have been few reports of sex steroid treatment to induce puberty in CF but this is a widely used and relatively simple treatment, which can be of considerable psychological benefit.

REFERENCES

1. Haeusler G, Frisch H, Waldhor T, Gotz M. Perspectives of longitudinal growth in cystic fibrosis from birth to adult age. *Eur J Pediatr* 1994; **153**:158–163.
2. Morison S, Dodge JA, Cole TJ *et al.* Height and weight in cystic fibrosis: a cross sectional study. *Arch Dis Child* 1997; **77**:497–500.
3. Taylor AM, Bush A, Thomson A *et al.* Relation between insulin-like growth factor-I, body mass index, and clinical status in cystic fibrosis. *Arch Dis Child* 1997; **76**:304–309.
4. Aswani N, Taylor CJ, McGaw J *et al.* Pubertal growth and development in cystic fibrosis: a retrospective review. *Acta Paediatr* 2003; **92**:1029–1032.
5. Peterson ML, Jacobs DR, Milla CE. Longitudinal changes in growth parameters are correlated with changes in pulmonary function in children with cystic fibrosis. *Pediatrics* 2003; **112**:588–592.
6. Zemel BS, Jawad AF, Fitzsimmons S, Stallings VA. Longitudinal relationship among growth, nutritional status, and pulmonary function in children with cystic fibrosis: Analysis of the Cystic Fibrosis Foundation National CF Patient Registry. *J Pediatr* 2000; **137**:374–380.
7. Konstan MW, Butler SM, Wohl MEB *et al.* Growth and nutritional indexes in early life predict pulmonary function in cystic fibrosis. *J Pediatr* 2003; **142**:624–630.
8. McNaughton SA, Stormont DA, Shepherd RW *et al.* Growth failure in cystic fibrosis. *J Paediatr Child Health* 1999; **35**:86–92.
9. Johannesson M, Gottlieb C, Hjelte L. Delayed puberty in girls with cystic fibrosis despite good clinical status. *Pediatrics* 1997; **99**:29–34.
10. Laursen EM, Koch C, Petersen JH, Muller J. Secular changes in anthropometric data in cystic fibrosis patients. *Acta Paediatr* 1999; **88**:169–174.
11. Nir M, Lanng S, Johansen HK, Koch C. Long-term survival and nutritional data in patients with cystic fibrosis treated in a Danish center. *Thorax* 1996; **51**:1023–1027.
12. Johannesson M, Landgren BM, Csemiczky G *et al.* Female patients with cystic fibrosis suffer from reproductive endocrinological disorders despite good clinical status. *Hum Reprod* 1998; **13**:2092–2097.
13. Laursen EM, Lanng S, Rasmussen MH *et al.* Normal spontaneous and stimulated GH levels despite decreased IGF-I concentrations in cystic fibrosis patients. *Eur J Endocrinol* 1999; **140**:315–321.
14. Hochberg Z, Hertz P, Colin V *et al.* The distal axis of growth hormone (GH) in nutritional disorders: GH-binding protein, insulin-like growth factor-I (IGF-I), and IGF-I receptors in obesity and anorexia nervosa. *Metabolism* 1992; **41**:106–112.
15. Taylor AMA, Thomson C, Bruce-Morgan ML *et al.* The relationship between insulin, IGF-I and weight gain in cystic fibrosis. *Clin Endocrinol* 1999; **51**:659–665.
16. Lebl J, Zahradnikova M, Bartosová J *et al.* Insulin-like growth factor-I and insulin-like growth factor-binding protein-3 in cystic fibrosis: a positive effect of antibiotic therapy and hyperalimentation. *Acta Paediatr* 2001; **90**:868–872.
17. Clayton KL, Holly JM, Carlsson LM *et al.* Loss of the normal relationships between growth hormone, growth hormone-binding protein and insulin-like growth factor-I in adolescents with insulin-dependent diabetes mellitus. *Clin Endocrinol* 1994; **41**:517–524.
18. Edge JA, Dunger DB, Matthews DR *et al.* Increased overnight growth hormone concentrations in diabetic compared with normal adolescents. *J Clin Endocrinol Metab* 1990; **71**:1356–1362.
19. Moran A, Doherty L, Wang X *et al.* Abnormal glucose metabolism in cystic fibrosis. *J Pediatr* 1998; **133**:10–17.
20. Yung B, Noormohamed FH, Kemp M *et al.* Cystic fibrosis-related diabetes: the role of peripheral insulin resistance and beta-cell dysfunction. *Diabet Med* 2002; **19**:221–226.

21. Ripa P, Robertson I, Cowley D *et al.* The relationship between insulin secretion, the insulin-like growth factor axis and growth in children with cystic fibrosis. *Clin Endocrinol* 2002; **56**:383–389.

22. Nousia-Arvanitakis S, Galli Tsinopoulou A, Karamouzis M. Insulin improves clinical status of patients with cystic-fibrosis-related diabetes mellitus. *Acta Paediatr* 2001; **90**:515–519.

23. Ballinger A. Fundamental mechanisms of growth failure in inflammatory bowel disease. *Hormone Res* 2002; **58**:7–10.

24. Street ME, Miraki Moud F, Sanderson IR *et al.* Relationships between serum IGF-1, IGFBP-2, interleukin-1beta and interleukin-6 in inflammatory bowel disease. *Hormone Res* 2004; **61**:159–164.

25. De Benedetti F. Role of interleukin-6 in growth failure: an animal model. *Hormone Res* 2002; **58**:24–27.

26. Wolf M, Bohm S, Brand M, Kreymann G. Proinflammatory cytokines interleukin 1 beta and tumor necrosis factor alpha inhibit growth hormone stimulation of insulin-like growth factor I synthesis and growth hormone receptor mRNA levels in cultured rat liver cells. *Eur J Endocrinol* 1996; **135**:729–737.

27. Nixon LS, Yung B, Bell SC *et al.* Circulating immunoreactive interleukin-6 in cystic fibrosis. *Am J Respir Crit Care Med* 1998; **157**:1764–1769.

28. Hardin DS, Ellis KJ, Dyson M *et al.* Growth hormone decreases protein catabolism in children with cystic fibrosis. *J Clin Endocrinol Metab* 2001; **86**:4424–4428.

29. Hardin DS, Leblanc A, Marshall G *et al.* Mechanisms of insulin resistance in cystic fibrosis. *Am J Physiol Endocrinol Metabol* 2001; **281**:E1022–E1028.

30. Senaris RM, Lago F, Coya R *et al.* Regulation of hypothalamic somatostatin, growth hormone-releasing hormone, and growth hormone receptor messenger ribonucleic acid by glucocorticoids. *Endocrinology* 1996; **137**:5236–5241.

31. Magiakou MA, Mastorakos G, Gomez MT *et al.* Suppressed spontaneous and stimulated growth hormone secretion in patients with Cushing's disease before and after surgical cure. *J Clin Endocrinol Metabol* 1994; **78**:131–137.

32. Lai HC, Fitzsimmons SC, Allen DB *et al.* Risk of persistent growth impairment after alternate-day prednisone treatment in children with cystic fibrosis. *N Engl J Med* 2000; **342**:851–859.

33. Doull IJM. The effect of asthma and its treatment on growth. *Arch Dis Child* 2004; **89**:60–63.

34. Bircan Z, Soran M, Yildirim I *et al.* The effect of alternate-day low-dose prednisolone on bone age in children with steroid dependent nephrotic syndrome. *Int Urol Nephrol* 1997; **29**:357–361.

35. Dobson L, Hattersley AT, Tiley S *et al.* Clinical improvement in cystic fibrosis with early insulin treatment. *Arch Dis Child* 2002; **87**:F430–F431.

36. Allen DB, Julius JR, Breen TJ, Attie KM. Treatment of glucocorticoid induced growth suppression with growth hormone. *J Clin Endocrinol Metab* 1998; **83**:2824–2829.

37. Hardin DS, Rice J, Ahn C *et al.* Growth hormone treatment enhances nutrition and growth in children with cystic

38. Bourguignon JP. Growth and timing of puberty: reciprocal effects. *Hormone Res* 1991; **36**:131–135.

39. Crowne EC, Shalet SM, Wallace WH *et al.* Final height in boys with untreated constitutional delay in growth and puberty. *Arch Dis Child* 1990; **65**:1109–1112.

40. Llop-Vinolas D, Vizmanos Lamotte B, Areste Pitzalis A *et al.* Onset of puberty at eight years of age in girls determines a specific tempo of puberty but does not affect adult height. *Acta Paediatr* 2004; **93**:874–879.

41. Houchin LD, Rogol AD. Androgen replacement in children with constitutional delay of puberty: the case for aggressive therapy. *Baillière's Clin Endocrinol Metabol* 1998; **12**:427–440.

42. Mobbs EJ. The psychological outcome of constitutional delay of growth and puberty. *Hormone Res* 2005; **63** (Suppl 1):1–66.

43. Sawyer SM, Rosier MJ, Phelan PD, Bowes G. The self-image of adolescents with cystic fibrosis. *J Adoles Hlth* 1995; **16**:204–208.

44. Pfeffer PE, Pfeffer JM, Hodson ME. The psychosocial and psychiatric side of cystic fibrosis in adolescents and adults. *J Cyst Fibros* 2003; **2**:61–68.

45. Krupa B, Miazgowski T. Bone mineral density and markers of bone turnover in boys with constitutional delay of growth and puberty. *J Clin Endocrinol Metab* 2005; **90**:2828–2830.

46. Ujhelyi R, Treszl A, Vasarhelyi B *et al.* Bone mineral density and bone acquisition in children and young adults with cystic fibrosis: a follow-up study. *J Pediatr Gastroenterol Nutr* 2004; **38**:401–406.

47. Buckler JM. Skeletal age changes in puberty. *Arch Dis Child* 1984; **59**:115–119.

48. Landon C, Rosenfeld RG. Short stature and pubertal delay in male adolescents with cystic fibrosis: androgen treatment. *Am J Dis Child* 1984; **138**:388–391.

49. Hutler M, Schnabel D, Staab D *et al.* Effect of growth hormone on exercise tolerance in children with cystic fibrosis. *Med Sci Sports Exerc* 2002; **34**:567–72.

50. Schibler A, von der Heiden R, Birrer P, Mullis PE. Prospective randomised treatment with recombinant human growth hormone in cystic fibrosis. *Arch Dis Child* 2003; **88**:1078–1081.

51. Darmaun D, Hayes V, Schaeffer D *et al.* Effects of glutamine and recombinant human growth hormone on protein metabolism in prepubertal children with cystic fibrosis. *J Clin Endocrinol Metab* 2004; **89**:1146–1152.

52. Hardin DS, Ahn C, Prestidge C *et al.* Growth hormone improves bone mineral content in children with cystic fibrosis. *J Pediatr Endocrinol* 2005; **18**:589–595.

53. Hardin DS, Ferkol T, Ahn C *et al.* A retrospective study of growth hormone use in adolescents with cystic fibrosis. *Clin Endocrinol* 2005; **62**:560–566.

fibrosis receiving enteral nutrition. *J Pediatr* 2005; **146**:324–328.

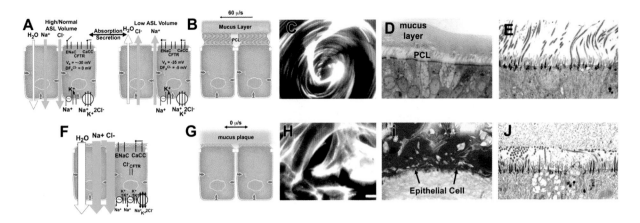

Plate 4.1 Ion and mucus transport in CF and non-CF airway epithelia. **(A)** Non-CF airway epithelia can exhibit both absorptive and secretory modes to regulate airway surface liquid (ASL) height. In the presence of an excess of liquid on airway surfaces, the dominant mode is Na^+-dependent volume absorption (active transcellular Na^+ transport with apical ingress via ENaC channels and passive paracellular Cl^- transport). In contrast, when ASL is depleted, ENaC is inhibited and a more negative membrane potential favors apical secretion of Cl^- via CFTR or the CaCC. **(B)** Schema illustrating optimal hydration of non-CF airway surfaces. Note that the adequate periciliary liquid (PCL) layer allows cilia to stretch upward and touch the underside of the mucus blanket, which floats above. **(C)** This optimal situation allows for rotational mucus transportation on primary cultures of non-CF airway epithelium (the image represents time lapse photograph of fluorescent beads within an aggregation of rotating mucus upon the polarized culture surface). **(D)** Mucus layer in fixed specimen of a primary culture preparation of non-CF airway epithelia. **(E)** Electron microscopic imaging demonstrating normal PCL height and ciliary orientation in a primary cultured airway epithelial preparation grown at an air–liquid interface. **(F)** Schema illustrating ion-transport pathways in CF airway epithelial cells. Note that Na^+ absorption, via ENaC, is augmented and unopposed by Cl^- secretion via CFTR, although the CaCC pathway remains intact. This results in adherence of mucus plaques to apical cell surfaces **(G)**, absent rotational mucus transport on cultured airway epithelial cells **(H)** and adherence and stagnation of mucus plaques on CF airway surfaces *in vitro* **(I)** and flattening and abnormal ciliary orientation in CF culture preparations **(J)**. Adapted from [124] and [125].

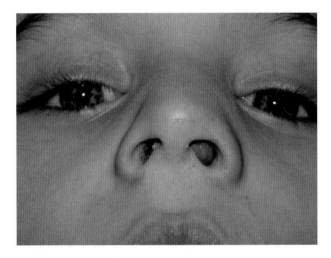

Plate 14.1 Photograph demonstrating nasal polyposis with complete occlusion of left nasal airway and broadening of nasal dorsum secondary to extensive anterior ethmoid polyposis.

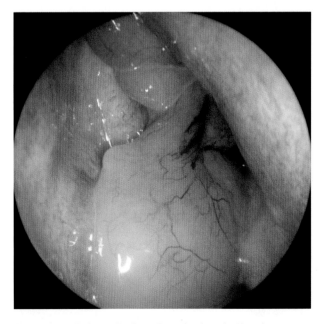

Plate 14.2 Endoscopic view of nasal polyposis, shrunken following application of vasonstricting agent.

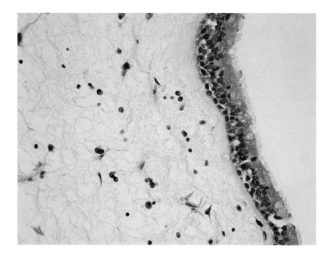

Plate 14.6 Area of polypoid mucosa showing sub-surface oedema with chronic inflammatory cells (few eosinophils). H&E × 200.

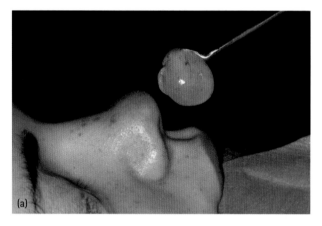

(a)

Plate 14.7 Nasal polyp on delivery.

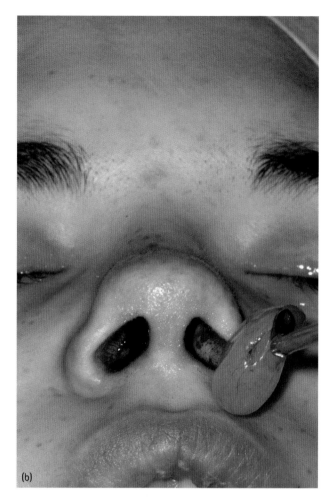

(b)

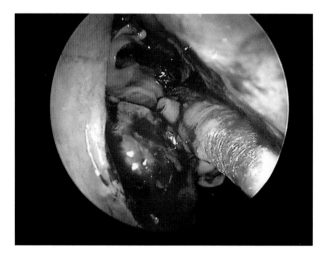

Plate 14.8 Endoscopic photograph showing both polyp and release of pocket of *Pseudomonas* pus from infected ethmoid air cell.

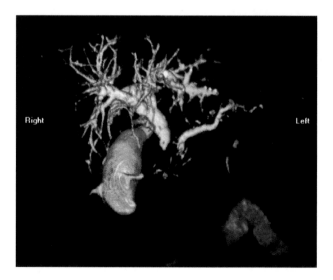

Plate 15.12 A workstation-constructed 3-D MRCP scan showing stricturing of both the distal pancreatic duct and common bile duct in a patient with established symptomatic chronic pancreatitis. Both strictures were managed by endoscopic stenting.

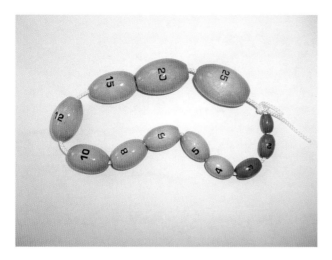

Plate 17.1 Prader orchidometer. The numbers are volume in milliliters, with a testicular volume of 4 mL or over marking the onset of puberty. Assessment of testicular volume is helpful in monitoring pubertal progress in boys.

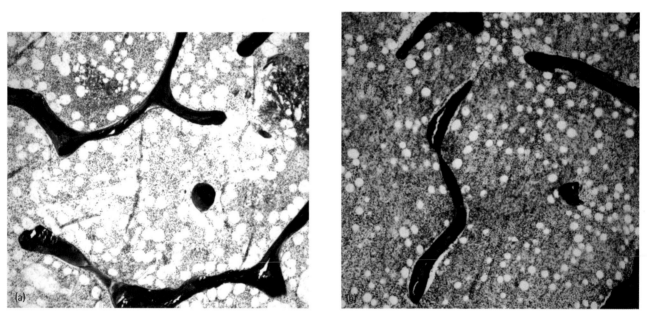

Plate 18.2 Toluidine blue-stained sections of iliac crest bone biopsy from adult patients with cystic fibrosis demonstrating decreased connectivity and bone area.

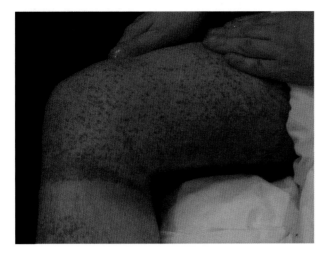

Plate 19.1 CF patient with recurrent vasculitic rash of the lower limbs.

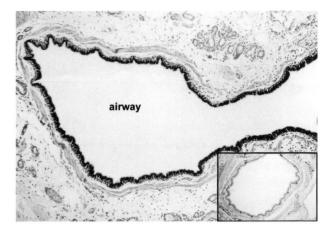

Plate 33.5 Efficient Sendai virus (SeV)-mediated transfection of airway epithelial cells in an animal model. Ferrets were transduced with SeV carrying a β-galactosidase reporter gene, which turn transduced cells blue. Insert shows untransduced control for comparison.

18

Cystic-fibrosis-related low bone mineral density

SARAH L. ELKIN AND CHARLES S. HAWORTH

INTRODUCTION

Low bone mineral density was first recognized to occur in patients with cystic fibrosis (CF) in the late 1970s. Since the first reports by Mischler and Hahn [1,2] much research has been performed investigating the prevalence, natural history, prevention and treatment of CF-related low bone mineral density (BMD). Prevention and recognition of low BMD is important as the clinical consequence of fragility fracture can impact adversely on the health of individuals by causing pain and interfering with chest physiotherapy. Furthermore, it is becoming increasingly common for patients to be refused transplantation if they have low BMD. Healthcare professionals now require an understanding of bone health issues to provide optimal care to their patients.

Definitions

Osteoporosis is a systemic skeletal disease characterized by low bone mass and microarchitectural deterioration of bone tissue with a consequent increase in bone fragility and susceptibility to fracture [3]. *Osteomalacia* is a disorder where there is an increase in the proportion of non-mineralized bone, in contrast to osteoporosis where there is a reduction in bone mass in the absence of a change in the ratio of mineralized to non-mineralized bone. Patients with CF are at risk of developing both osteoporosis and osteomalacia as a result of various risk factors (Table 18.1), including pancreatic insufficiency and the consequent malabsorption of the fat-soluble vitamins D and K.

BONE PHYSIOLOGY

Bone is a living tissue that undergoes constant remodelling throughout life. This process serves to maintain the mechanical integrity of the skeleton and provides a means by which calcium homeostasis may be maintained. Bone remodelling occurs at discrete sites called bone remodelling units and consists of the removal of a quantum of bone by osteoclasts followed by the formation of a similar amount of new bone by the osteoblasts [4]. Under normal circumstances this is a balanced process, but bone loss may occur as a result of remodelling imbalance. This occurs when the amount of bone formed is less than that resorbed. During normal growth, bone formation exceeds resorption up to the time of peak bone mass, which is reached at between 25 and 30 years of age. There is then a period of stabilization before age-related bone loss occurs in both sexes, at which time bone resorption exceeds formation (Fig. 18.1). Around the menopause, women sustain a phase of accelerated loss.

MEASUREMENT OF BONE MINERAL DENSITY

Several techniques are available to assess bone mass including dual energy x-ray absorptiometry (DXA), quantitative computed tomography (QCT) and broadband ultrasound attenuation. DXA is most commonly used because it is non-invasive, quick, highly reproducible and delivers an extremely low dose of radiation.

Table 18.1 Risk factors for the development of low BMD in patients with cystic fibrosis.

Delayed puberty
Low body mass index
Moderate/severe lung disease – increased cytokines
Decreased physical activity
Systemic glucocorticoid use
Malabsorption – vitamins D and K and calcium
Hypogonadism
CF-related diabetes
Drugs – e.g. depot medroxyprogesterone acetate (DepoProvera), Heparin
Transplantation

The purpose of performing bone densitometry is to identify individuals at risk of developing a fragility fracture, as fracture risk appears to be inversely related to the standard deviation (SD) score in postmenopausal populations. Bone mineral density values are usually expressed in relation to reference data as standard deviation scores. A Z score represents the number of standard deviations above or below the age- and sex-matched mean reference value. A T score is similarly expressed in relation to reference values for young adults at peak bone mass. Peak bone mass is normally achieved during the third decade of life, at which time Z and T scores are similar.

The WHO working definition of osteoporosis based on bone densitometry T scores is shown in Table 18.2. This system is validated in postmenopausal women but the relationship between BMD and fracture risk has not been established in other groups. How accurately this assessment of fracture risk translates into people with cystic fibrosis is therefore unknown. However, it is likely that the fracture risk for each SD reduction in BMD will be less in a young adult population than in an aging postmenopausal population. Due to these uncertainties within the CF population, the authors recommend that BMD values should be

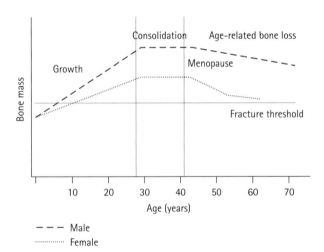

Figure 18.1   Age-related changes in bone mass.

Table 18.2   World health Organization (WHO) working definition of osteoporosis.

Normal	BMD not >1 SD below the mean value for young adults
Low bone mass	BMD 1–2.5 SD below the young adult mean
Osteoporosis	BMD > 2.5 SD below the young adult mean
Established osteoporosis	Osteoporosis with fragility fractures and BMD > 2.5 SD below young adult mean

BMD, bone mineral density; SD, standard deviation.

expressed as Z scores in premenopausal females and males aged under 50 years, and as T scores thereafter. The term 'osteoporosis' should be confined to those with a history of fragility fracture and the term 'low BMD' applied to children or adults with a BMD Z score below −2.

It is also important to appreciate the potential limitations of DXA measurements within the CF population.

- DXA is a two-dimensional rather than three-dimensional measurement, which can lead to erroneous assessments of depth of bone and result in falsely low BMD readings in patients with small bones. This must be considered when interpreting BMD data in patients with a small body habitus.
- There is a paucity of robust normative BMD data for children and so Z scores should be interpreted in the light of the best available pediatric reference data and the reference database should be cited in the report. Serial BMD scans and analysis of the raw data (bone mineral content in grams) may be more informative than single scans. Serial scans should ideally be performed on the same scanner and by the same technician to optimize precision.
- Both osteomalacia and osteoporosis cause low BMD and so the two conditions must be distinguished as their treatments are quite different.

PREVALENCE OF LOW BONE MINERAL DENSITY

Some reports suggest that well-nourished children with normal lung function have normal BMD [5,6]. However, low BMD has been reported in children in a number of studies. For example, there was a 10% lower bone density in 57 patients (mean age 12 years) when compared to local controls using quantitative computed tomography [7]. This finding was confirmed in a DXA study of 62 patients with mean age of 10.7 years [8]; the authors reported mean BMD Z scores of −1.03 at the lumbar spine and −0.71 at the femoral neck. Both studies found that BMD values correlated with disease severity.

Numerous studies have reported low BMD in adults with CF [6,9–13]. Earlier studies tended to investigate small numbers or concentrate on patients with end-stage pulmonary disease. One study found mean BMD Z scores of −1.7 at the lumbar spine and −1.9 at the femoral neck in 49 CF patients with a mean age of 20.6 years (range 8.4–48.5 years, 43% younger than 18) [14]. Another group studied 60 adult CF patients whom had been referred for lung transplantation; they found mean BMD Z scores of −2.17 at the lumbar spine and −2.02 at the femoral neck [15].

Three larger prevalence studies have been performed in the UK. The Royal Brompton Hospital reported 38% of 107 patients to have Z scores of under −1, with 13% having Z scores of under −2 in the lumbar spine or proximal femur [12]. The Manchester group reported a higher prevalence with 34% (48 of 143) of adults having a BMD Z score of under -2 in the lumbar spine, proximal femur or distal forearm [10]. The Leeds group reported 66% of 114 patients to have T scores of under -1.5, with 27% having T scores below -2.5 [11]. In a cross-sectional study involving 153 subjects aged 5–56 years with CF and 149 local healthy controls, there was a significant reduction in axial and total body BMD in adults, normal axial BMD (after correction for height) in adolescents, and normal BMD in children and adolescents [6]. This study suggests that the BMD loss in occurs during late adolescence and early adulthood.

In summary, it appears that approximately 25% of CF adults have reduced BMD and this figure increases to 75% in some series.

CHANGE IN BMD WITH AGE

There are limited data available from longitudinal studies. In a prospective study of 41 patients over one year the Z scores of younger patients with CF reduced over 18 months [16]. These data indicate failure to gain bone mineral density at the expected rate. The authors also found adult males ($n = 6$) to show a reduction of 1.2% at the femoral neck. The latter finding was corroborated in another prospective study that measured the BMD of 114 CF adults; there was an annual loss of approximately 2% in the proximal femur, but BMD in the lumbar spine did not change significantly [17]. More recently, similar findings have been reported in a retrospective review of BMD measurements over a 3- to 4-year period [18].

BONE HISTOMORPHOMETRY

Bone histomorphometry has helped to characterize the bone disease in CF and has found adult patients with low BMD measured by DXA to have significantly lower cancellous bone area, confirming that the low BMD identified by densitometry is real (Fig. 18.2). An in-depth analysis of iliac crest bone biopsies revealed a reduction in bone formation rate, wall width and mineral apposition rate when compared to controls, indicating that a reduction in bone formation to be the predominant cause of measured low BMD [19]. A study of autopsy bone samples reported a reduction in osteoblastic activity, increased osteoclastic activity and increased resorption [20]. This was not a significant finding in the Elkin *et al.* study, but there was heterogeneity in the size of the resorption cavities. It is likely, therefore, that increased bone resorption occurs in some patients during periods of ill-health or secondary hyperparathyroidism and this is supported by bone turnover data [21,22].

CLINICAL RELEVANCE OF LOW BMD

The increased prevalence of low BMD in children and adults with CF is likely to predispose to fracture, in view of the inverse relationship between BMD and fracture risk demonstrated in population-based studies. However, the prevalence of fragility fracture in children and adults with cystic fibrosis remains unclear. It was reported that females with CF aged between 6 and 16 years had higher fractures rates than controls or male CF patients [23]. It is unclear if this increase was statistically significant. In 70 patients awaiting

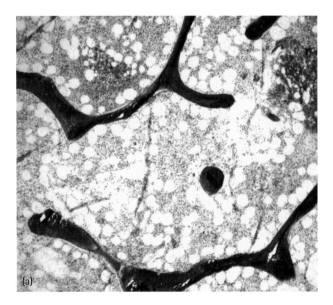
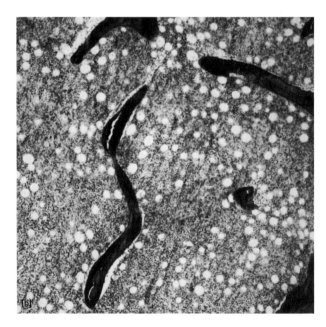

Figure 18.2 Toluidine blue-stained sections of iliac crest bone biopsy from adult patients with cystic fibrosis demonstrating decreased connectivity and bone area. *See also Plate 18.2.*

lung transplantation, a 2-fold increase was reported in fractures in females aged 16–34 and in males aged 25–45. Rib and vertebral fractures were reported as being respectively 10- and 100-fold more common than in a general US population [9]. In this series the majority of the vertebral wedge fractures were relatively mild with 60% of the fractures showing anterior height loss of 10–25%, but 6% of fractures showed anterior height loss of over 40%. Elkin and co-workers [12] reported that 35% of adults had a history of fracture, 9% of which were rib fractures; 17% of patients had evidence of vertebral deformity (>20% reduction in height). Although this prevalence is lower than that of Aris *et al.*, it is still higher than would be expected, considering the prevalence of vertebral fracture in 50- to 79-year-old Europeans is 12% [24]. More recently, vertebral deformities have been reported in 26.7% of 191 adult CF patients, with a slightly higher prevalence in males (32%) than in females (21%; $p = 0.058$) [25].

Transplant physicians are increasingly wary of listing patients with low BMD as lung transplantation may further increase bone loss and fracture risk in these patients [26]. It is therefore important to optimize BMD prior to transplant referral [26,27].

ETIOLOGY AND RISK FACTORS

Disease severity

There is little doubt that low BMD is associated with the severity of CF disease with many studies demonstrating a relationship between BMD and forced expiratory volume in one second (FEV_1), body mass index, intravenous antibiotic days and activity. It also appears that well-nourished patients with near-normal weight and lung function have normal BMD [5] while those listed for transplantation invariably have low BMD or osteoporosis [15]. Elevated levels of pro-inflammatory cytokines as a consequence of pulmonary sepsis probably adversely effect bone metabolism, thereby explaining the link between CF disease severity and BMD in this patient population [28,29].

Vitamin D

The majority of patients with CF are pancreatic-insufficient and malabsorb fat-soluble vitamins (D, E, A, K). Vitamin D deficiency can lead to osteomalacia while subclinical deficiency can lead to secondary hyperparathyroidism and consequently osteoporosis by increasing bone turnover. Although 1,25-dihydroxyvitamin D is the active form, 25-hydroxyvitamin D (25-OHD) gives a better measure of vitamin D stores having a longer half-life of 3–4 weeks. Most textbooks quote optimum serum levels as being in the range 20–60 ng/mL (50–150 nmol/L) and this wide reference range is due to differences in latitude and season. Hypovitaminosis D has been reported as a common occurrence in patients with CF despite vitamin supplementation of 600–800 IU/day (Table 18.3) [10,12,30–32]. A study in Washington, USA, found average values of 18.9 ng/L with 63% of the 87 patients having levels below 20 ng/L [33]. There have also been reports from areas with higher sun exposure such as North Carolina [9] with 20% of patients having subnormal 25 OHD levels (mean 20.9 ng/L). More recently, a significant BMD deficit in the presence of vitamin D sufficiency was reported in a large Australian cohort suggesting that low BMD in CF can occur independently of vitamin D insufficiency [34]. Despite the later report, it is likely that low vitamin levels are contributing to the decreased bone mass found in some populations by increasing bone turnover.

Vitamin D absorption appears to vary considerably among individuals with cystic fibrosis. CF adults absorbed less than one-half of the amount of oral vitamin D_2 given as a one-off dose in comparison to non-CF controls [35]. The 25-OHD levels in the CF group as a whole did not rise in response to the vitamin D_2, contrary to the control group who showed a doubling of serum levels. However, there was a wide variability in the individual absorption curves of the CF subjects, with three subjects actually exceeding the average of the controls. This observation has been confirmed more recently; it was reported that only 8% of patients with serum 25-OHD levels <30 ng/mL increased the serum level with high-dose ergocalciferol (50 000 IU/week for 8 weeks)

Table 18.3   Vitamin D levels in patients with cystic fibrosis.

Reference	No. Hypovitaminosis % ng/mL	Age (years)	Location	Serum 25-OHD (ng/mL ± SD)	Hypovitaminosis % ng/mL
[6]	141	5.3–55.8	Australia	24	25 <20
[11]	98	18–29	Leeds	18	40 <15
[12]	104	18–60	London	15 ± 11	83 <20
[10]	151	15–52	Manchester	19 ± 11.1	38 <15
[32]	71	18–57	Seattle	19 ± 10	63 <20
[14]	49	8–48	California		52 <18
[26]	11	>18	New York	17 ± 13	36 <10
[30]	31	17–52	London	10 ± 6	26 <15
[29]	20	14–25	Dublin	10	75 <13

OHD, hydroxy vitamin D.

[36]. It therefore appears that a subpopulation of patients with CF have difficulty in absorbing adequate vitamin D and it may be that increasing exposure to sunlight in these individuals would be a better therapeutic approach.

Calcium

Cystic fibrosis patients are at risk of a negative calcium balance from gastrointestinal malabsorption, low vitamin D levels and increased gastrointestinal excretion. In one study, CF subjects absorbed less calcium that controls; this appeared to improve but was not completely reversed by pancreatic supplements [37]. Low serum calcium could lead to low BMD, especially if intake is insufficient during periods of bone acquisition, for example during the pubertal growth spurt [38]. It is recommended that healthy adolescents and young adults should consume between 1200 and 1500 mg of calcium/day, so CF patients should receive this as a minimum [39].

Vitamin K

Vitamin K malabsorption may be a significant contributor in the multifactorial etiology of CF-related low BMD. Osteocalcin (OC), the major non-collagenous protein of the bone matrix, undergoes a vitamin K-dependent, post-transcriptional γ-carboxylation of the glutamic acid residues, which results in a higher mineral binding coefficient with the calcium ions in the new bone-forming matrix. It is therefore feasible that vitamin K deficiency may in part be causing the abnormal bone formation reported in histomorphometry studies. There is evidence suggesting that many patients with CF have inadequate levels of vitamin K. A prospective study investigating 98 patients and 62 healthy controls reported that 78% of pancreatic-insufficient patients and all those with CF liver disease had raised PIVKA-II levels (proteins formed in vitamin K absence) [40].

A cause–effect relationship between vitamin K deficiency and low BMD has not been proven, although authors speculate that, through its role in the carboxylation of OC, vitamin K deficiency might be associated with an uncoupling of the balance between bone resorption and bone formation [41,42].

Physical activity

At present it is unknown whether weight-bearing exercise can lead to increases in peak bone mass, help preserve BMD, or improve bone mass in CF patients found to have low BMD. However, it is known that total immobilization leads to bone loss in the general population due to increased resorption and decreased formation, and that bone health can be maintained with weight-bearing exercise. Therefore it seems sensible to encourage weight-bearing activity (with

varying strains) in the CF population to improve bone and muscle mass.

Delayed puberty and hypogonadism

It is known that adolescents with CF can enter puberty late and this is usually linked to malnutrition. However, recent longitudinal data from Australia involving 85 children and adolescents with CF and 100 age- and sex-matched controls showed normal pubertal progression as indicated by clinical pubertal staging and age of menarche [43]. Testosterone replacement therapy can be given to males with delayed puberty, but it should not be given too early as it can encourage epiphyseal closure and thus prevent further bone growth. Estrogen therapy can be considered in women with delayed puberty.

Hypogonadism is likely to be detrimental to bone health as androgens have a protective effect on the skeleton. Hypogonadism can occur in adults with CF and is probably under-recognized. In males, low serum testosterone levels have been reported to occur with normal gonadotrophins [12]; this is in keeping with suppression of the hypothalamic–pituitary–testicular axis (central hypogonadism). Many studies have found testosterone levels to be normal [10,11], but Elkin and co-workers [12] found 31 of 58 males to have low total serum testosterone, with 18% having low free values. The latter correlated with total body BMD. A recent study investigated 191 adults (100 males) and found serum estradiol levels to be below the normal range in 27% of males and 23% of females [25]. Levels were significantly related to femur BMD in both sexes. Interestingly, significantly lower free testosterone levels were observed in males with vertebral fractures.

Glucocorticoid therapy

Glucocorticoids decrease bone formation and increase bone resorption by decreasing calcium absorption, increasing renal calcium excretion, increasing parathyroid hormone concentrations, depressing gonadal function, decreasing osteoblast number and increasing osteoclastic activity. In the general population, glucocorticoids are the commonest cause of secondary osteoporosis. Most of the larger cross-sectional studies have detected an association between oral glucocorticoid usage and low BMD. The cumulative dose of steroids was reported to be a predictor of BMD in patients awaiting transplantation [15], and there was a negative correlation between usage and femoral neck BMD [12]. In another study, steroid use was reported to be inversely related to change in BMD over a 1-year period [17]. These data have recently been corroborated; it was reported that steroid use was a significant predictor of bone loss at the femoral neck over 3 years [18]. It therefore appears that oral glucocorticoid use contributes to bone loss in patients with CF.

Influence of mutant CFTR

It is most likely that bone health deteriorates due to the secondary complications of cystic fibrosis transmembrane conductor regulator (CFTR) dysfunction rather than a direct effect on bone cells. There are, however, some data suggesting that mutant CFTR may play a direct role on bone. CFTR-mutant mice had reduced cortical bone in the absence of obvious nutritional differences [44], and the analysis of dynamic parameters showed a reduction in bone formation. King et al. reported lower BMD in patients with the F508del genotype [13] and Haworth et al. reported high levels of bone turnover in F508del homozygotes compared to non-homozygotes [10]. To date, it is not known whether CFTR is expressed in osteoblasts or osteoclasts or other organs where mutant CFTR could potentially affect bone metabolism.

SCREENING

The optimal age for commencing DXA screening is not known. Some authorities suggest performing DXA from 8 years of age if risk factors for low BMD have been identified. Most clinicians feel that DXA should be performed before puberty and repeated every 1–3 years depending on the initial result to ensure bone accrual is occurring at a satisfactory rate. Peak bone mass can be identified in this way, after which treatment can be considered if premature bone loss occurs. The present authors recommend that a DXA scan be performed at transition to adult services if not already performed.

MANAGEMENT OF LOW BONE MINERAL DENSITY

The following recommendations are based on the CF Foundation consensus document on bone health [39] and the soon to be published CF Trust bone health guidelines.

General principles

Problems with bone health are likely to have origins in childhood. Pediatric care workers should therefore optimize factors that are likely to affect bone health to enable their patients to reach a normal peak bone mass – and this is especially important during puberty.

- Check vitamin D level at least annually. Autumn is the optimal time to measure serum levels, as it is reasonable to assume that levels will reduce during the winter months due to reduced solar exposure. The CFF and CF Trust guidelines recommend that serum 25-OHD levels should be 30–60 ng/mL. In practice, these high serum levels are hard to achieve in northern latitudes and it is likely that many patients will require vitamin D doses greater than the usual 800–2000 IU ergocalciferol/day. Alternative strategies to treat vitamin D insufficiency include the prescription of calcitriol or UVB therapy.
- Consider vitamin K supplementation in patients with low BMD.
- Ensure that dietary intake contains at least the recommended daily intake of calcium. The CFF consensus statement recommends intakes of 1300–1500 mg/day from the age of 18 years.
- Encourage weight-bearing exercise, especially during the pubertal growth spurt.
- Tanner staging should be performed in children and adolescents to ensure normal pubertal development. An endocrine referral may be appropriate for patients with pubertal delay or hypogonadism.
- Check testosterone levels in adult males annually and consider correction of low levels.
- An oral glucose tolerance test should be performed annually in adolescents and adults to screen for CF-related diabetes.
- Use glucocorticoids only when necessary and at the lowest dose possible.

Bisphosphonates

Bisphosphonates are potent inhibitors of osteoclastic bone resorption and are also thought to inhibit osteoblast apoptosis.

The effect of intravenous pamidronate was assessed in a randomized controlled trial involving 28 CF adults with low BMD [45]. Pamidronate-treated patients received pamidronate 30 mg every 3 months and both groups were prescribed calcium (1 g/day) and vitamin D (800 IU/day). After 6 months the pamidronate group ($n = 13$) showed a significant increase in absolute BMD compared with the control group ($n = 15$) in the lumbar spine (mean difference 5.8%; CI 2.7–8.9%) and total hip (mean difference 3.0%; CI 0.3–5.6%). Several patients developed severe bone pain after pamidronate but patients taking oral glucocorticoids and patients who had recently completed intravenous antibiotic treatment were asymptomatic suggesting that these measures had a protective effect [46]. Severe musculoskeletal pain was also experienced by 3 of 5 participants in a study investigating the effect of annual intravenous zoledronic acid (Boyle et al., personal communication). Although the study was stopped prematurely, the zoledronic acid-treated patients demonstrated a significant increase in lumbar spine BMD compared to placebo after 6 months.

The effect of alendronate (10 mg/daily) was assessed in a 1-year randomized double-blind placebo-controlled trial in 48 CF adults with low BMD [47]. All patients were prescribed cholecalciferol 800 IU/day and calcium 1000 mg/day. In the alendronate group compared to the control group, the mean ± SD change in bone density was 4.9 ± 3.0% versus −1.8 ± 4.0% in the lumbar spine ($p < 0.001$) and 2.8 ± 3.2% versus −0.7 ± 4.7% in the femur ($p = 0.003$).

The effect of intravenous pamidronate (30 mg every 3 months) was evaluated in a 2-year randomized controlled study in 34 CF patients following lung transplantation. All patients were prescribed cholecalciferol 800 IU/day and calcium 1000 mg/day. The patients treated with pamidronate gained 8.8 ± 2.5% and 8.2 ± 3.8% in the lumbar spine and femur, respectively, after 2 years compared to controls who gained 2.6 ± 3.2% and 0.3 ± 2.2%, respectively ($p \leq 0.015$ for both) [48]. None of the patients in this study developed bone pain, further suggesting that glucocorticoids reduce the risk of pamidronate-associated bone pain in people with CF.

In the present authors' opinion, bisphosphonate treatment in CF *adults* should be considered in the following circumstances.

- The patient has sustained a fragility fracture.
- The lumbar spine or total hip Z score is less than −2 *and* the patient has sustained significant bone loss despite implementation of the general measures to optimize bone health. The significance of bone loss is determined by the coefficient of variation of the measurement, and this varies according to the type of densitometer used, the skeletal site and the experience of the operator.
- The patient is starting a prolonged (>3 months) course of oral glucocorticoid treatment and has a BMD Z score of less than −1.5.
- The patient is listed for or has received a solid organ transplant and has a BMD Z score of less than −1.5.

There are no published data reporting the outcome of bisphosphonate use in CF children. Bisphosphonates may be beneficial in children with a history of fragility fracture and those listed for, or after, solid organ transplantation. Some authorities suggest bisphosphonates for children who have lost bone mass despite implementing the general measures for optimizing bone health, but we would strongly recommend seeking the advice of a pediatric bone specialist before commencing treatment.

The choice of bisphosphonate depends on clinical circumstances and patient preference. Intravenous bisphosphonates overcome some of the problems associated with the oral bisphosphonates such as poor oral bioavailability, upper gastrointestinal intolerance and adherence, but are associated with severe bone pain. However, in the authors' experience, oral alendronate and risedronate can also cause bone discomfort when first used in people with CF. A 3- to 5-day course of prednisone prior to administering intravenous pamidronate may prevent or reduce the bone pain associated with intravenous bisphosphonates.

Bisphosphonates cross the placenta and even if bisphosphonates have been discontinued prior to conception there is a theoretical risk that they could be released from bone during pregnancy. Thus patients who may wish to become pregnant should be fully informed of the potential risks to the fetus and females should use adequate contraception while prescribed bisphosphonates.

We would suggest repeating BMD measurements initially annually. If patients continue to lose bone mass while taking oral bisphosphonates and poor adherence or poor gut absorption are thought to be contributing factors, changing to intravenous bisphosphonates is advisable. Vitamin D insufficiency and osteomalacia should be excluded before commencing bisphosphonates through measuring the serum corrected calcium, 25-hydroxyvitamin D and parathyroid hormone (PTH) levels, and annual levels should be measured thereafter.

CONCLUSIONS

Approximately 25% of young adults with cystic fibrosis have low bone mineral density. As life expectancy increases, poor skeletal health can add significant morbidity. Much has been learnt about the pathogenesis of CF-related low BMD over the last decade and further research is required to ensure that the skeletal health of CF patients is sufficient to support them as their survival increases.

REFERENCES

1. Mischler EH, Chesney PJ, Chesney RW, Mazess RB. Demineralization in cystic fibrosis detected by direct photon absorptiometry. *Am J Dis Child* 1979; **133**:632–635.
2. Hahn TJ, Squires AE, Halstead LR, Strominger DB. Reduced serum 25-hydroxyvitamin D concentration and disordered mineral metabolism in patients with cystic fibrosis. *J Pediatr* 1979; **94**:38–42.
3. Andersson GB, Bostrom MP, Eyre DR *et al.* Consensus summary on the diagnosis and treatment of osteoporosis. *Spine* 1997; **22**(24 Suppl):63S–65S.
4. Ralston S, Compston JE (eds). *Osteoporosis: New Perspectives on Causes, Prevention and Treatment.* London, Royal College of Physicians of London, 1996, pp31–38.
5. Hardin DS, Arumugam R, Seilheimer DK *et al.* Normal bone mineral density in cystic fibrosis. *Arch Dis Child* 2001; **84**:363–368.
6. Buntain HM, Greer RM, Schluter PJ *et al.* Bone mineral density in Australian children, adolescents and adults with cystic fibrosis: a controlled cross sectional study. *Thorax* 2004; **59**:149–155.
7. Gibbens DT, Gilsanz V, Boechat MI *et al.* Osteoporosis in cystic fibrosis. *J Pediatr* 1988; **113**:295–300.
8. Henderson RC, Madsen CD. Bone density in children and adolescents with cystic fibrosis. *J Paediatr* 1996; **128**:28–34.
9. Aris RM, Renner JB, Winders AD *et al.* Increased rate of fractures and severe kyphosis: sequelae of living into adulthood with cystic fibrosis. *Ann Intern Med* 1998; **128**:186–193.
10. Haworth CS, Selby PL, Webb AK *et al.* Low bone mineral density in adults with cystic fibrosis. *Thorax* 1999; **54**:961–967.
11. Conway SP, Morton AM, Oldroyd B *et al.* Osteoporosis and osteopenia in adults and adolescents with cystic fibrosis: prevalence and associated factors. *Thorax* 2000; **55**:798–804.

12. Elkin SL, Fairney A, Burnett S *et al*. Vertebral deformities and low bone mineral density in adults with cystic fibrosis: a cross-sectional study. *Osteoporos Int* 2001; **12**:366–372.

13. King SJ, Topliss DJ, Kotsimbos T *et al*. Reduced bone density in cystic fibrosis: ΔF508 mutation is an independent risk factor. *Eur Respir J* 2005; **25**:54–61.

14. Bhudhikanok GS, Lim J, Marcus R *et al*. Correlates of osteopenia in patients with cystic fibrosis. *Pediatrics* 1996; **97**:103–111.

15. Aris RM, Neuringer IP, Weiner MA *et al*. Severe osteoporosis before and after lung transplantation. *Chest* 1996; **109**:1176–1183.

16. Bhudhikanok GS, Wang MC, Marcus R *et al*. Bone acquisition and loss in children and adults with cystic fibrosis: a longitudinal study. *J Pediatr* 1998; **133**:18–27.

17. Haworth CS, Selby PL, Horrocks AW *et al*. A prospective study of change in bone mineral density over one year in adults with cystic fibrosis. *Thorax* 2002; **57**(8):719–723.

18. Tomlinson GS, MacGregor G, Fairhurst M *et al*. A longitudinal study of bone mineral density change in adults with cystic fibrosis. *J Cyst Fibros* 2006; 5(Suppl 1):S109.

19. Elkin SL, Vedi S, Bord S *et al*. Histomorphometric analysis of bone biopsies from the iliac crest of adults with cystic fibrosis. *Am J Respir Crit Care Med* 2002; **166**:1470–1474.

20. Haworth CS, Webb AK, Egan JJ *et al*. Bone histomorphometry in adult patients with cystic fibrosis. *Chest* 2000; **118**:434–439.

21. Aris RM, Ontjes DA, Buell HE *et al*. Abnormal bone turnover in cystic fibrosis adults. *Osteoporosis Int* 2002; **13**: 151–157.

22. Baroncelli GI, De Luca F, Magazzu G *et al*. Bone demineralization in cystic fibrosis: evidence of imbalance between bone formation and degradation. *Pediatr Res* 1997; **41**:397–403.

23. Henderson RC, Specter BB. Kyphosis and fractures in children and young adults with cystic fibrosis. *J Pediatr* 1994; **125**:208–212.

24. O'Neill TW, Felsenberg D, Varlow J *et al*. The prevalence of vertebral deformity in european men and women: the European Vertebral Osteoporosis Study. *J Bone Miner Res* 1996; **11**:1010–1018.

25. Rossini M, Del Marco A, Dal Santo F *et al*. Prevalence and correlates of vertebral fractures in adults with cystic fibrosis. *Bone* 2004; **35**:771–776.

26. Spira A, Gutierrez C, Chaparro C *et al*. Osteoporosis and lung transplantation: a prospective study. *Chest* 2000; **117**:476–481.

27. Shane E, Silverberg SJ, Donovan D *et al*. Osteoporosis in lung transplantation candidates with end-stage pulmonary disease [see comments]. *Am J Med* 1996; **101**:262–269.

28. Aris RM, Stephens AR, Ontjes DA *et al*. Adverse alterations in bone metabolism are associated with lung infection in adults with cystic fibrosis. *Am J Respir Crit Care Med* 2000; **162**:1674–1678.

29. Haworth CS, Selby PL, Webb AK *et al*. Inflammatory related changes in bone mineral content in adults with cystic fibrosis. *Thorax* 2004; **59**:613–617.

30. Hanly JG, McKenna MJ, Quigley C *et al*. Hypovitaminosis D and response to supplementation in older patients with cystic fibrosis. *Quart J Med* 1985; **56**:377–385.

31. Stead RJ, Houlder S, Agnew J *et al*. Vitamin D and parathyroid hormone and bone mineralisation in adults with cystic fibrosis. *Thorax* 1988; **43**(3):190–194.

32. Donovan DSJ, Papadopoulos A, Staron RB *et al*. Bone mass and vitamin D deficiency in adults with advanced cystic fibrosis lung disease. *Am J Respir Crit Care Med* 1998; **157**:1892–1899.

33. Ott SM, Aitken ML. Osteoporosis in patients with cystic fibrosis. *Clin Chest Med* 1998; **19**:555–567.

34. Buntain HM, Greer RM, Schluter PJ *et al*. Bone mineral density in Australian children, adolescents and adults with cystic fibrosis: a controlled cross-sectional study. *Thorax* 2004; **59**(2):149–155.

35. Lark RK, Lester GE, Ontjes DA *et al*. Diminished and erratic absorption of ergocalciferol in adult cystic fibrosis patients. *Am J Clin Nutr* 2001; **73**:602–606.

36. Boyle MP, Noschese ML, Watts SL *et al*. Failure of high-dose ergocalciferol to correct vitamin D deficiency in adults with cystic fibrosis. *Am J Respir Crit Care Med.* 2005; **172**:212–217.

37. Aris RM, Lester GE, Dingman S, Ontjes D. Altered calcium homeostasis in adults with cystic fibrosis. *Osteoporos Int* 1999; **10**:102–108.

38. Johnston CCJ, Miller JZ, Slemenda CW *et al*. Calcium supplementation and increases in bone mineral density in children [see comments]. *N Engl J Med* 1992; **327**:82–87.

39. Aris RM, Merkel PA, Bachrach LK *et al*. Consensus Conference Report: Guide to bone health and disease in cystic fibrosis. *J Clin Endocrinol Metab* 2005; **90**(3):1888–1896.

40. Rashid M, Durie P, Andrew M *et al*. Prevalence of vitamin K deficiency in cystic fibrosis. *Am J Clin Nutr* 1999; **70**:378–382.

41. Conway SP. Vitamin K in cystic fibrosis. *J R Soc Med* 2004; **97**(Suppl 44):48–51.

42. Aris RM, Ontjes DA, Brown SA *et al*. Carboxylated osteocalcin levels in cystic fibrosis. *Am J Respir Crit Care Med* 2003; **168**:1129.

43. Buntain HM, Schluter PJ, Bell SC *et al*. Controlled longitudinal study of bone mass accrual in children and adolescents with cystic fibrosis. *Thorax* 2006; **61**:146–154.

44. Dif F, Marty C, Baudoin C *et al*. Severe osteopenia in CFTR-null mice. *Bone* 2004; **35**:595–603.

45. Haworth CS, Selby PL, Adams JE *et al*. Effect of intravenous pamidronate on bone mineral density in adults with cystic fibrosis. *Thorax* 2001; **56**:314–316.

46. Haworth CS, Selby PL, Webb AK *et al*. Oral corticosteroids and bone pain after pamidronate in adults with cystic fibrosis. *Lancet* 1999; **353**:1886.

47. Aris RM, Lester GE, Caminiti M *et al*. Efficacy of alendronate in adults with cystic fibrosis with low bone density. *Am J Respir Crit Care Med* 2004; **169**(1):77–82.

48. Aris RM, Lester GE, Renner JB *et al*. Efficacy of pamidronate for osteoporosis in patients with cystic fibrosis following lung transplantation. *Am J Respir Crit Care Med* 2000; **162**(3 Pt 1):941–946.

19

Other system disorders in cystic fibrosis

KHIN MA GYI

This chapter discusses vasculitis, arthropathies, renal problems, electrolyte disorders, neurological, hematological and ocular problems, and oral health in cystic fibrosis (CF).

VASCULITIS

Vasculitis is a well-recognized but uncommon complication of CF. The estimated frequency is about 2–3% [1–3]. Although it can occur in childhood, the majority of cases occur in adult CF patients over 20 years of age. Vasculitis mainly involves the small vessels, arterioles, capillaries or venules. A common histological finding is leukocytoclastic vasculitis [1,4]. There is vascular and perivascular infiltration by neutrophils, endothelial swelling and fibrinoid necrosis of the vessel wall. Cutaneous vasculitis is the usual presentation but systemic involvement can rarely occur, affecting the renal, gastrointestinal and central nervous systems [2,3,5]. In some cases of renal involvement, biopsy showed changes similar to those of Henoch–Schönlein purpura [1,3].

The etiology of vasculitis is not well understood. Circulating immune complexes have been frequently reported in CF patients with vasculitis, indicating underlying immune mechanisms [2,6]. Multiple factors, including chronic persistent bacterial infections and medications, may provide a source of potential antigen [1–3,6]. Many cases of vasculitis have been associated with hyperglobulinemia [2,7]. Purpura due to cryoglobulinemia has been described in one patient [8]. Anti-neutrophilic cytoplastic antibody (ANCA) against bacterial/permeability-increasing protein (BPI) has been described in sera of 55–90% of CF patients [1,2,9–11]. BPI is an important host defense protein with bactericidal and anti-endotoxin properties. It has protective activity against lipopolysaccharide-induced vascular endothelial cell injury [12]. Therefore, it is postulated that anti-BPI antibody may predispose to vascular inflammation. Whether this particular mechanism is responsible for CF vasculitis is not established. Anti-BPI is correlated with pseudomonal load,

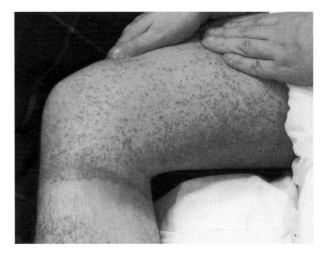

Figure 19.1 CF patient with recurrent vasculitic rash of the lower limbs. *See also Plate 19.1.*

severity of lung disease and the presence of vasculitis in adult CF patients [9,11].

Cutaneous vasculitis presents as a petechial or maculopapular rash, commonly involving the lower limbs, around the ankles and on the dorsum of the feet (Fig. 19.1). It may extend to the upper limbs, trunk and face. It is non-blanching, sometimes palpable, painful and can be itchy. Constitutional symptoms including fever, malaise and myalgia may be present. Arthralgia, and arthritis involving the ankles or knees, occurs in about 50% of cases. Hematuria and proteinuria are present in cases of renal involvement [1,3]. Recurrent iron deficiency anemia and intestinal bleeding can be presenting features of vasculitis involving the gastrointestinal tract [5,6,13]. Central nervous system involvement has been described in at least one case [1]. In the majority of cases, purpura disappears within a few days to a few weeks, but in a few cases this is recurrent and episodic.

Treatment for cutaneous vasulitis without systemic involvement is symptomatic with non-steroidal anti-inflammatory agents and antihistamine if necessary. In recurrent, severe or persistent vasculitis, and in cases of systemic involvement, corticosteroids, azathioprine and methotrexate have been used. Plasmapheresis has been described in cases of severe hyperglobulinemic purpura [7]. Any suspected medications should be withdrawn.

The majority of CF vasculitis occurs in the presence of CF lung disease. Many reported cases show increased mortality after the appearance of vasculitis. It is not certain whether the deleterious effect of vasculitis contributes to the poor prognosis or simply reflects the severity of the underlying CF lung disease.

Other skin involvement in CF includes acrodermatitis enteropathica-like eruptions and aquagenic wrinkling of the palms (AWP). Infants with CF may present with the former which is a rash consisting of extensive, dry, scaly, fissured, itchy erythematous plaques involving the perioral area, diaper region and extremities. It is thought to be due to malnutrition with deficiency of zinc, essential fatty acids and protein [14]. AWP is characterized by the rapid and transient formation of edematous whitish plaques on the palms on exposure to water. It is suggested that exposure of the skin to an abnormally high concentration of salt may play a role in the pathogenesis [15].

ARTHROPATHIES

Symptoms related to the joints occur in up to 12% of CF patients [4,16,17]. They may be directly related to CF, a complication of drug treatment or due to the presence of coincidental disease involving the joints. The most common arthropathies related to cystic fibrosis are: episodic arthritis (EA) and hypertrophic pulmonary osteoarthropathy (HPOA). They can occur at any age, but more commonly affect adults in the second decade of life.

Episodic arthritis (EA)

This is the most common form of arthritis in CF and affects 2–8% of adults. It is characterized by acute onset of mono- or polyarticular arthritis affecting large joints such as knees, ankles, wrists, hips and shoulders. Occasionally the small joints of the hands and feet may be affected. It is usually asymmetrical and can present as arthralgia or sometimes be associated with swelling and disabling pain. Episodes are transient and subside spontaneously within 7–10 days. Some cases may evolve into relapsing and remitting courses, which may last for weeks to years. Episodes may be associated with high fever, vasculitis rash, and erythema nodosum [3,4,17] Characteristically, episodic arthritis is non-erosive with negative rheumatoid factor, and the x-rays are normal. However, progression to erosive, chronic destructive polyarthritis has been reported in small subgroups of patients [17].

The underlying etiology is unknown but immunological mechanisms may play a role. Chronic, persistent bacterial infection with excessive antigen load can cause immune stimulation resulting in the formation of immune complexes [18,19]. It is speculated that arthritis may be due to a spillover of immune complexes from the respiratory tract into the circulation and subsequent deposition in the joints. High levels of circulating immune complexes are reported in CF arthropathy patients, compared to CF patients with no arthropathy. Immunoglobulins and complement deposition have been found in synovial blood vessels in biopsies taken during an exacerbation of episodic arthritis [4]. There is no evidence of an association with any specific HLA types [4,20].

Unlike in HPOA, there is no consistent relationship between episodic arthritis and the severity of underlying pulmonary disease or infective exacerbation. Treatment is usually symptomatic, with non-steroidal anti-inflammatory agents. Oral corticosteroids are occasionally used to control the inflammation. Very rarely, azathioprine, sulfasalazine and hydroxychloroquine have been tried [17,21].

Hypertrophic pulmonary arthropathy (HPOA)

HPOA was the first joint disease described in cystic fibrosis. It occurs in 2–7% of CF patients, predominantly affecting younger adults [22,23], but the median age of onset is about 20, and it rarely occurs before 10 years of age. It is characterized by clubbing and chronic periostitis of the long bones with or without periosteal new bone formation (Fig. 19.2).

Most patients present with an insidious onset of asymmetrical polyarthritis with pain, swelling and effusions, involving knees, ankles, wrists, and associated tenderness

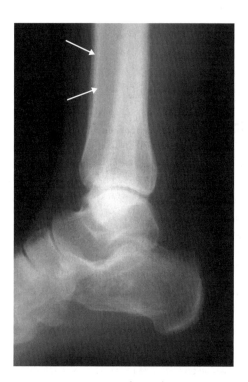

Figure 19.2 Periosteal reaction (arrows) of tibia and fibula in a CF patient with hypertrophic pulmonary arthropathy (HPOA).

of the ends of the long bones. It rarely involves the small joints of the hands or feet. Large joint effusions can sometimes occur. Gynecomastia and mastalgia may be present [24]. In contrast to episodic arthritis, HPOA is associated with more severe underlying lung disease and it accompanies or worsens during acute pulmonary exacerbations [16,17]. The etiology of HPOA is unknown. Theories have included neurogenic and humoral mechanisms and a hyperactive immune system as a result of acute infection. HPOA can regress after vagotomy and lung transplantation. Another theory relates to platelet function. This proposes that in the presence of some lung disease megakaryocytes accumulate in the small vessels of the distal long bones, inappropriately releasing some mediators, which can cause inflammation and new bone formation. In one study, PDGF (platelet-derived growth factor) was significantly higher in HPOA patients compared with healthy controls [25].

Management includes intensive treatment of underlying lung disease and acute exacerbations, non-steroidal anti-inflammatory agents for pain, and occasionally corticosteroids are used. In severe, refractory cases, intravenous pamidronate can be useful [26]. The onset of HPOA is associated with increased mortality [21].

Other systemic diseases involving the joints in CF

A few cases of rheumatoid arthritis (RA) have been reported in CF patients (Fig. 19.3) [16,27,28]. RA occurs more frequently in CF than can be attributed to chance alone. It has been postulated that CF episodic arthritis may be a mild form of RA with the potential for progressing to full-blown RA after several years of antigen stimulation, related to episodes

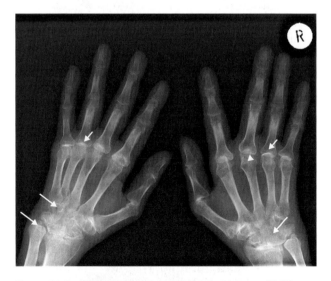

Figure 19.3 Severe rheumatoid arthritis in 23-year-old CF female showing erosions (long arrows); loss of joint space and ulnar deviation of metacarpophalangeal joints (arrow head); and juxta-articular osteopenia (short arrows).

of infective exacerbations [29]. Clinical presentation includes symmetrical polyarthritis with nodules, joint erosion and positive rheumatoid factor.

Other causes of arthropathy include sarcoidosis [30], amyloidosis [31,32] and secondary to hyperuricemia. The most common group of drugs responsible for arthritis in CF patients are the quinolones, ciprofloxacin causing acute tenosynovitis of knees and ankles [33]. However, this is rare when the numbers of courses of ciprofloxacin prescribed are considered.

RENAL PROBLEMS

Cystic fibrosis transmembrane conductance regulator (CFTR) is abundantly expressed in all nephron segments [34]. Despite this, in CF patients, there is no renal phenotype and no major primary renal dysfunction. In polycystic kidneys the secretion of chloride through CFTR is responsible for cyst enlargement [35]. However, the exact role of CFTR in renal physiology is still not fully understood [36]. There are subtle abnormalities of renal capacity to dilute and concentrate urine, excrete salt load and renal handling of some drugs [37,38]. CF patients have enhanced excretion of penicillin and aminoglycosides in their urine [39].

Renal abnormalities in CF are due either to secondary causes or to associated conditions. These include exposure to aminoglycosides and other nephrotoxic antibiotics and drugs, immune complex mediated injury in the presence of chronic bacterial infection, diabetes mellitus, liver disease, cor pulmonale, malabsorption and steatorrhea. Hypoxemia in severe lung disease may increase the nephrotoxic potentials of these risk factors.

Histological abnormalities from autopsy or biopsy material showed tubulointerstitial pathology related to antibiotics or nephrotoxic drugs, glomerular enlargement which is a non-specific finding in heart failure, mesengial immunoglobulin and complement deposition [40] and changes consistent with nodular glomerulosclerosis both in the presence or absence of diabetes [41,42]. A high incidence of microscopic nephrocalcinosis was reported in the autopsy of the kidneys in CF patients [43]. Renal amyloid deposition is found in CF patients with secondary amyloidosis and it could be one of the causes of nephrotic syndrome. Cases of IgA nephropathy has also been described in CF patients [44].

Clinical presentation of renal problems in CF patients includes nephrolithiasis, urolithiasis, hydronephrosis, nephrotic syndrome, progressive renal insufficiency and antibiotic-induced renal dysfunction or acute renal failure.

Nephrolithiasis

CF patients have increased rates of nephrocalcinosis and nephrolithiasis [43,45–47]. The incidence of renal stones in CF patients is higher than in an age-matched control population [45]. It is reported that up to 6.3% of CF patients are affected with renal stones, mainly in adolescence and early adulthood (Fig. 19.4).

There are multifactorial causes of stone formation in CF. Absorptive hyperoxaluria is one of the major factors for renal calcium oxalic stone formation. In the presence of malabsorption, calcium binds to fatty acids in the intestinal lumen rather than to oxalate, which leads to increased absorption of free oxalate [48]. Malabsorped bile salts also facilitate greater colonic oxalate permeability [49]. Frequent antibiotic treatment can cause absence or reduction of intestinal oxalate-degrading bacteria such as *Oxalobacter formigenes*, resulting in increased oxalate absorption. Normally up to 70% of daily oxalate intake is degraded by this bacterium [50,51]. A prospective study of 37 patients demonstrated that increased intestinal oxalate absorption was the cause of hyperoxaluria in 79% of the patients studied [52].

Citrate is the stone inhibitory substance. It slows stone formation by reducing calcium concentration in the urine and inhibits crystallization of calcium oxalate. Therefore hypocitraturia is a risk factor for a renal stone formation in the presence of hyperoxaluria [52]. It is a common finding in CF patients with oxalate stone formation compared to CF patients without stones [45,53]. Hypocitraturia in CF could be due to dietary acid load caused by high protein diet and pancreatic enzymes. Another cause is metabolic acidosis as a result of stool losses of bicarbonate, which, in turn, stimulates the proximal tubules reabsorption of citrate [45].

There is no definite evidence of a primary defect in renal calcium handling in CF patients [45]. Hypercalciuria rarely occurs in CF patients and it is usually due to glucocorticoid administration and immobilization. Hypercalciuria if present may contribute to the overall risk of stone formation. Hyperuricosuria can be a factor for calcium oxalate stone

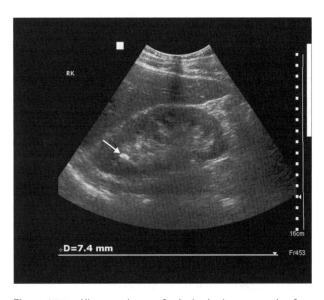

Figure 19.4 Ultrasound scan of calculus in the upper pole of the right kidney (arrow) in CF patient presenting with recurrent renal colic.

formation. It has been associated with high doses of pancreatic enzymes in some CF patients [54]. Low urine volume as the result of extracellular fluid volume contraction caused by sodium and chloride loss in sweat and feces may also contribute to stone formation. Therefore, in CF, hyperoxaluria, hypocitraturia and low urine volume act in combination to promote stone formation [55].

The patient may present with renal colic, hematuria and recurrent urinary tract infection. The diagnosis is confirmed by a plain abdominal film, renal ultrasound, intravenous pyelogram and helical CT. Treatment includes lithotripsy, ureteral stent, percutaneous nephrostomy and ureteroscopy. Other treatment includes increased fluid intake, oral potassium citrate supplement, avoidance of high oxalate diet (e.g. spinach, chocolate) and intestinal recolonization with *Oxalobacter* or treatment with other oxalate-degrading bacteria [56].

Antibiotic-induced renal impairment

Aminoglycosides are the most commonly used antibiotics associated with renal toxicity in CF patients. Acute toxicity is usually due to excess levels resulting in acute tubular necrosis. This can be potentiated by dehydration and nonsteroid anti-inflammatory drugs. Repeated, long-term use of intravenous aminoglycosides has been strongly associated with decreasing renal function in CF patients with previously normal renal function. The cumulative lifetime dose is negatively correlated with glomerular filtration rate (GFR) in CF [57]. In these patients the annual measurement of creatinine clearance is recommended. This effect is potentiated by co-administration of Colomycin. Proximal tubular activity can be assessed by urinary *N*-acetyl-beta-D-glucosaminidase (NAG) activity. Long-term gentamicin inhalation therapy may predispose to renal toxicity as there is positive correlation between urinary NAG activity and cumulative dose of gentamicin [58]. Acute renal failure as a result of acute tubular necrosis has been reported in a few CF patients treated with a combination of ceftazidime and gentamicin [59,60]. This is thought to be direct tubular toxicity by the combined effect of the drugs or ceftazidime causing interstitial nephritis. Management includes withdrawal of the drug, supportive treatment for acute renal failure and dialysis in some severe cases. Hypomagnesemia is also a common finding after repeated courses of aminoglycosides and is frequently associated with hypocalcemia and hypokalemia.

Nephrotic syndrome and progressive renal insufficiency

Nephrotic syndrome and progressive renal insufficiency has been reported in CF patients with systemic amyloidosis, diabetic nephropathy and glomerulonephritis [31,41].

ELECTROLYTE DISORDERS

Metabolic alkalosis

Acute or chronic metabolic alkalosis is described as an initial presentation or complication of cystic fibrosis in infants and children but rare in adults [61]. Mutations in CFTR cause abnormal epithelial chloride transport. As a result of dysfunctional CFTR there is a loss of fluid high in chloride from the sweat glands (Fig. 19.5), bronchial mucosa, gastrointestinal mucosa, pancreatic secretion, salivary glands and tear glands [62,63]. Renal tubular handling of chloride is usually normal.

In infants and young children there is normally a rather low dietary chloride intake with consistent loss in sweat and gastrointestinal tract and daily retention is high. Chloride depletion leads to an excessive reabsorption of bicarbonate in the distal renal tubules, resulting in metabolic alkalosis. Urinary chloride excretion was quite low in these cases [61,64]. However, in some adult CF patients with metabolic alkalosis there is lack of avid urinary chloride retention for which the reason is unknown [65]. Urinary chloride/creatinine ratio discriminates between extrarenal and renal origin of metabolic alkalosis. This is low in the former and normal or higher in the latter [66]. Albumin is a weak acid

and hypoalbuminemia associated with chronic malnutrition may also contribute to metabolic alkalosis [67]. CFTR is known to alter bicarbonate transport thus it may play a role in acid–base disturbance [68]. Acute or chronic metabolic alkalosis with hypochloremia, hyponatremia and hypokalemia – sometimes referred to as pseudo-Bartter syndrome – is not an uncommon presentation in infants and young children with CF [61,69–71]. Usually anorexia, nausea, vomiting, respiratory exacerbations, fever and weight loss precede metabolic alkalosis. Sometimes it may be the initial presentation which results in the diagnosis of CF. Chronic metabolic alkalosis is fairly frequent in young CF patients with severe respiratory involvement, poor nutritional status and a high intake of pancreatic enzyme supplements [64]. After correction of salt deficiency and metabolic abnormalities, failure to thrive resolves and rapid weight gain has been achieved [69].

In adults, vigorous exercise in a hot climate causes excessive sweating with loss of sweat electrolytes and dehydration. In combination with an intake of unsalted water this could result in heat exhaustion with severe hyponatremia, hypokalemia and metabolic alkalosis [72,73]. These patients responded well to rehydration and electrolyte replacement.

In metabolic alkalosis, hypoventilation with hypercapnia may occur as a compensatory response to restore pH towards normal. This can contribute to acute hypercapnic respiratory failure in adult CF with infective exacerbation [74]. In these cases, without correction of the underlying electrolyte abnormalities, hypercapnia may respond less well to assisted ventilation. Clinical features of severe alkalemia include arrythmias, hypoventilation with hypoxia and hypercapnia, hypokalemia, hypocalcemia and cerebral manifestations including tetany, seizures, delirium and stupor [75].

Investigations includes serum urea and electrolytes, blood gases, serum bicarbonate and urinary electrolytes. Urinary sodium and chloride are typically low (<10 mmol/L). Management consists of adequate volume replacement, sodium and chloride supplements in the form of normal saline, and potassium supplements. Total body potassium can be low despite normal serum level. In hot weather and in the presence of excess sweating the CF patient should take salty snacks or salt tablets and adequate fluids.

Syndrome of inappropriate ADH secretion (SIADH)

SIADH is a common manifestation of bacterial and viral pneumonias and its occurrence has been observed occasionally in CF patients during acute exacerbations of chronic pulmonary disease [76]. This is another cause of hyponatremia in CF patients, in addition to salt loss. The urine sodium concentration is typically greater than 40 mmol/L (compared with pseudo-Bartter's syndrome, <10 mmol/L). Symptoms and signs of hyponatremia include headache, lethargy, dizziness, ataxia, confusion, psychosis, seizures and

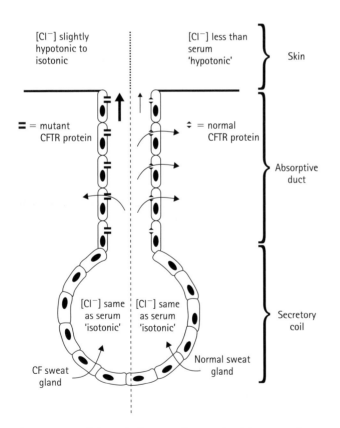

Figure 19.5 Schematic diagram of sweat gland. In a normal sweat gland CFTR drives Cl⁻ reabsorption, so normal sweat is hypotonic. CF patient has reduced Cl⁻ permeability and increased Cl⁻ in sweat. Modified from [97].

coma. Treatment includes fluid restriction, demeclocycline, in severe cases in combination with hypertonic saline and diuretics.

NEUROLOGICAL PROBLEMS

Several neurological symptoms and manifestations have been described in CF patients. Seizures and epilepsy occurred in relation to electrolyte abnormalities (i.e. hyponatremia, hypochloremia, metabolic alkalosis, hypoglycemia) and also due to drug reactions (e.g. ciprofloxacin and theophylline interaction, due to both drugs being metabolized by the same cytochrome P450 metabolic pathway). Cases of brain abscess have been reported in adolescent CF patients with advanced pulmonary disease. The organisms responsible include aerobic and anaerobic bacteria of low virulence and fungi, but *Pseudomonas* is rarely identified [77,78].

Acute onset of neurological deficits resembling strokes or transient ischemic attacks have been reported in some CF patients [79–81]. These could result from paradoxical embolization which can occur due to left-to-right shunt through a patent foramen ovale during coughing episodes or a Valsalva maneuver. These patients frequently have a totally implantable venous access device (TIVAD) with a thrombus formation around the catheter from which the emboli originate. The neurological episode can be confirmed by brain MRI, and transesophageal echocardiogram (TEE) is a sensitive method for detection of patent foramen ovale.

Coughing paroxysms are common in many CF patients as a result of underlying lung disease. Stern and co-workers [82] described neurological symptoms developing in these patients, including light-headedness, headaches, visual disturbances, speech abnormalities, movement disorders and syncope. CF patients who develop neurological symptoms have more severe obstructive lung disease than patients who do not experience such symptoms [82]. One of the underlying mechanisms could be due to cerebral hypoperfusion. During coughing, increased intrathoracic pressure is transmitted via valveless veins to the intracranial compartment, causing a transient increase in intracranial pressure, resulting in impairment of cerebral blood flow. Increased intrathoracic pressure also obstructs venous outflow causing reduced cardiac output and blood pressure, resulting in cerebral hypoperfusion [83,84]. In addition, hypoxia can occur during prolonged episodes of coughing paroxysm. In advanced lung disease, extreme pressure changes in the thoracic cavity during inspiration can cause physiological tamponade which may interfere with cardiac output and cerebral perfusion [85].

Rao and co-workers [86] described two CF patients who developed cough-induced hemiplegic migraine resulting in acute neurological symptoms and altered consciousness. The symptoms responded to treatment with verapamil. The CFTR channel is abundantly expressed in the brain [84]. Hemiplegic migraine is one of the disorders characterized under channelopathy [87]. Since CFTR is responsible for regulating other channels, it is suggested that it may indirectly contribute to the production of migraine [86].

Headache is common and in one study 55% of CF children had chronic headache and the main etiology was hypercarbia, hypoxia, sinusitis or migraine [88]. Severe vitamin E deficiency causes muscle weakness, hyporeflexia, ataxia, and reduced vibration and position sense [89].

Investigations for neurological symptoms include a detailed neurological history and examination, blood tests including electrolytes and vitamin levels, glucose monitoring, neurological imaging with CT and MRI scan, EEG, 24-hour ECG monitoring, echocardiogram with a shunt study, carotid Doppler and overnight oxygen saturation monitoring.

HEMATOLOGICAL PROBLEMS

Iron deficiency is common in CF and is thought to be due to chronic inflammation. It was found to be directly related to the increased severity of suppurative lung disease associated with *Pseudomonas aeruginosa* [90]. Thrombophilic abnormalities were described in some CF patients at screening but most abnormalities were inconsistent. The clinical significance is not clear but it may be relevant in TIVAD-related thrombosis [91,92]. Severe hemolytic anemia and clotting disorders due to vitamin E and vitamin K deficiency, respectively, may be the first presenting signs of CF in infants [93].

OCULAR PROBLEMS

Endogenous endopthalmitis caused by *Pseudomonas aeruginosa* rarely occurs in CF patients after lung transplantation and has also been reported in patients who have not undergone a transplant. The visual prognosis is poor and usually enucleation is necessary despite aggressive surgical intervention and appropriate antibiotic therapy [94,95]. Vitamin A deficiency can cause xerophthalmia, night blindness and poor dark adaptation. Severe vitamin E deficiency is associated with abnormal eye movement and visual field restrictions [89].

ORAL HEALTH

A decreased prevalence of dental caries was observed in CF children, which is thought to be due to long-term antibiotic usage and pancreatic enzyme supplements. However, enamel opacities are more common [96].

REFERENCES

1. Finnegan MJ, Hinchcliffe J, Russell-Jones D *et al.* Vasculitis complicating cystic fibrosis. *Quart J Med* 1989; **72**:609–621.
2. Hodson ME. Vasculitis and arthropathy in cystic fibrosis. *J R Soc Med* 1992; **85**(Suppl 19):38–40.

3. Schidlow DV, Goldsmith DP, Palmer J *et al*. Arthritis in cystic fibrosis. *Arch Dis Child* 1984; **59**:377–379.

4. Bourke S, Rooney M, Fitzgerald M *et al*. Episodic arthropathy in adult cystic fibrosis. *Quart J Med* 1987; **64**:651–659.

5. Parameswaran K, Keaney NP, Veale D. A case of chronic gastrointestinal blood loss in cystic fibrosis. *Respir Med* 1995; **89**:577–579.

6. Soter NA, Mihm MC, Colten HR. Cutaneous necrotizing venulitis in patients with cystic fibrosis. *J Pediatr* 1979; **95**:197–201.

7. Nielsen HE, Lundh S, Jacobsen SV *et al*. Hypergammaglobulinemic purpura in cystic fibrosis. *Acta Paediatr Scand* 1978; **67**:443–447.

8. Garty BZ, Scanlin T, Goldsmith DP *et al*. Cutaneous manifestations of cystic fibrosis: possible role of cryoglobulins. *Br J Dermatol* 1989; **121**:655–658.

9. Mahadeva R, Dunn AC, Westerbeek RC *et al*. Anti-neutrophil cytoplasmic antibodies (ANCA) against bactericidal/permeability-increasing protein (BPI) and cystic fibrosis lung disease. *Clin Exp Immunol* 1999; **117**:561–567.

10. Sediva A, Kolarova I, Bartunkova J. Antineutrophil cytoplasmic antibodies in children. *Eur J Pediatr* 1998; **157**:987–991.

11. Zhao MH, Jayne DR, Ardiles LG *et al*. Autoantibodies against bactericidal/permeability-increasing protein in patients with cystic fibrosis. *Quart J Med* 1996; **89**:259–265.

12. Arditi M, Zhou J, Huang SH *et al*. Bactericidal/permeability-increasing protein protects vascular endothelial cells from lipopolysaccharide-induced activation and injury. *Infect Immun* 1994; **62**:3930–3936.

13. McFarlane H, Holzel A, Brenchley P *et al*. Immune complexes in cystic fibrosis. *Br Med J* 1975; **1**:423–428.

14. Hansen RC, Lemen R, Revsin B. Cystic fibrosis manifesting with acrodermatitis enteropathica-like eruption: association with essential fatty acid and zinc deficiencies. *Arch Dermatol* 1983; **119**:51–55.

15. Katz KA, Yan AC, Turner ML. Aquagenic wrinkling of the palms in patients with cystic fibrosis homozygous for the delta F508 CFTR mutation. *Arch Dermatol* 2005; **141**:621–624.

16. Dixey J, Redington AN, Butler RC *et al*. The arthropathy of cystic fibrosis. *Ann Rheum Dis* 1988; **47**:218–223.

17. Rush PJ, Shore A, Coblentz C *et al*. The musculoskeletal manifestations of cystic fibrosis. *Semin Arthritis Rheum* 1986; **15**:213–225.

18. Moss RB, Lewiston NJ. Immune complexes and humoral response to *Pseudomonas aeruginosa* in cystic fibrosis. *Am Rev Respir Dis* 1980; **121**:23–29.

19. Wisnieski JJ, Todd EW, Fuller RK *et al*. Immune complexes and complement abnormalities in patients with cystic fibrosis: increased mortality associated with circulating immune complexes and decreased function of the alternative complement pathway. *Am Rev Respir Dis* 1985; **132**:770–776.

20. Rush PJ, Gladman DD, Shore A *et al*. Absence of an association between HLA typing in cystic fibrosis arthritis and hypertrophic osteoarthropathy. *Ann Rheum Dis* 1991; **50**:763–764.

21. Phillips BM, David TJ. Pathogenesis and management of arthropathy in cystic fibrosis. *J R Soc Med* 1986; **79** (Suppl 12):S44–S50.

22. Cohen AM, Yulish BS, Wasser KB *et al*. Evaluation of pulmonary hypertrophic osteoarthropathy in cystic fibrosis: a comprehensive study. *Am J Dis Child* 1986; **140**:74–77.

23. Johnson S, Knox AJ. Arthropathy in cystic fibrosis. *Respir Med* 1994; **88**:567–570.

24. Braude S, Kennedy H, Hodson M *et al*. Hypertrophic osteoarthropathy in cystic fibrosis. *Br Med J* 1984; **288**:822–823.

25. Silveri F, De Angelis R, Argentati F *et al*. Hypertrophic osteoarthropathy: endothelium and platelet function. *Clin Rheumatol* 1996; **15**:435–439.

26. Garske LA, Bell SC. Pamidronate results in symptom control of hypertrophic pulmonary osteoarthropathy in cystic fibrosis. *Chest* 2002; **121**:1363–1364.

27. Gardiner PV, Roberts SD, Bell AL. Cystic fibrosis and rheumatoid arthritis. *Br J Rheumatol* 1989; **28**:179.

28. Lawrence JM, Moore TL, Madson KL *et al*. Arthropathies of cystic fibrosis: case reports and review of the literature. *J Rheumatol Suppl* 1993; **38**:12–15.

29. Botton E, Saraux A, Laselve H *et al*. Musculoskeletal manifestations in cystic fibrosis. *Joint Bone Spine* 2003; **70**:327–335.

30. Soden M, Tempany E, Bresnihan B. Sarcoid arthropathy in cystic fibrosis. *Br J Rheumatol* 1989; **28**:341–343.

31. Gaffney K, Gibbons D, Keogh B *et al*. Amyloidosis complicating cystic fibrosis. *Thorax* 1993; **48**:949–950.

32. Ristow SC, Condemi JJ, Stuard ID *et al*. Systemic amyloidosis in cystic fibrosis. *Am J Dis Child* 1977; **131**:886–888.

33. Warren RW. Rheumatologic aspects of pediatric cystic fibrosis patients treated with fluoroquinolones. *Pediatr Infect Dis J* 1997; **16**:118–122.

34. Riordan JR, Rommens JM, Kerem B *et al*. Identification of the cystic fibrosis gene: cloning and characterization of complementary DNA. *Science* 1989; **245**:1066–1073.

35. Sullivan LP, Wallace DP, Grantham JJ. Chloride and fluid secretion in polycystic kidney disease. *J Am Soc Nephrol* 1998; **9**:903–916.

36. Morales MM, Carroll TP, Morita T *et al*. Both the wild type and a functional isoform of CFTR are expressed in kidney. *Am J Physiol* 1996; **270**(6 Pt 2):F1038–F1048.

37. Donckerwolcke RA, Diemen-Steenvoorde R, van der LJ *et al*. Impaired diluting segment chloride reabsorption in patients with cystic fibrosis. *Child Nephrol Urol* 1992; **12**:186–191.

38. Stenvinkel P, Hjelte L, Alvan G *et al*. Decreased renal clearance of sodium in cystic fibrosis. *Acta Paediatr Scand* 1991; **80**:194–198.

39. Touw DJ. Clinical pharmacokinetics of antimicrobial drugs in cystic fibrosis. *Pharm World Sci* 1998; **20**(4):149–160.

40. Abramowsky CR, Swinehart GL. The nephropathy of cystic fibrosis: a human model of chronic nephrotoxicity. *Hum Pathol* 1982; **13**:934–939.

41. Scott AI, Clarke BE, Healy H *et al*. Microvascular complications in cystic fibrosis-related diabetes mellitus: a case report. *JOP* 2000; **1**(4):208–210.

42. Westall GP, Binder J, Kotsimbos T et al. Nodular glomerulosclerosis in cystic fibrosis mimics diabetic nephropathy. Nephron Clin Pract 2004; 96:c70–c75.

43. Katz SM, Krueger LJ, Falkner B. Microscopic nephrocalcinosis in cystic fibrosis. N Engl J Med 1988; 319:263–266.

44. Stirati G, Antonelli M, Fofi C et al. IgA nephropathy in cystic fibrosis. J Nephrol 1999; 12:30–31.

45. Gibney EM, Goldfarb DS. The association of nephrolithiasis with cystic fibrosis. Am J Kidney Dis 2003; 42:1–11.

46. Matthews LA, Doershuk CF, Stern RC et al. Urolithiasis and cystic fibrosis. J Urol 1996; 155:1563–1564.

47. Strandvik B, Hjelte L. Nephrolithiasis in cystic fibrosis. Acta Paediatr 1993; 82:306–307.

48. Dharmsathaphorn K, Freeman DH, Binder HJ et al. Increased risk of nephrolithiasis in patients with steatorrhea. Dig Dis Sci 1982; 27:401–405.

49. Dobbins JW, Binder HJ. Importance of the colon in enteric hyperoxaluria. N Engl J Med 1977; 296:298–301.

50. Bohles H, Gebhardt B, Beeg T et al. Antibiotic treatment-induced tubular dysfunction as a risk factor for renal stone formation in cystic fibrosis. J Pediatr 2002; 140:103–109.

51. Sidhu H, Hoppe B, Hesse A et al. Absence of Oxalobacter formigenes in cystic fibrosis patients: a risk factor for hyperoxaluria. Lancet 1998; 352:1026–1029.

52. Hoppe B, von Unruh GE, Blank G et al. Absorptive hyperoxaluria leads to an increased risk for urolithiasis or nephrocalcinosis in cystic fibrosis. Am J Kidney Dis 2005; 46:440–445.

53. Bohles H, Michalk D. Is there a risk for kidney stone formation in cystic fibrosis? Helv Paediatr Acta 1982; 37:267–272.

54. Hoppe B, Hesse A, Bromme S et al. Urinary excretion substances in patients with cystic fibrosis: risk of urolithiasis? Pediatr Nephrol 1998; 12:275–279.

55. von der HR, Balestra AP, Bianchetti MG et al. Which factors account for renal stone formation in cystic fibrosis? Clin Nephrol 2003; 59:160–163.

56. Hoppe B, von Unruh G, Laube N et al. Oxalate degrading bacteria: new treatment option for patients with primary and secondary hyperoxaluria? Urol Res 2005; 33:372–375.

57. Al Aloul M, Miller H, Alapati S et al. Renal impairment in cystic fibrosis patients due to repeated intravenous aminoglycoside use. Pediatr Pulmonol 2005; 39:15–20.

58. Ring E, Eber E, Erwa W et al. Urinary N-acetyl-beta-D-glucosaminidase activity in patients with cystic fibrosis on long-term gentamicin inhalation. Arch Dis Child 1998; 78:540–543.

59. Kennedy SE, Henry RL, Rosenberg AR. Antibiotic-related renal failure and cystic fibrosis. J Paediatr Child Health 2005; 41:382–383.

60. Stephens SE, Rigden SP. Cystic fibrosis and renal disease. Paediatr Respir Rev 2002; 3:135–138.

61. Mauri S, Pedroli G, Rudeberg A et al. Acute metabolic alkalosis in cystic fibrosis: prospective study and review of the literature. Min Electrolyte Metab 1997; 23:33–37.

62. Gilljam H, Ellin A, Strandvik B. Increased bronchial chloride concentration in cystic fibrosis. Scand J Clin Lab Invest 1989; 49:121–124.

63. Johansen PG, Anderson CM, Hadorn B. Cystic fibrosis of the pancreas: a generalised disturbance of water and electrolyte movement in exocrine tissues. Lancet 1968; 1:455–460.

64. Pedroli G, Liechti-Gallati S, Mauri S et al. Chronic metabolic alkalosis: not uncommon in young children with severe cystic fibrosis. Am J Nephrol 1995; 15:245–250.

65. Baird JS, Walker P, Urban A et al. Metabolic alkalosis and cystic fibrosis. Chest 2002; 122:755–756.

66. Mersin SS, Ramelli GP, Laux-End R et al. Urinary chloride excretion distinguishes between renal and extrarenal metabolic alkalosis. Eur J Pediatr 1995; 154:979–982.

67. Figge J, Rossing TH, Fencl V. The role of serum proteins in acid–base equilibria. J Lab Clin Med 1991; 117:453–467.

68. Choi JY, Lee MG, Ko S et al. Cl(−)-dependent HCO_3 transport by cystic fibrosis transmembrane conductance regulator. JOP 2001; 2(4 Suppl):243–246.

69. Kennedy JD, Dinwiddie R, Daman-Willems C et al. Pseudo-Bartter's syndrome in cystic fibrosis. Arch Dis Child 1990; 65:786–787.

70. Sojo A, Rodriguez-Soriano J, Vitoria JC et al. Chloride deficiency as a presentation or complication of cystic fibrosis. Eur J Pediatr 1994; 153:825–828.

71. Yalcin E, Kiper N, Dogru D et al. Clinical features and treatment approaches in cystic fibrosis with pseudo-Bartter syndrome. Ann Trop Paediatr 2005; 25:119–124.

72. Bates CM, Baum M, Quigley R. Cystic fibrosis presenting with hypokalemia and metabolic alkalosis in a previously healthy adolescent. J Am Soc Nephrol 1997; 8:352–355.

73. Smith HR, Dhatt GS, Melia WM et al. Cystic fibrosis presenting as hyponatraemic heat exhaustion. Br Med J 1995; 310:579–580.

74. Holland AE, Wilson JW, Kotsimbos TC et al. Metabolic alkalosis contributes to acute hypercapnic respiratory failure in adult cystic fibrosis. Chest 2003; 124:490–493.

75. Adrogue HJ, Madias NE. Management of life-threatening acid–base disorders [second of two parts]. N Engl J Med 1998; 338:107–111.

76. Cohen LF, di Sant'Agnese PA, Taylor A et al. The syndrome of inappropriate antidiuretic hormone secretion as a cause of hyponatremia in cystic fibrosis. J Pediatr 1977; 90:574–578.

77. Cooper DM, Russell LE, Henry RL. Cerebral abscess as a complication of cystic fibrosis. Pediatr Pulmonol 1994; 17:390–392.

78. Fischer EG, Shwachman H, Wepsic JG. Brain abscess and cystic fibrosis. J Pediatr 1979; 95:385–388.

79. Espiritu JD, Kleinhenz ME. Paradoxical embolization in an adult patient with cystic fibrosis. Mayo Clin Proc 2000; 75:1100–1102.

80. Playfor SD, Smyth AR. Paradoxical embolism in a boy with cystic fibrosis and a stroke. Thorax 1999; 54:1139–1140.

81. Sritippayawan S, MacLaughlin EF, Woo MS. Acute neurological deficits in a young adult with cystic fibrosis. Pediatr Pulmonol 2003; 35:147–151.

82. Stern RC, Horwitz SJ, Doershuk CF. Neurologic symptoms during coughing paroxysms in cystic fibrosis. J Pediatr 1988; 112:909–912.

83. Mattle HP, Nirkko AC, Baumgartner RW *et al.* Transient cerebral circulatory arrest coincides with fainting in cough syncope. *Neurology* 1995; **45**(3 Pt 1):498–501.

84. Mulberg AE, Resta LP, Wiedner EB *et al.* Expression and localization of the cystic fibrosis transmembrane conductance regulator mRNA and its protein in rat brain. *J Clin Invest* 1995; **96**:646–652.

85. Ketchell RL, Gyi KM, Badawi R. Cardiac compromise in end-stage cystic fibrosis. *Pediatr Pulmonol* 2004; **38**(S27):312.

86. Rao DS, Infeld MD, Stern RC *et al.* Cough-induced hemiplegic migraine with impaired consciousness in cystic fibrosis. *Pediatr Pulmonol* 2006; **41**:171–176.

87. Surtees R. Inherited ion channel disorders. *Eur J Pediatr* 2000; **159**(Suppl 3):S199–S203.

88. Ravilly S, Robinson W, Suresh S *et al.* Chronic pain in cystic fibrosis. *Pediatrics* 1996; **98**(4 Pt 1):741–747.

89. Sitrin MD, Lieberman F, Jensen WE *et al.* Vitamin E deficiency and neurologic disease in adults with cystic fibrosis. *Ann Intern Med* 1987; **107**:51–54.

90. Reid DW, Withers NJ, Francis L *et al.* Iron deficiency in cystic fibrosis: relationship to lung disease severity and chronic *Pseudomonas aeruginosa* infection. *Chest* 2002; **121**:48–54.

91. Barker M, Thoenes D, Dohmen H *et al.* Prevalence of thrombophilia and catheter-related thrombosis in cystic fibrosis. *Pediatr Pulmonol* 2005; **39**:156–161.

92. Balfour-Lynn IM, Malbon K, Burman JF *et al.* Thrombophilia in children with cystic fibrosis. *Pediatr Pulmonol* 2005; **39**:306–310.

93. ter Avest PC, Tytgat GA, Westra M *et al.* [Haemolytic anaemia and a clotting disorder as first signs of cystic fibrosis in two infants]. *Ned Tijdschr Geneeskd* 2005; **149**:2125–2128.

94. Motley WW, Augsburger JJ, Hutchins RK *et al. Pseudomonas aeruginosa* endogenous endophthalmitis with choroidal abscess in a patient with cystic fibrosis. *Retina* 2005; **25**:202–207.

95. Detering K, Jenney A, Hall A *et al.* Metastatic choroidal abscess due to *Pseudomonas aeruginosa* in patients with cystic fibrosis. *Clin Infect Dis* 1997; **24**:525–526.

96. Narang A, Maguire A, Nunn JH *et al.* Oral health and related factors in cystic fibrosis and other chronic respiratory disorders. *Arch Dis Child* 2003; **88**:702–707.

97. Lyczak JB, Cannon CL, Pier GB. Lung infections associated with cystic fibrosis. *Clin Microbiol Rev* 2002; **15**(2):194–222.

20

Sexual and reproductive health

SUSAN M. SAWYER

INTRODUCTION

An important result of improving survival in people with cystic fibrosis (CF) is that the significance of particular CF-related issues or complications differs physiologically as well as psychologically as children become adolescents and mature as adults. In most large CF centers today, the majority of children are expected to survive through adolescence to face the array of sexual and reproductive health issues negotiated by healthy young people as they mature. Additionally, however, there are significant sexual and reproductive complications of CF itself. Improved survival in CF now results in sexual and reproductive health issues being of greater significance to a greater proportion of people with CF, with wide-ranging repercussions for individuals with CF, their families and their healthcare professionals.

People with CF risk not being fully informed about sexual and reproductive health issues for a range of reasons. Participation in a specialty CF clinic may be at the expense of primary care involvement which may reduce opportunities for access to universally important sexual and reproductive health education and screening opportunities (e.g. safe sex, PAP smears) [1]. Studies continue to highlight that people with CF, both male and female, are not optimally informed about the specific sexual and reproductive health aspects of CF [2–5]. This may reflect that the attention and expertise of health professionals is on promoting disease stability and survival. However, an integral part of CF management is to ensure that young people are informed of the various impacts of CF at developmentally appropriate times. While there are many unanswered questions deserving further research in this area, the difficulty that health professionals have in discussing sexual and reproductive health topics is another reason why young people are not fully informed [6]. Reliable clinical information – plus strong communication skills – should underpin these discussions.

MALE SEXUAL AND REPRODUCTIVE HEALTH

Men with CF are azoospermic due to congenital bilateral absence of the vas deferens [7–9]. Most males with CF, regardless of the severity of their respiratory or gastrointestinal disease, have aberrant development of the reproductive portion of the mesonephric (Wolffian) duct, accounting for absence or atrophy of the vas deferens, seminal vesicle, ejaculatory duct, and body and tail of the epididymis [10]. There can be variability in the clinical findings: in some men the epididymides are entire and the scrotal portion of one or both of the vasa may be present. Dysfunction (and often absence) of the seminal vesicles accounts for the much lower volume and acidic ejaculate in men with CF; the volume of ejaculate in men with CF is generally less than 1 mL compared to 3.5 mL in other men [7,8,11]. Many males with CF do not experience nocturnal emissions [3], presumably as a consequence of variably reduced semen volume from atretic seminal vesicles. Testicular histology is normal and active spermatogenesis occurs, as in men who have undergone a vasectomy. Occasionally sperm antibodies develop. Sexual potency is not affected by these abnormalities. However, acute and chronic ill-health can impair testicular function and coincidental defective spermatogenesis is relatively common.

Infertility is thought to occur in at least 98% of men with CF. Bilateral absence of the vas is an easy clinical diagnosis to make, as the normal epididymis and vas is palpable. Retroversion of the testis in which the epididymis and vas are anterior to the testis instead of posterior is relatively common and may cause confusion. Semen analysis will confirm azoospermia or identify the small number of men with CF who are potentially fertile. This is more likely in men with particular genotypes such as the $3849 - 10\,\text{kb}$ $C \rightarrow T$ mutation [12,13].

We are gradually understanding more about the sexual and reproductive health knowledge of men with CF, the significance of infertility in adolescent and adult life, and

Table 20.1 The age (in years) at which males with CF report is the most appropriate to be informed about male infertility, compared with the age reported first heard.

	Number	Appropriate age to be informed (mean and SD)	Actual age informed (mean and SD)
Adult males	40	14.2 (2.6)	16.0 (4.7)
Adult males	93	14.4 (2.8)	16.4 (4.1)
Adolescent males	10	–	13.9 (1.6)
Parents	10	13.9 (2.6)	–

Data are combined from [3] and [5].

the use of assisted reproductive technologies. The earliest studies to explore any aspect of the sexual and reproductive health needs of men with CF date only from the 1980s. These initial studies suggested widespread lack of knowledge of male infertility in both adolescent and adult males, as well as parents [14,15]. More recent studies from New England, USA [3], Scotland [16], Birmingham, UK [17] and Melbourne, Australia [4] show increasing awareness of infertility in men with CF. Indeed, only 1 of 93 adult Australian men were unaware that CF commonly affects male fertility [4].

It appears that men are now better informed about infertility than previous generations. However, they continue to report hearing about infertility later than they would have wished (Table 20.1) [3,4,18]. For example, the mean (and SD) age of first hearing about infertility was 16.4 (4.1) years in comparison to their preferred age of 14.4 (2.8) years [4]. This suggests that health professionals experience barriers to more timely discussion of infertility – as well as other topics. Reported barriers include doctor as well as patient embarrassment, insufficient time and insufficient training [6]. However, a major barrier resulting in delayed discussions about male infertility is a common concern by doctors of how negatively this information might be received by young men [6].

Few studies have directly assessed the impact of future infertility on adult men, let alone in teenagers. Indeed, apart from a qualitative US study [3] that included 10 teenage males, of whom 5 were unaware of male infertility, our knowledge of the impact of infertility in adolescence is obtained only from the retrospective reflections of young adult men with CF. However, the few studies we have suggest that it is far less overwhelming for adolescents than might be expected, with 90% of adult men reporting they were not distressed when they first heard about infertility during adolescence [3]. Typical comments were 'There was no real effect at the time. I just took it as part of CF', by a 29-year-old who first heard about infertility when aged 12, and 'I didn't really think about it much. At the time I wasn't upset', by a 27-year-old who first heard when aged 15. Ten percent described a significant impact in adolescence,

saying 'It took me by surprise, I was shocked' (25-year-old who was first told when aged 12) [19]. Those who hear about infertility when older are more likely to be upset than those hearing when younger [3,4]. Doctors should thus feel encouraged to discuss these issues with young adolescents.

However, careful attention should be paid to language. For example, adolescents reported confusing the meaning of infertility with impotence [3,4]. One teenager said 'My mother told me I couldn't have kids but I wasn't sure what she meant, whether it was having kids or having sex.' There is no evidence that men with CF delay commencement of sexual activity in comparison to other teenagers. It is therefore especially concerning that one-third of adolescent males with CF fail to differentiate aspects of contraception from other sexual health risks, namely sexually transmitted infections [3,4]. For example, one young man said 'I don't have to use condoms because I don't have to worry about contraceptives' [19]. This highlights the importance of ensuring that young people (and their parents) have an appropriate level of knowledge and skills to protect themselves from common sexual health risks unrelated to CF.

The impact of infertility appears to increase with age [3,4]. This is not surprising as young people form more intimate and committed relationships as they mature, with an increasing expectation of parenting. A 20-year-old man reported: 'At first it went in one ear and out the other, but then I thought about it.' Another 19-year-old underlined the potential significance, stating: 'At the moment it's not a concern. It's like it hasn't really hit me yet. Later, it could be devastating.' Infertility was reported as insignificant by only 10% of adult men with CF [3].

The increasing significance of infertility with maturity and the need to broaden discussions of sexual and reproductive health to include protection from sexually transmitted infections reinforces that sexual and reproductive health is another theme within CF care that cannot be dealt with in a single consultation. Rather, as with other aspects of CF care, these issues need to be revisited repeatedly as the young person matures. Studies have consistently shown than men want more information about their sexual and reproductive health [4,16–18]. As few men with CF feel comfortable initiating these discussions [16,18], the responsibility rests with health professionals to take the lead with these discussions.

Infertility in men with CF is expected, but not universal. This highlights the importance of semen analysis. In an Australian study, 53% of Australian men report having had semen analysis but two-thirds of those who had not been tested wanted confirmation of their fertility status [4]. In a US study, the value of semen analysis is reinforced by the fact that 17% of men obtained testing without a recommendation by their CF doctor [3]. The most appropriate age to offer semen analysis is unclear. In a small UK study, 5 of 18 males had undergone semen analysis at a median age of 26 years; 17 of these 18 felt that semen analysis should be offered universally to all men with CF [18]. In a larger

Australian study, universal testing was also supported, with 95% of men supporting testing under 20 years (73% of men suggested 17–18 years, 22% suggested 19–20 years). While only 5% suggested testing be undertaken at over 20 years, the earliest age of testing in this population was 24 years [4]. The value of the test appears independent of relationship status. Men who are not in a current relationship should still be offered semen analysis.

However, semen analysis should be sensitively undertaken. Some men produce such small ejaculate volumes that testing itself may be highly embarrassing if this has not been discussed in advance. The embarrassment experienced by most men in producing a specimen by masturbation (at a novel adult fertility clinic), and the disappointment and sadness of the likely negative result, suggests that the process of semen analysis will at the very least be confronting for men. Careful discussion is required both prior to the test as well as after azoospermia is confirmed. Testing should not be within 3–4 months of serious illness as sperm production is affected by illness.

In summary, while there is no single 'right' or 'best' age to talk about infertility, parents need to be well informed before their sons reach puberty so that they can have appropriate discussions with their sons. Health professionals, parents and young people themselves are in general agreement that discussions by health professionals should commence no later than mid-adolescence (approximately 14 years) with every reason to think that even earlier discussion is indicated [3,4,6]. While no clinical guidelines have yet been developed, suggested topics to discuss include infertility (including differentiating infertility from impotence, encouraging safe-sex practices and the importance of condoms), small-volume ejaculates, the role of semen analysis, and reproductive options, with the emphasis varying with maturity.

Reproductive options

Men with CF are increasingly interested in parenting. In a recent Australian study, 84% of men without children reporting wanting children in the future and 8 of the 17 men who already had children wanted more [4]. The reproductive options for infertility when the male has CF are: adoption; artificial insemination by donor sperm; and assisted reproductive techniques that harvest sperm and combine them with retrieved oocytes using in-vitro approaches. Most adoption agencies will not accept parents with illnesses likely to reduce their life span, while in other countries, long waiting lists for adoption agencies may limit its appropriateness. However, there are options for short-term fostering in many countries.

Few data are available about how often any reproductive options are used by men with CF. In one Australian study, 17 of 93 men (18%) had children, ranging in number from 1 to 4. Six men had used assisted reproductive technologies, nine had used artificial insemination by donor

sperm, one had stepchildren and one was presumed to be fertile having conceived naturally [4]. In the UK at least, very few men with CF seek fertility treatment [20].

The assisted reproductive technology known as MESA, or microsurgical epididymal sperm aspiration, is a surgical technique to harvest epididymal and testicular spermatozoa. Other techniques include percutaneous epididymal sperm aspiration, and testicular sperm aspiration (TESA). Use of aspiration techniques to yield epididymal spermatozoa is the preferred method because the large numbers of spermatozoa obtained can be easily frozen and used in multiple cycles. MESA can be performed under a general anesthesia or local anesthesia and IV sedation. Men are generally able to return to work within a few days.

Combining sperm harvesting approaches with intracytoplasmic sperm injection (ICSI) is now standard procedure. ICSI consists of microinjection of either epididymal or testicular sperm directly into the oocyte [21–23] and significantly higher rates of fertilization have been achieved than with previous conventional in-vitro fertilization techniques [23]. Neither CF genotype nor sperm morphology has an adverse effect on fertilization or pregnancy rates using ICSI [24]. Multiple pregnancies are frequent, occurring in approximately 30% of IVF conceptions (25% twins, 5% triplets or more), with greater rates of low birth weight, cerebral palsy and major birth defects following use of assisted reproductive technologies [25].

Concerns have recently been raised about whether assisted reproductive technologies such as ICSI might effect the epigenetics of early embryogenesis and cause increased birth defects [25]. Disruption of imprinted genes are responsible for Beckwith–Wiedemann, Angelman and Prader–Willi syndromes [26], and there are now reports of children born with Beckwith–Wiedemann and Angelman syndrome following ICSI procedures [27–29]. Increased rates of Y chromosome microdeletions are also described, although the significance of this is uncertain [25].

Because of the increased risk of CF in the offspring, both partners undergoing MESA–ICSI should be extensively screened for CFTR mutations in addition to karyotyping. If the female partner is positive for a CFTR mutation, a good outcome can be achieved when MESA–ICSI is coupled with preimplantation genetic diagnosis with transfer of embryos that are either free of the mutation or carriers [30–32]. However, misdiagnosis is known to have occurred and preimplantation genetic diagnosis remains a technical challenge.

The use of MESA and TESA in association with ICSI in couples affected by CF has resulted in pregnancy rates of 30–35% per cycle, with 62.5% couples achieving pregnancy following treatment [11,33]. For example, McCallum and co-workers [11] reported 13 couples who underwent infertility assessment where the male had CF. Eight of the 13 couples chose to use assisted reproductive technologies (MESA–ICSI), with five of the eight becoming pregnant. Pregnancy occurred within the first ICSI cycle in three and in the second cycle in two of the five couples, with seven live births (three sets of twins and one singleton). It must be remembered that these are expensive technologies (with the expense often bourne by the couple) that have limited availability internationally.

Congenital bilateral absence of the vas deferens

In contrast to male infertility which is fundamental to the clinical picture of CF, congenital bilateral absence of the vas deferens (CBAVD) can occur in otherwise healthy men without coexistent pulmonary or gastrointestinal disease. CBAVD accounts for up to a quarter of men with obstructive azoospermia, which itself accounts for 1–2% of male infertility [34]. Once thought to be a distinct clinical entity, the genetic link between men with CF and those with CBAVD that was first postulated by Holsclaw and co-workers [35], has been confirmed. Genetic similarities between the two conditions are now well described [36–41]. A small proportion of men with obstructive azoospermia will be found to have the more complete clinical phenotype of CF on more thorough assessment [42]. However, the majority of otherwise healthy men with CBAVD have no clinical evidence of CF apart from infertility [42].

The genetic similarities between CF and CBAVD suggest that *CFTR* mutations are important in the etiology of infertility in both conditions. *CFTR* mRNA is present in the male genital tract from 18 weeks' gestation with variable expression in different anatomical regions [43–45]. In a large French study of 327 men with CBAVD, detailed analysis of the *CFTR* gene revealed mutations in nearly 80% of *CFTR* genes: 71% of patients carried a mutation on both *CFTR* genes; 16% carried a mutation on one gene; no mutation was found on either *CFTR* gene in 13% [41]. In those with two mutant *CFTR* genes, at least one was a mild (class IV or V) *CFTR* mutation. The most frequent *CFTR* mutation conferring a mild phenotype in men with CBAVD is the T5 polymorphism [46]. T5 is one of the alleles found at the polymorphic Tn locus in intron 8 of the *CFTR* gene. Either 5, 7 or 9 thymidine residues are found at this locus. Less efficient splicing occurs with a lower thymidine number, resulting in transcripts that lack exon 9 sequences [47]. This results in CFTR proteins that do not mature. When T5 is found in compound heterozygosity with a severe mutation, or even T5, pathology might be observed such as CBAVD. However, not all male compound heterozygotes for a severe *CFTR* mutation and T5 develop CBAVD, such as some fathers of CF children. The T5 polymorphism is classified as a disease mutation with partial penetrance. Whether the T5 polymorphism is pathologic or benign appears to depend on the number of TG repeats at an adjacent locus, the TGm locus [48]. At this locus, the higher the number of repeats, the less efficient the exon 9 splicing. Thus, apparently innocent polymorphisms can, in particular combinations, result in mutant *CFTR* genes with partial production of CFTR protein explaining the presence of clinical features of CBAVD without more overt features of CF [49].

It had been thought that the 20% of men with CBAVD who also have renal malformations did not have *CFTR* mutations [50]. However, in a more recent study, two of four men with CBAVD and a single kidney were carriers of a *CFTR* mutation, including a compound heterozygote for F508 and T5 [51].

In summary, there is more complex regulation or modulation of currently known *CFTR* alleles and other unknown alleles than has previously been recognized. In this widening spectrum of CFTR-associated disease, a dichotomy is emerging between the perspective of the scientist and that of the clinician and patient. While it is highly appropriate for the scientist to consider CBAVD as part of the spectrum of CFTR-related disorders, it is important to make distinctions between etiology, nosology and the clinical interface. The clinically relevant question is whether CBAVD as an isolated finding should be classified within the spectrum of CF disease or defined as CFTR-associated but distinguishable from clinical CF. While the importance of genetic studies in this area cannot be overstated, caution is advocated in describing CBAVD alone as a mild version of CF in the clinical setting.

FEMALE SEXUAL AND REPRODUCTIVE HEALTH

Women with CF have anatomically normal reproductive tracts [52], but abnormalities of cervical mucus have been described. The water content of cervical mucus is reduced in comparison to control subjects, resulting in the formation of thick, tenacious cervical mucus without cyclic variation with ovulation [53]. The success of intrauterine insemination suggests cervical mucus abnormalities may contribute to infertility in some women [54]. However, while it was widely reported that women with CF have significantly reduced fertility [55,56], the basis of the original report of fertility rates as low as 20% of normal is obscure [53]. Recent studies have shown that three in four women who tried to conceive became pregnant [2,57]. A Canadian study described that 13 of 29 women (45%) took more than 2 years to conceive [58], while a Scandinavian study of pregnancy reported that 12 of 80 pregnancies (15%) were facilitated using assisted reproductive technologies (7 used intrauterine insemination; 5 used IVF) [57]. However, reports of unplanned pregnancy [59,60] reinforce that women with CF should assume they have relatively normal fertility.

Women with CF with severe disease and very poor nutritional status are at risk of secondary amenorrhea and anovulatory cycles, although pregnancy is described in even the most unwell women [61,62]. The combination of improved respiratory function, better nutrition and longer survival means that contemporary young women with CF will have higher fertility rates than previous generations of

Table 20.2   Pregnancy outcomes among pregnant women with CF, 1990–94 (US CFF registry data).

	Year				
	1990	**1991**	**1992**	**1993**	**1994**
Number of reported pregnancies	114	127	119	133	140
Number of completed pregnancies	70	99	74	99	87
– Live birth (%)[a]	45 (64)	72 (73)	54 (73)	74 (75)	62 (71)
– Still birth (%)[a]	1 (1)	10 (10)	7 (9)	2 (2)	0 (0)
– Termination (%)[a]	24 (34)	17 (17)	13 (18)	23 (23)	25 (29)
Pregnancy continuing	35	28	39	31	50
Pregnancy outcome uncertain	9	0	6	3	3

[a] Percentage of completed pregnancies.
Modified from [86].

women (Table 20.2). Indeed, the annual number of pregnancies reported to the CF Foundation Data Registry in the United States doubled between 1986 and 1990 [60].

Most young women with CF commence sexual activity at a similar age as their healthy peers [2]. Indeed, a number of studies of young people with a range of chronic conditions suggest they may commence sexual activity at an earlier age [63–66] and report more sexually transmitted infections [67]. Some sexually active young women with CF continue to erroneously believe that they have reduced fertility and therefore do not need to use contraception [2]. Continuing high rates of termination of pregnancy in women with mild as well as severe lung disease suggests that greater effort is required by health professionals to ensure that women with CF fully understand that contraception should be used if pregnancy is to be avoided.

As with young men, studies show that young women with CF have unmet sexual and reproductive health needs, with two in three young women wanting more information about sexual and reproductive health [5]. In one Australian study, nearly 100% of mothers of teenage girls wanted more information about a range of sexual and reproductive health topics – before their daughters reached puberty [5]. While mothers viewed the CF team as the best source of CF-specific sexual and reproductive health information, few had ever discussed these topics with their daughter's CF specialist.

In summary, women with CF should be considered fertile. Contraception should be offered to all sexually active women who do not want to become pregnant and approaches to avoiding sexually transmitted diseases should be discussed. As with young men, discussions with girls (and their parents) and women with CF about various aspects of sexual and reproductive health in young women should be incorporated into routine CF care.

Contraception

The range of available contraceptive devices is wider now than ever before; different factors will determine the most

appropriate contraceptive agent for each woman. Barrier methods are safe and effective in motivated patients but are associated with high failure rates in the adolescent population. The oral contraceptive pill (OCP) is the most common method of contraception in women with CF [2]. Depot progesterone may also suit some women. Tubal ligation is an option to consider for mature women who have clearly decided against pregnancy.

There are theoretical concerns about the OCP in women with CF if complicated by diabetes, cholelithiasis, liver disease, poorly controlled malabsorption, or indwelling intravenous access [68]. However, avoiding unplanned pregnancy is a priority, and the risks of contraception need to be balanced with the physiological and psychosocial risks of unplanned pregnancy. In complex cases, referral to a gynecologist is recommended. Higher pill failure occurs with both short- and long-term antibiotic use [69], although this is less significant than previously believed [70]. Pregnancy from antibiotic-related OCP failure has not been reported in CF. Malabsorption, ileal resection, active liver disease and poor adherence can all be associated with reduced serum steroid levels and reduced contraceptive reliability. These factors, together with the altered pharmacokinetics of CF, raise concerns that low-dose estrogen preparations will be less reliable in some patients [71]. Fifty-microgram estrogen preparations may provide more reliable hormonal contraception.

Urinary incontinence

Daytime urinary incontinence is common among healthy women, increasing in frequency with age and parity. Adult women with chronic respiratory disease have increased rates of urinary incontinence with repeated coughing thought to promote the earlier development of the anatomic and pressure transmission abnormalities that are associated with the development of stress incontinence [72].

Recent studies have demonstrated higher rates of urinary incontinence in both adult women with CF [73–75] as well as adolescents [76]. The first study in 29 adult Australian women reported a prevalence of urinary incontinence of

38%, with 22% reporting at least twice-monthly symptoms [73]. An Italian study of 176 women aged 15–41 years found an overall prevalence of 59%, with 24% experiencing incontinence twice or more a month [74]. Adolescent girls appear to have similar rates, with 22% reporting small-volume daytime incontinence twice a month or more [76]. In both adolescent and adult women, urinary incontinence is generally unreported unless specific enquire is made. While this might reflect low symptom impact, it is concerning that nearly half of those reporting urinary incontinence also reported it caused significant interference with their performance of chest physiotherapy. The lack of association with age, lung function, body mass index or menarchal status suggests that coughing, whether spontaneously or through positive pressure physiotherapy, may be an explanation [76]. Pelvic floor muscle exercises have been shown to be effective at improving endurance and reducing urinary leakage in adult women with CF [77]. Approaches to stabilizing pelvic floor muscles while participating in positive pressure physiotherapy should be routine for all women with CF.

Vaginal yeast infections

High rates of symptoms consistent with vaginal yeast infections are reported in women with CF [78], which is likely to reflect frequently changing systemic antibiotics. Diabetes mellitus may be another risk factor, as could an intrinsic alteration of vaginal flora. Enquiring about the frequency of vaginal symptoms prior to changing antibiotics is recommended, as is concurrent prescription of topical treatment for yeast infections for those women who commonly suffer from vaginal yeast infections when antibiotics are changed. Nebulized antibiotics may be an appropriate alternative for women who suffer from frequent infections.

It may also be expected that women with CF, especially those with severe disease who are anovulatory, will have hypo-estrogenized vaginal epithelium and be at greater risk of dyspareunia. The use of lubricant gels may assist, as might topical and systemic estrogens.

Pregnancy

There have been multiple single reports of pregnancy in women with CF following the first case report in 1960 [79]. Two and three decades later, two large series described 129 pregnancies from multiple centers [80], and 38 pregnancies from a single center [81]. A number of smaller case series have been reported from single centres [82–85], while recently a number of case series, case–control and cohort studies have provided fresh insights [20,57,86–91].

High rates of spontaneous abortion, preterm delivery and maternal death reported in early series raised serious concerns about the safety of pregnancy for both women and their offspring [80,84,86]. However, accumulated clinical experience is now more positive and pregnancy is generally well tolerated by women with mild disease ($FEV_1 > 70\%$ predicted). Increasing numbers of women with CF are becoming pregnant (Table 20.3), and over 100 pregnancies are reported annually to the US Cystic Fibrosis Data Registry [60,89].

A review of 111 pregnancies reported to the Cystic Fibrosis Data Registry in 1990 revealed that all severities of lung function were represented in pregnant women: 37% had mild lung function with $FEV_1 > 70\%$ predicted, 26% had more moderate disease with FEV_1 50–69% predicted, and 36% had severe disease with $FEV_1 > 50\%$ predicted. Women who delivered a live birth at term had the highest level of lung function. Approximately a quarter of completed pregnancies resulted in a preterm delivery. Women with moderate to severe lung disease were more likely to deliver prematurely or to terminate pregnancy.

An important question is whether pregnancy adversely affects the long-term health of the mother. The largest study uses data from the US CFF database to assess the impact of pregnancy on survival of women, from 1985 to 1997 [89]. At study entry, the 680 women who reported pregnancy were more likely to have a higher FEV_1 percentage (67.5 vs 61.7%) and higher weight (52.9 vs 46.4 kg). The 10-year survival rate in pregnant women was higher (77%) than in those who did not become pregnant (58%). After adjustment of the figures for the initial severity of

Table 20.3 Comparison of pregnancy outcomes among women with CF in different developed.

Country	Time period	Number of pregnancies	Live births	Full–term pregnancies	Pre–term pregnancies	Spontaneous miscarriages	Therapeutic abortions	Other[a]
UK [91]	1977–96	72	48 (67%)	26 (36%)	22 (30%)	7 (10%)	14 (20%)	3 (4%)
Canada [58]	1963–80	92	74 (80%)	68 (74%)	6 (6%)	11 (12%)	7 (7%)	0
France [88]	1980–99	75	64[b] (85%)	45 (60%)	10 (18%)	5 (7%)	5 (7%)	1 (1%)
Scandinavia [90]	1977–98	33	33 (100%)	25 (76%)	8 (24%)	0	0	0
Scandinavia [57]	1977–98	80	60 (75%)	Not reported		11 (14%)	8 (10%)	1 (1%)
US [89]	1985–97	680	455 (67%)	Not reported		39 (6%)	103 (15%)	83 (12%)
UK [20]	2001	84	76 (90%)	62 (74%)	14 (17%)	8 (10%)	0	0

[a] 'Other' combines those currently pregnant, maternal deaths, extra-uterine pregnancies, and those lost to follow-up.
Modified from [20].
[b] Documentation is only available for 55 of the 64 live births.

illness, women who became pregnant did not have a significantly shortened survival. During the 12-year observation period, there were 96 deaths (14%) in the pregnant women and 23% in the non-pregnant women. The rate of solid organ transplantation did not differ between pregnant and non-pregnant women (1.2% and 1.5%, respectively). These data are reassuring and consistent with other more recent reports of pregnancy outcomes in women with CF in other developed countries [20,57,58,88,90]. However, therapeutic abortion rates up to 20% and preterm pregnancy rates up to 30% underline the seriousness of pregnancy [91], as does the stark commentary by Goss and co-workers [89] that 20% of mothers with CF will be dead before their child's tenth birthday, increasing to 40% if the FEV$_1$ is less than 40% of predicted. By way of balance, Gilljam and co-workers [58] report that a Canadian woman with a pre-pregnancy FEV$_1$ of 35% predicted was well with stable pulmonary function 9 years after delivery, while another woman lived 25 years after delivery with a pre-pregnancy FEV$_1$ of 35% predicted.

A number of recommendations and commentaries have been made in regard to pregnancy and CF [92,93]. It is generally accepted that pregnancy is less hazardous in those with milder disease. These women can be reassured that they should tolerate pregnancy relatively well, although the potential for pregnancy to significantly affect the health of any women with CF, even for those with mild disease, needs to be understood [92,94]. It is worrying that a significant proportion of young women with CF do not know that pregnancy has the potential to detrimentally affect their respiratory status [3]. Pregnancy cannot be recommended for those with severe lung disease, especially those with pulmonary hypertension, significant liver disease, poor nutritional status or diabetes. Despite this, a significant proportion of pregnancies occur in those with severe respiratory disease and therapeutic termination of pregnancy continues to be a relatively common outcome of pregnancy.

Pregnancy is possible following lung transplantation [95,96]. A case series of 29 heart and 3 heart–lung transplants described 27 live births [95]. While 41% were born pre-term, no fetal abnormalities were reported. Experience is limited, but current opinions suggest that pregnancy is ideally delayed until at least 2 years following transplantation. Pregnancy appears not to result in additional risk of rejection, organ failure or fetal abnormalities [92].

Pregnancy in women with CF is best managed when it is a planned event and where there is close collaboration between the medical and obstetric teams. A strong emphasis needs to be placed on achieving the best possible respiratory and nutritional status prior to pregnancy. Pregnancy counselling should include genetic counselling and carrier screening. If the woman's partner is not a CF carrier, the risk of an affected child is 1 in 50, with all unaffected children being carriers. If her partner is a CF carrier, the risk of a child with CF is 1 in 2. Antenatal screening using chorionic villus sampling can be performed at 8–12 weeks' gestation. In addition to genetic counselling, topics to discuss

include the increased risks to the mother, the increased risks to the fetus, and the complex short- and long-term issues surrounding parenthood in CF.

Regular monitoring and early treatment of complications will help minimize the risks of pregnancy for both the mother and fetus. Monitoring of pulmonary status should include serial pulmonary function tests, with close monitoring of cardiovascular status. Different approaches to physiotherapy may be required as the pregnancy progresses. A woman's usual exercise regimen may need modifying during pregnancy, with increasing reliance on specific physiotherapy techniques. Increased gastro esophageal reflux is expected in pregnancy generally which will have repercussions for any physiotherapy regimen involving positioning.

Close involvement with an experienced nutritionist before, during and after pregnancy is recommended for all women with CF considering pregnancy. Close attention should be paid to maternal weight gain. Women with CF are advised to reach 90% of their ideal body weight prior to pregnancy and a weight gain during pregnancy of 12.5 kg is recommended [87]. Consideration should be given to nutritional supplementation for poor weight gain during pregnancy. Nasogastric feeds are better tolerated early rather than later in pregnancy, and women better tolerate continuous rather than bolus feeds [87]. Close monitoring of fetal growth is also required. In addition to regularly monitoring maternal weight gain, regular monitoring of blood glucose, glucose tolerance test, hemoglobin, liver function tests, protein production and coagulation profile is recommended, with periodic monitoring of vitamins A and E.

Hospital admission may be required for a range of reasons, including management of hyperemesis, respiratory infection, nutritional supplementation or rest. Consideration of the teratogenic effects of maternal drug use, especially systemic antibiotics, will result in the avoidance of particular drugs during pregnancy if at all possible, although the priority needs to be the mother's health. Review of all medications with an appropriate reference text is recommended (Table 20.4) [97]. The β-lactam class of antibiotics is generally considered safe during pregnancy. There are no controlled studies of the safety of gentamicin in pregnancy, although there are few concerning case reports. Intravenous gentamicin is safer than some other aminoglycosides, although aerosolized antibiotics will be safer than intravenous administration due to reduced systemic availability. There are few safety data concerning vancomycin and ciprofloxacin, although they have been associated with good fetal outcomes.

Close monitoring of the mother is recommended during labor with a low threshold for supplemental oxygen. A vaginal delivery is actively encouraged.

The first analysis of breast milk from a mother with CF was found to be hypernatremic [98] and led to the widespread but erroneous belief that this was a universal finding. The amount of sodium and protein is in fact normal [99–101]. Although a low-normal lipid content has been reported [102,103], analysis of the specific lipid content of

Table 20.4 Drug safety in pregnancy.

Drug category	Drug name or type	Fetal risk category[a]
Antibiotics	Aztreonam	B
	Cephalosporins	B
	Chloramphenicol	C
	Clavulanate potassium	B
	Gentamicin	C
	Penicillins	B
	Quinolones	C
	Tetracyclines	D
	Tobramycin	C
	Trimethoprim	C
	Vancomycin	C
Anti-fungals	Amphotericin B	B
	Clotrimazole	B
	Ketoconazole	C
	Nystatin	B
Non-steroidal anti-inflammatory drugs	Ibuprofen	B (D if used in third trimester)
	Indomethacin	B (D if used for longer than 48 hours, after 34 weeks' gestation or close to delivery)
Sedatives	Chloral hydrate	C
	Diazepam	D
	Ethanol	D (X if used in large amounts)
	Temazepam	X
Anti-secretory agents	Cimetidine	B
	Ranitidine	B
Gastrointestinal stimulant	Cisapride	C
Adrenal steroids	Prednisolone	B
	Beclometasone	C
	Dexamethasone	C
Bronchodilators	Salbuterol	C
	Theophylline	C
Anti-diabetic agents	Insulin	B
Immunosuppressive agents	Ciclosporin	C
	Azathioprine	D
Vitamins	Vitamin A	A (if taken above recommended daily allowance)
	Vitamin E	A (C if taken above recommended daily allowance)
Pancreatic supplementation		Not reported in text, but the enteric coating diethylphthalate is known to be teratogenic in rats.

[a] Categories: **A**: Controlled studies in women fail to demonstrate a risk to the fetus in the first trimester (and there is no evidence of risk in later trimesters) and the possibility of fetal harm appears remote. **B**: Either animal-reproduction studies have not demonstrated a fetal risk but there are no controlled studies in pregnant women or animal-reproduction studies have shown an adverse effect (other than a decrease in fertility) that was not confirmed in controlled studies in women in the first trimester (and there is no evidence of a risk in later trimesters). **C**: Either studies in animals have revealed adverse effects on the fetus (teratogenic or embryocidal or other) and there are no controlled studies in women or controlled studies in women and animals are not available. Drugs should be given only if the potential benefit justifies the potential risk to the fetus. **D**: There is positive evidence of human fetal risk but the benefits from use in pregnant women may be acceptable despite the risk. **X**: Studies in animals or humans have demonstrated fetal abnormalities or there is evidence of fetal risk based on human experience or both, and the risk of the drug in pregnant women clearly outweighs any possible benefit. The drug is contraindicated in women who are or may become pregnant.
Adapted from [97].

milk from six women with CF revealed that in all cases they supplied the energy needs of nursing infants. Breast-feeding in women with CF can supply sufficient infant energy without deleterious affect on maternal nutritional status [103], although the additional energy requirements imposed by breast-feeding may be difficult to achieve for some women and many women cease breast-feeding early [90]. Possible drug transmission through breast milk needs to be considered when prescribing medication for the breast-feeding mother, and review of all medications with an appropriate reference text is recommended [97].

RELATIONSHIPS AND SEXUAL FUNCTION

Young people with chronic illnesses such as CF are at increased risk of low emotional and social well-being, with body image, family connectedness and concern about peer relations being salient explanatory variables [104]. The physical burdens of CF, such as prominent coughing, growth and pubertal delay, surgical scars, and the visibility of permanent intravenous access ports may complicate the development of relationships, or the perception of physical attractiveness and self-worth. Both physical and emotional factors may result in young people being less well connected socially to a peer group than other young people, with less opportunity for the development of social skills and intimate relationships. Family attitudes, whether real or perceived, realistic or not, are likely to influence young people's thoughts about themselves as people deserving loving, intimate relationships, despite CF. And it is worth remembering that expectations and attitudes that are formed about future relationships and parenting roles can be subjectively refined through the lens of what is said, as much as by what is left unsaid, whether by parents or by CF teams.

There is no evidence of delayed onset of sexual activity in young people with CF. However, studies report avoidance of close relationships in adolescence and a delay in intimacy due to concerns about their partner's reactions to their illness [105]. It is noteworthy that a greater proportion of girls and boys with invisible conditions, such as CF, report a history of sexual abuse than those without chronic illness [64].

As respiratory illness progresses and exercise capacity declines it is normal for interest in sexual activity as well as sexual function to be reduced, at least to some extent. Greater planning and preparation for sexual activity may reduce the spontaneity but increase the enjoyment. Consideration of different sexual positions (because of pain or the effect of their partner's body weight, for example), optimizing the time of day to when the person with CF is least fatigued, and the use of supplemental oxygen may all improve the enjoyment of sexual activity as well as improving sexual function. While sexual function may decline, the need for intimacy does not. This provides a challenge for individuals with CF and their partners, as well as for those without partners.

PARENTING DECISION-MAKING

Decisions about reproductive options may come more easily to some individuals and couples than to others. A proportion will elect to conceive regardless of any potential health risks; others will try to conceive having made an informed decision. For some, a decision against parenting may be made independently of CF; for others the lack of a partner (which may be due, at least in part, to CF) will reduce the chance of parenthood. However, for many couples living with CF, the added challenge that CF brings to daily life will result in a decision against parenthood. A decision against parenthood will not necessarily alter the sadness associated with known infertility for many men, or the sadness that many women experience knowing they will never be well enough to parent children.

Any decision to proceed with a pregnancy rests with the patient and partner, not the health professional. However, it is important that the array of issues surrounding conception, antenatal screening, pregnancy and parenting is explicitly and sensitively discussed. Topics need to include the amount of time and energy required to parent children, a frank discussion of likely survival in the face of CF and the implications for the partner and child following the premature death of a parent. These topics are probably as difficult for health professionals to discuss as they are for couples affected by CF.

Health professionals should discuss the range of reproductive options in a balanced manner. It is important to ensure that patients are fully informed of new technologies. However, there is a risk that discussion of a newly available technical intervention such as MESA subtly changes the focus from a complex and emotional discussion of infertility and its consequences to a more typical medical consultation where information is provided to 'fix' a problem. We should recognize that in the very situation where we most want patients to maturely and realistically reflect on the personal risks of parenthood and the future of those children, our own (professional) need to offer technological solutions (that we may find easier to discuss and that may reduce our personal level of discomfort) may also reduce the opportunities for people with CF, both men and women, to start to come to terms with the reality that they may not be well enough to parent children for very long.

SUMMARY

Cystic fibrosis has both specific and broad impacts upon the sexual and reproductive health of individuals. The significance of these issues to individuals, as well as the impact on parents, partners and families, changes as the person matures. A single discussion about any of these issues is therefore insufficient. Rather, as with other aspects of CF care, reviewing these topics and tailoring the content to the individual's life stage and level of maturation is an integral component of complete CF care. As young people with CF face the same range of sexual and reproductive health issues as other people, it is important that sexuality education is comprehensive of the range of issues faced by all young people.

Discussions about many of these issues are as difficult for physicians as they are for patients and their families. It is important that physicians themselves be fully informed of the sexual and reproductive health issues that affect people with CF. It is, however, equally important that these issues be communicated to young people in an appropriate manner. Sensitivity, empathy and confidentiality should be key components of these consultations.

REFERENCES

1. Carroll G, Massarelli E, Opzoomer A et al. Adolescents with chronic disease: are they receiving comprehensive health care? J Adolesc Health Care 1983; 4:261–265.

2. Sawyer SM, Bowes G, Phelan PD. Reproductive health in young women with cystic fibrosis: knowledge, attitudes and behaviour. J Adolesc Health 1995; 17:46–50.

3. Sawyer SM, Tully MA, Dovey M, Colin AA. Reproductive health in males with cystic fibrosis: knowledge, attitudes, and experiences of patients and their parents. Pediatr Pulmonol 1998; 25:226–230.

4. Sawyer SM, Farrant B, Cerritelli B, Wilson J. A survey of sexual and reproductive health in men with cystic fibrosis: new challenges for adolescent and adult services. Thorax 2005; 60:326–330.

5. Nixon GM, Glazner JA, Martin JM, Sawyer SM. Female sexual healthcare in cystic fibrosis. Arch Dis Child 2003; 88:265–266.

6. Sawyer SM, Tully MA, Colin AA. Reproductive and sexual health in men with CF: a case for professional education and training. J Adolesc Health 2001; 28:36–40.

7. Denning CR, Sommers SC, Quigley HJ. Infertility in male patients with cystic fibrosis. Pediatrics 1968; 41:7–17.

8. Kaplan E, Shwachman H, Perlmutter AD et al. Reproductive failure in males with cystic fibrosis. N Engl J Med 1968; 279:65–69.

9. Landing BH, Wells TR, Wang C-I. Abnormality of the epididymis and vas deferens in cystic fibrosis. Arch Pathol 1969; 88:569–580.

10. Oppenheimer EH, Esterley JR. Observations on cystic fibrosis of the pancreas. V: Developmental changes in the male genital system. J Pediatr 1969; 75:806–811.

11. McCallum TJ, Milunsky JM, Cunningham DL et al. Fertility in men with cystic fibrosis: an update on current surgical practices and outcomes. Chest 2000; 118:1059–1062.

12. Stern RC, Doershuck CF, Drumm M. 3849 + 10 kb C-T mutation and disease severity in cystic fibrosis. Lancet 1995; 346:274–276.

13. Dreyfus DH, Bethel R, Gelfand EW. Cystic fibrosis 3849 + 10 kb C-T mutation associated with severe pulmonary disease and male fertility. Am J Resp Crit Care Med 1996; 153:858–860.

14. Nolan T, Desmond K, Herlich R, Hardy S. Knowledge of cystic fibrosis in patients and their parents. Pediatrics 1986; 77:229–235.

15. Hames A, Beesley J, Nelson R. Cystic fibrosis: what do patients know and what else would they like to know? Respir Med 1991; 85:389–392.

16. Fair A, Griffiths K, Osman LM. Attitudes to fertility among adults with cystic fibrosis in Scotland. Thorax 2000; 55:672–677.

17. Thickett KM, Stableforth DE, Davis RE et al. Awareness of infertility in men with cystic fibrosis. Fertil Steril 2001; 76:407–408.

18. Rodgers HC, Baldwin DR, Knox AJ. Questionnaire survey of male infertility in cystic fibrosis. Respir Med 2000; 94:1002–1003.

19. Farrant B, Sawyer S. Sexual and reproductive health in adolescents with CF: hard to talk about but too important to ignore. In: Balen R, Crawshaw M (eds) Sexuality and Fertility in Ill Health and Disability from Early Adolescence to Adulthood. London, Jessica Kingsley Publishers, 2006.

20. Boyd JM, Mehta A, Murphy DJ. Fertility and pregnancy outcomes in men and women with cystic fibrosis in the United Kingdom. Hum Reprod 2004; 19:2238–2243.

21. Palermo G, Joris H, Devroey P, Van Steirteghem A. Pregnancies after intracytoplasmic injection of single spermatozoon into an oocyte. Lancet 1992; 340:17–18.

22. Palermo G, Joris H, Derde M et al. Sperm characteristics and outcome of human assisted fertilization by subzonal insemination and intracytoplasmic sperm injection. Fertil Steril 1993; 59:826–835.

23. Van Steirteghem AC, Nagy Z, Joris H et al. High fertilization and implantation rates after intracytoplasmic sperm injection. Hum Reprod 1993; 8:1061–1066.

24. Schlegel PN, Cohen J, Goldstein M et al. Cystic fibrosis gene mutations do not affect sperm function during in-vitro fertilisation with micromanipulation for men with bilateral congenital absence of vas deferens. Fertil Steril 1995; 64:421–426.

25. Kurinczuk JJ. Safety issues in assisted reproductive technology. Hum Reprod 2003; 18:925–931.

26. Surani MA. Immaculate conception. Nature 2000; 416:491–493.

27. Cox GF, Burger J, Lip V et al. Intracytoplasmic sperm injection may increase the risk of imprinting defects. Am J Hum Genet 2002; 71:162–164.

28. DeBaun MR, Niemitz EL, Feinberg AP. Association of in-vitro fertilization with Beckwith–Wiedemann syndrome and epigenetic alterations of LIT1 and H19. Am J Hum Genet 2003; 72:156–160.

29. Maher ER, Brueton LA, Bowdin SC et al. Beckwith–Wiedemann syndrome and assisted reproductive technology (ART). J Med Genet 2003; 40:62–64.

30. Harper JC, Handyside AH. The current status of preimplantation diagnosis. Curr Obstet Gynecol 1994; 4:143–149.

31. Handyside AH, Lesko JG, Tarin JJ et al. Birth of a normal girl after in-vitro fertilization and preimplantation

diagnostic testing for cystic fibrosis. *N Engl J Med* 1992; **327**:905–909.

32. Liu J, Lissens W, Silber SJ *et al.* Birth after preimplantation diagnosis of the cystic fibrosis delta F508 mutation by polymerase chain reaction in human embryos resulting from intracytoplasmic sperm injection with epididymal sperm. *J Am Med Assoc* 1994; **23**:1858–1860.

33. Rosenlund B, Sjoblam P, Dimitrakopoulos A, Hillensjo T. Epididymal and testicular sperm injection in the treatment of obstructive azospermia. *Acta Obstet Gynecol Scand* 1997; **75**:135–139.

34. Hull MGR, Glazener CMA, Kelly NJ *et al.* Population study of causes, treatment and outcome of infertility. *Br Med J* 1985; **291**:1693–1697.

35. Holsclaw DS, Perlmutter AD, Jockin H, Shwachman H. Congenital abnormalities in male patients with cystic fibrosis. *J Urol* 1971; **106**:568–574.

36. Dumur V, Gervais R, Rigot JM *et al.* Abnormal distribution of CF delta F508 allele in azoospermic men with congenital aplasia of epididymis and vas deferens. *Lancet* 1990; **336**:512.

37. Rigot JM, Lafitte JJ, Dumur V *et al.* Cystic fibrosis and congenital absence of the vas deferens. *N Eng J Med* 1991; **325**:64–65.

38. Anguiano A, Oates RD, Amos JA *et al.* Congenital bilateral absence of the vas deferens: a primarily genital form of cystic fibrosis. *J Am Med Assoc* 1992; **267**:1794–1797.

39. Oates RD, Amos JA. The genetic basis of congenital bilateral absence of the vas deferens. *J Androl* 1994; **15**:1–8.

40. Osborne LR, Lynch M, Middleton PG *et al.* Nasal epithelial ion transport and genetic analysis of infertile men with congenital bilateral absence of the vas deferens. *Hum Mol Genet* 1993; **2**:1605–1609.

41. Claustres M, Guittard C, Bozon D *et al.* Spectrum of CFTR mutations in cystic fibrosis and congenital absence of the vas deferens in France. *Hum Mutat* 2000; **16**:143–156.

42. Colin AA, Sawyer SM, Mickel JE *et al.* Pulmonary function and clinical observations in males with congenital bilateral absence of the vas deferens. *Chest* 1996; **110**:440–445.

43. Tizzano EF, Chitayat D, Buchwald M. Cell-specific localization of CFTR mRNA shows developmentally regulated expression in human fetal tissues. *Hum Mol Genet* 1993; **2**:219–224.

44. Trezise AE, Chambers JA, Wardle CJ *et al.* Expression of the cystic fibrosis gene in human foetal tissues. *Hum Mol Genet* 1993; **2**:213–218.

45. Tizzano EF, Silver MM, Chitayat D *et al.* Differential cellular expression of cystic fibrosis transmembrane regulator in human reproductive tissues: clues for the infertility in patients with cystic fibrosis. *Am J Pathol* 1994; **144**:906–914.

46. Chillon M, Casals T, Mercier B *et al.* Mutations in the cystic fibrosis gene in patients with congenital absence of the vas deferens. *N Engl J Med* 1995; **332**:1475–1480.

47. Chu C-S, Trapnell BC, Curristin S *et al.* Genetic basis of variable exon 9 skipping in cystic fibrosis transmembrane conductance regulator mRNA. *Nat Genet* 1993; **3**:151–156.

48. Groman JD, Hefferon TW, Casals T *et al.* Variation in a repeat sequence determines whether a common variant of the cystic fibrosis transmembrane regulator gene is pathogenic or benign. *Am J Hum Genet* 2004; **74**:176–179.

49. Cuppens H, Cassiman JJ. CFTR mutations and polymorphisms in male infertility. *Int J Androl* 2004; **27**:251–256.

50. Augarten A, Yaha Y, Kerem BS *et al.* Congenital bilateral absence of the vas deferens in the absence of cystic fibrosis. *Lancet* 1994; **344**:1473–1474.

51. Daudin M, Bieth E, Bujan L *et al.* Congenital bilateral absence of the vas deferens: clinical characteristics, biological parameters, cystic fibrosis transmembrane conductance regulator gene mutations, and implications for genetic counselling. *Fertil Steril* 2000; **74**:1164–1174.

52. Oppenheimer EH, Esterly JR. Observations on cystic fibrosis of the pancreas.VI: The uterine cervix. *J Pediatr* 1970; **77**:991–995.

53. Kopito LE, Kosasky HJ, Shwachman H. Water and electrolytes in cervical mucus from patients with cystic fibrosis. *Fertil Steril* 1973; **24**:512–516.

54. Kredentser JV, Pokrant C, McCoshen JA. Intrauterine insemination for infertility due to cystic fibrosis. *Fertil Steril* 1996; **45**:425–426.

55. Brugman SM, Taussig LM. The reproductive system. In: Taussig LM (ed.) *Cystic Fibrosis.* New York, Thieme-Stratton, 1984, pp323–337.

56. Stern RC. Cystic fibrosis and the reproductive system. In: Davis PB (ed.) *Cystic Fibrosis.* New York, Marcel Dekker, 1993, pp381–400.

57. Odegaard I, Stray-Pedersen B, Hallberg K *et al.* Prevalence and outcome of pregnancies in Norwegian and Swedish women with cystic fibrosis. *Acta Obstet Gynecol Scand* 2002; **81**:693–697.

58. Gilljam M, Antoniou M, Shin J *et al.* Pregnancy in cystic fibrosis: fetal and maternal outcome. *Chest* 2000; **118**:85–91.

59. Hull SC, Kass NE. Adults with cystic fibrosis and infertility: how has the health care system responded? *J Androl* 2000; **21**:809–813.

60. Kotloff RM, FitzSimmons, Fiel SB. Fertility and pregnancy in patients with cystic fibrosis. *Clin Chest Med* 1992; **13**:623–635.

61. Parry E, O'Carroll M, Bass E. Successful pregnancy in a woman with cystic fibrosis and type 2 respiratory failure. *Aust NZ J Obstet Gynecol* 2004; **44**:481–482.

62. Bose D, Yentis SM, Fauvel NJ. Caesarian section in a parturient with respiratory failure caused by cystic fibrosis. *Anaesthesia* 1997; **52**:578–582.

63. Choquet M, Du Pasquier Fediaevsky L *et al.* Sexual behaviour among adolescents reporting chronic conditions: a French national survey. *J Adolesc Health* 1997; **30**:62–67.

64. Suris JC, Resnick MD, Cassuto N, Blum RW. Sexual behavior of adolescents with chronic disease and disability. *J Adolesc Hlth* 1996; **19**:124–131.

65. Wager MD, Neuspiel DR, Coupey SM. Sexual behavior of chronically ill adolescents: evidence of unmet health needs. *Pediatr Res* 1986; **20**:158A.

66. Alderman EM, Lauby JL, Coupey SM. Problem behaviours in inner-city adolescents with chronic illness. *J Dev Behav Pediatr* 1995; **16**:339–344.

67. Valencia LS, Cromer BA. Sexual activity and other high-risk behaviors in adolescents with chronic illness: a review. *J Pediatr Adolesc Gynecol* 2000; **13**:53–64.

68. FitzPatrick SB, Stokes DC, Rosenstein BJ *et al.* Use of oral contraceptives in women with cystic fibrosis. *Chest* 1984; **86**:863–867.

69. Hughes BR, Cunliffe WJ. Interactions between the oral contraceptive pill and antibiotics. *Br J Dermatol* 1990; **122**:717–718.

70. Archer JSM, Archer DF. Oral contraceptive efficacy and antibiotic interaction: a myth debunked. *J Am Acad Dermatol* 2002; **46**:917–923.

71. Stead RJ, Grimmer SFM, Rogers SM *et al.* Pharmacokinetics of contraceptive steroids in patients with cystic fibrosis. *Thorax* 1987; **42**:59–64.

72. Bump RC, Norton PA. Epidemiological and natural history of pelvic floor dysfunction. *Obstet Gynecol Clin N Am* 1998; **254**:723–746.

73. White D, Stuiller K, Roney F. The prevalence and severity of symptoms of incontinence in adult cystic fibrosis patients. *Physiother Theory Pract* 2000; **16**:35–42.

74. Cornacchia M, Zenorini A, Perobelli S *et al.* Prevalence of urinary incontinence in women with cystic fibrosis. *BJU Int* 2001; **88**:44–48.

75. Orr A, McVean RJ, Webb AK, Dodd ME. Questionnaire survey of urinary incontinence in women with cystic fibrosis. *Br Med J* 2001; **322**:1521.

76. Nixon GM, Glazner JA, Martin JM, Sawyer SM. Urinary incontinence in female adolescents with cystic fibrosis. *Pediatrics* 2002; **110**:e22.

77. McVean RJ, Orr A, Webb AK *et al.* Treatment of urinary incontinence in cystic fibrosis. *J Cystic Fibros* 2003; **2**:171–176.

78. Sawyer SM, Bowes G, Phelan PD. Vulvovaginal candidiasis in young women with cystic fibrosis. *Br Med J* 1994; **308**:1690.

79. Siegal B, Siegal S. Pregnancy and delivery in a patient with cystic fibrosis of the pancreas. *Obstet Gynecol* 1960; **16**:438–440.

80. Cohen LF, di Sant'Agnese PA, Friedlander J. Cystic fibrosis and pregnancy: a national survey. *Lancet* 1980; **2**:842–844.

81. Canny GJ, Corey M, Livingstone RA *et al.* Pregnancy and cystic fibrosis. *Obstet Gynecol* 1991; **77**:850–853.

82. Grand RJ, Talamo RC, di Sant'Agnese PA, Shwartz RH. Pregnancy in cystic fibrosis of the pancreas. *J Am Med Assoc* 1966; **195**:993–1000.

83. Corkey CWB, Newth CJL, Corey M, Levison H. Pregnancy in patients with cystic fibrosis: a better prognosis in patients with pancreatic function? *Am J Obstet Gynecol* 1981; **140**:737–742.

84. Palmer J, Dillon-Baker C, Tecklin JS *et al.* Pregnancy in patients with cystic fibrosis. *Ann Int Med* 1983; **99**:596–600.

85. Metz O, Metz S. Cystic fibrosis and pregnancy. *Monatsschrift Kinderheilkunde* 1991; **139**:409–412.

86. Hilman BC, Aitken ML, Constantinescu M. Pregnancy in patients with cystic fibrosis. *Clin Obstet Gynecol* 1996; **39**:70–86.

87. Frangolias DD, Nakielna EM, Wilcox PG. Pregnancy and cystic fibrosis: a case–controlled study. *Chest* 1997; **111**:963–969.

88. Gillet D, de Braekeleer M, Bellis G, Durieu I. Cystic fibrosis and pregnancy: report from French data (1980–1999). *BJOG* 2002; **109**:912–918.

89. Goss CH, Rubenfeld GD, Otto K, Aitken ML. The effect of pregnancy on survival in women with cystic fibrosis. *Chest* 2003; **124**:1460–1468.

90. Odegaard I, Stray-Pedersen B, Hallberg K *et al.* Maternal and fetal morbidity in pregnancies of Norwegian and Swedish women with cystic fibrosis. *Acta Obstet Gynecol Scand* 2002; **81**:698–705.

91. Edenborough FP, Mackenzie WE, Stableforth DE. The outcome of 73 pregnancies in 55 women with cystic fibrosis in the UK 1977–1996. *BJOG* 2000; **107**:254–261.

92. Edenborough FP. Pregnancy in women with cystic fibrosis. *Acta Obstet Gynecol Scand* 2002; **81**:689–692.

93. Edenborough FP. Women with cystic fibrosis and their potential for reproduction. *Thorax* 2001; **56**:649–655.

94. Fiel SB, FitzSimmons S. Pregnancy in patients with cystic fibrosis. *Pediatr Pulmonol* 1995; Suppl 12:S4.2.

95. Wagoner LE, Taylor DPO, Olsen SL *et al.* Immunosupressive therapy, management and outcome of heart transplant recipients during pregnancy. *J Heart Lung Transplant* 1994; **12**:993–1000.

96. Armenti VT, Gertner GS, Eisenberg JA *et al.* National Transplant Pregnancy Registry: outcomes of pregnancies in transplant recipients. *Transplant Proc* 1998; **30**:1528–1530.

97. Briggs GE, Freeman RK, Yaffe SJ. *Drugs in Pregnancy and Lactation: A Reference Guide to Fetal and Neonatal Risk*, 5th edn. Baltimore, Williams & Wilkins, 1998.

98. Whitelaw A, Butterfield A. High breast milk sodium in cystic fibrosis. *Lancet* 1977; **2**:1288.

99. Alpert SE, Cormier AD. Normal electrolyte and protein content in milk from mothers with cystic fibrosis: an explanation for the initial report of elevated milk sodium concentration. *J Pediatr* 1983; **102**:77–80.

100. Welch MJ, Phelps DL, Osher AB. Breast-feeding by a mother with cystic fibrosis. *Pediatrics* 1981; **67**:664–666.

101. Shiffman ML, Seale TW, Flux M *et al.* Breast-milk composition in women with cystic fibrosis: report of two cases and a review of the literature. *Am J Clin Nutr* 1989; **49**:612–617.

102. Bitman J, Hamosh M, Wood DL *et al.* Lipid composition of milk from mothers with cystic fibrosis. *Pediatrics* 1987; **80**:927–932.

103. Michel SH, Mueller DH. Impact of lactation on women with cystic fibrosis and their infants: a review of five cases. *J Am Diet Assoc* 1994; **95**:159–165.

104. Wolman C, Resnick MD, Harris LJ, Blum RW. Emotional well-being among adolescents with and without chronic conditions. *J Adolesc Hlth* 1994; **15**:199–204.

105. Johannessen M, Carlson M, Bruicefors AS, Hjelte L. Cystic fibrosis through a female perspective: psychological issues and information concerning puberty and motherhood. *Pt Edu Couns* 1998; **34**:115–123.

21

Transplantation

PAUL AURORA, KHIN GYI AND MARTIN CARBY

INTRODUCTION

Lung transplantation (LTx) is a well-established treatment for both adults and children with end-stage lung disease in cystic fibrosis (CF). The number of transplants performed worldwide per year in adults is now approximately 1700, with this being split almost equally between double- and single-lung transplants (Fig. 21.1a) [1]. This number increased dramatically through the 1990s, but has now stabilized because of limited donor availability. The majority of transplants performed in the 1980s were heart–lung transplants, where both heart and lungs are transplanted while the recipient is on cardiopulmonary bypass. The explanted heart could then be transplanted into another patient with terminal cardiac disease (the domino procedure). Over the last 10 years there has been a worldwide shift away from heart–lung transplantation in favor of bilateral or double-lung transplantation (Fig. 21.1b). Single-lung transplantation maximizes use of donor organs, but is not suitable in subjects with suppurative lung diseases such as CF. Approximately one-third of double-lung transplants are performed in patients with CF (Fig. 21.1c), though very few single-lung transplants are performed for this indication.

Lung transplantation is far less common in children, with 60–70 procedures performed each year worldwide [2]. Most of these procedures, particularly in adolescence, are performed in children with CF (Figs 21.2a,b).

Although both short-term and long-term outcomes are improving, they still lag behind outcomes for other solid-organ transplants (Fig. 21.3) [1,2]. In addition, there is a disparity between the number of subjects waiting for transplants and the number of donor organs that are available. It is essential, therefore, that the optimal time for referral for a lung transplant assessment, and for subsequent listing, is carefully considered both by the referring CF center and by the transplant team [3–6]. This chapter will review the criteria for the selection of lung transplant candidates, post-transplant management, and outcomes. We will also discuss issues that are particular to pediatric patients, and summarize important research in this field.

SELECTION FOR LUNG TRANSPLANTATION

International guidelines describing criteria for referral of patients to a specialist lung transplant center and the selection of recipients for lung transplantation were published in 1998 [7–9]. These guidelines were based upon limited data. The suitability of an individual for lung transplantation is still decided on following detailed discussion by a multidisciplinary team in designated transplant centers. The following section discusses these criteria. However, the authors suggest that early communication by the referring physician directly with the transplant center about individual cases is the most effective means of decision-making regarding suitability of an individual for lung transplantation. Early referral of a patient is rarely a problem, as the transplant center can delay the assessment if necessary, or assess the patient and then arrange to review the person some months later. Late referral of a patient is much more of a problem. At best, the patient will not have sufficient time to consider the decision; at worst he or she may miss out on a transplant altogether.

Lung transplantation is indicated for patients with end-stage CF-related lung disease, whose lung function parameters and quality of life are declining despite maximal medical therapy [3–9]. The potential longevity and quality of life benefits of lung transplantation for these individuals must be offset against the individual risk of perioperative mortality and both short- and long-term complications. An individual's suitability for lung transplantation may change according to clinical status during the pre-transplant period.

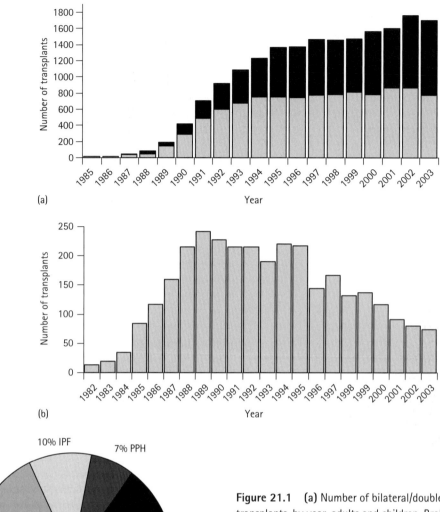

Figure 21.1 **(a)** Number of bilateral/double-lung and single-lung transplants, by year, adults and children. Broken bars represent single-lung transplants, solid bars represent bilateral and double-lung transplants. Reproduced, with amendment, from [1]. **(b)** Number of heart–lung transplants, by year, adults and children. Note that fewer than 100 procedures are now performed per year. Reproduced, with amendment, from [1]. **(c)** Indications for lung transplantation in adults. 'Other' includes sarcoidosis, bronchiectasis, congenital heart disease, and re-transplantation, amongst others. ATD, anti-trypsin deficiency; PPH, primary pulmonary hypertension; IPF, idopathic pulmonary fibrosis; COPD, chronic obstructive pulmonary disease. These charts include all data submitted to the Registry of the International Society for Heart and Lung Transplantation (ISHLT).

Patients will usually be considered for lung transplantation if:

- the patient has a predicted life expectancy, without transplant, of 2 years or less;
- the patient has a poor quality of life, which is likely to be improved by transplant;
- there are no specific contraindications to transplant;
- the patient is fully informed about the procedure, and is committed to proceeding.

The first criterion is that the patient should have a predicted life expectancy of 2 years or less despite maximal medical therapy. This is in consideration of the likely waiting time for a suitable organ for use in lung transplantation into any individual to become available. Assessment of prognosis is based on the results of a number of large survival studies. One of the first of these was a seminal paper by Kerem and colleagues, published in 1992 [10]. This retrospective analysis identified patients with an FEV_1 of less than 30% predicted, PaO_2 less than 55 mmHg (7.3 kPa) or $PaCO_2$ greater than 50 mmHg (6.7 kPa) as having a 2-year mortality rate above 50%. FEV_1 was the most significant predictor of mortality. Studies in adult populations [11–15], and one study in a pediatric population, have sought to

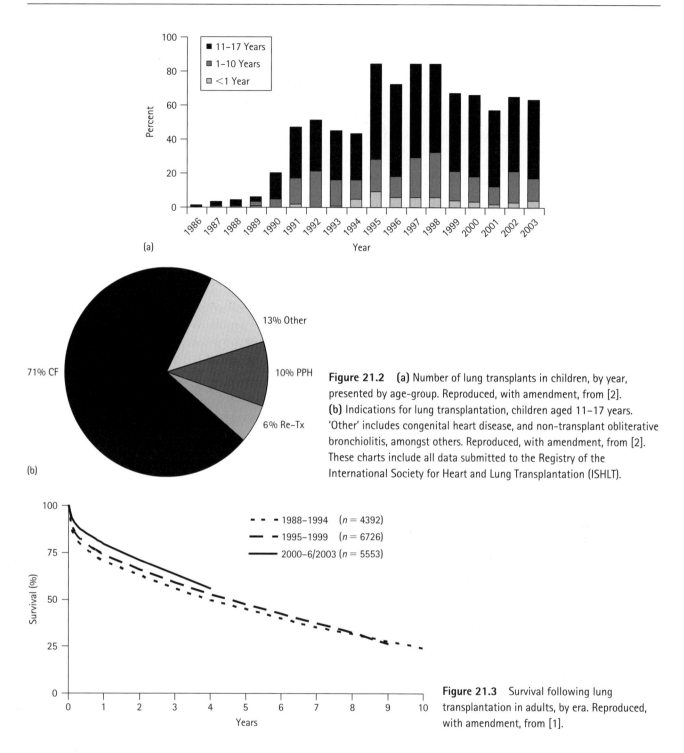

Figure 21.2   **(a)** Number of lung transplants in children, by year, presented by age-group. Reproduced, with amendment, from [2]. **(b)** Indications for lung transplantation, children aged 11–17 years. 'Other' includes congenital heart disease, and non-transplant obliterative bronchiolitis, amongst others. Reproduced, with amendment, from [2]. These charts include all data submitted to the Registry of the International Society for Heart and Lung Transplantation (ISHLT).

Figure 21.3   Survival following lung transplantation in adults, by era. Reproduced, with amendment, from [1].

further refine this analysis [16], and a large number of individual variables have now been identified as independent predictors of prognosis (Table 21.1).

The proposals made by Kerem and colleagues still apply, with minor elaboration. Namely, subjects with an FEV_1 of 30% predicted or less, who have poor nutritional status and poor exercise tolerance, should be considered for a transplant assessment. However, females, very young patients, subjects declining quickly and subjects who have other relevant clinical factors such as a history of massive hemoptysis or increasing frequency of respiratory exacerbations

should be considered for transplant referral before they reach this point.

A number of cautions in the prediction of life expectancy are warranted. None of these models are perfect predictors of survival. All have to make a practical compromise between accuracy and practicality. There are many complications that physicians know to be important determinants of survival, which are not considered in these models. If, for example, the patient has recurrent pneumothoraces, then he or she should be considered to be in a poorer prognostic category than would otherwise be predicted by a survival model.

Table 21.1 Predictors of prognosis in CF.[a]

Domain	Parameter
Spirometry	FEV_1
	FVC
Poor exercise tolerance	Reduced 6-minute walk distance
	Desaturation on exercise
	Reduced maximal oxygen consumption
Poor blood gases	Resting hypercarbia
	Resting hypoxia
Poor nutrition	Hypoalbuminemia
	Anemia
	Short stature
	Poor weight for height
Rapid decline	Rapid rate of fall of FEV_1
	Frequent exacerbations
	Young age
Female sex	
Increased energy expenditure	Resting tachycardia
Multisystem involvement	Liver disease
	Diabetes mellitus

[a] A large number of parameters have been identified as being of prognostic value in CF. Here they are presented in domains for ease of reference, but it should be noted that many are inter-related, even across domains. The list is not exhaustive.

Second, some of the published models are derived from the entire CF population, rather than specifically from patients with severe lung disease who are being considered for transplant. This generates selection bias, and it is likely that such models will overestimate the survival of true lung transplant candidates. Third, these models should not be extrapolated outside the populations from which they were derived. Therefore models derived from adult data sets are suitable for predicting prognosis in adult patients, whereas models derived from pediatric populations should be used for predicting prognosis in children. Fourth, the medical management of CF is changing and mean survival is increasing. These models are based on historical data, and that needs to be factored into interpretation.

Patients with end-stage CF-related lung disease have a reduced quality of life (QoL) due to the restrictions caused by breathlessness, recurrent infections requiring hospitalization, limitation of exercise capacity and dependence on oxygen or non-invasive ventilation. Despite having to cope with continued medication and medical follow-up, there is a clear quality-of-life benefit for individuals following lung transplantation as judged by the St Georges Respiratory Questionnaire, Short Form-36, and the Hospital Anxiety and Depression Scale. This is especially so for individuals transplanted for CF versus other indications for lung transplantation [17].

Assessment of QoL is particularly difficult in children, as there are no widely accepted measures of QoL in childhood. Recent studies have attempted to objectively measure QOL

in children with CF [18–20], but as yet these scoring systems have not been applied to transplant assessment. In the UK, assessment is made by the clinician in combination with other members of the transplant team, and takes account of ability to partake in daily activities such as schooling or social activity, exercise tolerance, time spent in hospital, and requirement for oxygen and intravenous antibiotic therapy. As far as possible this assessment is taken from the child's perspective rather than from the parents', and detailed information from the referring center is of great value. Although inexact, assessment of quality of life is an essential component of the risk assessment. A child with an FEV_1 of 30% is unlikely to be accepted for transplantation if he still maintains a quality of life acceptable to that child.

The transplant assessment process aims to assess not only whether lung transplantation is justifiable in terms of quality of life and survival benefits, but also whether the individual has any features that would contraindicate lung transplantation. Any individual considering lung transplantation should have a satisfactory psychological profile and social support network to allow recovery and rehabilitation following surgery. He or she must also be willing to make the necessary lifestyle adjustments following lung transplantation and adhere strictly to the medication regimen. The issue of informed consent is relatively straightforward in a competent adult, but becomes more complex with a young child.

There are few absolute contraindications to lung transplantation [6–9], and consideration of relative contraindications is most often made on a case-by-case basis (Table 21.2). Factors most often regarded as contraindications include the presence of major dysfunction in another organ system, for instance the heart or kidneys, an acutely ill or unstable patient, the presence of any active malignancy, unacceptable nutritional status (body mass index less than 18 or greater than 25), drug or alcohol abuse, or evidence of HIV, hepatitis B or C virus infection. Other factors that are considered include the potential for rehabilitation, previous thoracic surgery, osteoporosis, severe musculoskeletal disease, presensitization to HLA antigens, long-term high-dose corticosteroid treatment and sputum microbiology. The presence in the sputum of *Burkholderia cenocepacia* is no longer considered an absolute contraindication to lung transplantation [21,22].

DONOR ALLOCATION

A discrepancy exists between the number of subjects who might benefit from lung transplantation and the number of lung donors available. In the United Kingdom and the United States there are approximately three times as many patients awaiting transplant as there are transplant operations performed each year [21,23]. The lungs are unique among body organs in that they are continuously exposed to the external environment. For this reason only approximately 20–30% of lungs offered for use in organ transplantation are usable. Others have been damaged by trauma,

Table 21.2 Contraindications to transplantation.

Absolute contraindications	Relative contraindications[a]
Active malignancy	Ventilator-dependent respiratory failure[b]
Hepatitis B or C infection	Obesity (BMI > 25)
Severe acute illness	Gross under-nutrition (BMI < 18)
Mycobacterium tuberculosis infection	HIV infection
Major psychiatric illness	*Burkholderia cenocepacia* infection
Major dysfunction of other organs (e.g. severe cardiac, renal or hepatic disease)[c]	Multiresistant non-tuberculous mycobacteria infection
	HLA antigen pre-sensitization
	Previous thoracic surgery
	Long-term high-dose corticosteroid therapy
	Psychosocial difficulties
	Severe osteoporosis or musculoskeletal disease
	Minor dysfunction of other organs

[a] Many of the factors listed as relative contraindications may be amenable to pre-transplant intervention. It is important for the referring center to discuss these issues with the transplant center as early as possible.
[b] Ventilator-dependent respiratory failure is considered an absolute contraindication by most UK centers, but this is not true in other countries.
[c] In the presence of major second organ dysfunction a double organ transplant may be possible.

infection or fluid overload or have become consolidated. Attempts are being made both to allocate this scarce resource most appropriately to give the maximum benefit to the greatest number of people and to maximize the numbers of lungs that are usable in transplantation.

Orens and colleagues recently reviewed standard donor criteria on behalf of the pulmonary council of the International Society for Heart and Lung Transplantation (ISHLT) [24]. Their conclusion was that the criteria that had traditionally been applied were probably too strict. In particular, there are limited data that a history of smoking in the donor, a prolonged period of ventilation prior to harvesting, or even minor abnormalities on chest x-ray have major adverse effects on subsequent outcome. Research in this area currently focuses on more detailed physiological assessment of donor lungs, rather than the more crude clinical criteria that have been traditionally used [25–38]. As with other aspects of lung transplant practice, there is variation between centers on how strictly donor criteria are applied. In addition, many centers are willing to use so-called marginal donors for patients who are in extremis, as long as the patients themselves have given informed consent.

Transplant teams in the United States have recently implemented a major change in how donor lungs are allocated to individuals. Rather than just basing allocation

on waiting list seniority, subjects are now given a survival benefit score that calculates their predicted survival without transplant, and their predicted post-transplant survival [26]. The aim is to direct scarce lungs toward patients who will derive the most benefit from them. Children are excluded from this allocation process as there are so few data on survival modelling in this age group. Interestingly, for adult subjects, it is likely that the new system will result in more lungs being allocated to subjects with cystic fibrosis. This is because subjects with CF are known to have a poorer waiting list survival than subjects with emphysema or chronic obstructive pulmonary disease, but conversely have a better post-transplant survival [39]. At the time of writing it is too early to determine what impact this new allocation system will have.

In the UK donor lungs are allocated according to compatible donor/recipient blood group matching and size matching and according to the clinical conditions of recipients on the waiting list at the zonal center. Furthermore, attempts are being made to optimize the management of organ donors following brain death to maintain lungs in the optimal condition prior to retrieval [40,41]. Alternative sources of donor organs are being sought [27,29,30]. Living donor lobar transplantation provides similar benefit to cadaveric lung donation for those with family and close friends willing to undergo lobectomy to provide tissue for use in organ transplantation [42–45]. This remains a second-line treatment due to the inevitable risk of lobectomy to the donors. Non-heart-beating donors are individuals who do not meet brain-stem death criteria but for whom the attending physicians and family agree that further medical intervention is futile. If the next of kin agree to organ donation then organs can be rapidly retrieved after certification of death following withdrawal of support and asystole. This process is already a well-recognized treatment in renal transplantation and is becoming recognized in lung transplantation also [27,40,41].

PREOPERATIVE MANAGEMENT

The aim of the CF center should be to keep the patient as healthy as possible while waiting for transplantation. Essentially this means continuing aggressive holistic care. The importance of maintaining good nutrition and bone density should not be underestimated [46]. These factors will have a major impact during post-transplant rehabilitation. If the patient is deteriorating, the use of non-invasive positive pressure ventilation (NIPPV) may be considered as a means of bridging the patient to transplantation [47]. The use of invasive ventilation is more controversial. There is no doubt that patients who are invasively ventilated have a significantly poorer post-transplant outcome than patients who are not ventilated. In addition, the shortage of donors means that a suitable organ is unlikely to become available in the necessary time frame for most patients. For this reason centers in the UK normally recommend against invasive ventilation in this scenario. However, this practice varies between different countries. An important ethical point to consider at this time is that the possibility of transplantation should not override a need for palliative care. If it is clear that a patient is reaching the last days of life, and the possibility of lung transplantation is remote, then the option of removing the patient from the transplant list, and concentrating on providing a dignified death, should be considered.

PERIOPERATIVE MANAGEMENT

The aim of management in the early transplant period is to initiate effective immunosuppression, to minimize the risk of infection, to rehabilitate the patient as rapidly as possible, and to protect other organ systems (such as renal). This requires close liaison between transplant physicians, surgeons and intensive care staff, together with experienced nursing staff and support from pathologists and radiologists experienced in thoracic organ transplantation. Detailed information on donor management, organ retrieval and preservation, and surgical techniques, is beyond the scope of this text.

Immunosuppression

Prior to transplantation the subject receives loading doses of maintenance immunosuppression, this being either tacrolimus or ciclosporin, and either azathioprine or mycophenolate mofetil (MMF). Tacrolimus and ciclosporin are calcineurin inhibitors (CIs) – metabolites of these drugs bind to cytoplasmic calcineurin, and therefore interfere with the transcription of various cytokines, including IL-2, -3, -4 and -5, tumor necrosis factor-α, interferon-γ, and granulocyte/macrophage colony stimulating factor, and therefore inhibit T-cell stimulation [48,49]. Cell cycle inhibitors (azathioprine, MMF) interfere with DNA and RNA synthesis, and purine synthesis, thereby inhibiting proliferation of T and B lymphocytes.

During the transplant procedure the subject receives high-dose methylprednisolone. There is no universal agreement on the administration of further induction of immunosuppression. Some transplant centers give a monoclonal antibody (basiliximab or daclizimab), which binds irreversibly to the IL-2 receptor on T-cells, while other centers give antithymocyte globulin [50,51]. These additional agents may reduce the risk of rejection during the first month posttransplant, but this may be at the expense of increased severity of infection or later increased incidence of malignancy.

Anti-infective therapy

Appropriate intravenous antibiotic prophylaxis is essential at the time of lung transplantation for CF and these will normally be continued until the patient is mobilizing and able to clear secretions [21,22,52–59]. Care must be taken when explanting lungs to guard against contamination of the thoracic cavity by airway secretions. It may be prudent at explantation to electively wash out the thoracic cavity, either with saline or with a weak antibiotic solution. The use of antifungal prophylaxis for those known to be colonized with fungi pre-transplant can reduce the postoperative rate of fungal infections.

Intensive care management and rehabilitation

The patient is invariably ventilated for a few hours posttransplant. At this time inotropic support is also usually necessary, particularly if the operation was performed on cardiopulmonary bypass. It is important at this stage that the patient be kept relatively hypovolemic, so that pulmonary edema does not develop. Careful monitoring of renal function is necessary, particularly as the patients will be receiving a calcineurin inhibitor. Most patients will have a temporary paralytic ileus early after transplant. If this is allowed to progress to distal ileal obstruction syndrome then the consequences can be disastrous. For this reason most centers commence small volumes of enteral feeds very early post-transplant, and some centers also give lact-ulose or *N*-acetyl cysteine during the early postoperative period [60].

Most patients can be extubated within the first 24 hours after transplant. It is then essential that they begin to mobilize, and in particular that they clear respiratory secretions. Delay in extubation can occur for a number of reasons. The most important is development of primary graft failure (PGF), which is clinically, physiologically and radiologically similar to adult respiratory distress syndrome (ARDS) (Fig. 21.4) [61–66]. PGF occurs in approximately 10% of

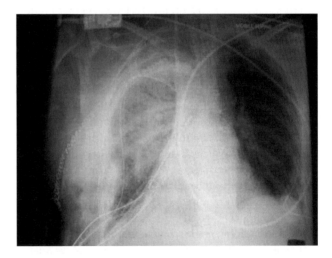

Figure 21.4 Primary graft failure in a subject who recently received a right single-lung transplant for emphysema. The right lung shows diffuse pulmonary infiltrates, similar to those seen in ARDS.

transplant recipients. Incidence is increased in marginal donors and in situations when the graft ischemic time is greater than 6 hours, but it is also seen in lungs from supposedly low-risk donors. Diagnosis is based on clinical pattern and exclusion of other diagnoses (particularly acute rejection). The pathophysiology of PGF is related to alveolar capillary leak, but no specific treatments have been demonstrated to show great benefit. Management is supportive [67].

Following extubation, the goal is to rehabilitate the patient – to simplify his or her complicated treatment regimen and ready the individual for discharge. It is also essential to monitor for complications, the most common of which are lower respiratory infection and acute rejection. Most centers will perform at least one bronchoscopic biopsy and lavage prior to the patient being discharged. The typical inpatient stay following an uncomplicated transplant is 2–3 weeks, though this is usually slightly longer in children and in subjects who have other medical conditions.

POST-TRANSPLANT MANAGEMENT

The goal of post-transplant management is to maintain adequate immunosuppression, to protect the graft from non-immune insults, to protect other organ systems from the consequences of immunosuppressive therapy (particularly renal failure), and to monitor for complications.

Immunosuppression

The great majority of lung transplant recipients remain on three maintenance immunosuppressive agents life-long [1,2]. Typically, one of these will be a calcineurin inhibitor, one will be a cell-cycle inhibitor, and the third will be prednisolone. The most important side-effect of these agents is that they cause immunosuppression, and the incidence of severe infection and malignancy are greatly increased. In addition, however, they have a number of specific side-effects, which are listed in Table 21.3.

Calcineurin inhibitors have a narrow therapeutic window and significant side-effects. Absorption after oral administration is poor, and can be even poorer in patients with CF. Both drugs are given twice daily, and dosage adjustment is performed dependent on trough blood levels. However, there is increasing evidence that trough levels do not reflect systemic exposure, as assessed by a full pharmacokinetic profile over 12 hours (area under the curve AUC 0–12) [68,69].

Recently there has been a trend to use tacrolimus instead of ciclosporin in some transplant centers. Evidence for superior efficacy mostly comes from studies in renal transplant recipients [70–72], but studies in lung transplant recipients are ongoing. One clear difference between the drugs is in their side-effect profile. Ciclosporin frequently causes hirsutism and gingivism, which some patients find unacceptable, and which causes particular distress in girls and young women. If the psychological impact of these side-effects is

considered to be affecting drug adherence, then thought should be given to switching to tacrolimus. Conversely, a much higher incidence of post-transplant diabetes mellitus has been recorded with tacrolimus than with ciclosporin, and this obviously has implications for patients with cystic fibrosis. MMF (versus azathioprine) is reported to reduce the incidence of acute rejection in renal and cardiac patients [73,74]. The one multicenter trial that has been reported in lung transplant recipients showed no benefit of MMF over azathioprine at 6 months in survival or incidence of acute rejection [75].

Anti-infective therapy

The use of anti-infective prophylaxis varies widely between centers. The authors advocate continued use of nebulized anti-pseudomonal antibiotics (usually colistin) for at least 6 months. All patients receive some form of antifungal prophylaxis (either oral itraconazole or nebulized amphotericin,

Table 21.3 Common side-effects of maintenance immunosuppression.

Drug	Side-effects
Ciclosporin	Nephrotoxicity
	Tremor
	Paresthesia/hypersensitivity
	Hypertension
	Hypercholesterolemia
	Hypertrichosis
	Gingival hypertrophy
Tacrolimus	Nephrotoxicity
	Tremor
	Paresthesia/hypersensitivity
	Hypertension
	Hypercholesterolemia
	Neurotoxicity
	Diabetes mellitus
	Alopecia
Prednisolone	Cushing's syndrome
	Dyspepsia
	Peptic ulceration
	Osteoporosis
	Proximal myopathy
	Increased appetite
	Neuropsychiatric effects
	Glaucoma, papilledema, cataracts
	Skin atrophy, striae, bruising, acne
Azathioprine	Bone marrow suppression
	Hypersensitivity reactions
Mycophenolate mofetil (MMF)	Bone marrow suppression
	Nausea, dyspepsia, diarrhea, constipation
	Hyperglycemia
	Hypercholesterolemia

and oral nystatin) [76–82]. Patients who are at high or medium risk for CMV activation receive prophylactic valganciclovir for approximately 3 months [83–85].Co-trimoxazole is also given for approximately 3 months or longer as prophylaxis against *Pneumocystis carinae* pneumonia [86,87].

Graft monitoring

After discharge, patients are recommended to monitor their own health, and to report to the transplant center if they have any untoward symptoms. Patients are provided with portable spirometers and asked to record spirometry daily, and report if their FEV_1 falls by 10% or more.

When a patient presents with acute respiratory symptoms, rapid diagnosis and treatment is essential. The clinical picture of early acute rejection is non-specific, and indistinguishable from an infection. Patients who have cough, malaise, low-grade pyrexia or minor drop in lung function should be thoroughly evaluated [88,89]. Chest x-ray may be normal in the presence of rejection, but even if changes are seen they do not distinguish between rejection and infection. Although fractional exhaled nitric oxide measurement has been proposed as a non-invasive marker of acute rejection, the sensitivity and specificity of this marker is still unclear [90–93]. In most cases an urgent bronchoscopy, lavage and transbronchial biopsy is indicated. The biopsy is graded for the presence of rejection using a scoring system developed by the ISHLT [94]. The presence of perivascular and interstitial mononuclear cell infiltrates are graded from A0 (no acute rejection) up to grade A4 (severe rejection). In addition, the presence of airway inflammation is graded from B0 (no airway inflammation) to B4 (severe airway inflammation). If the biopsy shows moderate to severe rejection (A3 or A4), then this can usually be cleared with a 3- to 5-day course of high-dose methylprednisolone. Occasionally, more aggressive therapy with polyclonal anti-lymphocyte antibodies (antithymocyte globulin, ATG) is necessary. The correct approach to grade A2 rejection is more controversial, and some centers will treat this with a short course of oral prednisolone [95–99]. Grade A1 rejection is usually not treated.

The importance of airway inflammation in the absence of interstitial changes is uncertain. There is some evidence that airway inflammation is associated with subsequent development of bronchiolitis obliterans syndrome [100], but this inflammation does not always respond well to high-dose steroid treatment. The presence of infection on lavage should always be taken seriously [101–104]. Positive bacterial or fungal cultures warrant antibiotic or antifungal treatment respectively. Presence of respiratory viruses in bronchoalveolar lavage (BAL) is more problematic since few specific antiviral agents are available.

Many transplant centers have traditionally performed surveillance bronchoscopies and biopsies in asymptomatic patients during the first year post-transplant. The value of these surveillance biopsies is uncertain. While there is no doubt that surveillance bronchoscopy frequently shows asymptomatic mild rejection and asymptomatic mild infection, it is not yet clear whether the treatment of these abnormal findings has a positive impact on long-term outcome. In practice there may be relatively little difference in the way patients are managed. In 1997, Tam and colleagues in the UK reported a post-hoc analysis of patients transplanted in the Papworth center [99]. After surveillance biopsies were suspended they described no difference in outcome for 75 patients who did not have surveillance biopsies compared with historical controls who did. However, the non-surveillance biopsy group had just as many biopsies in their first year as the historical controls, presumably because more frequent biopsies were performed during symptomatic episodes. The pickup rate of surveillance transbronchial biopsy has differed between published studies. Experience in a pediatric population at Great Ormond Street, London, suggests that the detection rate for infection or rejection is as high as 40% in asymptomatic subjects (author's own data).

The clinical significance of low-grade rejection is unknown. Hopkins and co-workers [96] have prospectively analyzed 1159 transbronchial biopsies in 128 patients: 24% of these biopsies showed A1 rejection, of which the great majority were in asymptomatic patients; 34.5% of these patients progressed to develop either high-grade acute rejection or lymphocytic bronchiolitis. In addition, 68% of patients who had multiple A1 lesions subsequently developed bronchiolitis obliterans syndrome (BOS; see later), compared with 43% of patients, who had one or fewer lesions.

Non-infectious complications

Different complications exist in the early and late post-transplant periods. Early complications are usually related to the bronchial anastomosis [105–109]. In the absence of bronchial artery circulation, healing of the anastomosis is dependent on a retrograde blood supply from pulmonary collaterals. This healing can be further hampered by corticosteroids, or by post-transplant infections. In the early days of lung transplantation early necrosis leading to subsequent stenosis, or even dehiscence, were important complications. Improvement in surgical techniques, particularly performing the anastomosis more distally, has reduced the incidence of these complications. The commonest time for bronchial stenosis to develop is 2–4 months post-transplant. Treatment of choice is balloon dilatation, which often needs to be repeated to have a long-lasting effect [105–113]. If the stenosis is caused by granuloma formation, then repeated laser treatment may also be of benefit. If these techniques are unsuccessful, an expandable bronchial stent can be placed [113]. This has the disadvantage of interrupting ciliary transport and has a negative effect on long-term results.

Other early complications are damage to the phrenic nerve, leading to impairment of diaphragmatic function, and damage to the vagus nerve, which contributes to delayed gastric emptying.

Late complications following lung transplantation include an increased incidence of malignancy and calcineurin inhibitor-induced renal impairment. Post-transplant lymphoproliferative disease (PTLD) is a heterogeneous condition that varies from a relatively benign proliferation of B lymphocytes to monoclonal lymphoma. Although the majority of PTLD tumors are of B-cell origin, rare T-cell and other cell type tumors have been diagnosed. The incidence is higher in lung transplant recipients than in other solid-organ recipients [114,115], and is higher in children than in adults, with a lifetime prevalence of 7% in pediatric lung transplant recipients [114]. The majority of disorders are caused by a clonal expansion of B-cells infected with Epstein–Barr virus (EBV), because of loss of normal T-cell surveillance due to immunosuppression. Historically, PTLD has carried a high mortality, with 1-year survival as low as 50%. With the introduction of anti B-cell monoclonal antibody (rituximab), outcomes are improving.

Lifelong immunosuppression results in a higher incidence of other malignancies in transplant recipients, and also contributes to these malignancies being more aggressive [116]. In addition to PTLD, the most common cancers in cardiothoracic transplant recipients are skin cancers, lung cancers, prostate cancer and Kaposi's sarcoma. The usual risk factors for developing such cancers apply to transplant recipients also. Therefore it is important to give transplant patients advice about sunlight exposure, etc.

Renal impairment is extremely common after transplantation, because of long-term treatment with calcineurin inhibitors [1,2]. There is no difference in nephrotoxicity between ciclosporin and tacrolimus. Patients with cystic fibrosis are particularly at risk, because many of them have impaired renal function before they come to transplant probably due to repeated courses of aminoglycoside antibiotic treatment. Although this was previously seen mostly in adult CF transplant recipients, our recent experience has been that the majority of children with CF coming to transplant also have impaired renal function (author's own data). Treatment of renal failure can be extremely difficult. One approach has been to withdraw the calcineurin inhibitor and give sirolimus or everolimus as an alternative immunosuppressant. Snell and colleagues have reported improved renal function in adult lung recipients with renal failure managed by this approach [117]. However, there are no data regarding the long-term efficacy of sirolimus in the maintenance of lung allografts, and such patients may therefore be at risk of acute rejection or bronchiolitis obliterans syndrome.

Other non-infectious complications are listed in Table 21.4.

Non-transplant complications

Subjects with cystic fibrosis who have transplants must still be monitored for all other CF-related complications.

Table 21.4 Common non-infectious complications after lung transplantation.

Early
Anastomotic dehiscence or stenosis
Phrenic nerve injury
Vagal nerve injury

Intermediate and late
Malignancy, particularly lymphoproliferative disease
Nephrotoxicity
Hypertension
Osteoporosis
Growth failure (children)
Diabetes mellitus
Hyperuricemia/gout
Warts

In particular, bone disease, diabetes mellitus and growth failure are more common in transplant recipients than in the general CF population.

LONG-TERM OUTCOMES

Compared to other solid-organ transplant recipients, lung transplant recipients have a higher incidence of complications. Outcomes are slowly improving with time, but this change is not dramatic when viewed from a worldwide perspective (see Fig. 21.3) [1]. In addition, there is some evidence that outcome in children is even poorer than outcome in adults, though this may be in part because most pediatric centers inevitably perform a small volume of transplants [2]. Children awaiting transplantation at Great Ormond Street are currently quoted a median survival of 5–6 years, while adults considering lung transplantation at Harefield Hospital are quoted an average 1-year survival of 75% and average 5-year survival of 45%.

Post-transplant obliterative bronchiolitis

In the first year post-transplant the leading cause of mortality is overwhelming infection. This is often because infection is the final insult following surgical complications, severe rejection or primary graft dysfunction [1,2]. After 1 year, the commonest cause of death is obliterative bronchiolitis (OB) [1,2]. This develops in up to 70% of survivors by 5 years after transplantation, and eventually progresses to respiratory failure. True OB is diagnosed histologically, but such confirmation is not always easy to obtain. It is rarely possible to get adequate tissue samples from transbronchial biopsy, and open lung biopsy is a hazardous procedure in patients who are already in respiratory compromise. Therefore the transplant community has adopted the term 'bronchiolitis obliterans syndrome' (BOS) as the clinical correlate of obliterative bronchiolitis [118,119]. BOS is defined by an irreversible fall in lung function when other

Table 21.5 Bronchiolitis obliterens syndrome (BOS) grading.

Grade	Definition
BOS 0	FEV_1 >90% of baseline and FEF_{25-75} >75% of baseline
BOS 0-P	FEV_1 81–90% of baseline and/or FEF_{25-75} ≤75% of baseline
BOS 1	FEV_1 66–80% of baseline
BOS 2	FEV_1 51–65% of baseline
BOS 3	FEV_1 ≤50% of baseline

causes have been excluded, and is graded from BOS 0P to BOS 3 (Table 21.5) [119]. OB and BOS have previously been described as a form of chronic rejection. However, it is likely that there are many factors that contribute to the development of BOS. In particular, non-immune insults such as gastroesophageal reflux or airway infection may lead to graft dysfunction, and aggressive treatment of these complications can reverse this dysfunction. Specifically, a number of centers have now reported a very high prevalence of gastroesophageal reflux in transplant recipients [120–124], and a gratifying improvement in outcomes following surgical treatment of this reflux [125–128].

In addition, reports from more than one center have described how low-dose macrolide therapy can improve graft function in many patients [129–131]. The mechanism is not fully understood, but the observation that patients who respond are usually those who have evidence of neutrophilic airway inflammation suggests that the anti-inflammatory properties of macrolides are responsible. Strictly speaking, the patients who benefit from such interventions did not really have BOS (or OB) but rather had reversible airway dysfunction related to inflammation.

Patients who have established OB/BOS, which does not respond to such measures, are in far more difficulty, as by definition there is no effective treatment. Some of these patients stabilize, and can continue for many years with limited lung function. Others develop steadily worsening graft dysfunction and progress to respiratory failure. OB/BOS is the commonest cause of late death following transplantation and is the main reason why long-term outcome is only slowly improving [1,2]. The current focus is on development of techniques for early detection of airway dysfunction, with the intention of preventing the development of BOS [132].

Re-transplantation

Repeat lung transplantation is rarely performed [1,2]. The main reason for this is because of the shortage of donor organs and potential additional risks involved in re-transplantation [133–136]. In particular, repeat surgery may be more difficult because of previous thoracotomy, and other systemic complications such as renal dysfunction are more prevalent. With donor shortage denying many subjects a first transplant it is difficult to justify repeat transplantation for others.

Does lung transplantation confer benefit to the patient?

There is increasing evidence that lung or heart–lung transplantation significantly increases life expectancy in appropriately selected patients. Testing this hypothesis has not been straightforward, as randomized controlled trials would not be acceptable in this situation. However, hazards modelling techniques can be employed to calculate the survival benefit from transplantation [137,138]. There have now been a large number of published studies that have employed these methods and obtained similar results [139–141]. The one study that has been performed in a pediatric population calculated a hazard ratio for transplantation of 0.31, equating to a reduction in risk of death of 69% (95% confidence interval 28–87%) [142]. Two recent studies from the CF Foundation database in the United States have calculated a lower survival benefit for the procedure [143,144], but these two studies employed a different analysis method from all others cited [137,138,145], and this probably explains the discrepancy in results.

Despite the negative impact of OB/BOS, functional outcome for the majority of lung transplant recipients is very good. Data from the ISHLT registry suggest that more than 80% report no limitation to activity at 1, 3 and 5 years post-transplant [1,2]. Similar results are seen in pediatric transplantation. In adult subjects there is evidence that transplantation produces a dramatic improvement in quality of life [146–150], and unpublished data from Great Ormond Street, London, suggest that the same applies to pediatric recipients. As post-transplant outcomes continue to improve, the potential benefit of the procedure is no longer an area of controversy.

SPECIFIC PEDIATRIC ISSUES

There are number of small but important differences between how monitoring is performed in children compared to adults.

Lung function testing

Most children over the age of 4 years are able to perform spirometry successfully, provided they are given adequate training. It may be necessary to modify the outcome measures that are used (e.g. by reporting $FEV_{0.75}$ rather than FEV_1) [151]. As well as performing spirometry on every clinic visit, most transplant centers provide the family with a portable spirometer which the child should use daily at home. A drop in FEV_1 (or $FEV_{0.75}$) of greater than 10%, which lasts for more than 24 hours, should be referred for medical advice. Exhaled nitric oxide (eNO) measurement may provide a non-invasive means for detecting airway inflammation post-transplant. Data are limited in adults and non-existent in children, but it is known that eNO measurement can be successfully performed in young children [152]. There are intriguing data from Estenne and colleagues [132] suggesting that gas mixing techniques may provide earlier indication of airway dysfunction than spirometry. A modified version of the multiple-breath washout technique can be used in children, including those in the infant and pre-school age groups [153]. There are as yet no published data on gas mixing studies following lung transplantation in children.

Transbronchial biopsy

If a child is suspected of having rejection or lower respiratory infection then bronchoscopy and transbronchial biopsy should nearly always be performed. Preferably this should be done as early as possible, prior to starting treatment. The technique employed varies between centers, with some preferring general anesthesia, and others using sedation [154]. General anesthesia with a laryngeal mask airway allows the use of adult-size (e.g. 4.9 mm) bronchoscopes even in pre-school children. This allows adequate samples to be obtained.

Radiology

The new generation of multislice CT scanners allows rapid acquisition of high-resolution (HR) images with relatively little radiation exposure [155]. General anesthesia is rarely necessary for this investigation, even in the youngest children. If a HRCT is to be used for monitoring of graft structure in asymptomatic children, then it is essential that the protocol be modified from the normal adult settings so that the radiation dose is minimized.

Infections

This is one area where pediatric practice differs from adult practice. Many children will not have had previous exposure to common viruses, and the incidence of primary infection is much higher than for adults. It is therefore essential that immunization status be optimized prior to listing for transplantation [156]. Following transplantation the family should be given advice to keep their child away from outbreaks of measles, varicella etc., and to seek advice if their child has been in contact with other children who may be infectious. Post-transplant lymphoproliferative disease (PTLD) is far more common in children than in adults [157], and in most cases is related to reactivation of EBV infection. Although there are many centers that now monitor quantitative EBV load post-transplant, there is little evidence that viral load is related to subsequent development of PTLD [158].

Side-effects of immunosuppressive therapy

The approach to this is similar as for adult patients. The most important points are to monitor renal function, as ciclosporin and tacrolimus are both nephrotoxic; to monitor for bone marrow suppression from azathioprine and MMF; to monitor for hyperglycemia, particularly in children with CF; and to monitor bone mineral density [159]. Related to this, it should also be remembered that all children with CF may still get non-respiratory complications, such as fat-soluble vitamin deficiency, salt depletion in hot weather, nasal polyps, distal ileal obstruction, etc.

Growth and development

Many children who are referred for lung transplantation have growth failure secondary to chronic illness. Even if a transplant is successful, the use of maintenance corticosteroids post-transplant also affects linear growth [158,160]. If the child has had no episodes of rejection it is important to reduce the steroid dose to the lowest possible to allow catch-up growth. The use of growth hormone in these situations is controversial, as there is some laboratory evidence that it may trigger acute rejection [161]. The transplanted lungs themselves grow as the child grows. There is some evidence from lung function testing and from CT that the airways of transplanted lungs grow with the child [162], but it is still unclear as to whether graft alveoli continue to multiply, or whether they simply distend.

Psychosocial issues

As mentioned above, many children coming to transplant are physically and emotionally immature because of their chronic illness. A successful transplant allows a child to transform his or her life and to catch up on many of the activities that were previously denied. Some children find this change in lifestyle difficult, particularly if it coincides with puberty [163].

Anecdotal reports from a number of centers suggest that survival rates are steadily improving. Non-adherence to therapy is therefore becoming a proportionately greater cause of poor outcomes. This problem is particularly seen in teenage patients, and appears worst in those who have a chronic illness like cystic fibrosis. There is limited evidence as to the best approach for assisting children in this position. However, most centers stress that adolescents should steadily take more responsibility for their own care and are given practical assistance to boost adherence to therapy. In addition, it is important to encourage adolescents to develop long-term goals and ambitions, so that they have positive aims for the future [164].

Table 21.6 Key areas of research in lung transplantation.

Humoral rejection
Innate immune response
New immunosuppressant agents (e.g. sirolimus, everolimus)
Aerosolized delivery of ciclosporin
Use of marginal donors
Monitoring of calcineurin inhibitor dosage
Alternative methods for monitoring graft function
Non-invasive detection of rejection or infection

KEY AREAS FOR RESEARCH IN LUNG TRANSPLANTATION

Space limitations prevent a full discussion of current research in lung transplantation, but a list of some of the most important fields of research is presented in Table 21.6.

CONCLUSIONS

Lung transplantation is now an established, accepted treatment option for children and adults with end-stage CF lung disease, which extends life and improves quality of life in appropriately selected patients. Outcomes are steadily improving, but they remain poorer than for other solid-organ transplants. Lung transplant recipients are committed to lifelong medication and monitoring. As outcomes continue to improve, and the number of long-term survivors increases, more CF physicians and pediatricians will need to be involved with the shared care of these patients.

REFERENCES

1. Trulock EP, Edwards LB, Taylor DO *et al*. Registry of the International Society for Heart and Lung Transplantation: twenty-second official adult lung and heart–lung transplant report, 2005. *J Heart Lung Transplant* 2005; **24**:956–967.

2. Boucek MM, Edwards LB, Keck BM *et al*. Registry of the International Society for Heart and Lung Transplantation: eighth official pediatric report, 2005. *J Heart Lung Transplant* 2005; **24**:968–982.

3. Aurora P, Lynn IM. Lung transplantation and end of life issues in cystic fibrosis. *Paediatr Respir Rev* 2000; **1**:114–120.

4. Aurora P. When should children be referred for lung or heart–lung transplantation? *Pediatr Pulmonol Suppl* 2004; **26**:116–118.

5. Minai OA, Budev MM. Referral for lung transplantation: a moving target. *Chest* 2005; **127**:705–707.

6. Steinman TI, Becker BN, Frost AE *et al*. Guidelines for the referral and management of patients eligible for solid organ transplantation. *Transplantation* 2001; **71**:1189–1204.

7. American Society for Transplant Physicians (ASTP) / American Thoracic Society (ATS)/European Respiratory Society (ERS)/ International Society for Heart and Lung Transplantation (ISHLT). International guidelines for the selection of lung transplant candidates. *Am J Respir Crit Care Med* 1998; **158**:335–339.

8. Maurer JR, Frost AE, Estenne M *et al*. for the International Society for Heart and Lung Transplantation, the American Thoracic Society, the American Society of Transplant Physicians, and the European Respiratory Society. International guidelines for the selection of lung transplant candidates. *Transplantation* 1998; **66**:951–956.

9. Yankaskas JR, Mallory GBJ. Lung transplantation in cystic fibrosis: consensus conference statement. *Chest* 1998; **113**:217–226.

10. Kerem E, Reisman J, Corey M *et al*. Prediction of mortality in patients with cystic fibrosis. *N Engl J Med* 1992; **326**:1187–1191.

11. Mayer-Hamblett N, Rosenfeld M, Emerson J *et al*. Developing cystic fibrosis lung transplant referral criteria using predictors of 2-year mortality. *Am J Respir Crit Care Med* 2002; **166**(12 Pt 1):1550–1555.

12. Noone PG, Egan TM. Cystic fibrosis: when to refer for lung transplantation – is the answer clear? *Am J Respir Crit Care Med* 2002; **166**(12 Pt 1):1531–1532.

13. Powers PM, Gerstle R, Lapey A. Adolescents with cystic fibrosis: family reports of adolescent health-related quality of life and forced expiratory volume in one second. *Pediatrics* 2001; **107**:E70.

14. Studer SM, Krishnan JA, Orens JB. Indications for lung transplant referral: physician attitudes. *J Heart Lung Transplant* 2002; **21**:716–717.

15. Vizza CD, Yusen RD, Lynch JP *et al*. Outcome of patients with cystic fibrosis awaiting lung transplantation. *Am J Respir Crit Care Med* 2000; **162**:819–825.

16. Aurora P, Wade A, Whitmore P, Whitehead B. A model for predicting life expectancy of children with cystic fibrosis. *Eur Respir J* 2000; **16**:1056–1060.

17. Smeritschnig B, Jaksch P, Kocher A *et al*. Quality of life after lung transplantation: a cross-sectional study. *J Heart Lung Transplant* 2005; **24**:474–480.

18. Modi AC, Quittner AL. Validation of a disease-specific measure of health-related quality of life for children with cystic fibrosis. *J Pediatr Psychol* 2003; **28**:535–545.

19. Quittner AL. Measurement of quality of life in cystic fibrosis. *Curr Opin Pulm Med* 1998; **4**:326–331.

20. Quittner AL, Buu A, Messer MA *et al*. Development and validation of the Cystic Fibrosis Questionnaire in the United States: a health-related quality-of-life measure for cystic fibrosis. *Chest* 2005; **128**:2347–2354.

21. Aris RM, Routh JC, LiPuma JJ *et al*. Lung transplantation for cystic fibrosis patients with *Burkholderia cepacia* complex: survival linked to genomovar type. *Am J Respir Crit Care Med* 2001; **164**:2102–2106.

22. De Soyza A, McDowell A, Archer L *et al*. *Burkholderia cepacia* complex genomovars and pulmonary transplantation outcomes in patients with cystic fibrosis. *Lancet* 2001; **358**:1780–1781.

23. Miranda B, Canon J, Cuende N *et al*. Organ shortage and the organisation of organ allocation. In: Boe J, Estenne M, Weder W (eds) *European Respiratory Monograph 26: Lung Transplantation*. Sheffield, UK, ERS Journals Ltd, 2006; ch. 6.

24. Orens JB, Boehler A, de Perrot M *et al.* A review of lung transplant donor acceptability criteria. *J Heart Lung Transplant* 2003; **22**:1183–1200.

25. Koukoulis G, Caldwell R, Inokawa H *et al.* Trends in lung pH and PO$_2$ after circulatory arrest: implications for non-heart-beating donors and cell culture models of lung ischemia–reperfusion injury. *J Heart Lung Transplant* 2005; **24**:2218–2225.

26. Egan TM, Kotloff RM. Pro/Con debate: lung allocation should be based on medical urgency and transplant survival and not on waiting time. *Chest* 2005; **128**:407–415.

27. Egan TM. Non-heart-beating donors in thoracic transplantation. *J Heart Lung Transplant* 2004; **23**:3–10.

28. Paik HC, Hoffmann SC, Egan TM. Pulmonary preservation studies: effects on endothelial function and pulmonary adenine nucleotides. *Transplantation* 2003; **75**:439–444.

29. Kiser AC, Ciriaco P, Hoffmann SC, Egan TM. Lung retrieval from non-heart beating cadavers with the use of a rat lung transplant model. *J Thorac Cardiovasc Surg* 2001; **122**:18–23.

30. Hoffmann SC, Bleiweis MS, Jones DR *et al.* Maintenance of cAMP in non-heart-beating donor lungs reduces ischemia–reperfusion injury. *Am J Respir Crit Care Med* 2001; **163**:1642–1647.

31. Jones DR, Becker RM, Hoffmann SC *et al.* When does the lung die? Kfc, cell viability, and adenine nucleotide changes in the circulation-arrested rat lung. *J Appl Physiol* 1997; **83**:247–252.

32. D'Armini AM, Tom EJ, Roberts CS *et al.* When does the lung die? Time course of high energy phosphate depletion and relationship to lung viability after 'death'. *J Surg Res* 1995; **59**:468–474.

33. Sundaresan S, Semenkovich J, Ochoa L *et al.* Successful outcome of lung transplantation is not compromised by the use of marginal donor lungs. *J Thorac Cardiovasc Surg* 1995; **109**:1075–1079.

34. Bhorade SM, Vigneswaran W, McCabe MA, Garrity ER. Liberalization of donor criteria may expand the donor pool without adverse consequence in lung transplantation. *J Heart Lung Transplant* 2000; **19**:1199–1204.

35. Pierre AF, Sekine Y, Hutcheon MA *et al.* Marginal donor lungs: a reassessment. *J Thorac Cardiovasc Surg* 2002; **123**:421–427.

36. Ware LB, Wang Y, Fang X *et al.* Assessment of lungs rejected for transplantation and implications for donor selection. *Lancet* 2002; **360**:619–620.

37. de Perrot M, Bonser RS, Dark J *et al.* Report of the ISHLT Working Group on Primary Lung Graft Dysfunction. III: Donor-related risk factors and markers. *J Heart Lung Transplant* 2005; **24**:1460–467.

38. Fisher AJ, Donnelly SC, Pritchard G *et al.* Objective assessment of criteria for selection of donor lungs suitable for transplantation. *Thorax* 2004; **59**:434–437.

39. Hosenpud JD, Bennett LE, Keck BM *et al.* Effect of diagnosis on survival benefit of lung transplantation for end-stage lung disease. *Lancet* 1998; **351**:24–27.

40. Williams TJ, Snell GI. Organ procurement: strategies to optimize donor availability. *Semin Respir Crit Care Med* 2001; **22**:541–550.

41. Studer SM, Orens JB. Cadaveric donor selection and management. *Respir Care Clin N Am* 2004; **10**:459–471.

42. Barr ML, Schenkel FA, Bowdish ME, Starnes VA. Living donor lobar lung transplantation: current status and future directions. *Transplant Proc* 2005; **37**:3983–3986.

43. Wells WJ, Barr ML. The ethics of living donor lung transplantation. *Thorac Surg Clin* 2005; **15**:519–525.

44. Starnes VA, Barr ML, Cohen RG *et al.* Living-donor lobar lung transplantation experience: intermediate results. *J Thorac Cardiovasc Surg* 1996; **112**:1284–1290.

45. Goldsmith MF. Mother to child: first living donor lung transplant. *J Am Med Assoc* 1990; **264**:2724.

46. Snell GI, Bennetts K, Bartolo J *et al.* Body mass index as a predictor of survival in adults with cystic fibrosis referred for lung transplantation. *J Heart Lung Transplant* 1998; **17**:1097–1103.

47. Madden BP, Kariyawasam H, Siddiqi AJ *et al.* Noninvasive ventilation in cystic fibrosis patients with acute or chronic respiratory failure. *Eur Respir J* 2002; **19**:310–313.

48. Calne RY, Rolles K, White DJ *et al.* Cyclosporin A initially as the only immunosuppressant in 34 recipients of cadaveric organs: 32 kidneys, 2 pancreases, and 2 livers. *Lancet* 1979; **2**:1033–1036.

49. Calne RY, White DJ, Thiru S *et al.* Cyclosporin A in patients receiving renal allografts from cadaver donors. *Lancet* 1978; **2**:1323–1327.

50. Brock MV, Borja MC, Ferber L *et al.* Induction therapy in lung transplantation: a prospective, controlled clinical trial comparing OKT3, anti-thymocyte globulin, and daclizumab. *J Heart Lung Transplant* 2001; **20**:1282–1290.

51. Garrity ER, Villanueva J, Bhorade SM *et al.* Low rate of acute lung allograft rejection after the use of daclizumab, an interleukin 2 receptor antibody. *Transplantation* 2001; **71**:773–777.

52. Dobbin C, Maley M, Harkness J *et al.* The impact of pan-resistant bacterial pathogens on survival after lung transplantation in cystic fibrosis: results from a single large referral centre. *J Hosp Infect* 2004; **56**:277–282.

53. De Soyza A, Archer L, Wardle J *et al.* Pulmonary transplantation for cystic fibrosis: pre-transplant recipient characteristics in patients dying of peri-operative sepsis. *J Heart Lung Transplant* 2003; **22**:764–769.

54. Helmi M, Love RB, Welter D *et al. Aspergillus* infection in lung transplant recipients with cystic fibrosis: risk factors and outcomes comparison to other types of transplant recipients. *Chest* 2003; **123**:800–808.

55. Palmer SM, Alexander BD, Sanders LL *et al.* Significance of blood stream infection after lung transplantation: analysis in 176 consecutive patients. *Transplantation* 2000; **69**:2360–2366.

56. Snell GI, Kotsimbos TC, Levvey BJ *et al.* Pharmacokinetic assessment of oral ganciclovir in lung transplant recipients with cystic fibrosis. *J Antimicrob Chemother* 2000; **45**:511–516.

57. Kesten S, Chaparro C. Mycobacterial infections in lung transplant recipients. *Chest* 1999; **115**:741–745.

58. Nunley DR, Ohori P, Grgurich WF *et al.* Pulmonary aspergillosis in cystic fibrosis lung transplant recipients. *Chest* 1998; **114**:1321–1329.

59. Nunley DR, Grgurich W, Iacono AT *et al.* Allograft colonization and infections with *Pseudomonas* in cystic fibrosis lung transplant recipients. *Chest* 1998; **113**:1235–1243.

60. Egan JJ, Woodcock AA, Webb AK. Management of cystic fibrosis before and after lung transplantation. *J Roy Soc Med* 1997; **90**(Suppl 31):47–58.

61. Meyers BF, de la Morena M, Sweet SC *et al.* Primary graft dysfunction and other selected complications of lung transplantation: a single-center experience of 983 patients. *J Thorac Cardiovasc Surg* 2005; **129**:1421–1429.

62. Christie JD, Sager JS, Kimmel SE *et al.* Impact of primary graft failure on outcomes following lung transplantation. *Chest* 2005; **127**:161–165.

63. Christie JD, Kotloff RM, Pochettino A *et al.* Clinical risk factors for primary graft failure following lung transplantation. *Chest* 2003; **124**:1232–1241.

64. de Perrot M, Liu M, Waddell TK, Keshavjee S. Ischemia–reperfusion-induced lung injury. *Am J Respir Crit Care Med* 2003; **167**:490–511.

65. Thabut G, Vinatier I, Stern JB *et al.* Primary graft failure following lung transplantation:predictive factors of mortality. *Chest* 2002; **121**:1876–1882.

66. Hoffman TM, Spray TL, Gaynor JW *et al.* Survival after acute graft failure in pediatric thoracic organ transplant recipients. *Pediatr Transplant* 2000; **4**:112–117.

67. Hartwig MG, Appel JZ, Cantu E *et al.* Improved results treating lung allograft failure with venous extracorporeal membrane oxygenation. *Ann Thorac Surg* 2005; **80**:1872–1879.

68. Levy G, Thervet E, Lake J, Uchida K. Patient management by Neoral C(2) monitoring: an international consensus statement. *Transplantation* 2002; **73**:S12–S18.

69. Nashan B, Cole E, Levy G, Thervet E. Clinical validation studies of Neoral C(2) monitoring: a review. *Transplantation* 2002; **73**:S3–S11.

70. Knoll GA, Bell RC. Tacrolimus versus cyclosporin for immunosuppression in renal transplantation: meta-analysis of randomised trials. *Br Med J* 1999; **318**:1104–1107.

71. Treede H, Klepetko W, Reichenspurner H *et al.* Tacrolimus versus cyclosporine after lung transplantation: a prospective, open, randomized two-center trial comparing two different immunosuppressive protocols. *J Heart Lung Transplant* 2001; **20**:511–517.

72. Keenan RJ, Konishi H, Kawai A *et al.* Clinical trial of tacrolimus versus cyclosporine in lung transplantation. *Ann Thorac Surg* 1995; **60**:580–584.

73. Halloran P, Mathew T, Tomlanovich S *et al.* for the International Mycophenolate Mofetil Renal Transplant Study Groups. Mycophenolate mofetil in renal allograft recipients: a pooled efficacy analysis of three randomized, double-blind, clinical studies in prevention of rejection. *Transplantation* 1997; **63**:39–47.

74. Kobashigawa J, Miller L, Renlund D *et al.* for the Mycophenolate Mofetil Investigators. A randomized active-controlled trial of mycophenolate mofetil in heart transplant recipients. *Transplantation* 1998; **66**:507–515.

75. Palmer SM, Baz MA, Sanders L *et al.* Results of a randomized, prospective, multicenter trial of mycophenolate mofetil versus azathioprine in the prevention of acute lung allograft rejection. *Transplantation* 2001; **71**:1772–1776.

76. Shitrit D, Ollech JE, Ollech A *et al.* Itraconazole prophylaxis in lung transplant recipients receiving tacrolimus (FK 506): efficacy and drug interaction. *J Heart Lung Transplant* 2005; **24**:2148–2152.

77. Dummer JS, Lazariashvilli N, Barnes J *et al.* A survey of anti-fungal management in lung transplantation. *J Heart Lung Transplant* 2004; **23**:1376–1381.

78. Monforte V, Roman A, Gavalda J *et al.* Nebulized amphotericin B concentration and distribution in the respiratory tract of lung-transplanted patients. *Transplantation* 2003; **75**:1571–1574.

79. Minari A, Husni R, Avery RK *et al.* The incidence of invasive aspergillosis among solid organ transplant recipients and implications for prophylaxis in lung transplants. *Transpl Infect Dis* 2002; **4**:195–200.

80. Casey P, Garrett J, Eaton T. Allergic bronchopulmonary aspergillosis in a lung transplant patient successfully treated with nebulized amphotericin. *J Heart Lung Transplant* 2002; **21**:1237–1241.

81. Monforte V, Roman A, Gavalda J *et al.* Nebulized amphotericin B prophylaxis for *Aspergillus* infection in lung transplantation: study of risk factors. *J Heart Lung Transplant* 2001; **20**:1274–1281.

82. Palmer SM, Drew RH, Whitehouse JD *et al.* Safety of aerosolized amphotericin B lipid complex in lung transplant recipients. *Transplantation* 2001; **72**:545–548.

83. Humar A, Kumar D, Preiksaitis J *et al.* A trial of valganciclovir prophylaxis for cytomegalovirus prevention in lung transplant recipients. *Am J Transplant* 2005; **5**:1462–1468.

84. Fellay J, Venetz JP, Aubert JD *et al.* Treatment of cytomegalovirus infection or disease in solid organ transplant recipients with valganciclovir. *Transplant Proc* 2005; **37**:949–951.

85. Danziger-Isakov LA, Faro A, Sweet S *et al.* Variability in standard care for cytomegalovirus prevention and detection in pediatric lung transplantation: survey of eight pediatric lung transplant programs. *Pediatr Transplant* 2003; **7**:469–473.

86. Faul JL, Akindipe OA, Berry GJ *et al.* Recurrent *Pneumocystis carinii* colonization in a heart–lung transplant recipient on long-term trimethoprim–sulfamethoxazole prophylaxis. *J Heart Lung Transplant* 1999; **18**:384–387.

87. Kramer MR, Stoehr C, Lewiston NJ *et al.* Trimethoprim–sulfamethoxazole prophylaxis for *Pneumocystis carinii* infections in heart–lung and lung transplantation: how effective and for how long? *Transplantation* 1992; **53**:586–589.

88. De Vito DA, Hoffman LA, Iacono AT *et al.* Are symptom reports useful for differentiating between acute rejection and pulmonary infection after lung transplantation? *Heart Lung* 2004; **33**:372–380.

89. Morlion B, Knoop C, Paiva M, Estenne M. Internet-based home monitoring of pulmonary function after lung transplantation. *Am J Respir Crit Care Med* 2002; **165**:694–697.

90. Brugiere O, Thabut G, Mal H *et al.* Exhaled NO may predict the decline in lung function in bronchiolitis obliterans syndrome. *Eur Respir J* 2005; **25**:813–819.

91. Verleden GM, Dupont LJ, Van Raemdonck DE, Vanhaecke J. Accuracy of exhaled nitric oxide measurements for the diagnosis of bronchiolitis obliterans syndrome after lung transplantation. *Transplantation* 2004; **78**:730–733.

92. Verleden GM, Dupont LJ, Delcroix M *et al.* Exhaled nitric oxide after lung transplantation: impact of the native lung. *Eur Respir J* 2003; **21**:429–432.

93. Gabbay E, Walters EH, Orsida B *et al.* Post-lung transplant bronchiolitis obliterans syndrome (BOS) is characterized by increased exhaled nitric oxide levels and epithelial inducible nitric oxide synthase. *Am J Respir Crit Care Med* 2000; **162**:2182–2187.

94. Yousem SA, Berry GJ, Cagle PT *et al.* for the Lung Rejection Study Group. Revision of the 1990 working formulation for the classification of pulmonary allograft rejection. *J Heart Lung Transplant* 1996; **15**:1–15.

95. Hachem RR, Khalifah AP, Chakinala MM *et al.* The significance of a single episode of minimal acute rejection after lung transplantation. *Transplantation* 2005; **80**:1406–1413.

96. Hopkins PM, Aboyoun CL, Chhajed PN *et al.* Association of minimal rejection in lung transplant recipients with obliterative bronchiolitis. *Am J Respir Crit Care Med* 2004; **170**:1022–1026.

97. Chhajed PN, Aboyoun C, Malouf MA *et al.* Risk factors and management of bleeding associated with transbronchial lung biopsy in lung transplant recipients. *J Heart Lung Transplant* 2003; **22**:195–197.

98. Hopkins PM, Aboyoun CL, Chhajed PN *et al.* Prospective analysis of 1235 transbronchial lung biopsies in lung transplant recipients. *J Heart Lung Transplant* 2002; **21**:1062–1067.

99. Tamm M, Sharples LD, Higenbottam TW *et al.* Bronchiolitis obliterans syndrome in heart–lung transplantation: surveillance biopsies. *Am J Respir Crit Care Med* 1997; **155**:1705–1710.

100. Husain AN, Siddiqui MT, Holmes EW *et al.* Analysis of risk factors for the development of bronchiolitis obliterans syndrome. *Am J Respir Crit Care Med* 1999; **159**:829–833.

101. Lehto JT, Koskinen PK, Anttila VJ *et al.* Bronchoscopy in the diagnosis and surveillance of respiratory infections in lung and heart–lung transplant recipients. *Transpl Int* 2005; **18**:562–571.

102. Starobin D, Fink G, Shitrit D *et al.* The role of fiberoptic bronchoscopy evaluating transplant recipients with suspected pulmonary infections: analysis of 168 cases in a multi-organ transplantation center. *Transplant Proc* 2003; **35**:659–660.

103. Chan KM, Allen SA. Infectious pulmonary complications in lung transplant recipients. *Semin Respir Infect* 2002; **17**:291–302.

104. Mallory GB. Inflammation in lung transplantation for CF: immunosuppression and modulation of inflammation. *Clin Rev Allergy Immunol* 2002; **23**:105–122.

105. Choong CK, Sweet SC, Zoole JB *et al.* Bronchial airway anastomotic complications after pediatric lung transplantation: incidence, cause, management, and outcome. *J Thorac Cardiovasc Surg* 2006; **131**:198–203.

106. Mughal MM, Gildea TR, Murthy S *et al.* Short-term deployment of self-expanding metallic stents facilitates healing of bronchial dehiscence. *Am J Respir Crit Care Med* 2005; **172**:768–771.

107. Paulson EC, Singhal S, Kucharczuk JC *et al.* Bronchial sleeve resection for posttransplant stricture. *Ann Thorac Surg* 2003; **76**:2075–2076.

108. Aigner C, Jaksch P, Seebacher G *et al.* Single running suture: the new standard technique for bronchial anastomoses in lung transplantation. *Eur J Cardiothorac Surg* 2003; **23**:488–493.

109. Herrera JM, McNeil KD, Higgins RS *et al.* Airway complications after lung transplantation: treatment and long-term outcome. *Ann Thorac Surg* 2001; **71**:989–993.

110. Mayse ML, Greenheck J, Friedman M, Kovitz KL. Successful bronchoscopic balloon dilation of nonmalignant tracheobronchial obstruction without fluoroscopy. *Chest* 2004; **126**:634–637.

111. Mulligan MS. Endoscopic management of airway complications after lung transplantation. *Chest Surg Clin N Am* 2001; **11**:907–915.

112. Chhajed PN, Malouf MA, Glanville AR. Bronchoscopic dilatation in the management of benign (non-transplant) tracheobronchial stenosis. *Intern Med J* 2001; **31**:512–516.

113. Orons PD, Amesur NB, Dauber JH *et al.* Balloon dilation and endobronchial stent placement for bronchial strictures after lung transplantation. *J Vasc Interv Radiol* 2000; **11**:89–99.

114. Craig FE, Gulley ML, Banks PM. Posttransplantation lymphoproliferative disorders. *Am J Clin Pathol* 1993; **99**:265–276.

115. Ho M, Jaffe R, Miller G *et al.* The frequency of Epstein–Barr virus infection and associated lymphoproliferative syndrome after transplantation and its manifestations in children. *Transplantation* 1988; **45**:719–727.

116. Kotloff RM, Ahya VN. Medical complications of lung transplantation. *Eur Respir J* 2004; **23**:334–342.

117. Snell GI, Levvey BJ, Chin W *et al.* Sirolimus allows renal recovery in lung and heart transplant recipients with chronic renal impairment. *J Heart Lung Transplant* 2002; **21**:540–546.

118. Cooper JD, Billingham M, Egan T *et al.* for the International Society for Heart and Lung Transplantation. A working formulation for the standardization of nomenclature and for clinical staging of chronic dysfunction in lung allografts. *J Heart Lung Transplant* 1993; **12**:713–716.

119. Estenne M, Maurer JR, Boehler A *et al.* Bronchiolitis obliterans syndrome 2001: an update of the diagnostic criteria. *J Heart Lung Transplant* 2002; **21**:297–310.

120. Hartwig MG, Appel JZ, Li B *et al.* Chronic aspiration of gastric fluid accelerates pulmonary allograft dysfunction in a rat model of lung transplantation. *J Thorac Cardiovasc Surg* 2006; **131**:209–217.

121. Button BM, Roberts S, Kotsimbos TC *et al.* Gastroesophageal reflux (symptomatic and silent): a potentially significant problem in patients with cystic fibrosis before and after lung transplantation. *J Heart Lung Transplant* 2005; **24**:1522–1529.

122. Benden C, Aurora P, Curry J *et al.* High prevalence of gastroesophageal reflux in children after lung transplantation. *Pediatr Pulmonol* 2005; **40**:68–71.

123. Young LR, Hadjiliadis D, Davis RD, Palmer SM. Lung transplantation exacerbates gastroesophageal reflux disease. *Chest* 2003; **124**:1689–1693.

124. Rinaldi M, Martinelli L, Volpato G *et al.* Gastro-esophageal reflux as cause of obliterative bronchiolitis: a case report. *Transplant Proc* 1995; **27**:2006–2007.

125. Hartwig MG, Appel JZ, Davis RD. Antireflux surgery in the setting of lung transplantation: strategies for treating gastroesophageal reflux disease in a high-risk population. *Thorac Surg Clin* 2005; **15**:417–427.

126. O'Halloran EK, Reynolds JD, Lau CL *et al.* Laparoscopic Nissen fundoplication for treating reflux in lung transplant recipients. *J Gastrointest Surg* 2004; **8**:132–137.

127. Davis RD, Lau CL, Eubanks S *et al.* Improved lung allograft function after fundoplication in patients with gastroesophageal reflux disease undergoing lung transplantation. *J Thorac Cardiovasc Surg* 2003; **125**:533–542.

128. Palmer SM, Miralles AP, Howell DN *et al.* Gastroesophageal reflux as a reversible cause of allograft dysfunction after lung transplantation. *Chest* 2000; **118**:1214–1217.

129. Shitrit D, Bendayan D, Gidon S *et al.* Long-term azithromycin use for treatment of bronchiolitis obliterans syndrome in lung transplant recipients. *J Heart Lung Transplant* 2005; **24**:1440–1443.

130. Yates B, Murphy DM, Forrest IA *et al.* Azithromycin reverses airflow obstruction in established bronchiolitis obliterans syndrome. *Am J Respir Crit Care Med* 2005; **172**:772–775.

131. Verleden GM, Dupont LJ. Azithromycin therapy for patients with bronchiolitis obliterans syndrome after lung transplantation. *Transplantation* 2004; **77**:1465–1467.

132. Estenne M, Van Muylem A, Knoop C, Antoine M. Detection of obliterative bronchiolitis after lung transplantation by indexes of ventilation distribution. *Am J Respir Crit Care Med* 2000; **162**:1047–1051.

133. Brugiere O, Thabut G, Castier Y *et al.* Lung retransplantation for bronchiolitis obliterans syndrome: long-term follow-up in a series of 15 recipients. *Chest* 2003; **123**:1832–1837.

134. Kotloff RM. Lung retransplantation:all for one or one for all? *Chest* 2003; **123**:1781–1782.

135. Huddleston CB, Mendeloff EN, Cohen AH *et al.* Lung retransplantation in children. *Ann Thorac Surg* 1998; **66**:199–203.

136. Novick RJ. Heart and lung retransplantation: should it be done? *J Heart Lung Transplant* 1998; **17**:635–642.

137. Cox DR, Oakes D. *Analysis of Survival Data*. London, Chapman & Hall, 1984.

138. Turnbull BW, Brown BW, Hu M. Survivorship analysis of heart transplant survival data. *J Am Stat Assoc* 1974; **69**:74–80.

139. Charman SC, Sharples LD, McNeil KD, Wallwork J. Assessment of survival benefit after lung transplantation by patient diagnosis. *J Heart Lung Transplant* 2002; **21**:226–232.

140. Groen H, van der Bij W, Koeter GH, TenVergert EM. Cost-effectiveness of lung transplantation in relation to type of end-stage pulmonary disease. *Am J Transplant* 2004; **4**:1155–1162.

141. Sharples L, Hathaway T, Dennis C *et al.* Prognosis of patients with cystic fibrosis awaiting heart and lung transplantation. *J Heart Lung Transplant* 1993; **12**:669–674.

142. Aurora P, Whitehead B, Wade A *et al.* Lung transplantation and life extension in children with cystic fibrosis. *Lancet* 1999; **354**:1591–1593.

143. Liou TG, Adler FR, Cahill BC *et al.* Survival effect of lung transplantation among patients with cystic fibrosis. *J Am Med Assoc* 2001; **286**:2683–2689.

144. Liou TG, Adler FR, Huang D. Use of lung transplantation survival models to refine patient selection in cystic fibrosis. *Am J Respir Crit Care Med* 2005; **171**:1053–1059.

145. Kalbfleisch JD, Prentice RL. *The Statistical Analysis of Failure Time Data*. New York, Wiley, 1980.

146. Rodrigue JR, Baz MA. Are there sex differences in health-related quality of life after lung transplantation for chronic obstructive pulmonary disease? *J Heart Lung Transplant* 2006; **25**:120–125.

147. Kugler C, Fischer S, Gottlieb J *et al.* Health-related quality of life in two hundred-eighty lung transplant recipients. *J Heart Lung Transplant* 2005; **24**:2262–2268.

148. Gerbase MW, Spiliopoulos A, Rochat T *et al.* Health-related quality of life following single or bilateral lung transplantation: a 7-year comparison to functional outcome. *Chest* 2005; **128**:1371–1378.

149. Rodrigue JR, Baz MA, Kanasky WF, MacNaughton KL. Does lung transplantation improve health-related quality of life? The University of Florida experience. *J Heart Lung Transplant* 2005; **24**:755–763.

150. Smeritschnig B, Jaksch P, Kocher A *et al.* Quality of life after lung transplantation: a cross-sectional study. *J Heart Lung Transplant* 2005; **24**:474–480.

151. Aurora P, Stocks J, Oliver C *et al.* Quality control for spirometry in pre-school children with and without lung disease. *Am J Respir Crit Care Med* 2004; **169**:1152–1159.

152. Baraldi E, de Jongste JC. Measurement of exhaled nitric oxide in children, 2001. *Eur Respir J* 2002; **20**:223–237.

153. Gustafsson PM, Aurora P, Lindblad A. Evaluation of ventilation maldistribution as an early indicator of lung disease in children with cystic fibrosis. *Eur Respir J* 2003; **22**:972–979.

154. Faro A, Visner G. The use of multiple transbronchial biopsies as the standard approach to evaluate lung allograft rejection. *Pediatr Transplant* 2004; **8**:322–328.

155. Kuhn JP, Slovis TL, Haller JO. *Caffey's Pediatric Diagnostic Imaging*, 10th edn. Philadelphia, Mosby, 2004.

156. Stark K, Gunther M, Schonfeld C *et al.* Immunisations in solid-organ transplant recipients. *Lancet* 2002; **359**:957–965.

157. Green M, Webber S. Posttransplantation lymphoproliferative disorders. *Pediatr Clin N Am* 2003; **50**:1471–1491.

158. Benden C, Aurora P, Burch M *et al.* Monitoring of Epstein–Barr viral load in pediatric heart and lung transplant recipients by real-time polymerase chain reaction. *J Heart Lung Transplant* 2005; **24**:2103–2108.

159. Saland JM. Osseous complications of pediatric transplantation. *Pediatr Transplant* 2004; **8**:400–415.

160. Fine RN. Growth following solid-organ transplantation. *Pediatr Transplant* 2002; **6**:47–52.

161. Acott PD, Pernica JM. Growth hormone therapy before and after pediatric renal transplant. *Pediatr Transplant* 2003; **7**:426–440.

162. Cohen AH, Mallory GBJ, Ross K *et al.* Growth of lungs after transplantation in infants and in children younger than 3 years of age. *Am J Respir Crit Care Med* 1999; **159**:1747–1751.

163. Wray J, Radley-Smith R. Beyond the first year after pediatric heart or heart–lung transplantation: changes in cognitive function and behavior. *Pediatr Transplant* 2005; **9**:170–177.

164. Durst CL, Horn MV, MacLaughlin EF *et al.* Psychosocial responses of adolescent cystic fibrosis patients to lung transplantation. *Pediatr Transplant* 2001; **5**:27–31.

PART 5

MONITORING

22 Using databases to improve care   311
    Sheila G. McKenzie and Margaret E. Hodson

23a Infant and pre-school children: lung function   321
    Sarath Ranganathan

23b Infant and pre-school children: role of bronchoscopy   331
    Gary Connett

23c Infant and pre-school children: imaging the lungs   337
    Samatha Sonnappa and Catherine M. Owens

24 Physiological monitoring of older children and adults   345
    Mark Rosenthal

25a Exercise: testing   353
    David M. Orenstein and Wolfgang Gruber

25b Exercise: use in therapy   361
    David M. Orenstein and Linda W. Higgins

26 Clinical outcome measures to assess new treatments for CF lung disease 375
    Jane C. Davies and Eric W.F.W. Alton: on behalf of the UK CF Gene Therapy Consortium

22

Using databases to improve care

SHEILA G. MCKENZIE AND MARGARET E. HODSON

OBSERVATIONAL DATA VERSUS RANDOMIZED CONTROLLED TRIALS

Although randomized controlled clinical trials (RCTs) are the gold standard in assessing the efficacy of any medical intervention, these can be impractical in cystic fibrosis (CF) for several reasons:

- The number of patients required to provide the statistical power necessary to detect the difference between treatment and control groups may be so large that a multicenter study is required, with the attendant logistic difficulties.
- The desired outcome measure may be attained only after long-term follow-up of individual patients, implying that the rigors of a controlled trial must be maintained for many years.
- The protocol for a long-term trial must be flexible enough to accommodate the changing medical needs of patients over time, but rigorous enough to maintain the integrity of the hypothesis being tested.
- Results from RCTs can properly be extrapolated only to the population of CF patients with the same characteristics as those entering the trial. In a rapidly changing field like CF the entry characteristics of trial subjects may be irrelevant by the time a long-term trial is completed.

For these reasons it appears that some of the most crucial questions on the efficacy of interventions in improving the quality and duration of life for CF patients are scarcely amenable to RCT. Observational data are therefore particularly valuable in CF because they provide the opportunity to assess the association between changes in outcomes and changes in treatment regimens without subjecting patients to specific trial protocols.

Study design

Observational databases can document treatments and outcomes and, to a limited extent, the relationships between them. The principal difference from RCTs is that patients are not randomized to treatments and this shortcoming cannot be overcome. On the other hand, readily accessible observational data can be analyzed relatively quickly and cheaply to highlight apparent associations and generate hypotheses for further testing. The key is not to over-interpret associations as implying causality, but to test any hypotheses generated in future studies. The hierarchy of different research designs to answer a clinical question convincingly, from case reports as the least powerful to RCTs at the top of the hierarchy, is shown in Table 22.1 [1].

The value of observational databases lies in their non-exclusivity; i.e. all eligible patients are included regardless of specific interventions or outcomes. While a small database can yield valuable information on the population of patients included in it (e.g. all those from a particular clinic), multicenter data gain validity for the CF population at large and the largest databases can arguably represent the entire CF

Table 22.1 Hierarchy of study designs from highest to lowest.

Analytic studies
Randomized controlled trials (RCTs)
Observational studies
– cohort analysis
  • prospective
  • retrospective
– case–control studies

Descriptive studies
Population correlational studies
Cross-sectional surveys (sample or whole population)
Case reports and case series (selected individuals)

Adapted from [1].

population. The intent of CF registries is to include, within a single database, the entire population of CF patients within a defined geographical area. It should be noted that the disadvantage of such an approach is that treatment differences between centers may mask disease effects.

Prospectively collected data are items that are entered into a database routinely as they occur and may include only items that are considered to be of specific interest (see later under Choice of data items for collection). Retrospective data collection implies a search through medical records for data that were not routinely collected in one source. As opposed to prospective data, retrospectively collected data may be incomplete and subject to ascertainment bias; i.e. uncontrolled factors may influence whether or not the event was recorded at all. Therefore, prospectively collected data have a higher intrinsic value than retrospectively collected data.

Because observational studies are not randomized, they are unable per se to ascribe a cause-and-effect relationship between a specific intervention and an outcome. In real life (which observational databases can describe very well) many factors, some of which are unsuspected, contribute to a particular outcome. Descriptive (cross-sectional or correlational) studies provide a 'snapshot' in time about disease status and exposure to risks and/or treatments that cannot distinguish between cause and effect. However, they can discover significant correlations and generate useful hypotheses.

Case–control studies begin by identifying a series of patients with a specific outcome (cases) and a matched group of similar patients without that outcome (controls). Previous exposure to specified risks or treatments is then compared between the groups. The critical assumption in this type of analysis is that all potential risk factors are identified in advance and the control group is well matched in all respects other than exposure to the factor(s) under investigation. The odds ratio (OR) is the change in risk that is calculated to be caused by exposure to the investigational factor(s) if the assumptions of the analysis are valid. Because case–control analysis depends more on existing concepts of what is relevant to the outcome under study, it is lower in the hierarchy than cohort analysis.

Cohort analyses compare outcomes in groups of patients known to have been previously exposed versus unexposed to a specific risk or treatment. This is the highest form of observational analysis and most closely resembles RCT design except that assignment to treatment is not at random. A database containing all relevant data collected prospectively is the ideal source for this type of study, but retrospectively collected data may also be used even if it is less reliable. Other factors that may contribute to outcome(s) of interest, if they are reliably recorded, can be assessed in the statistical analysis (see later under Data analysis options). The relative risk is the change in likelihood of a particular outcome that is calculated to be due to the specific exposure if all other risk factors have been accounted for in the analysis. For example, a perfect analysis of the impact of a specific drug treatment on survival would consider all other factors contributing to mortality in CF; in an adequately powered RCT these can be assumed to be randomly distributed between treatment and control groups.

Both case–control and cohort analyses attempt to create credible treatment and control groups by matching cofactors that may contribute to the outcome(s) in question. Ultimately, however, no observational study can compensate for its lack of randomization because prescription of any treatment in daily practice is the result of a series of circumstances that depends in large part on the patient's status, and outcomes depend to some extent on unrecorded and possibly unrecognized factors including the 'placebo effect'. If, for example, a specific antibiotic is routinely prescribed upon acquisition of a particular micro-organism, it will be impossible from observational data to distinguish the result of antibiotic prescription from that of organism acquisition. This problem is called confounding, and confounding by indication is the situation whereby a treatment and the reason for its initiation are inextricably linked. Because of confounding by indication and undocumented factors that influence outcomes, RCTs remain the gold standard for assessing treatment efficacy. However, observational analyses gain validity to the extent that their conclusions have a plausible mechanistic cause and are reproducible from independent observational sources; until these characteristics have been established, conclusions (e.g. differences in prognosis between male and female CF patients) must be considered tentative at best. While it is likely that observational data will ultimately provide much of the rationale for future CF treatment, newly introduced therapies must be subjected to adequately powered RCTs before their use becomes routine and the opportunity for rigorous assessment is lost.

Data quality

A second important difference between RCTs and observational data is that, whereas the former must be documented and assessed according to *good clinical practice* (GCP) [2], for understandable reasons this is not generally true of the contents of observational databases. Data entry is a time-consuming task that may become an added chore to busy clinic personnel if it is inadequately resourced. The GCP standard of double data entry, whereby two independent individuals enter the data separately before final data consolidation, may be unthinkable in a busy clinic routine. Furthermore, it is unlikely in routine practice that human resources will be assigned to checking the data's validity after they have been entered into the database. Finally, it is unlikely that data collection was specifically planned to meet the needs of all analyses ultimately performed. For these reasons, observational databases are often suspected to be rather unreliable sources of information. However, with the assistance of computers, it is possible today for the quality of observational data to approach GCP standards.

POTENTIAL OBJECTIVES OF OBSERVATIONAL DATABASES

Despite their admitted shortcomings, observational databases can reveal a great deal about current practice and its relative success, as well as ideas that may impact on standards of care. The objective of any database may range from the purely local desire to optimize patient care to the international goal of identifying critical factors influencing the survival of CF patients. Legitimate objectives of even the largest registries may include simple descriptive studies. The implication of overall objectives on the content of individual databases is outlined below. Although aspiring to GCP standards [2] is most important for more ambitious projects, quality assurance is an important issue for even the smallest database.

Monitoring individual patient progress

The simplest objective for an observational database is to collect in one source all the information required to assess the progress of an individual patient. Since this objective does not imply comparison among patients, it can accommodate any uncoded language that may be helpful in assessing the patient. Although planning a database to meet this objective has the fewest constraints, confidence in the quality of collected data is clearly desirable. Publishable output is limited to individual case reports or possibly case series if uncoded data can be summarized manually. However, if it is intended that patients attending the same clinic be automatically compared by computer, additional considerations are required.

Clinic management and quality assurance

Objectives for this type of database are defined by the goals of the clinic entering the data. These may include planning local resources, identifying patients with particular characteristics or conditions, or bench-marking clinical outcomes. If the clinic is large enough its database may support limited analytical studies, but the impact of pervasive local assumptions cannot be assessed.

Since individual patient data are intended to be pooled into an aggregate for the clinic, some consideration must be given to preferred terms that describe similar conditions or treatments. This allows a computer to generate groups of patients who are similar in certain important respects. A simple database like this can document the frequency of treatments actually prescribed and important clinical outcomes that may be compared informally with national or international norms, such as the annual report of the US Cystic Fibrosis Foundation (CFF). It can also be used to monitor the result of interventions designed to change routine practice within the clinic. However, if the intention is to compare treatments and outcomes directly with those of another clinic or group of clinics, then a common documentation procedure (as described later under Data standards) should be implemented to ensure that comparable data have been systematically collected.

In comparing its treatments and outcomes to other clinics or the wider norm, each clinic must remain aware of the demographics of its particular CF patient population. For example, if it exclusively sees all patients in its catchment area, then its outcomes may be expected to be similar to other clinics in areas with similar social demographics. However, if a clinic commonly receives referrals for specific interventions (e.g. lung transplantation), then its treatments and outcomes are expected to deviate from the norm and should properly be compared with similar centers. Although an unrepresentative patient population may be construed as an argument against a clinic's participation in a registry, large registries are the only opportunity for similar clinics to identify each other and compare practices.

Formal documentation of comparative data can be of tremendous value in generating support for needed change. For example, after the French CF community published a comparison of the country's CF practices and outcomes with those in Europe as a whole [3], it was able to justify the formal establishment in France of specialized CF clinics and a national consensus on practice guidelines [4]. Note that this national quality assurance effort required the participation of many French clinics in an international registry and the resultant database objectives described later. Since national planning of health care resources requires data sharing, individual clinics should seriously consider applying the requirements of their national registry to their local database. By analogy, national registries in Europe should consider transnational European registry requirements to permit comparison directly with each other and indirectly with other large jurisdictions such as the USA, where CF patients tend to be of mixed European stock.

Epidemiological studies

The intent of patient registries is to collect data from individual clinics into a large multicenter database that contains the preponderance of data from an entire CF population. Therefore, it is essential that data from each individual clinic conform with the expectations of the central registry. Clear definitions are necessary of the nature of the data to be contributed as well as its required format.

Whenever text is used, a registry must implement a reliable preferred term dictionary to encode such things as treatments, gene mutations, microbiology, medical diagnoses, etc. Therefore, it is preferable to avoid text completely by offering foreseeable alternatives and recording simple yes/no answers. Small databases can also benefit from this concept.

The larger the volume of data and the more diverse the treatment strategies it encompasses, the more suited a registry is to performing analytic studies. This is because large numbers of patients undergoing different treatment regimens are required to adequately reflect the multiplicity of factors that can influence patient outcomes. However, the downside to collecting huge amounts of data may be a lack of completeness, as participants lose enthusiasm for a laborious task, and it may be necessary to compromise on a smaller, but more complete, data set. In single clinics, local demographics or established practice patterns may obscure correlations that are of practical importance to other clinics.

ENSURING THE SECURITY OF ELECTRONIC DATA

Medical databases should be accessible only to authorized persons logging in with a recognized password. After data have been entered it is advisable that any changes be tracked, together with the identity of the person making each change. Regular backups should be made on a removable medium (e.g. CD or DVD) and the backup stored under lock and key in a location distant from the computer holding the original data.

Data privacy laws must be respected when data on individual patients are shared, especially electronically, with another site. There is concern that data may be intercepted by unauthorized persons and that cross-linkage of electronic databases may easily lead to the identification of individual patients. The primary international directive is that shared medical data may *not* be identifiable as to the person concerned, either within a single database or by linkage with another database. This implies that common personal identifiers such as name, address, social insurance number, hospital admission number, may not be used in shared databases. Pooled data that obliterate the possibility of identifying individual patients are not considered to be personal medical data.

In order to comply with these regulations, it is recommended that disease registries assign to each participating patient a unique number that identifies the patient for the purpose of the registry but which is unrelated to national or local patient identifiers. If data are transmitted using the Internet, including e-mail, then this must be in encrypted form. Acceptable encryption procedures can be performed on most computers.

Clinics intending to share medical data with other sites are advised to consult their Institutional Review Board (or Ethics Committee) and Research Office. As with all research, governance issues must be addressed. In particular, written informed consent may be required from each patient or guardian before data are shared. For new patients, documenting this consent should become a routine procedure that is displayed prominently in the patient's clinical record.

ENSURING THE QUALITY OF ELECTRONIC DATA

The Epidemiologic Registry of Cystic Fibrosis (ERCF) ran for 7 years and included almost 16 000 patients from nine European countries. In acknowledgment of the fact that the quality of data in observational databases is generally of concern, ERCF initially attempted to approach GCP standards for data quality by having data double-entered and checked by the clinical research organization, Quintiles. However, it soon became apparent that, without personal on-site monitoring of the quality of data collection, the cost of checking and correcting a large volume of complicated data from so many sites was prohibitive, even for the industrial sponsor. Practical innovation became necessary to preserve the ERCF project. As a first step, data fields for which there was no planned use were excluded from the checking routine and data handling rules were defined to permit justifiable completion of some empty fields. (For example, although height at the time of each spirometric measurement is required to calculate percentage predicted values, actual height may not be recorded at each clinic visit. For adults, a rule was developed that permitted use of the most recently recorded height in such calculations.) The remaining checks were fully automated. Ultimately, a highly innovative but rather cumbersome system for Internet-based data entry was built and maintained by Spider AG, to perform over 300 routine checks before accepting data into ERCF, and to feed results back to the person entering the data.

ERCF experience illustrates the need to keep data collection as simple as possible and emphasizes both the need for routine checks of data contributed to central registries by multiple sites and the extremely high cost of data correction. Therefore, an important feature of data checks is that they be performed prior to acceptance of data into a registry, preferably during the process of data entry. Indeed, high data quality cannot be assumed in single-center databases under most practical situations – i.e. when data entry is delegated to a staff member unfamiliar with the details of patients' condition and treatment. Staff who coordinate and enter data are so important to data quality that they must be well trained in the objectives, practical value and significant details of their task. Written detailed instructions should be available and all questions answered promptly. If problems arise, a mutually acceptable solution should be found and the need for retraining considered. Because accurate data entry is crucial, sufficient time and therefore financial resources must be allocated to the task.

The completeness of data in an observational database cannot be checked by computer. For example, a patient who has no follow-up beyond a certain date may have died, moved to another clinic that may or may not continue to enter his data into the same registry, or may have dropped out of routine follow-up for any reason. It is therefore necessary to take stock periodically of patients without the expected degree of follow-up and to update these patients' status in the database as necessary. This requirement argues in favor of compulsory longitudinal follow-up of all patients enrolled in any large registry at probably no more than annual frequency. It is with gratitude that ERCF acknowledges the conscientious completeness that was found during source data verification in seven participating UK clinics [5].

Computerized checks

In the absence of double data entry and on-site study monitors, both of which are routine in RCTs, the quality of observational data is best checked automatically by computer. The design of these checks should take account, not only of the clinical importance of specific data fields, but also of common errors recognized by data entry professionals (Table 22.2).

Automated checks are logical algorithms with a yes/no answer that are designed specifically for each data field (Table 22.3). Routine checks should be specified at the same time as the database is defined, and require clinical input to define acceptable ranges for each field and the inter-relationships among different fields. A rule of thumb is that if a piece of data is important it should be checked; if it cannot be easily checked, then perhaps it is not worth collecting ('check it or forget it').

If a check reveals a potential problem (i.e. generates a 'no' answer) it must trigger an action, such as a message on the data entry screen describing the problem and offering

Table 22.2 Common data entry errors.

Entry of new data into the wrong patient record
Omission of compulsory data fields
Transposition of dates
Confusion of the year of an observation, especially during the first months of a new year
Transposition of height and weight data
Transposition of digits in a quantitative measurement
Inconsistency if interrelated data are to be entered in more than one data field

Table 22.3 Examples of automated checks for logic and consistency used by ERCF.

Are all compulsory fields completed?
Do completed fields contain the correct form of data (alphabetic, numeric, date, etc.)?
Are data within the accepted range of values for each field?
Is the ratio of interrelated data values within the accepted range?
Where there is a sequence of dates, is it logical?
Where optional data fields are interrelated, have all relevant fields been completed?
Is there an unexpected difference between currently and previously entered data?

the opportunity to correct it. The speed of modern computers is such that most checks can be performed instantaneously. Exceptions may be checks of consistency with previously entered data (longitudinal checks) if new data are kept in a separate file until all checks are complete. It is recommended that final data acceptance into a registry be delayed until all potential problems have been satisfactorily resolved.

Source data verification (SDV)

In RCTs, verification of at least a sample of all data collection and case report forms against the patient's medical records is routine practice. This procedure is intended to ensure that the data collected for submission to the trial database truly reflects the patient's medical history. When an epidemiological study is performed using observational data, a proportion of the contents of the database is also usually compared to original medical records (source data). SDV assesses the fitness of a specific database to address a particular epidemiological question in terms of the reliability of the relevant data.

Whereas participants in RCTs are required to give informed consent to the SDV procedure, patients whose personal medical data are incorporated into a database as part of routine clinic business may not have consented to an independent third party reviewing their medical history. Therefore, SDV may become an additional duty of busy clinic personnel. Fortunately, SDV is not necessary as a routine measure but only as part of a specific observational study protocol.

CONSTRUCTING A NEW DATABASE

Experience with ERCF has provided insight into the factors likely to contribute to a new registry's success or failure. The following advice is aimed at those who have the opportunity to plan and implement a new registry from scratch and is not intended as criticism of any past or present project.

The key ingredient for success is careful planning, not only of the database itself, but also of the financial and human resources necessary to implement and maintain it. For the reasons outlined elsewhere in this chapter, construction and implementation of a successful observational database is expected to be both labor- and cost-intensive. The more attention to detail is invested in planning, the more accurate the resulting resource estimates will be; available resources may well constrain the quantity of data that can realistically be collected. Although intended to define the steps necessary to validate formal drug efficacy trials, GCP [2] can provide guidance on factors to consider when planning observational studies. Because constructing a new patient registry presents the greatest planning challenge, most of this section is devoted to that subject.

Table 22.4 Some possible major objectives of a patient registry.

Provide regular summaries of outcomes and patterns of care for the entire patient population of the registry

Compare outcomes and patterns of care in different subgroups of the patient population

Allow centers to compare their own performance with other comparable clinics, to identify areas where a change in practice may be needed

Summarize how patient care and outcomes have changed over time

Attempt to identify factors that improve or worsen patient survival and/or other outcomes

Encourage voluntary participation in the registry

Objectives and scope

The first planning step is to be confident of the objectives and scope of the project. For the simplest objective of monitoring individual patient progress, there is no constraint beyond the limits of human capacity on how much data can be stored electronically for each patient. Constraints occur primarily when data have to be recorded comparably and consistently for different patients and in different clinics, particularly for large disease registries.

Some potential major objectives of a patient registry are listed in Table 22.4. Although most are driven by the organization holding the registry data, if it is necessary to encourage centers to participate, then fulfilling each center's unmet needs may be a very important goal. Each major objective should be subdivided into individual projects that are achievable within the first 5–10 years of registry operation, and an analysis plan constructed for each project before the registry's core data set is defined (see Choice of data items for collection).

Choice of software

While simple projects may be easily manageable using simple software, large registry projects must consider purchasing commercial specialist software. In general it is much more efficient to purchase existing commercial software than to rely on home-made or untested solutions. Although the purchase may represent substantial capital investment, the manufacturer or supplier of specialist software will provide the expertise necessary to tailor it to specific needs and to correct any problems encountered.

Purchased software should include a user-friendly interface, user-specified database-checking routines, and features to track the source of any changes made to the existing database. User-friendly data entry screens facilitate data entry substantially, especially if data coordinators receive or can compile data on a paper form that mimics the screen. Screens and corresponding forms can also

be translated into several languages for international projects.

Optional extras include automatic and secure transmission of newly entered data to a designated remote computer. The number of licenses necessary for the project should be estimated in advance so that economies of scale can be realized.

Choice of data items for collection

While the temptation to collect as much data as possible is almost irresistible to clinicians, the most reliable patient registries adopt the opposite approach. The complexities of data management, which are substantial in any registry, are compounded as the number of data fields expands. Again, planning is key.

A detailed data analysis plan should be prepared in advance, outlining the specific analyses that a new registry realistically plans to perform within its first 5–10 years of operation and mock tables of the results that it expects to produce. Longer-term planning seldom reflects reality. The data items required for these analyses will define the core set of data that must be collected.

Once the core data set has been defined, it should be altered only on predefined occasions (milestones) and for easily justifiable reasons. The implications of redefining core data include adjustment of the database definition and specifications, communicating the changes effectively to all participants, and implementing the changes successfully on all contributing computers. As soon as the change has been implemented, all future analyses must be redesigned to account for the fact that core data may be missing for certain patients. These tasks are time-consuming and costly.

Data standards

Definitions must be established for the format in which data are to be recorded – e.g. date format, weight in pounds or kilograms, etc. In many instances a simple computer program can perform the necessary conversion before transmission of clinic data to a central registry. Other information, such as how drug dosages are to be recorded, may require adoption of specific data fields in a clinic's own database for the express purpose of data sharing.

Database design

If the analysis plan requires details on genetic mutations, organisms cultured, treatments given, intercurrent diagnoses or causes of death, then it is highly recommended that the most common responses be anticipated and offered in check boxes or pull-down lists so that text data is kept to a minimum. Computers still cannot interpret text, and even humans have difficulty if text is presented in a foreign language. Where responses do not conform to those anticipated, it is important to decide in advance whether or not 'other' data are relevant. If so, then preferred term dictionaries must be implemented and maintained. Even although this process can be semi-automated, human resources are required to deal with all novel entries, including abbreviations and typographical errors.

Recruiting centers into a registry

Assuming that most clinics today maintain their own patient database, when a new registry is planned with the intention of capturing data from all CF patients in a wide geographic region, there are two basic approaches it may take to recruiting centers. If the holder of the registry has financial or other compelling authority over all clinics in the region, it may choose to design its own data collection device and require that the data it needs be entered afresh in its own system. In circumstances where the registry holder has less direct authority, sites are more likely to participate voluntarily if the effort involved is small and they perceive a direct benefit from the partnership. Ideally, data already collected in local databases should be imported automatically into the registry. Some potential incentives to registry participation, other than financial, are suggested in Table 22.5.

Since core registry data may be only a small proportion of the information contained in a clinic's own database, a simple data extraction procedure may be developed for each center provided that the quality of the original data is adequate. However, the registry's responsibility to ensure the quality of its own data implies that it should ultimately aim to replace each center's private database with a state-of-the-art alternative. This approach also has the advantage that registry-defined, optional data fields can be incorporated into local systems gradually, in a format that is easily uploaded if the registry later decides to expand its definition of core data. This process opens the possibility of natural expansion of the registry over time, as new interests emerge.

Table 22.5 Suggested non-financial incentives for registry participation.

Provision of a state-of-the-art, user-friendly database that fulfills all of a clinic's needs from a clinic management system

Provision of non-core data fields for the clinic's own purposes, and instruction in how to use them

Instruction in how a clinic can evaluate its own data for its own purposes

Assistance to transfer data from any previous database to the registry's new system

Quick and easy uploading (preferably automated) of core data into the registry

Regular feedback of useful information from the registry

Data analysis options

As described earlier, observational data cannot provide definitive answers to specific questions in the same way as RCTs. Instead, general acceptance of the results of observational studies depends on their reproducibility and there being a plausible mechanism to explain the findings. While some clinicians may interpret the result of sophisticated analyses as the best estimate given the current state of knowledge, others may subscribe to the philosophy that 'there are lies, damned lies and statistics'. Therefore, although good observational data can make very powerful statements, a registry should seriously consider its credibility, especially before its reputation is established, when preparing its initial analysis plan.

Descriptive analyses present data in a non-judgmental manner and invite interpretation of results. Powerful examples of descriptive registry data include cross-sectional descriptions of the entire registry population and of subpopulations from individual clinics or geographic areas, as epitomized in the annual national and center reports of the CFF, ERCF and the Epidemiologic Study of Cystic Fibrosis (ESCF). Cross-sectional studies can also identify apparent correlations within a diverse population (Table 22.6). Often, a probable explanation is obvious and so a hypothesis can be generated for further testing if required. However, descriptive analyses cannot establish a cause and effect relationship.

Analytic studies rely on building a mathematical model, which is intended to simulate a match between treatment (or case) and control groups, to clarify cause-and-effect relationships. Cohort and case–control studies attempt to document all relevant factors in the cause-and-effect relationship under study and assess their potential importance one by one by simple regression analysis. Potentially significant factors are subsequently included in a mathematical model that takes account of the inter-relationship among factors (multiple regression analysis) and yields an estimate of the likelihood that each factor plays a role in the relationship, and the potential magnitude of that role. While analytic studies are the next best thing to RCTs, their conclusions depend on the validity of the study's assumptions.

In order to permit a new registry and its public to gain confidence in its data, it should consider performing descriptive analyses before it addresses more sophisticated problems. Established registries publish useful analyses of both types (see Table 22.6).

Project management

A project with the complexity of a new patient registry requires a team of people with diverse skills and a coordinator to ensure that all tasks are planned and performed in good time and within budget.

Table 22.6 Some examples of registry publications.

Registry	Type of analysis	Topic	Author	Reference
CFF	A	2-year survival model	Mayer-Hamblett N et al.	[6]
CFF	A	5-year survival model	Liou TG et al.	[7]
ERCF	D	Pulmozyme prevents PFT decline at 1 and 2 years and reduces exacerbation frequency	Hodson ME et al.	[8]
ERCF	D	Impact of diabetes	Koch C et al.	[9]
ERCF	D	Factors affecting pulmonary function at enrolment (cross-sectional analysis)	Navarro J et al.	[10]
ERCF	D	Effect of genotype on disease expression	Koch C et al.	[11]
ERCF (Germany)	D	Continuous anti-staph therapy increases risk of Pseudomonas colonization	Ratjen F et al.	[12]
ERCF	D, A	ABPA	Mastella G et al.	[13]
ERCF (France)	D	French vs European practice and outcomes	Delaisi B et al.	[14]
ERCF	D	Practice patterns	Koch C et al.	[15]
ESCF	D	Maternal pregnancy outcomes	McMullen AH et al.	[16]
ESCF	D	Characteristics of patients with diabetes	Marshall BC et al.	[17]
ESCF	D	Clinical characteristics associated with treatment for exacerbation	Rabin HR et al.	[18]
ESCF	D	Nutritional parameters at age 3 predict pulmonary function at age 6	Konstan MW et al.	[19]
ESCF	D	Center comparison: frequent monitoring and use of meds improve outcomes	Johnson C et al.	[20]
ESCF	D	Methods description	Morgan WJ et al.	[21]
ESCF	D	ABPA	Geller DE et al.	[22]
ESCF	D	Practice patterns, part 1	Konstan MW et al.	[23]
ESCF	D	Practice patterns part 2: prescribing	Konstan MW et al.	[24]
ESCF	A	Pulmozyme 12 mo effectiveness	Johnson CA et al.	[25]
ESCF	D	Survey of microbiology practice	Shreve MR et al.	[26]

ABPA, Allergic Bronchopulmonary Aspergillosis; CFF, Cystic Fibrosis Foundation; ERCF, Epidemiologic Registry of Cystic Fibrosis; ESCF, Epidemiologic Study of Cystic Fibrosis.
A, analytic; D, descriptive.

CONCLUSION

Because it is unlikely that randomized controlled trials can be designed to answer all questions concerning the optimal care of cystic fibrosis patients, observational data are likely to be an extremely important source of new knowledge. Provided that their limitations are recognized and managed appropriately, CF patient registries are likely to improve patient care at both local and international levels.

REFERENCES

1. Hennekens CH, Buring JE. *Epidemiology in Medicine.* Boston, Little, Brown, 1987, pp16–29.
2. European Agency for the Evaluation of Medicines. *ICH Topic 6: Guideline for Good Clinical Practice.* CPMP/ICH/135/95, January 1997. Available at www.emea.eu.int/pdfs/human/ich/013595en.pdf.
3. Delaisi B, Grosskopf C, Reignault E et al. Register international sur la mucoviscidose: comparison des données françaises avec les données européennes pour 1995. *Arch Pediatr* 1998; **5**:384–388.
4. Marguet C, Bellon G, de Blic J et al. Conférence de consensus. Prise en charge du patient atteint de mucoviscidose. Recommandations (versions courtes). *Arch Pediatr* 2003; **10**:280–294.
5. Strobl J, Enzer I, Bagust A et al. Using disease registries for pharmaco-epidemiological research: a case study of data from a cystic fibrosis registry. *Pharmacoepidemiol Drug Safety* 2003; **12**:467–473.
6. Mayer-Hamblett N, Rosenfeld M, Emerson J et al. Developing cystic fibrosis lung transplant referral criteria using predictors of 2-year mortality. *Am J Respir Crit Care Med* 2002; **166**:1550–1555.
7. Liou TG, Adler FR, FitzSimmons SC et al. Predictive 5-year survivorship model of cystic fibrosis. *Am J Epidemiol* 2001; **153**:345–352.

8. Hodson ME, McKenzie S, Harms HK *et al.* Dornase alfa in the treatment of cystic fibrosis in Europe: a report from the Epidemiologic Registry of Cystic Fibrosis. *Pediatr Pulmonol* 2003; **36**:427–432.

9. Koch C, Rainisio M, Madessani U *et al.* Presence of cystic fibrosis-related diabetes mellitus is tightly linked to poor lung function in patients with cystic fibrosis: data from the European Epidemiologic Registry of Cystic Fibrosis. *Pediatr Pulmonol* 2001; **32**:343–350.

10. Navarro J, Rainisio M, Harms HK *et al.* Factors associated with poor pulmonary function: cross-sectional analysis of data from the ERCF. European Epidemiologic Registry of Cystic Fibrosis. *Eur Respir J* 2001; **18**:298–305.

11. Koch C, Cuppens H, Rainisio M *et al.* European Epidemiologic Registry of Cystic Fibrosis (ERCF): comparison of major disease manifestations between patients with different classes of mutations. *Pediatr Pulmonol* 2001; **31**:1–12.

12. Ratjen F, Comes G, Paul K et al. Effect of continuous antistaphylococcal therapy on the rate of P. aeruginosa acquisition in patients with cystic fibrosis. *Pediatr Pulmonol* 2001; **31**:13–16.

13. Mastella G, Rainisio M, Harms HK *et al.* Allergic bronchopulmonary aspergillosis in cystic fibrosis. A European epidemiological study. *Eur Respir J* 2000; **16**:464–471.

14. Delaisi B, Grosskopf C, Reignault E et al. Registre international sur la mucoviscidose: comparaison des données françaises avec les données européennes pour 1995. *Arch Pediatr* 1998; **5**:384–388.

15. Koch C, McKenzie SG, Kaplowitz H *et al.* International practice patterns by age and severity of lung disease in cystic fibrosis. Data from the Epidemiologic Registry of Cystic Fibrosis (ERCF). *Pediatr Pulmonol* 1997; **24**:147–154.

16. McMullen AH, Pasta DJ, Frederick PD *et al.* Impact of pregnancy on women with cystic fibrosis. *Chest* 2006; **129**:706–711.

17. Marshall BC, Butler SM, Stoddard M *et al.* Epidemiology of cystic fibrosis-related diabetes. *J Pediatr* 2005:**146**:681–687.

18. Rabin HR, Butler SM, Wohl MEB *et al.* Pulmonary exacerbations in cystic fibrosis. *Pediatr Pulmonol* 2004; **37**:400–406.

19. Konstan MW, Butler SM, Wohl MEB *et al.* Growth and nutritional indexes in early life predict pulmonary function in cystic fibrosis. *J Pediatr* 2003; **142**:624–630.

20. Johnson C, Butler SM, Konstan MW *et al.* Factors influencing outcomes in cystic fibrosis. A center-based analysis. *Chest* 2003; **123**:20–27.

21. Morgan WJ, Butler SM, Johnson CA *et al.* Epidemiologic Study of Cystic Fibrosis: design and implementation of a prospective, multicenter, observational study of patients with cystic fibrosis in the U.S. and Canada. *Pediatr Pulmonol* 1999; **28**:231–241.

22. Geller DE, Kaplowitz H, Light MJ *et al.* Allergic bronchopulmonary aspergillosis in cystic fibrosis. Reported prevalence, regional distribution, and patient characteristics. *Chest* 1999; **116**:639–646.

23. Konstan MW, Butler SM, Schidlow DV *et al.* Patterns of medical practice in cystic fibrosis: Part I. Evaluation and monitoring of health status of patients. *Pediatr Pulmonol* 1999; **28**:242–247.

24. Konstan MW, Butler SM, Schidlow DV *et al.* Patterns of medical practice in cystic fibrosis: Part II. Use of therapies. *Pediatr Pulmonol* 1999; **28**:248–254.

25. Johnson CA, Butler SM, Konstan MW *et al.* Estimating effectiveness in an observational study: a case study of dornase alfa in cystic fibrosis. *J Pediatr* 1999; **134**:734–739.

26. Shreve MR, Butler S, Kaplowitz HJ *et al.* Impact of microbiology practice on cumulative prevalence of respiratory tract bacteria in patients with cystic fibrosis. *J Clin Microbiol* 1999; **37**:753–757.

Infant and pre-school children: lung function

SARATH RANGANATHAN

INTRODUCTION

Measurement of lung function is a central part of the clinical assessment of older children and adults with cystic fibrosis (CF). Serial tests provide longitudinal information about the extent of abnormality, progression of disease and individual response to treatment. Respiratory disease is responsible for much of the morbidity occurring in childhood, and neutrophil-dominated inflammation similar to that seen in older subjects with CF has been identified in the lungs of affected infants [1,2]. It is important to recognize that the disease process commences early in infancy even in those whom clinicians consider to be asymptomatic. Although the evolution of airway pathology in infancy remains poorly understood, the need to evaluate lung function early is self-evident. The limiting factors, however, are that infant lung function is technically difficult to perform, expensive, time-consuming and requires sedation and thus has been performed in only a few specialist centers. Furthermore, between infancy and school age, toddlers are too old to sedate and too young to cooperate with most testing. Consequently, many studies have been difficult to interpret due to the small numbers of subjects, lack of appropriate control data from prospectively studied healthy infants, and the use of relatively insensitive techniques [3]. However, joint efforts between the European Respiratory Society and American Thoracic Society to provide standards for equipment and procedures for infant lung function testing have ensured that findings in subjects with CF can be related to normative data and confirmed in other centers. Such collaborative efforts have been meticulous in their adherence to standards of data collection and quality control and have ensured great scientific progress and advances in our knowledge of the 'missing link' in lung function before conventional spirometry becomes feasible at school age [4].

In older patients with CF, spirometry – for example, forced expiratory volume in one second (FEV_1) and maximal expiratory flow at low lung volumes (e.g. MEF_{25}) – is most frequently used to assess airway function. MEFs are considered better at detecting earlier changes but are too variable to be useful for monitoring lung function longitudinally; FEV_1 is used conventionally for this purpose. Partial forced expiratory maneuvers have been performed in infants for almost 30 years using the tidal rapid thoraco-abdominal compression technique (RTC) to measure MEF from the partial flow–volume curve measured at the volume landmark of functional residual capacity. In this technique an inflatable jacket is used to apply a rapidly rising external pressure to the chest wall and abdomen at the end of a tidal inspiration in order to generate forced expiratory flow–volume curves. Methods to assess forced expiration over an extended volume range in infants, and therefore to provide expiratory curves that are more like those of conventional spirometry, have been described only recently [5,6]. This raised-volume rapid thoraco abdominal technique ('raised-volume technique', RVRTC) involves using a pump or augmented manual inflations to increase the volume of inspiration prior to forcing expiration. The infant becomes briefly apneic, and can be passively inflated to near total lung capacity before a forced squeeze is applied as above [7]. From the RVRTC flow–volume curves (Fig. 23.1) it is possible to derive parameters comparable to those obtained in older subjects such as forced expiratory volume in 0.4 or 0.5 seconds ($FEV_{0.4}$ or $FEV_{0.5}$, which are used because lung emptying is complete in less than 1 second, rendering FEV_1 meaningless) and MEF_{25} [8].

Most recent studies of infant lung function in those with CF have used the raised-volume technique.

AIRWAY FUNCTION

Early changes

Airway function of infants newly diagnosed with CF was measured in a recent cohort study. The RTC and RVRTC

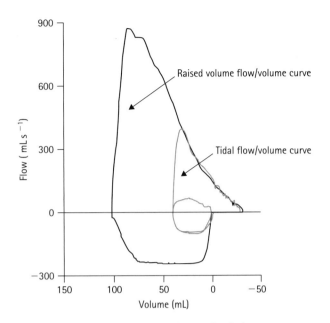

Figure 23.1 Overlay of forced expiratory flow/volume curves obtained from raised and tidal volumes. The raised volume flow/volume curve is similar to that obtained using conventional spirometry in older subjects and similar parameters such as $FEV_{0.5}$ and MEF_{25} can be calculated.

were used to compare the airway function of newly diagnosed infants with CF with healthy controls in order to test the hypothesis that lung function is diminished shortly after diagnosis independent of clinically recognized lower respiratory illness [9,10]. The association between FVC, $FEV_{0.5}$ and $FEV_{0.5}/FVC$ and length according to disease status is shown in Fig. 23.2. On average the decrement in $FEV_{0.5}$ in those with CF was 40 mL ($p < 0.001$) when their median (range) age was 30 (6–93) weeks. A subgroup of CF infants within this cohort without any clinical evidence of prior lower respiratory illness (LRI) of median age 12 weeks had a similar decrement in airway function.

Approximately a third of infants with CF had an $FEV_{0.5}$ below two z scores [10]. The data suggest a distribution of z scores for $FEV_{0.5}$ in those with CF below that for healthy infants (Fig. 23.3). Seventeen of the 47 CF infants were assessed as having normal clinical respiratory status by their specialist, but $FEV_{0.5}$ was diminished by more than one standard deviation. There were four infants whose airway function was below two z scores for healthy infants. The RVRTC identified diminished airway function in more infants with CF than RTC, suggesting that the RVRTC is more sensitive at detecting early changes.

Thus airway function was diminished early in the course of disease in those with CF, was more likely to be detected by the raised-volume technique than the tidal forced expiratory technique, and occurred irrespective of clinical evidence of prior LRI and even when specialist physicians identified infants with CF as having normal respiratory status. In this study, infants were diagnosed with CF following a clinical presentation of the disease and so those without clinical evidence of prior LRI usually had

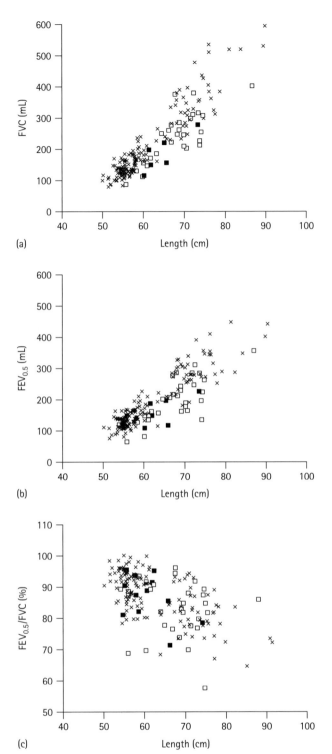

Figure 23.2 FVC, $FEV_{0.5}$ and $FEV_{0.5}/FVC$ plotted against length. Crosses indicate airway function of healthy infants. The open and closed squares indicate infants with CF with and without prior lower respiratory illness, respectively. Infants with CF have evidence of diminished airway function. From [10].

presented with meconium ileus in the newborn period, or had evidence of failure to thrive when airway function was assessed. Whether there is a reduction in airway function evident during the first months of life in those diagnosed

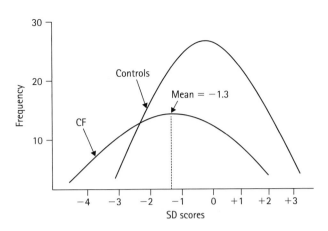

Figure 23.3 Overlay of the distribution of Z scores for $FEV_{0.5}$ for healthy infants and infants with CF. As a group, infants with CF have diminished airway function. Although the majority of individual infants have lung function within the distribution calculated from measurements made in healthy infants, $FEV_{0.5}$ is below the 2.5th centile in up to a third.

CF by neonatal screening and without failure to thrive remains unknown.

Evolution of airway function

The evolution of airway function has been assessed by measuring $FEV_{0.5}$ using the RVRTC soon after diagnosis (median age 28 weeks) and 6 months later in subjects with CF, and on two occasions 6 months apart (median age 7.4 and 33.7 weeks) in healthy infants. Repeated measurements were successful in 34 CF and 32 healthy subjects. After adjustment for age, length, sex and exposure to maternal smoking, mean $FEV_{0.5}$ was significantly lower in infants with CF both shortly after diagnosis and at second test, with no significant difference in rate of increase in $FEV_{0.5}$ with growth between the two groups despite treatment in specialist CF centers (Fig. 23.4). When compared with published reference data, $FEV_{0.5}$ was reduced by an average of two z scores on both test occasions in those with CF. On average, $FEV_{0.5}$ was reduced by 20% in those with CF [11].

These data show that airway function is diminished soon after diagnosis in infants with CF and does not catch-up (or deteriorate) over a 6-month period during infancy and early childhood despite treatment in centers specializing in the management of CF. This result needs confirmation, but does highlight the potential value of such measurements for future clinical research and the implications for early interventions in CF. The pivotal importance of early changes is emphasized in follow-up studies in older children and adults (see Chapter 24).

Airway obstruction

In older subjects, chronic inflammation and infection lead to airway obstruction. Identification of an obstructive

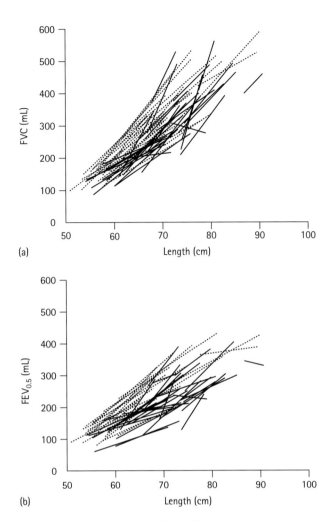

Figure 23.4 Association of FVC and $FEV_{0.5}$ with length. The dashed and solid lines indicate airway function of healthy infants and infants with CF, respectively, and demonstrate that airway function in infants with CF remains diminished when re-tested in later infancy. From [11].

process in infancy would suggest similar pathophysiology. This could be indicated by a reduction in the ratio of forced expiratory volume to forced vital capacity. Although this appears to be the case (see Fig. 23.2), the mean reduction in $FEV_{0.5}/FVC$ appears to be small in infants with CF, approximately 3% ($p = 0.015$), and such a small reduction is unlikely to be clinically significant and clearly does not definitively confirm an important obstructive process. The ratio is in the normal range in the vast majority of infants with CF, even those in whom $FEV_{0.5}$ is reduced. Moreover, interpretation of this ratio in infancy is especially difficult due to the rapid increase in the forced expiratory time with age or length and the fact that $FEV_{0.5}/FVC$ is so close to unity in early life [8].

In a recent study of infants with CF [12], gas-trapping (as an indication of airway obstruction) was assessed by a combination of plethysmography to determine functional residual capacity and the raised-volume technique to determine forced vital capacity (FVC) and the expiratory reserve volume. Gas-trapping was indicated by a significant increase in the ratio of residual volume to total lung capacity in those with CF (mean z score 0.18) compared with healthy infants (mean z score -0.73) ($p = 0.013$). These data provide further evidence that diminished airway function identified in infants with CF is indeed obstructive in nature.

ELASTIC PROPERTIES OF THE LUNG

Measurements of the compliance of the respiratory system (C_{rs}) in infants with CF have yielded conflicting results [3]. Most studies have been limited to the lung volume range of tidal breathing which may result in underestimation of C_{rs} due to airway closure. A recent study evaluated C_{rs} in healthy infants and infants with CF using passive deflation pressure–volume curves from a lung volume at an airway pressure of 30 cmH$_2$O to functional residual capacity [13]. The investigators were able to standardize volume history, theoretically open up closed airways by use of augmented inflations, and obtain measurements over an extended range of lung volumes. In comparison to age-matched healthy infants, C_{rs} was not significantly different in those with CF – suggesting that, unlike older subjects with CF, measured in an era when severe pulmonary disease was more likely to be present at an earlier age and in whom decreased pulmonary elastic recoil was found to contribute to airway obstruction [14,15], infants with CF have normal elastic properties of the respiratory system. This finding is consistent with the concept that the early pathophysiology of CF is limited to the airways and that the reduction in forced expiratory flows is not contributed to by decreased elastic recoil.

MARKERS OF INFLAMMATION OR INFECTION AND EARLY LUNG FUNCTION

As the gold standard for determining airway inflammation or lower respiratory tract infection is bronchoscopy and bronchoalveolar lavage (BAL) usually under general anesthesia, few investigators have combined assessments of inflammation or infection and infant lung function in the same study. In one recent study, specific respiratory system compliance was measured using the single-breath occlusion technique and lung volumes by nitrogen washout in CF children of median age 23 months [16]. Diminished lung function correlated with BAL markers of both inflammation (interleukin-8 and neutrophil percentage) and infection. However, for the majority of subjects, lung function remained within the normal range and only very little of the variability in lung function was explained by either inflammation or infection. As C_{rs} is most likely to be normal in infants with CF compared with healthy infants, studies using measurements of airway function rather than assessments of mechanics are indicated. In another study, recruitment commenced in infancy but measurements in 40 subjects were made initially at a mean of 13 months of age [17]. No association between lung function and IL-8

concentration, neutrophil density or pathogen load was demonstrated. However, due to the invasive nature of the assessments, not all parameters were measured simultaneously, BAL being performed annually and infant lung function every 6 months. An association of borderline significance between FEV$_{0.5}$ measured using RVRTC and infection (defined as at least 10^5 colony-forming units of bacterial respiratory pathogens per milliliter of BAL fluid) and no association between FEV$_{0.5}$ and pulmonary inflammation was identified in a third study in 36 CF children during the second year of life [18].

No studies have been able to address this association during the first year of life. Although it is highly likely that the early functional abnormalities identified are the result of inflammation and infection, as is the case in older subjects, further studies are required in order to clarify these relationships in infants with CF.

STRUCTURAL CHANGES AND EARLY LUNG FUNCTION

Using controlled ventilation similar to that used for the RVRTC technique, high-resolution CT scans in 34 infants and young children with CF of mean age 2.4 years (10 weeks to 5.5 years) demonstrated that the airways of minimally symptomatic subjects have thickened airway walls and more dilated airways than those of subjects without CF. These structural changes appear to be present in both smaller and larger airways and at least one thickened airway was identified in over 50% of patients, suggesting that bronchiectasis begins very early in life [19]. Another recent study [20] also used high-resolution CT imaging to determine airway caliber in 13 infants and young children with CF of mean age 17 months (range 8–33 months) in comparison to measurements obtained in 13 age- and length-matched children without pulmonary disease. In this study, overall airway area following adjustment for airway size was similar between the two groups, but patients with CF had thicker airway walls and smaller airway lumens than the controls (Fig. 23.5), suggesting that the airway wall had encroached upon the airway lumen to produce airway narrowing in the CF subjects. The raised-volume technique was used to assess FEV$_{0.5}$, MEF$_{50}$ and MEF$_{25}$ in 11 patients of the group with CF. There were significant negative correlations ($p < 0.002$ for all) between the ratio of wall area to lumen area and the measures of airway function; the larger the ratio of wall area to lumen area, the lower the z score for airway function (FEV$_{0.5}$: $r^2 = 0.66$; MEF$_{50}$: $r^2 = 0.41$; MEF$_{25}$: $r^2 = 0.4$), suggesting that diminished airway function in infants and young children is likely to be a consequence of airway narrowing.

The finding of an increase in diameter of the airway lumen in the study of Long and colleagues [19] seems to contradict the finding of a smaller airway lumen area in that of Martinez and colleagues [20] and could be a consequence of assessing significantly older subjects in the former

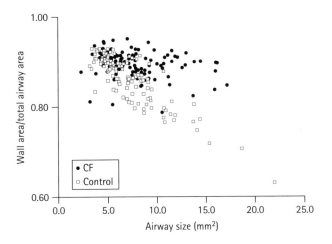

Figure 23.5 Wall area/total airway area against airway size for airways measured from control subjects (open squares) and subjects with CF (solid circles). Total airway area is similar in controls and those with CF but those with CF have thickened airway walls, reduced luminal area and diminished airway function. From [20].

study, or technical differences in the methodology such as selection of airways, airway distending pressures and software analysis. It is possible that narrowing of the airway lumen precedes the tortuous luminal dilatation associated with frank bronchiectasis and that the different findings are a consequence of disease progression. The study of Martinez, however, is the first to demonstrate structural/functional relationships in infants with CF. Further studies are required to study the possibility of similar relationships in the first few months of life and their subsequent progression over the first few years of life.

INFLUENCE OF EXPOSURE TO ENVIRONMENTAL TOBACCO SMOKE

The adverse effects associated with indirect or passive cigarette smoke exposure during early life are evident in terms of immediate and long-term health problems [21,22]. Exposure to maternal smoking during pregnancy and/or postnatally is independently associated with diminished airway function in infants with CF, the effect size being approximately 50% of that associated with CF [9,10]. The relative contributions of pre- and postnatal exposure on diminished airway function is, however, unknown and whether parents of those with CF are any more successful than parents of healthy children in adhering to smoking cessation programs is doubtful.

EARLY LUNG FUNCTION AND GENOTYPE/PHENOTYPE

Infants with pulmonary hyperinflation had a different genotype from those without in one study [23]: infants who

were compound heterozygote *3905insT/F508del* ($n = 9$) had a mean *z* score for functional residual capacity of 8.4 (SD 4.9) above the mean of a reference population, whereas 8 infants who were compound heterozygotes for the nonsense mutation *R553X* were not significantly different from normal. However, as weight gain was abnormally low in the former (58% predicted) the elevated values for functional residual capacity may at least in part reflect inappropriate comparison in underweight infants with CF to the reference population of healthy infants. In any case, the numbers studied are small. Repeating the study in CF infants identified by neonatal screening and without failure to thrive and comparing functional residual capacity with age-matched healthy controls is indicated. In another study, in which infants were grouped into those homo- or heterozygous for *F508del*, a washout technique and the single-breath technique were used to assess lung volume and respiratory mechanics, respectively [24]. Infants homozygous for *F508del* had elevated respiratory system resistance measured in this way and a positive bronchodilator response. Studies in which airway function has been measured, however, failed to demonstrate any association between CF genotype and results of infant lung function probably due to insufficient power. Much larger multicenter collaborations are required before such associations can be confirmed or negated in infants with CF.

Probably also due to lack of power, no studies in infants have confirmed impairment of lung function in association with infection with *Pseudomonas aeruginosa*.

DETECTING AND MONITORING EARLY LUNG FUNCTION CHANGES USING SIMPLER METHODS

The RVRTC appears to be a sensitive test to detect early changes in lung function in those with CF but the test is relatively invasive. Since the Tucson study suggested that time to reach peak tidal expiratory flow in relation to total expiratory time (the tidal breathing ratio, $t_{PTEF}:t_E$) was diminished in symptom-free male infants who subsequently wheezed, several groups have examined tidal flow patterns in both healthy infants and those with airway disease [25–27]. Recording of tidal breathing is technically simple and potentially allows measurements to be undertaken at the patient's bedside during natural quiet sleep, without the need for sedation. Consequently, evaluation of the 'tidal breathing ratio' and other related parameters has continued to attract interest. The relationship between tidal breathing parameters and $FEV_{0.4}$ in infants with CF has been assessed and compared with a prospectively recruited population of healthy infants [28]. There was no difference in $t_{PTEF}:t_E$ and tidal volume between healthy infants and those with CF. Minute ventilation was significantly greater in infants with CF due to a mean increase in respiratory rate of 5.8 per minute (95% CI 3.2–8.4). Thirteen infants (28%) with CF had a respiratory rate elevated by more than two *z* scores.

Unlike for $FEV_{0.4}$, there was clear discrimination in respiratory rate between those with and without prior LRI, suggesting that an elevated respiratory rate may be due in part to ventilation inhomogeneities. As no association between respiratory rate and $FEV_{0.4}$ could be identified, respiratory rate was poorly predictive of diminished airway function measured by forced expiration. The use of more sophisticated techniques such as multiple-breath inert-gas washout (see later), which can also be performed during tidal breathing, but which give detailed information on ventilation distribution, could be used in the future to evaluate the relative contribution of impaired gas mixing to alterations in respiratory rate in infants with CF.

PRE-SCHOOL LUNG FUNCTION

The long-term implications of early lung function findings in those with CF will only be known when lung function is measured longitudinally until school age and beyond, when conventional measurements using spirometry become possible. The years between 2 and 6 provide several challenges to those wishing to measure lung function. In many centers, pre-school children with CF do not undergo lung function testing until they are able to perform reproducible forced expiratory maneuvers. In order to bridge the 'silent years', international efforts have focused on standardization of techniques for measuring lung function in pre-schoolers.

Resistance interrupter technique

The resistance interrupter technique (R_{int}) requires minimal cooperation, is quick, easy and effort-independent and can be performed in the ambulatory setting in pre-school children [29]. R_{int} is based on the assumption that, during an imperceptibly brief interruption of airflow during tidal breathing, the pressure changes at the airway opening can be used to determine the alveolar pressure at the moment of interruption; hence, knowing the flow immediately prior to interruption, resistance can be calculated (resistance = pressure/flow). The assumption that mouth pressure is equal to alveolar pressure is invalid if there is severe airway obstruction. Resistance measured by this technique was significantly elevated in 40 subjects with CF aged between 3 and 8 years (z score of 1.31 compared with 0.19 in healthy controls) [30]. Those with a history of prior LRI or exposure to environmental tobacco smoke had significantly elevated expiratory resistance. Although measurements in those with CF were no more variable than those made in healthy subjects, the overall variability of the resistance measurements was high, limiting its use in assessing response to interventions and disease progression. Expiratory resistance measured by the interrupter technique depends on the proximal airways and so physiologically it would not appear to be the ideal test to measure peripheral airway function associated with early pulmonary disease.

Incentive spirometry

Using incentives such as blowing games, spirometry can be undertaken in pre-school children and suggests that tracking of lung function is likely to persist through the pre-school years (that is, those with the lowest airway function in infancy maintain this position with growth). When infants with CF, who had been tested using the raised-volume technique and found to have diminished airway function, were retested at a mean age of 3.9 years, mean (SD) z scores were -0.55 (0.85) for $FEV_{0.5}$, with only one child with CF still having an abnormal $FEV_{0.5}$. These data suggest that either airway function may improve through the pre-school years or alternatively that incentive spirometry is less able to identify diminished airway function in pre-school subjects than the raised-volume technique in infants [31].

A recent study reported that 33 of 38 children with CF (including four of six 3-year-olds and nine of eleven 4-year-olds) were able to perform either two or three conventional spirometry maneuvers (without incentive) and fulfill study acceptability and reproducibility criteria when tested by skilled pediatric pulmonary function technicians who regularly work with pre-school children [32]. Children with CF had significantly lower FVC, FEV_1 and MEF_{75-25} than healthy subjects. Those homozygous for $\Delta F508$ had significantly lower FVC and FEV_1 than heterozygotes. Subjects were well at the time of lung function and so the feasibility and variability of performing spirometry during exacerbations is not known.

RVRTC had been performed previously in 14 subjects during infancy in this study and again tracking of lung function occurred through to the pre-school assessments [32]. In those with lung function in the normal range as infants (z score for $MEF_{75-25} > -2$) there was no significant change in z score for the same parameter measured using spirometry. However, z scores increased significantly between infancy and childhood in four subjects with diminished MEF_{75-25} as infants. Similarly, these data would suggest that either airway function genuinely improves with age or that the raised-volume technique is better able to detect diminished airway function in infants than spirometry in pre-school children. The reasons for improvement could include the result of treatment, normal lung development, or an increase in airway luminal diameter such that obstruction is less severe in older subjects. The process of augmenting inflations, the effects of sedation and testing in the supine as opposed to upright position in infants may alter airway and lung mechanics, increasing detection of functional abnormalities by the raised-volume technique when compared with older children tested using spirometry.

The reliability of measurements of forced expiration depends on strict quality control. No internationally agreed guidelines exist for pre-school children currently and adult criteria do not apply [33]. Further assessment of those with CF is limited by the need for standardization of spirometry in this age group, but the studies outlined suggest that obtaining data using incentives or by skilled workers is feasible.

Tracking of pre-school lung function to school age

In a prospective study in which lung function was measured serially over 3 years in 30 young children with CF aged 2–8 years, specific airway resistance (sR_{aw}) measured using whole-body plethysmography was compared with measurements of respiratory system resistance obtained using R_{int} and the impulse oscillometry technique, respectively [34]. Mean sR_{aw} was consistently elevated at the start of the study (mean z score 2.52) and remained so at the end of the study (mean z score 2.74). Neither respiratory resistance by the interrupter technique nor the impulse oscillation technique demonstrated consistent abnormal levels. In contrast, 37–57% of subjects exhibited significantly elevated sR_{aw}, and in approximately two-thirds of subjects lung function tracked such that sR_{aw} remained elevated at each assessment. When FEV_1 could be measured in these subjects there was significant correlation between sR_{aw} and FEV_1 ($r^2 = 0.8$). These data indicate that sR_{aw} is elevated in early childhood, that measurements of sR_{aw} track between pre-school age and school age, and that measurements of sR_{aw} are significantly correlated with those of FEV_1. One limitation of this study, however, is that only 13 of the subjects were under 6 years of age at the time of the first lung function test. Further longitudinal studies in which measurements of sR_{aw} are measured in those aged less than 6 years are therefore indicated.

NEWER LUNG FUNCTION TECHNIQUES

The wider acceptability of tests of airway function in infancy is limited due to the necessity for sedation of the subject. The repeatability of measurements following a short interval, such as 2 weeks, is unknown and will be difficult to determine because of reluctance to repeat sedation. This will have an impact on study design where short-term interventions, such as a 2-week course of intravenous antibiotics, are being assessed. Newer techniques may prove more suitable for the early detection of lung function abnormalities in CF and offer further insights into the pathophysiology of pulmonary disease.

Multiple-breath inert-gas washout

This technique is performed during tidal breathing and therefore requires minimal cooperation. Subjects breathe in inert gases, such as helium and sulphur hexafluoride, until wash-in is complete when gas concentrations within the lung reach a steady state. Following disconnection from the gas source, the concentrations of the gases are evaluated as they are washed out during ensuing tidal breathing. Several parameters can be measured, the commonest being measures of the efficiency of expiration such as the lung clearance index (calculated as the cumulative expired volume, expressed as a ratio to functional residual capacity, required to reduce the concentration of the inert gas 40-fold, arbitrarily, from a starting concentration of 4% to 0.1%) and the mixing index (Fig. 23.6). The technique has the advantage that it is quick and easy to perform, that the lung clearance index appears to be stable throughout life in healthy subjects, and that the use of multiple gases of different densities may provide insights into the site of inhomogeneity within the lung.

During inspiration, two mechanisms contribute to gas transport: convection (bulk flow) predominates in the conducting airways as far as the bronchioles, and diffusion predominates in the alveolus. Between the conducting airways and alveoli there is a transition zone termed the 'diffusion front'. Because of their different molecular weights, helium (light) and sulphur hexafluoride (heavy) have different diffusivities. For helium the diffusion front is thought to be located near the terminal and respiratory bronchioles (pre-acinar) and that for sulphur hexafluoride around the alveolar ducts (intra-acinar). The location of the diffusion front contributes to the phase III slope of a standard gas washout curve, another measure of inhomogeneity. Theoretically, comparing the phase III slopes for gases of different molecular weights could be used to estimate the anatomical site affected by disease.

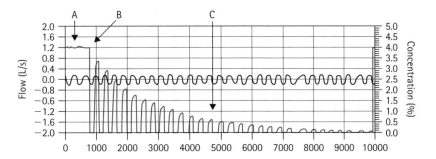

Figure 23.6 Expired gas concentration during multiple-breath inert-gas washout performed during tidal breathing. During the wash-in phase **(A)** a steady-state gas concentration (in this example 4%) indicates that wash-in is complete at which time the subject is disconnected from the test gas and breathes air **(B)**. Subsequently the concentration of test gas in expired air decreases exponentially **(C)**. The lung clearance index is calculated as the cumulative expired volume, expressed as a ratio to functional residual capacity, required to reduce the concentration of the inert gas 40-fold, arbitrarily, from a starting concentration of 4% to 0.1%.

As reductions in flow from obstructed lung regions appear to be compensated by increases in flow from unobstructed regions, during measurements of forced expiration upstream (peripheral) non-uniformities may be masked [35]. For this reason, the maximum forced expiratory flow–volume curve is not considered the ideal tool for the detection of early non-uniform airway disease, while the multiple-breath inert-gas washout technique should be more sensitive at detecting such inhomogeneities.

Measurements using the technique have been obtained in CF subjects of all ages. Multiple-breath inert-gas washout disclosed airway dysfunction in the majority of children with CF aged 3–18 years who had normal lung function assessed by spirometry, suggesting that multiple-breath inert-gas washout is indeed of greater value than spirometry in detecting early CF lung disease [36]. These findings have recently been confirmed in younger subjects [37,38]. In the more recent study [38], 40 children with CF aged 2–5 years and 37 age-matched healthy control subjects performed multiple-breath inert-gas washout, plethysmography and spirometry. Thirty children in each group successfully completed all measures, with success on first visit being between 68% and 86% for all three measures. Children with CF had significantly higher mean lung clearance index (2.7; 95% CI 1.9–3.6, $p < 0.001$) and higher specific airway resistance (z score 1.65; 95% CI 0.96–2.33, $p < 0.001$), and significantly lower $FEV_{0.5}$ (z score -0.49; 95% CI -0.95 to -0.03, $p < 0.05$). Abnormal lung function results were identified in 22 of 30 children (73%) with CF by multiple-breath washout, compared with 14 of 30 (47%) by plethysmography, and 4 of 30 (13%) by spirometry, suggesting that the technique is indeed more sensitive at detecting airway disease in pre-school children with CF. Results of studies in infants using the multiple-breath technique are due to be published soon.

It is not known if multiple-breath washout will be more or less useful than parameters of forced expiration to monitor lung function longitudinally or the response to therapeutic interventions, so further studies are required in order to determine its role. As measurements in infants have so far been incorporated into studies with protocols including more invasive and complex tests, they have been performed following sedation of the infant. It is possible that, when used alone, a period of natural sleep without sedation would be sufficient to enable successful performance of the test. This would significantly enhance the ability of investigators to obtain longitudinal data during the first months of life.

Forced oscillation technique

Although no advantage of the forced oscillation technique (FOT) over conventional spirometry has been identified in older subjects with CF [39,40], the FOT requires minimal cooperation and, when performed at low frequencies, has the theoretical advantage of being able to determine early

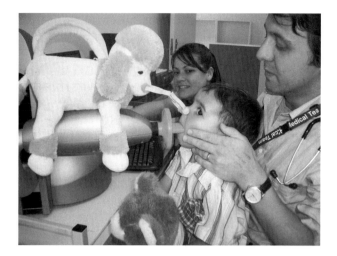

Figure 23.7 Forced oscillation technique (FOT) performed during tidal breathing in a pre-school child aged 2 years. The child is able to maintain a seal around the mouthpiece. The cheeks and chin are supported by the investigator to decrease the influence of upper airway shunt impedance. A second observer is vigilant for technical problems, such as glottic closure and leaks, and any signs of distress in the child.

peripheral functional abnormalities in the alveolar ducts, alveoli and interstitium and its progression more centrally into those parts of the respiratory tree where bulk flow occurs (airway opening to the terminal bronchioles) and could therefore provide further information regarding the pathophysiology and location of very early functional abnormalities in cystic fibrosis. The FOT is easy to perform in pre-school children during tidal breathing using commercially available equipment (Fig. 23.7).

In one longitudinal study, in which FOT, R_{int} and plethysmographic airway resistance were measured serially in pre-school children with CF, only resistance was abnormal in the CF group [34]. FOT at low frequencies (LFFOT) has been used to measure the lung function of infants. The airway is occluded at the end of an augmented inflation in order to invoke the Hering–Breuer inflation reflex, resulting in a short period of apnea during which a pressure wave is applied to the airway opening. Impedance is calculated as the ratio of pressure to flow measured at the airway opening at each frequency of the applied pressure and represents the complex viscoelastic resistance of the respiratory system. Modelling in animals has confirmed both frequency-dependent and independent components of impedance which are considered to provide separate estimates of airway and parenchymal function. Impedance is contributed to by resistance and inertance, attributed to airway function, and coefficients of tissue damping, elastance and hysteresivity (the ratio of tissue damping to inertance), which provide a component of parenchymal function. In one study of 24 children with CF of median age 1.58 years in which LFFOT was performed during an anesthetic for BAL, a significant relationship between lung function parameters which reflect parenchymal mechanics and markers of pulmonary inflammation obtained by BAL was identified [41]. There were significant correlations between measurements of tissue damping and markers of total cell burden, neutrophil number and total cell count per milliliter of fluid retrieved at BAL. Tissue hysteresivity was also significantly related to total cell count and neutrophil number. As lung disease in CF is thought to begin in the distal airways and should therefore be reflected in abnormalities of parenchymal mechanics, measurements made with LFFOT hold promise for detection of lung disease early in the clinical course of young children with CF. Adaptation may make it possible to perform the test in unsedated infants with CF during natural sleep [42].

CONCLUSIONS

Evidence is accumulating that lung function is diminished early in infancy in those with CF and that lung function is associated with structural airway abnormalities and pulmonary inflammation. These findings suggest that the neutrophil-dominated airway pathophysiology and chronic infection, whose progression results in structural alterations, bronchiectasis and ultimately respiratory failure and death, has its onset in infancy. Further studies are required to clarify these associations. Early detection of pre-symptomatic changes in lung function, together with the ability objectively to assess response to treatment, should strengthen our competence at evaluating the effectiveness of therapeutic interventions which aim to minimize or prevent such lung damage in subjects with CF during the critical period of somatic and lung growth and development in infancy. This in turn could increase longevity and contribute to an improved quality of life for these children. Full forced expiratory maneuvers provide useful information regarding airway status in infants with CF and recommendations are available for their standardized performance [7]. Further evaluation is required to determine the appropriateness and feasibility of their use as outcome measures in multicenter studies. However, if exciting newer techniques can be performed in unsedated subjects, then this would signify a major advance in the assessment of infants and pre-school children with cystic fibrosis.

REFERENCES

1. Balough K, McCubbin M, Weinberger M *et al.* The relationship between infection and inflammation in the early stages of lung disease from cystic fibrosis. *Pediatr Pulmonol* 1995; **20**:63–70.

2. Khan TZ, Wagener JS *et al.* Early pulmonary inflammation in infants with cystic fibrosis. *Am J Respir Crit Care Med* 1995; **151**:1075–1082.

3. Gappa M, Ranganathan SC, Stocks J. Lung function testing in infants with cystic fibrosis: lessons from the past and future directions. *Pediatr Pulmonol* 1995; **32**:228–245.

4. Gustafsson PM. Pre-school lung function: the missing link. *Paediatr Respir Rev* 2005; **6**:237–238.

5. Feher A, Castile R, Kisling J *et al.* Flow limitation in normal infants: a new method for forced expiratory maneuvers from raised lung volumes. *J Appl Physiol* 1996; **80**:2019–2025.

6. Turner DJ, Stick SM, Lesouef KL *et al.* A new technique to generate and assess forced expiration from raised lung volume in infants. *Am J Respir Crit Care Med* 1995; **151**:1441–1450.

7. Lum S, Stocks J, Castile R *et al.* ATS/ERS Statement. Raised Volume Forced Expirations in Infants: Guidelines for Current Practice. *Am J Respir Crit Care Med* 2005; **172**:1463–1471.

8. Ranganathan SC, Hoo AF *et al.* Exploring the relationship between forced maximal flow at functional residual capacity and parameters of forced expiration from raised lung volume in healthy infants. *Pediatr Pulmonol* 2002; **33**:419–428.

9. Ranganathan S, Dezateux CA, Bush A *et al.* Airway function in infants newly diagnosed with cystic fibrosis. *Lancet* 2001; **358**:1964–1965.

10. Ranganathan SC, Bush A, Dezateux C *et al.* Relative ability of full and partial forced expiratory maneuvers to identify diminished airway function in infants with cystic fibrosis. *Am J Respir Crit Care Med*, 2002; **66**:1350–1357.

11. Ranganathan SC, Stocks J, Dezateux C *et al.* The evolution of airway function in early childhood following clinical diagnosis of cystic fibrosis. *Am J Respir Crit Care Med* 2004; **169**:928–933.

12. Castile RG, Iram D, McCoy KS. Gas trapping in normal infants and in infants with cystic fibrosis. *Pediatr Pulmonol* 2004; **37**:461–469.

13. Tepper RS, Weist A, Williams-Nkomo T, Kisling J. Elastic properties of the respiratory system in infants with cystic fibrosis. *Am J Respir Crit Care Med* 2004; **170**:505–507.

14. Landau LI, Phelan PD. The spectrum of cystic fibrosis: a study of pulmonary mechanics in 46 patients. *Am Rev Respir Dis* 1973; **108**:593–602.

15. Mansell A, Dubrawsky C, Levison H *et al.* Lung elastic recoil in cystic fibrosis. *Am Rev Respir Dis* 1974; **109**:190–197.

16. Dakin CJ, Numa AH, Wang H *et al.* Inflammation, infection, and pulmonary function in infants and young children with cystic fibrosis. *Am J Respir Crit Care Med* 2002; **165**:904–910.

17. Rosenfeld M, Gibson RL, McNamara S *et al.* Early pulmonary infection, inflammation, and clinical outcomes in infants with cystic fibrosis. *Pediatr Pulmonol* 2001; **32**:356–366.

18. Nixon GM, Armstrong DS, Carzino R *et al.* Early airway infection, inflammation, and lung function in cystic fibrosis. *Arch Dis Child* 2002; **87**:306–311.

19. Long FR, Williams RS, Castile RG. Structural airway abnormalities in infants and young children with cystic fibrosis. *J Pediatr* 2004; **144**:154–161.

20. Martinez TM, Llapur CJ, Williams TH *et al.* High-resolution computed tomography imaging of airway disease in infants with cystic fibrosis. *Am J Respir Crit Care Med* 2005; **172**:1133–1138.

21. Cook DG, Strachan DP. Health effects of passive smoking. 10: Summary of effects of parental smoking on the respiratory

health of children and implications for research. *Thorax* 1999; **54**:357–366.

22. Le Souef PN. Pediatric origins of adult lung diseases. 4: Tobacco-related lung diseases begin in childhood. *Thorax* 2000; **55**:1063–1067.

23. Kraemer R, Birrer P, Liechti-Gallati S. Genotype–phenotype association in infants with cystic fibrosis at the time of diagnosis. *Pediatr Res* 1998; **44**:920–926.

24. Mohon RT, Wagener JS, Abman SH *et al.* Relationship of genotype to early pulmonary function in infants with cystic fibrosis identified through neonatal screening. *J Pediatr* 1993; **122**:550–555.

25. Banovcin P, Seidenberg J, von der Hardt H. Assessment of tidal breathing patterns for monitoring of bronchial obstruction in infants. *Pediatr Res* 1995; **38**:218–220.

26. Bates J, Schmalisch G, Filbrun D, Stocks J. Tidal breath analysis for infant pulmonary function testing. *Eur Respir J* 2000; **16**:1180–1192.

27. Dezateux CA, Stocks J, Dundas I *et al.* The relationship between t_{PTEF}:t_E and specific airways conductance in infancy. *Pediatr Pulmonol* 1994; **18**:299–307.

28. Ranganathan SC, Goetz I, Hoo AF *et al.* Assessment of tidal breathing parameters in infants with cystic fibrosis. *Eur Respir J* 2003; **22**:761–766.

29. Bridge PD, Ranganathan S, McKenzie SA. Measurement of airway resistance using the interrupter technique in preschool children in the ambulatory setting. *Eur Respir J* 1999; **13**:792–796.

30. Beydon N, Amsallem F, Bellet M *et al.* Pulmonary function tests in preschool children with cystic fibrosis. *Am J Respir Crit Care Med* 2002; **166**:1099–1104.

31. Kozlowska WJ, Aurora P, Lum S *et al.* Longitudinal assessment of lung function in infants and pre-school children with cystic fibrosis. *Arch Dis Child* 2004; **89**(Suppl 1):A38.

32. Marostica PJ, Weist AD, Eigen H *et al.* Spirometry in 3- to 6-year-old children with cystic fibrosis. *Am J Respir Crit Care Med* 2002; **166**:67–71.

33. Aurora P, Stocks J, Oliver C *et al.* Quality control for spirometry in preschool children with and without lung disease. *Am J Respir.Crit Care Med* 2004; **169**:1152–1159.

34. Nielsen KG, Pressler T, Klug B *et al.* Serial lung function and responsiveness in cystic fibrosis during early childhood. *Am J Respir Crit Care Med* 2004; **169**:1209–1216.

35. McNamara J, Castile R, Ludwig M. Interdependent regional emptying during forced expiration. *J Appl Physiol* 1994; **76**:356–360.

36. Gustafsson PM, Aurora P, Lindblad A. Evaluation of ventilation maldistribution as an early indicator of lung disease in children with cystic fibrosis. *Eur Respir J* 2003; **22**:972–979.

37. Aurora P, Gustaffson P, Bush A *et al.* Multiple-breath inert gas washout as a measure of ventilation distribution in children with cystic fibrosis. *Thorax* 2004; **59**:1068–1073.

38. Aurora P, Bush A, Gustafsson P *et al.* Multiple-breath washout as a marker of lung disease in preschool children with cystic fibrosis. *Am J Respir Crit Care Med* 2005; **171**:249–256.

39. Hellinckx J, De Boeck K, Demedts M. No paradoxical bronchodilator response with forced oscillation technique in children with cystic fibrosis. *Chest* 1998; **113**:55–59.

40. Lebecque P, Stanescu D. Respiratory resistance by the forced oscillation technique in asthmatic children and cystic fibrosis patients. *Eur Respir J* 1997; **10**:891–895.

41. Brennan S, Hall GL, Horak F *et al.* Correlation of forced oscillation technique in preschool children with cystic fibrosis with pulmonary inflammation. *Thorax* 2005; **60**:159–163.

42. Pillow JJ, Stocks J, Sly PD, Hantos Z. Partitioning of airway and parenchymal mechanics in unsedated newborn infants. *Pediatr Res* 2005; **58**:1210–1215.

Infant and pre-school children: role of bronchoscopy

GARY CONNETT

INTRODUCTION

Health professionals caring for patients with cystic fibrosis (CF) over the last 30–40 years have witnessed major improvements in the outcome for individuals who are diagnosed with this condition. The consensus view is that this has largely been achieved as a result of improved nutritional management and the aggressive use of measures to treat lung infection.

A complete understanding of the pathophysiology of CF-related lung disease remains frustratingly elusive, but a number of prospective studies of diagnosed infants detected through newborn screening programs have consistently demonstrated that, while the lungs are structurally normal at birth, significant infection and inflammation commonly occurs in early infancy. These important data underline the need to consider early interventions to interrupt or prevent these processes that are almost certainly relevant to the occurrence of lung damage in later life.

Unfortunately, the optimal strategy for the use of antimicrobial therapies and other measures to enhance the clearance of abnormal secretions in early childhood has yet to be defined. There are considerable differences in the approach to microbial surveillance and the use of antibiotics between and even within specialist centers. Such differences might reasonably be a result of differences in disease phenotype, local availability of services and various social factors determining each family's ability to achieve recommendations for care. Despite these variations in practice there is no doubt that fiberoptic bronchoscopy is an essential part of the modern management of CF and should be readily available to all patients. This chapter will review the insights bronchoscopy studies have given us about the early events within the airways of CF children and the use of bronchoscopy in managing the pre-school age group.

RESEARCH STUDIES

The Denver pediatric CF service was one of the first to investigate the early onset of infection in CF [43]. The group initially published their findings from throat swabs in a cohort of infants identified through newborn screening and reported high rates of *Staphylococcus aureus* and *Haemophilus influenzae* isolates in infants (43% and 62%, respectively). *Pseudomonas aeruginosa* was isolated in a quarter of children by a mean age of 20 months. Those with *P. aeruginosa* commonly had preceding *S. aureus* infection and were more symptomatic. Subsequently the group reported their bronchial lavage studies and found increased numbers of neutrophils and increased levels of the pro-inflammatory cytokine IL-8 from infants as young as 4 weeks [44]. These results have been confirmed in other studies [45]. While indices of inflammation were increased in some non-infected CF patients compared with non-CF controls, the amount of inflammation was much higher in those who were culture-positive.

The early onset of a neutrophil-dominated inflammatory process before the detection of bacterial pathogens in some of the CF infants led to speculation about a causal association between the basic gene defect and the initiation of an inflammatory process starting shortly after birth. Serial bronchial lavage studies have shown continued neutrophil-dominated inflammation, several weeks after successful eradication of infecting organisms. These findings have led researchers to suggest that defects in CFTR function might cause the perpetuation of a relentless inflammatory process, irrespective of ongoing infection, once triggered within the airways [46]. The relationship between infection and inflammation in the CF airway remains controversial. The most recently reported bronchoscopy study of lower airways inflammation in infants with cystic fibrosis identified by screening showed similar findings comparing newly diagnosed, asymptomatic, uninfected infants and a non-CF control group. However, once infection had occurred, this precipitated a sustained inflammatory process within the lung [47].

Unfortunately suitable anti-inflammatory agents for use in infancy have not come to clinical trials and subsequent bronchoscopy studies have focused on the use of sequential bronchoscopies to characterize the development of lower respiratory infection during early life.

The Melbourne pediatric CF service was one of the first units to report the results of repeated annual bronchial lavage cultures performed under general anesthesia in a pre-school CF population identified through newborn screening [48–50]. *Pseudomonas aeruginosa* infection diagnosed on the basis of quantitative culture ($>10^5$ colony-forming units/mL) was common and found in up to 43% of their cohort. This threshold level of detection was identified as being associated with a significant step up in measures of airways inflammation. Unfortunately the center had cross-infection problems with a particularly virulent pseudomonad within the unit that is of relevance to their findings, and may limit the generalizability of some of their conclusions. However, the group provided good evidence that early acquisition of *Pseudomonas* was associated with increased morbidity and mortality.

A larger longitudinal study, performed in three US CF centers, reported similar findings [51]. This group found that *H. influenzae* was the most common pathogen in infancy but that *S. aureus* and *P. aeruginosa* were more prevalent at ages 2 and 3 years. *P. aeruginosa* occurred at any density in one-third of children and in $>10^5$ colony-forming units/mL in 20% of children at 2 and 3 years of age. The density of CF pathogens and markers of airway inflammation increased over time in association with subtle indices of worsening respiratory status. However, it was difficult to identify infected individuals on the basis of symptoms alone. Surprisingly, antibiotic treatment prior to bronchoscopies did not appear to impact on culture results.

The most important finding from these studies is the recognition that many infants with little or no symptomatic lung disease have significant lower respiratory infection at the time of routine bronchoscopies. Those children with *P. aeruginosa* infection tended to be more symptomatic, and did less well subsequently. These results raise important issues about the recommended frequency and methods of routine microbial surveillance. Clearly there are practical limitations in carrying out very frequent bronchoscopies and so subsequent studies have examined the use of less invasive culture techniques to guide antibiotic choices in this age group.

OROPHARYNGEAL CULTURES VERSUS BRONCHOALVEOLAR LAVAGE

Cystic fibrosis centers have used a number of different microbiological specimens to identify the cause of lower respiratory infection in young children. It is unusual for children to expectorate sputum before the age of 6 years and if they can this generally implies the early development of significant airway complications. Sputum induction with hypertonic saline is difficult under the age of 8 years in CF patients, although these specimens have been obtained in much younger children as part of the diagnostic work-up of tuberculosis [52,53]. Oropharyngeal cough swabs and, in some centers laryngeal aspirates, are the most commonly used culture specimens. Oropharyngeal specimens in particular have been investigated in a number of studies to determine their usefulness in detecting lower respiratory infection detected by bronchoscopy[54–56].

In older children, oropharyngeal cultures have high positive predictive value for lower respiratory infection, but in one study less than half of *P. aeruginosa* infections were detected among those who could not expectorate [54]. The combined results of three studies in early childhood suggest that oropharyngeal cultures have high specificity and high negative predictive value for *P. aeruginosa* [56] This means that if culture results are negative, lower airway infection is unlikely. This finding must be treated with caution. The high specificity in young children is because the prevalence of *Pseudomonas* infection is relatively low at an early age (around 20%) and so most swabs will be negative anyway. The positive predictive value – the ratio of true positives to (true positives + false positives) – is a more clinically relevant statistic and in early childhood this figure is around 44% for *Pseudomonas* in the first 18 months of life, with a similarly low sensitivity of less than 50%. Not surprisingly, oropharyngeal cultures are more sensitive when there is a higher density of infecting organisms in the lower airway and so become more informative as children grow older.

Similar findings are reported for *S. aureus* and *H. influenzae*. These bacteria are more prevalent and so, while they also have high negative predictive value when not grown, the specificity of a positive culture is low. For example, positive upper airway cultures for *S. aureus* tend to over-diagnose lower respiratory infection by a factor of approximately 2. The presence of symptoms has not been found to be of use in improving the specificity of the culture results for these organisms.

One problem when trying to interpret these studies is that they have been carried out in clinically stable patients and there is little information about the relative usefulness of bronchoscopy and upper airway cultures in diagnosing the cause of acute symptoms. Furthermore, the oropharyngeal cultures used in these studies were obtained by swabbing the oropharyngeal wall and tonsillar pillars. In many centers cough swabs are used. A swab is placed in the oropharynx to capture aerosolized secretions without touching the upper airway walls if possible. The relative benefits of this type of specimen have not been studied in detail.

When the genotypes of bacterial species are considered, the clinical picture becomes more complicated. Studies that have compared the type of *Pseudomonas* strains from the upper and lower airway have found that in many cases they are unrelated and, when studied longitudinally, genetically different strains appear at different times in the same airway [55,57].

CLINICAL CONSIDERATIONS

It appears from these data that the greatest potential for the use of bronchoscopy in young children is in the early detection of *Pseudomonas* infection in situations where there is clinical concern about the progression of lung complications but no evidence for infection using other microbial samples. Early infection with *Pseudomonas* species might be anticipated more commonly during winter months occurring concomitantly with and persisting after viral respiratory illnesses that typically occur at this time of year [58]. When pseudomonads are initially identified in young patients they are typically present in small numbers, nonmucoid in type, pan-sensitive to anti-pseudomonal antibiotics and, provided there are no local cross-infection issues with highly transmissible trains, unique to that individual.

Treating *Pseudomonas* infection when detected at this early stage is commonly regarded as a useful intervention during a 'window of opportunity' before progression to chronic infection and associated lung damage. Unfortunately we have little information about what constitutes the best antibiotic treatment regimen for these early isolates, and recurrent infection with different *Pseudomonas* strains is common. A cohort study that looked hard for *Pseudomonas* in the first three years of life found recurrent isolates on lavage and/or the presence of positive serological markers to exotoxin A and whole-cell membrane proteins in nearly all of the patients studied [59]. These findings raise issues about how to balance the use of early interventions to prevent the onset of chronic infection against the overuse of antibiotics and invasive investigations with their concomitant risk of potentially harmful side-effects.

There are practical considerations that limit the extent to which bronchoscopy can be considered as the gold standard for detecting infection.

One of the most important considerations is determining whereabouts in the lung bronchoalveolar lavage should be performed. While secretions, if present in the major branches of the tracheobronchial tree, might usefully be collected for culture during bronchoscopy, bronchoalveolar lavage will sample washings obtained only from the subsegmental bronchi within which the bronchoscope is wedged. For reasons that are not understood, upper lobes and the right upper lobe in particular are typically involved with early focal bronchiectasis, but there is endless variability in the pattern of bronchial damage; so an individualized approach, based on each child's clinical circumstances, is recommended.

Bronchoscopy studies where lavage specimens have been obtained from more than one site clearly demonstrate variability in the organisms cultivated, irrespective of the extent to which there is inflammation in different parts of the lung. These findings emphasize the need for careful planning prior to bronchoscopy to maximize the probability of yielding clinically useful information and to consider lavage in more than one site [60].

Chest x-rays can be particularly difficult to interpret in this age group. Localized changes are not always readily identifiable, but there is some evidence that ventilation scans can usefully detect regional defects that are missed on plain films. High-resolution chest CT studies can also usefully demonstrate whether there are early focal structural changes or a more diffuse disease process affecting all lung areas [61].

BRONCHOSCOPY TECHNIQUE

In general the largest bronchoscope that can be tolerated by the child should be used, to minimize the occurrence of blockage of the suctioning channel with mucopurulent secretions. Suctioning of the upper airway through the bronchoscope should be avoided to prevent contamination of lavage samples by upper airway organisms. In centers using general anesthesia for their bronchoscopies, placement of a laryngeal mask airway can help minimize upper airway contamination, Aliquots of warmed normal saline should be used for lavage. Although there is no consensus on the optimal volumes to use, a return of 40% or more of the volume instilled is generally judged as technically satisfactory. Occasionally, in severely affected CF patients, lavage returns are low in volume because of recurrent blockage of the suction channel. Suctioning pressures might need to be individually titrated to maximize returns without causing complete collapse of the bronchial lumen.

If cytological studies are available, the first aliquot, which is of more bronchial origin, tends to have a higher cell count and is perhaps therefore more usefully indicative of the airway disease process [62]. The relative merits of general anesthesia versus sedation continue to be debated. Children bronchoscoped under sedation tend to cough more during the bronchoscopy but this can usefully identify where abnormal secretions are coming from and thus where the bronchoscope should be best placed for diagnostic lavage. Occasionally, the child's coughing achieves short-term therapeutic benefits as a result of improved airway clearance during the procedure. The retention of lidocaine in the bronchoscope can contaminate lavage samples and this drug has the potential to inhibit bacterial growth [63,64].

WHEN TO PERFORM BRONCHOSCOPY: RECOMMENDATIONS

Given the available evidence, the following recommendations relate to how bronchoscopy might best be used for diagnosis of microbial infection and to detect other pathology in this age group (Table 23.7).

Table 23.7   Indications for bronchoscopy.

Acute respiratory exacerbation, uniformative cultures and poor
    response to empirical broad-spectrum antibiotic treatment
Acute respiratory exacerbation poorly responsive to treatment of
    positive oropharyngeal/cough swab cultures
Persistent focal atelectasis despite aggressive medical
    treatment
Atypical symptoms such as recurrent or persistent wheezing
New radiological abnormalities, declining lung function or any
    other deterioration in respiratory status with uninformative
    cultures
Investigation for histological evidence of atypical mycobacteria
    infection
Investigation for reflux/aspiration pneumonitis

Bronchoscopy as part of microbial surveillance

It is difficult to justify the *routine* use of bronchoscopy in all pre-school children, irrespective of whether or not they have symptoms, solely for the purpose of microbiological studies. Opportunistic culture results from bronchoscopies performed just once yearly, and not necessarily at times when the need for more detailed clinical information is specifically indicated, are unlikely to result in major benefits to the individuals concerned. However, routine bronchoscopies are justified in this age group if they are carried out within the constructs of ethically approved research studies with the informed consent of each child's parents. Indeed, such a randomized controlled trial is currently ongoing in Australasia, although the results will take some years to accrue. More studies, around the time when lung inflammation first occurs in childhood, are critical to our future understanding of the pathophysiology of CF lung damage and how best to treat it.

Within current best practice, there is clearly a need for closer surveillance of respiratory status during the pre-school years to identify early any deterioration in lower respiratory status and bronchoscopy has an important role in this area. As well as careful questioning about the occurrence of symptoms, clinical examination and chest x-rays, CF centers should also consider the use of supplementary investigations such as ventilation scans, chest computed tomography and lung function testing [23] to improve detection of lung complications. When abnormal findings are detected, routine microbial cultures should be obtained. If these do not identify CF pathogens, or if there is a poor response to antimicrobial treatment of the pathogens identified on upper airway culture, bronchoscopy should be performed to clarify the cause of lower respiratory symptoms. Specimens must be sent for viral as well as bacterial isolation. Lower respiratory viral infection during an acute exacerbation is an important risk factor for early acquisition of chronic *Pseudomonas* infection [66].

Bronchoscopy to investigate the cause of atypical symptoms

A wealth of clinical experience has established that bronchoscopy has an important role in identifying the cause of lower respiratory symptoms when the clinical picture is atypical [67]. In particular, bronchoscopy should be considered in young children when recurrent wheezing is a predominant feature. CF children with a wide variety of comorbidities have been identified. These include tracheomalacia, subglottic stenosis, bronchomalacia, and aortic arch anomalies. Differential cell counts can also be useful to identify the predominant cell types involved if there is inflammation.

Occasionally mucoid plugs extending into the large airways can be a cause of segmental atelectasis and cause persistent radiological abnormalities despite rigorous physiotherapy and intravenous antibiotics. Endobronchial aspergillosis can also cause this complication. Plugs can be effectively cleared from the bronchial lumen after suctioning with or without the local instillation of rhDNase [68]. Such problems are more likely to be encountered in older children.

Infection with atypical mycobacteria can occur in this age group but it can be difficult to determine the clinical relevance of positive airway cultures. Bronchoscopy to obtain histological evidence for lung infection can usefully help identify those cases for whom aggressive antituberculous chemotherapy would be appropriate [69].

Bronchial lavage specimens can also be analyzed to measure the quantity of lipid in alveolar macrophages. This has been suggested as a potentially useful marker of aspiration. Unfortunately, studies in CF suggest that the lipid laden macrophage index is very non-specific in identifying when aspiration is the cause of inflammation [70].

THE FUTURE

Further bronchoscopy studies are critical to our increased understanding of cystic fibrosis. Gene therapy research is ongoing and bronchoscopic techniques have been developed for measuring potential differences in the lower airways of children as young as 12 months, making this a potentially useful end-point assay [71]. Such measurements might find application in assessing the direct benefits of other novel therapies.

REFERENCES

43. Abman SH, Ogle JW, Harbeck RJ *et al.* Early bacteriologic, immunologic, and clinical courses of young infants with cystic fibrosis identified by neonatal screening. *J Pediatr* 1991; **119**:211–217.
44. Khan TZ, Wagener JS, Bost T *et al.* Early pulmonary inflammation in infants with cystic fibrosis. *Am J Respir Crit Care Med* 1995; **151**:1075–1082.

45. Balough K, McCubbin M, Weinberger M *et al.* The relationship between infection and inflammation in the early stages of lung disease from cystic fibrosis. *Pediatr Pulmonol* 1995; **20**:63–70.

46. Konstan MW, Berger M. Current understanding of the inflammatory process in cystic fibrosis: onset and etiology. *Pediatr Pulmonol* 1997; **24**:137–142.

47. Armstrong DS, Hook SM, Jamsen KM *et al.* Lower airway inflammation in infants with cystic fibrosis detected by newborn screening. *Pediatr Pulmonol* 2005; **40**:500–510.

48. Armstrong DS, Grimwood K, Carzino R *et al.* Lower respiratory infection and inflammation in infants with newly diagnosed cystic fibrosis. *Br Med J* 1995; **310**:1571–1572.

49. Armstrong DS, Grimwood K, Carlin JB *et al.* Lower airway inflammation in infants and young children with cystic fibrosis. *Am J Respir Crit Care Med* 1997; **156**:1197–1204.

50. Nixon GM, Armstrong DS, Carzino R *et al.* Clinical outcome after early *Pseudomonas aeruginosa* infection in cystic fibrosis. *J Pediatr* 2001; **138**:699–704.

51. Rosenfield M, Gibson RL, McNamara S *et al.* Early pulmonary infection, inflammation, and clinical outcomes in infants with cystic fibrosis. *Pediatr Pulmonol* 2001; **32**:356–366.

52. Reinhardt N, Chen CI, Loppow D *et al.* Cellular profiles of induced sputum in children with stable cystic fibrosis: comparison with BAL. *Eur Resp J* 2003; **22**:497–502.

53. Zar HJ, Hanslo D, Apolles P *et al.* Induced sputum versus gastric lavage for microbiological confirmation of pulmonary tuberculosis in infants and young children: a prospective study. *Lancet* 2005; **365**:130–134.

54. Ramsey BW, Wentz KR, Smith AL *et al.* Predictive value of oropharyngeal cultures in identifying lower airway bacteria in cystic fibrosis patients. *Am Rev Respir Dis* 1991; **144**:331–337.

55. Armstrong DS, Grimwood K, Carlin JB *et al.* Bronchoalveolar lavage of oropharyngeal cultures to identify lower respiratory pathogens in infants with cystic fibrosis. *Pediatr Pulmonol* 1996; **21**:267–275.

56. Rosenfield M, Emerson J, Accurso F *et al.* Diagnostic accuracy of oropharyngeal cultures in infants and young children with cystic fibrosis. *Pediatr Pulmonol* 1999; **28**:321–328.

57. Jung A, Kleinau I, Schonian G *et al.* Sequential genotyping of *Pseudomonas aeruginosa* from upper and lower airways of cystic fibrosis patients. *Eur Resp J* 2002; **20**:1457–1463.

58. Rosenfeld M, Ramsey BW, Gibson RL. *Pseudomonas* acquisition in young patients with cystic fibrosis: pathophysiology, diagnosis and management. *Curr Opin Pulm Med* 2003; **9**:492–497.

59. Johansen HK, Hoiby N. Seasonal onset of initial colonisation and chronic infection with *Pseudomonas aeruginosa* in patients with cystic fibrosis. *Thorax* 1992; **47**:109–111.

60. Gutierrez JP, Grimwood K, Armstrong DS *et al.* Interlobar differences in bronchoalveolar lavage from children with cystic fibrosis. *Eur Respir J* 2001; **17**:281–286.

61. Bush A, Davies J. Early detection of lung disease in pre-school children with cystic fibrosis. *Curr Opin Pulm Med* 2005; **11**:534–538.

62. Ratjen F, Rietschel E, Griese M *et al.* Fractional analysis of bronchoalveolar lavage in cystic fibrosis patients with normal lung function: bronchoalveolar lavage for the evaluation of anti-inflammatory treatment (BEAT study group). *Eur Resp J* 2000; **15**:141–145.

63. Schmidt RM, Rosenkranz HS. Antimicrobial activity of local anaesthetics: lidocaine and procaine. *J Infect Dis* 1970; **121**:597–607.

64. Ravin CE, Latimer JM, Matsen JM. In-vitro effects of lidocaine on anaerobic respiratory pathoens and strains of *Haemophilus influenzae*. *Chest* 1977; **72**:439–441.

65. Ragnanathan SC, Dezeateux C, Bush A *et al.* Airway function in infants newly diagnosed with cystic fibrosis. *Lancet* 2001; **358**:1964–1965.

66. Armstrong D, Grimwood K, Carlin JB *et al.* Severe viral respiratory infections in infants with cystic fibrosis. *Pediatr Pulmonol* 1998; **26**:371–379.

67. Connett GJ, Doull I, Keeping K, Warner JO. Flexible fibre optic bronchoscopy in the management of lung complications in cystic fibrosis. *Acta Paediatr* 1996; **85**:675–678.

68. Slattery DM, Waltz DA *et al.* Bronchoscopically administered recombinant human DNase for lobar atelectasis in cystic fibrosis. *Pediatr Pulmonol* 2001; **31**:383–388.

69. Quittell LM. Management of non-tuberculous mycobacteria in patients with cystic fibrosis. *Paediatr Respir Rev* 2004; **5**(Suppl A):S217–S219.

70. Kazachkov MY, Muhlebach MS, Livasy CA, Noah TL. Lipid laden macrophage index and inflammation in bronchoalveolar lavage fluids in children. *Eur Resp J* 2001; **18**:790–795.

71. Davies JC, Davies M, McShane D *et al.* Potential difference measurements in the lower airway of children with and without cystic fibrosis. *Am J Resp Crit Care Med* 2005; **171**:1015–1019.

Infant and pre-school children: imaging the lungs

SAMATHA SONNAPPA AND CATHERINE M. OWENS

INTRODUCTION

Chest radiography is the primary imaging modality and the most widely used diagnostic method for assessing and following progression of cystic fibrosis (CF) lung disease. The Cystic Fibrosis Foundation recommends annual chest radiographs to assess serial changes in all CF patients [72–74]. Chest radiography is simple, inexpensive, widely available and involves relatively little radiation exposure. Hence, at the current time the chest radiograph remains the most widely used diagnostic method for assessing progression of CF lung disease outside of research institutions.

Global measures of pulmonary function may not accurately depict lung involvement particularly in the early stages in CF due to the heterogeneity of the disease process. More sensitive imaging studies, in particular computed tomography (CT), and high-resolution CT (HRCT) scans which display regional variation in CF lung disease, have been shown to have a higher sensitivity in detecting minor pulmonary abnormalities in CF and have a role in the early detection of CF lung disease as demonstrated by several recent studies [75–81].

The first report of CT scanning to monitor CF-related lung disease was published in 1986 [82], and since then further publications have ensued. In recent years the fact that morphological changes seen with CT scanning have been shown to precede functional changes identified with conventional spirometry, accompanied by the need for more sensitive outcome measures to assess novel therapies, has caused a resurgence of interest in this imaging technique.

Despite the availability of more sensitive tools, current recommendations for imaging in CF include chest radiography for surveillance and as needed for pulmonary exacerbations [72]. However, challenges in managing CF include early detection and treatment before irreversible lung damage occurs, with emphasis on potential benefits. Hence it is important to assess the potential benefits of more sensitive tools for diagnosis and surveillance with a careful risk–benefit analysis.

At the present time newborn screening and gene therapy promise potential improvement in morbidity. Therapeutic options that are being developed for the treatment of CF lung disease include gene therapy, compounds that target the mutated CF protein, alternate chloride channel stimulators, newer antibiotics and anti-inflammatory agents. Sensitive methods for evaluating effectiveness of these novel therapies in patients are an important priority in order to deliver better healthcare to patients with CF. This represents an important potential role for imaging [83]. CT scanning has the potential to offer information that may be complimentary to that provided by pulmonary function tests, both in understanding the pathophysiology of CF lung disease and in evaluating patients clinically.

EVOLUTION OF CF LUNG DISEASE IN THE EARLY YEARS

The development of early lung disease in patients with CF remains poorly defined. CF lung disease is predominantly located in the airways. Several papers have shown that the lungs are essentially normal at birth, but histological abnormalities are detectable in the airways within the first few days of life. Submucosal gland hypertrophy, duct obstruction and mucus cell hyperplasia of the trachea and major bronchi have been demonstrated even before there is evidence of clinical infection [84]. Quantitative evaluation of the tracheobronchial mucus glands in infants with CF has shown a significant dilatation of acini compared to controls [85]. Inflammation is usually present in the airways of minimally symptomatic infants and pre-school children with CF, often even in the absence of infection with bacteria traditionally identified as CF lung pathogens [86,87]. Infection becomes established with bacteria such as *Staphylococcus aureus*, *Haemophilus influenzae* and *Pseudomonas aeruginosa*. The CF lung is constantly undergoing an onslaught of severe proteolytic attack even during 'well' periods, resulting in persistent lung infection and inflammation [88]. This ultimately destroys the airways causing bronchiolectasis and bronchiectasis [89].

MONITORING LUNG DISEASE

Monitoring the onset and progression of lung disease closely is essential for effective individualized management. Lung function and lung structure are important aspects in the assessment of respiratory disease progression in CF patients.

Standard pulmonary function testing (PFT) in CF includes forced expiratory maneuvers and measurement of lung volumes usually performed in children older than 5 years of age [90]. Forced expiratory volume in one second (FEV$_1$) has been shown to reflect progression of pulmonary disease in CF, and to correlate with mortality [91]. However, FEV$_1$ is not very sensitive to early disease. Sensitive, non-invasive methods of assessing early pulmonary changes that can be used from birth have recently been developed in a research context. These studies have shown that airway function is diminished soon after diagnosis in infants with CF and does not catch up during infancy and early childhood [92,93]. Other recently published studies have demonstrated that abnormal ventilation distribution measured by multiple breath washout (MBW) studies is found in most pre-school children with CF, including many with normal spirometry and normal plethysmography [94]. These findings suggest that destructive processes in the airways of children with CF may start early in life and that these changes are not always readily detected by commonly used measures of lung function. Lung function changes are discussed in more detail in Chapter 23a.

CHEST RADIOGRAPHY

Conventional chest radiographs are widely used both for monitoring acute exacerbations and for annual reviews [74]. In the newborn with cystic fibrosis the lungs are initially radiographically normal, but in those with early disease progression substantial small airway mucus plugging, inflammation and infection develop. This is reflected radiographically as hyperinflation of the lungs [95,96]. Peribronchial cuffing of end-on bronchi (bronchial wall thickening) and mucus plugging of small airways are manifest as nodular or reticulonodular patterns on chest radiography [97]. With advancing disease, large airways bronchiectasis develops which is the hallmark of established CF. Bronchial wall thickening is common in bronchiectasis and may precede bronchial dilatation and it is this abnormal wall thickening that allows

visualization of the pathologically thickened airways in the periphery of the lung beyond the level of the segmental bronchi, which are not normally visible. With further progression of bronchiectasis larger cysts form [97]. Mucoid impaction of the bronchi appears as rounded or band-like opacities of increased density following the course of the dilated bronchi. Lobar and segmental atelectasis may result, most frequently seen in the upper and middle lobes. Interestingly, and unlike in the normal host where infection manifests as lobar pneumonia, this pattern is unusual in CF, where patchy areas representing peribronchial consolidation occur.

Standard posteroanterior (PA) radiographs are performed to clinically evaluate and exclude complications such as atelectasis, consolidation, pneumothorax or cor pulmonale on regular follow-ups or during exacerbations. Conventional radiography remains the primary imaging technique for following the progression of disease and assessing serial change. However, the chest x-ray is less sensitive at detecting early disease compared with other modalities such as computed tomography (CT) scanning (Fig. 23.8a).

Various chest radiographic scoring systems exist to assess the severity of respiratory disease in CF, based either on chest radiography alone or in combination with clinical status [98–103]. The commonly used scoring systems are Shwachman–Kulczycki [98], Chrispin–Norman [99], modified Chrispin–Norman [104], Brasfield [100], Wisconsin (designed particularly for early-stage disease [102]) and Northern [103]. Most of these systems require both PA and lateral chest x-rays, with the exception of the Northern and the modified Chrispin–Norman systems. The limitation of the scoring systems is the inability to discriminate between milder disease forms in infants and young children.

The European CF Consensus Committee recently recommended that CF patients should have a chest x-ray as part of their annual assessment and advised the use of a scoring system that requires only a PA film [74].

The distinct advantage of chest radiography over other more sensitive imaging techniques such as CT scanning is the lower radiation exposure to the patient and the low financial cost. Conventional chest radiographs are usually adequate to detect the salient radiographic features of CF and to provide objective parameters for longitudinal qualitative disease progression. However there are limitations, including difficult interpretation of the precise nature of structural lung abnormalities, poor prognostic value, and structural changes not obvious in the early stages. Also as the pulmonary disease progresses the chest x-ray becomes less sensitive to change [82,105].

USE OF CT IN CLINICAL CARE OF THE PATIENT

Some studies have shown a poor association between relatively good spirometry compared to the abnormalities detected on more sensitive imaging tools such as CT [80].

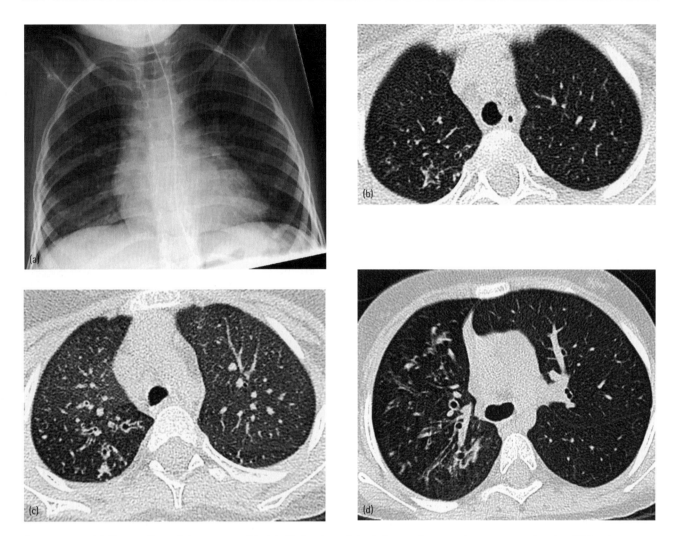

Figure 23.8 (a) Chest radiograph in a 3-year-old with CF showing minimal abnormality secondary to mucus plugging. (b) Inspiratory and (c) expiratory high-resolution CT (HRCT) in the same patient at the same level. Expiratory view shows air trapping (hyper-transradiant lung) more clearly, associated with bronchiectatic changes. (d) HRCT in the same patient at the level of carina showing right upper lobe

Substantial structural lung damage was demonstrated in some children who had normal spirometry [106], and more recently a study in older children and adults with CF found that MBW measurements correlated more closely to HRCT changes than did spirometry [107]. HRCT is clearly more sensitive and accurate than conventional chest radiography in delineating the extent and severity of bronchiectasis and other parenchymal and airway lesions in CF [77,108]. While CT scanning has been shown to reflect improvement in patients treated for respiratory tract exacerbations, no clinical advantage has been shown for this evaluation [109,110].

In summary, functional lung changes can be absent when structural changes are present. Thin-slice CT scanning appears to be a more sensitive method than conventional spirometry to detect structural changes and disease progression. However, whether using CT in routine patient management improves the health and outcome of patients has yet to be proven. There is an additional risk of radiation-induced morbidity and mortality with routine annual

CT scanning, particularly as survival rates for patients with CF is improving [111].

CT techniques

The two CT techniques that have been used for the evaluation of CF lung disease are high-resolution CT (HRCT) and volumetric (or spiral) CT. Conventional (incremental) HRCT uses thin sections (<2 mm) obtained at discontiguous intervals through the lungs. The technique was developed to provide thin sections necessary for detailed parenchymal evaluation at a time when an extensively long breath hold (>60 seconds) and higher radiation dose would be required if contiguous thin sections were obtained through the entire chest [112].

The development of helical and multislice CT scanners, resulting in faster scan acquisition times, enables images of diagnostic quality to be obtained in children during quiet respiration, obviating the need for sedation[113–115].

However, since the greatest impediment to high-quality CT studies in children is respiratory and other motion, sedation may be required in uncooperative children between the ages of 6 months and 6 years. Children less than 6 months old usually fall asleep after a feed and wrap, and sedation is rarely required after the age of 5 years.

The HRCT technique involves the use of the narrowest available sections. As children are more radio sensitive than adults and have a longer life span in which to develop radiation-induced disease, great care must be taken with the use of radiation and the HRCT protocol should be designed to provide the best image quality at the lowest possible radiation dose. It has been shown that as compared to a 180-mA s technique, a lower-dose HRCT technique results in a significant dose reduction of 72% for 50 mA s and 80% for 34 mA s; good-quality images were obtained with 50 mAs in uncooperative children and with 34 mA s in cooperative children and young adult patients [116]. Low-dose HRCT has been reported to have a radiation dose as low as that required for several chest radiographs [112,117]. The use of even lower doses in children such as the use of 25 mA and 1-second scan time has been reported [115,118]. Some authors advocate that section spacing differs slightly from that used in adult examinations (i.e. 10 mm) due to the smaller thoracic volume that has to be scanned and recommend obtaining inspiratory examinations with 5 mm interspacing for children under 2 years of age, 7 mm interspacing in children from 2 to 10 years, and 10 mm interspacing in children over 10 years (as for adults) [114]. A set of expiratory images can be obtained using twice the interval of the inspiratory images; we however recommend only three expiratory sections, one through the upper lobes, one through the middle lobe/lingula and one through the lower lobes (Figs 23.8b, c and d) [118]. In uncooperative patients we perform decubitus images where the dependent lung represents the 'expiratory' and the non-dependent lung the 'inspiratory' lung (Fig. 23.9). A high-frequency reconstruction algorithm (bone) is used to increase edge enhancement and improve visualization of pulmonary parenchymal detail. The use of the smallest field of view possible optimizes spatial resolution. Scan acquisition time is crucial, and needs to be as short as possible in order to minimize motion artefacts [114]. Electron-beam CT (EBCT) scanners with a 0.1-second scan time and the new multisection helical CT scanners with subsecond scanning are optimal in this respect and are particularly useful for imaging children [113]. It is important to bear in mind that image noise (giving a granular appearance) produced by the use of thinner slices is higher with helical CT than with the conventional axial technique [118], so some authors advocate axial (non-helical) acquisition [119].

The chief benefit of incremental HRCT scanning is an approximately 3-fold reduction in radiation dose for HRCT studies compared to volumetric scanning, due primarily to the interval (discontiguous) rather than complete exposure of the lungs to the CT x-ray beam. HRCT involves several separate single-slice acquisitions and takes significantly longer than volumetric CT which is done in a single

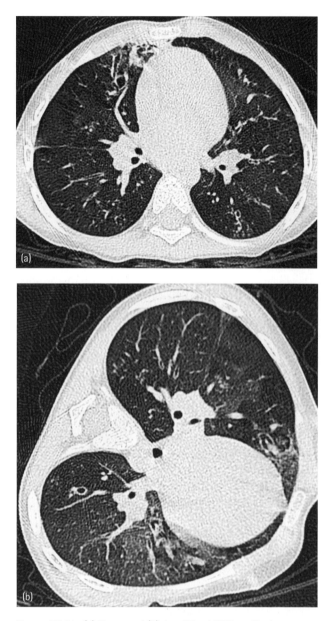

Figure 23.9 (a) Prone and (b) decubitus HRCT confirming air trapping in the superior segment of left lower lobe (the dependent lung is expiratory and the non-dependent lung is inspiratory).

spiral data acquisition (approx 4–7 seconds) so cooperation is better and the movement artefacts minimized.

If used as an outcome measure HRCT is suitable for qualitative evaluation using particular scoring systems, but poses problems for semi-automated quantitative analysis and for longitudinal comparison (when volumetric data are required). Using volumetric CT, the lungs can be viewed in three dimensions with true isotropic resolution, allowing more distal airways to be measured accurately anywhere along their course. Serial volumetric scanning will allow reproducible measurements of the same airway at the same point for more precise longitudinal assessment. Diagnostic images require the scan to be taken during a breath-hold at near full inflation and exhalation volumes.

This helps to eliminate motion artefacts, hence improves resolution, increases reproducibility and so optimizes the detection of abnormalities [120]. Older children breath-hold at full inflation and deflation, or one can resort to spirometer-controlled scan acquisitions at defined full inspiratory and expiratory lung volumes [121].

The extent and distribution of the lung disease needs to be considered when determining the number of images required for the evaluation of a specific lung disease as early CF lung disease may affect any lobe and is patchy in distribution, rather than evenly distributed through the lungs [122]. A recent study has shown that incremental HRCT images at intervals greater than 10 mm will underestimate the severity of CF lung disease.

Quantitative CT air-trapping measurement is a promising new technique for providing standardized quantitative CT measures similar to quantitative spirometric air-flow measurements. This method has the potential advantage of serving as a sensitive quantitative measure looking at airway structure during therapeutic trials to discriminate differences in treatment effect, particularly in subjects with minimal disease [123].

Controlled ventilation technique is another method, described in young children and infants who cannot cooperate with breath-holding. This is accomplished by hyperventilating a sedated child with positive pressure applied by a face-mask to produce a brief pause for CT scanning. During the pause, the lungs are at either full lung inflation or end exhalation. This technique has the potential to be considered as an alternative to general anesthesia for CT and enhance the diagnostic power of CT [120,124].

To summarize, while conventional HRCT allows lower-dose CT scanning and may be useful for qualitative evaluation, volumetric CT is necessary for optimal longitudinal evaluation and for quantitative analysis.

CT as a clinical research tool

CT must be shown to provide a valid outcome surrogate in order to monitor CF lung disease in clinical trials. The criteria for bronchiectasis were developed from pathological correlation studies [125] as CT images are similar to pathological specimens. HRCT is a sensitive indicator of early CF lung disease and has provided evidence of bronchiectasis, peribronchial thickening, mosaic perfusion, and mucus plugging in infants and children with CF [76,126,127]. Multiple cross-sectional studies of patients with CF show that HRCT correlates with other evaluations including clinical status and spirometry, indicating that higher CT scores occur in subjects with worse spirometry despite the frequent poor association of CT scores and spirometry in individual subjects and in longitudinal studies [76,77,79,81,109,126–130].

There is increasing emphasis on the detection and aggressive treatment of early CF lung disease, resulting in increased interest in detecting lung disease in infants and pre-school children with CF.

NEWER TECHNIQUES

Magnetic resonance imaging

Hyperpolarized noble-gas magnetic resonance imaging (MRI) of the lung is a relatively new, versatile imaging modality that depicts both lung function and morphology [131]. With this technique, it is possible to acquire images of the lung with relatively high temporal and spatial resolution. Helium (^{3}He) and xenon (^{129}Xe) are the two non-radioactive isotopes of noble gases that can be hyperpolarized, but ^{3}He has been primarily used for hyperpolarized MRI of the lungs in humans [131,132]. Mucus plugging and airway obstruction result in ventilation inhomogeneity in CF lungs and hyperpolarized ^{3}He MRI of the lung reflects these functional changes as shown in older children and adults [133,134]. HRCT is the imaging modality of choice to assess structural CF lung disease but its ability to assess lung function is limited. The other major limitation is the level of radiation exposure, particularly for longitudinal assessment of disease progression, which requires repeated scans. ^{3}He MRI involves no ionizing radiation, which makes it an ideal imaging tool in children [135]. Although ^{3}He MRI has the potential to serve as a biomarker for assessment of severity of lung disease and to follow disease progression in children with CF, this technique is still in its infancy and has yet to be evaluated in pre-school children. The current major limitation with this technique is that the technology to polarize noble gases is not widely available. The other potential limitation is that MRI in children under 5 years of age requires either sedation or a general anesthetic and can be claustrophobic.

Molecular imaging techniques

Molecular imaging is distinct from structural or functional imaging and aims to non-invasively characterize and quantify cellular and subcellular events. These techniques include optical imaging and radionuclide-based methods such as planar gamma scintigraphy, single-photon emission computed tomography (SPECT) and positron emission tomography (PET). These modalities offer the possibility of monitoring and quantifying molecular and cellular processes non-invasively. However, they are still limited to the research laboratory and the potential impact on clinical research and practice is yet undetermined [136].

REFERENCES

72. Cystic Fibrosis Foundation Center Committee and Guidelines Subcommittee. Cystic Fibrosis Foundation guidelines for patient services, evaluation, and monitoring in cystic fibrosis centers. *Am J Dis Child* 1990; 144:1311–1312.

73. Schidlow DV, Taussig LM, Knowles MR. Cystic Fibrosis Foundation consensus conference report on pulmonary

complications of cystic fibrosis. *Pediatr Pulmonol* 1993; **15**:187–198.

74. Kerem E, Conway S, Elborn S, Heijerman H. Standards of care for patients with cystic fibrosis: a European consensus. *J Cyst Fibros* 2005; **4**:7–26.

75. Brody AS, Molina PL, Klein JS *et al.* High-resolution computed tomography of the chest in children with cystic fibrosis: support for use as an outcome surrogate. *Pediatr Radiol* 1999; **29**:731–735.

76. Marchant JM, Masel JP, Dickinson FL, Masters IB, Chang AB. Application of chest high-resolution computer tomography in young children with cystic fibrosis. *Pediatr Pulmonol* 2001; **31**:24–9.

77. Demirkazik FB, Ariyurek OM, Ozcelik U *et al.* High resolution CT in children with cystic fibrosis: correlation with pulmonary functions and radiographic scores. *Eur J Radiol* 2001; **37**:54–59.

78. Nasr SZ, Kuhns LR, Brown RW *et al.* Use of computerized tomography and chest x-rays in evaluating efficacy of aerosolized recombinant human DNase in cystic fibrosis patients younger than age 5 years: a preliminary study. *Pediatr Pulmonol* 2001; **31**:377–382.

79. Santamaria F, Grillo G, Guidi G *et al.* Cystic fibrosis: when should high-resolution computed tomography of the chest be obtained? *Pediatrics* 1998; **101**:908–913.

80. de Jong PA, Ottink MD, Robben SG *et al.* Pulmonary disease assessment in cystic fibrosis: comparison of CT scoring systems and value of bronchial and arterial dimension measurements. *Radiology* 2004; **231**:434–439.

81. de Jong PA, Nakano Y, Lequin MH *et al.* Progressive damage on high resolution computed tomography despite stable lung function in cystic fibrosis. *Eur Respir J* 2004; **23**:93–97.

82. Jacobsen LE, Houston CS, Habbick BF *et al.* Cystic fibrosis: a comparison of computed tomography and plain chest radiographs. *Can Assoc Radiol J* 1986; **37**:17–21.

83. Brody AS. Scoring systems for CT in cystic fibrosis: who cares? *Radiology* 2004; **231**:296–298.

84. Oppenheimer EH, Esterly JR. Pathology of cystic fibrosis review of the literature and comparison with 146 autopsied cases. *Perspect Pediatr Pathol* 1975; **2**:241–278.

85. Sturgess J, Imrie J. Quantitative evaluation of the development of tracheal submucosal glands in infants with cystic fibrosis and control infants. *Am J Pathol* 1982; **106**:303–311.

86. Balough K, McCubbin M, Weinberger M *et al.* The relationship between infection and inflammation in the early stages of lung disease from cystic fibrosis. *Pediatr Pulmonol* 1995; **20**:63–70.

87. Khan TZ, Wagener JS, Bost T *et al.* Early pulmonary inflammation in infants with cystic fibrosis. *Am J Respir Care Med* 1995; **151**:1075–1082.

88. Cantin A. Cystic fibrosis lung inflammation: early, sustained, and severe. *Am J Respir Crit Care Med* 1995; **151**:939–941.

89. Konstan MW, Berger M. Current understanding of the inflammatory process in cystic fibrosis: onset and etiology. *Pediatr Pulmonol* 1997; **24**:137–142.

90. Gappa M, Ranganathan SC, Stocks J. Lung function testing in infants with cystic fibrosis: lessons from the past and future directions. *Pediatr Pulmonol* 2001; **32**:228–245.

91. Kerem E, Reisman J, Corey M *et al.* Prediction of mortality in patients with cystic fibrosis. *N Engl J Med* 1992; **326**:1187–1191.

92. Ranganathan SC, Dezateux C, Bush A *et al.* Airway function in infants newly diagnosed with cystic fibrosis. *Lancet* 2001; **358**:1964–1965.

93. Ranganathan SC, Stocks J, Dezateux C *et al.* The evolution of airway function in early childhood following clinical diagnosis of cystic fibrosis. *Am J Respir Crit Care Med* 2004; **169**:928–933.

94. Aurora P, Bush A, Gustafsson P *et al.* Multiple-breath washout as a marker of lung disease in preschool children with cystic fibrosis. *Am J Respir Crit Care Med* 2005; **171**:249–256.

95. Wood BP. Cystic fibrosis: 1997. *Radiology* 1997; **204**:1–10.

96. Oikonomou AHD. Recent advances in imaging. In: *Cystic Fibrosis in the 21st Century*, Cape Town, Karger, 2006.

97. Tomashefski JF, Bruce M, Stern RC *et al.* Pulmonary air cysts in cystic fibrosis: relation of pathologic features to radiologic findings and history of pneumothorax. *Hum Pathol* 1985; **16**:253–261.

98. Shwachman H, Kulczycki LL. Long-term study of one hundred five patients with cystic fibrosis: studies made over a five- to fourteen-year period. *AMA J Dis Child* 1958; **96**:6–15.

99. Chrispin AR, Norman AP. The systematic evaluation of the chest radiograph in cystic fibrosis. *Pediatr Radiol* 1974; **2**:101–105.

100. Brasfield D, Hicks G, Soong S, Tiller RE. The chest roentgenogram in cystic fibrosis: a new scoring system. *Pediatrics* 1979; **63**:24–29.

101. Taussig LM, Kattwinkel J, Friedewald WT, Di Sant'Agnese PA. A new prognostic score and clinical evaluation system for cystic fibrosis. *J Pediatr* 1973; **82**:380–390.

102. Weatherly MR, Palmer CG, Peters ME *et al.* Wisconsin cystic fibrosis chest radiograph scoring system. *Pediatrics* 1993; **91**:488–495.

103. Conway SP, Pond MN, Bowler I *et al.* The chest radiograph in cystic fibrosis: a new scoring system compared with the Chrispin–Norman and Brasfield scores. *Thorax* 1994; **49**:860–862.

104. van der Put JM, Meradji M, Danoesastro D, Kerrebijn KF. Chest radiographs in cystic fibrosis: a follow-up study with application of a quantitative system. *Pediatr Radiol* 1982; **12**:57–61.

105. Greene KE, Takasugi JE, Godwin JD *et al.* Radiographic changes in acute exacerbations of cystic fibrosis in adults: a pilot study. *Am J Roentgenol* 1994; **163**:557–562.

106. Brody AS, Klein JS, Molina PL *et al.* High-resolution computed tomography in young patients with cystic fibrosis: distribution of abnormalities and correlation with pulmonary function tests. *J Pediatr* 2004; **145**:32–38.

107. Lindblad A, de Jong PA, Brink M *et al.* Measurements of ventilation inhomogeneity correlates better to structural

changes on high resolution CT than conventional spirometry. *Pediatr Pulmonol* 2005; **40**:310–311.

108. Tiddens HA. Detecting early structural lung damage in cystic fibrosis. *Pediatr Pulmonol* 2002; **34**:228–231.

109. Shah RM, Sexauer W, Ostrum BJ *et al.* High-resolution CT in the acute exacerbation of cystic fibrosis: evaluation of acute findings, reversibility of those findings, and clinical correlation. *Am J Roentgenol* 1997; **169**:375–380.

110. Robinson TE, Leung AN, Northway WH *et al.* Spirometer-triggered high-resolution computed tomography and pulmonary function measurements during an acute exacerbation in patients with cystic fibrosis. *J Pediatr* 2001; **138**:553–559.

111. de Jong PA, Mayo JR, Golmohammadi K *et al.* Estimation of cancer mortality associated with repetitive computed tomography scanning. *Am J Respir Crit Care Med* 2006; **173**:199–203.

112. Mayo JR, Jackson SA, Muller NL. High-resolution CT of the chest: radiation dose. *Am J Roentgenol* 1993; **160**:479–481.

113. Copley SJ, Padley SP. High-resolution CT of paediatric lung disease. *Eur Radiol* 2001; **11**:2564–2575.

114. Kuhn JP, Brody AS. High-resolution CT of pediatric lung disease. *Radiol Clin N Am* 2002; **40**:89–110.

115. Garcia-Pena P, Lucaya J. HRCT in children: technique and indications. *Eur Radiol* 2004; **14**(Suppl 4):L13–L30.

116. Lucaya J, Piqueras J, Garcia-Pena P *et al.* Low-dose high-resolution CT of the chest in children and young adults: dose, cooperation, artifact incidence, and image quality. *Am J Roentgenol* 2000; **175**:985–992.

117. Owens C. Radiology of diffuse interstitial pulmonary disease in children. *Eur Radiol* 2004; **14**(Suppl 4):L2–L12.

118. Brody AS. Thoracic CT technique in children. *J Thorac Imaging* 2001; **16**:259–268.

119. Donnelly LF, Frush DP. Pediatric multidetector body CT. *Radiol Clin N Am* 2003; **41**:637–655.

120. Long FR, Castile RG, Brody AS *et al.* Lungs in infants and young children: improved thin-section CT with a noninvasive controlled-ventilation technique: initial experience. *Radiology* 1999; **212**:588–593.

121. Robinson TE, Leung AN, Moss RB *et al.* Standardized high-resolution CT of the lung using a spirometer-triggered electron beam CT scanner. *Am J Roentgenol* 1999; **172**:1636–1638.

122. Helbich TH, Heinz-Peer G, Eichler I *et al.* Cystic fibrosis: CT assessment of lung involvement in children and adults. *Radiology* 1999; **213**:537–544.

123. Robinson TE, Goris ML, Zhu HJ *et al.* Dornase alfa reduces air trapping in children with mild cystic fibrosis lung disease: a quantitative analysis. *Chest* 2005; **128**:2327–2335.

124. Long FR, Castile RG. Technique and clinical applications of full-inflation and end-exhalation controlled-ventilation chest CT in infants and young children. *Pediatr Radiol* 2001; **31**:413–422.

125. Kang EY, Miller RR, Muller NL. Bronchiectasis: comparison of preoperative thin-section CT and pathologic findings in resected specimens. *Radiology* 1995; **195**:649–654.

126. Stiglbauer R, Schurawitzki H, Eichler I *et al.* High resolution CT in children with cystic fibrosis. *Acta Radiol* 1992; **33**:548–553.

127. Maffessanti M, Candusso M, Brizzi F, Piovesana F. Cystic fibrosis in children: HRCT findings and distribution of disease. *J Thorac Imaging* 1996; **11**:27–38.

128. Helbich TH, Heinz-Peer G, Fleischmann D *et al.* Evolution of CT findings in patients with cystic fibrosis. *Am J Roentgenol* 1999; **173**:81–88.

129. Bhalla M, Turcios N, Aponte V *et al.* Cystic fibrosis: scoring system with thin-section CT. *Radiology* 1991; **179**:783–788.

130. Nathanson I, Conboy K, Murphy S *et al.* Ultrafast computerized tomography of the chest in cystic fibrosis: a new scoring system. *Pediatr Pulmonol* 1991; **11**:81–86.

131. Altes TA, de Lange EE. Applications of hyperpolarized helium-3 gas magnetic resonance imaging in pediatric lung disease. *Top Magn Reson Imaging* 2003; **14**:231–236.

132. Kauczor HU. Hyperpolarized helium-3 gas magnetic resonance imaging of the lung. *Top Magn Reson Imaging* 2003; **14**:223–230.

133. Koumellis P, van Beek EJ, Woodhouse N *et al.* Quantitative analysis of regional airways obstruction using dynamic hyperpolarized 3He MRI-preliminary results in children with cystic fibrosis. *J Magn Reson Imaging* 2005; **22**:420–426.

134. Mentore K, Froh DK, de Lange EE *et al.* Hyperpolarized HHe 3 MRI of the lung in cystic fibrosis: assessment at baseline and after bronchodilator and airway clearance treatment. *Acad Radiol* 2005; **12**:1423–1429.

135. Puderbach M, Kauczor HU. Assessment of lung function in children by cross-sectional imaging: techniques and clinical applications. *Pediatr Radiol* 2006; **36**:192–204.

136. Richard JC, Chen DL, Ferkol T, Schuster DP. Molecular imaging for pediatric lung diseases. *Pediatr Pulmonol* 2004; **37**:286–296.

Physiological monitoring of older children and adults

MARK ROSENTHAL

This chapter deals with lung function testing in cystic fibrosis (CF) at two different levels:

- how lung function should be monitored and interpreted on a day-to-day basis in the clinic, and used as part of routine decision-making (e.g. whether a course of intravenous antibiotics is warranted);
- how lung function (in particular spirometry) appears to decline as the CF patient gets older and the relationship of spirometry and its rate of change over time until death.

The final parts deal with other physiological tests. Fitness-to-fly tests are dealt with in Chapter 11.

THE ROUTINE CLINIC

As 95% of people with CF die of respiratory failure, monitoring lung function and responding to decrements as far as possible is crucial. A short-term decline in forced expired volume in one second (FEV_1) of above 10% is a key part of the definition of a pulmonary exacerbation (see later). A slower decline but over a longer period demands close attention, including consideration of additional diagnoses such as allergic bronchopulmonary aspergillosis (ABPA), new treatments such as a trial of rhDNase or azithromycin, and the management of adherence to current and future treatment. A precipitous decline in lung function demands immediate attention, hospital admission, diagnostic endeavor and aggressive treatment. Forced vital capacity is far less sensitive to both acute and indeed chronic change. The terms 'slower decline' and 'precipitous decline' need definition. Opinions differ; but objectively, the variability in spirometry in subjects with CF is considerable. Cooper and co-workers [1] reported in stable CF subjects that FEV_1 varies by 10% and mid-expiratory flow by 20%, and then Fuchs and co-workers [2] used this

as part of the definition of a pulmonary exacerbation. Chavasse and co-workers [3] found that FEV_1 variability was less in CF children (5%) and reduced further when using nose-clips (3.2%). So an absolute reduction of more than 10% in FEV_1 or 20% in mid-expiratory flow, whether over a short or longer (6-month) period certainly merits close attention. Clearly other measurements have a role in outpatient assessment and oxygen saturation is one. Our clinic has regularly seen subjects whose lung function is 'a little down', and who are trying to minimize their symptoms but their oxygen saturation is under 94%. Other factors such as weight loss are important in considering what action is needed. Clinical geneticists use the German term *Gestalt* meaning form or face, and unquestionably the biggest service a regular CF clinic with stable personnel, serving patients over a long period, can give is to detect that indefinable quality that 'all is not right with the patient's Gestalt'.

It is widely recommended that, annually, plethysmographic measures of lung volume (total lung capacity, residual volume and functional residual capacity, FRC) should be made, as well as airway resistance, specific airways conductance and carbon monoxide gas transfer. However, there is no published evidence that any of these measurements are of clinical value, with the possible exception of FRC [4], either in the evaluation of short-term change – as it is too complex and time-consuming to routinely perform especially in children – or in long-term prediction of prognosis.

In summary, spirometry should be measured at every clinic visit in every child who is able to perform the maneuver, and the results should be an important part of the clinical evaluation. Oxygen saturation should be measured in all children at every visit. The evidence for the clinical utility of any other measurement of lung function presently does not exist.

LONGITUDINAL STUDIES OF LUNG FUNCTION, AND PREDICTION OF SURVIVAL

Lung function

However valuable spirometry is in the individual clinic setting, the evidence that lung function is a reliable indicator of long term-health, prognosis and life expectancy is much more doubtful. Three vignettes illustrate this. A 16-year-old girl who had spent the last 2 months in hospital receiving intensive treatment and who had an FEV_1 resolutely fixed at 18% of predicted survived 8.5 years. An undernourished 10-year-old who initially refused a gastrostomy, and had an FEV_1 of 37% predicted, became a strapping 18-year-old with a gastrostomy whose FEV_1 was still 37%. A girl who at 13 years had an FEV_1 of 85% and a 50th centile body mass index received a lung transplant 15 months later.

An important issue is what lung function to measure and what constitutes a relevant change. Although FEV_1 is unquestionably the commonest single measure of lung function used and is discussed extensively below, forced vital capacity (FVC), mid-expiratory flow (MEF), transfer factor (DL_{CO}) and the ratio of residual volume to total lung capacity (RV/TLC) have also all been studied. Newer measures such as the lung clearance index, LCI (which is discussed more extensively in the context of infants and pre-school children in Chapter 23c) are also being used. A longitudinal cohort study extending throughout childhood has demonstrated that abnormalities in LCI occur some 2.3 years earlier than changes in FEV_1 and that an abnormal LCI was present in 52% of children with a normal FEV_1, while for the converse (normal LCI, abnormal FEV_1) the rate was only 0.5% – confirming the reports in the pre-school child [4]. The next most useful measure was forced expired flow at 50% of forced vital capacity, and third was plethysmographically measured FRC. It is also true that CT scanning appears to be more sensitive to change in structure than spirometry; there is a need for comparisons between CT scanning and other, more sensitive tests of lung function (the role of HRCT is discussed in Chapter 23c).

The factors that may be relevant to the absolute lung function, and rate of change over time, include: gender; genotype (at the CFTR locus and modifier genes); pancreatic status; CF-related diabetes, and pre-diabetic insulin deficiency; microbiology; markers of nutrition such as weight for age or body mass index; and education and social class.

Gender is a factor that has been extensively explored to try to explain the reduced female life expectancy. As an example, a 2-year survivorship study in 2001 of 181 children referred for transplant demonstrated that female gender consistently led to a reduced 2-year survivorship by 15%, irrespective of FEV_1 [5]. Unfortunately, as with so many such models, it has not been validated in a second population. This is a prerequisite for genetic association studies to be taken seriously; it would appear that physiologists and epidemiologists are less rigorous in this context.

It could be that there is something about the effect of CFTR dysfunction or absence per se in girls which makes them die earlier, or it could be that they are more prone to particular complications, and it is the earlier onset of these complications that shorten life. In another study, acquisition of mucoid *Pseudomonas* in children under 6 years of age led to a greater rate of death over the next 10 years in girls than boys (40% vs 20%), implying that girls are more vulnerable to the effects of infection with *P. aeruginosa*. The drawback of the study is that the data set was acquired over such a along period (1954 to 1990) that other confounders cannot be discounted.

However, this difference would disappear if effective antipseudomonal treatment was in place. The subject of gender differences is discussed in more detail in Chapters 16 and 24.

EPIDEMIOLOGY

Although epidemiological studies have always demonstrated that life expectancy for girls with CF was consistently worse than for boys [7], multicenter studies by definition involve centers with likely different treatment policies, which may make interpretation difficult. A large single-center longitudinal study has shown that, since 1993, if anything lung function in girls is now superior to that of boys [8]. Thus female sex, at least in childhood (including the teenage years), does not seem necessarily to convey a worse prognosis as regards lung function. However, whether this will translate into a life expectancy that does not differ between the sexes remains to be seen.

An important point is that as clinicians we are interested in the prognosis for an individual, but the data on which the prognosis is based comes from large mixed longitudinal cohorts. Epidemiological data may help us understand mechanisms of disease, but as is well known when considering the prognosis in a given individual, it is not good for guiding decision-making, for example in transplant referral. So, for example, even the most accurate group prognostic indicator, spirometry, is no better than flipping a coin for an individual (50% death within 2 years, 50% survival with $FEV_1 < 30\%$ predicted) [9].

This is also illustrated by longitudinal data in children from the US national CF patient registry which demonstrate the curvilinear reduction in FEV_1 (more rapid in girls compared with boys) and the negative interaction with weight (nutritional status as judged by weight Z score and percentage weight for height influences lung function decline) [10]. Interestingly those with the best initial lung function declined more quickly than those with a lower initial lung function. Whether this illustrates the phenomenon of regression to the mean or is a real biological phenomenon cannot be determined from this study alone. However, in either case children in mid childhood had a decline in lung function that settled to a very slow rate (about 1% per year).

The second paper, published only in abstract form, reviewed the 30 deaths occurring in Melbourne, Australia, in a single center and in particular the lung function in the years before death [11]. Table 24.1 shows the median FEV_1 2 years prior to death. At least a third of subjects had an FEV_1 above 75% predicted 2 years before death, demonstrating that even a normal FEV_1 cannot be absolutely reassuring as a precipitate and seemingly unstoppable decline remains a real if small threat.

Milla and Warwick [12] tried to determine whether an FEV_1 of <30% occurring on at least three occasions within 12 months predicted mortality. This hypothesis was on the previous observation that an FEV_1 <30% predicted more than 50% mortality within 2 years [9]. Of the 49 (of 56) deceased patients with an FEV_1 <30% close to death, only 17 had entered this range in the previous 2 years, the rest having had similar lung function for between 2 and 14 years.

Gender, nutrition (whether above or below 85% weight for height), presence of diabetes treated with insulin, or decade (1975–84 or 1985–94) in which the lung function first reached 30% had no effect on outcome, and rate of decline of FVC was no different between survivors and non-survivors. The conclusion was that patients who had an FEV_1 that continued to decline rapidly had a greater risk of death that those whose FEV_1 was low (<30%) but declined slowly. Looking at young adults as a whole, Que and co-workers [13] demonstrated the steady slowing of FEV_1 decline over time at one institution, so that for those born between 1985 and 1989 the rate of decline was now 0.8% per year (Table 24.2). They also tabulated the rates of decline from other studies (placebo arm) and cohorts and these are summarized in Table 24.3. This clearly demonstrates the variability depending on institution, year of birth and study.

The largest study on the decline of lung function comes from the European CF database which examined 12 500 subjects between 1993 and 1997, mainly to examine the effects of allergic bronchopulmonary aspergillosis (ABPA) [14]. Fig. 24.1 is a reproduction of their mixed longitudinal data depending on the initial entry FEV_1 and the initial age group at measurement. What it illustrates is that, regardless of the starting FEV_1, the rate of subsequent decline was remarkably similar (and largely unaffected by ABPA) and independent of age. The crucial conclusion of this is that the starting FEV_1 is determined much earlier in childhood

Table 24.1 Data showing very wide range of FEV_1 2 years prior to death, in Melbourne, Australia [11].

	Number	Median age at death (in months) (range in brackets)	Median FEV_1 (% predicted) (range in brackets)
Male	13	176 (62–233)	69 (31–90)
Female	17	171 (89–225)	47 (24–102)
Overall	30	172 (62–233)	52.5 (24–102)

Table 24.2 Lung function decline in young adults aged 18–22 years [13].

	Birth cohort					
	1960–64	1965–69	1970–74	1975–79	1980–84	1985–89
Follow-up to:	1978	1983	1988	1993	1998	2003
Study (n)	132	120	114	90	90	108
FEV_1 slope/year	−2.1	−2.6	−2.5	−1.8	−1.1	−0.8

Table 24.3 Published rates of decline in percentage predicted FEV_1 in CF from cohort studies or the placebo arms of clinical trials.

Reference	n	Age (years)	Follow-up (years)	Annual decline in FEV_1 (% predicted)	
				Mean	SE
Corey et al. [35]	132	5–27	7	−1.87 (male) −2.71 (female)	NS[a]
Kerem et al. [36]	39	7–40	2	−2.2	1.67
Kovesi et al. [37]	325	4–28	15	−1.25	0.14
Konstan et al. [38]	43	5–39	4	−3.6	0.55
Eigen et al. [39]	95	6–14	4	−1.5	NS
Corey et al. [40]	366	18–32 (born 1960–74)	15	−2.72	NS
Davis et al. [41]	215	–	2–5	−2.3	0.28
Milla et al. [20]	152	–	4	−0.8	NS
Merkus et al. [42]	52	Children	3.9	−2.2	NS
Merkus et al. [17]	53	Children	3.8	−1.8	NS

[a] Not stated.
Modified from [13].

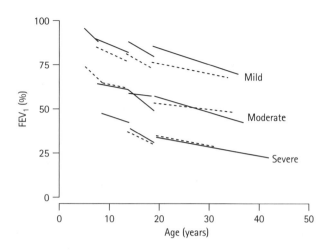

Figure 24.1 Mixed model regression lines of forced expiratory volume in one second (FEV_1) versus age for allergic bronchopulmonary aspergillosis (ABPA) (- - -) and non-ABPA (—) patients. The data are divided into three disease severity categories determined on the basis of FEV_1 at enrolment, and each severity category is subdivided into four age classes at enrolment (from left to right: <6 years; 6–12 years; 13–17 years, ≥18 years). Reproduced with permission from [14].

Table 24.4 Annual rate of decline of FEV_1 in 420 Swedish CF patients up to 40 years of age.

	Rate of decline of FEV_1 (%/yr)	Significance of difference compared with top line of each box
ΔF508/ΔF508	0.8	
Two severe mutations	0.9	0.6
One or two missense mutations	0.04	0.01
Male	0.6	
Female	0.9	0.16
PS	0.2	
PI	0.9	0.01
Dead/transplanted	2.0	
Alive/not transplanted	0.6	0.00001
PI/PA	1.0	
PI/no PA	0.5	0.03
PS/PA	0.3	
PS/no PA	0.2	0.83
PI/diabetes	1.2	
PI/no diabetes	0.7	0.02
PI/cirrhosis	0.8	
PI/no cirrhosis	0.8	0.84

Confidence intervals were not stated. PS, pancreatic-sufficient; PI, pancreatic-insufficient; PA, chronically infected with *Pseudomonas aeruginosa* (3 positive in 6 months).
Data adapted from [15].

and that, once a low FEV_1 is established, although the rate of decline appears similar, inevitably the ones with the low initial FEV_1 run into trouble sooner. These observations tie in with the studies in infancy and pre-school children (Chapter 24c), which suggests that lung function tracks from diagnosis until school age at least. One unexpected consequence of the slowing rate of decline in FEV_1 is that new treatments are becoming increasingly difficult to evaluate as the use of the end-point, change in rate of decline of FEV_1 is now so low that a trial is going to require each arm to have more than 200 patients studied over several years to establish a significant difference. This is similar to the study size required when exacerbation rate is used as the primary end-point.

Schaedel and co-workers [15] studied the entire CF Swedish population alive in 1998 and born prior to 1993 and in addition included 25 patients who died in the 1990s, nine from the 1980s and 21 (16 alive) who had been transplanted, to minimize bias. Table 24.4 shows the significant effect association of in particular chronic infection with *Pseudomonas aeruginosa* and the diagnosis of diabetes mellitus, such that in the 19–24-year age group the relative risk of an FEV_1 <60% was increased 2.6-fold (95% CI 1.1–6.5) if the patient was pancreatic-insufficient (PI), 1.7-fold (95% CI 1.1–2.8) if chronically infected with *P. aeruginosa*, and 1.5-fold (95% CI 1.1–2.2) if a diagnosis of diabetes had been given (CFRD). The authors do not state whether these factors are additive, but the implication from Table 24.4 is that diabetes in someone with PI had increased the rate of decline by an extra 50%. None of the above explains why certain individuals decline so much faster than the average. Schaedel's methodology proposed an intercept at age 5 years when lung function could be reasonably performed.

Those who died or were transplanted had a considerable inferred absolute reduction in FEV_1 at 5 years (63%) compared to the rest (89%; $p < 0.001$), again emphasizing the crucial importance of early life events, and aggressive management of the disease in the pre-school years. This underscores the imperative to develop better monitoring tools for clinical, as opposed to research use.

Paradoxically for an obstructive condition, an increase in carbon monoxide transfer has been observed in a cross-sectional study of CF patients [16]. This may be due to redistribution of blood flow to the best-ventilated regions of the lung, or to the increased bronchial circulatory flow secondary to inflammation. However, a longitudinal study of 53 children over an average 4 years showed that, while FEV_1 declined (with again maximum declines in the youngest age groups), gas transfer remained constant as indeed did the ratio of residual volume to total lung capacity, another measure of gas trapping [17].

DIABETES MELLITUS

It is clear that CFRD has a significant impact on lung function. A study in 1988 demonstrated that only 25% of CF patients with CFRD were alive aged 30 years compared

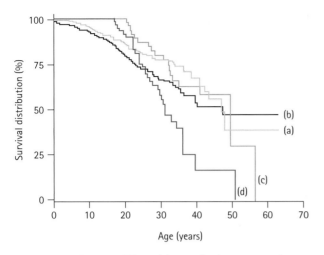

Figure 24.2 Data on differential mortality between genders depending on the presence of CF-related diabetes (a) males without CFRD; (b): females without CFRD; (c): males with CFRD; (d): females with CFRD.

with 60% of the non-diabetics, and that the clinical decline predated diagnosis by at least 2 years [18]. This underscores the need for active detection strategies of the early phases of insulin deficiency. Clinicians should certainly perform a glucose tolerance test in any subject with an unexplained clinical deterioration, and, if this is normal, undertake a period of home glucose monitoring. Koch and colleagues's analysis in 2001 of the European CF database demonstrated that in every age cohort CFRD subjects had an FEV_1 10% lower than non-CFRD subjects [19]. However, there is an inconsistency stemming from the rates of decline of FEV_1. If from Koch *et al.*'s data the average FEV_1 in the 20–24-year age group was 49%, and the annual rate of decline is 1.2% [15], 2.5% [20] or 0.8% [13], then for 75% of CF/CFRD subjects to be dead at aged 30 years (as suggested in [18]) they would die with an FEV_1 ranging from about 42% through 39% to 29%, assuming linear rates of decline. This assumption is of course not always valid (see later). If CFRD is ignored, from Que *et al.*'s data the 1980–84 birth cohort had a mean FEV_1 of 64% at age 22 years and declined by 0.8% per year. Given the median life expectancy of this cohort is 30–35 years, and assuming that 10% were already dead, then a further 40% will be predicted to die in the next 13 years. However, by extrapolation, their FEV_1 would be expected to be around 51% at the time of death. Thus a linear decline is certainly convenient for analysis and statistics, but highly unlikely in reality.

What was not analyzed in the previous studies but is clear in Milla *et al.*'s [21] and Sims *et al.*'s [22] studies is the differential effect of CFRD on females. Milla and co-workers studied the 1081 patients from a single US clinic which performed annual oral glucose tolerance tests, with complete follow-up data from 1987 to 2002 or death. The median survivals for male subjects without and with CFRD were respectively 49.5 and 47.4 years, while for females they were

respectively 47.0 and 30.7 years ($p < 0.001$) – not confounded by genotype, microbiology, nutrition, pregnancy or steroid usage (Fig. 24.2). This difference accounted for 89% of the excess female mortality over males. In the cross-sectional part of a study from the UK database, Sims and co-workers showed that female subjects were 12-fold (3 to 59 times) more likely to have CFRD than males. Females with CFRD but without *P. aeruginosa* had an FEV_1 20% (12–28%) lower than non-CFRD females; in chronically infected subjects the FEV_1 difference was 14% (8–19%). Interestingly the FEV_1 decline in female CFRD subjects did *not* occur in the first year after diagnosis, suggesting an opportunity for intervention, though this is at odds with the observation of lung function decline before CFRD diagnosis [23]. However, it should be stated that the completeness and quality of the UK data, in terms of ascertainment of the diagnosis of CFRD at least, is below that of the US study.

COMPOSITE MODELS PREDICTING SURVIVAL

The ideal study from a statistical standpoint should have at least 2000 subjects of varying ages followed for a minimum of 8 (and ideally 15) years, all being treated in a uniform way. The results should then be validated on a second matched contemporaneous cohort. Inevitably by the time such results have been produced, treatments and their applications have changed, and because of the effects of secular trends the results lose much of their future applicability.

In 1993, Liou and co-workers [24] produced a validated 5-year survivorship model built from 5810 patients from the US CF registry, and tested on a further 5810 patients. The model is shown in Table 24.5. It emphasizes the persisting survivorship disadvantage of female gender and the relatively low contribution from FEV_1. It is interesting to note the factors *not* significant for the model included *rate of decline of FEV_1*, height, presence of *Pseudomonas aeruginosa*, or presence/absence of $\Delta F508$ genes. Liou and co-workers did not analyze other measures of lung function such as FVC, but these are unlikely to relate to outcome. It has been argued that the reason FEV_1 appears to play a comparatively minor role in prognosis may be due to its insensitivity in detecting changes in particular in distal airway resistance until more than 90% of the distal airways are occluded. For this reason, more sensitive techniques such as LCI are becoming increasingly important. However, until these methods become more generally available, and there are more data on within-subject and over-time reproducibility, there are unlikely to be sufficient data to build them into survival models, let alone validate them in a second population.

Whether these models, even if validated, translate into other settings (countries, treatment practices or indeed into the future) is debatable. We used Liou *et al.*'s data on a cohort of our patients where data were available from the 1993 era – a minimum of 4 years' lung function data, $n = 126$ (69 males, 67 with previously isolated *P. aeruginosa*, 54 with

Table 24.5   Predictive 5-year survivorship model for cystic fibrosis [24].

Covariate	Coefficient		Odds ratio
(X_{0-10})	β_{1-10}	SE	
(Intercept)	1.93	0.27	6.88
Age (per year)	−0.028	0.0060	0.97
Gender (male = 0, female = 1)	−0.23	0.10	0.79
FEV$_1$% (per %)	0.038	0.0028	1.04
Weight-for-age z score	0.40	0.053	1.50
Pancreatic sufficiency (0 or 1)	0.45	0.31	1.58
Diabetes mellitus (0 or 1)	−0.49	0.15	0.61
Staphylococcus aureus (0 or 1)	0.21	0.12	1.24
Burkerholderia cepacia (0 or 1)	−1.82	0.30	0.16
No. of acute exacerbations (0–5)	−0.46	0.031	0.63
No. of acute exacerbations × *B. cepacia*	0.40	0.12	1.49

The conditional probability of 5-year survival by logistic regression analysis is: $x = \exp(X)/[1 + \exp(X)]$

where $X = \beta_0 + \beta_1(\text{age}) + \beta_2(\text{gender}) + \beta_3(\text{FEV}_1\%) + \beta_4(Z \text{ score}) + \beta_5(\text{pancreatic sufficiency}) + \beta_6(\text{diabetes}) + \beta_7(S.\ aureus) + \beta_8(B.\ cepacia) + \beta_9(\text{exacerbations}) + \beta_{10}(\text{exacerbations} \times B.\ cepacia)$.
For a more detailed explanation, see [24].

S. aureus, 4 with *Burkholderia cepacia*, 7 pancreatic-sufficient, and 10 taking insulin). There were five deaths (three male, none with *B. cepacia*) in patients where the *lowest* prior recorded probability of surviving 5 years was calculated at 71%, and there were twelve living patients whose lowest recorded probability of surviving 5 years had been below 71% in the preceding years. One possible reason for the discrepancy may be socioeconomic. While Liou *et al.*'s data showed that education was not significant, there were insufficient data to test either employment, insurance status (in the US) or marital status.

Schechter and co-workers [25] looked at the US CF database from 1986 to 1994. The relative risk of death if on Medicaid (a proxy for poverty) – adjusted for race, age, sex and pancreatic enzyme usage – was 3.65-fold (95% CI 3.03–4.40) that of insured patients. However, when the *initial* FEV$_1$ on entry to the database was included the effect of Medicaid disappeared. Again, the importance of early life events is emphasized. The average FEV$_1$ of Medicaid patients was 9.1% (7.2–11.0%) lower than insured patients and was present from age 5 years, and they were 2.3 times (2.0–2.5) more likely to have a weight for age below the 5th centile. However, they did not have fewer outpatient attendances and if anything were diagnosed earlier (median 131 days) than non-Medicaid patients (median 157 days). The influence of socioeconomic class is discussed further in Chapter 6b.

So how can we predict prognosis? Fig. 24.3 hypothesizes at least a three-stage – and probably a five-stage – model lettered A to F based on a combination of the evidence cited and personal experience. The stage AB is the early rapidly declining FEV$_1$ but rapidly decelerating velocity of fall in FEV$_1$ (data from [10] and hinted at in Fig. 24.1). The next stage (BC) is from mid childhood onwards where the

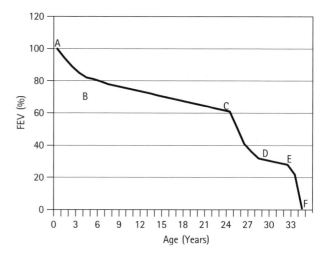

Figure 24.3   Highly stylized model of the decline in FEV$_1$ in an individual from birth to death divided into stages AB, BC, CD, DE. For description of the stages see text.

great majority of children are healthy and lung function decline is indeed very slow. Point C represents some event or combination of circumstances where there is a precipitate fall in lung function which either naturally or by dint of aggressive treatment is temporarily halted at D for a variable period, if at all, before final decline (E) and death (F). Clearly the prediction of, and intervention to prevent the decline at C is crucial but there is no objective evidence concerning this except that an accelerated decline in lung function precedes the diagnosis of CFRD by 2–4 years. Inevitably for an individual this graph is not very useful, as with all the other models discussed. However, it is to be hoped that it will emphasize the non-linearity of progression of lung function changes. C of course can occur much earlier and stage DE can quite commonly persist for many years. The US data imply that the inflection point (B) is lower rather than earlier with indices of poverty and may be *higher* if the patient is diagnosed by screening. C may be reached earlier if CFRD develops, or infection with some strains of *Burkholderia cepacia* is acquired. Lung function differences between the sexes at least in childhood and adolescence may now be insignificant, but whether that will result in equalization of mortality cannot be determined.

OTHER PHYSIOLOGICAL MEASUREMENTS

Bronchial responsiveness

Bronchial hyper-responsiveness is certainly common in CF, but it is variable between individuals, within individuals over time, and dependent on the stimulus. The stimuli that have been studied can be divided into direct challenges (histamine, methacholine) and indirect (exercise, cold air, saline and adenosine). Reactivity is surprisingly not related to a history of wheeze, allergic disease or indeed positive skin prick tests [26]. Bronchial hyper-reactivity measurement may be useful at it is the responsive group that seemed to do well with 2 months of bronchodilator therapy [27]. However, this relationship does not hold throughout the course of the disease, as late on more patients exhibit bronchial responsiveness but fewer respond to bronchodilators [28].

Exercise challenge universally led to bronchodilation and not bronchoconstriction in one study [29], and in another bronchodilation was maximal in the most severely affected subjects [30]. Cold air challenge also led to paradoxical bronchodilation in 10 of 34 patients [31], while in a 4-year longitudinal study in children aged 2–8 years there was a positive response to cold air in about 10% of patients, the same rate as in controls [32]. Hypertonic saline (HS), now promulgated as a new adjunctive treatment, produces varying effects [33]. In about a third of patients there was a progressive fall in FEV_1 with increasing doses of HS in a manner similar to in asthmatics. In another third, there was a transient fall and then restoration of FEV_1 by the end of the challenge; and in the final third, the post-challenge FEV_1 after 10% challenge was greater than the pre-challenge FEV_1 with no prior factors to predict the result.

Thus depending on the disease severity, age at challenge and stimulus, the CF airway will constrict or dilate; there may be a positive response to bronchodilators. The many possible mechanisms underlying variable response possibilities are beyond the scope of this chapter, but clearly there is airway instability of an inconsistent nature; whether this is inflammatory in origin, with uncoupling of the airway wall from the adventitial guy-ropes, or a failure of the smooth muscle to maintain a consistent tone, is conjectural. However, the impressive variation in lung function in adult CF women during the menstrual cycle may be indicative of a smooth muscle problem [34]. The practical consequences are that, if the use of bronchodilators is contemplated, then

the response should be formally tested. Perhaps bronchodilators before physiotherapy may be more appropriate in mildly affected subjects, and such exercise as can be undertaken prior to physiotherapy in more severely affected patients; however there is no substitute for testing this in the individual concerned.

CONCLUSIONS

It remains virtually impossible to predict accurately an individual's life expectancy in childhood. FEV_1 is not as useful as might be thought and the persisting female survival disadvantage does not appear related to FEV_1 but is likely to be due to abnormal glucose metabolism. In short, the presence of CF-related diabetes at any age, and poor lung function (a low FEV_1 or high LCI) at age 5 years, will be the two most likely adverse factors. The importance of early life events cannot be over-emphasized. Measurement of the lung clearance index needs to become routine practice in the CF clinic, but assessment of 'Gestalt' should not be ignored.

REFERENCES

1. Cooper PJ, Robertson CF, Hudson IL, Phelan PD. Variability of pulmonary function tests in cystic fibrosis. Pediatr Pulmonol 1990; **8**:16–22.
2. Fuchs HJ, Borowitz DS, Christiansen DH *et al.* for the Pulmozyme Study Group. Effect of aerosolized recombinant human DNase on exacerbations of respiratory symptoms and on pulmonary function in patients with cystic fibrosis. *N Engl J Med* 1994; **331**:637–642.
3. Chavasse R, Johnson P, Francis J *et al.* To clip or not to clip? Noseclips for spirometry. *Eur Respir J* 2003; **21**:876–878.
4. Kraemer R, Blum A, Schiler A *et al.* Ventilation inhomogeneities in relation to standard lung function in patients with cystic fibrosis. *Am J Respir Crit Care Med* 2005; **171**:371–378.
5. Aurora P, Whitehead B, Wade A *et al.* Lung transplantation and life extension in children with cystic fibrosis. *Lancet* 1999; **354**:1591–1593.
6. Demko CA, Byard PJ, Davis PB. Gender differences in cystic fibrosis: *Pseudomonas aeruginosa* infection. *J Clin Epidemiol* 1995; **148**:1041–1049.
7. Rosenfeld M, Davis R, FitzSimmons S *et al.* Gender gap in cystic fibrosis mortality. *Am J Epidemiol* 1997; **145**:794–803.
8. Verma N, Bush A, Buchdahl R. Is there still a gender gap in cystic fibrosis? *Chest* 2005; **128**:2824–2834.
9. Kerem E, Reisman J, Corey M *et al.* Prediction of mortality in patients with cystic fibrosis. *N Engl J Med* 1992; **326**:1187–1191.
10. Zemel BS, Jawad AF, FitzSimmons S, Stallins VA. Longitudinal relationship among growth nutritional status and pulmonary function in children with cystic fibrosis: analysis of the Cystic

Fibrosis Foundation national CF patient registry. *J Pediatr* 2000; **137**:374–380.

11. Robinson PJ, Meehan J, Sawyer SM, Vyas J. Forced expiratory volume in 1 second is an unreliable marker of risk of death in the next 2 years. *Pediatr Pulmonol* 1999; **19**(Suppl): A452.

12. Milla CE, Warwick WJ. Risk of death in cystic fibrosis patients with severely compromised lung function. *Chest* 1998; **113**:1230–1234.

13. Que C, Cullinan P, Geddes D. Improving rates of decline of FEV₁ in young adults with cystic fibrosis. *Thorax* 2005; Epub doi:10.1136/thx2005.043372.

14. Mastella G, Rainisio M, Harms HK *et al.* Allergic bronchopulmonary aspergillosis in cystic fibrosis: a European epidemiological study. *Eur Respir J* 2000; **16**:464–471.

15. Schaedel C, de Monestrol I, Hjelte L *et al.* Predictors of deterioration of lung function in cystic fibrosis. *Pediatr Pulmonol* 2002; **33**:483–491.

16. Keens TG, Mansell A, Krastins IR *et al.* Evaluation of the single-breath diffusing capacity in asthma and cystic fibrosis. *Chest* 1979; **76**:41–44.

17. Merkus PJ, Govaere ES, Hop WH *et al.* Preserved diffusion capacity in children with cystic fibrosis. *Pediatr Pulmonol* 2004; **37**:56–60.

18. Finkelstein SM, Wielinski CL, Elliott GR *et al.* Diabetes mellitus associated with cystic fibrosis. *Pediatrics* 1988; **112**:373–377.

19. Koch C, Cuppens H, Rainisio M *et al.* European Epidemiologic Registry of Cystic Fibrosis: comparison of major disease manifestations between patients with different classes of mutations. *Pediatr Pulmonol* 2001; **31**:1–12.

20. Milla CE, Warwick WJ, Moran A. Trends in pulmonary function in patients with cystic fibrosis correlate with the degree of glucose intolerance at baseline. *Am J Respir Crit Care Med* 2000; **162**:891–895.

21. Milla CE, Billings J, Moran A. Diabetes is associated with dramatically decreased survival in female but not male subjects with cystic fibrosis. *Diabetes Care* 2005; **28**:2141–2144.

22. Sims EJ, Green MW, Mehta A. Decreased lung function in female but not male subjects with established cystic fibrosis related diabetes. *Diabetes Care* 2005; **28**:1581–1587.

23. Koch C, Rainisio M, Madessani U *et al.* Presence of cystic fibrosis related diabetes mellitus is tightly linked to poor lung function in patients with cystic fibrosis. *Pediatr Pulmonol* 2001; **32**:343–350.

24. Liou TG, Adler FR, FitzSimmons SC *et al.* Predictive 5 year survivorship model of cystic fibrosis. *Am J Epidemiol* 2001; **153**:345–352.

25. Schechter MS, Shelton BJ, Margolis PA, FitzSimmons SC. The association of socioeconomic status with outcomes in cystic fibrosis patients in the United States. *Am J Respir Crit Care Med* 2001; **163**:1331–1337.

26. Eggleston PA, Rosenstein BJ, Stackbone CM, Alexander MF. Airway hyperreactivity in cystic fibrosis: clinical correlates and possible effects of the disease. *Chest* 1988; **94**:360–365.

27. Eggleston PA, Rosenstein BJ, Stackbone CM *et al.* A controlled trial of long term bronchodilator therapy in cystic fibrosis. *Chest* 1991; **99**:1088–1092.

28. Van Haren EHJ, Lammers JWJ, Festen J, van Herwaarden CLA. Bronchodilator response in adult patients with cystic fibrosis: effects on large and small airways. *Eur Respir J* 1991; **4**:301–307.

29. Van Haren EH, Lammers JW, Festen J, van Herwaarden CL. Bronchial vagal tone and responsiveness to histamine exercise and bronchodilators in adult patients with cystic fibrosis. *Eur Respir J* 1992; **5**:1083–1088.

30. Macfarlane PI, Heaf D. Changes in airflow obstruction and oxygen saturation in response to exercise and bronchodilators in cystic fibrosis. *Pediatr Pulmonol* 1990; **8**:4–11.

31. Darga LL, Eason LA, Zach MS, Polgar G. Cold air provocation of airway hyperreactivity in patients with cystic fibrosis. *Pediatr Pulmonol* 1986; **2**:82–88.

32. Nielson KG, Pressler T, Klug B *et al.* Serial lung function and responsiveness in cystic fibrosis during early childhood. *Am J Respir Crit Care Med* 2004; **169**:1209–1216.

33. Rodwell LT, Anderson SD. Airway responsiveness to hyperosmolar saline challenge in cystic fibrosis: a pilot study. *Pediatr Pulmonol* 1996; **21**:282–289.

34. Johannesson M, Ludviksdottir D, Janson C. Lung function changes in relation to menstrual cycle in females with cystic fibrosis. *Respir Med* 2000; **94**:1043–1046.

35. Corey M, Levison H, Crozier D. Five- to seven-year course of pulmonary function in cystic fibrosis. *Am Rev Respir Dis* 1976; **114**:1085–1092.

36. Kerem E, Corey M, Gold R *et al.* Pulmonary function and clinical course in patients with cystic fibrosis after pulmonary colonization with *Pseudomonas aeruginosa*. *J Pediatr* 1990; **116**:714–719.

37. Kovesi T, Corey M, Levison H. Passive smoking and lung function in cystic fibrosis. *Am Rev Respir Dis* 1993; **148**:1266–1271.

38. Konstan MW, Byard PJ, Hoppel CL, Davis PB. Effect of high-dose ibuprofen in patients with cystic fibrosis. *N Engl J Med* 1995; **332**:848–854.

39. Eigen H, Rosenstein B, FitzSimmons S *et al.* A multicenter study of alternate-day prednisone therapy in patients with cystic fibrosis. *J Pediatr* 1995; **126**:515–523.

40. Corey M, Edwards L, Levison H *et al.* Longitudinal analysis of pulmonary function decline in patients with cystic fibrosis. *J Pediatr* 1997; **131**:809–814.

41. Davis PB, Byard PJ, Konstan MW. Identifying treatments that halt progression of pulmonary disease in cystic fibrosis. *Pediatr Res* 1997; **41**:161–165.

42. Merkus PJ, Tiddens HA, de Jongste JC. Annual lung function changes in young patients with chronic lung disease. *Eur Respir J* 2002; **19**:886–891.

Exercise: testing

DAVID M. ORENSTEIN AND WOLFGANG GRUBER

INTRODUCTION

Exercise testing has become an important tool in the continuing evaluation and care of patients with cystic fibrosis (CF). Among the reasons that exercise testing has become common in CF centers is the evidence that survival is strongly correlated with exercise test results, particularly peak oxygen uptake ($VO_{2\ peak}$). CF patients with a high peak VO_2 have a much better long-term survival than patients with a lower peak VO_2 [1,2].

Exercise capacity in CF in general is deficient, and correlates with lung function. However, patients with CF have a wide range of physical fitness, from nearly bedridden to extremely athletic [3,4]. Several factors, including nutritional status, genetics, ventilatory and musculoskeletal factors, and habitual physical activity, influence exercise capacity in CF [5–8].

In healthy people, exercise is limited by circulatory factors and fatigue of peripheral muscles, rather than ventilatory mechanics. Patients with CF often have a ventilatory demand that is greater than normal, with reference to both total workload and resting ventilatory capacity. At maximum effort, healthy people employ minute ventilation (V_E) of no more than 50–80% of their resting maximum voluntary ventilation (MVV) [9]. In contrast, patients with CF may use minute ventilation of greater than 80% of their resting MVV, suggesting a ventilatory limitation of exercise capacity [10,11].

With progression of lung disease, the ability to exercise decreases. In general, exercise capacity correlates with lung function, but there is a tremendous interindividual variation with a wide range of physical fitness (Fig. 25.1). Therefore it is not possible to predict exercise tolerance from resting lung function [12,13].

For this reason, exercise testing (XT) is a useful and important tool to assess exercise capacity, to identify functional limits, and to detect oxygen desaturation, which occurs in some patients with advanced lung disease (Tables 25.1 and 25.2) [12,14]. Information gained from exercise

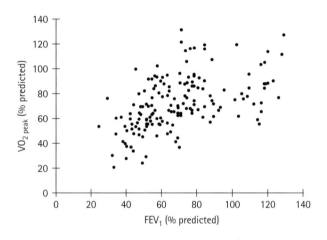

Figure 25.1 Peak VO_2 vs FEV_1 in patients with CF, showing statistically significant correlation between pulmonary function and aerobic fitness, and also showing wide interindividual variation. Reproduced from [40].

Table 25.1 Indications for exercise testing, even if testing is not standard in a CF clinic.

FEV_1 or FVC lower than 60% predicted
SaO_2 lower than 94% at rest
Fear of exercise or physical activity
Evidence of cor pulmonale

Table 25.2 Uses of exercise test results.

Determine submaximal and maximal exercise capacity
Helping design an exercise training program
Evaluating the effects of an exercise training program
Assessing the course of progressive pulmonary disease and its
     treatment

testing is useful in designing and assessing the success of a training program or regular physical exercise [5,15] (see also Chapter 25b), as well as following disease progression or judging the success of any therapeutic intervention.

Table 25.3 Components of the medical history and physical exam.

Medical history	Physical exam/laboratory tests
Symptoms	Body weight, height, BMI
Recent illness, hospitalization, surgical procedures, i.v. antibiotics, etc.[a]	Resting pulse rate
	Auscultation of heart and lungs
	Inspection/palpation of lower
Orthopedic problems[a]	extremities for edema
Medications	
Exercise history	Orthopedic exam, focusing on areas of reported injury that would exclude testing[a]
School/work history	Oximetry
	Pulmonary function tests

[a] Exercise testing should be delayed until the acute illness, post-surgical, or orthopedic condition has resolved, at least back to the patient's own baseline.
BMI, body mass index.

Table 25.4 Contraindications to exercise testing.

Acute infections
Uncontrolled asthma
Uncontrolled diabetes
Acute cardiac disease
Acute injury to lower extremity

When exercise capacity is tested, one has to consider a number of factors that will influence the procedure and the interpretation of results [16].

Before any patient (CF or other) undergoes an exercise test, a medical evaluation should be done to rule out any contraindications to testing [17]. This medical evaluation should include a history, physical examination, measurement of resting oxygen saturation, electrocardiogram and a resting lung function. Components of the medical history and physical examination are given in Table 25.3. Patients with CF seldom need to be excluded from exercise testing.

There are risks of exercise testing for patients with CF in some circumstances. An exercise test should not be performed if one of these risks exists. The contraindications are shown in Table 25.4.

We do not consider severe pulmonary disease, including oxyhemoglobin desaturation, to be a contraindication to exercise testing.

MEASUREMENT OF EXERCISE CAPACITY

Patients with CF may perform the same tests as healthy persons of the same age. The choice of test protocol depends on the aim of the test and the aspect of exercise capacity of interest, age and disease status of the patient, and the resources of the laboratory.

Tests to determine exercise capacity in CF can be divided into two main categories: the laboratory-based exercise test and the field exercise test. Exercise laboratory personnel should obtain training and certification in basic life support [16,19]. At least one of the staff should be a physician, and emergency equipment should be available. To minimize anxiety, especially when young patients are tested, the environment should be private and quiet. Room temperature should be 18–23 degrees Celsius (64–74°F) and humidity should be 40–60%.

The two most commonly used platforms for exercise testing in CF are the cycle ergometer and the treadmill. Since the early 1970s the gold standard of exercise testing has included the collection of inspired and expired gases for the measurement of minute ventilation and determination of oxygen consumption and carbon dioxide production [10].

Field tests are used when laboratory tests are impractical or impossible. Compared to the laboratory test, a field test is inexpensive and easy to administer. With field tests it is not always possible to determine the maximal exercise capacity, but the test can yield valuable information about the patient's functional abilities and limitation [16].

MAXIMAL AEROBIC AND ANAEROBIC EXERCISE TESTING

Aerobic testing

Maximum oxygen uptake ($VO_{2\,max}$) is considered to be the single best index for aerobic fitness. The most commonly used protocol to determine $VO_{2\,max}$ on a cycle ergometer is the Godfrey protocol (Table 25.5) [19].

In this test, the subject begins to pedal at a low workload; then with each minute, the workload increases, until the subject can no longer maintain the prescribed pedaling rate (60/min). The power increase depends on the height of the patient or disease severity. When patients with severe disease ($FEV_1 < 30\%$ predicted) or with very low weight are tested it is appropriate to individualize the Godfrey protocol and to reduce the incremental workload. Reference values for peak power and $VO_{2\,max}$ are available [20,21]. A technical point is worth mentioning here. Most physiologists require that VO_2 reaches a plateau (VO_2 remains unchanged despite increased workload) before calling the final value $VO_{2\,max}$. As this is seldom accomplished in children, with or without CF, most physiologists refer to the highest VO_2 recorded (or, the VO_2 for the last full minute, or last full workload), in a progressive exercise test, as the *peak* VO_2 ($VO_{2\,peak}$), or *symptom-limited* VO_2.

There are a number of protocols to test the maximal aerobic fitness on a treadmill. The most commonly used are the Bruce protocol and the Balke protocol [5,18] (Tables 25.6 and 25.7). Normal values for the Bruce

Table 25.5 Godfrey protocol [10].

Apparatus: cycle ergometer
Time at each stage: 1 minute
Workload increments:
− 10 watts/min (for subjects shorter than 125 cm)
− 15 watts/min (125–150 cm)
− 20 watts/min (>150 cm)
Test termination: subject cannot maintain pedalling frequency of 60 r.p.m.

Table 25.6 Bruce protocol for treadmill exercise testing [5].

Step	Speed		Grade (%)	Duration (min)
	(km/h)	(mile/h)		
1	2.7	1.7	10	3
2	4.0	2.5	12	3
3	5.5	3.4	14	3
4	6.8	4.2	16	3
5	8.0	5.0	18	3
6	8.8	5.5	20	3
7	9.7	6.0	22	3

Test termination: subject cannot maintain walking/jogging speed of treadmill; or subject requests termination.

Table 25.7 Modified Balke protocol for exercise testing [15].

Subject	Speed		Initial grade 9 (%)	Increment (%)	Duration (min)
	(km/h)	(mile/h)			
Poorly fit	4.8	3.0	6	2	2
Sedentary	5.2	3.25	6	2	2
Active	7.9	5.00	0	2–2.5	2
Athlete	8.3	5.25	0	2–2.5	2

Test termination: subject cannot maintain walking/jogging speed of treadmill; or subject requests termination.

protocol for children aged from 4 to 14 years have been published [22].

Whichever protocol is used, certain procedures are followed:

- *Resting phase.* This should least 3–5 minutes to make the patient familiar with the test procedure and the equipment.
- *Warm-up phase.* This consists of 3–5 minutes of unloaded cycling or walking on the treadmill with low speed and grade.
- *Testing-phase.* Immediately after the warm-up phase the incremental exercise test starts. The duration of the aerobic exercise test should be between 6 and 10 minutes to avoid premature muscle fatigue or boredom.

Table 25.8 Criteria for maximum effort on aerobic exercise test.

Heart rate > age-predicted maximum (200 + 10 b.p.m., for most children/adolescents)
Minute ventilation >70% of resting maximum voluntary ventilation
Respiratory exchange ratio >1.05
Surpassing ventilatory threshold
Blood lactate level > resting value

- *Resting phase.* The duration of this phase should be 3–5 minutes with unloaded pedaling or walking on the treadmill, to avoid problems of decreased cerebral and cardiac blood flow from venous pooling in the vasodilated legs.

$VO_{2\text{ peak}}$ measurement requires the maximal effort of the patient [23]. It may be difficult to determine if the patient has given a maximal effort. Some pointers can help determine maximum efforts (Table 25.8).

Any patient who reaches a heart rate greater than his or her age-predicted maximum (200 ± 10 beats/min for most children, adolescents and adults) can be assumed to be giving a maximum effort. Further, the ventilatory anaerobic threshold (VAT) or lactate threshold (LT) can be used. The VAT is the point above which V_E increases out of proportion to VO_2. Although it may be an oversimplification, most physiologists understand the basis for this change to be as follows. With increasingly intense aerobic exercise (i.e. exercise performed with adequate oxygen for the exercising muscle), oxygen consumption and carbon dioxide production (VCO_2) increase proportionally. Since the main stimulus for ventilation is carbon dioxide, V_E increases in direct proportion to VCO_2. As the metabolic demand of the exercising muscles outstrips the oxygen supply, further energy is supplied in greater part via anaerobic pathways. Anaerobic metabolism results in the generation of lactic acid, which in turn is buffered, with water and carbon dioxide the byproducts. Thus, with the onset of anaerobic metabolism, there is an abrupt increase in VCO_2 and V_E. The VAT can be determined non-invasively during an incremental exercise test as the point where VCO_2 and V_E abruptly increase, or show an inflection point (Fig. 25.2).

Furthermore, several other indicators, V_E/VCO_2, RER (respiratory exchange ratio, VCO_2/VO_2) can help to determine the ventilatory anaerobic threshold [9,24]. The lactate threshold is determined from blood lactate measurement during the exercise test. In the past a fixed cutoff for lactate concentration was used. Today the individual LT, defined as the first increase of lactate concentration – sometimes referred to OBLA, for onset of blood lactate accumulation – is used by most investigators. The correlation between VAT and $VO_{2\text{ peak}}$ is high, and in cystic fibrosis the VAT seems to be a useful indicator of a submaximal exercise intensity to be used during aerobic training sessions [25]. Reference values for children have been published [26].

During incremental exercise tests the information in Table 25.9 can be obtained for maximal or submaximal

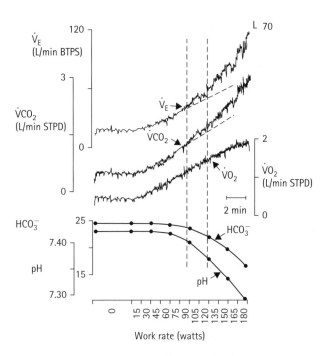

Figure 25.2 Ventilatory anaerobic threshold, shown by an increase in V_E and VCO_2, out of proportion to VO_2. Modified from [63].

exercise capacity. Table 25.10 shows predicted values. An abnormal response is considered to be an individual $VO_{2\,peak}$ less than 80% of the predicted value [9].

Anaerobic testing

Another component of exercise capacity is anaerobic capacity. Anaerobic exercise is that performed without adequate oxygen supply to the exercising muscle. This situation occurs with very intense exercise (all-out sprinting, lifting very heavy loads), but also with relatively low-intensity exercise at the onset of activity, before blood supply has redistributed to the newly exercising muscle. Anaerobic exercise is part of daily physical activity (playing soccer, running to the bus) (Table 25.11).

There are several testing protocols for anaerobic performance (for more details see [27]). The most used is the Wingate anaerobic test [28]. After a warm-up phase of 3 minutes, the patient has to pedal as fast as possible against a high constant resistance. With this test three parameters are determined: peak power (PP, in watts or watts per kg of body weight), mean power (MP, same units) and percentage fatigue. Reproducibility of the test is high, as is the correlation between the test and performance in sprint running or high jumping [28]. To carry out the Wingate anaerobic test (WAnT) an ergometer with a constant resistance mode is required.

Oxyhemoglobin saturation, SaO_2, is measured in nearly every exercise test in every exercise lab around the world, and in fact is an important measure in that it can serve as

Table 25.9 Outcome measurements.

VO_2 (L/min, mL/min or mL/kg per min)
$VCO_{2\,max}$ (L/min, mL/min or mL/kg per min)
Power (watts or watts/kg body weight)
RER (respiratory exchange ratio) = VCO_2/VO_2
Oxygen pulse (VO_2/HR, mL)
V_E (L/min)
V_E/MVV (L/min)
f (breaths/min)
V_T (L, mL)
Oxygen saturation (SaO_2) (%)
Heart rate (b/min)
Heart rate reserve (HRR)
Assessment of breathlessness (Borg, VAS)
Perceived muscular effort (Borg, OMNI scale)
Test time of onset of V_T or L_T
Highest stage of onset of V_T or L_T
Duration of test
Highest stage
Speed (km/h, mile/h, m/min, mile/min, m/s)
Grade (%)

$VO_{2\,peak}$ = peak oxygen uptake, indicating the highest oxygen uptake achieved in an exercise test from inspired gas in a given period of time; $VCO_{2\,peak}$ = carbon dioxide output per minute from exhaled gas in a given period of time; RER = respiratory exchange ratio: the ratio of carbon dioxide output to oxygen uptake per unit time; O_2 pulse = oxygen uptake divided by the heart rate HR; V_E = minute ventilation: the minute ventilation achieved during an exercise test; V_E/MVV = ratio of ventilation to maximum voluntary ventilation; f = breathing frequency: frequency of respiratory cycles per minute (breaths); V_T = tidal volume: the volume of a single breath; BR = breathing reserve: difference between maximal voluntary ventilation and the maximum exercise ventilation; SaO_2 (oxygen saturation) = estimated arterial blood oxygen saturation achieved during a incremental exercise test; HRR = heart rate reserve = difference between predicted highest heart rate and heart rate achieved during a maximum exercise test; power = rate of performing work achieved in an incremental exercise test on a bicycle; stage = step: achieved during an incremental exercise test on a bicycle or treadmill; speed = velocity: reflects the speed achieved during a exercise test, grade = slope: reflects the grade achieved during an exercise test on a treadmill; Borg = RPE (rating of perceived exertion) scale, a scale to determine the extent of breathlessness during exercise, intensity of a physical activity, effort and pain; VAS = visual analogue scale; OMNI scale = a scale which combines numbers, words and pictures to estimate strain of an physical activity.

Table 25.10 Normal predicted peak values and submaximal values for VO_2 (from [26]).

Normal predicted peak values for children [21]
 Girls: $VO_{2\,peak}$ (L/min) = 0.0308806 × height (in cm) − 2.877
 Boys: $VO_{2\,peak}$ (L/min) = 0.044955 × height (in cm) − 4.64

Normal predicted peak values for adults [16]
 Females: $VO_{2\,peak}$ (mL/kg) = 42.83 − (0.371 × age)
 Males: $VO_{2\,peak}$ (mL/kg) = 50.02 − (0.394 × age)

Submaximal values VT as % of $VO_{2\,peak}$
 Girls: 61–70% or 24–29 mL/min; females: 58–74%
 Boys: 58–74% or 29–35 mL/min; males: 61–70%

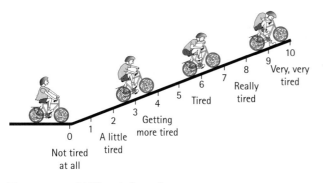

Figure 25.3   OMNI scale [31,34].

Table 25.11   Anaerobic testing: normal values for peak power.

Maximal values for peak power can calculated as follows [20]:
   Girls: P_{max} (in watts) = 2.38 × length (in cm) − 238
   Boys: P_{max} (in watts) = 2.87 × length (in cm) − 291

one measure of disease severity. Oxyhemoglobin *desaturation* with exercise is very uncommon in patients with CF and resting FEV_1 above 50% predicted [12]. Even in patients with severe disease and SaO_2 below 50%, many will not desaturate; but some of these sicker patients will desaturate during exercise. Supplemental oxygen will allow these patients to exercise without desaturating, and with lower heart rates and minute ventilation than if they breathed room air for the same external load [29]. Many of these sicker patients will also breathe more comfortably with supplemental oxygen. On the other hand, there are no data proving that brief periods of oxyhemoglobin desaturation during exercise is harmful to patients with CF.

Perceived exertion

Many laboratories attempt to gauge the subject's perception of exertion during, or immediately following, exercise [30,31]. Subjects are asked to rate the level of difficulty, for their whole body, for their legs, or for their breathing, using one of several available scales. One of the most commonly used scales (the Borg) ranges from 6 ('no exertion at all') to 20 ('maximal exertion'), with a very rough correlation between the point on the scale ×10 and the heart rate at that level of exertion (HR of 60 beats/min at rest, 200 at maximal effort). More recently, the modified Borg scale is used, with ratings from 0 to 10 [32]. Alternatively, some laboratories use a visual analogue scale (VAS) [33], where subjects indicate a point on a 10-cm continuous line that best represents their feeling of exertion. Most promisingly, Robertson has introduced the OMNI scale, which uses both pictorial verbal cues and anchors to aid the child in identifying varying levels of perceived exertion (Fig. 25.3). The OMNI scale also ranges from 0 to 10, and has been shown to have excellent validity and reliability [31,34].

Table 25.12   Walk test outcome measurements.

Walking distance (m)
Heart rate before and after the test
Oxygen saturation before and after the test
Measures of breathlessness (VAS or Borg)
Perceived muscular effort (Borg or OMNI scale)

FIELD TESTS

While the gold-standard of exercise testing includes the online analysis of expired air and ventilation, a number of field tests can determine a subject's exercise response in a non-laboratory setting. These tests are inexpensive, easy to administer and non-invasive. The choice depends on the practical consideration of the test, the required assessment and the facilities. Furthermore the patient's disease state and age have an influence on the choice of the test. Most of the field tests are submaximal, and prediction of $VO_{2\,peak}$ is not the primary goal of these tests [35,36]. However, most activities of daily life are performed at submaximal levels, and walking tests may better reflect the functional exercise level of daily physical activities.

Walking tests

In the last decade walking tests have been used to assess the individual's response to exercise (Table 25.12). The most frequently used are the 12-minute test (12-MWT) and the 6-minute test (6-MWT) [16,35,36]. Both represent submaximal exercise [37]. Reproducibility and validity of these tests are high [18,36]. However, the 6-MWT is easier to carry out, causes less boredom and better reflects the activities in daily life [38].

Both walking tests are used to help determine when to list a patient for transplantation; walking distance is a more informative with respect to survival than single parameters such as FEV_1, body mass index or SaO_2 [39]. In one study in children with severe pulmonary disease, including some with CF, the 6-MWT uncovered greater oxyhemoglobin desaturation than a standard progressive cycle ergometer test [40].

The 6-MWT and the 12-MWT require no equipment or advanced training for the staff. A hallway (30–50 m long) or gym hall is needed with a flat and hard surface. The turn-around points of the course should be marked with a cone and the walking course on the corridor should be marked every 3 m.

Recent published studies have been shown a high correlation between the $VO_{2\,peak}$ and the walking distance in children with mild to moderate CF and healthy children [36,41]. However, if a walking test is used to assess the effects of a training program, or disease progression, it is important to consider that walking distance is influenced by several factors including learning effect, encouragement during test and improvement in walking economy [16,37,42,43]. Reference

Table 25.13 Step test outcome measurements.

Heart rate before and after the test
Oxyhemoglobin saturation (SaO_2)
Measures of breathlessness (VAS or Borg)
Perceived muscular effort (Borg or OMNI scale)
Number of steps if the test is stopped before the time limit

Table 25.14 Shuttle test outcome measurements.

Walking or running distance (m)
Heart rate before and after the test
Oxygen saturation before and after the test
Measures of breathlessness (VAS or Borg)
Perceived muscular effort (Borg or OMNI scale)

values for the walking distance of the 6- and 12-MWT have been published only for adults, not for children [44].

Step tests

Step tests are one of the oldest aerobic exercise tests (Table 25.13) [5]. In CF, a 3-minute step test was introduced in the late 1990s which is modified from the original Master two-step test [45]. In this test the patient has to step up and down on a single 15-cm (6-inch) step with a stepping rate of 30 per minute for 3 minutes. In comparison to a 6-MWT, the step test elicits a higher heart rate and perceived exertion (Borg score). Oxyhemoglobin saturation fall was similar in both tests, except in those with severe lung disease, who had a great fall in SaO_2 with the step test [46] and reproducibility for both tests was similar. The 3-minute step test has been used to determine changes in exercise tolerance in children with CF after a course of intravenous antibiotics [47].

There are some limitations of the step test. The workload is not reproducible because of the different height and weight and different motor skill ability of the person who is tested [23,48].

Shuttle test

Shuttle walk or running tests are incremental, externally paced maximal exercise tests that overcome many of the problems associated with other exercise tests. The subject has to walk (10 m) or run (20 m) between two markers; walking or running speed is increased every minute (Table 25.14) [45,49,50]. The test is terminated if muscular fatigue or symptoms occur or the patient cannot reach the turn-around within the required time. The pace during the test is set by audio signals emitted from a recorded tape; with this signal the patient has to reach the end of the course. The original test has 12 levels, and the modified shuttle test includes 15 levels. For clinical application the running or walking distance is reduced to 10 m per shuttle.

Shuttle tests show a strong correlation between walking or running distance and peak VO_2 and good reproducibility, reliability and sensitivity in children and adult patients with CF [51–53]. However, this test measures more than just aerobic exercise capacity, as it has been shown that muscle strength is related to the incremental shuttle walking distance [54]. Therefore, weak, deconditioned patients may stop the test very early due to fatigue of the peripheral muscles.

Muscular strength

Another component of the exercise capacity is muscular strength. Patients with CF have less muscular strength than their healthy peers [6,55–57]. However, muscular strength, endurance and function are as important in daily life as in sports activities. Muscular strength enables the patients to perform activities without fatigue and encourages patients to participate in sport activities.

Strength is defined as 'the maximal force or torque developed by a muscle or muscle group, during one maximal voluntary action of unlimited duration at a specific velocity of movement'. Muscle endurance is the 'ability of a muscle or muscle group to generate force repeatedly or for an extended period of time' [58]. Strength can be measured during isometric, concentric and eccentric and isokinetic action and strength endurance can be determined by measuring time or repetitions at a specific resistance [5].

While testing the strength or endurance of specific muscle group it is possible to gain information about functional capacity or impairment of the strength capacity, progression of the disease, and changes of muscle function through medication, physical therapy, strength training and rehabilitation [17].

The selection of a strength testing method depends on the purpose for testing, the available equipment, and age and disease severity of the patient. A number of test methods are described for laboratory testing (e.g. isokinetic test with a Cybex dynamometer) and field testing (e.g. sit-up test). For more details see references [5] and [58].

Motor performance

Motor performance is important in daily physical activity and sport activities; therefore factors of motor performance are concerned with health and well-being of an individual. Motor performance includes cardiorespiratory fitness and body composition and strength, muscular endurance, flexibility agility and coordination. The quality of movements depends on the individual conditions of the patient's motor performance.

Motor performance testing has a long tradition, and test batteries have great popularity in many countries. Generally the tests are used to determine the factors of motor performance and to motivate children to improve fitness.

In recent years many test batteries have been developed and normative scales have been published. In general, tests of motor performance are field tests, inexpensive and easy to administer.

Several test batteries have been described, and reference values have been published [59]. The most commonly used are the AAHPERD (American Alliance for Health, Physical Education, Recreation and Dance), CAHPERD (Canadian Association for Health, Physical Education, Recreation and Dance), Canada Fitness Award [59], and in Europe the EUROFIT [60]. Reliability and validity of most of the test batteries is good and most patients can perform these tests.

Fitness components measured in these tests are manifold and examine several aspects of physical fitness. Most tests investigated attributes like flexibility (e.g. sit and reach test), strength (e.g. standing broad jump, vertical jump, push-ups) and muscular endurance (e.g. sit-ups). Furthermore other attributes such as agility (e.g. shuttle-run, 50-m dash), cardiorespiratory fitness (e.g. 12-minute run, 9-minute run) and static or dynamic balance (e.g. flamingo balance) are included in most motor–fitness–performance testing.

Only little is known about motor performance in CF. If inactivity in daily life increases, exercise capacity decreases [61]. One can speculate that motor performance is impaired in CF, and with increase in the severity of disease and inactivity in daily life motor performance will suffer.

For that reason it is important to include a test of motor performance as an additional diagnostic and therapeutic tool in children and adults with CF. Such tests are useful for diagnosis and assessment of functional impairment to design and to evaluate the effects of a training program [62]. Furthermore, a better result after a training program can motivate the CF patient to maintain or achieve a higher level of fitness, and include the most advantageous amount of physical activity in his or her present and future lifestyle.

REFERENCES

1. Nixon PA, Orenstein DM, Kelsey SF et al. The prognostic value of exercise testing in patients with cystic fibrosis. *N Engl J Med* 1992; **327**:1785–1788.

2. Pianosi P, LeBlanc J, Almudevar A. Peak oxygen uptake and mortality in children with cystic fibrosis. *Thorax* 2005; **60**:50–54.

3. Boas SR. Exercise recommendation for individuals with cystic fibrosis. *Sports Med* 1997; **24**:17–37.

4. Orenstein DM, Rosenstein BJ, Stern RC. *Cystic Fibrosis: Medical Care*. Philadelphia, Lippincott Williams & Wilkins, 2000.

5. Bar-Or O, Rowland TW. *Pediatric Exercise Medicine: From Physiologic Principles to Health Care Application*. Champaign, IL, Human Kinetics, 2004.

6. Lands L, Heigenhauser GJ, Jones NL. Respiratory and peripheral muscle function in cystic fibrosis. *Am Rev Respir Dis* 1993; **147**:865–869.

7. Orenstein DM, Franklin BA, Doershuk CF et al. Exercise conditioning and cardiopulmonary fitness in cystic fibrosis: the effects of a three month supervised running program. *Chest* 1981; **80**:375–379.

8. Selvadurai HC, Allen J, Sachinwalla J et al. Muscle function and resting energy expenditure in female athletes with cystic fibrosis. *Am J Respir Crit Care Med* 2003; **168**:1476–1480.

9. Wasserman K, Hansen JE, Sue DY et al. *Principles of Exercise Testing and Interpretation*. Philadelphia, Lea & Febinger, 1994.

10. Godfrey S, Davies CTM, Wozniak E. Cardio-respiratory response to exercise in normal children. *Clin Sci* 1971; **40**:419–431.

11. Cerny F, Pullano TP, Cropp JA. Cardiorespiratory adaptations to exercise in CF. *Am Rev Respir* 1982; **126**:261–265.

12. Henke KG, Orenstein DM. Oxygen saturation during exercise in cystic fibrosis. *Am Rev Respir Dis* 1984; **129**:708–711.

13. Rogers D, Prasad A, Doull I. Exercise testing in children with cystic fibrosis. *J R Soc Med* 2003; **96**(Suppl 43):23–29.

14. Lebecque P, Lapierre JG, Lamarre A, Coates AL. Diffusion capacity and oxygen desaturation effects on exercise in patients with cystic fibrosis. *Chest* 1987; **91**:693–697.

15. Rowland TW. Aerobic exercise testing protocols. In: Rowland T (ed.) *Pediatric Laboratory Exercise Testing*. Champaign, IL, Human Kinetics, 1993, pp19–41.

16. Cooper CB, Storer TW. *Exercise Testing and Interpretation: A Practical Approach*. Cambridge, Cambridge University Press, 2001.

17. American College of Sports Medicine. *Guidelines for Exercise Testing and Prescription*, 3rd edn. Baltimore, Williams & Wilkins, 1995.

18. Tomassoni TL. Conducting the pediatric exercise test. In: Rowland T (ed.) *Pediatric Laboratory Exercise Testing*. Champaign, IL, Human Kinetics, 1993, pp1–17.

19. Hebestreit H, Bar-Or O. Differences between children and adults for exercise testing and exercise prescription. In: Skinner J (ed.) *Exercise Testing and Exercise Prescription for Special Cases: Theoretical Basis and Clinical Application*, 3rd edn. Philadelphia, Lippincott Williams & Wilkins, 2005, pp68–84.

20. Godfrey S, Mearns M. Pulmonary function and response to exercise in cystic fibrosis. *Arch Dis Child* 1971; **46**:144–151.

21. Orenstein DM. Assessment of exercise pulmonary function. In: Rowland T (ed.) *Pediatric Laboratory Exercise Testing*. Champaign, IL, Human Kinetics, 1993, pp141–163.

22. Cumming GR, Everat D, Hastman L. Bruce treadmill test in children: normal values in a clinical population. *Am J Cardiol* 1978; **4**:69–75.

23. Hollmann W, Hettinger T. *Sportmedizin: Grundlagen für Arbeit, Training und Prevention*, 4th edn. Stuttgart, Schattauer Verlag, 2004.

24. Hebestreit H, Staschen B, Hebestreit A. Ventilatory threshold: a useful method to determine aerobic fitness in children? *Med Sci Sports Exerc* 2000; **32**:1964–1969.

25. Gruber W, Kiosz D, Braumann KM. The respiratory anaerobic threshold as a possibility to determine exercise intensity in

patients with cystic fibrosis [in German]. *Atemwegs-Lungenk* 1999; **9**:488–496.

26. Washington RL, Van Gundy JC, Cohen C *et al*. Normal aerobic and anaerobic exercise data for North American school-age children. *J Pediatr* 1988; **112**:223–233.

27. Bar-Or O. Anaerobic performance. In: Docherty D (ed.) *Measurement in Paediatric Exercise Science*. Champaign, IL, Human Kinetics, 1996, pp161–182.

28. Inbar O, Bar-Or O, Skinner JS. *The Wingate Anaerobic Test*. Champaign, IL, Human Kinetics, 1996.

29. Nixon PA, Orenstein DM, Curtis SA, Ross EA. Oxygen supplementation during exercise in cystic fibrosis. *Am Rev Respir Dis* 1990; **142**:807–811.

30. Mahon AD, Ray ML. Ratings of perceived exertion at maximal exercise in children performing different graded exercise test. *J Sports Med Phys Fitness* 1995; **35**(1):38–42.

31. Robertson RJ. *Perceived Exertion for Practitioners*. Champaign, IL, Human Kinetics, 2004.

32. Borg G. *Borg's Perceived Exertion and Pain Scales*. Champaign, IL, Human Kinetics, 1998.

33. Swinburn CR, Wakefield JM, Jones PW. Relationship between ventilation and breathlessness during exercise in chronic obstructive airways disease is not altered by prevention of hypoxemia. *Clin Sci* 1984; **67**:515–519.

34. Robertson RJ *et al*. Children's OMNI Scale of Perceived Exertion: mixed gender and race validation. *Med Sci Sports Exerc* 2000; **32**:452–458.

35. ATS Statement. Guidelines for the six-minute walk-test. *Am J Respir Crit Care Med* 2002; **166**:111–117.

36. Li AM, Yu CCW, Tsang T *et al*. The six-minute walk test in healthy children: reliability and validity. *Eur Respir J* 2005; **25**:1057–1060.

37. Kervio G, Carre F, Ville NS. Reliability and intensity of a six minute walk test in healthy elderly subjects. *Med Sci Sports Exerc* 2003; **35**:169–174.

38. Solway S, Brooks D, Lacasse Y *et al*. A qualitative systematic overview of the measurement properties of functional walking test used in the cardiorespiratory domain. *Chest* 2001; **119**:256–270.

39. Ruter K, Staab D, Magdorf K. The 12 minute walk test as an assessment criterion for lung transplantation in subjects with cystic fibrosis. *J Cyst Fibros* 2003; **2**:8–13.

40. Nixon PA. Role of exercise in the evaluation and management of pulmonary disease in children and youth. *Med Sci Sports Exerc* 1996; **28**:414–420.

41. Gulmans VAM, van Veldoven NHM, de Meer K *et al*. The six-minute walk test in children with cystic fibrosis: reliability and validity. *Pediatr Pulmonol* 1996; **22**:85–89.

42. Beneke R, Meyer K. Walking performance and economy in chronic heart failure patients pre and post exercise training. *Eur J Appl Physiol* 1997; **75**:246–251.

43. Iriberri M, Galdiz JB, Gorostiza A *et al*. Comparison of the distances covered during a 3 and 6 min walking test. *Respir Med* 2002; **96**:812–816.

44. Enright PL, Sherill DL. Reference equations for the six minute walk in healthy adults. *Am J Respir Crit Care Med* 1998; **158**:1384–1387.

45. Bradley J, Howard J, Wallace E *et al*. Validity of a modified shuttle test in adult cystic fibrosis. *Thorax* 1999; **54**:437–439.

46. Aurora P, Prasad SA, Balfour-Lynn IM *et al*. Exercise tolerance in children with cystic fibrosis undergoing lung transplantation assessment. *Eur Respir J* 2001; **18**:293–297.

47. Pike S, Prasad SA, Balfour-Lynn IA. Effect of intravenous antibiotics on exercise tolerance (3-Min Step Test) in cystic fibrosis. *Pediatr Pulmonol* 2001; **32**:38–43.

48. Orenstein D. Exercise testing in cystic fibrosis. *Pediatr Pulmonol* 1998; **25**:223–225.

49. Leger L, Mercier D, Gadoury C *et al*. The multistage 20 meter shuttle test for aerobic fitness. *J Sport Sci* 1988; **6**:93–101.

50. Singh SJ, Morgan MD, Scott S *et al*. Development of a shuttle walking test of disability in patients with chronic airway obstruction. *Thorax* 1992; **47**:1019–1024.

51. Bradley J, Howard J, Wallace E *et al*. Reliability, repeatability, and sensitivity of the modified shuttle test in adult cystic fibrosis. *Chest* 2000; **117**:1666–1671.

52. Singh JH, Morgan MDL, Hardman AE *et al*. Comparison of oxygen uptake during a conventional treadmill test and the shuttle walking test in chronic airflow limitation. *Eur Respir J* 1994; **7**:2016–2020.

53. Selvadurai HC, Cooper PJ, Meyers N *et al*. Validation of shuttle tests in children with cystic fibrosis. *Pediatr Pulmonol* 2003; **35**:133–138.

54. Steiner MC, Singh SJ, Morgan MD. The contribution of peripheral muscle function to shuttle walking performance in patients with chronic obstructive pulmonary disease. *J Cardiopulm Rehab* 2005; **25**:43–49.

55. Barry SC, Gallagher CG. Corticosteroids and skeletal muscle function in cystic fibrosis. *J Appl Physiol* 2003; **95**:1379–1384.

56. de Meer K, Gulmans VAM. Peripheral muscle weakness and exercise capacity in children with cystic fibrosis. *Am J Crit Care Med* 1999; **159**:748–754.

57. Sahlberg ME, Svantesson U, Thomas EM *et al*. Muscular strength and function in patients with cystic fibrosis. *Chest* 2005; **125**:1587–1592.

58. Gaul CA. Muscular strength and endurance. In: Docherty D (ed.) *Measurement in Pediatric Exercise Science*. Champaign, IL, Human Kinetics, 1996, pp225–283.

59. Docherty D. Field test and test batteries. In: Docherty D (ed.) *Measurement in Pediatric Exercise Science*. Champaign, IL, Human Kinetics, 1996, pp285–334.

60. Committee of Experts on Sports Research. *Handbook for the Eurofit Tests of Physical Fitness*. Rome, Edigraf Editoriale Grafica, 1988.

61. Gruber W, Braumann KM, Paul K *et al*. Is motor performance reduced in CF patients? *Pediatr Pulmonol Suppl* 2005; **28**:320.

62. Gruber W, Braumann KM, Paul K *et al*. Effects of an exercise program on motor performance in CF patients. *Pediatr Pulmonol Suppl* 2005; **28**:311.

63. Wasserman K. The anaerobic threshold measurement in exercise testing. *Clin Chest Med* 1984; **5**(1):85.

Exercise: use in therapy

DAVID M. ORENSTEIN AND LINDA W. HIGGINS

INTRODUCTION

The hallmark of cystic fibrosis (CF), progressive and inevitable loss of pulmonary function, is typically accompanied by progressive loss of exercise tolerance. Because the primary disease process in CF cannot yet be reversed, treatment efforts have been largely directed at preservation of lung function. In the past decade, maintaining or even improving exercise tolerance through exercise training has been added to the list of standard therapeutic CF regimens. This can take the form of aerobic training, anaerobic training, or resistance training of specific muscle groups, including the ventilatory muscles. Regimens of each of these, sometimes in combination, have been shown to be both physiologically and psychologically beneficial to patients with CF. In this chapter, we review the response of CF patients to single bouts of exercise, how exercise and regular physical activity are related to and can promote health in these patients, and guidelines for exercise prescription.

RESPONSE TO SINGLE BOUTS OF EXERCISE

The response to exercise in patients with CF can be explained largely in terms of three systems: cardiovascular, pulmonary and muscle/metabolic. During a single bout of exercise, the cardiovascular response of CF patients with mild to moderate lung disease tends to be similar to that of healthy individuals, where cardiac output increases with increasing workloads, as a result of increased stroke volume at low intensities followed by an increase in heart rate at higher exercise intensities [64]. However, age-predicted maximal heart rates are seldom achieved, except in those with the mildest disease [65], because ventilatory factors limit exercise capacity well before the heart can be driven to its physiological potential [66,67]. In some patients with severe lung dysfunction, stroke volume may be reduced [68].

Both gas exchange and pulmonary mechanics may be abnormal in exercise. Patients with CF have increased dead space (ventilated, but no gas exchange). During exercise, CF patients increase minute ventilation more through higher breathing frequencies than increases in tidal volume, to meet the demands of exercise and attempt to overcome the disease-related dead space [64,66]. Not unlike healthy subjects, patients with CF are able to increase their tidal volume to about 50% of their vital capacity; however, especially in sicker patients, their vital capacity may be reduced, and the resulting tidal volume inadequate, requiring further increases in respiratory rate to achieve higher minute ventilation [69]. It is likely that sicker patients are unable to increase tidal volume because their inspiratory muscles are at a mechanical disadvantage, caused by pulmonary over-inflation [70]. The diaphragm is depressed and its fibers shortened below the ideal portion of the length/tension curve. When increases in minute ventilation are not sufficient to compensate for the increased dead space and when airway obstruction is severe, arterial oxygen desaturation and CO_2 retention may occur with exercise. This is true for many, but not all, patients with an FEV_1 below 50% of predicted (Fig. 25.4) [71], or diffusing capacity of the lung for CO (DLCO) <80% [72]. In cases where oxygen desaturation occurs during exercise, supplemental oxygen for submaximal exercise may be warranted to maintain sufficient oxygenation. At peak exercise, the minute ventilation for many CF patients may approach or even exceed maximal voluntary ventilation, indicating a mechanical ventilatory limitation to exercise. This contrasts with healthy individuals, who have ventilatory reserve even during maximal exercise efforts and whose minute ventilation typically does not surpass 70% of their maximal capacity [66].

The role of arterial oxygen desaturation in limiting exercise tolerance among patients with more severe disease is unclear. During submaximal exercise, supplemental oxygen prevents oxygen desaturation [73,74], decreases heart rate and minute ventilation [74] and increases exercise time [73], particularly in patients who desaturate during room-air exercise. The effect of oxygen on maximal exercise tolerance is less clear. Two groups of investigators administered maximal exercise tests to patients with CF; one found that

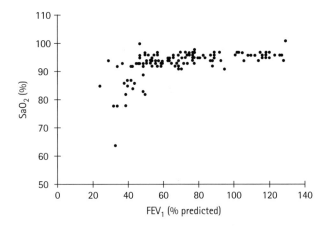

Figure 25.4 Relationship of pulmonary function (FEV₁% predicted) and oxyhemoglobin saturation (SaO₂%) at peak exercise in 130 patients with cystic fibrosis. Reprinted with permission from [168].

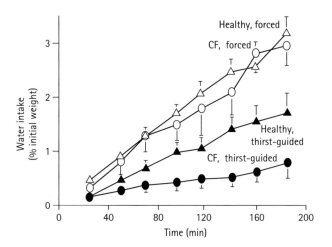

Figure 25.5 Mean (SEM) cumulative water intake during exercise in the heat, comparing forced drinking with thirst-guided drinking sessions. Reprinted with permission from [84].

supplemental oxygen decreased oxyhemoglobin desaturation and increased exercise time and maximal oxygen consumption [75], while the other found decreased oxyhemoglobin desaturation, minute ventilation and heart rate, but no increase in maximal exercise time or peak oxygen uptake [74]. One elegant study [76] examined the effects of both supplemental oxygen and added dead space on exercise capacity, and found that patients with CF actually had greater exercise capacity when they breathed 38% oxygen through added dead space than when they breathed the supplemental oxygen without increased dead space. The authors concluded that hypoxemia, rather than mechanical ventilatory factors, was the cause of exercise limitation.

Other exercise limitations in patients with CF may be related to reductions in muscle mass and respiratory muscle strength [77–79]. This muscle weakness may [77–79] or may not [80] be explained by nutritional deficiency, pulmonary status or habitual activity. Patients with more severe disease may also have elevated lung volumes ('dynamic hyperinflation') during exercise [81] which might interfere with cardiac output [82].

Exercise in the heat

Because of the sweat defect in CF, exercising in the heat presents a unique challenge to CF patients. Under moderate environmental conditions, patients with CF have higher than normal concentrations of sodium and chloride in their sweat, and, when exposed to exercise and heat stress, they have been shown to lose significantly more sodium and chloride than normal; if patients are encouraged to drink plain water, these sweat losses are reflected in decreased serum concentrations of the ions [83]. If CF patients drink only as guided by thirst, they underestimate their fluid losses, and drink significantly less water than healthy controls [84], a situation referred to as 'voluntary dehydration' (Fig. 25.5).

Thirst is regulated by hypothalamic osmoreceptors. During exercise in the heat, healthy controls lose more fluid than salt, rendering their serum hyperosmolar, thus triggering thirst. In contrast, patients with CF lose relatively more solutes (sodium and chloride) than fluid, rendering their serum relatively hypo-osmolar; as a result, the hypothalamic osmoreceptors do not stimulate thirst [85]. If patients are offered flavored water, with additional salt, they are more likely to drink than if they are offered only water [85]. After eight days of daily sessions of exercise in the heat, patients with CF are able to tolerate the exercise and heat stress better than they did on day one, with lower heart rate and lower core body temperature, but, unlike healthy control subjects, they do not produce a more dilute sweat than they did on day one [86].

Exercise and CFTR

Three recent studies have suggested that exercise might affect the basic cellular defect in CF. Two groups [87,88] measured nasal bioelectrical potential difference (PD) during exercise in patients with CF and healthy controls, and found that the PD of the patients progressively increased towards normal during exercise. Further studies of the effects of amiloride and low-chloride perfusates on the nasal PD during exercise suggested that the differences seen in nasal PD were the result of decreased sodium absorption, and not chloride conductance [88]. Work in cell culture [89] points to a possible mechanism for these observations: when CF cells are subjected to phasic shear stress, as might happen with deep breathing (as during exercise), ATP is released, with the nucleotides inhibiting sodium transport. Thus, evidence is beginning to emerge from basic science labs to explain some of the long-recognized benefits of exercise in patients with CF.

Table 25.15 Therapeutic uses of exercise.[a]

	Type of training/activity							
	Aerobic		Anaerobic		Inspiratory muscle		Peripheral muscle	
	Children	Adults	Children	Adults	Children	Adults	Children	Adults
Aerobic fitness	[92] [94-98] [102] [103] [105]	[92] [94] [96] [98] [104-106]	[107]		[109]	[110]	[103]	
Anaerobic fitness			[107]					
Pulmonary function	[92] [97] [107] [116-119]	[92] [93] [105] [106]			[109]	[110]	[97] [121]	[121]
Sputum clearance	[116]	[104] [122]				[123]		
Ease of breathing		[106] [124]						[124]
Inspiratory muscle Strength/endurance	[92] [108]	[92]			[108] [109] [125] [126]	[110] [125] [126]		
Peripheral muscle Strength	[92] [102] [103]	[92]					[97] [103] [121]	[121]
Urinary continence								[130][b]
Nutritional status		[93]					[97] [121]	[121]
Health-related QoL	[97] [105]	[105]	[107]					
Psychosocial status	[102]					[110]		

[a] The table provides a summary of published exercise intervention studies in patients with CF. The number in each cell gives the reference for the study employing a given type of intervention resulting in the specific benefit. For example, reference [109] was a study using inspiratory muscle training in children that showed improved aerobic fitness, pulmonary function, and inspiratory muscle endurance.
[b] The muscle training in this study involved the pelvic floor muscles.

BENEFITS OF EXERCISE AND HABITUAL PHYSICAL ACTIVITY

See Table 25.15.

Increased cardiopulmonary fitness

The most fundamentally important use of exercise therapy for patients with CF is to improve aerobic fitness, as higher peak oxygen consumption ($\dot{V}O_2$) has been correlated with significantly lower 5- to 8-year mortality (Fig. 25.6) [90,91]. (No studies have yet shown that changing $\dot{V}O_2$ changes mortality, but it is clear that (a) patients with higher $\dot{V}O_2$ have better survival than those with lower $\dot{V}O_2$, and (b) it is possible to improve patients' $\dot{V}O_2$.) Although other exercise parameters – namely, peak power output (PO) and peak working capacity (PWC) – and lung function indices (specifically FEV_1 and FVC) are reflected in, and related to, $\dot{V}O_{2\,peak}$, $\dot{V}O_2$ appears to be a marker that is something greater than the sum of its parts. For patients with CF, improvements in $\dot{V}O_{2\,peak}$ are certainly most desirable because of the suggestion that they could extend life, but increases in related measures (whose exact relationships may be unclear) also have merit. With improved exercise tolerance, CF patients can do more physical work, at a lower physiological cost, and with less distress.

AEROBIC TRAINING

Over the past 25 years, a number of intervention studies have shown that aerobic exercise training can improve peak V̇O₂, peak power output, and PWC in adults and children with CF. The training programs have been diverse in terms of exercise modality, duration and supervision, with short-term supervised interventions showing the greatest

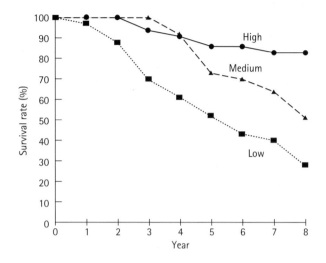

Figure 25.6 Survival among 109 patients with cystic fibrosis, according to fitness level. Reprinted with permission from [91].

success. Supervised running [92], biking [93], swimming [94], trampolining [95], multi-modal [96] and in-hospital cycle ergometer and treadmill training [97,98] programs have all been implemented. For all of these supervised programs, follow-up has been short or absent. Some of these programs are summarized in Table 25.16.

Other researchers have employed partial or no supervision of longer training programs, and these are also found in the table. While supervised programs present advantages in terms of ensuring exercise adherence and improving fitness, they are often burdensome to maintain, and it is unknown whether their benefits can be sustained in the long term without continued participation in the structured activity. Unsupervised exercise programs pose fewer logistical concerns but are likely to be dependent on patients' intrinsic motivation, and only a few published studies [104–106] have documented improvements in exercise tolerance with unsupervised training. It is difficult to ascertain why training effects have not been evident in more of the unsupervised studies. It may be that (a) the training was not maintained; (b) the training stimulus was insufficient; (c) the subjects were relatively healthy and/or active with little potential for improved fitness; or (d) some combination of these factors.

Table 25.16 Aerobic exercise interventions in CF.

Exercise mode	Program specifics	Outcome	Reference
Running	Supervised/controlled/non-random; 30-mins, three times a week for 3 months	↑ peak V̇O₂; ↑ PWC; ↓ HR at submax; no change in controls	[92]
Cycling	Adults; oxygen-assisted; 3–13 weeks	↑ peak V̇O₂; ↑ W$_{max}$;	[93]
Cycle ergometer/treadmill	In-hospital; children; controlled two control groups – no exercise, resistance exercise; 30 mins, five times a week for 18 days	↑ peak V̇O₂; no change in controls	[97]
Treadmill	In-hospital; adolescents/young adults;12 weeks	↑ peak V̇O₂	[98]
Swimming		↑ treadmill time	[94]
Multimodal	Camp (mountain climbing, swimming, 'ball games', trampoline; three times a week	↑ peak V̇O₂; ↑ PWC	[96]
Trampoline	Three times a week for 8 weeks	↑ peak V̇O₂	[95]
Cycling	At home; semi-supervised; 6 months	↑ peak V̇O₂	[102]
Stair-stepping	Controlled/randomized; 1 year	↑ PWC	[103]
Cycling	At home; 2 months	↑ peak V̇O₂; ↑ PWC	[104]
Cycling	At home; 3 months	↑ peak V̇O₂; ↑ PWC	[105]
Multimodal	Upper body weights; walk/jog, cycling; swimming, sport; adults	↓ blood lactate	[106]

PWC, peak working capcity; V̇O₂, oxygen consumption.

ANAEROBIC TRAINING

Daily activities of adults and especially children frequently entail repeated bouts of anaerobic exercise rather than sustained aerobic efforts. Although an understanding of the positive outcomes of anaerobic exercise performance is of practical importance, little attention has been given to the effects of anaerobic training programs for individuals with CF. One group [107] found that, after a 3-month supervised anaerobic training program, aerobic performance was increased in a sample of children with CF and mild-to-moderate pulmonary disease severity. The training group showed significant increases in $\dot{V}O_{2peak}$ and W_{max}, and decreases in serum lactate levels at the end of the training period, compared to controls. They also demonstrated significantly improved anaerobic fitness, as measured by peak power (PP) and mean power (MP), PP and MP per kilogram of body weight , and PP and MP per kilogram of fat-free mass (see Chapter 25a). Unfortunately, as is often true in any population, the training benefits were not maintained after the intervention.

INSPIRATORY MUSCLE TRAINING

As ventilatory factors may be central to exercise limitation in CF, it seems reasonable to think that ventilatory muscle training might help overall exercise tolerance, but few studies have addressed this question directly. Keens and colleagues [108] were the first to examine the effects of any exercise training program in patients with CF; they focused on upper body (canoeing and swimming) exercise and specific ventilatory muscle training (of which more later). They found increased ventilatory muscle endurance, but no change in overall exercise tolerance, with 4 weeks of either approach. Despite the Keens study's groundbreaking work, the impact of inspiratory muscle training (IMT) on exercise tolerance in patients with CF has been largely overlooked. One study [109] examined the effect of a 10-week program using an inspiratory threshold loading device, and reported increased treadmill time in the intervention group and no change in controls. A more recent study [110] addressed inadequacies of previous IMT research by fixing the workload and resetting it (according to maximal inspiratory pressure generated) before each training session. CF patients were randomly assigned to three groups (training intensity of 80% of maximal inspiratory effort, 20% of maximal inspiratory effort, or control). High-intensity (80% of maximum) IMT significantly improved physical working capacity. Unfortunately, no follow-up was conducted after the 8-week, at-home, supervised training period.

HABITUAL PHYSICAL ACTIVITY

Although habitual physical activity (HPA) of children with CF has not been experimentally manipulated, correlational studies have shown relationships between HPA and exercise tolerance parameters. Habitual activity levels of CF children have been monitored by various methods, including motion-sensing devices and questionnaires [111–113] and in general have been described as being equal to [112] or lower than [113] those of healthy peers, with boys with CF reporting greater activity than girls [112,114]. One study looking at gender differences in HPA in CF children [115] found that the activity levels of the children, with varying levels of disease severity, correlated significantly and most strongly with anaerobic power and aerobic capacity. In addition, two studies have shown relationships between activity levels and $\dot{V}O_{2peak}$ [113,114]. Schneiderman-Walker's group [114] reported a significant correlation between weekday total activity and $\dot{V}O_{2peak}$ in 109 boys and girls with CF, and Nixon's [113] analyses for a subgroup of patients ($n = 10$) with the worst lung function (those in the lowest tertile; FEV_1 <80% predicted) revealed strong and significant correlations between hours per week spent in vigorous activity and VO_{2peak}.

SUMMARY

The results of these training interventions and correlational analyses continue to substantiate the use of exercise programs to improve exercise tolerance in patients with CF. For further validation, studies are needed with longer follow-up, ideally with more patients, and with more emphasis on the best ways to assure continued patient participation.

Improvement and maintenance of pulmonary function

In a smaller number of studies, exercise has also been shown to preserve and even improve lung function in individuals with CF. Several investigators have reported that pulmonary function improves in patients with CF after implementation of swimming [116], cycling [93,105] and combined exercise regimens [117]. One of the earliest studies documented improvements in pulmonary function during an intensive multimodal exercise program, but did not include non-exercise control groups [117]. Another uncontrolled study found improvements in FEV_1 in 16 patients with CF after a cycle training program [93]. And, with 10 patients with CF serving as their own controls in a cycling intervention trial, a different group found increases in FEV_1 values as well [102]. In our 3-month jogging study [92], no pulmonary function measure changed significantly in either exercise or control patients, except that FEV_1 fell significantly in the controls.

In randomized, controlled studies of exercise as part of in-hospital treatment of pulmonary exacerbations, Cerny [118] and Selvadurai and colleagues [97] reported improvements in FEV_1. In Cerny's study of moderately-to-severely ill patients, pulmonary function increased for both the exercise and control group. The intent of this study was not to see if exercise by itself could improve pulmonary function, but rather if daily exercise could be substituted for standard airway clearance (chest physiotherapy) during in-hospital treatment of pulmonary exacerbations. Selvadurai and colleagues performed a similar study, but with patients assigned to different exercise regimens during their in-patient treatment of pulmonary exacerbation. The exercise conferred a differential effect: FEV_1 increased more among the exercise groups (resistance > aerobic) than it did for the controls. Patients in both of these studies received aggressive intravenous antibiotic therapy throughout their hospital stays.

Changes in pulmonary function were reported in two unsupervised aerobic training studies. One three-times-per-week program [119] consisted of a variety of exercise modalities, including running, swimming, cycling and soccer. In the control group, there was a greater annual decline in FVC and a trend for the same in FEV_1 compared to the exercise group. Patients maintained participation with the regimen over the long study period of 3 years. Similarly, in another individualized, 1-year exercise training program of upper and lower body exercise in adults with CF [106], exercising patients showed a trend for better preservation of lung function (FEV_1) and a significant improvement in FVC compared to controls.

The length of the trial is particularly important in studies of patients with CF because the goal is to prevent deterioration in function. The expected annual decline in pulmonary function in patients with CF is as low as 1% [120]. This suggests that studies of patients with CF may be unable to detect a difference in pulmonary function between control and intervention subjects if the study period is less than 1 year, unless very large numbers of patients are included.

There is also some support for the use of weight training and inspiratory muscle training (IMT) to achieve pulmonary benefits in CF patients. One early study [121] employed largely upper-body variable weight training in 12 teenagers and adults with cystic fibrosis for 6 months. Compared to a 3-month control period, the subjects demonstrated significant decreases in residual volume and RV/TLC after training (suggesting less air trapping). More recently, CF patients showed improved lung volumes after an 8-week controlled, randomized program of IMT in which the training intensity was set at either 80% or 20% of maximal effort [110]. Significant increases in vital capacity (VC) and total lung capacity (TLC) were evident only in the 80% IMT group. These findings supported previous work [109] that tested inspiratory muscle training in 20 children with CF and found significant increases in VC and TLC in the experimental group that trained at a high-pressure load ($\geq 29\,cmH_2O$) compared to the control group that trained at a minimal pressure load ($< 15\,cmH_2O$). The effects of exercise training on ventilatory muscle function are discussed later.

Most recently, habitual physical activity has been correlated with pulmonary function. Schneiderman-Walker's group [114] evaluated unsupervised habitual physical activity in children with CF and its relationship to lung function decline. They found that, in girls with CF, those in the two lowest activity quartiles had a significantly more rapid rate of decline in FEV_1 than those in the two highest activity quartiles. This adds to the increasing evidence for the benefits of exercise training and physical activity on respiratory health, and possibly survival, in patients with CF, although it leaves unanswered the question of the direction of causality. Might those girls with better lung function be more active because they feel better, rather than the activity slowing pulmonary decline?

Increased sputum clearance

Many patients and families report that exercise stimulates cough and sputum expectoration, and many teenaged patients with CF ask if they can substitute physical activity for the drudgery of airway clearance. Whole-body training regimens and inspiratory muscle training (IMT) have been examined alone and as adjuncts to standard physiotherapy to enhance sputum expectoration in CF patients. Salh and colleagues [104] assessed the roles of physiotherapy and home cycle ergometer exercise in sputum production and found that exercise contributed to expectoration but that more sputum was produced during and after physiotherapy than during and after exercise. Similarly, Bilton and colleagues [122] found that physiotherapy and the combination of exercise and physiotherapy produced a significantly higher sputum weight than did exercise alone. However, perhaps not surprisingly, patients preferred exercise as the treatment option for use at home. A recent study evaluated the impact of repeated maximum inspiratory vital capacity maneuvers against a fixed resistance on sputum clearance compared to standard physiotherapy that included postural drainage with percussion and active cycle of breathing techniques [123]. Twenty CF patients were randomly allocated to alternate-day treatment (with inspiratory maneuvers or standard physiotherapy) for the first 4 days of hospitalization and antibiotic therapy for pulmonary exacerbation. All patients received both treatments twice, on days one and three or on days two and four. The resistive inspiratory maneuvers increased the weight of the sputum 2-fold compared to the standard approach, independent of treatment order or day. Exercise appears to have some value in facilitating sputum expectoration in CF patients, but in order to determine its exact role more investigation is required.

Decreased breathlessness

Breathlessness, likely the most distressing symptom experienced by patients with CF, can be diminished by exercise training. O'Neill and colleagues [124] assessed breathlessness with a visual analogue scale in 8 patients with CF before and after a 2-month daily exercise program, and documented a significant decrease in breathlessness after the program. Moorcroft and colleagues [106] also showed a trend for a small reduction in breathlessness in their active group during submaximal arm ergometry exercise, compared to controls. Improvements in the subjective experience of dyspnea may facilitate daily living in CF patients who are limited in what they can do by difficult breathing.

Increased peripheral and ventilatory muscle strength and endurance

Efforts to increase muscular strength and endurance in CF patients have focused on both inspiratory and peripheral muscles. In the earliest such study, Keens and colleagues [108] showed that 4 weeks of upper-body exercise (swimming and canoeing) or specific ventilatory exercise (daily sessions breathing against resistance) could each induce an increase in ventilatory muscle endurance in patients with CF; the study did not include a non-exercise control group. Similar improvements in ventilatory muscle endurance were seen after a 6-week low-intensity (40% of maximal static inspiratory pressure) inspiratory threshold loading program [125]. Further, 8 weeks of inspiratory muscle training at 80% and 20% intensity resulted in significant increases in maximal inspiratory pressure and sustained maximal inspiratory pressure compared to controls but without differences between the training groups [110], and 10 weeks of high- and low-pressure load inspiratory muscle training produced significant increases in inspiratory muscle strength in the high-pressure load group [109]. Increases in inspiratory muscle strength and endurance have been shown following even shorter programs of inspiratory muscle training (4 weeks) [126]. A 3-month supervised running program also resulted in increased ventilatory muscle endurance in the training group, compared to a non-exercise control group [92], presumably because of the increased minute ventilation required for the metabolic demands of the leg exercise. Preservation of inspiratory muscle function and averting inspiratory muscle fatigue may delay dyspnea [125].

Peripheral muscle strength changes have been reported after a 6-month cycling program, where 14 CF patients serving as their own controls demonstrated significant increases in muscle strength of knee extensors and ankle dorsiflexors [102] and following a 6-month variable weight training program in which the CF patients, serving as their own controls, showed significant improvements in upper-arm muscle size and strength [121]. Similarly, CF children who received weight training in a more recent randomized, controlled study achieved better leg strength than the children in the aerobic training or control group [97]. In another recent study, both those who received weight training and those randomly assigned to stair-stepping aerobic exercise increased peripheral muscle strength [103].

Urinary incontinence treatment

Urinary incontinence can be embarrassing and underreported. It has only recently been recognized as a problem in women with CF. It can reduce their quality of life and may interfere with their ability to perform adequate pulmonary function testing, and, more importantly, carry out airway clearance routines. Over the past 15 years, a small number of studies have explored the incidence of urinary incontinence in women with CF [127–129], and one has investigated treatment options [130]. Prevalence of urinary incontinence in CF women has been reported as ranging from 37.9% [129] to 59% [127] or even 68% [128]. As pelvic floor muscle exercises have been shown to be effective in the treatment of urinary incontinence in other groups of patients, McVean and colleagues [130] tested individualized pelvic floor muscle exercise. The 19 women with CF in the study were those who requested help for their urinary incontinence. At the end of the 3-month program, endurance (hold time) had increased significantly, but pelvic floor muscle strength remained unchanged. Continued study of how exercise can be used as a therapeutic modality for this problem is warranted.

Enhanced nutritional status

Several cross-sectional studies [77,131,132] and one longitudinal study [133] have shown that aerobic fitness in patients with CF is associated with nutritional status. Anaerobic performance in CF patients also has been reported to correlate with fat-free mass [134–137]. Independent of aerobic performance, nutritional status is associated with prognosis and survival in this population [138,139]. Exercise burns calories and acutely stimulates appetite, and in non-CF populations has been shown to improve nutritional status, both in those who are above [140] or below [141] their ideal body weight. Data are lacking, however, regarding the effects of exercise training on nutritional status in CF patients. One sample of 16 adult CF patients with advanced lung disease [93] showed a statistically significant improvement in body weight after a 3-week oxygen-assisted cycle ergometer program; however, some patients who were considered to be malnourished also received hyperalimentation (a possible confounding variable) during the training period, and no controls were used. Significant increases in weight gain have also been demonstrated after 6 months of variable weight training in 12 adolescents and adults with CF [121]. Two recent studies provide further reassurance that caloric expenditure during exercise need not be detrimental to patients with CF. Gulmans and colleagues [142] carried out a 3-month exercise (cycle ergometer) study with 10 patients age 12–17 years, all with $FEV_1 < 80\%$ predicted. After each of the five-times-weekly training sessions, patients drank a high-carbohydrate drink, in doses calculated to replace calories expended during the exercise. Subjects began the program with lower-than-normal levels of insulin-like growth factors I and II, yet experienced significant increases in these important anabolic hormones over the course of the study. In a study comparing aerobic and resistance training in hospitalized children with CF, Selvadurai and colleagues [97] found that the children who received resistance training had better weight gain at discharge and at 1-month follow-up than children in the aerobic training or control groups. All patients received nutritional supplementation as part of standard care.

The relationship between habitual physical activity and nutritional status has also been explored. Boucher and colleagues [112] evaluated the relationship between activity level as measured by the Habitual Activity Estimation Scale and nutritional status as measured by body mass percentile (BMP) in 36 CF children. These researchers showed that time spent active or somewhat active was significantly related to BMP in the patients with significant lung disease ($FEV_1 \leqslant 75\%$ predicted). As with many correlational studies, this finding does not answer the question of the direction of causality. Are better nourished patients better able to be active, and does activity help contribute to overall health, including nutrition? However, the correlation at least suggests that activity is not associated with worse nutritional status.

Increased bone mineral density

Decreased bone mineral density (BMD) and increased risk of fractures have been documented in children [143–145] and adults [146–148] with CF. The pathophysiology of bone disease is discussed in more detail in Chapter 18. In non-CF children, physical activity and weight-bearing exercise have been shown to be important for optimal bone health [149]. Correlational support can also be found for the relationship between physical activity and BMD in individuals with CF [150–152]. In a descriptive study of 68 CF adults [152], exercise capacity ($VO_{2\,peak}$) was shown to be a significant predictor of BMD. Similarly, in a controlled cross-sectional study of Australian children, adolescents and adults, an activity questionnaire score was the only significant predictor for lumbar spine BMD in the regression model for the adults with CF [151]. For all ages of CF patients, there were significant associations between BMD and activity questionnaire scores. Positive correlations were also shown between hours of physical activity and lumbar spine BMD in the children and adolescents with CF, and between the activity questionnaire score and physical/sedentary ratio and lumbar spine BMD in the adult CF subjects. Physical activity was found to be one of the most important predictors of change in BMD Z scores over a 1.5-year period in pediatric and adult patients with CF [150].

Although pharmacotherapy has been used for improving BMD in CF, not all medications are suitable for children [153]. Weight-bearing exercise and physical activity appear to represent safe and promising treatment options to promote bone health is this population. Randomized clinical trials are needed to assess the impact of exercise training programs on BMD in patients with CF and to help define treatment guidelines.

Enhanced health–related quality of life

Cystic fibrosis patients are faced with long-term, burdensome daily treatment routines as well as new health challenges that may affect a number of physical and psychosocial domains. Health-related quality-of-life (HRQoL) measures can provide a broad picture of this impact over time. Although some progress has been made over the past two decades in defining and measuring HRQoL, methodologically sound studies examining HRQoL and CF are limited. The crux of the problem is that there is no 'gold standard' against which to validate HRQoL measures. Both generic and disease-specific questionnaires have been applied to patients with CF and continued use of both in future studies will provide meaningful information. Instrument selection should be developmentally appropriate and based on specific study aims as well as sound psychometric properties.

Some researchers have found correlations between HRQoL and exercise performance [154,155], and a few studies have shown improvements in HRQoL after exercise training [97,107]. Our group [155] along with de Jong's [154] used generic measures to assess HRQoL. We administered the Quality of Well-Being (QWB) scale [156] to 44 patients (aged 7–36 years) with CF and found that QWB scores were significantly related to $VO_{2\,peak}$ values. Also, with 15 similarly aged patients (16–40 years), de Jong and colleagues [154] used the Sickness Impact Profile (SIP) [157] and showed that the overall SIP score had a significant correlation to maximal exercise capacity.

In the randomized three-group, in-hospital exercise study [67] (aerobic training, resistance training, control), only the children who received aerobic training showed significant improvements in quality of life as measured by the QWB scale. These changes correlated better with changes in $VO_{2\,peak}$ than changes in FEV_1. In another randomized, controlled trial [107], effects of an anaerobic training program were evaluated using a disease-specific measure of HRQoL, the Cystic Fibrosis Questionnaire (CFQ) [158]. CF children in the training group achieved significantly higher scores in the domain of physical functioning, while there was no change in the controls. The regression analysis revealed that peak power accounted for 41% of the variance in this domain. Finally, a 3-year, home-based trial [119] explored patients' feelings about being involved in regular exercise compared to not being involved. Of those who responded, from both the training and control groups, 88% gave positive responses, including feeling better about themselves with more energy and less chest congestion.

Physical training may help patients with CF improve their ability to perform normal daily activities. It is difficult to isolate the mechanism by which this enhancement occurs. Improvements in abilities to implement daily routines are most likely nested within other results of exercise, such as increased exercise tolerance, improved pulmonary function, and increased muscle strength. De Jong and colleagues [105] studied 10 adolescent CF patients who participated in a semi-supervised, 3-month home cycling program. Pretraining assessment was done during the 2 months prior to the start of the exercise program; a 1-month follow-up period in which the patients were instructed to continue exercising without supervision was also included in the study. At the end of the training period, patients had significantly less limitation in carrying out activities of daily living, with no significant differences between post-training and follow-up values, indicating maintenance of the benefits. What patients with CF can actually do from day to day makes a difference to how they live their lives, and because they are living longer, exploration of ways to improve the quality of this increased quantity of life is becoming increasingly important. Exercise seems to be a prime candidate for bringing about such improvements. The mechanism by which this can occur is not completely clear. Exercise may directly affect some of the physical components of HRQoL, and/or it may influence psychosocial functioning indirectly. More training studies are needed that include generic and CF-specific quality-of-life outcome measures so that a comprehensive picture of the full effects of the exercise interventions can be gained.

Improved psychosocial status

The effects of exercise on a few other psychosocial variables have also been assessed in children and adults with CF. In a 6-month home cycling program, Gulmans and colleagues [102] examined perceived competence using the Dutch version [159] of the Self-Perception Profile for Children [160] in 12 children with CF who served as their own controls. After training, they found significant improvements in total perceived competence scores as well as in subscale scores for feelings about physical appearance and general self-worth. After 8 weeks of a randomized, controlled trial of IMT (without an aerobic training component) [110] in 29 adults with CF, depression and anxiety scores measured by the Hospital Anxiety and Depression Questionnaire [161] were significantly lower in the high-intensity IMT (at 80% of maximal effort) intervention group than in the control group. These findings begin to highlight the multidimensional benefits of exercise on the complex and interrelated physical and psychosocial sequelae of CF. Other areas worthy of investigation might include health beliefs, social support, coping, self-image, self-management strategies, and attitudes as they relate to exercise.

Comparison to non-CF populations

Similar to its positive influences on people with CF, exercise has multiple benefits for healthy people too. With the right amount, intensity and type of exercise, healthy people can increase their cardiorespiratory fitness and strength and can also enhance their emotional well-being. However, the pulmonary benefits of exercise in CF patients are not evident in their non-CF counterparts.

EXERCISE PRESCRIPTION

See Table 25.17.

There is substantial evidence to support the use of exercise as a therapy for CF patients. Because of its numerous benefits, known or suggested, the most compelling being improved survival, exercise must be emphasized as part of comprehensive treatment for children and adults with CF. Several considerations influence how best to prescribe this treatment. First, it depends on the overall health of the patient, and second, it depends on the desired outcome. In patients with severe disease (those with resting FEV_1 below 50% predicted), an exercise test should be performed prior to the prescription of any exercise regimen [162]. The purpose of this test is primarily to ascertain whether, and at what intensity of exercise, the patient develops hypoxemia (see Chapter 25a for more on exercise testing). In patients who experience oxyhemoglobin desaturation, exercise can be prescribed at an intensity (measured most readily by heart rate, perhaps by the patient's own perception of exertion, or by direct pulsoximetry) below that at which SaO_2 fell during the test. Alternatively, especially for those with profound desaturation, exercise can be prescribed with supplemental oxygen. It is worth noting, perhaps, that recommendations to avoid desaturation are nearly universal, yet based more on emotion than data. We are aware of no data that brief periods of desaturation are detrimental, and in fact in our laboratory we never stop an exercise test because of hypoxemia. In addition, since maintaining weight is a concern

Table 25.17 Guidelines for exercise prescription in cystic fibrosis.

- *Pre-training exercise test*: required for those with $FEV_1 < 50\%$ predicted to identify patients who require oxygen supplementation
- *Selection of type of exercise*: encourage several different forms of exercise to avoid boredom and overuse injury
- 'FIT' (Frequency, Intensity, Time)
  Frequency: 3–5 times per week
  Intensity: 'pleasantly tired' (see text)
  – 4 to 7 on 10-point scale
  – 70–85% of patient's own maximum heart rate
  Time: goal = 30 minutes per session
  1st week: 10 minutes per session
  2nd week: 12 minutes per session
  3rd week: 14 minutes per session, etc.
- *Exercising in the heat*: drink more than thirst calls for; drink electrolyte-rich sports drinks [167]
- *Safety*: similar to exercise in non-CF populations

for people with CF, and since exercise burns calories, it is important to emphasize that mealtimes should not be compromised by exercise activity.

For most CF patients with mild to moderate airway obstruction, programs with traditional guidelines for frequency and duration of exercise, identical to those that are prescribed for healthy people, are appropriate. The intensity of aerobic exercise prescribed for non-CF populations to bring about improved exercise tolerance is usually expressed in terms of target heart rates (HR), equivalent to a given percentage (typically 70–85%) of the individual's age-predicted maximum heart rate. As many patients with CF are limited in exercise by their ventilatory capacity well before they are able to achieve age-predicted maximal heart rates, HR-based exercise prescriptions should be founded on the patient's own maximum heart rate as measured in a formal progressive exercise test, rather than healthy norms. Even this method is imperfect, as changes in fitness resulting from exercise training or deteriorations in clinical status could render target HRs derived from baseline graded exercise tests inaccurate.

Ideally, exercise intensity could be regulated on the basis of something other than heart rate. Perceived exertion is a prime candidate for determining the appropriate intensity of exercise for an exercise training program for patients with CF, for several reasons:

- Exercise that is unpleasantly intense is unlikely to be sustained, or repeated, and therefore unlikely to result in improved fitness.
- Exercise that is too easy is likely to be inadequate to improve fitness.
- Exercise that is in the 'in-between' range, specifically between 4 and 7 on a 10-point scale of perceived exertion, where 1 is 'very, very easy' and 10 is 'as difficult as it ever could be', is likely to be sustainable and adequate to result in improved fitness [163].

Both healthy children [164] and those with CF [165] are capable of learning to produce exercise at intensities graded on a 1 to 10 scale. Until CF centers become comfortable with teaching this formal system of regulating exercise programs based on perceived exertion scales, we have had success asking children with CF to strive for feeling 'pleasantly tired' during and following exercise sessions. We stress that exercise programs are useful only if they can be sustained in the long term, so if the patient is only tired he or she is working harder than necesary and won't want to repeat the exercise. Conversely, exercise that is just pleasant is unlikely to be accomplishing anything. Exercise does burn calories, so exercise sessions should not compete with mealtimes.

Other tricks to enhance long-term maintenance of an exercise treatment program include providing a program that is home-based, enjoyable, has a choice of activities, and includes a self-care component balanced with available support from healthcare professionals and family. Having an exercise partner is also useful. Moreover, patients and families must be educated about the benefits of exercise so that they understand the rationale for the treatment and are motivated to adhere to it. It has been shown that patient and parent knowledge of prescribed CF therapies can enhance compliance with treatments [166]. It certainly is encouraging that with exercise we (caregivers, patients and families) have a tool with the potential to make a big difference in patient comfort, satisfaction, ability to participate in normal essential and recreational activities, and perhaps even extend longevity. We should make every effort to use that tool.

REFERENCES

64. Cerny FJ, Pullano TP, Cropp GJ. Cardiorespiratory adaptations to exercise in cystic fibrosis. *Am Rev Respir Dis* 1982; **126**:217–220.

65. Cropp GJ, Pullano TP, Cerny FJ. Nathanson IT. Exercise tolerance and cardiorespiratory adjustments at peak work capacity in cystic fibrosis. *Am Rev Respir Dis* 1982; **126**:211–216.

66. Godfrey S, Mearns M. Pulmonary function and response to exercise in cystic fibrosis. *Arch Dis Child* 1971; **46**:144–151.

67. Marcotte JE, Grisdale RK, Levison H *et al.* Multiple factors limit exercise capacity in cystic fibrosis. *Pediatr Pulmonol* 1986; **2**:274–281.

68. Hortop J, Desmond KJ, Coates A. The mechanical effects of expiratory airflow limitation on cardiac performance in cystic fibrosis. *Am Rev Respir Dis* 1988; **137**:132–137.

69. Orenstein DM, Nixon PA. Exercise performance and breathing patterns in cystic fibrosis: male–female differences and influence of resting pulmonary function. *Pediatr Pulmonol* 1991; **10**:101–105.

70. Cerny FJ. Ventilatory control during exercise in children with cystic fibrosis. *Am Rev Respir Dis* 1981; **123**:195.

71. Henke KG, Orenstein DM. Oxygen desaturation during exercise in cystic fibrosis. *Am Rev Respir Dis* 1984; **129**:708–711.

72. Lebecque P, Lapierre JG, Lamarre A, Coates AL. Diffusion capacity and oxygen desaturation effects on exercise in patients with cystic fibrosis. Chest 1987; **91**: 693–697.

73. McKone EF, Barry SC, Fitzgerald MX, Gallagher CG. The role of supplemental oxygen during submaximal exercise in patients with cystic fibrosis. *Eur Respir J* 2002; **20**:134–142.

74. Nixon PA, Orenstein DM, Curtis SA *et al.* Oxygen supplementation during exercise in cystic fibrosis. *Am Rev Respir Dis* 1990; **142**:807–811.

75. Marcus CL, Bader D, Stabile MW *et al.* Supplemental oxygen and exercise performance in patients with cystic fibrosis with severe pulmonary disease. *Chest* 1992; **101**:52–57.

76. McKone EF, Barry SC, Fitzgerald MX, Gallagher CG. Role of arterial hypoxemia and pulmonary mechanics in exercise limitation in adults with cystic fibrosis. *J Appl Physiol* 2005 **99**:1012–1018.

77. Coates AL, Boyce P, Muller D *et al.* The role of nutritional status, airway obstruction, hypoxia, and abnormalities in serum lipid composition in limiting exercise tolerance in children with cystic fibrosis. *Acta Paediatr Scand* 1980; **69**:353–358.

78. Lands L, Heigenhauser GJ, Jones NL. Analysis of factors limiting maximal exercise performance in cystic fibrosis. *Clin Sci* 1992; **83**:391–397.

79. Lands L, Heigenhauser GJ, Jones NL. Respiratory and peripheral muscle function in cystic fibrosis. *Am Rev Respir Dis* 1993; **147**:865–869.

80. de Meer K, Gulmans VAM, van der Laag J. Peripheral muscle weakness and exercise capacity in children with cystic fibrosis. *Am J Respir Crit Care Med* 1999; **159**:748–754.

81. Alison JA, Regnis JA, Donnelly PM *et al.* End-expiratory lung volume during arm and leg exercise in normal subjects and patients with cystic fibrosis. *Am J Respir Crit Care Med* 1998; **158**:1450–1458.

82. Hortop J, Desmond KJ, Coates AL. The mechanical effects of expiratory airflow limitation on cardiac performance in cystic fibrosis. *Am Rev Respir Dis* 1988; **137**:132–137.

83. Orenstein DM, Henke KG, Costill DL *et al.* Exercise and heat stress in cystic fibrosis patients. *Ped Res* 1983; **17**:267–269.

84. Bar-Or O, Blimkie CJ, Hay JD *et al.* Voluntary dehydration and heat intolerance in cystic fibrosis. *Lancet* 1992; **339**:696–699.

85. Kriemler S, Wilk B, Schurer W *et al.* Preventing dehydration in children with cystic fibrosis who exercise in the heat. *Med Sci Sports Exerc* 1999; **31**:774–779.

86. Orenstein DM, Henke KG, Green CG. Heat acclimation in cystic fibrosis. *J Appl Physiol* 1984; **57**:408–412.

87. Alsuwaidan S, Li Wan Po A, Morrison G *et al.* Effect of exercise on the nasal transmucosal potential difference in patients with cystic fibrosis and normal subjects. *Thorax* 1994; **49**:1249–1250.

88. Hebestreit A, Kersting U, Basler B *et al.* Exercise inhibits epithelial sodium channels in patients with cystic fibrosis. *Am J Respir Crit Care Med* 2001; **164**:443–446.

89. Tarran R, Button B, Picher M *et al.* Normal and cystic fibrosis airway surface liquid homeostasis: the effects of phasic shear stress and viral infections. *J Biol Chem* 2005; **280**:35751–35759.

90. Pianosi P, LeBlanc J, Almudevar A. Peak oxygen uptake and mortality in children with cystic fibrosis. *Thorax* 2005; **60**:50–54.

91. Nixon PA, Orenstein DM, Kelsey SF, Doershuk CF. The prognostic value of exercise testing in patients with cystic fibrosis. *N Engl J Med* 1992; **327**:1785–1788.

92. Orenstein DM, Franklin BA, Doershuk CF *et al.* Exercise conditioning and cardiopulmonary fitness in cystic fibrosis: the effects of a three-month supervised running program. *Chest* 1981; **80**:392–398.

93. Heijerman HG, Bakker W, Sterk PJ, Dijkman JH. Oxygen-assisted exercise training in adult cystic fibrosis patients with pulmonary limitation to exercise. *Int J Rehabil Res* 1991; **14**:101–115.

94. Edlund LD, French RW, Herbst JJ *et al.* Effects of a swimming program on children with cystic fibrosis. *Am J Dis Child* 1986; **140**:80–83.

95. Stanghelle JK, Hjelnes N, Bangstad HJ, Michalsen H. Effect of daily short bouts of trampoline exercise during 8 weeks on the pulmonary function and the maximal oxygen uptake of children with cystic fibrosis. *Int J Sports Med* 1988; **9**(Suppl 1):32–36.

96. Blau H, Mussaffi-Georgy H, Fink G *et al.* Effects of an intensive 4-week summer camp on cystic fibrosis. *Chest* 2002; **121**:1117–1122.

97. Selvadurai H, Blimkie C, Meyers N *et al.* Randomized controlled study of in-hospital exercise training programs in children with cystic fibrosis. *Pediatr Pulmonol* 2002; **33**:194–200.

98. Turchetta A, Salerno T, Lucidi V *et al.* Usefulness of a program of hospital-supervised physical training in patients with cystic fibrosis. *Pediatr Pulmonol* 2004; **38**:115–118.

99. Prasad SA, Cerny FJ. Factors that influence adherence to exercise and their effectiveness: application to cystic fibrosis. *Pediatr Pulmonol* 2002; **34**:66–72.

100. Barak A, Wexler ID, Efrati O *et al.* Trampoline use as physiotherapy for cystic fibrosis patients. *Pediatr Pulmonol* 2005; **39**:70–73.

101. American Academy of Pediatrics Committee on Injury and Poison Prevention and Committee on Sports Medicine and Fitness. Policy Statement: Trampolines at home, school, and recreational centers. *Pediatrics* 1999;**103**:1053–1056. (Reaffirmed: *Pediatrics* 2006;**117**:1846–1847.)

102. Gulmans VA, de Meer K, Brackel HJ *et al.* Outpatient exercise training in children with cystic fibrosis: physiological effects, perceived competence, and acceptability. *Pediatr Pulmonol* 1999; **28**:39–46.

103. Orenstein DM, Hovell MF, Mulvihill M *et al.* Strength vs aerobic training in children with cystic fibrosis: a randomized controlled trial. *Chest* 2004; **126**:1204–1214.

104. Salh W, Bilton D, Dodd M, Webb AK. Effect of exercise and physiotherapy in aiding sputum expectoration in adults with cystic fibrosis. *Thorax* 1989; **44**:1006–1008.

105. de Jong W, Grevink RG, Roorda RJ *et al.* Effect of a home exercise training program in patients with cystic fibrosis. *Chest* 1994; **105**:463–468.

106. Moorcroft AJ, Dodd ME, Morris J, Webb AK. Individualised unsupervised exercise training in adults with cystic fibrosis: a 1-year randomized controlled trial. *Thorax* 2004; **59**:1074–1080.

107. Klijn PHC, Oudshoorn A, van der Ent CK *et al.* Effects of anaerobic training in children with cystic fibrosis. *Chest* 2004; **125**:1299–1305.

108. Keens TG, Krastins IR, Wannamaker EM *et al.* Ventilatory muscle endurance training in normal subjects and patients with cystic fibrosis. *Am Rev Respir Dis* 1977; **116**:853–860.

109. Sawyer EH, Clanton TL. Improved pulmonary function and exercise tolerance with inspiratory muscle conditioning in children with cystic fibrosis. *Chest* 1993; **104**:1490–149.

110. Enright S, Chatham K, Ionescu AA *et al.* Inspiratory muscle training improves lung function and exercise capacity in adults with cystic fibrosis. *Chest* 2004; **126**:405–411.

111. Orenstein DM, Nixon PA, Washburn RA, Kelsey SF. Measuring physical activity in children with cystic fibrosis: comparison of four methods. *Pediatr Exerc Sci* 1993; **5**:125–133.

112. Boucher GP, Lands LC, Hay JA, Hornby L. Activity levels and the relationship to lung function and nutritional status in children with cystic fibrosis. *Am J Phys Med Rehabil* 1997; **76**:311–315.

113. Nixon PA, Orenstein DM, Kelsey SF. Habitual physical activity in children and adolescents with cystic fibrosis. *Med Sci Sports Exerc* 2001; **33**:30–35.

114. Schneiderman-Walker J, Wilkes DL, Strug L *et al.* Sex differences in habitual physical activity and lung function decline in children with cystic fibrosis. *J Pediatr* 2005; **147**:321–326.

115. Selvadurai H, Blimkie C, Cooper PJ *et al.* Gender differences in habitual activity in children with cystic fibrosis. *Arch Dis Child* 2004; **89**:928–933.

116. Zach M, Purrer B, Oberwaldner B. Effect of swimming on forced expiration and sputum clearance in cystic fibrosis. *Lancet* 1981; **2**:1201–1203.

117. Zach M, Oberwaldner B, Hausler F. Cystic fibrosis: physical exercise versus chest physiotherapy. *Arch Dis Child* 1982; **57**:587–589.

118. Cerny FJ. Relative effects of bronchial drainage and exercise for in-hospital care of patients with cystic fibrosis. *Phys Ther* 1989; **69**:633–639.

119. Schneiderman-Walker J, Pollock SL, Corey M *et al.* A randomized controlled trial of a 3-year home exercise program in cystic fibrosis. *J Pediatr* 2000; **136**:304–310.

120. Hodson M, McKenzie S, Harms HK *et al.* Dornase alpha in the treatment of cystic fibrosis in Europe: a report from the Epidemiologic Registry of cystic fibrosis. *Pediatr Pulmonol* 2003; **36**:427–432.

121. Strauss GD, Osher A, Wang CI *et al.* Variable weight training in cystic fibrosis. *Chest* 1987; **92**:273–276.

122. Bilton D, Dodd ME, Abbot JV, Webb AK. The benefits of exercise combined with physiotherapy in the treatment of adults with cystic fibrosis. *Respir Med* 1992; **86**:507–511.

123. Chatham K, Ionescu AA, Nixon LS, Shale DJ. A short-term comparison of two methods of sputum expectoration in cystic fibrosis. *Eur Respir J* 2004; **23**:436–439.

124. O'Neill PA, Dodds M, Phillips B *et al.* Regular exercise and reduction of breathlessness in patients with cystic fibrosis. *Br J Dis Chest* 1987; **81**:62–69.

125. de Jong W, van Aalderen WMC, Kraan J *et al.* Inspiratory muscle training in patients with cystic fibrosis. *Respir Med* 2001; **95**:31–36.

126. Asher MI, Pardy RL, Coates AL *et al.* The effects of inspiratory muscle training in patients with cystic fibrosis. *Am Rev Respir Dis* 1982; **126**:855–859.

127. Cornacchia M, Zenorini A, Perobelli S *et al.* Prevalence of urinary incontinence in women with cystic fibrosis. *BJU Int* 2001; **88**:44–48.

128. Orr A, McVean RJ, Webb AK, Dodd ME. Questionnaire survey of urinary incontinence in women with cystic fibrosis. *Br Med J* 2001; **322**:1521.

129. White D, Stiller K, Rooney F. The prevalence and severity of symptoms of incontinence in adult cystic fibrosis patients. *Physiother Theor Pract* 2000; **16**:35–42.

130. McVean RJ, Orr A, Webb AK *et al.* Treatment of urinary incontinence in cystic fibrosis. *J Cyst Fibros* 2003; **2**:171–176.

131. Gulmans VA, de Meer K, Brackel HJ, Helders PJ. Maximal work capacity in relation to nutritional status in children with cystic fibrosis. *Eur Respir J* 1997; **10**:2014–2017.

132. Marcotte JE, Canny GJ, Grisdale R *et al.* Effects of nutritional status on exercise performance in advanced cystic fibrosis. *Chest* 1986; **90**:375–379.

133. Klijn PHC, van der Net J, Kimpen JL *et al.* Longitudinal determinants of peak aerobic performance in children with cystic fibrosis. *Chest* 2003; **124**:2215–2219.

134. Boas SR, Danduran MJ, McColley SA. Energy metabolism during anaerobic exercise in children with cystic fibrosis and asthma. *Med Sci Sports Exerc* 1999; **31**:1242–1249.

135. Boas SR, Joswiak ML, Nixon PA *et al.* Factors limiting anaerobic performance in adolescent males with cystic fibrosis. *Med Sci Sports Exerc* 1996; **28**:291–298.

136. Klijn PHC, Terheggen-Lagro SW, van der Ent CK *et al.* Anaerobic exercise in pediatric cystic fibrosis. *Pediatr Pulmonol* 2003; **36**:223–229.

137. Shah AR, Gozal D, Keens TG. Determinants of aerobic and anaerobic exercise performance in cystic fibrosis. *Am J Respir Crit Care Med* 1998; **157**:1145–1150.

138. Corey M, McLaughlin FJ, Williams M, Levison H. A comparison of survival, growth, and pulmonary function in patients with cystic fibrosis in Boston and Toronto. *J Clin Epidemiol* 1988; **41**:583–591.

139. Kraemer R, Rudeberg A, Hadorn B *et al.* Relative underweight in cystic fibrosis and its prognostic value. *Acta Paediatr Scand* 1978; **67**:33–37.

140. Stefanick ML. Exercise and weight control. *Exerc Sport Sci Rev* 1993; **21**:363–396.

141. Pupim LB, Flakoll PJ, Levenhagen DK, Ikizler TA. Exercise augments the acute anabolic effects of intradialytic parenteral nutrition in chronic hemodialysis patients. *Am J Physiol Endocrinol Metab* 2004; **286**:E589–E597.

142. Gulmans V, van der Laag J, Wattimena D *et al.* Insulin-like growth factors and leucine kinetics during exercise training in children with cystic fibrosis. *J Pediatr Gastroenterol Nutr* 2001; **32**:76–81.

143. Bhudhikanok GS, Lim J, Marcus R *et al.* Correlates of osteopenia in patients with cystic fibrosis. *Pediatrics* 1996; **97**:103–111.

144. Gibbens DT, Gilsanz V, Boechat MI *et al.* Osteoporosis in cystic fibrosis. *J Pediatr* 1988; **113**:295–300.

145. Henderson RC, Madsen CD. Bone density in children and adolescents with cystic fibrosis. *J Pediatr* 1996; **128**:28–34.

146. Bachrach LK, Loutit CW, Moss RB. Osteopenia in adults with cystic fibrosis. *Am J Med* 1994; **96**:27–34.

147. Grey AB, Ames RW, Matthews RD, Reid IR. Bone mineral density and body composition in adult patients with cystic fibrosis. *Thorax* 1993; **48**:589–593.

148. Baroncelli GI, De Luca F, Magazzu G *et al.* Bone demineralization in cystic fibrosis: evidence of imbalance between bone formation and degradation. *Pediatr Res* 1997; **41**:397–403.

149. Slemenda CW, Miller JZ, Hui SL *et al.* Role of physical activity in the development of skeletal mass in children. *J Bone Miner Res* 1991; **6**:1227–1233.

150. Bhudhikanok GS, Wang MC, Marcus R *et al.* Bone acquisition and loss in children and adults with cystic fibrosis: a longitudinal study. *J Pediatr* 1998; **133**:18–27.

151. Buntain HM, Greer RM, Schluter PJ *et al.* Bone mineral density in Australian children, adolescents and adults with cystic fibrosis: a controlled cross-sectional study. *Thorax* 2004; **59**:149–155.

152. Frangolias DD, Pare PD, Kendler DL *et al.* Role of exercise and nutrition status on bone mineral density in cystic fibrosis. *J Cyst Fibros* 2003; **2**:161–162.

153. Hecker TM, Aris RM. Management of osteoporosis in adults with cystic fibrosis. *Drugs* 2004; **64**:133–147.

154. de Jong W, Kaptein AA, van der Schans CP *et al.* Quality of life in patients with cystic fibrosis. *Pediatr Pulmonol* 1997; **23**:95–100.

155. Orenstein DM, Nixon PA, Ross EA, Kaplan RM. The quality of well-being in cystic fibrosis. *Chest* 1989; **95**:344–347.

156. Kaplan RM, Bush JW, Berry CC. The reliability, stability, and generalizability of a health status index. *ASA Proc Social Statist Sect* 1978; 704–709.

157. Bergner M, Bobbitt RA, Carter WB, Gilson BS. The Sickness Impact Profile: development and final revision of a health status measure. *Med Care* 1981; **19**:787–805.

158. Quittner AL, Sweeny S, Watrous M *et al.* Translation and linguistic validation for a disease-specific quality of life measure for cystic fibrosis. *J Pediatr Psychol* 2000; **25**:403–414.

159. Straathof MAE, Treffers PDA. *Translation of the Perceived Competence Scale for Adolescents.* Oegstgeest, University Centre for Psychiatry in Children and Youth Curriculum, 1988, p20.

160. Harter S. *Manual for the Self Perception Profile for Children.* Denver, CO, University of Denver, 1985, p87.

161. Zigmond AS, Snaith RD. The hospital anxiety and depression scale. *Acta Psychiatr Scand* 1983; **67**:361–370.

162. Rogers D, Prasad SA, Doull I. Exercise testing in children with cystic fibrosis. *J R Soc Med* 2003; **96**:23–29.

163. Robertson RJ, Goss FL, Boer NF *et al.* OMNI Scale perceived exertion at ventilatory breakpoint in children: normalized response. *Med Sci Sports Exerc* 2001; **33**:1946–1952.

164. Robertson RJ, Goss FL, Bell JA *et al.* Self-regulated cycling using the Children's OMNI Scale of Perceived Exertion. *Med Sci Sports Exerc* 2002; **34**:1168–1175.

165. Higgins LW, Robertson RJ, Kelsey SF *et al.* Validity of self-regulated exercise intensity in children with cystic fibrosis using the OMNI scale of perceived exertion. *Pediatr Pulmonol* 2004; **24**(Suppl 27):311.

166. Ievers CE, Brown RT, Drotar D *et al.* Knowledge of physician prescriptions and adherence to treatment among children with cystic fibrosis and their mothers. *J Dev Behav Pediatr* 1999; **20**:335–343.

167. Kriemler S, Wilk B, Schurer W *et al.* Preventing dehydration in children with cystic fibrosis who exercise in the heat. *Med Sci Sports Exerc* 1999; **31**:774–779.

168. Nixon PA. Role of exercise in the evaluation and management of pulmonary disease in children and youth. *Med Sci Sports Exerc* 1996; **28**:414–420.

26

Clinical outcome measures to assess new treatments for CF lung disease

JANE C. DAVIES AND ERIC W. F. W. ALTON
On behalf of the UK CF Gene Therapy Consortium

INTRODUCTION

The design of clinical trials in cystic fibrosis (CF) is becoming more complex and challenging. Whereas, several decades ago, patients deteriorated rapidly and had a short life expectancy, predicted survival of today's children is around 40 years and many live relatively healthy lives, albeit at the cost of time spent on multiple treatments. This means that certain previously appropriate outcome measures (rate of decline in lung function, mortality) are now inappropriate for the vast majority of trials, and that more sophisticated surrogate measures have to be designed and applied.

Which of these surrogates are chosen will depend in part on the intervention being applied, on the severity of the group being studied, and the time period available over which change can be measured. Certain assays are precluded in young children because of their reduced ability to cooperate or because the assays are invasive (bronchoscopy) or may pose a risk (radiation exposure), whereas others may be more sensitive in this age group. Outcome measures range right through from the most basic, molecular assays, to standard clinical measurements. Whereas the relationship between the latter and disease status might be clear, many of these assays are noisy (both within and between patients), leading to the requirement for higher patient numbers and a longer study duration. In contrast, it is hoped that some of the more basic assays, at the molecular and cellular levels, may be more sensitive to change, but for many of them the relationship with the clinical picture is poorly understood.

In this chapter, we outline the assays available for human studies, beginning with the most basic molecular and leading on to clinical measurements, illustrating with examples from trials where appropriate, although these examples are

by no means exhaustive. Finally, we mention briefly some potential assays that are, as yet, insufficiently developed to be useful clinically but which may hold promise for the future. As the majority of clinical trials are aimed at the lung, disease of which is the main cause of both morbidity and mortality in CF patients, we have concentrated on this organ. Assays involved in trials for example of liver, pancreas or bone disease will be mentioned, where relevant, in the chapters on these organs.

MOLECULAR ASSAYS

CFTR mRNA

Reverse transcriptase polymerase chain reaction (RT-PCR) based methods of quantifying mRNA are now readily available, for example using TaqMan technology [1]. mRNA levels are unlikely to be relevant for the majority of interventions, but have been used in studies of CFTR gene transfer, where, unlike detection of transgene DNA, detection confirms cell transfection and gene transcription. However, endogenous levels of CFTR in airway epithelial cells are very low [2] and detection of levels adequate for clinical benefit pose technical challenges related to assay sensitivity. Further, the assay is most commonly performed on either airway brushings or, less commonly, biopsies, both of which contain abundant cells of non-epithelial origin, including leukocytes and connective tissue cells. Gene transfer to such cells could lead to false positive results, making either enrichment of the sample for epithelial cells, or some method to render the assay epithelium-specific, highly desirable. Finally, the complex post-translational biogenesis of CFTR means that mRNA levels may not necessarily correlate with CFTR protein levels or function and so this assay should not be relied upon in isolation.

CFTR protein

Antibody-based assays to confirm the presence of CFTR protein, such as immunoblotting, immunoprecipitation and immunohistochemical staining, have been employed in the context of both preclinical drug development [3] and clinical trials including gene transfer agents, trafficking drugs [4,5] and aminoglycosides [6]. One of the major advantages of immunohistochemistry is the ability to visualize the localization of the protein on the apical surface and to co-stain for proteins such as cytokeratin, confirming epithelial expression. However, a paucity of specific, high-affinity anti-CFTR antibodies make these techniques and quantification difficult.

ASSAYS DIRECTLY MEASURING THE ION CHANNEL FUNCTIONS OF CFTR

Ex-vivo

HALIDE EFFLUX ASSAYS

In these assays, cells are loaded with halide-sensitive fluorescent dyes [7]. Intracellular fluorescence is quenched by the addition of high concentrations of halides, most commonly iodide, loaded into the cells by hypotonic shock. Subsequently, the response to drugs such as forskolin and isoproterenol, which stimulate CFTR channels to open, can be measured by the rate of increase in fluorescent signal. These assays thus directly measure CFTR ion transport function. However, although the techniques work well on cultured cells, they are technically much more challenging with non-adherent cells, such as those removed from the nose or lower airway by brushing, particularly in the presence of ciliary beating. The challenges are even greater with biopsy tissues where success has not been reported to date.

SHORT-CIRCUIT CURRENT MEASUREMENTS

Tissue pieces such as rectal biopsies have been successfully mounted in Using chambers and used to measure short circuit current (I_{sc}) [8]. In contrast to the potential difference measurements discussed below, which can be heavily influenced by a single corrected cell, changes in I_{sc} are more reflective of the numbers of cells corrected and may therefore be of more clinical relevance. However, the technique is technically challenging and time-consuming and has not been reported as possible with the necessarily small airway biopsies which might be of more interest in the context of most clinical lung trials.

In-vivo

POTENTIAL DIFFERENCE MEASUREMENTS

The passage of charged ions across an intact epithelial surface generates a measurable millivoltage potential difference (PD) across the epithelium, whereby the outside of the cell is negatively charged compared to the inside. For many years, measurement of nasal PD has been available as an aid to diagnosis in difficult cases: CF subjects have more negative baseline PD and a greater response to the sodium channel blocking agent, amiloride (both reflecting increased sodium absorption), with reduced or absent responses to attempts to induce chloride secretion [9]. The latter is conventionally done in two ways. First the outside of the cell is exposed to a low or zero chloride solution, which results in secretion of Cl$^-$ through any open channels. Second, CFTR channels are activated by the cAMP-agonist, isoproterenol, inducing further Cl$^-$ secretion. The combined response to these two interventions is widely accepted as providing the best distinguishing test between CF and non-CF epithelia. However, the limited data available suggest that patients with so-called 'mild' mutations, which appear to protect from severe lung disease, may have nasal PD measurements similar to more classic CF patients [10,11], raising questions over its clinical applicability and how much change should be enough. Nasal PD has been used as an outcome measure in clinical trials of CFTR gene therapy (reviewed in [12]), aminoglycosides in patients with class I (stop) mutations [6], and many novel pharmacological agents including those aimed at restoring CFTR function [13,14], stimulating chloride secretion [15,16] and blocking sodium absorption [17,18]. Recently, the technique has been adapted for use in the lower airway via a flexible bronchoscope, with similar CF/non-CF differences being observed as far out as seventh- or eighth-generation airways [19]. However, this technique does require a general anesthetic and is therefore less suitable for studies requiring repeated measurements. Rectal PD is also abnormal in CF patients and could be a useful surrogate in the context of a systemically applied drug; one small study showed changes in the rectal PD of children after systemic administration of N-acetyl-cysteine [20]; the chemical chaperone, TMAO (trimethylamine N-oxide), also resulted in changes in rectal PD when administered to CF mice [21].

SWEAT ELECTROLYTES

The sweat test is used as the gold standard diagnostic test for patients suspected of having CF. Abnormally raised levels of both sodium and chloride are detected, resulting in increased conductivity of the sweat, an alternative assay being used by some laboratories. Although limited in applicability to systemically applied drugs acting on the basic defect and predicted to influence ion channel activity, the test has the advantage of being easy, quick, relatively cheap and reproducible. It has been used as an outcome assay in clinical trials of 4-phenylbutyrate [22], CPX (8-cyclopentyl-1,3-dipropylxanthine) [14] and essential fatty acid supplements [23].

ASSAYS RELATED TO OTHER FUNCTIONS OF CFTR

Pseudomonas aeruginosa adherence

Pseudomonas aeruginosa adheres in greater numbers to the surface of epithelial cells of CF origin than to wild-type, related at least in part to increased abundance of one of its receptors, asialoGM1 [24]. Whether or not this is relevant in disease pathogenesis remains uncertain; if it is an important mechanism, it is likely only so in the early stages of acquisition, because in the end-stage lung the bacteria appear not to be in contact with the cell surface, but are present as microcolonies in the airway lumen [25]. However, we have previously shown that ex-vivo CFTR gene transfer reduced the numbers of *Pseudomonas* adhering to respiratory epithelial cells [26], and subsequently we explored this as an assay in a clinical trial of CFTR gene therapy [27]. The noise of the assay and the small numbers of samples studied led to no statistically significant differences being observed after treatment, although there was a trend towards a reduction in the active group. We have used the same assay, on nasal brushings, in a study exploring the mechanisms of macrolide antibiotics, where we concluded that the beneficial clinical effects were unlikely to relate to changes in bacterial adherence [28]. Macrolides have been shown to reduce adherence to buccal cells, however, although only after the bacteria were pre-incubated with the drug [29]. Thus, despite the uncertainty over pathogenic significance, this assay, or perhaps similar assays with other bacteria, could form a useful surrogate end-point.

Glutathione levels

There is some evidence in support of a role for CFTR in transport of glutathione, which is pivotal in the antioxidant response in the lungs. Attempts to boost levels with exogenous supplements have been explored [30], and recently a clinical trial of oral *N*-acetyl-cysteine was reported to lead to significant increases in both local and systemic glutathione levels which were associated with decreases in inflammatory markers including sputum cells and cytokines [31].

MUCOCILIARY CLEARANCE

The low-volume hypothesis of CF disease pathogenesis relates to reduced Cl^- secretion and hyperabsorption of Na^+ ions leading to osmotic dehydration and reduced volume of the airway surface liquid (ASL) [32]. This hypothesis is discussed in more detail in Chapter 4. The volume of ASL is maintained in normal health to facilitate optimal mucociliary clearance (MCC), one of the pivotal innate defence mechanisms of the lung. Impairment of this mechanism in CF is thought to lead to mucus stasis, with failure to clear inhaled particles, such as pollutants, viruses and bacteria, allowing infection and inflammation to ensue. Moreover, MCC may be further impaired by these secondary processes, as demonstrated by the abnormalities in lung MCC reported in patients with bronchiectasis of other etiologies [33]. The difficulties inherent in the techniques to measure lung MCC have resulted in a paucity of information about this process in early CF disease, so it is uncertain how much of the impaired MCC seen in older children and adults relates to the primary ion transport defect and how much to secondary damage. Studies in the nose have produced conflicting results, with some groups reporting preserved MCC in the absence of mucosal disease [34]. However, the fully ciliated epithelial surfaces of the nose may not reflect mechanisms in the sparsely ciliated distal small airways, where CF disease is thought to begin. For certain interventions, a full understanding of the relative contributions of primary and secondary mechanisms may be unimportant. For example, lung MCC has been improved by rhDNase [35], mannitol [36] and hypertonic saline (HS) [37]. Improvements in trials of ion channel-related drugs, amiloride and uridine triphosphate (UTP) [38,39], lend some support to the importance of the primary defect, although some recent clinical data suggest that – in the case of sodium channel blockers at least – these drugs may be ineffective [40]. The technique requires specialized skills and equipment and is time-consuming for the subject (most protocols requiring a scan at 24 hours), but involves relatively modest radiation levels and is thus likely to be considered ethically acceptable as a clinical trial end-point. Nasal MCC has also been assessed with the saccharin clearance technique in trials of saline and amiloride [41], gene therapy [27] and topically applied corticosteroid agents [42].

INFECTION

Quantification of bacterial load

Patients with CF are commonly chronically infected with a narrow range of organisms, in particular *P. aeruginosa*, *Staphylococcus aureus*, *Haemophilus influenzae* and less frequently *Burkholderia cepacia*. All of these organisms can infect the airways in huge numbers (up to 10^9 CFU/mL), often coexisting with other pathogens. Many conventional treatments are aimed at reducing the numbers of (or less frequently, eradicating) these pathogens, including continuous nebulized anti-pseudomonal antibiotics, systemic antibiotics and lung clearance techniques. Accurate quantification of bacterial load can be performed by serial dilution and culture allowing a reduction in infective load to be assessed as a treatment outcome. One caveat to this is that different numbers, and even varying pathogens, have been obtained from different areas of individual patients' lungs, making this measurement prone to noise. Despite this, significant reductions in CFU have been reported after intravenous antibiotics [43,44] and inhaled tobramycin [45].

Time to next positive culture

Once *P. aeruginosa* infection becomes chronic, it is rarely eradicated. However, studies have shown convincingly that, in the early stages of acquisition, the organism can be successfully cleared, sometimes for several years; so conventional management guidelines now include eradication regimens. The time until the second positive culture could therefore be used to assess additional interventions, and was employed in a clinical trial of anti-pseudomonal immunoglobulin (IgY) gargles [46]. Although the study was not performed in a randomized, controlled fashion, which limits interpretation of the findings, there appeared to be an increase in the time to next positive culture and a reduced proportion of patients experiencing a recurrence in the treated group. One potential downside to the use of this as a surrogate outcome is that most initial isolates of *P. aeruginosa* are experienced in childhood. Many clinical trials exclude children for safety and ethical reasons in the early stages, and those that do recruit them may experience problems with reliability of culture methods; many children cannot repeatedly and reproducibly expectorate sputum, and other methods of assessing airway infection, such as cough swabs or cough plates, may be limited in sensitivity or specificity. These caveats may also apply to adults with milder lung disease, and induction of sputum may be helpful in both groups.

Number of antibiotic courses or pulmonary exacerbations (including time to next exacerbation)

It should be relatively easy to collect information on the number of courses of antibiotics (both intravenous and oral) prescribed to patients over a given time period and look for a reduction in a trial intervention group. However, patients are prescribed antibiotics for a variety of reasons, including a true exacerbation, an impending exacerbation prior to an event such as an examination or a holiday, or even on occasions prophylactically for such events. It is unlikely that prescribing habits are consistent between centers or even clinicians within a center. This outcome measure will therefore be noisy and possibly prone to yielding false negative results. This has probably contributed to attempts by many investigators to quantify, instead, numbers of pulmonary exacerbations, which are usually defined by the presence of a set number of features in a list of symptoms and signs, including increasing cough, sputum production,

breathlessness, fever, weight loss, etc. Such 'protocol-defined' exacerbations have been shown to be reduced by rhDNase [47,48], azithromycin [49], inhaled tobramycin [45] and hypertonic saline [37]. However, in many cases, patients will be treated before becoming unwell enough to fulfil all these criteria, meaning that numbers experiencing an exacerbation may be smaller than initially anticipated, leading to underpowering. As a reflection of an outcome measure that would be of direct clinical relevance to the patient, however, it may be one of the best to choose.

INFLAMMATION

Sputum

CF sputum contains high levels of inflammatory cells, pro-inflammatory cytokines and proteolytic enzymes. Certain of these appear to correlate with other measures of pulmonary severity, such as spirometry, although whether they are causative of the pulmonary damage is less clear. There is also a well-described deficiency of anti-inflammatory cytokines, such as IL-10, and a relative deficiency of antiproteases. Cytokines can be measured reproducibly, even in sputum from young children [50], and several of these have been shown to be reduced by treatment with conventional intravenous antibiotics [51,52]. Studies of other agents including the cystenyl leukotriene receptor antagonist, montelukast, have also reported decreased levels of IL-8, eosinophil cationic protein (ECP) and myeloperoxidase (MPO), and increased IL-10 [53].

The effects of antibiotics and anti-inflammatory agents may not be surprising; more so perhaps are the results from studies of other agents. For example, decreased levels of sputum IL-8 were observed after a single dose of liposome-mediated CFTR gene therapy [27] and after the first, but not subsequent, doses of AAV-mediated CFTR gene therapy [54]. Nebulized heparin, which in addition to its anticoagulant properties thins sputum and is anti-inflammatory, was shown to decrease sputum cytokines after a 1-week period, over which time a change in spirometric parameters could not be detected [55]. This may either suggest that these measures are more sensitive to detect change than conventional lung function, or may simply reflect the fact that changes in lung function occur only later. RhDNase has also been shown to reduce levels of sputum neutrophil elastase over a 12-week time period, an effect that was significant despite the very small patient numbers included ($n = 15$) [56]. Although investigators have looked specifically, there has to date not been a consistent significant effect produced by either inhaled corticosteroid agents or the macrolide group of antibiotics. Encouragingly, results suggest that spontaneously expectorated sputum and samples obtained by induction methods based on nebulization of HS are not significantly different with respect to inflammatory markers, and this technique has been confirmed as safe in CF children, the group in which it is most likely to be required [57].

One limitation of the interpretation of these data is the varied, and often unvalidated, methodologies used in the processing stage. For example, mucolytics such as dithiothreitol (DTT) are often used. This substance, by cleaving disulphide bonds, affects the levels of many proteins [58]. A second concern relates to the lack of standardization with regard to the nature and concentration of protease inhibitors used. There is an urgent need for these methodological issues to be addressed, specifically for CF sputum, before results from different studies can be compared.

Bronchoalveolar lavage

Bronchoalveolar lavage (BAL) fluid is often considered the gold standard of airway sampling techniques. Similar patterns of inflammation have been described as in sputum, with an excess of proinflammatory cytokines, cells and proteases and relative deficiencies of anti-inflammatory cytokines and antiproteases, although there is a paucity of data comparing inflammation in the two types of sample. One recent study looking at inflammatory cell counts described a better correlation between sputum and the first aliquot of BAL (believed to sample bronchi and bronchioles) than pooled BAL (thought also to contain fluid from the alveolar region) [59]. The recently published BEAT study assessing anti-inflammatory effects of rhDNase described significant reductions in total neutrophil count in BAL from young children with early-stage disease after 18 months of treatment [60]. BAL, whether bronchoscopic or non-bronchoscopic, is however invasive and not easily repeated in a short time period. Side-effects such as fever have been reported, although this is rarely significant in our experience. Further limitations include the large and unknown dilution factor (markers for dilution are of limited use and recent guidelines suggest they are not helpful [61]), and the fact that the technique samples only a small part of the airway, which may be problematic in a disease known to be inhomogeneous [62].

Exhaled breath and breath condensate

Both exhaled breath and exhaled breath condensate (EBC) are easy and non-invasive to obtain, and can be used reproducibly even in young children as long as attention is paid to methodological detail. Much interest has focused on the observation that levels of exhaled nitric oxide (NO) are reduced in CF. Given the described anti-inflammatory and anti-infective properties of the compound, some consider that this may play an important primary role in the pathophysiology of the disease, a hypothesis supported by the finding of low levels of NO mRNA in relatively undamaged airways. An alternative view is that NO production is itself adversely affected by inflammation and that the low levels observed are secondary to CF lung disease [63]. Levels of NO are extremely low in primary ciliary dyskinesia (PCD),

a disease with a generally much better outlook than CF [64]. A recent clinical trial of orally administered L-arginine, an NO donor, used eNO as an outcome measure, reporting a sustained increase in NO production, which was not mirrored by any significant effect on lung function [65]. Condensate can be collected by asking the subject to exhale during tidal breathing into a cold tube. The resulting fluid contains a small (but variable and undetermined) volume of airway lining fluid. The pH of this fluid has been shown to be abnormally low in CF [66] and other inflammatory airway diseases [67], potentially providing an 'inflammamometer' to assess interventions. Attempts to measure other substances in CF have met with variable success, possibly related in part to methodological issues [68–70].

Blood

Serum inflammatory markers, including inflammatory cells and cytokines, acute phase reactants such as C-reactive protein (CRP) and immunoglobulin (Ig)G, have been used both as efficacy [71–73] and safety [74] outcome measures in CF clinical trials. In many studies in both these contexts they have proved useful, but although there are not the same methodological issues as exist with the airway sampling techniques described above, serum would probably be considered by most to be an adjunct to, rather than a substitute for, such direct measures.

Urine

Several groups have reported increased levels of tissue degradation products such as desmosine and isodesmosine in the urine of patients with chronic lung diseases including CF [75,76]. However, variable and rapidly fluctuating levels have been observed, which might limit applicability in the clinical trial context.

OTHER SPUTUM PROPERTIES

The main purpose of airway clearance techniques such as conventional chest physiotherapy is to clear the airways of the copious amounts of thick, viscous sputum produced in CF. If such sputum can be expectorated instead of swallowed, its weight or volume may provide a measure of success for the intervention applied, as has been the case in studies of physiotherapy [77]. In addition to simply measuring the amount of sputum produced, ratios of wet and dry weights [78], which could provide a measure of mucus hydration, could be particularly useful in trials of therapies aimed at restoring ion transport or providing an osmotic stimulus to rehydrate the airway surface. Sputum color is potentially a much more subjective outcome, but was used with success in a recent study of inhaled glutathione [79]. The mucus produced by CF patients is abnormally viscous and possesses reduced elasticity, both properties that can be measured in the laboratory. Significant effects on these properties have been reported in several clinical studies, including of physiotherapy [80], rhDNase [81] and azithromycin [82]. One of the reasons for this greatly increased viscosity of CF sputum is the extremely high levels of DNA, released by large numbers of necrotic inflammatory neutrophils. Measurement of DNA content could therefore provide a surrogate measure of airway inflammation and a direct measure of the efficacy of the enzymatic properties of rhDNase.

IMAGING

Chest radiographs

Chest x-rays (CXRs) have been employed as end-points in clinical trials, both independently [51] and as part of global disease scores [83]. The use of a variety of different scoring systems and the relative lack of sensitivity compared with other imaging modalities are significant limitations. However, the low levels of radiation employed and their low cost renders them useful, particularly perhaps in the context of safety studies, if required on a repeated basis.

Computerized tomography (CT)

The use of CT in cystic fibrosis has been the subject of several recent reviews and editorials [84–86]. Changes at different disease stages have been described (e.g. air trapping and bronchial wall thickening), some of which can be reversible, rendering them useful markers of clinical success in interventional trials [87,88]. Several scoring systems, of varying complexity, have been devised and reported, with some authors strongly favoring composite scores with, for example, spirometric indices [89]. Alternatively, CT could provide a sensitive safety measure, and has been employed in some studies of novel therapies to this end. The levels of radiation involved need of course to be borne in mind, although they may be significantly reduced by some of the more modern scanning equipment and by using protocols with limited cuts.

Other imaging

Ventilation/perfusion scanning, although not widely employed in CF, was reported as being useful in a clinical study examining the effects of both intravenous antibiotics and the sodium channel blocker, amiloride [90]. Magnetic resonance imaging (MRI) was until recently widely regarded as lacking sufficient resolution for imaging the lung; however, the additional use of hyperpolarized helium 3 (HHe) has recently been shown to improve sensitivity to such an extent that significant differences were visible after bronchodilator treatment in a small clinical trial [91].

PHYSIOLOGY

Spirometry/plethysmography

Many studies have used lung function parameters, in particular FEV_1, as primary end-points, a logical choice based on the correlation of this measurement with prognosis and life expectancy. The reproducibility, repeatability and limitations of spirometric measurements are well established; and for interventions predicted to produce an increase in lung function over a relatively short period (e.g. antibiotics, rhDNase or other mucus-clearing agents), inclusion of this end-point is likely appropriate and, based on a widespread familiarity with the technique, may facilitate interpretation of the findings. However, many novel therapeutic agents are more likely to lead to a slowing in the rate of decline, or at best stabilization, of lung function. Patients receiving medical care in specialist CF centers are now declining very slowly over time (between 1% and 3% of baseline FEV_1 annually), making it extremely difficult to power such studies to detect significant changes in response to treatment. (Davis and co-workers have recently calculated that up to 500 patients would need to be studied for a 2-year period [92].) However, even in studies unlikely to achieve this sort of power, spirometric assessment is likely to be included, perhaps more appropriately as a secondary end-point. Further, inclusion can help to exclude the possibility that a novel agent is detrimental, for example by triggering bronchospasm, and as such it has been included in many phase I safety studies. The requirement for specialized equipment, trained staff and the time-consuming nature of plethysmography probably explains the fact that these measurements are infrequently used in the context of clinical trials. Gas transfer measurements (KCO and TLCO) have been used in some, for example to assess potential toxicity of gene transfer agents [27].

Infant pulmonary function tests

Before the last decade, lung function measurements relied entirely on the cooperation of the individual, and were therefore rarely attempted on children under 6 or 7 years of age. More recently, equipment has been developed to allow reproducible measurements to be made in both infants [93] and pre-school children [94]. They are discussed in more detail in Chapter 23a.

Multiple–breath washout and lung clearance indices

Changes in spirometry reflect mainly the larger airways, and are insensitive to loss of distal airway function. Spirometric measurements that are believed to represent small airway function (such as $FEF_{25–75}$) have very high coefficients of variability, and are likely also measuring more proximal airways. In addition, it is well recognized that patients can maintain normal spirometry in the presence of significant airway inflammation and damage, and so there has been a search for tests representing both more distal airways and possessing greater sensitivity. Lung clearance tests measure the time taken to completely wash out an inert gas, this period increasing with increased inhomogeneity of ventilation, airway plugging, gas trapping etc. The earliest of these used 100% oxygen to wash out nitrogen, and newer techniques have been developed using gases such as sulphur hexafluoride (SF_6). The test can be reliably performed in even very young children, and is, at this stage of disease, significantly more sensitive to airway damage than FEV_1 [95]. It may be less useful in the later stages of disease, where it also becomes more cumbersome to administer, because of long wash-in and wash-out periods.

Exercise testing

A variety of tests ranging from simple timed walks and shuttle tests through to more complex techniques to monitor cardiopulmonary status and maximum oxygen consumption (VO_{2max}) have been used in CF patients in clinical trials. In general, such tests have proved, at best, complimentary to others such as spirometry, with little evidence of any increased sensitivity to change, although one might argue for their inclusion into study protocols on the basis of relevance to the patient themselves.

Weight gain

Although this chapter has focused on pulmonary outcome measures, one adverse effect of pulmonary disease, increased work of breathing and infection/inflammation, is poor weight gain. Thus, changes in body weight or mass index (BMI) could reflect an improvement in pulmonary status.

QUALITY-OF-LIFE AND SYMPTOM SCORES

Quality of life is becoming increasingly accepted as a relevant outcome measure of trials in many varying diseases. There are now CF- and age-specific questionnaires that have been well tested and validated [96,97] and translated into several languages, some of which have been used in CF clinical trials.

SUMMARY AND FUTURE DIRECTIONS

The focus of this chapter has been on assays that have been used in clinical trials, although as described, many of these could benefit from further refinement and standardization. Others are currently under investigation, either at the preclinical or early clinical stage, by several groups including the UK CF Gene Therapy Consortium (www.cfgenetherapy. org.uk). These may not yet have not yet been validated and published in the clinical trial context, but include measurements of airway surface liquid height, which is reduced in the CF murine nose, on human biopsy material; detection methods for novel protein markers, including the use of SELDI-TOF and proteomics; microarray technology to compare gene expression profiles in response to clinical change; molecular analysis of bacterial pathogens; and further non-invasive measures of inflammation such as assessment of bronchial blood flow, which is raised in asthma. The search continues for the ideal assay(s) that are (a) able to be accurately measured, (b) reproducible with little 'noise', (c) sensitive to change, (d) relatively non-interventional and can be performed, if required, on a repeated basis, and (e) known in some way to relate to clinical status. Determining which of these qualities are possessed by either individual assays or composite scores based on several assays will require the rigorous testing and comparison of multiple measures in the context of clinical trials. The development of multicenter groups following the same protocols for sample collection and analysis will allow the resulting data to be as widely applicable as possible and for progress in this field to be advanced most quickly.

REFERENCES

1. Rose AC, Goddard CA, Colledge WH *et al.* Optimisation of real-time quantitative RT-PCR for the evaluation of non-viral mediated gene transfer to the airways. *Gene Ther* 2002; **9**:1312–1320.

2. Engelhardt JF, Zepeda M, Cohn JA *et al.* Expression of the cystic fibrosis gene in adult human lung. *J Clin Invest* 1994; **93**:737–749.

3. Lim M, McKenzie K, Floyd AD *et al.* Modulation of deltaF508 cystic fibrosis transmembrane regulator trafficking and function with 4-phenylbutyrate and flavonoids. *Am J Respir Cell Mol Biol* 2004; **31**:351–357

4. Dormer RL, Derand R, McNeilly CM *et al.* Correction of delF508-CFTR activity with benzo(c)quinolizinium compounds through facilitation of its processing in cystic fibrosis airway cells. *J Cell Sci* 2001; **114**:4073–4081.

5. Dormer RL, Harris CM, Clark Z *et al.* Sildenafil (Viagra) corrects DeltaF508-CFTR location in nasal epithelial cells from patients with cystic fibrosis. *Thorax* 2005; **60**:55–59.

6. Wilschanski M, Yahav Y, Yaacov Y *et al.* Gentamicin-induced correction of CFTR function in patients with cystic fibrosis and CFTR stop mutations. *N Engl J Med* 2003; **349**:1433–1441.

7. Munkonge F, Alton EW, Andersson C *et al.* Measurement of halide efflux from cultured and primary airway epithelial cells using fluorescence indicators. *J Cyst Fibros* 2004; **3**(Suppl 2):171–176.

8. Veeze HJ, Sinaasappel M, Bijman J *et al.* Ion transport abnormalities in rectal suction biopsies from children with cystic fibrosis. *Gastroenterology* 1991; **101**:398–403.

9. Middleton PG, Geddes DM, Alton EW. Protocols for in-vivo measurement of the ion transport defects in cystic fibrosis nasal epithelium. *Eur Respir J* 1994; **7**:2050–2056.

10. Walker LC, Venglarik CJ, Aubin G *et al.* Relationship between airway ion transport and a mild pulmonary disease mutation in CFTR. *Am J Respir Crit Care Med* 1997; **155**:1684–1689.

11. Pradal U, Castellani C, Delmarco A, Mastella G. Nasal potential difference in congenital bilateral absence of the vas deferens. *Am J Respir Crit Care Med* 1998; **158**:896–901.

12. Griesenbach U, Geddes DM, Alton EW. Advances in cystic fibrosis gene therapy. *Curr Opin Pulm Med* 2004; **10**:542–546.

13. Zeitlin PL, Diener-West M, Rubenstein RC *et al.* Evidence of CFTR function in cystic fibrosis after systemic administration of 4-phenylbutyrate. *Mol Ther* 2002; **6**:119–126.

14. McCarty NA, Standaert TA, Teresi M *et al.* A phase I randomized, multicenter trial of CPX in adult subjects with mild cystic fibrosis. *Pediatr Pulmonol* 2002; **33**:90–98.

15. Zeitlin PL, Boyle MP, Guggino WB, Molina L. A phase I trial of intranasal Moli1901 for cystic fibrosis. *Chest* 2004; **125**:143–149.

16. Knowles MR, Clarke LL, Boucher RC. Activation by extracellular nucleotides of chloride secretion in the airway epithelia of patients with cystic fibrosis. *N Engl J Med* 1991; **325**:533–538.

17. Middleton PG, Geddes DM, Alton EW. Effect of amiloride and saline on nasal mucociliary clearance and potential difference in cystic fibrosis and normal subjects. *Thorax* 1993; **48**:812–816.

18. Rodgers HC, Knox AJ. The effect of topical benzamil and amiloride on nasal potential difference in cystic fibrosis. *Eur Respir J* 1999; **14**:693–696.

19. Davies JC, Davies M, McShane D *et al.* Potential difference measurements in the lower airway of children with and without cystic fibrosis. *Am J Respir Crit Care Med* 2005; **171**:1015–1019.

20. Ballke EH, Wiersbitzky S, Mahner B, Konig A. The effect of N-acetyl-cysteine (Mucosolvin) on the transmural potential difference of the mucosa in children. *Padiatr Grenzgeb* 1992; **31**(2):97–101.

21. Fischer H, Fukuda N, Barbry P *et al.* Partial restoration of defective chloride conductance in DeltaF508 CF mice by trimethylamine oxide. *Am J Physiol Lung Cell Mol Physiol* 2001; **281**:L52–L57.

22. Rubenstein RC, Zeitlin PL. A pilot clinical trial of oral sodium 4-phenylbutyrate (Buphenyl) in deltaF508-homozygous cystic fibrosis patients: partial restoration of nasal epithelial CFTR function. *Am J Respir Crit Care Med* 1998; **157**:484–490.

23. Dodge JA, Custance JM, Goodchild MC *et al.* Paradoxical effects of essential fatty acid supplementation on lipid profiles and sweat electrolytes in cystic fibrosis. *Br J Nutr* 1990; **63**:259–271.

24. Saiman L, Prince A. *Pseudomonas aeruginosa* pili bind to asialoGM1 which is increased on the surface of cystic fibrosis epithelial cells. *J Clin Invest* 1993; **92**:1875–1880.

25. Hoiby N. Understanding bacterial biofilms in patients with cystic fibrosis: current and innovative approaches to potential therapies. *J Cyst Fibros* 2002; **1**:249–254.

26. Davies JC, Stern M, Dewar A *et al.* CFTR gene transfer reduces the binding of *Pseudomonas aeruginosa* to cystic fibrosis respiratory epithelium. *Am J Respir Cell Mol Biol* 1997; **16**:657–663.

27. Alton EW, Stern M, Farley R *et al.* Cationic lipid-mediated CFTR gene transfer to the lungs and nose of patients with cystic fibrosis: a double-blind placebo-controlled trial. *Lancet* 1999; **353**:947–954.

28. Equi AC, Davies JC, Painter H *et al.* Exploring the mechanisms of macrolides in cystic fibrosis. *Respir Med* 2006; **100**:687–697.

29. Baumann U, Fischer JJ, Gudowius P *et al.* Buccal adherence of *Pseudomonas aeruginosa* in patients with cystic fibrosis under long-term therapy with azithromycin. *Infection* 2001; **29**:7–11.

30. Grey V, Mohammed SR, Smountas AA *et al.* Improved glutathione status in young adult patients with cystic fibrosis supplemented with whey protein. *J Cyst Fibros* 2003; **2**:195–198.

31. Abstracts of the 19th Annual North American Cystic Fibrosis Conference, Baltimore, MD, 20–23 October 2005. *Pediatr Pulmonol Suppl* 2005; **28**:263.

32. Matsui H, Grubb BR, Tarran R *et al.* Evidence for periciliary liquid layer depletion, not abnormal ion composition, in the pathogenesis of cystic fibrosis airways disease. *Cell* 1998; **95**:1005–1015.

33. Currie DC, Pavia D, Agnew JE *et al.* Impaired tracheobronchial clearance in bronchiectasis. *Thorax* 1987; **42**:126–130.

34. McShane D, Davies JC, Wodehouse T *et al.* Normal nasal mucociliary clearance in CF children: evidence against a CFTR-related defect. *Eur Respir J* 2004; **24**:95–100.

35. Robinson M, Hemming AL, Moriarty C *et al.* Effect of a short course of rhDNase on cough and mucociliary clearance in patients with cystic fibrosis. *Pediatr Pulmonol* 2000; **30**:16–24.

36. Robinson M, Daviskas E, Eberl S *et al.* The effect of inhaled mannitol on bronchial mucus clearance in cystic fibrosis patients. a pilot study. *Eur Respir J* 1999; **14**:678–685.

37. Donaldson SH, Bennett WD, Zeman KL *et al.* Mucus clearance and lung function in cystic fibrosis with hypertonic saline. *N Engl J Med* 2006; **354**:241–250.

38. Olivier KN, Bennett WD, Hohneker K *et al.* Acute safety and effects on mucociliary clearance of aerosolized uridine 5′-triphosphate±amiloride in normal human adults. *Am J Respir Crit Care Med* 1996; **154**:217–223.

39. Bennett WD, Olivier KN, Zeman KL *et al.* Effect of uridine 5′-triphosphate plus amiloride on mucociliary clearance in adult cystic fibrosis. *Am J Respir Crit Care Med* 1996; **153**(6 Pt 1):1796–1801.

40. App EM, King M, Helfesrieder R *et al.* Acute and long-term amiloride inhalation in cystic fibrosis lung disease: a rational approach to cystic fibrosis therapy. *Am Rev Respir Dis* 1990; **141**:605–612.

41. Middleton PG, Geddes DM, Alton EW. Effect of amiloride and saline on nasal mucociliary clearance and potential difference in cystic fibrosis and normal subjects. *Thorax* 1993; **48**:812–816.

42. Graham SM, Scott SN, Launspach J, Zabner J. The effects of fluticasone propionate on nasal epithelial potential difference. *Am J Rhinol* 2002; **16**:145–149.

43. Smith AL, Redding G, Doershuk C *et al.* Sputum changes associated with therapy for endobronchial exacerbation in cystic fibrosis. *J Pediatr* 1988; **112**:547–554.

44. Ordonez CL, Henig NR, Mayer-Hamblett N *et al.* Inflammatory and microbiologic markers in induced sputum after intravenous antibiotics in cystic fibrosis. *Am J Respir Crit Care Med* 2003; **168**:1471–1475.

45. Ramsey BW, Pepe MS, Quan JM *et al.* for the Cystic Fibrosis Inhaled Tobramycin Study Group. Intermittent administration of inhaled tobramycin in patients with cystic fibrosis. *N Engl J Med* 1999; **340**:23–30.

46. Kollberg H, Carlander D, Olesen H *et al.* Oral administration of specific yolk antibodies (IgY) may prevent *Pseudomonas aeruginosa* infections in patients with cystic fibrosis: a phase I feasibility study. *Pediatr Pulmonol* 2003; **35**:433–440.

47. Fuchs HJ, Borowitz DS, Christiansen DH *et al.* for the Pulmozyme Study Group. Effect of aerosolized recombinant human DNase on exacerbations of respiratory symptoms and on pulmonary function in patients with cystic fibrosis. *N Engl J Med* 1994; **331**:637–642.

48. Quan JM, Tiddens HA, Sy JP *et al.* for the Pulmozyme Early Intervention Trial Study Group. A two-year randomized, placebo-controlled trial of dornase alfa in young patients with cystic fibrosis with mild lung function abnormalities. *J Pediatr* 2001; **139**:813–820.

49. Saiman L, Marshall BC, Mayer-Hamblett N *et al.* for the Macrolide Study Group. Azithromycin in patients with cystic fibrosis chronically infected with *Pseudomonas aeruginosa*: a randomized controlled trial. *J Am Med Assoc* 2003; **290**:1749–1756.

50. Ordonez CL, Kartashov AI, Wohl ME. Variability of markers of inflammation and infection in induced sputum in children with cystic fibrosis. *J Pediatr* 2004; **145**:689–692.

51. Colombo C, Costantini D, Rocchi A *et al.* Cytokine levels in sputum of cystic fibrosis patients before and after antibiotic therapy. *Pediatr Pulmonol* 2005; **40**:15–21.

52. Ordonez CL, Henig NR, Mayer-Hamblett N *et al.* Inflammatory and microbiologic markers in induced sputum after intravenous antibiotics in cystic fibrosis. *Am J Respir Crit Care Med* 2003; **168**:1471–1475.

53. Stelmach I, Korzeniewska A, Stelmach W *et al.* Effects of montelukast treatment on clinical and inflammatory variables in patients with cystic fibrosis. *Ann Allergy Asthma Immunol* 2005; **95**:372–380.

54. Moss RB, Rodman D, Spencer LT *et al.* Repeated adeno-associated virus serotype 2 aerosol-mediated cystic fibrosis transmembrane regulator gene transfer to the lungs of patients with cystic fibrosis: a multicenter, double-blind, placebo-controlled trial. *Chest* 2004; **125**:509–521.

55. Ledson M, Gallagher M, Hart CA, Walshaw M. Nebulized heparin in *Burkholderia cepacia* colonized adult cystic fibrosis patients. *Eur Respir J* 2001; **17**:36–38.

56. Costello CM, O'Connor CM, Finlay GA *et al.* Effect of nebulised recombinant DNase on neutrophil elastase load in cystic fibrosis. *Thorax* 1996; **51**:619–623.

57. Suri R, Marshall LJ, Wallis C *et al.* Safety and use of sputum induction in children with cystic fibrosis. *Pediatr Pulmonol* 2003; **35**:309–313.

58. Woolhouse IS, Bayley DL, Stockley RA. Effect of sputum processing with dithiothreitol on the detection of inflammatory mediators in chronic bronchitis and bronchiectasis. *Thorax* 2002; **57**:667–671.

59. Reinhardt N, Chen CI, Loppow D *et al.* Cellular profiles of induced sputum in children with stable cystic fibrosis: comparison with BAL. *Eur Respir J* 2003; **22**:497–502.

60. Paul K, Rietschel E, Ballmann M *et al.* for the Bronchoalveolar Lavage for the Evaluation of Antiinflammatory Treatment Study Group. Effect of treatment with dornase alpha on airway inflammation in patients with cystic fibrosis. *Am J Respir Crit Care Med* 2004; **169**:719–725.

61. Haslam PL, Baughman RP. Report of ERS Task Force: guidelines for measurement of acellular components and standardization of BAL. *Eur Respir J* 1999; **14**:245–248.

62. Gutierrez JP, Grimwood K, Armstrong DS *et al.* Interlobar differences in bronchoalveolar lavage fluid from children with cystic fibrosis. *Eur Respir J* 2001; **17**:281–286.

63. de Winter-de Groot KM, van der Ent CK. Nitric oxide in cystic fibrosis. *J Cyst Fibros* 2005; **4**(Suppl 2):25–29.

64. Van Gravesande KS, Omran H. Primary ciliary dyskinesia: clinical presentation, diagnosis and genetics. *Ann Med* 2005; **37**:439–449.

65. Grasemann H, Grasemann C, Kurtz F *et al.* Oral L-arginine supplementation in cystic fibrosis patients: a placebo-controlled study. *Eur Respir J* 2005; **25**:62–68.

66. Tate S, MacGregor G, Davis M *et al.* Airways in cystic fibrosis are acidified: detection by exhaled breath condensate. *Thorax* 2002; **57**:926–929.

67. Carpagnano GE, Barnes PJ, Francis J *et al.* Breath condensate pH in children with cystic fibrosis and asthma: a new noninvasive marker of airway inflammation? *Chest* 2004; **125**:2005–2010.

68. Ojoo JC, Mulrennan SA, Kastelik JA *et al.* Exhaled breath condensate pH and exhaled nitric oxide in allergic asthma and in cystic fibrosis. *Thorax* 2005; **60**:22–26.

69. Carpagnano GE, Barnes PJ, Geddes DM *et al.* Increased leukotriene B4 and interleukin-6 in exhaled breath condensate in cystic fibrosis. *Am J Respir Crit Care Med* 2003; **167**:1109–1112.

70. Rosias PP, Dompeling E, Hendriks HJ *et al.* Exhaled breath condensate in children: pearls and pitfalls. *Pediatr Allergy Immunol* 2004; **15**:4–19.

71. Greally P, Hussain MJ, Vergani D, Price JF. Interleukin-1 alpha, soluble interleukin-2 receptor, and IgG concentrations in cystic fibrosis treated with prednisolone. *Arch Dis Child* 1994; **71**:35–39.

72. Schmitt-Grohe S, Eickmeier O, Schubert R *et al.* Anti-inflammatory effects of montelukast in mild cystic fibrosis. *Ann Allergy Asthma Immunol* 2002; **89**:599–605.

73. Konstan MW, Davis PB, Wagener JS *et al.* Compacted DNA nanoparticles administered to the nasal mucosa of cystic fibrosis subjects are safe and demonstrate partial to complete cystic fibrosis transmembrane regulator reconstitution. *Hum Gene Ther* 2004; **15**:1255–1269.

74. Davies JC, Alton EW. Airway gene therapy. *Adv Genet* 2005; **54**:291–314.

75. Starcher B, Green M, Scott M. Measurement of urinary desmosine as an indicator of acute pulmonary disease. *Respiration* 1995; **62**:252–257.

76. Bode DC, Pagani ED, Cumiskey WR *et al.* Comparison of urinary desmosine excretion in patients with chronic obstructive pulmonary disease or cystic fibrosis. *Pulm Pharmacol Ther* 2000; **13**:175–180.

77. Warwick WJ, Wielinski CL, Hansen LG. Comparison of expectorated sputum after manual chest physical therapy and high-frequency chest compression. *Biomed Instrum Technol* 2004; **38**:470–475.

78. Braggion C, Cappelletti LM, Cornacchia M *et al.* Short-term effects of three chest physiotherapy regimens in patients hospitalized for pulmonary exacerbations of cystic fibrosis. a cross-over randomized study. *Pediatr Pulmonol* 1995; **19**:16–22.

79. Bishop C, Hudson VM, Hilton SC, Wilde C. A pilot study of the effect of inhaled buffered reduced glutathione on the clinical status of patients with cystic fibrosis. *Chest* 2005; **127**:308–317.

80. App EM, Kieselmann R, Reinhardt D *et al.* Sputum rheology changes in cystic fibrosis lung disease following two different types of physiotherapy: flutter vs autogenic drainage. *Chest* 1998; **114**:171–177.

81. Griese M, App EM, Duroux A *et al.* Recombinant human DNase (rhDNase) influences phospholipid composition, surface activity, rheology and consecutively clearance indices of cystic fibrosis sputum. *Pulm Pharmacol Ther* 1997; **10**:21–27.

82. Baumann U, King M, App EM *et al.* Long term azithromycin therapy in cystic fibrosis patients: a study on drug levels and sputum properties. *Can Respir J* 2004; **11**:151–155.

83. Conway SP, Etherington C, Peckham DG, Whitehead A. A pilot study of zafirlukast as an anti-inflammatory agent in the treatment of adults with cystic fibrosis. *J Cyst Fibros* 2003; **2**:25–28.

84. Robinson TE. High-resolution CT scanning: potential outcome measure. *Curr Opin Pulm Med* 2004; **10**:537–541.

85. Brody AS. Scoring systems for CT in cystic fibrosis: who cares? *Radiology* 2004; **231**:296–298.

86. Sibtain NA, Padley SP. HRCT in small and large airways diseases. *Eur Radiol* 2004; **14**(Suppl 4):L31–L43.

87. Nasr SZ, Kuhns LR, Brown RW *et al.* Use of computerized tomography and chest x-rays in evaluating efficacy of aerosolized recombinant human DNase in cystic fibrosis patients younger than age 5 years: a preliminary study. *Pediatr Pulmonol* 2001; **31**:377–382.

88. Robinson TE, Goris ML, Zhu HJ *et al.* Dornase alfa reduces air trapping in children with mild cystic fibrosis lung disease: a quantitative analysis. Chest 2005; **128**:2327–2335.

89. Robinson TE, Leung AN, Northway WH *et al.* Composite spirometric-computed tomography outcome measure in early cystic fibrosis lung disease. *Am J Respir Crit Care Med* 2003; **168**:588–593.

90. Lagerstrand L, Hjelte L, Jorulf H. Pulmonary gas exchange in cystic fibrosis: a basal status and the effect of i.v. antibiotics and inhaled amiloride. *Eur Respir J* 1999; **14**:686–692.

91. Mentore K, Froh DK, de Lange EE *et al.* Hyperpolarized HHe 3 MRI of the lung in cystic fibrosis: assessment at baseline and after bronchodilator and airway clearance treatment. *Acad Radiol* 2005; **12**:1423–1429.

92. Davis PB. The decline and fall of pulmonary function in cystic fibrosis: new models, new lessons. *J Pediatr* 1997; **131**:789–790.

93. Stocks J, Godfrey S, Beardsmore C *et al.* for the ERS/ATS Task Force on Standards for Infant Respiratory Function Testing. Plethysmographic measurements of lung volume and airway resistance. *Eur Respir J* 2001; **17**:302–312.

94. Aurora P, Stocks J, Oliver C *et al.* for the London Cystic Fibrosis Collaboration. Quality control for spirometry in preschool children with and without lung disease. *Am J Respir Crit Care Med* 2004; **169**:1152–1159.

95. Aurora P, Bush A, Gustafsson P *et al.* for the London Cystic Fibrosis Collaboration. Multiple-breath washout as a marker of lung disease in preschool children with cystic fibrosis. *Am J Respir Crit Care Med* 2005; **171**:249–256.

96. Quittner AL, Buu A, Messer MA *et al.* Development and validation of the Cystic Fibrosis Questionnaire in the United States: a health-related quality-of-life measure for cystic fibrosis. *Chest* 2005; **128**:2347–2354.

97. Klijn PH, van Stel HF, Quittner AL *et al.* Validation of the Dutch cystic fibrosis questionnaire (CFQ) in adolescents and adults. *J Cyst Fibros* 2004; **3**:29–36.

PART **6**

MULTIDISCIPLINARY CARE

27   Cystic fibrosis center care   387
     Penny Agent and Susan Madge
28   Nursing care   399
     Susan Madge and Christine Hockings
29   Physiotherapy   407
     Craig Lapin, Anne Lapin and Jennifer A. Pryor
30   Nutritional aspects   421
     Sue Wolfe and Sarah Collins
31   Psychological aspects of cystic fibrosis   431
     Alistair J. A. Duff and Helen Oxley
32   Palliative care in cystic fibrosis   441
     Calherine E. Urch and Margaret E. Hodson

27

Cystic fibrosis center care

PENNY AGENT AND SUSAN MADGE

WHAT IS CYSTIC FIBROSIS CENTER CARE?

Cystic fibrosis (CF) is a multisystem disease that requires a holistic approach to care by a multidisciplinary team of CF specialist health professionals. The aims of CF care are to:

- prevent chronic infection;
- minimize deterioration;
- maintain independence;
- optimize quality of life;
- maximize life expectancy [1].

It is generally agreed that specialist CF centers provide the optimum approach to CF care, but shared care may be set up between the specialist CF center and a shared-care CF clinic, usually in pediatric services [2–6]. Whether a local shared-care CF clinic or specialist CF center provides CF care, regular communication is essential to ensure that individual care is optimized.

Specialist CF centers usually manage at least 50 adult or pediatric patients, with CF being the predominant specialist area of expertise of the staff who carry out research as well as clinical activity in this area. These major centers provide full care not only for all local patients with CF, but also for patients living further away who are prepared to travel [7]. Local shared-care CF clinics tend to manage fewer than 50 patients, so it is the specialist CF centers that link up with local hospitals to plan the provision of shared care (discussed later in this chapter). The functions of major specialist CF center care are summarized in Table 27.1.

In the last few years, standards of care have been produced by national and international committees [1,8] and are widely recognized and acknowledged as a benchmark for services. These standards provide an overview of complete CF care from staffing recommendations, services provided, and recommendations for all inpatient and outpatient clinical services.

THE MULTIDISCIPLINARY TEAM

Cystic fibrosis is complex and multisystem, so it is inevitable that care should be provided by a team of specialists. Multidisciplinary care is consequently generally accepted as essential in the management of long-term chronic diseases such as CF [9]. Staffing requirements of specialists involved in CF multidisciplinary teams have been developed by working parties in the UK, Europe and North America, but no two CF teams will be the same. Most teams will adapt the recommendations to meet the local needs of their patient group such as patient ages and patient numbers. Unfortunately most CF teams around the world are subject to a limitation of resources and therefore have to work within imposed boundaries. This section will briefly describe the roles of professionals in an *ideal* CF multidisciplinary team as other chapters discuss the roles in more detail (except the roles of the pharmacist, occupational therapist and social worker, whose roles will be discussed in more detail here).

The 'primary' CF multidisciplinary team

THE MEDICAL TEAM

The consultant leading a CF multidisciplinary team (usually the Clinical Director or Lead Clinician for CF) must have a major commitment to CF care. It is useful for the consultant to have a senior colleague with knowledge of CF who is able to take over during periods of absence. A junior team will support the consultant, with one or more specialist registrars fulfilling a more dedicated role such as CF

Table 27.1 Functions of a specialist CF center.

Local patients	Provide treatment and advice
	Regular clinic/hospital assessment
	Specialist multidisciplinary team (MDT)
24-hour access	Advice available from staff experienced in CF
	Patients made aware of other CF centers if travelling, out of area and require advice
Annual assessments	For all patients attending the center (unless performed at local CF center)
	Full discussion of results with consultant physician
	Specialist multidisciplinary team
Specialized procedures	Expertise in procedures common to CF:
	– insertion of totally implantable venous access devices
	– gastrostomy
	– non-invasive ventilation
	– bronchial artery embolization
	– fiberoptic bronchoscopy
	Diagnostic and specialized lab services
Neonatal screening	Coordination of CF neonatal screening program (if available)
	Coordination of care at diagnosis, usually by CF nurse specialist
Home care	Organization of home intravenous antibiotic therapy
	Regular assessment/follow-up
	Provision of home compressor/nebulizer equipment service
	Provision of home enteral feeding equipment
Transition	Coordination of a regular transition clinic by specialist CF MDT members
Shared care	Provision of specialist advice and consultation for patients who have:
	– infections >2 weeks unresponsive to conventional treatment
	– deteriorating pulmonary function unresponsive to conventional treatment
	– pneumothorax
	– significant hemoptysis (>20 mL)
	– allergic bronchopulmonary aspergillosis
	– persistent atelectasis
	– respiratory/cardiac failure
	– distal intestinal obstructive syndrome
	– failure to thrive/severe unexplained weight loss
	– new-onset glucose intolerance
	– vasculitis
	– CF arthropathy
	– pregnancy
	– serious psychological problems
Transplantation	Assessment of possible suitable patients prior to referral to transplant center (may not be at same center)
	Optimization of full medical treatment
Education	Comprehensive education and advice regarding all aspects of CF care from specialist multidisciplinary team
	Attendance of specialist staff at national and international CF meetings
Research	Database information, local and national
	Clinical trials
	Audit
	Reporting and presentation of experiences for peer review/discussion

Fellow. These doctors will manage the day-to-day needs of the patients and work closely with the specialist nurses [1].

THE SPECIALIST NURSE

The nurse provides a clinical, educational and support service for patients and their families. Living with a life-limiting disease impacts on all areas of life as balancing treatment regimens with school, employment, social and family life can become overwhelming. Parents of young children find living with CF intrusive, isolating and time-consuming. Adolescents and young adults share those feelings as well as finding it differentiating at a time when they want to fit in with a peer group. Through the provision of both practical and emotional support and advice, the nurse can help to minimize adherence issues, maintain independence and improve quality of life. The role of the specialist nurse is discussed further in Chapter 28.

THE SPECIALIST PHYSIOTHERAPIST

Assisting, teaching and supporting patients and their families in chest physiotherapy techniques is the primary role of the physiotherapist. There are, however, many other areas that the physiotherapist has become involved in, such as osteoporosis and posture management, urinary incontinence, exercise programs, pregnancy care (pre- and postnatally), nebulizer therapy and non-invasive ventilation. To find out more about the role of the physiotherapist, refer to Chapter 29.

THE SPECIALIST DIETITIAN

As with the physiotherapist, the role of the dietitian has developed over the years. At the same time as ensuring good nutritional status in patients, dietitians have found themselves offering advice and support in a number of different areas. The expanded role of the dietitian includes feeding problems, CF-related diabetes, distal intestinal obstructive syndrome (DIOS) and other gastrointestinal problems, enteral feeding and pregnancy. Good communication and referral within the team is essential as the role of the dietitian often overlaps with other team members such as the nurse, physiotherapist and psychologist. See Chapter 30 for further discussion of this role.

THE SPECIALIST PSYCHOLOGIST

The provision of psychological services to the management of CF is essential. Psychologists work closely with the CF team supporting colleagues in psychological aspects of care and providing advice and opinion on particular issues. Areas generally covered by a psychologist include adherence to treatment, quality of life, management of procedural distress, management of feeding and behavioral difficulties, learning to live with a secondary diagnosis, and end-of-life issues. Typically the psychologist identifies patient needs through referral from team members or during psychological assessment carried out at annual review. Problems are identified and then in discussion with the team the most appropriate methods of resolving these problems are planned.

The psychological service is often run in parallel with the CF service, with the psychologist working as a gatekeeper for the onward referral of patients to mental health services. Further discussion of the role of the psychologist can be found in Chapter 31.

THE PHARMACIST

The specialist pharmacist has started to play a major part in the multidisciplinary team in the care of both inpatients and outpatients. The overall role of the pharmacist in the CF team is to ensure safe, appropriate and cost-effective drug treatment, and this falls into three main areas: advice to the team, advice to the patient, and managing the availability of medicines.

Pharmacists offer advice to the team around issues such as the appropriateness of therapies, adverse drug reactions and alternative choices. The pharmacist is also involved with discharge planning, ensuring liaison with the primary healthcare team and providing an accurate discharge drug summary. Liaison with other members of the CF team is important and the pharmacist works closely with the CF nurse in the provision of home intravenous antibiotics and the equipment needed for administration.

The pharmacist also works behind the scenes, taking responsibility for issues such as the procurement of unlicensed and named-patient medicines as appropriate and ensuring the managed entry of new drug therapies. The introduction of new therapies can cause problems in a resource-stressed service, and the pharmacist is involved with collaborating in finding funding and the commissioning of new therapies.

Many services have introduced self-medication schemes and the pharmacist helps with these initiatives by supporting ward staff in the introduction and maintenance of the scheme and empowering patients to take control of their treatment. The pharmacist offers medication counselling and meets with individual patients to enhance knowledge and understanding of their treatment regimens. This is done through completion of an accurate drug history at admission or annual review; then through reviewing the medication with the patient the pharmacist provides education and support, often recommending changes where necessary such as a change in formulation or method of administration. This also helps patients with adherence issues and the pharmacist often works in partnership with the nurse and psychologist with these problems (www.cftrust.org.uk).

THE SOCIAL WORKER

The hospital-based social worker works closely with all members of the CF team, taking referrals directly from colleagues. The role will differ between centers depending on availability, need and particular patient groups. Although social workers are commonly used as a resource for their knowledge on support benefits and allowances, in most CF centers the social worker is available both for patients attending outpatients and for those who are admitted. In some centers the social worker will visit patients in their homes to undertake an assessment of needs.

The tasks of the social worker working in a CF team have been summarised as:

- assessment of psychological care needs, including discharge planning and risk assessment;
- planning care in the community;
- assisting and supporting parents, partners or informal carers;
- counselling for personal and family difficulties encountered as a result of illness, changing ability or needs;
- bereavement counselling;
- practical assistance and advice on welfare rights, employment, care of dependants, etc. [10].

Most of these tasks overlap with other members of the CF team, particularly the occupational therapist, psychologist and nurse. Good communication and close working relationships will ensure the patient and their family receive optimum care.

Most countries offer a benefit system for people struggling with disease or disability; unfortunately these systems are often difficult to access and subject to delays and bureaucracy. The social worker can be helpful in negotiating the system and advocating on behalf of the patients. The social worker is often the link person in organizing packages of care provided through social services by collating relevant assessments and letters from other professionals and liaising with the local authorities. As health deteriorates there is often a need for adaptations in the home, so the social worker and the occupational therapist will assess housing needs and organize support (financial or practical) to help with this.

When young people start school or college, the social worker works with the nurse specialist in liaising with schools and colleges about potential problems such as access, travel, computer use, time extensions for course work, etc. Likewise the social worker can also liaise with employers to discuss short- or long-term needs for individuals.

Social workers may also be involved with assessing a patient for transplantation. The social worker does not make recommendations as to suitability; instead coping strategies, emotional, financial and practical supports are identified. Preparing the patient for the results of the assessment is also important. Some will be accepted and have to deal with an uncertain waiting period, some will not be accepted and have to deal with loss of hope. Both groups will have deteriorating health and an increasing need for support.

As with other members of the CF team, the social worker can offer psychological support, particularly around issues such as acceptance of CF and the emotional and practical implications of the disease, adherence to treatment, relationship issues and end-of-life issues. Medical advances are improving the lives of people with CF, but to maximize quality of life patients must be supported in living life as independently as possible.

THE OCCUPATIONAL THERAPIST

Occupational therapy (OT) is focused on enabling the continued occupations of everyday life through adaptation, while living with an illness or disability. This may involve problem-solving new ways of carrying out activities of daily living or utilizing adaptive equipment to assist with independence and decrease energy requirements for the task.

The purpose of the OT role is to work together with patients and their families by identifying any areas of difficulty within the realm of work, self-care and leisure tasks that are currently impacting on daily life. The timing of intervention is important when working with a population with CF. It can be difficult for young adults to accept the need for adaptations in the home environment in order to enable an increased quality of life.

Introduction of OT is often during an admission where information on the role of the occupational therapist as a member of the CF team is provided. This allows the patient later to address any concerns, being already aware of what OT has to offer.

Assessment is carried out on the ward and an individualized treatment plan is devised in consultation with the patient that focuses on his or her current goals. Two of the main goals from this initial meeting include trial and practice of adaptive and new techniques. To start with patients are encouraged to practise personal and domestic activities of daily living in order to enhance confidence and learn adaptive techniques. Alternatively – or parallel to this – they are also encouraged in the trial of adaptive equipment that can aid in independence and decrease the endurance required for the task.

Advocacy is another key part of the OT role through liaison with local authorities and social service occupational therapists. This includes providing a detailed functional assessment report that will include information on the disease process and the demands of daily treatments regimens. This will provide the community therapists with sufficient information to meet the needs of the patient when he or she returns home.

The occupational therapist is an active member of the CF multidisciplinary team. Although all members of the CF team make referrals, most are made through the clinical nurse specialists who bridge the gap between hospital and home. As the adult CF population increases, so will their demands for more home support, so it is essential that the role of the occupational therapist in CF constantly evolves in order to meet needs of the patients, the CF team and the organization [11,12].

THE SECRETARIES

Secretaries working in CF teams often find themselves the hub of communication for the service, with the CF team, patients and families all finding themselves making contact throughout the day. As well as the usual secretarial duties (e.g. typing clinic letters/summaries, collating clinic lists, test results, etc.) the secretary will get to know patients and families, and perhaps be involved in database management and liaison between different services.

THE DATA MANAGER

To audit and research CF, and to follow the natural history of the disease, it is necessary that individual patient clinical data from all CF centers is recorded, collated and analyzed. In many countries around the world specialist CF services are requested to contribute to their national databases. The data are usually collected from annual reviews or outpatient attendances, but entry of such complex data can be time-consuming. Many centers have found it invaluable to employ a data entry manager who becomes an essential member of the CF team.

The 'secondary' CF multidisciplinary team

Owing to the complexities of CF it is often necessary to involve other specialist health professionals to manage the range of disorders that CF can present with, such as liver disease and diabetes. This may be viewed as a second tier of the multidisciplinary team; access to these team members will be by referral only. It is the combination of the primary and secondary multidisciplinary teams working collectively that ensures the patient with CF receives the best care.

SPECIALIZED LABORATORY SERVICES

Laboratory services that offer specialized (non-routine) testing for patients with CF are paramount to accurate treatment plans being instigated. They may include sputum culture sensitivities being reported for a large range of antibiotics, and occasionally synergistic antibiotic sensitivities, which can prove invaluable when faced with multi-resistant organisms. Molecular biology provides services such as DNA and genotyping studies. Biochemistry is particularly useful in CF-related investigations such as levels of fat-soluble vitamins (A, D and E), analyzing fecal fats and pancreatic elastase-1 in determining pancreatic sufficiency/insufficiency. Immunology provides services such as identifying *Pseudomonas* antibodies, *Aspergillus* precipitins, radioallergosocbut test (RAST) and total IgE.

THE GASTROENTEROLOGIST

Individuals with CF present with a multitude of gastrointestinal issues such as gastroesophageal reflux (GER), liver disease, pancreatitis and distal intestinal obstructive syndrome (DIOS), all requiring specialist gastroenterologist intervention. Gastroenterology services also carry out endoscopic investigations, and placement of gastrostomy tubes for supplementary feeding. Close liaison with the specialist dietitian and medical team is paramount. See Chapter 15a for further discussion of this.

THE TRANSPLANT TEAM/THORACIC SURGEON

Lung transplantation for people with CF is carried out in a few transplant centers in the UK. Specialist CF centers are encouraged to make early contact to plan referrals at an appropriate time. Ongoing communication is essential between the two teams as the transplant team requires constant updating on a patient's medical status and patients need constant reassurance that they are not forgotten.

With a variety of complications such as pneumothorax or the need for implantable venous access devices, thoracic surgeons can frequently be part of the 'secondary' multidisciplinary team – see Chapter 21 for further details.

THE DIABETOLOGIST

Most CF specialists have knowledge of CF-related diabetes (CFRD), which is commonly managed day-to-day with a CF specialist dietitian. However, regular review with a diabetologist is recommended, especially for some of the more complicated cases. Manipulation of different insulin preparations, and specialist diabetic monitoring (eyes and feet), are essential in a population who are growing older.

THE EAR NOSE AND THROAT (ENT) SPECIALIST

ENT complications such as rhinosinusitis, nasal obstruction and nasal polyps are common in CF and may require specialist medical intervention or surgery. The CF team should therefore have an active working relationship with the ENT department for the investigation and management of severe sinus disease [8]. This is particularly important when surgical techniques such as polypectomy and endoscopic submucus resection are indicated.

THE OBSTETRICIAN/GYNECOLOGIST/FERTILITY SPECIALIST

It is now thought that women with CF are probably as fertile as non-CF individuals [8]. The CF team can often provide contraceptive advice and pre-conception support. However, close liaison with an obstetrician with experience in CF is essential throughout pregnancy and around the time of delivery. As the female CF population grows older further complications arise either directly or indirectly related to CF, so the support of a gynecologist with knowledge of CF can be invaluable.

Male infertility in CF has been transformed with the introduction of sperm aspiration from the epididymis and intracytoplasmic injection into eggs [13]. In the UK, men with CF can request either the CF team or their family doctor for referral to an assisted conception unit.

ANNUAL REVIEW

An annual review is a comprehensive assessment of every aspect of an individual's condition and treatment (Table 27.2). It is used to assess progress and identify areas where treatment could be improved [14]. It is now accepted as being beneficial in achieving the best care managing this changing, progressive, complex, multisystem disorder, and is usually performed at a specialist CF center [15].

The aims of the review can be summarized as:

- a thorough review of all aspects of an individual's disease status;
- identification of suboptimal treatment that can be improved;
- formalization of an individual treatment strategy;

Table 27.2 Annual review.

CF multidisciplinary team review	
Review of medical history	Detailed assessment/review of medical history, progress, medically relevant life events since last review by an experienced CF clinician Includes assessment of patient/family's knowledge of own clinical condition
Assessment by a CF clinical nurse specialist	Detailed assessment/review of progress, social/family life events since last review – to include managing school, work, help with care, housing, benefits
Assessment by a CF specialist physiotherapist	To include: Assessment of airway clearance techniques (competence, frequency, appropriateness) Review of treatment strategy for inhaled medications Assessment/replacement of home nebulizer equipment Exercise test (shuttle walking test/modified shuttle test/3-min step test/cycle ergometry) Incontinence advice Postural advice
Nutritional assessment by a CF specialist dietitian	Current diet Assessment of need for nutritional supplementation Adequacy and knowledge of pancreatic enzyme replacement therapy Vitamin supplements Weight profile over time
Review by a psychologist and social worker	Conduct a psychological assessment, to include adherence to treatment, quality of life, living with CF
Clinical measurements	
In addition to those performed at standard clinic visit (height, weight, sputum culture, pulse oximetry, spirometry)	
Full clinical examination	
Pulmonary function testing	Full lung function including lung volumes, gas transfer in adolescents and adults Spirometry in children over age 5 years Bronchodilator reversibility testing Arterial/capillary blood gases in adults, if $SaO_2 < 92\%$ on air
Imaging	Chest x-ray (may use a recognized scoring system) Dual energy x-ray absorptiometry (DEXA) scanning to assess bone mineral density
Blood sampling	Full blood count and film Routine inflammatory markers (ESR, C-reactive protein, IgG) Serum electrolytes (including sodium, chloride, bicarbonate, calcium, magnesium levels) Renal and liver function including serum albumin Iron status Prothrombin time Fat-soluble vitamin A, D, and E (plus K if available) *Aspergillus* species RAST (radioallergosocbert test) and precipitins, IgA, IgG, IgM and IgE *Pseudomonas* antibodies if available

(Continued)

Table 27.2   (Continued)

Glucose	Oral glucose tolerance testing in non-diabetic pancreatic-insufficient patients aged over 10 years
	Serum glycosylated hemoglobin (HbA_{1c}) measured in those with established diabetes
Sputum	Culture for microbiology, culture and sensitivity
	Culture for non-tuberculous mycobacteria
Evaluation of intestinal absorption	Combination of clinical and laboratory methods (e.g. semi-quantitative estimation of fecal fat by microscopy)
	Further evaluation by 3-day fecal fat collection
Urine	Urinalysis for: glucose, protein and blood

Results

Fully reviewed – patient may be asked to return to the CF center on a different day to when the tests were completed to enable a comprehensive analysis and assessment to take place after collation of all the results

Full discussion with patient/family with relevant follow-up as appropriate

Full annual review report and recommendations (preferably written by the CF consultant) sent to patient's general practitioner, local CF center (if applicable) and patient/parent (if requested)

Collection of data for audit and research (specialist CF center and national CF database)

- review by CF multidisciplinary team specialists;
- provision of information for center and national CF databases.

If the annual review includes the first visit to the specialist CF center, the following should be included [1,7]:

- diagnosis review – to include repeat sweat test, genotyping;
- confirmation of pancreatic status – by fecal pancreatic elastase-1;
- introduction to CF multidisciplinary team members and facilities;
- provision of local CF information and literature.

DISCHARGE PLANNING

The majority of CF care is managed in the home, with admission only for management of exacerbation of problems, for example chest infection, CF-related diabetes, commencement of enteral feeding or DIOS. During a hospital admission, a complete review of all aspects of the ongoing medical and psychological care should take place prior to discharge [1]. It is essential that individuals be provided with a clear treatment plan (from relevant multidisciplinary team members), including all medications and follow-up clinic/homecare arrangements [1]. It is hoped that there will be a return to baseline of clinical parameters such as spirometry and weight. If there has been deterioration or new therapies instigated, such as home oxygen therapy, non-invasive ventilation or nocturnal gastrostomy feeding, it is important that the relevant team members give adequate instruction and support both during admission and at discharge, with the opportunity for this to continue after discharge (either through continued contact with the CF center or local community services if appropriate).

Maintaining regular communication with the patient's general practitioner (GP) and other local community services is important, as these may be the first-line contact for patients. The primary healthcare teams need to be adequately informed regarding the complexities of medications recommended and receive timely discharge, clinic attendance and annual review summaries to ensure continuity of care. The inpatient team needs to liaise closely with any homecare, community services or home antibiotic support services to ensure appropriate notifications of discharge are given and that the process is a smooth transition.

As CF is a chronic, multisystem disorder requiring daily medications and treatments, it is imperative that the individual (or his/her carer/family) be competent in managing the daily maintenance program. This can be assessed during any admission, but particularly after initial diagnosis or any change in the overall treatment plan. Key elements of maintenance therapy are medications, physiotherapy and nebulized antibiotics; adherence to treatment needs to be emphasized during every admission and clinic visit.

TRANSITION FROM PEDIATRIC TO ADULT CARE

Adolescence is both a frightening and exciting time, full of many transitions as the young person develops from a dependent child to an independent young adult. For young people with CF this extra transition can interrupt a natural progression to self-sufficiency experiencing life as their peers with all the same concerns, problems and desires. There are issues that are of concern to all young adults but are of particular concern to those with CF such as further education, employment, fertility and pregnancy [16]. Likewise, some risk-taking behavior such as recreational drug use or smoking, otherwise normal teenage behaviors, can have a detrimental effect on CF. The CF team therefore plays an essential role in supporting both parents and young people with CF to survive this transition period and to make the move from pediatric to adult care [17].

Nowadays the majority of children with CF will have their care transferred to adult services. A successful transition plays a key role in disease management and understanding of the treatment regimens. It can be argued that the period of transition influences coping for many years into the future, so with early involvement of the patient and family, planning and good communication between the pediatric and adult CF teams and the patient and family, this can be a smooth process (Table 27.3).

Transition takes time, planning and the full support of both the pediatric and adult multidisciplinary teams. Recommendations suggest the formal planning of guidelines that have been agreed by both the pediatric and adult CF teams. Although CF populations differ between centers in a number of patients, geographical position of the adult CF center and staff available to coordinate the process, all guidelines should include the following:

- identity of the coordinators, both pediatric and adult;
- the age when discussions should start to take place;
- the upper age limit by which transition should have taken place;

Table 27.3 A formal plan for transition of care.

A formal plan of transition must be in place	Planned and agreed by the pediatric and adult teams
Discussion about transition to adult care with patient and carer must take place	Carried out before the age of 16 years and regularly discussed
Pediatric and adult teams must have coordinators who work together	The coordinators meet regularly to plan either individual patient transition or transition clinics Dates and times of clinics are agreed Suitable patients are identified (usually by age) and invited to meet the adult CF team. Invitations are sent to patients for transition (clinic) dates
The coordinators inform both the pediatric and adult teams of transition clinic dates in advance	It is recommended that pediatric and adult CF teams both attend the transition clinics
A referral letter/form about each patient is to be completed and sent to the adult team in preparation of the transition clinic	This is an introduction of each patient to the adult team and should include: – demographic data including siblings with and without CF – date and method of diagnosis with results – date of insertion of gastrostomy/indwelling venous access device – microbiological status – physiotherapy techniques used – details of surgical procedures – medication – lung function – height, weight and BMI (or equivalent) – details of CF-related complications – details of non-CF-related problems – general medical update
Preparation with each patient can be made in advance	Has the patient decided where to go for their adult care (if there is a choice)? Will they be moving away from home (college/work)? Do they know the names and doses of all their medication? Do they know how to obtain more when they run out? Have boys had a discussion about infertility? Have boys and girls had a discussion about contraception?
At the transition clinic the same professionals in each team should work together	This allows the patient and their family to see that: – the teams communicate – information about each patient is shared – there can be joint discussion about treatment – the patient and their family can talk about their concerns
Clinic letters should be sent to the adult team and the patient	This allows all present to have a record of what was discussed, especially questions asked and their answers
The follow up appointment will be made at the adult service	Following the transition clinic the adult team will deal with all queries from patients. If the patient or their family contact the pediatric team they will be asked to call the adult team instead

- information about the process and about the adult center available to the adolescent and his/her parent;
- evidence of good communication between pediatric and adult teams.

Without this structure and commitment from professionals, parents and adolescents find themselves reluctant to accept the inevitable. What should be welcomed as recognition of adulthood becomes something that is feared and avoided [18]. Problems in this process can be due to a number of issues:

- no formal plan of transition agreed between the pediatric and adult services;
- no coordinator;
- patient/family's reluctance to move;
- no obvious adult service to liaise with;
- concern about the potential adult service.

The process of transition does not end after the transition clinic. Follow-up during the changeover period must be handled carefully between the pediatric and adult teams, with an agreement as to which team takes responsibility. During the first few outpatient visits to the adult clinic familiarity is important and the patient and their family must meet the CF team members who were introduced to them during the transition clinic. Likewise, if the patient requires an admission soon after moving, the ward staff need to be informed of their status so that the admission can be handled sensitively.

A well-planned transition program, with good coordination and communication between the pediatric and adult teams, will ensure a successful move from pediatric to adult care for most patients [19]. There will be some young people, however, who cannot be managed within guidelines. These include siblings who are close in age, the terminally ill and those who do not attend appointments. Siblings who are close in age often go through the transition process together when they are both near an appropriate age. This often means keeping the older one past the guideline age and moving the younger at an early age; nevertheless, flexibility is important as families usually find this preferable.

Over the years a close relationship develops between patients, families and CF teams, especially when the disease deteriorates. Moving the young person and his or her family to an unknown team and unknown surroundings at such a vulnerable time should not be considered.

Finally, some patients, despite everyone's best efforts, fail to attend transition clinics. Unfortunately this group of young people miss out on the process and usually find that their next outpatient appointment is with the adult team. The adult team in this instance must spend time acquainting the individual with the changes.

HOMECARE

From diagnosis parents are encouraged to learn procedures such as chest physiotherapy, how to administer oral and inhaled medication and pay attention to diet so that children can be at home living as normal a life as possible. As children grow older they are supported in becoming independent in all aspects of their treatment including how to carry out chest physiotherapy and manage their diet. Support in the home environment therefore helps both children and young adults to fully participate in school, work and family life while maintaining their health.

The treatment demands of CF are burdensome and stressful. When a child or adult with CF is in good health this may take a few hours a day, but when they become more unwell treatment times will increase substantially. With decreasing health comes increasing needs – nebulizer therapy, home intravenous therapy, enteral feeding, oxygen therapy, physiotherapy aids, wheelchairs and non-invasive ventilation for example. Arranging delivery or collection, storage and maintenance of this extra equipment also places enormous practical and psychosocial demands on parents, carers and patients. Parents of children with CF may have other children, work, or care for other family members. Adults with CF may themselves have a family, be in employment or full-time education or care for other family members. Leading a busy and active life while maintaining CF treatment regimens is a major undertaking.

Most specialist CF services in the UK offer a home-based care service. The CF clinical nurse specialist usually provides this service, but in some places CF specialist physiotherapists and dietitians are also involved (Table 27.4). A comprehensive service therefore can often make a difference with adherence to treatment, hospital admissions, and coping with the day-to-day demands of CF [20].

Much of the equipment needed in home care today is readily available, easy to use and often disposable – for example, physiotherapy adjuncts, intravenous delivery systems or nebulizer pots. Technological advancements make communication with the CF team much easier. Developments such as webcams, online monitoring, telephone messaging and SMS texting means that the patient and the professional can discuss problems and check clinical measurements such as lung function in real time. Patients today live in a technology-driven society and have no problem in adapting their knowledge of electrical game devices or mobile telephones to using clinical equipment.

Advantages and disadvantages of homecare

Although a homecare service may appear an obvious model, CF teams need to evaluate its usefulness in relation to each patient at every exacerbation and be sensitive to the needs of the carers. For some families admitting a patient to hospital is important as a respite for carers, to prevent home becoming hospital, employment pressures of the carer, isolation of the adult patient, issues with non-adherence, or because of demands from other family members [21]. In some centers, resources will dictate and perhaps limit the level of service available, so it is essential in these instances that the homecare offered is appropriate for each

Table 27.4 Provision of CF specialist care in the home.

Nurses	Physiotherapists	Dietitians
Clinical assessments at home	Optimizing airway clearance techniques	Monitoring and advising on feeding problems
Support for patients/family	Problem-solving with non-invasive ventilation and liaising with respiratory support services	Advice on adherence issues
Health education	Lung function/oxygen saturation monitoring	Advice on oral supplements
Blood tests during an intravenous course of antibiotics	Encouraging exercise programs when well and after long hospital admissions	Advice on vitamins
Maintaining intravenous access during a course of intravenous antibiotics	Discussing posture	Problem-solving and giving advice with the administration of pancreatic enzyme therapy
Lung function/oxygen saturation	Discussing continence issues monitoring	Problem-solving and giving advice with managing CF-related diabetes
Flushing of implantable venous access devices	Problem-solving with nebulizers	Problem-solving and giving advice on the management of enteral feeding
Liaison with multidisciplinary hospital team including doctors, nurses, physiotherapists, dietitians, occupational therapists, social worker	Support for patients and family	Advising on pre- and post-pregnancy nutrition including breast-feeding
Liaison with GP/local healthcare providers	Liaison with multidisciplinary hospital team including doctors, nurses, physiotherapists, dietitians, occupational therapists, social worker	Problem-solving and advice about distal intestinal obstructive syndrome (DIOS)
Liaison with community services such as social services and housing departments		
Support to women planning pregnancy and during pregnancy		
Post-natal support		
Support to patients waiting for a transplant		
Bereavement support to family members		

patient. For the CF team an admission can provide an opportunity to monitor treatment closely, especially if there has been a problem with previous homecare treatment.

On a clinical level, homecare may not always be suitable. For example, reports indicate that treatment for exacerbations is more effective in hospital than at home – although more expensive for the health service [22]. Equally, when treated in the home there are economic savings for the patients in terms of being able to continue at work (for both parents or adults with CF) [23]. There is no doubt that patients and families prefer treatment at home and much of the literature supports the psychosocial benefits of homecare – such as ability to sleep, mood and overall energy

levels [21,24]. As with all CF treatment, care has to be individualized: in exploring methods to improve outcome for home treatment, patients and family preference must be balanced between home visiting and hospital attendance.

The homecare professional

From diagnosis onwards, parents and eventually the young person are involved in a collaboration of care with the CF team. Treatment decisions are planned with the involvement of parent and patient; their views and comments are important in final decision-making. It is inevitable, therefore, that an often close and trusting relationship develops between parents, patient and CF team members. Where the CF team member is involved with providing homecare this relationship may become stronger and over many years can become difficult to manage on an emotional level. Crossing professional boundaries can become a risk for the patient, the family and the professional, and the CF team have a responsibility to be aware of colleagues and their workload.

The term 'burnout' is commonly used to describe the overloading of an emotional and physical burden. It is almost inevitable that professionals involved over many years with children, distraught parents and young adults – often peers – who have a life-limiting disease can become 'burnt out'. CF care is palliative with no cure, and working with a patient population that will die may unavoidably lead to emotional involvement. This may not be a problem in itself, but over-involvement can lead to serious problems. Individuals must be conscious of their working relationships and be alert to potential issues.

Managing a homecare team

Paying for a homecare service can often stretch the financial restrictions of many of CF centers. However, for managers of the service it is essential to make sure that it is properly resourced and include funding for such extras as secretarial support, professional development, and computer/printers. Individuals providing a homecare service can find their work rewarding. Meeting families in their own homes leads to a greater understanding of disease management and how families have adapted their lives to cope. However, the role can also be isolating and dangerous, especially when travel is over large areas. Safety is an issue – many of the professionals carrying out this role are women who are driving through busy traffic or visiting families in remote on dangerous areas. Planning a visiting program so that the visiting timetable is know by team members based in the hospital, keeping in contact throughout the day, and carrying personal alarms can reduce many of the problems.

WHY CF CENTER CARE IS RECOMMENDED

Cystic fibrosis is a multisystem disease requiring the expertise of a multidisciplinary team of experts working together in a specialist center [25–27]. Patients with CF may present with a variety of both physical and psychological complications that often increase with age. CF care aims to prevent these complications for as long as possible through the minimization of risks and optimization of health status – mainly respiratory and nutritional. The members of a CF multidisciplinary team work together with often overlapping roles, but communication between all professionals within the team ensures that patients receive optimum care with a good quality of life. Children and adults with CF would like to have all the resources of a specialist CF center at their local

hospital, but unfortunately this will never be possible. Consensus throughout the world is for CF center care, while shared-care strategies have been adopted in some places [28]. Shared care is primarily used to optimize CF care in children.

Many specialist CF centers, owing to the number of patients and particular expertise of staff, are able to use and maintain specialist equipment. Resourcing such equipment, maintaining it and training operators may not be a priority in local hospitals. However, good communication and liaison between both services ensures that the patient receives the best of both.

In most specialist CF centers the multidisciplinary team attends the local hospital's Outpatients department two or more times a year to hold a clinic with the host consultant. For patients, these outreach clinics are alternated with a visit to the specialist CF center. Although this is the model of choice, in some instances only the consultant visits the outreach center; however this is usually due to resource limitations rather than preference.

When the specialist CF center is in a large area, it is essential that support be provided by the local hospital. This local service should meet the same requirements and standards as a specialist CF center and must be supported and supervised in liaison with staff from the specialist center [1].

CONCLUSION

Cystic fibrosis is not the only disease to have benefited from a more vigorous approach to treatment by specialized teams. Many other chronic conditions of childhood such as hemophilia have found that a team approach to delivering complex care increases efficiency and effectiveness. The initial success of these specialist pediatric teams has led to increased survival over the years and the adoption of this model in the provision of adult care.

Individuals with CF are now surviving well into adulthood, so CF can no longer be regarded as a fatal disease of childhood. Improving prognosis in can without a doubt be attributed to medical and scientific advances. However, the attention to detail in day-to-day management, the evaluation and introduction of more effective treatment regimens and the specialist knowledge of professionals working in large centers has also made a significant contribution to increasing survival.

REFERENCES

1. Cystic Fibrosis Trust Clinical Standards and Accreditation Group. *Standards for the Clinical Care of Children and Adults with Cystic Fibrosis in the UK.* Bromley, Kent, CF Trust, 2001.
2. Neilsen OH, Schoitz PO. Cystic fibrosis in Denmark in the period 1945–81: evaluation of centralised treatment. *Acta Paediatr Scand Suppl* 1982; **301**:107–119.
3. Phelan P, Hey E. Cystic fibrosis mortality in England and Wales and in Victoria, Australia. *Arch Dis Child* 1984; **59**:71–83.

4. Walters S, Hodson ME, Britton J. Hospital care for adults with cystic fibrosis: an overview and comparison between special cystic fibrosis clinics and general clinics using a patient questionnaire. *Thorax* 1994; **49**:300–306.

5. Frederiksen B, Laang S, Koch C, Holby N. Improved survival in the Danish center-treated cystic fibrosis patients: results of aggressive treatment. *Pediatr Pulmonol* 1996; **21**:153–158.

6. Mahadeva R, Webb K, Westerbeek RC *et al.* 1998. Clinical outcome in relation to care in centers specialising in cystic fibrosis: cross-sectional study. *Br Med J* 1998; **316**:1771–1775.

7. Littlewood J. Good care for people with cystic fibrosis. *Paediatr Resp Rev* 2000; **1**:179–189.

8. Kerem E, Conway S, Elborn S, Heijerman H. Standards of care for patients with cystic fibrosis: a European consensus. *J Cyst Fibros* 2005; **4**:7–26.

9. Madge S, Khair K. Multi-disciplinary teams in the United Kingdom: problems and solutions. *J Pediatr Nurs* 2000; **15**(2):131–134.

10. Cloutman N. Social work. In: Hodson ME, Geddes DM (eds) *Cystic Fibrosis*, 2nd edn. London, Arnold, 2000, pp413–418.

11. Otley Groom V. Occupational therapy. In: Hodson ME, Geddes DM (eds) *Cystic Fibrosis*, 2nd edn. London, Arnold, 2000, pp419–424.

12. Hagedorn R. Foundations for practice. In: *Occupational Therapy*, 3rd edn. London, Churchill Livingstone, 2001.

13. McCallum PJ, Milunski JM, Cunningham DL. Fertility in men with cystic fibrosis. *Chest* 2000; **118**:1059–1062.

14. Crozier DN. Cystic fibrosis: a not so fatal disease. *Pediatr Clin N Am* 1974; **21**:935–948.

15. Carr SB, Dinwiddie R. Annual review or continuous assessment? *J R Soc Med* 1996; **89**(Suppl 27):3–7.

16. Boylard DR. Sexuality and cystic fibrosis. *MCN Am J Matern Child Nurs* 2001; Jan/Feb:26.

17. Bryon M, Madge S. Transition from paediatric to adult care: psychological principles. *J R Soc Med* 2001; **94**(Suppl 40):5–7.

18. Madge S, Bryon M. A model for transition of care in cystic fibrosis. *J Pediatr Nurs* 2002; **17**:283–288.

19. Madge SL. National consensus standards for nursing children and young people with cystic fibrosis. *Paediatr Nurs* 2002; **14**(1):32–35.

20. Barnes R. Why home healthcare is so important for patients with cystic fibrosis. *Br J Home Healthcare* 2000; **1**(1):14–15.

21. Bramwell E, Harvey H. Care of cystic fibrosis in the community. *Commun Nurs* 1998; **3**:16–17.

22. Thornton J, Elliott RA, Tully MP *et al.* Clinical and economic choices in the treatment of respiratory infections in cystic fibrosis: comparing hospital and homecare. *J Cyst Fibros* 2005; **4**:239–247.

23. Strandvik B, Hjelte L, Malmborg AS, Widen B. Home intravenous antibiotic treatment of patients with cystic fibrosis. *Acta Paediatr* 1992; **81**:340–344.

24. Kuzemko JA. Home treatment of pulmonary infection in cystic fibrosis. *Chest* 1988; **94**(Suppl 2):162S–166S.

25. British Paediatric Association. Cystic fibrosis in the United Kingdom 1977–85: an improving picture. *Br Med J* 1988; **17**:1599–1602.

26. Clinical Standards Advisory Group. *Cystic Fibrosis: Access to and Availability of Specialist Services*. London, Her Majesty's Stationary Office, 1993.

27. Royal College of Physicians. *Cystic Fibrosis in Adults: Recommendations for Care of Patients in the United Kingdom*. London, RCP, 1990.

28. Dodge J. Patient-centered cystic fibrosis services. *J Soc Med* 2005; **98**(Suppl 45):2–6.

Nursing care

SUSAN MADGE AND CHRISTINE HOCKINGS

INTRODUCTION

Advances in medical management over the last few years have improved both quality of life and longevity for people with cystic fibrosis (CF). The multidisciplinary team works together to ensure a holistic approach to the care of these complex patients. All specialist CF centers in the UK have a clinical nurse specialist (CNS) with expert knowledge of cystic fibrosis. The role of the CNS is varied but in general offers care and support to patients attending hospital and those at home. In some centers the CNS coordinates and facilitates community care in liaison with local or generic community nursing teams. However, other centers have a dedicated CNS who is able to offer direct care to patients in the community. The CNS, whether based in the community or in hospital, can provide skilled support, advice and care directly to the patient and family wherever it is needed. Nurses working in hospitals where there is no opportunity to work with a CF team are strongly advised to make contact with the nearest specialist CF center, both for their own support and to assure optimum care for their patients [1].

This chapter will first discuss the role of the CNS – providing both the hospital service and the homecare service – and then describe the various key events throughout the life of a child and young adult where the role of the nurse is important in ensuring optimum clinical and psychosocial care. Further information on the role of the nurse (particularly the provision of a homecare service) can be found in Chapter 27.

THE ROLE OF THE CLINICAL NURSE SPECIALIST

Nurses looking after children or adults with CF have a variety of responsibilities, not only to patients and their families but also to other staff involved in the care of those patients [2,3]. These roles include the following:

- support, advocacy and communication;
- service planning;
- clinical skills and practice (e.g. teaching intravenous therapy, care of intravascular devices – Tables 28.1 and 28.2);
- education and research;
- professional skills and development.

Specialist CF centers and patient groups have differing requirements, so the CNS role varies not only between countries but also between centers within countries. It is inevitable that the CNS role will develop to meet the needs of the local CF population [4].

The CNS working with cystic fibrosis has a unique role in being involved with the patient and the family throughout a lifetime – from helping them to come to terms with the diagnosis to supporting them with end-of-life management. There are, however, certain key times in the patient's and family's life when more intensive support is required, such as at diagnosis, at first admission, planning transition from pediatric to adult care, discussion about lung transplantation, and planning care at the end of life. The CNS should also be involved in providing support and information in areas such as dealing with adolescence, adherence issues, fertility and pregnancy or following a secondary diagnosis (e.g. CF-related diabetes).

Cystic fibrosis is a demanding disease to manage for the patient, the family and the CF team. Patient well-being and satisfaction are principal aims of the CNS and providing support and advocacy to the patient and family helps to achieve this. The CNS is actively involved in treatment decisions and monitoring care. In addition to the practical care that they support (e.g. intravenous therapy, nebulizer and inhaler therapy and enteral feeding), the CNS has a responsibility to ensure that every patient receives optimum care

Table 28.1 Knowledge and skills required for a nurse working in CF.

Psychosocial issues	Diagnosis
	Living with a life-limiting disorder
	Adherence to treatment
Respiratory symptoms	Chest physiotherapy
	Nebulizer therapy
	Oxygen therapy
	Spirometry
	Oxygen saturation
	Collection of samples for sputum microbiology
	Cross-infection policies
Nutritional requirements	Measuring height and weight accurately
	Knowledge of nutritional supplements available
	Enteral feeding (nasogastric, gastrostomy)
	Administration of pancreatic enzyme therapy
	Care of CF-related diabetes
Intravenous therapy	Care of venous access
	Care of indwelling venous access devices
	Administration of intravenous antibiotics
	Teaching self-administration of intravenous antibiotics
	Monitoring of safe antibiotic plasma levels
Adolescence	Transition from pediatric to adult care
Adulthood	Fertility and contraception
	Pregnancy/pre- and post-natal care
	Further education/employment
	Smoking/substance abuse
Advanced disease	Support in decision-making
	Pre- and post-transplantation management
	Care of chest drains
	Pain management and symptom control
	Dealing with complications
	Options for and management of respiratory support
	Bereavement support

Table 28.2 Recommendations for best nursing practice: nursing care.

Inpatient care	Nurses caring for patients with CF will have access to a CF clinical nurse specialist
Outpatient care	Ensure that the patient has access to a CF team
Community care	Assess, plan, implement and monitor care according to the needs of each patient ensuring equity of care between hospital and home
	Ensure a partnership of care between the patient/family/carers
	Ensure continued psychosocial advice, support, counselling and education for the patient and family
	Ensure discharge planning with special reference to the GP, primary healthcare team, shared care center and school/work where appropriate
Surgical management For example: insertion of gastrostomy, indwelling venous access device, chest drains	Ensure appropriate postoperative monitoring with special attention to respiratory status
	Ensure suitable pain management to allow continuation of chest physiotherapy and early mobilization
	Monitor wound healing (potentially influenced by diabetes, compromised respiratory status, etc.)
	Ensure timely removal of sutures

for his or her individual needs. The CNS coordinates care between patient and family, community services and hospital, both practically and through support and advice. Attention to these aspects of a nursing role should help to ensure patients receive lifelong support and quality care [5].

COPING WITH STRESS AND PROFESSIONAL BOUNDARIES

Commonly there are two models of care adopted by professionals in the healthcare setting, the *expert model* where the carer assumes responsibility and the *partnership model* where professionals and patients negotiate care through mutual trust and collaboration. Management of CF demands a partnership model of care, and working with a population of patients who have a life-limiting disease demands a certain intensity of involvement. Supporting day-to-day management and managing acute crises requires a constant level of communication. It is inevitable and often helpful that a relationship of friendship and trust develops between not only the CNS and the patient/family but also other members of the CF team.

There is a danger that this relationship may change from a caring one to one that becomes more intense and intimate. Maintaining professional, caring boundaries and coping with stress for any member of the CF team can be difficult. The UK Nursing and Midwifery Council states that a nurse should 'maintain appropriate professional boundaries in relationships you have with patients and clients' [6]. Of course this may be true for any member of the CF team, so good support and regular communication within the team and supervision from colleagues outside the team will ensure that a caring relationship is maintained and that no member of the CF team is put at risk.

Table 28.3 Recommendations for best nursing practice: diagnosis.

Ensure that pre-diagnosis support and counselling is available.
Be present when the diagnosis is given
Help determine the appropriate timing for the introduction of new information
Offer continued psychosocial advice, support, counselling and education to the patient and family

DIAGNOSIS

Diagnosis through postnatal screening is common in many countries throughout the world. In the UK the CNS plays an active role in talking to parents at diagnosis and then offering ongoing support and continuing education following the initial discussion (Table 28.3). Where screening is not available most babies are diagnosed within the first year of life, through identification of meconium ileus at birth (or suspected prenatally on ultrasound), failure to thrive or repeated respiratory problems. Again, the CNS plays a similar role in offering ongoing support and education to the parents.

Although professionals can be relatively positive in talking to parents about CF, it is inevitable that parents will initially focus on the life-limiting nature of the disease. Receiving a diagnosis of CF is therefore devastating for parents, as it can be perceived as a death sentence for their newborn baby. Most parents will never have heard of CF and may not fully understand the implications of genetic inheritance; blame, guilt and confusion are often the most frequent reactions at this time.

Not only will parents have been given devastating news, from diagnosis onwards they will have to learn clinical skills that will become part of their daily lives. Performing chest physiotherapy or administering medication routinely to an infant may feel unnatural and the parenting role can become confused with a more medicalized role at this early time. Individuals experience different reactions on an emotional and practical level at different times. The support, education, advice and understanding that the nurse offers has therefore got to be individualized at a level and frequency to meet differing needs. Frequent contact between the nurse and the new parent is essential, either in hospital, through home visiting or by telephone.

The impact of this diagnosis on families – immediate and extended – cannot be exaggerated. Reproductive issues for both the new parents and their siblings become an issue, and nurses provide ongoing education and genetic counselling for both the parents and their families.

Although the majority of individuals with CF are diagnosed within the first year of life, there remains a minority who are diagnosed later. Diagnosis in adolescence and young adulthood is not uncommon, but there are also a very small number of older adults often with rare mutations who are being diagnosed in general respiratory or infertility clinics.

Receiving a diagnosis of CF in adolescence, early or later adulthood can be devastating. For the adolescent or young adult the introduction of the medicalized treatment regimens can be complicated. Much of the CF literature reports a life expectancy of approximately 30 years [7]; many late-diagnosed young adults report feeling alarmed of this prognosis and, however well they feel, expect to die at that age. Young adults from various age groups find dealing with a much shortened life expectancy, coupled with a complex treatment regimen, very hard to cope with and the nurse needs to spend a great deal of time supporting this particular group of individuals.

BEFORE SCHOOL

For many, after coming to terms with the diagnosis and learning how to carry out treatment regimens while adjusting back to family life, the early years can become almost normal. However, there are a few areas where CF management remains a nagging reminder of the disease.

Armed with the knowledge that the recommended treatment regimens are planned to optimize their child's health, many parents follow a family routine that is centered around CF care. For many parents the child with CF may not be their first, so not only are they having to organize life with a new baby and the demands of CF treatment, they are also looking after their other children. The CNS can be very helpful in supporting and guiding parents through the preschool period particularly with issues such as:

- nutrition;
- pancreatic enzyme replacement therapy (judging the correct amount or refusal to take the enzymes) in conjunction with the dietitian;
- early treatment of chest infections and making decisions about when to ask for advice or start treatment;
- management of chest physiotherapy in conjunction with the physiotherapist and clinical psychologist;
- starting nursery;
- dealing with siblings;
- planning further children.

AT SCHOOL AGE

A child starting school for the first time can be a traumatic experience for any parent – control is suddenly lost and trust of other adults is demanded. As a parent of a child with CF this loss of control is even greater. Parents will have been exclusively carrying out CF treatment and monitoring their child's every cough up until this point. Once at school another adult will have to be trusted to continue with this close monitoring. Issues such as eating properly at school, forgetting to take pancreatic enzymes and involvement of a school nurse need to be considered in advance.

Starting school is often not the only concern for parents at this time; there are mixed feelings about their child growing up and staying well. Starting school may also coincide with a change in treatment – for example the introduction of nebulizer therapy, an admission to hospital for intravenous antibiotic therapy or the commencement of overnight enteral feeding. Coupled with additional treatments their child will be starting to assert his or her own independence, so that issues surrounding non-adherence can start to become more of a problem, especially with eating and physiotherapy.

An established and trusting relationship with the nurse can be helpful for parents. Homecare particularly can be useful as it gives parents time away from the clinical setting and allows them to discuss their anxieties in a safe environment. The nurse may also, with or without parents (but always with their permission), go to the school to talk about CF and how it relates to the child in particular, with teachers and school nurses.

Most school-age children with CF are relatively well and take part in all the academic, sporting and social activities provided by the school. Being an accepted part of a peer group is important, and taking time off for outpatient visits or hospital admissions can interrupt this. Children have reported feelings of isolation and losing friends after repeated hospital admissions. Supporting treatment in the home such as intravenous therapy or enteral feeding often allows children to carry on at school. The provision of a homecare service can help as routine checks and early identification of problems can be carried out by the nurse in the patient's home, often after school has ended for the day. Some children, however, have to continue with their academic studies during admission to hospital. The hospital school teacher is invaluable as a liaison between hospital and school and as a support for ongoing school work.

ADOLESCENCE

Adolescents with CF go through the same physical and emotional changes, experience the same rites of passage and have the same expectations as their healthy peers. This expectation is irrespective of the severity of lung disease [8]. To this end the nurse should be able to have open and honest discussions about such issues as recreational drug use and the effects on CF, sexuality and safe sex, fertility, pregnancy, university, employment, body image, self-esteem and adherence to treatment regimens [9,10]. Relationships between adolescents and parents can become difficult and it is often left to the nurse to encourage and support the promotion of self-care and responsibility, as well as answer some difficult questions.

Becoming accountable for self-treatment involves young people with CF having access to accurate information about their disease and its treatment, and with this knowledge comes a greater understanding of their prognosis. Nurses need to be sensitive and honest when giving information to young people with CF. Much of the information they (and their families) receive is from peers, the media and the Internet, so nurses caring for this group of patients have a responsibility to ensure that the information they receive is correct. Preparing for complications such as hemoptysis, monitoring diabetes, the introduction of new drugs into the current treatment regimen and pregnancy are just a few of the possible topics where clear and accurate information is important. The CNS therefore plays a major role in the education of both the adolescent and the family of new treatments and complications that are part of adult life with CF.

Most children with CF will move from pediatric to adult care and it has been widely recognized that the transition process is important to get right (Table 28.4). Adolescents with CF have to deal not only with the usual challenges of growing up, but also with the challenges of assuming responsibility of care from their parents and transitioning of their care from a pediatric to an adult center [11]. Transition from pediatric to adult care happens at a time when the young person with CF is moving into adulthood in other areas of life, such as further education or employment, forming relationships and taking more responsibility for his or her own lifestyle. Transition therefore can be difficult for many reasons. Nurses involved with the transition process need to be aware of the many barriers that can prevent this process being successful [12]. See Chapter 27 for further information.

Nowadays children with CF are generally quite well and some adolescents have never needed an inpatient admission

Table 28.4 Recommendations for best nursing practice: adolescence and transition.

Adolescence and adulthood	Promotion of self-care and responsibility
	Support and advice to parents
	Liaison with schools and colleges to support continuing education
	Ensure the adolescent receives appropriate knowledge regarding issues such as: fertility, pregnancy, contraception, safe sex, cross-infection, further education, employment, smoking and substance abuse
	Allow opportunity for discussion between patient, parent and CF team members when problems arise
Transition	Use experience and knowledge to advise on the most appropriate time for transition
	Assist in the coordination of joint transition clinics
	Provide information and ongoing support for patients and parents during the transition period
	Consider the implications for the future such as further education, employment, families, housing, mortgages, etc

prior to transferring to adult services. However, it often happens that the age of transition coincides with deterioration in health status and many young people find their first admission is to an unfamiliar ward where they do not know anyone. Many parents and young people consider the first admission for any kind of deterioration in health a 'life event'; this, coupled with a change in hospital and CF team, can often exacerbate their anxiety. For these individuals and their families, the first inpatient admission requires an increase in awareness and sensitivity from the ward staff and further support to both the patient and the family from the CNS.

Cross-infection has become an important topic in CF care, with most young people and their families aware of the problems and associated risks. All specialist CF centers have policies that have been written to meet the needs of a particular patient population [13]. As young people become more independent, education about good hygiene and cross-infection practices are essential, with particular emphasis on hand-washing, covering their mouths when coughing and the risks of close, intimate contact with others who have CF.

Death in the pediatric setting is rare due to the advances in CF care over the last 30 years. Hence moving to an adult center not only brings these young people with CF into an environment where they will see others much sicker than themselves, it also signifies a step closer to death. Nurses need to be aware of the impact that a death can have on other patients in the ward. It is important to allow patients time to discuss their feelings and worries about their own mortality and be aware that these events can also impact on future hospital admissions [14].

ADULTHOOD

Cystic fibrosis is no longer a disease of childhood. Today, half the population of people with CF in the UK are adults and this number is increasing. Data from the UK CF database show that, of the 6861 patients registered in 2003, 51% were 16 years or older, and 9% were 35 years or older [15].

As with adolescents, adults with CF have the same anxieties and worries as their healthy peers. Studies from the UK, Canada and Australia have all identified health, family and financial matters as being concerns in the adult CF population [16,17]. As people with CF live longer a greater number of them will live away from their parents, marry, become parents, own homes, work full time and may also become carers themselves of their aging parents. They will do all of these things while their disease progresses and their treatments become more complex and time-consuming [18]. Nurses play a vital role in helping adults maintain a balance between treatment and lifestyle, recognizing the need to help individuals to adapt treatment regimens to suit them. This is most effectively done in collaboration with the multidisciplinary team.

The CNS working with adult patients can have a varied role, which often includes:

- educating employers and work colleagues;
- liaison with government agencies and the workplace to ensure maximum support (financial and practical) to enable patients to stay employed or retrain;
- advocating on a patient's behalf with local social services;
- educating family doctors;
- educating local pharmacists;
- negotiating easier access to classes at school or university;
- advising patients on how to access services such as life insurance and mortgages, which may not have been such an issue in previous generations;
- increasingly, working in collaboration with the family doctor, social services and the CF team to support patients caring for their aging parents.

As the adult CF population continues to increase it is to be expected that more will become parents. Nurses working with adults with CF need to be aware of the reproduction options available to both males and females with CF to ensure that both men and women are able to make informed choices and are supported whatever their decision. These discussions should also involve the extended family if they plan to be involved with the care of future children in later years.

It has previously been thought that motherhood was a significant risk factor in the morbidity and mortality in women with CF. However, research has shown that, with close monitoring, liaison with an obstetric team and a reasonable lung function before conception, the outcome for both baby and mother can be good [19,20]. The nurse not only helps to coordinate this multidisciplinary approach to care, but often carries out the care needed for a successful outcome [21]. Where possible, regular visits by the CNS in the community can provide invaluable support for the mother with CF both pre- and postnatally. These visits can be arranged to compliment regular appointments with the obstetric team, allowing for close monitoring of the mother as well as improving communication between the two teams, thereby optimizing the care given.

Parents with CF who have children involve them in CF in a variety of ways. Some try to keep the reality of the disease hidden away by carrying out treatments in separate rooms, not talking about CF and not taking the children to the hospital with them. Others involve their children from an early age through talking about the disease, carrying out treatment with the children around – often with the children helping – and taking them to hospital appointments with them. When providing care for adults with CF who have children, nurses need to recognize the individual beliefs and attitudes of patients and support them with a plan of care that will only involve their children if they wish it.

ADVANCED DISEASE

It is widely recognized that complications such as pneumothorax, hemoptysis and CF-related diabetes occur more commonly in older patients with CF [22–24]. Other complications in aging patients include osteoporosis, liver disease, cancer of the gastrointestinal tract and arthropathy. These complications develop at the same time as lung function starts to deteriorate, increasing the daily treatment requirements individuals have to maintain to continue with their level of health. Nurses providing a homecare service may have to manage one or more of these complications in the home. Complicated medication regimens and organizing care to help maintain a lifestyle/treatment balance requires nurses to plan care on an individual basis using their expert knowledge.

Respiratory disease is the main cause of morbidity and mortality in CF [25]. Oxygen therapy and non-invasive ventilation (NIV) are all commonly employed in advanced disease to combat decreased lung capacity. These new treatments are not always readily accepted, so part of the nurse's role is to investigate the barriers to accepting these treatments and educate patients about the potential benefits to promote independence.

When admissions become more frequent, longer in duration and the burden of treatment increases, patients or their families may wish to raise the issue of lung transplantation. The initial discussion can be a shock for both the patient and their families, and nurses should allow plenty of opportunity to encourage discussion of these thoughts and feelings with various members of the team [14]. Early discussion with the team can raise many questions and concerns, for both patients and their families, individually or together – they may come to the nurse with queries or to seeking further information and support. The nurse's role as advocate and educator for the patient is vital in this decision process.

Once the decision has been made, the CNS is heavily involved in the assessment process as well as supporting patients and families whether or not they have been accepted onto the transplant list. Home visiting allows regular monitoring of patients without the ordeal of attending outpatient appointments with NIV, oxygen or a wheelchair. Often when patients are waiting for a lung transplant, a trip to the hospital can leave them physically exhausted for the following two or three days. Assessment at home by the nurse allows for fewer hospital visits and regular physical and psychosocial assessment; it also facilitates early admission.

END OF LIFE

Cystic fibrosis continues to be a life-limiting disease, so that many young people with CF die before their thirtieth birthday [26]. Unlike other chronic diseases, the end stages of CF can be difficult to recognize, and during the terminal stages treatment can often be both active and palliative. Although CF teams have traditionally provided a lifetime of care, palliative care specialists are starting to augment CF care by becoming usefully involved in end-of-life management.

Although patients and their families have known about the prognosis of CF since diagnosis, even with some preparation and expectation every death brings shock and great pain. Individuals with CF – children and adults – know when they are dying. They often need opportunities to discuss their fears and anxieties but may feel uncomfortable or protective talking about these issues with their family for fear of upsetting them or 'letting them down'. Advocacy allows the nurse to facilitate discussion between the patient and family, providing an opportunity for final words and goodbyes. Early discussion about an individual's wishes for the terminal stage of his or her disease is essential to aid appropriate care planning. Issues that may be raised include transplantation, a will, funeral arrangements, writing of letters or diaries to the family and where they would like to be when they die (Table 28.5). For some patients early discussion may be upsetting, but for others it can be a relief. The nurse needs to use judgment to assess each patient and family member individually when starting such conversations. When these discussions are well organized patients' wishes can be documented and filed away until needed. Nurses also need to be sensitive to the possibility that there may be more than one member of the family with the disease who may be affected by the end-of-life plans [27,28].

Occasionally there can be a lack of understanding between the patient and the CF team; again this is often due to a degree of protection. This can sometimes prevent the patient and family from making their wishes known about any last requests. The nurse can play an important role by ensuring the provision of accurate information for both the patient and the family, enabling them to make choices, providing practical and emotional support for the patient and caregivers and liaising between the medical team and the patient.

Although the option of dying at home or in hospital is discussed with the patient (however old) and their family, the majority of both children and adults with CF are in hospital at the time of death. The ward has been described as a place of familiarity and security and children and

Table 28.5 Recommendations for best nursing practice: end-stage care.

Transplantation	Be aware of the concerns involved with transplantation as a treatment option Ensure the patient and family receives sufficient knowledge to make informed decisions
End stage	Advocate on the patient and family's behalf Recognize the patient's complexity of care and changing needs and be able to offer support to the patient and family to help them come to terms with and adapt to the changes

adults have often said that they feel most comfortable spending their last days on the ward they have been admitted to frequently in the past. Due to the complex nature of CF it can often be difficult to determine when patients are in the final stages of their disease, with patients often receiving active treatment and medication until the last few hours of life. Nurses caring for patients at this stage are delivering a combination of preventive, therapeutic and palliative care. These treatment regimens can be quite complex and the family may not be able to cope with such regimens in the home.

End-of-life management is a collaboration of care between the patient and the family, the nurse on the ward and the CF team. The nurse administering these regimens must combine regular assessment of the patient's condition and regular discussion with the multidisciplinary team. This collaboration provides optimum care for the patient and the family. It can also be helpful to access specialist advice providing the nurse with further ideas with which to offer better care for the patient [29].

In the UK, hospice facilities are not always available or appropriate for people with CF, with most based on an oncology model of care. However, unlike other patients with life-limiting diseases, people with CF may choose the security of hospital as a place to die. Many children and adults prefer the familiar surroundings of the ward with care being provided by staff who they may have known for many years. For the few who choose to die at home it is occasionally possible to liaise with local community symptom-care teams. For this to be successful the nurse plays a collaborative role, working closely with the symptom-care team, the patient and family, and the CF team. Wherever the patient and family choose for the end stages of life, the nurse offers emotional and practical support allowing the individual to die in comfort and dignity. See Chapter 32 on palliative care for further information.

BEREAVEMENT

Parents and carers of a child or adult with CF develop a close and trusting relationship with the CF team, often over many years. Although the CF team have a primary responsibility for the patient, there is no doubt that the sudden cessation of this relationship at death can cause additional feelings of loss to already bereaved families. It is now widely accepted that ongoing bereavement care can be provided by the CF team – often through the CNS.

People cope with grief in different ways. At a time when families most need support from each other, there can be difficulty in recognizing and accepting different reactions. Men and women respond differently, especially when their child has died (at whatever age). Mothers are more likely to experience a wide range of emotions including anxiety, anger, guilt and despair. Fathers are more likely to focus their grief, experiencing social isolation and hostility. As well as feeling different there may well be a mismatch in the

highs and lows of coping and unfortunately this can lead to feelings of irritation and anger towards each other. The nurse plays a key role in these circumstances by providing individual emotional support and by helping parents to understand each other's grief reaction, thereby allowing them to support each other.

Although some families are willing to return to the hospital following a death, many find this very difficult. Visiting the family at home allows bereavement support to be offered in a safe and comfortable environment. Home visiting also allows other family members, siblings or grandparents for example, to receive some support. Unfortunately, although bereavement support is regarded as a role that nurses or clinical psychologists take on, workload excludes this as a long-term commitment. Instead nurses and clinical psychologists must be aware of alternatives and be ready to refer on to other agencies at an appropriate time.

THE FUTURE

The population of adults with CF is increasing as deaths in childhood become rare and adults survive longer. The need for nurses with expertise in CF will increase as the adult population demand increasing support and intervention allowing them to live full and active lives away from the hospital setting. Pharmaceutical and technological advances will improve the management of CF care in the future; and with greater access to information, people with CF are also exploring alternative options available to them. Nurses will have to become familiar not only with the current research and potential new therapies, but also the options of complementary and alternative therapies.

Unfortunately, CF will continue to remain a life-limiting disease for many years to come. An increasing life expectancy inevitably leads to an older and sicker group of adults. Nurses will find a rise in the numbers of older patients they have to support through the end of their lives. Many of these adults will have partners, children and maybe grandchildren and bereavement care and support will become an important part of the nurse's role.

Nurses in the future will find themselves providing a service that will include increased support in the home, college and workplace. This service, however, may not always be face to face – nurses will be have to become familiar with the developing e-technology of telemedicine, using webcams, SMS texting and video phones. However, whether consulting by video-link or face to face, nurses will continue to offer both practical and emotional support to children and adults with CF, their parents, partners and families.

REFERENCES

1. Madge S, Khair K. Multi-disciplinary teams in the United Kingdom: problems and solutions. *J Pediat Nurs* 2000; **15**:131–134.

2. Dyer J. Cystic fibrosis nurse specialist: a key role. *J Roy Soc Med* 1997; **90**(Suppl 31):21–25.

3. Benner P. *From Novice to Expert: Excellence and Power in Clinical Nursing Practice.* California, Addison–Wesley, 1984.

4. Kerem E, Conway S, Elborn S, Heijerman H. Standards of care for patients with cystic fibrosis: a European consensus. *J Cyst Fibros* 2005; **4**:7–26.

5. Madge SL. National consensus standards for nursing children and young people cystic fibrosis. *Paediatr Nurs* 2002; **14**:32–35.

6. UK Nursing and Midwifery Council. *The NMC Code of Professional Conduct: Standards for Conduct, Performance and Ethics.* London, 2004.

7. Dodge JA, Lewis PA. Cystic fibrosis is no longe an important cause of childhood death in the UK. *Arch Dis Child* 2005; **90**:547.

8. Webb AK. Flying with cystic fibrosis: getting there and back. *Thorax* 2001; **56**:821–822.

9. Bolyard DR. Sexuality and cystic fibrosis. *MCN Am J Matern Child Nurs* 2001; Jan/Feb:26.

10. Roberts S, Green P. Sexual health of adolescents with cystic fibrosis. *J R Soc Med* 2005; **98**(Suppl 45):7–16.

11. Nasr SZ. Cystic fibrosis in adolescents and young adults. *Adolesc Med* 2000; **11**:589–603.

12. Flume PA, Taylor LA, Anderson DL *et al.* Transition programs in cystic fibrosis centers: perceptions of team members. *Pediatr Pulmonol* 2004; **37**:4–7.

13. Henskens JE, VonNessen SK. *Burkholderia cepacia* in cystic fibrosis: implications for nursing practice. *Pediatr Nurs* 2000; **26**:325–328.

14. Conway SP, Littlewood JM. *Cystic Fibrosis in Children and Adults: The Leeds Method of Management.* Forest Laboratories UK Ltd, 2003.

15. www.cystic-fibrosis.org.uk/ [Accessed 2005].

16. de Launiere L, Paquet F, Hébert Y. Socio-economic profile of the adult cystic fibrosis population of Quebec [abstract]. *J Cyst Fibros.* 2004; **3**(Suppl 1):109.

17. www.cysticfibrosiswa.org/[Accessed 2005].

18. Dobbin CJ, Bye PT. Adults with cystic fibrosis: meeting the challenge. *Intern Med J* 2003; **33**:593–597.

19. Pernaut J, Audra P, Mossan C, Gaucherand P. Cystic fibrosis and pregnancy: report of twin pregnancy and review of the literature. *J Gynecol Obstet Biol Reprod* 2005; **34**:716–720.

20. Boyd JM, Metha A, Murphy DJ. Fertility and pregnancy outcomes in men and women with cystic fibrosis in the United Kingdom. *Hum Reprod* 2004; **19**:2238–2243.

21. Connors PM, Ulles MM. The physical, psychosocial and social implications of caring for the pregnant patient and newborn with cystic fibrosis. *J Perinat Neonat Nurs* 2005; **19**:301–315.

22. Flume PA, Yankaskas JR, Ebeling M *et al.* Massive hemoptysis in cystic fibrosis. *Chest* 2005; **128**:729–738.

23. Flume PA, Strange C, Ye X *et al.* Pneumothorax in cystic fibrosis. *Chest* 2005; **28**:720–728.

24. Mackie AD, Thornton SJ, Edenborough FP. Cystic fibrosis related diabetes. *Diabet Med* 2003; **20**:425–436.

25. Hodson ME. Treatment of cystic fibrosis in the adult. *Respiration* 2000; **67**:595–607.

26. Tonelli MR. End of life care in cystic fibrosis. *Curr Opin Pul Med* 1998; **4**:332–336.

27. Robinson WM, Ravilly S, Berde C *et al.* End of life care in cystic fibrosis. *Pediatrics* 1997; **100**(2 Pt 1):205–209.

28. Robinson W. Palliative Care in cystic fibrosis. *J Palliat Med* 2000; **3**(2):187–192.

29. *National Consensus Standards for the Nursing Management of Cystic Fibrosis.* London, Cystic Fibrosis Trust, 2001.

Physiotherapy

CRAIG LAPIN, ANNE LAPIN AND JENNIFER A. PRYOR

INTRODUCTION

Physiotherapy or physical therapy for people with cystic fibrosis (CF) has historically been associated with postural drainage and percussion (PD&P), but today there are numerous effective and efficient airway clearance techniques (ACTs). Airway clearance techniques are an important component in the management of people with CF, but the physiotherapist's role goes beyond that of airway clearance alone. Additional and important aspects of the role of the physiotherapist, and as a member of the multidisciplinary team, include exercise prescriptions (Chapters 25a and 25b), inhalation therapy (Chapter 13), non-invasive ventilation (Chapter 12), continence management and support during pregnancy (Chapter 20), exacerbations of pulmonary infection, terminal care, body awareness and posture, as well as liaison between CF center, school and the community for physiotherapy issues and delivery.

Hypersecretion and lung disease

Inflammation and infection start to occur shortly after birth in children with cystic fibrosis, usually long before the development of any respiratory symptoms. Beginning therapy, including airway clearance from infancy, is therefore logical (see later section on infants and young children), although efficacy is unproven. Adherence to the multiple modalities of CF care is problematic, and in airway clearance is known to be poor [1,2]. Starting airway clearance in infancy makes it part of a daily routine and the toddler or young child will be less likely to rebel than if started later. There is, however, active debate regarding the initiation of airway clearance in asymptomatic infants and young children.

Airway clearance techniques have been shown to improve mucociliary clearance in some studies. Hypothetically airway clearance techniques can decrease mucus plugging and aid the removal of secretions containing inflammatory cells and by-products, thus decreasing damage to epithelia. Removal of secretions containing bacteria, especially *Pseudomonas*, may decrease local inflammatory responses and delay the change of *Pseudomonas* to mucoid morphology.

Mucociliary clearance factors

Mucociliary clearance is affected by quantity of mucus, viscosity of mucus, size of bronchi or bronchiolar aperture, ciliary beat frequency and the shear forces generated by airflow from breathing. The greater the shear force, the more movement of mucus. A very important corollary is, therefore, that without airflow airway clearance techniques cannot enhance secretion clearance [3]. It has also been suggested that mucus viscoelasticity will be decreased due to the strain caused on mucus cohesitivity from these shear forces [4]. Factors that can affect airflow include airway resistance, expiratory pressures, bronchial wall stability and elastic recoil. Airway clearance techniques employ maneuvers that can affect airflow by physiological means.

In health and in people with CF with minimal disease, ciliary action is normal, moving mucus up the smaller airways at a rate of 3–5 mm/min, and at a rate of 20 mm/min in the trachea. Later in the disease process, mucociliary clearance is impaired with tracheal transit being 3–5 mm/min [5] but approaches normal when patients are placed in the head-down position.

Medications can affect the viscosity of mucus (dornase alfa, hypertonic saline), airway caliber and possibly ciliary beat frequency (bronchodilators). The only study to examine whether dornase alfa is more effective given before or after airway clearance found no significant difference in FEV_1, $VO_{2\,max}$ or quality of well-being, although patients chronically infected with *Pseudomonas aeruginosa* may have more improvement in FEV_1 if delivered after physiotherapy [6].

Airway clearance physiology

Mucus is produced by bronchial glands in the bronchi and goblet cells in bronchioles. Terminal and respiratory bronchioles have little to no mucus-producing capacity. Elastic recoil pressure is affected by thoracic expansion and lung compliance. Bronchial wall stability is determined by cartilage and 'elastic resistance' and, while bronchioles lack cartilage, tethering by alveoli adds to elastic resistance. These oppose the tendency of positive pleural pressures during cough and forced exhalation to collapse the airway. Larger airways have more cartilage which helps combat collapse. Bronchi of the sixth to seventh generation lie within lung parenchyma, have muscular walls and may be less compressible but subject to bronchospasm.

Many techniques utilize the concepts of asynchronous ventilation, collateral ventilation channels and the equal pressure point (EPP). Asynchronous ventilation refers to different filling times for different regions of the lung – faster for healthier and unobstructed areas, slower for more diseased and obstructed regions. Alternate or collateral ventilation channels exist between bronchi and/or alveoli [7], but are not present in infants and toddlers. In healthy lungs and with regular breathing, little gas movement occurs through these channels. By performing breath-holding maneuvers, patients can improve aeration in obstructed, less healthy areas by maximizing filling time for slow-filling regions, promoting ventilation through collateral channels and interdependence (*Pendelluft* – see later) [8]. The EPP is the site at which the pressure within the airway is equal to the pleural (extramural) pressure and hence the pressure difference across the airway wall is zero. With tidal volume breathing to functional residual capacity (FRC), the EPP lies in the trachea and main bronchi. As exhalation moves into lower lung volumes (expiratory reserve volume), the point at which dynamic compression takes place moves more peripherally [9,10].

Coughing is the body's natural mechanism for airway clearance. Usually, a deeper inspiration is followed by closure of the glottis. High intrapulmonary pressures build up behind the glottis and, when the glottis opens, supramaximal expiratory, turbulent airflows (flow transients) are generated. The EPP plays an extremely important part in the effectiveness of cough, because a significant jump in airflow velocity occurs at the points of narrowing (choke points). High linear airflow velocity is associated with turbulent flow, high shearing forces at the airway walls and high kinetic energies. These conditions are ideal for suspending and moving secretions adhering to the airway walls.

Another technique to produce supramaximal airflow and high linear velocities is a 'huff'. This is a forced expiratory maneuver, usually initiated from mid to low lung volumes and is performed with an open glottis [11,12]. The EPP augments the linear velocities occurring with this maneuver. Although a huff does not produce the same magnitude

of flow transients as a cough, it may have several other advantages. A cough is generated by the build-up of extremely high pressures, both intra- and extraluminal. The potential for more significant airway collapse at the EPP exists, especially if airway stability is lacking. Cartilaginous support decreases from the trachea and larger bronchi to the smaller bronchi, and is probably minimal within bronchioles. Although smooth muscle may aid in maintaining the patency of these smaller airways, a cough may compress these airways so much that effective clearance is not possible. Another mechanism contributing to markedly impaired cough clearance is dynamic collapse which may occur in disease states with increased compliance of the airways. The larger airways may become unstable where constant coughing (barotrauma) and potentially inflammation from infection has damaged the cartilage (chronic bronchitis, CF).

Another advantage of huff over cough is that coughing is mostly reflexive (although it can be 'directed') and as such allows less significant conscious control of starting lung volume or pressures developed than a huff. This advantage means the patient and therapist can adjust a huff to balance the potential of airway collapse against expiratory force. A huff may also be instituted at different lung volumes, allowing the shift of the EPP into more peripheral airways and maximizing airflow.

The question arises as to whether flows generated by a huff or by moving the EPP would be sufficient to promote mucus clearance. Studies have shown that mucus can be mobilized with expiratory airflow velocities of 1–2.5 m/s for annular flow, or greater than 2.5 m/s for mist flow moving sputum droplets suspended as an aerosol [13]. Airflows of sufficient magnitudes to mobilize secretions, and mucus transport itself, can occur during forced exhalations (huffs) or even with tidal breathing in some circumstances [14]. Bennett and Zeman determined that airway clearance with huff was faster than control, and similar to that generated by voluntary cough (Fig. 29.1) [15].

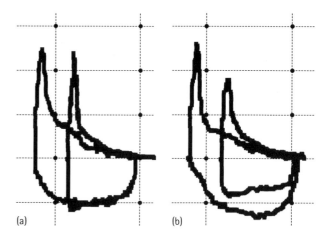

Figure 29.1 Flow/volume loops with superimposed flow transients of (a) cough and (b) huff.

AIRWAY CLEARANCE TECHNIQUES

Airway clearance techniques were limited to postural drainage and percussion for decades, but since the late 1970s other effective and efficient regimens have evolved and are now practised internationally. The techniques of postural drainage and percussion require help from an assistant, and remain the easiest to deliver to infants, toddlers and some young children. The other effective regimens can be undertaken independent of an assistant, used in the sitting position and may be preferred by the patient [16]. It is likely that the regimens of the active cycle of breathing techniques (ACBT), autogenic drainage (AD), positive expiratory pressure (PEP), oscillating PEP (OscPEP) and high-frequency chest compression (HFCC) are equally effective [17,18]. Each regimen can be adapted to suit the individual patient and modified, by the patient, for each treatment session and within a treatment session as necessary. The most effective regimen for an individual patient may depend on personal preference, as this may increase adherence to treatment. Selection of a regimen is also likely to be influenced by the knowledge and familiarity of the physiotherapist, and the culture and health economics of the patient's country. A change of regimen at intervals may increase adherence to treatment, but this is as yet unknown.

Postural drainage and percussion

PD&P for decades has been synonymous with chest physical therapy (CPT). Postural drainage consists of placing the patient in a position that allows gravity to enhance mucus movement centrally from the bronchopulmonary segment to the larger airways. There are 12 different positions in which a patient may be placed, either over the caregiver's lap or, for children and adults, over a postural drainage or foam board. Percussion, vibration and shaking may be used as an adjunct. In each position the chest is percussed for 2–10 minutes, usually followed by deep breathing exercises and huffing on exhalation.

The theory of PD&P hypothesizes that percussion over the bronchopulmonary segment increases intrathoracic pressure [19], transmitting vibration through the chest wall and loosening secretions in the airways. As mentioned earlier, postural drainage is hypothesized to assist airway clearance secondary to gravity assistance and subsequent improved secretion transit [5]. An alternative theory speculates that the redistribution of ventilation that occurs with changes in body position could alter the local airway patency and gas/liquid movements [20]. Positioning can be used for drainage of the uppermost lung segments or to increase ventilation to the dependent lung in an adult and the uppermost lung regions in a child. The study by Lannefors and Wollmer [21] demonstrated, in adults, an increase in mucus clearance from the dependent lung rather than uppermost lung, suggesting that the effect of the increase in regional lung ventilation may be greater than the direct effect of gravity on mucus in mucus clearance.

Studies have shown PD&P to be an effective technique in clearing excessive bronchial secretions in patients with cystic fibrosis [22–25]. Indeed, many of the studies of airway clearance over the past two decades have compared the newer alternative techniques to PD&P. If gravity-assisted positioning is indicated, it is likely that the lying positions without a head-down tip will be as effective as those with a head-down tip and will be preferred by the patient [26].

Problems associated with PD&P may include time and energy used, discomfort and pain, hypoxemia [27], arrhythmias [28] and bronchospasm [29]. Recently, the head-down tip has become controversial due to concerns over gastroesophageal reflux and increased pulmonary disease [30,31]. Modified PD&P excludes this position unless a specific focal lesion warrants it, for example lung abscess, and it is now suggested that modified PD&P (omitting the head-down position) be used, especially for those with symptoms of gastroesophageal reflux.

Active cycle of breathing techniques

The ACBT is a cycle of breathing control, thoracic expansion exercises and the forced expiration technique (huffing combined with breathing control) (Fig. 29.2) [12]. It can be introduced as huffing games from about 18–24 months of age.

- *Breathing control* is tidal breathing, at the patient's own rate and depth, encouraging use of the lower chest with relaxation of the upper chest and shoulders, to minimize the work of breathing. It is used in between the more active parts of the cycle.

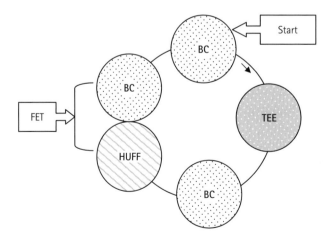

Figure 29.2 Components of the active cycle of breathing techniques (ACBT): BC – breathing control, TEE – thoracic expansion exercises, FET – forced expiration technique, HUFF – see text for explanation.

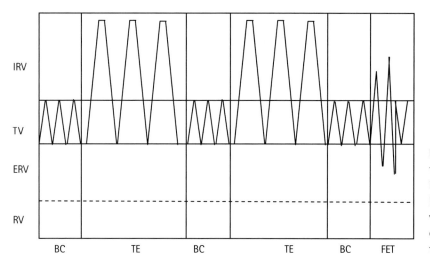

Figure 29.3 Physiological representation of the active cycle of breathing techniques: IRV – inspiratory reserve volume, TV – tidal volume, ERV – expiratory reserve volume, RV – residual volume, BC – breathing control, TE – thoracic expansion exercises, FET – forced expiration technique.

- *Thoracic expansion exercises* are deep breathing exercises emphasizing inspiration with a 3-second breath hold at the end of inspiration. Exhalation is quiet and relaxed. It is probable that there is an increase in airflow to less well ventilated parts of the lungs with the increase in lung volume and this is likely to be via the collateral ventilatory channels [7]. Patients may be encouraged to maintain an open glottis with the breath hold as this may augment airflow through these channels [32].

- *Forced expiration technique* is one or two huffs (forced expirations) combined with periods of breathing control [33]. Huffing to low lung volumes will assist in mobilizing and clearing the more peripherally situated secretions, and when secretions have reached the larger proximal upper airways, a huff or cough from a high lung volume can be used to clear them.

The regimen (Fig. 29.3) must be used flexibly. Patients should understand how the different components work and be trained to use the thoracic expansion exercises to get air in behind secretions to loosen the mucus. Huffing combined with breathing control (forced expiration technique) is used to move the secretions from different parts of the airways, utilizing the appropriate lung volume. If the patient has an asthmatic component to his or her lung problem or is tired, the length of the periods of breathing control (breathing around tidal volume) should be increased. The movement of secretions can be influenced from the choke point, the point just proximal to the equal pressure point [9,10,34,35] where collapse and compression, or the squeezing of the airways, begins. The increase in airflow, as the air passes through these narrowed segments of airways, may reduce the viscosity of the mucus [34] and this would facilitate the movement of the mucus up the airway. In addition to the squeezing action of the airways there is also an inbuilt oscillatory action of the airway wall [36].

The ACBT can be used in the sitting position or in modified postural drainage positions.

Autogenic drainage

The underlying concept of AD is to achieve high, optimal expiratory flow rates in different generations of bronchi by controlled breathing, but to avoid coughing or significant airway closure [37–39]. The incorporation of a breath-hold at the end of inspiration may improve asynchronous ventilation by lengthening the time for airflow via the collateral ventilatory channels. Autogenic drainage also involves breathing at different lung volumes, changing the position of the EPP to improve secretion clearance. The technique of AD requires feedback to the patient until he or she becomes attuned to the auditory and chest sensations to facilitate mucociliary clearance.

The treatment is initiated with an inspiration performed slowly through the nose and completed with a breath-hold of 2–3 seconds. Slowly breathing through the nose provides optimal humidification, warming of the inspired air and decreased turbulent airflow, all of which help to prevent coughing. The breath-hold and slow inspiration will provide optimal filling of obstructed lung segments while at the same time avoiding excessive intrapleural pressure.

Autogenic drainage consists of three phases (Fig. 29.4):

- The first phase is 'unsticking' the peripheral mucus by breathing tidal lung volumes (TVs) with an open glottis, down to low lung volume (into the expiratory reserve volume, ERV) but not to residual volume. Exhalation should be active, but without generating wheeze, bronchospasm or compression of collapsible segments of airways. Repeated tidal volume breaths, each with a 2- to 3-second breath-hold, are performed in this manner. After breathing at this level, the patient may feel and hear peripheral secretions as they move into the more central airways.

- The next phase, 'collecting', begins to gather central secretions. The patient gradually moves his or her breathing from low lung volumes to mid lung volumes

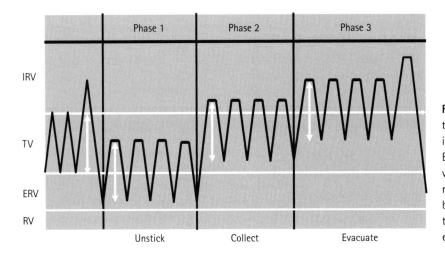

Figure 29.4 Physiological representation of the three phases of autogenic drainage: IRV – inspiratory reserve volume, TV – tidal volume, ERV – expiratory reserve volume, RV – residual volume. White arrows indicate size of respirations are similar to normal tidal volume breaths. Although four breaths are shown in this diagram, more will usually be required for each phase for an actual treatment.

(above the functional residual capacity and into the lower inspiratory reserve volume (TV-IRV)). Inspiration of tidal-volume sized breaths continues to be punctuated by the breath-hold. Exhalation should be active, but not so great that there is compression of airways. Coughing or expectorating should be discouraged if at all possible.

- The final 'evacuation' phase is accomplished by moving the secretions proximally using tidal volume breaths with a breath-hold at mid to high lung volumes (low to mid-IRV) followed by a forced expiratory maneuver from high lung volume or gentle clearing of the throat.

The optimal expiratory airflow must be individually adjusted at each phase, depending on the viscosity of the mucus and the reactivity of the airways. Unproductive coughing with forced exhalation is undesirable at this or any other stage [14,15,39].

Unfortunately there have been few published studies of AD. In the cystic fibrosis literature, Pfleger and co-workers [40] compared AD to high pressure PEP (Hi-PEP) and both regimens significantly improved pulmonary function. AD caused the most significant change, although it produced the least amount of sputum. An abstract [41] addressed patient preference for AD, a complicated technique, to PD&P. In a planned 2-year cross-over study there was no difference in clinical status or pulmonary function and the measures improved in both groups. Compliance was strictly monitored. At the end of the first year, almost half the AD group refused to change over to PD&P because they felt AD was more effective [41]. One study comparing AD, the ACBT and PD&P demonstrated improved ventilation by nuclear medicine scans, with AD having an improved airway clearance rate centrally and for the whole lung compared with ACBT. There was no significant effect on pulmonary function or oxygen saturation [42].

A comparison of AD to PD&P showed a small but statistically significant desaturation with PD&P, and a small but statistically significant improved saturation with AD

[43]. Comparison of sputum rheology following flutter and AD showed no improvement with AD [44].

This technique and its instruction make it difficult to teach successfully to young children under the age of 5 years, although 'passive' AD is used in some countries on infants. The therapist uses his/her hands to guide the thorax and respiratory movements to accomplish the goals of AD. The treatment is passive, non-violent and is not uncomfortable.

Positive expiratory pressure

PEP probably increases airflow via the collateral ventilatory channels [7]. Andersen and Jespersen [45] demonstrated the existence of these channels in all lobes in normal lungs, but it is unknown as to when, in the developmental process, these channels become patent. In the presence of lung disease, at high lung volumes and when breathing out against a positive expiratory pressure, it is possible that these channels would enlarge, the resistance to airflow would fall and air would flow along collateral channels, building up behind secretions to assist in loosening and mobilizing them. More slowly ventilating lung units may receive part of their inspired volume, from the more rapidly ventilating units, via the collateral channels. This is the *Pendelluft* flow [8]. From in-vitro work, a lower respiratory frequency and larger tidal volume should increase collateral ventilation [46]. The positive expiratory pressure may also reduce dynamic compression of unstable airways during expiration [47].

The definitive paper on PEP [48] demonstrated its effectiveness as an airway clearance regimen and revolutionized the management of patients with excess bronchial secretions in Denmark, including those with cystic fibrosis. The device consists of a mask and one-way valve system. A mouthpiece may be used if the patient does not like a mask, but this should be in conjunction with a nose-clip. A resistor is attached to the expiratory limb and this is adjusted to give a pressure of 10–20 cmH$_2$O in mid-expiration (Fig. 29.5d).

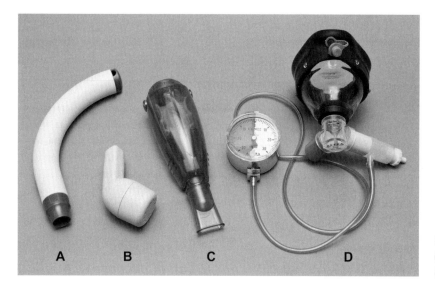

Figure 29.5 (a) Cornet, (b) Flutter, (c) Acapella, (d) positive expiratory pressure (PEP) mask and manometer.

The technique is one of tidal breathing, with a slightly active expiration, and the lung volume is kept up by avoiding complete expiration. Usually about 12 breaths are taken through the mask and this is followed by the forced expiration technique. The sequence is repeated as necessary. The PEP mask is available in small sizes and the technique can be introduced in infancy.

Mortensen and co-workers [49] demonstrated improved central and peripheral radioaerosol clearance with both PEP and the ACBT compared with controls. A 1-year study [50] showed improvements in lung function (FEV_1 and forced vital capacity) with PEP, compared with a decline in lung function in the group using PD&P. An added advantage of the PEP regimen was that of independence for the patient. A Cochrane review of PEP [51] concluded that there was no clear evidence that PEP was a more or less effective intervention than other forms of physiotherapy.

High-pressure PEP (Hi-PEP) is a modification [52] in which eight to ten breaths against a fixed resistor with pressures 10–20 cmH$_2$O, similar to regular PEP, is followed by one to two huffs or forced exhalations through the resistor. The pressures generated are usually between 50 and 120 cmH$_2$O, and the resistor selected is the one that maximizes forced vital capacity. The regimen of Hi-PEP requires close and ongoing monitoring, using flow/volume loops to select the resistor which optimizes the flow/volume loop for the highest vital capacity. Care must be taken to ensure exhalation continues to residual volume for the Hi-PEP maneuver. This modality has been shown to be effective in airway clearance in cystic fibrosis [53].

Oscillating positive expiratory pressure

This technique combines positive expiratory pressure with high-frequency oscillations generating intermittent acceleration of expiratory airflow. When the positive expiratory pressure build-up exceeds the device's resistance to flow, air escapes, pressure decreases and the device obstructs

airflow again. Oscillatory endobronchial pressure pulses cause flow transients within the airway. Flow transients are microsecond (transient) periods when flow exceeds the maximal expiratory flow able to be generated by a forced expiratory maneuver. Coughing and huffing generate flow transients (see Fig. 29.1). The flow transients generated occur in oscillatory frequency from 2 to 32 Hz, with transient positive expiratory pressure 5–25 cmH$_2$O (Fig. 29.6).

Endobronchial oscillating pressures are thought to act as 'micro-coughs', transiently increasing the airflow and shear forces over the mucus layer, thus promoting mucus clearance [54]. It is also proposed that the positive expiratory pressure generated decreases dynamic collapse of unstable airways, and endobronchial vibrations help to dislodge secretions from the airway lumen [55]. Additionally, studies have shown high-frequency oscillations are capable of breaking mucus bonds and decreasing viscosity [44]. Finally, it is hypothesized that the oscillations may enhance ciliary beat frequency as well as disrupting mucus adhesion to airway walls.

The three main devices used in OscPEP are the Flutter®, RC Cornet® and the Acapella® (see Fig. 29.5). The oscillation frequency with the first two devices is modulated by adjusting the position of the Flutter® or the 'twist' of the rubber hose in the Cornet®. The Acapella® oscillation is dependent solely on expiratory flow, and the Acapella® may also be set to deliver a fixed exogenous positive expiratory pressure beneath the endobronchial pressure pulses. In-vitro comparative studies of the Flutter® and Cornet® showed that the Flutter® generated a higher peak pressure at a higher frequency, but a lower amplitude of endobronchial pulse. Comparison of the Flutter® versus Acapella® showed small, but possibly not clinically relevant, differences [56,57]. Both devices produced similar waveforms at median flows, but at lower flows the Acapella® generated a more stable wave form with lower frequency, higher amplitude and wider range of positive expiratory pressure than Flutter® [58].

OscPEP technique is performed in the sitting position. Patients are instructed to take an active inhalation (usually

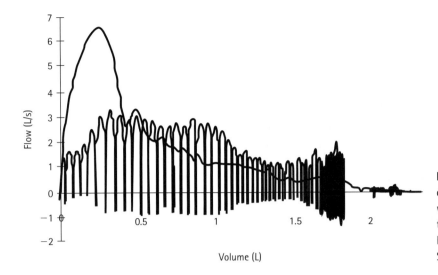

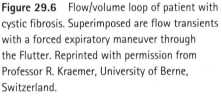

Figure 29.6 Flow/volume loop of patient with cystic fibrosis. Superimposed are flow transients with a forced expiratory maneuver through the Flutter. Reprinted with permission from Professor R. Kraemer, University of Berne, Switzerland.

through the nose) into the inspiratory reserve (but not to total lung capacity), a breath-hold of 2–3 seconds is incorporated and then an active exhalation into the expiratory reserve volume (but not to residual volume) is performed over a 3- to 4-second period. After repeating 10 to 15 breaths through the device to loosen secretions, the patient is instructed to huff (a faster and larger inhalation and exhalation) through the device to initiate expectoration [59]. Oscillation is maximized by tilting the Flutter® or twisting the rubber tubing of the Cornet®, if these devices are used. If PEP is desired it may be set on the Acapella® to maintain pressure at between 10 and 20 cmH$_2$O; the Acapella® may also be used without setting on exogenous PEP.

The Flutter® has been the subject of several studies in cystic fibrosis showing equivalent or improved outcomes compared with PD&P [60,61], but it did not improve results when added to the active cycle of breathing (ACBT) [62]. Individual patients may in the short term prefer OscPEP over some of the other airway clearance regimens (PD&P [63] and ACBT [64]). Although one study comparing Flutter® with PEP showed no significant difference [65], another demonstrated less effectiveness of the Flutter® versus PEP [66]. The decreased efficacy was found only after 6 months into the study, whereas almost all other oscillatory PEP studies have been short-term (days to weeks). The authors hypothesize that lack of end-expiratory pressure at low lung volumes with the Flutter® may lead to airway closure and air trapping. Theoretically, therapy with the Acapella® would not encounter this problem.

OscPEP can be introduced as soon as a child can use the device, usually around 4–6 years of age, as it is important for the patient to exhale into expiratory reserve volume to achieve oscillation of the smaller airways.

High-frequency chest compression

Mechanical ventilation via high-frequency oscillation had been noted to cause an increase in bronchial secretions.

King and co-workers [67,68] in a set of early experiments established that high-frequency chest wall oscillation increased tracheal mucus clearance rates by as much as 240–340% of controls. These observations led to the development of 'The Vest®'.

HFCC is proposed to increase mucociliary clearance by increasing an expiratory flow bias. This cephalad flow bias is purported to be the main mechanism of mucus clearance in smaller airways with ventilation (as opposed to convection) airflow. It is associated with a tendency towards shearing mucus and movement centrally [69,70]. Rubin and co-workers [71] compared a percussor to an oscillator. The percussor produced an expiratory flow rate of 0.25 L/s at 40 Hz but no significant change in mucus velocity, whereas the oscillator caused a 2–3 L/s flow with an unbiased sine wave at 13 Hz and increased mucus velocity by 204% ($p < 0.003$) [72]. Another mechanism by which HFCC theoretically enhances secretion clearance is by decreasing the viscoelasticity of mucus. Tomkiewicz and co-workers [72] and App and colleagues [44] demonstrated that high-frequency oscillation applied *in vitro* to mucus or mucus analogues caused a decrease viscoelasticity, and the higher the frequency the greater the decrease.

Multiple versions of HFCC vests exist, but each consists of a compressor system which delivers large volumes of air at high frequencies attached to a non-stretchable inflatable vest which is worn by the patient over the thorax (Fig. 29.7). The waveform of the pressure pulse delivered varies with the vest device used (square wave for ThAirPy, ABI and Hill-Rom 101 and 102; sine wave for 103, 104, MedPulse and Smart-Pulse; and triangular wave for inCourage System®). Detailed reading of the airway clearance technique literature is critical, as variations and misinterpretations of techniques are common and possible differences due to wave form from the device used should also be considered. Review and evaluation of the literature on HFCC requires careful attention to the device used [73,74].

Pressure pulses that inflate the vest and frequencies that vibrate the chest wall are controlled by the patient. Pulse

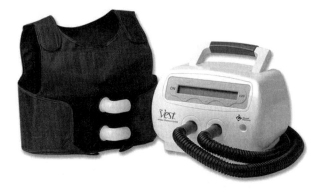

Figure 29.7 The Vest® Airway Clearance System. © 2005 Hill-Rom Services, Inc. Reprinted with permission – all rights reserved.

frequency is adjustable from 5 to 25 Hz, with pressure settings varying from zero to 19 cmH_2O. For most vests, although lower frequencies oscillate more volume for a given pressure setting, higher frequencies cause higher oscillating flow rates and higher flows cause more shear force. Increasing pressure settings increases both flow and volume, but is usually associated with greater discomfort.

For HFCC from vests generating sine waveforms, therapy is performed by fitting the vest snuggly but with enough room to slide the flat of the hand between vest and chest. The vest is set to oscillate for 5 minutes at frequencies of 6, 8, 9, 18, 19 and 20 Hz (30 minutes) at the highest pressure comfortable for the patient. At the conclusion of each 5 minutes the tubing is disconnected from the vest to allow it to deflate and to allow the patient to take a deeper breath. The patient should then cough or huff for 1–2 minutes to clear secretions mobilized at that frequency setting. The vest is then reconnected and the frequency advanced. The advantage of the newest (inCourage System) vests is the delivery of triangular waveform pulse pressures and reportedly the largest airflows and air volumes both occur over the same frequency range of 5–11 Hz [74].

HFCC was found to provide clinically effective airway clearance in a retrospective comparison trial in cystic fibrosis by FEV_1 and sputum production [75]. A randomized, controlled study showed increased sputum production with HFCC compared with PD&P [76], although the PD&P intervention appeared to be shorter than standard therapy, and possibly shorter than the HFCC treatment in this study. Arens and co-workers [77] evaluated HFCC and PD&P in hospitalized patients, reporting equivalence in efficacy and safety (HFCC produced significantly greater wet-weight sputum). For some patients, perhaps especially those with end-stage disease or low vital capacities, the inflated vest may cause a sense of constriction and inability to inhale an adequate breath. Decreased end-expiratory lung volumes have been documented with use of the vest [78], raising the concern of developing atelectasis (although no reports of these complications have been published). Studies have documented improved oscillatory flows with HFCC and positive end-expiratory pressure in CF [79,80]. A recent small,

short-term study showed improved pulmonary function and sputum weight following ACBT compared with HFCC using the Hayek Oscillator® (waveform not reported) [81]. There are patients who also object to the device because of discomfort or pain from the inflated vest (compressing breast tissue, surgical sites, indwelling catheters). Concern has been voiced regarding the cost of the device (US$15 000), but a cost analysis showed an actual decrease in aggregate healthcare cost following institution of HFCC [82]. This apparent improvement may be overstated as pre-healthcare cost included home PD&P treatments.

There are no studies of HFCC in infants, but the treatment is usually well tolerated by young children who often laugh through it. The vest comes in several sizes, pediatric to adult. The smallest vest will fit a child with a measured chest circumference of 48 cm.

Intrapulmonary percussive ventilation (IPV)

Because of the aforementioned mobilization of secretions during ventilation with high-frequency oscillation, IPV was developed. IPV delivers continuous oral oscillating pressures during both inhalation and exhalation (whereas OscPEP occurs only during exhalation). Treatment involves the setting of proximal pressure (inspiratory peak and expiratory peak pressures, usually for a ΔP of approximately 10 cm), percussive frequency which may vary from 6 to 24 Hz (usually 6–12 Hz) and the inspiratory/expiratory (I:E) ratio (usually 1:1.5 to 1:2.5). Duration of therapy is generally recommended to be shorter than other airway clearance modalities: 1–7 minutes.

In theory, the modality improves airway clearance by several means. Mucus viscosity is decreased with exposure to high-frequency oscillation. During inspiration, high-frequency air pulses expand the lungs, vibrate and enlarge the airways, and deliver gas into distal lung segments beyond accumulated mucus [83]. It is further hypothesized that, due to the percussive amplitude of shaking airways, mucus is dislodged. In a similar way to high-frequency oscillation, IPV should decrease asynchronous ventilation and improve gas exchange by oscillatory movement and migration of oxygen (room air).

Studies on IPV are not extensive and it is not commonly used as other techniques should be considered first, but the literature does support its efficacy. Its cost is less than for HFCC, but still significant (US$1600). Comparison of IPV to PD&P over 6 months showed no significant difference in pulmonary function, number of hospital admissions or courses of antibiotics, with the conclusion of equal efficacy [84]. Evaluation of IPV and flutter versus PD&P showed no difference between sputum production or pulmonary function. All showed a trend to decrease lung volumes, suggesting less gas trapping [85]. A study comparing IPV, HFCC and PD&P in hospitalized patients revealed increased wet sputum weight from IPV and HFCC compared with PD&P, but no change in dry sputum weight or pulmonary function

[86]. Patient preference for IPV was equal to PD&P and less than HFCC. There was no statistically significant difference in group preference. IPV is usually delivered via mouthpiece, although a mask can be used. Reports of its use in infants or younger children have yet to be published.

Anecdotal reports of adverse events suggest an increased incidence of pneumothorax. However, there are no large series, and pneumothoraces occur spontaneously in cystic fibrosis, so it is unclear whether IPV was causative or coincidental. There are also anecdotal reports of dilated bronchiectatic airways in CF patients using IPV [87]. Until larger, longer, prospective studies of IPV delineate the true risks of adverse events with this therapy, care providers should remain vigilant for signs of complications and adverse events.

Resistive inspiratory maneuvers

Repeated maximum inspiratory vital capacity maneuvers against a fixed resistance have been shown to improve inspiratory muscle function when used for an 8-week period in people with cystic fibrosis [88]. The same technique has also been used for airway clearance and more sputum was expectorated with resistive inspiratory maneuvers than with the ACBT in some [89] but not other [90] patients.

Chatham and co-workers [89] acknowledge that airway clearance techniques have aimed to increase expiratory flow with resultant high shearing forces, to loosen and mobilize excess secretions from the smaller peripheral to the larger more central airways. With the resistive inspiratory maneuvers method the subject is required to carry out a full inspiratory vital capacity maneuver at 80% of maximal pressure by breathing against a fixed resistance. The maximum pressure is that developed between residual volume and total lung capacity. This increases inspiratory time, and it is hypothesized that resistive inspiratory maneuvers may increase inspiratory airflow to more peripheral airways, with consequent shearing forces acting on airway secretions during the inspiratory phase. This may reduce the need for higher expiratory flows. Further work needs to be undertaken in this area.

EXERCISE

Exercise is discussed in detail in Chapters 25a and 25b. Exercise has been identified as an adjunct to airway clearance and is sometimes used as an alternative to airway clearance. A meta-analysis of PEP, forced expiration technique (FET), AD, exercise and 'standard physical therapy' (PD&P) looked at outcomes of FEV_1, sputum weight or sputum clearance. PD&P significantly increased sputum expectoration above no treatment, and only exercise and PD&P increased FEV_1 above PD&P alone [24]. There are few data to suggest precisely how it improves clearance. Recently, exercise was shown to inhibit epithelial sodium channels in patients with CF, causing a partial normalization of potential difference, and therefore improved ion and water movement into airway secretions [91]. Weight-bearing exercise is also important in increasing bone mineral density (Chapter 18).

THE INFANT AND YOUNG CHILD

There is debate as to when airway clearance should be instigated in the asymptomatic infant [92]. In countries with neonatal screening, cystic fibrosis can be diagnosed at birth and the dilemma is whether or not to introduce airway clearance before the infant becomes symptomatic. There are several studies that document early signs of disease even in infants [93–95], but few studies that have looked at airway clearance at this age [96–98]. Traditionally postural drainage using the head-down tipped position and chest clapping was introduced at the time of diagnosis, but this regimen has been questioned because of worries about reflux disease in the young child [30]. Internationally there is support for treatment of the asymptomatic infant and young child, but PD&P is not the only available regimen. ACBT, PEP, HFCC and exercise can be introduced early in life and, as soon as the child is able to cooperate, other airway clearance regimens can be used.

CONTINENCE

Urinary incontinence, the involuntary loss of urine, is associated with adverse effects on quality of life [99] and for people with cystic fibrosis it is likely to reduce the effectiveness of and adherence to an airway clearance regimen. It is a problem that affects not only women, but also men and children with CF. A valid way in which to assess the problem is from the patient's perspective using psychometrically robust self-completion questionnaires [100]. The prevalence of incontinence in women with CF ranges from 38% to 68% [100–102], in men 16% [103], and in children (6–17 years of age) 14% to 33% [104,105], with a higher prevalence in females. The prevalence of urinary incontinence in the population without cystic fibrosis increases with increasing age up to 46% in women and 34% in men aged over 80 years [99]. For people with CF additional risk factors include coughing and, for some, poor nutrition of the perineal muscles [106]. There is the factor of pregnancy for women, and for both men and women with cystic fibrosis urinary incontinence increases with age and is inversely proportional to FEV_1 [102].

Treatment using pelvic floor muscle exercises has been shown to increase endurance of the pelvic floor muscles and consequently subjective improvement in symptoms, reduction in leakage, without improvement in pelvic floor muscle strength [106]. Urinary leakage is receiving increasing recognition in clinical practice leading to appropriate management for those willing to participate in treatment.

PREGNANCY

With increasing longevity and quality of life, the number of pregnancies in women with cystic fibrosis has increased. Modifications in airway clearance techniques and exercise may be required pre-partum and post-partum until lung function and exercise capacity return to normal. Dodd and Webb [107] have highlighted the implications of importance to physiotherapists including hormonal changes which may result in an increase in airway obstruction, breathlessness and bronchial wall instability, the reduction in functional residual capacity which may lead to early airway closure especially at the lung bases with a consequent increase in the retention of secretions, and hypoxemia which may result from ventilation–perfusion mismatch. Although debatable, loss of lung function as a consequence of pregnancy may not be permanent [108].

SPECIAL SITUATIONS

Hemoptysis

Blood streaking of sputum is a frequent occurrence in people with CF, but is not usually a reason to alter the physiotherapy regimen. In cases of frank hemoptysis, it is appropriate to discontinue airway clearance temporarily until the bleeding begins to settle. It is important to restart treatment using airway clearance techniques as soon as possible to avoid the accumulation of old blood in the airways and retention of sputum. Theoretically, since AD and ACBT minimize coughing they may be less likely to dislodge new clot formation. If embolization is necessary, physiotherapy can be restarted soon after the procedure.

Pneumothorax

A small pneumothorax is not a contraindication to physiotherapy, but when a large pneumothorax requires intercostal drainage, physiotherapy should be withheld until the drain has been inserted.

If surgical intervention is undertaken and a patent throcotomy tube is present, physiotherapy is important preoperatively and should be restarted as soon as possible postoperatively. High humidification, probably combined with oxygen therapy, should assist the clearance of secretions. Effective analgesia is essential.

Chest wall stiffness and changes in posture

Chronic lung disease leads to structural and functional changes in the muscles and connective tissues of the chest wall, abdomen, spine and pelvis. Chest strength and mobility training can lead to improvements in posture, chest wall mobility and body strength in addition to subjective improvements in well-being [109].

Critical care

If a patient is admitted for critical care management, physiotherapy for both airway clearance and rehabilitation should be continued.

Transplantation

The physiotherapist should be involved both before and after lung transplantation. Cardiopulmonary rehabilitation programs have demonstrated improvements in exercise ability and quality of life in patients awaiting transplantation surgery. Postoperatively, rehabilitation is essential to gain maximum benefit from surgery and to improve quality of life [110].

Due to denervation of the lungs below the tracheal anastomosis, the normal awareness of excess bronchial secretions is lost and cilial function is less effective. Early recognition of signs of a chest infection is important to prevent pooling of secretions in the transplanted lung, which may lead to bronchiectasis. A short, daily assessment should be undertaken and an airway clearance regimen reinstated during periods of chest infection.

Terminal care

Physiotherapy and the physiotherapist become integral to the lives of people with cystic fibrosis and it is important that the physiotherapist continues to support the patient through the terminal stages of the disease. Initially this may be the setting up of nocturnal non-invasive ventilation, modifying the exercise program, and assessing and adapting as necessary the patient's airway clearance techniques. Near the end of life it is still important that the physiotherapist has a presence and does not withdraw from the terminal stages of care. The physical management, together with input from nursing and other members of the multidisciplinary team, may include the effective administration of inhaled drugs, management of non-invasive ventilation, positioning to optimize breathing and comfort, and pain control. If the patient is on non-invasive ventilation, alteration of the ventilator settings to support airway clearance during physiotherapy may be indicated. A device such as intermittent positive pressure breathing may be used to reduce the work of breathing and to assist airway clearance. Nasotracheal suction is not indicated as it would cause distress and serve no useful purpose in terminal care.

EVIDENCE-BASED MEDICINE

The sound physiological reasons and theories upon which the airway clearance techniques discussed are based, as well as scientific studies, support their use in cystic fibrosis. There are significant costs involved in the performance of airway clearance techniques – not just for the therapist's time in performance of a technique or training a patient or family, but perhaps even more significantly in the time that patients or families expend. Two excellent reviews have questioned the evidence supporting the use of any type of airway clearance [111,112]. Many studies show no significant change between a treated group or the control. In CF, most of the studies compare one technique with another because airway clearance has become standard care, and the ethical question of withholding treatment has almost eliminated true controls. The majority of studies are short or have small numbers of patients, thus decreasing their ability to determine a difference; and the consideration of statistical significance versus clinical significance must be considered. For example, a study showing $p < 0.005$ for an FEV_1 change of 3% from baseline is obviously statistically important, but is it of clinical importance?

Two approaches are necessary. Improved randomized, controlled trials of longer duration and larger sample size are essential. Until such studies are performed, the care provider (therapist and physician) is in a quandary as to whether and as to which ACT is appropriate for their patients. Until larger, randomized controlled studies are available, the care provider should use the 'n = 1' approach, where the patient acts as his or her own control. If an airway clearance seems appropriate, baseline values and observations of respiratory health should be obtained. An ACT should then be initiated and evaluated. The length of time before re-evaluation will vary dependent on the chronicity or acuteness of the disease process. If there has been no clinical improvement, the intervention should be discontinued and another trialled. If the patient has improved, the regimen should be continued.

EDUCATION AND ADHERENCE

Education on the part of the physiotherapist and patient must be an ongoing process. It starts at the time of diagnosis and continues lifelong. Adapting airway clearance and continuing education as the patient grows and the disease changes is imperative. The therapist must remain at the forefront of new techniques, medications and regimens. Time must be built into clinic, outpatient and inpatient settings to allow individual assessment and education sessions. As the patient's lung disease alters, so should airway clearance regimens. Therapists should take into account the developmental stage of the patient and family when prescribing or altering therapy.

Adherence with airway clearance is variable, but usually reported as low [1,2]. Reasons vary from 'time-consuming', 'boring', 'no immediate improvement' to 'I forgot!' Adherence is strongly related to education. It is important that the patient understands the basic concepts behind his or her airway clearance technique. The patient should also be trained at an early age to assess his or her own chest, respond

to subtle symptoms and report these findings to care providers. The therapist should develop open communication between the patient and the family. Consideration must be given to the cultural needs, socioeconomic status, psychology and lifestyle of the patient and family, understanding that certain techniques may be suited at one point in time, but will change with the demands of school or work, or as the disease alters.

CONCLUSION

Cystic fibrosis continues to be an unrelenting, progressive lung disease – highly variable from patient to patient, and within individual patients. Because of this, daily airway clearance should, until evidence indicates otherwise, be established at the time of diagnosis. Patients and their families should be given the educational tools necessary to make a choice with regard to airway clearance techniques and how and which techniques best fit into their daily routine. The emphasis should be on helping the family to lead as normal a life as possible. Fortunately there are now many choices of airway clearance techniques that can be tailored to the specific lung disease and lifestyle of the patient. There is no single 'ideal' airway clearance technique that is best for all patients. Frequent re-evaluation of the patient's disease and needs enables the therapist to vary, alter and 'fine tune' techniques, taking into account changing lung physiology and patient/family situation throughout the patient's lifetime.

Today's CF physiotherapists should have a toolbox that includes an individualized, evidence-based, creative, holistic approach, with frequent reassessments and fine-tuning of techniques in order to optimize lung health and general physical fitness.

REFERENCES

1. Muszynski-Kwan AT, Perlman R, Rivington-Law BA. Compliance with and effectiveness of chest physiotherapy in cystic fibrosis: a review. *Physiother Can* 1988; **40**:28–32.

2. Geiss SK, Hobbs SA, Hammersley-Maercklein G *et al.* Psychosocial factors related to perceived compliance with cystic fibrosis treatment. *J Clin Psychol* 1992; **48**:99–103.

3. Lapin CD. Airway physiology, autogenic drainage, and active cycle of breathing. *Respir Care* 2002; **47**:778–785.

4. Lopez-Vidriero MT, Reid L. Bronchial mucus in health and disease. *Br Med Bull* 1978; **34**:63–74.

5. Wood RE, Wanner A, Hirsch J, Farrell PM. Tracheal mucociliary transport in patients with cystic fibrosis and its stimulation by terbutaline. *Am Rev Respir Dis* 1975; **111**:733–738.

6. Fitzgerald DA, Hilton J, Jepson B, Smith L. A cross-over, randomized, controlled trial of dornase alfa before versus after physiotherapy in cystic fibrosis. *Pediatrics* 2005; **116**:e549–e554.

7. Menkes HA, Traystman RJ. Collateral ventilation. *Am Rev Respir Dis* 1977; **116**:287–309.

8. Mead J, Takishima T, Leith D. Stress distribution in lungs: a model of pulmonary elasticity. *J Appl Physiol* 1970; **28**:596–608.

9. Mead J, Turner JM, Macklem PT, Little JB. Significance of the relationship between lung recoil and maximum expiratory flow. *J Appl Physiol* 1967; **22**:95–108.

10. Zach MS, Oberwaldner B. Chest physiotherapy. In: Taussig L, Landau L (eds) *Textbook of Pediatric Respiratory Medicine*. St Louis, Mosby, 1999, pp299–311.

11. Rossman CM, Waldes R, Sampson D, Newhouse MT. Effect of chest physiotherapy on the removal of mucus in patients with cystic fibrosis. *Am Rev Respir Dis* 1982; **126**:131–135.

12. Pryor JA, Webber BA, Hodson ME, Batten JC. Evaluation of the forced expiration technique as an adjunct to postural drainage in treatment of cystic fibrosis. *Br Med J* 1979; **2**:417–418.

13. Clarke SW, Jones JG, Oliver DR. Resistance to two-phase gas-liquid flow in airways. *J Appl Physiol* 1970; **29**:464–471.

14. Sackner MA, Kim CS. Phasic flow mechanisms of mucus clearance. *Eur J Respir Dis* 1987; **153**(Suppl):159–164.

15. Bennett WD, Zeman KL. Effect of enhanced supramaximal flows on cough clearance. *J Appl Physiol* 1994; **77**:1577–1583.

16. Main E, Prasad A, van der Schans C. Conventional chest physiotherapy compared to other airway clearance techniques for cystic fibrosis (Cochrane review). In: *The Cochrane Library, Issue 2*. Chichester, John Wiley, 2005.

17. Accurso FJ, Sontag MK, Koenig M, Quittner AL. Multi-center airway secretion clearance study in cystic fibrosis. *Pediatr Pulmonol* 2004; Suppl 27:314.

18. Pryor JA. A comparison of five airway clearance techniques in the treatment of people with cystic fibrosis. Thesis submitted for the degree of Doctor of Philosophy, Imperial College London, 2005.

19. Flower KA, Eden RI, Lomax L *et al.* New mechanical aid to physiotherapy in cystic fibrosis. *Br Med J* 1979; **2**:630–631.

20. Menkes H, Britt J. Physical therapy rationale for physical therapy. *Am Rev Respir Dis* 1980; **122**(Suppl 2):127–131.

21. Lannefors L, Wollmer P. Mucus clearance with three chest physiotherapy regimes in cystic fibrosis: a comparison between postural drainage, PEP and physical exercise. *Eur Respir J* 1992; **5**:748–753.

22. Desmond KJ, Schwenk WF, Thomas E *et al.* Immediate and long-term effects of chest physiotherapy in patients with cystic fibrosis. *J Pediatr* 1983; **103**:538–542.

23. Reisman JJ, Rivington-Law B, Corey M *et al.* Role of conventional physiotherapy in cystic fibrosis. *J Pediatr* 1988; **113**:632–636.

24. Thomas J, Cook DJ, Brooks D. Chest physical therapy management with cystic fibrosis: a meta-analysis. *Am J Respir Care Med* 1995; **151**:846–850.

25. Van der Schans C, Prasad A, Main E. Chest physiotherapy compared to no chest physiotherapy for cystic fibrosis. *Cochrane Database of Systematic Reviews* 2003; **1**:1–36.

26. Cecins NM, Jenkins SC, Pengelley J, Ryan G. The active cycle of breathing techniques: to tip or not to tip? *Respir Med* 1999; **93**: 660–665.

27. McDonnell T, McNicholas WT, FitzGerald MX. Hypoxaemia during chest physiotherapy in patients with cystic fibrosis. *Irish J Med Sci* 1986; **155**:345–348.

28. Laws AK, McIntyre RW. Chest physiotherapy: a physiological assessment during IPPV in respiratory failure. *Can Anaest Soc J* 1969; **16**:487–493.

29. Wollmer P, Ursing K, Midgren B, Eriksson L. Inefficiency of chest percussion in the physical therapy of chronic bronchitis. *Eur J Respir Dis* 1985; **66**:233–239.

30. Button BM, Heine RG, Catto-Smith AG *et al.* Chest physiotherapy in infants with cystic fibrosis: to tip or not? A five-year study. *Pediatr Pulmonol* 2003; **35**:208–213.

31. Phillips GE, Pike SE, Rosenthal M, Bush A. Holding the baby: head downwards positioning for physiotherapy does not cause gastro-oesophageal reflux. *Eur Respir J* 1998; **12**:954–957.

32. Chevaillier J. Thoracic expansion exercises. Personal communication, 2000.

33. Thompson B, Thompson HT. Forced expiration exercises in asthma and their effect on FEV_1. *NZ J Physiother* 1968; **3**:19–21.

34. Selsby D, Jones JG. Some physiological and clinical aspects of chest physiotherapy. *Br J Anaesth* 1990; **64**:621–631.

35. West JB. *Pulmonary Pathophysiology*, 5th edn. Baltimore, Williams & Wilkins, 1997.

36. Freitag L, Bremme J, Schroer M. High frequency oscillation for respiratory physiotherapy. *Br J Anaesth* 1989; **63** (Suppl 1):44S–46S.

37. Chevaillier J. Autogenic drainage. In: Lawson D (ed.) *Cystic Fibrosis Horizons*. Chichester, John Wiley, 1984, p235.

38. Schöni MH. Autogenic drainage: a modern approach to chest physiotherapy in cystic fibrosis. *J R Soc Med* 1989; **82** (Suppl 16):32–37.

39. Dab I, Alexander F. The mechanism of autogenic drainage studied with flow volume curves. *Monogr Paediat* 1979; **10**:50–53.

40. Pfleger A, Theissl B, Oberwalder B, Zach MS. Self-administered chest physiotherapy in cystic fibrosis: a comparative study of high-pressure PEP and autogenic drainage. *Lung* 1992; **170**:323–330.

41. Davidson AGF, Wong LTK, Pirie GE, McIlwaine PM. Long-term comparative trial of conventional percussion and drainage physiotherapy to autogenic drainage in in cystic fibrosis. *Pediatr Pulmonol* 1992; Suppl 8:A235.

42. Miller S, Hall DO, Clayton CB, Nelson R. Chest physiotherapy in cystic fibrosis: a comparative study of autogenic drainage and the active cycle of breathing techniques with postural drainage and percussion. *Thorax* 1995; **50**:165–169.

43. Giles DR, Wagener J, Accurso F, Butler-Simon N. Short-term effects of postural drainage with clapping vs autogenic drainage on oxygen saturation and sputum recovery in patients with cystic fibrosis. *Chest* 1995; **108**:952–954.

44. App EM, Kieselmann R, Reinhardt D *et al.* Sputum rheology changes in cystic fibrosis lung disease following two

different types of physiotherapy: flutter vs autogenic drainage. *Chest* 1998; **114**:171–177.

45. Andersen JB, Jespersen W. Demonstration of intersegmental respiratory bronchioles in normal human lungs. *Eur J Respir Dis* 1980; **61**:337–341.

46. Elad D, Schochat A, Shiner RJ. Computational model of oscillatory airflow in a bronchial bifurcation. *Respir Physiol* 1998; **112**:95–111.

47. Zach MS, Oberwaldner B, Forche G, Polgar G. Bronchodilators increase airway instability in cystic fibrosis. *Am Rev Respir Dis* 1985; **131**:537–543.

48. Falk M, Kelstrup M, Andersen JB et al. Improving the ketchup bottle method with positive expiratory pressure, PEP, in cystic fibrosis. *Eur J Respir Dis* 1984; **65**:423–432.

49. Mortensen J, Falk M, Groth S, Jensen C. The effects of postural drainage and positive expiratory pressure physiotherapy on tracheobronchial clearance in cystic fibrosis. *Chest* 1991; **100**:1350–1357.

50. McIlwaine PM, Wong LT, Peacock D, Davidson AG. Long-term comparative trial of conventional postural drainage and percussion versus positive expiratory pressure physiotherapy in the treatment of cystic fibrosis. *J Pediatr* 1997; **131**:570–574.

51. Elkins MR, Jones A, van der Schans C. Positive expiratory pressure physiotherapy for airway clearance in people with cystic fibrosis (Cochrane review). In: *The Cochrane Library, Issue 4.* Chichester, John Wiley, 2004.

52. Oberwaldner B. High-pressure PEP. In: International Physiotherapy Group for Cystic Fibrosis (ed.) *Physiotherapy in the Treatment of Cystic Fibrosis* 2002, pp20–23. Available at www.cfww.org/IPG-CF/index.asp.

53. Oberwaldner B, Evans JC, Zach MS. Forced expirations against a variable resistance: a new chest physiotherapy method in cystic fibrosis. *Pediatr Pulmonol* 1986; **6**:358–367.

54. Schibler A, Casaulta C, Kraemer R. Rationale of oscillatory breathing as chest physiotherapy performed by the Flutter in patients with cystic fibrosis. *Pediatr Pulmonol* 1992; Suppl 2:301.

55. Lindeman H. The value of physical therapy with VRP1 Destin (Flutter). [in German]. *Pneumologie* 1992; **46**:626–630.

56. Volsko TA, DiFiore JM, Chatburn RL. Performance comparison of two oscillating positive pressure devices: Acapella versus Flutter. *Respir Care* 2003; **48**:124–130.

57. Cegla UH. Physiotherapy with oscillating PEP systems (RC-Cornet, VRP1) [in German]. *Pneumologie* 2000; **54**:440–446.

58. Blackney DA, Chipps B. Comparison of airway pressure and oscillation frequency of four airway clearance devices. *Pediatr Pulmonol* 1999; Suppl 16:430.

59. Althaus P. Oscillating PEP – Flutter therapy. In: International Physiotherapy Group for Cystic Fibrosis (ed.) *Physiotherapy in the Treatment of Cystic Fibrosis* 2002, pp24–26. Available at www.cfww.org/IPG-CF/index.asp.

60. Konstan MW, Stern RC, Doershuk CF. Efficacy of the flutter device for airway mucus clearance in patients with cystic fibrosis. *J Pediatr* 1994; **124**:689–693.

61. Gondor M, Nixon PA, Mutich R et al. Comparison of the Flutter device and chest physical therapy in the treatment of

cystic fibrosis pulmonary exacerbation. *Pediatr Pulmonol* 1999; **28**:255–260.

62. Pryor JA, Webber BA, Hodson ME, Warner JO. The Flutter VRP1 as an adjunct to chest physiotherapy in cystic fibrosis. *Respir Med* 1994; **88**:677–681.

63. Oermann CM, Sockrider MM, Giles D et al. Comparison of high frequency chest wall oscillation and oscillatory positive expiratory pressure in the home management of cystic fibrosis: a pilot study. *Pediatr Pulmonol* 2001; **32**:372–377.

64. Patterson JE, Bradley JM, Hewitt O et al. Airway clearance in bronchiectasis: a randomized crossover trial of active cycle of breathing techniques versus Acapella. *Respiration* 2005; **72**:239–242.

65. van Winden CM, Visser A, Hop W et al. Effects of flutter and PEP mask physiotherapy on symptoms and lung function in children with cystic fibrosis. *Eur Respir J* 1998; **12**:143–147.

66. McIlwaine PM, Wong LT, Peacock D, Davidson AGF. Long-term comparative trial of positive expiratory pressure versus oscillating positive expiratory pressure (flutter) physiotherapy in the treatment of cystic fibrosis. *J Pediatr* 2001; **138**:845–850.

67. King M, Phillips DM, Gross D et al. Enhanced tracheal mucus clearance with high frequency chest wall compression. *Am Rev Respir Dis* 1983; **128**:511–515.

68. King M, Phillips DM, Zidulka A, Chang HK. Tracheal mucus clearance in high frequency oscillation. II: Chest wall versus mouth oscillation. *Am Rev Respir Dis* 1984; **130**:703–706.

69. Chang HK, Weber ME, King M. Mucus transport by high-frequency nonsymmetrical oscillatory airflow. *J Appl Physiol* 1988; **65**:1203–1209.

70. Gross D, Zidulka A. Peripheral mucociliary clearance with high frequency chest wall compression. *J Appl Physiol* 1985; **58**:1157–1163.

71. Rubin E, Scantlen GE, Chapman GA et al. Effect of chest wall oscillation on mucus clearance: comparison of two vibrators. *Pediatr Pulmonol* 1989; **6**:122–126.

72. Tomkiewicz RP, Biviji AA, King M. Effects of oscillating air on the rheological properties and clearability for mucus gel simulant. *Biorheology* 1994; **124**:689–693.

73. Milla CM, Hansen LG, Weber A, Warwick WJ. High frequency chest compression: effect of the third generation compression waveform. *Biomed Instrum Technol* 2004; **38**:32–38.

74. Warwick WJ. High-frequency chest compression. In: Button B, McIlwaine M (eds) *Airway Clearance Techniques Training Class*. North American Cystic Fibrosis Conference, 2005.

75. Warwick WJ, Hansen LG. The long-term effect of high-frequency chest compression therapy on pulmonary complications of cystic fibrosis. *Pediatr Pulmonol* 1991; **11**:265–271.

76. Kluft J, Beker, L, Castagnino M et al. A comparison of bronchial drainage treatments in cystic fibrosis. *Pediatr Pulmonol* 1996; **22**:271–274.

77. Arens R, Gozal D Omlin KJ et al. Comparison of high frequency chest compression and conventional chest physiotherapy in hospitalized patients with cystic fibrosis. *Am J Respir Crit Care Med* 1994; **150**:1154–1157.

78. Jones RL, Lester RT, Brown NE. Effects of high frequency chest compression on respiratory system mechanics in normal and cystic fibrosis patients. *Can Respir J* 1995; **2**:40–46.

79. Perry RJ, Man GCW, Jones RL. Effects of positive end-expiratory pressure on oscillated flow rate during high frequency chest compression. *Chest* 1998; **113**:1028–1033.

80. Dosman CF, Zuberbuhler PC. Effects of positive end-expiratory pressure on oscillated flow rate during high frequency chest compression in children with cystic fibrosis. *Can Respir J* 2003; **10**:94–98.

81. Phillips GE, Pike SE, Jaffe A, Bush A. Comparison of active cycle of breathing and high-frequency oscillation jacket in children with cystic fibrosis. *Pediatr Pulmonol* 2004; **37**:71–75.

82. Ohnsorg F. A cost analysis of high-frequency chest wall oscillation in cystic fibrosis. *Am J Resp Crit Care Med* 1994; **149**:A669.

83. Langenderfer B. Alternatives to percussion and postural drainage, autogenic drainage, positive expiratory pressure, flutter valve, intrapulmonary percussive ventilation, and high frequency chest compression with the ThAIRpy vest. *J Cardiopulmon Rehabil* 1998; **18**:283–289.

84. Homnick DN, White F, deCastro C. Comparison of the effects of an intrapulmonary percussive ventilator to standard aerosol and chest physiotherapy in cystic fibrosis. *Pediatr Pulmonol* 1995; **20**:50–55.

85. Newhouse PA, White F, Marks JH, Homnick DN. The intrapulmonary percussive ventilator and flutter device compared to standard chest physiotherapy in patients with cystic fibrosis. *Clin Pediatr* 1998; **37**:427–432.

86. Varekojis SM, Douce FH, Flucke RL *et al.* A comparison of the therapeutic effectiveness of and preference for postural drainage and percussion, intrapulmonary percussive ventilation, and high-frequency chest compression in hospitalized cystic fibrosis patients. *Respir Care* 2003; **48**:24–28.

87. Wagener JS, Headley AA. Cystic fibrosis: current trends in respiratory care. *Respir Care* 2003; **48**:234–245.

88. Enright S, Chatham K, Ionescu AA *et al.* Inspiratory muscle training improves lung function and exercise capacity in adults with cystic fibrosis. *Chest* 2004; **126**:405–411.

89. Chatham K, Ionescus AA, Nixon LS, Shale DJ. A short-term comparison of two methods of sputum expectoration in cystic fibrosis. *Eur Respir J* 2004; **23**:435–439.

90. Patterson JE, Bradley JM, Elborn JS. Airway clearance in bronchiectasis: a randomized crossover trial of active cycle of breathing techniques (incorporating postural drainage and vibration) versus test of incremental respiratory endurance. *Chron Respir Dis* 2004; **1**:127–130.

91. Hebestreit A, Kerstin U, Basler B *et al.* Exercise inhibits epithelial sodium channels in patients with cystic fibrosis. *Am J Respir Crit Care Med* 2001; **164**:443–446.

92. Pryor JA, Main E, Agent P, Bradley JM. Physiotherapy. In Bush A *et al.* (eds) *Cystic Fibrosis.* Basel, Karger, 2006.

93. Abman SH, Ogle JW, Harbeck RJ *et al.* Early bacteriologic, immunologic, and clinical courses of young infants with cystic fibrosis identified by neonatal screening. *J Pediatr* 1991; **119**:211–217.

94. Frederick R, Long MD, Roger S *et al.* Structural airway abnormalities in infants and young children with cystic fibrosis. *J Pediatr* 2004; **144**:154–161.

95. Davis S, Jones M, Kisling J *et al.* Comparison of normal infants and infants with cystic fibrosis using forced expiratory flow breathing air and heliox. *Pediatr Pulmonol* 2001; **31**:17–23.

96. Ratjen F, Paul K, Van Koningsbruggen S *et al.* DNA concentrations in BAL fluid of cystic fibrosis patients with early lung disease:influence of treatment with dornase alpha. *Pediatr Pulmonol* 2005; **39**:1–4.

97. Hardy KA, Wolfson MR, Schidlow DV, Shaffer TH. Mechanics and energetics of breathing in newly diagnosed infants with cystic fibrosis: effect of combined bronchodilator and chest physical therapy. *Pediatr Pulmonol* 1989; **6**:103–108.

98. Maayan C, Bar-Yishay E, Yaacobi T *et al.* Immediate effect of various treatments on lung function in infants with cystic fibrosis. *Respiration* 1989; **55**:144–151.

99. Scottish Intercollegiate Guidelines Network. *Management of Urinary Incontinence in Primary Care,* 2004, p79. Available at www.sign.ac.uk/pdf/sign.

100. White D, Stiller K, Roney F. The prevalence and severity of symptoms of incontinence in adult cystic fibrosis patients. *Physiother Theory Pract* 2000; **16**:35–42.

101. Orr A, McVean RJ, Webb AK, Dodd ME. Questionnaire survey of urinary incontinence in women with cystic fibrosis. *Br Med J* 2001; **322**:1521.

102. Cornacchia M, Zenorini A, Perobelli S *et al.* Prevalence of urinary incontinence in women with cystic fibrosis. *BJU Int* 2001; **88**:44–48.

103. Gumery L, Lee J, Whitehouse J, Honeybourne D. The prevalence of urinary incontinence in adult cystic fibrosis males. *J Cyst Fibros* 2005; **4**(Suppl 1):S97.

104. Prasad A, Francis J, Johnson P *et al.* A comparison of the prevalence of urinary incontinence in girls with cystic fibrosis and asthma. *Pediatr Pulmonol* 2002; Suppl 24:316.

105. Moraes T, Carpenter S, Taylor L. Cystic fibrosis incontinence in children. *Pediatr Pulmonol* 2002; Suppl 24:315.

106. McVean RJ, Orr A, Webb AK *et al.* Treatment of urinary incontinence in cystic fibrosis. *J Cyst Fibros* 2003; **2**:171–176.

107. Dodd ME, Webb AK. Bronchiectasis, primary cilia dyskinesia, and cystic fibrosis. In: Pryor JA, Prasad SA (eds) *Physiotherapy for Respiratory and Cardiac Problems,* 3rd edn. Edinburgh, Churchill Livingstone, 2002, p608.

108. Goss CH, Rubenfeld GD, Otto K, Aitken ML. The effect of pregnancy on survival in women with cystic fibrosis. *Chest* 2003; **124**:1460–1468.

109. Demry A, Ben Ami S, Levi M *et al.* Chest strength and mobility training: a new approach to airways clearance. *J Cyst Fibros* 2006; **5**(Suppl 1):S82.

110. Bray CE. Cardiopulmonary transplantation. In: Pryor JA, Prasad SA (eds) *Physiotherapy for Respiratory and Cardiac Problems,* 3rd edn. Edinburgh, Churchill Livingstone, 2002, pp517–535.

111. Wallis C, Prasad A. Who needs chest physiotherapy? Moving from anecdote to evidence. *Arch Dis Child* 1999; **80**:393–397.

112. Hess DR. The evidence for secretion clearance techniques. *Respir Care* 2001; **46**:1276–1292.

30

Nutritional aspects

SUE WOLFE AND SARAH COLLINS

INTRODUCTION

The dietetic management of cystic fibrosis (CF) is an important and integral part of modern care. In the past, malnutrition and poor growth were inevitable consequences of the condition [1]. Reduced respiratory muscle function [2], decreased exercise tolerance [3] and immunological impairment contributed to an increased susceptibility to infections and higher morbidity and mortality rates. Over the last few decades there have been many advances in both the respiratory and nutritional management of CF and most patients should now be well nourished. Long-term nutritional support has been shown to improve nutritional status [4] and stabilize (or slow) the rate of decline in lung function [5,6]. Recent studies have also shown that nutritional status has an important prognostic significance, with poor body weight [7] and height [8] being independent risk factors for early death.

In order to optimize nutritional status it is essential that all patients receive regular expert dietetic review. Advice should be age-specific, and nutritional care plans and interventions must suit the patient's needs, lifestyle and clinical status. The aims of dietetic management are to ensure patients achieve normal weight gain, growth, body composition and bone health, pubertal development and vitamin, mineral and essential fatty acid (EFA) status. The improvement in life expectancy has also created new nutritional challenges such as the treatment of CF-related diabetes (CFRD), osteoporosis, pregnancy and transplantation.

NUTRITIONAL REQUIREMENTS

Energy requirements vary widely and depend on age, gender, nutritional status, lung function and presence of pancreatic insufficiency. Energy needs are generally quoted to be 120–150% of those required by healthy individuals of the same age and gender [9]. Undernutrition results from an unfavorable energy balance between increased energy expenditure and losses and a reduced energy intake.

Increased energy expenditure

Infection, inflammation, deteriorating lung function and possibly a genetic component of CF [10,11] increase resting energy expenditure (REE). An abnormal adaptive response to malnutrition results in an increase in muscle protein catabolism and poor tolerance to acute infections [12]. Drugs such as salbutamol may also increase REE [13].

Increased energy losses

Despite pancreatic enzyme replacement therapy (PERT) maldigestion and malabsorption may still contribute to increased energy losses [14]. Undiagnosed or inadequately treated CFRD may also increase energy losses through glycosuria.

Reduced energy intakes

Many patients fail to meet recommended energy intakes with dietary fat providing approximately 35–40% of the energy [15,16]. Anorexia is often present and dietary intakes may be inadequate to maintain or support normal weight gain and growth. Other factors such as food dislikes, gastroesophageal reflux (GER), increased sputum production, abdominal pain, vomiting and psychosocial problems may contribute.

In order to promote growth and development, a diet high in energy and protein with adequate PERT should be advised. In practice, if high energy intakes are achieved sufficient dietary protein is usually provided. It is important that children and adults with CF receive regular dietary reviews and assessment throughout their life to ensure optimal nutritional status is maintained both when well and during periods of infection.

Monitoring growth

Serial data on weight, height and – in children under 5 years of age – head circumference should be recorded on appropriate centile charts. The recommended frequency of recordings are shown below [17]:

- *children:* weight and height at each clinic visit;
- *adults:* weight at each clinic visit, height at each clinic visit until growth has ceased then annually.

When interpreting growth charts it is important to take into account the effects of delayed puberty (see Chapter 20). Body mass index (BMI) is also used to assess nutritional status in adults and children [18]. For children, BMI must be plotted on centile charts or converted to standard deviation (SD) values. The possibility of nutritional stunting must also be considered. The increasing use of dual-energy x-ray absorptiometry (DEXA) for detecting bone mineralization problems has provided the opportunity for more accurate and detailed assessment of body composition.

PANCREATIC ENZYME REPLACEMENT THERAPY

In northern Europe, approximately 95% of patients are pancreatic-insufficient (PI) [14] and require pancreatic enzyme replacement therapy (PERT) to control the symptoms of malabsorption, achieve adequate weight gain and maintain a good nutritional status. If uncontrolled, malabsorption results in abdominal pain, frequent oily pale and offensive stools, poor growth, malnutrition and deficiencies of fat-soluble vitamins and EFA [14]. In addition to lack of pancreatic enzymes there are many other factors that contribute to maldigestion and malabsorption of nutrients (see Chapter 15a).

Pancreatic enzymes should be started if symptoms of malabsorption are obvious and PI should then be confirmed using fecal pancreatic elastase-1 [19]. If clinical symptoms of malabsorption are absent, PI should be confirmed before PERT is commenced (see Chapter 15b). Fecal pancreatic elastase-1 is also useful for annual monitoring of pancreatic-sufficient patients to identify the onset of PI [20].

All patients should receive enteric-coated acid-resistant pancreatic enzyme preparations (Table 30.1). Powdered and uncoated enzymes are largely ineffective and should

Table 30.1 Recommendations for pancreatic enzyme replacement therapy.

General
- Enzymes should be stored at room temperature and humidity
- The expiry date should not be exceeded – enzymes that have expired are less potent
- Pill cases are convenient for keeping enzymes in a pocket or bag
- Enzymes should be kept at places that are frequently visited

Infants
- Microsphere or mini-microsphere preparations should be used
- For every 120 mL of infant formula or breast milk an initial dose of one-half scoop of Creon Micro (2500 IU lipase) or one-quarter or one third capsule of Creon 10 000 (2500–3333 IU lipase) or one-half capsule Pancrease (2500 IU lipase) should be given. These doses equate to approximately 400–800 IU lipase/g of dietary fat
- Enzymes should be mixed with a small amount of formula, expressed breast milk or fruit pureé and given from a spoon. Exposure to hot food or food with a pH greater than 5.5 will reduce enzyme efficacy. The dose should be divided throughout the feed depending on symptoms
- The dose should be gradually increased according to clinical symptoms, appearance of the stools and objective assessment of weight gain, growth and absorption
- Once solid food is introduced, PERT should be adjusted according to fat intake. Regular advice from a dietitian is mandatory

Older children
- An initial dose of one or two capsules of Creon 10 000 (10 000–20 000 IU lipase) or two capsules of Pancrease (10 000 IU lipase) per meal and one-half to a full capsule Creon/Pancrease with fat-containing snacks should be given
- Enzymes should be given with all fat-containing foods. The dose should be worked out individually according to fat intake. 500–4000 IU lipase/g dietary fat is usually required
- Capsules can usually be swallowed whole at 3 or 4 years of age. If capsules are opened, the microspheres should be mixed with a small amount of fluid or solid and given from a spoon. They must not be crushed or chewed, as this will destroy the enzymatic activity
- The ideal timing of enzyme administration varies according to the individual. In general if meals are eaten quickly enzymes are best given at the beginning and middle of the meal. If meals are take over 30 minutes PERT is best given before, during and towards the end of the meal. Dividing the dose also avoids overdosing if food is refused half way through
- PERT should be gradually increased until symptoms of malabsorption are controlled
- Patients should be aware of foods/drinks that do not require PERT, such as fruit pastilles and vegetables
- Adherence problems should be openly discussed and advice should be given to help overcome these problems

PERT, pancreatic enzyme replacement therapy.

not be used routinely. In general, standard-strength enzymes containing 5000–10 000 IU of lipase per scoop/capsule are given to infants and children. High-strength preparations containing 25 000–40 000 IU of lipase per capsule may be used for adolescents and adults. The dose of enzymes required depends on the fat content of the food or drink taken. Educating patients about dose adjustment and timing of PERT is essential to achieve optimal absorption.

In the early 1990s following the occurrence of fibrosing colonopathy [21] the safety of some high-strength enzyme preparations was questioned (see Chapter 15a). The Committee on Safety of Medicines in the UK advised that preparations containing the copolymer Eudragit L30 D55 should not be given to children aged 15 years or less. They also advised that for any patient the daily dose of lipase should not usually exceed 10 000 IU/kg per day, regardless of the preparation used [22]. In practice, if the dietary fat intake is very high enzyme requirements may be slightly greater than this. If excessively high doses appear necessary, enzyme efficacy may be improved by using H_2 antagonists or proton pump inhibitors [23] to reduce gastric acid output. Using an alternative enzyme preparation may help as all enzymes have different pharmacological characteristics that affect their efficacy. Changing the timing of enzyme administration may also improve absorption because of individual variation in the rate at which enzymes and food leave the stomach [24]. If symptoms persist, a full gastrointestinal investigation should be performed to rule out other conditions, such as celiac disease, pancreatitis, bacterial overgrowth and cows' milk protein intolerance [14].

Monitoring and adherence with PERT

Regular dietetic assessment is essential to achieve optimal PERT [25]. Using symptoms alone to adjust doses may lead to both over- and underdosing as patients may fail to recognize malabsorption. A detailed review of the biochemical assessment of PERT is given in Chapter 15a and in a review by Borowitz and colleagues [19].

Poor adherence to enzyme therapy is relatively common and may be the cause of persisting malabsorption despite apparently optimal enzyme dosing. Patients may be embarrassed and reluctant to take enzymes in front of their friends. A persistently low fecal chymotrypsin level will help to identify this problem. Non-adherence to other medications (e.g. low fat-soluble vitamin levels despite the prescription of an adequate supplemental dose) also suggests non-adherence.

Constipation and distal intestinal obstructive syndrome

Constipation is relatively common in CF and in a few cases can result in distal intestinal obstructive syndrome (DIOS) [26]. Inconsistent or excessive enzyme doses can contribute to the problem [14]. These patients should receive a thorough assessment of the adequacy of PERT and titration of dose according to dietary fat intake. Enzyme doses should not be increased unless malabsorption is documented. Improving the patient's fluid and fiber intake may also help [27].

Ventilation and PERT

Enteric-coated pancreatic enzymes cannot be put down standard nasogastric (NG) and gastrostomy tubes. If a patient is unable to take enzymes orally a powdered preparation may be used. If the patient is fed continuously, small doses of powdered enzymes should be mixed with fluid and flushed down the tube every 2–3 hours. Alternatively enteric-coated enzymes can be dissolved in sodium bicarbonate solution and given in the same way. Giving a proton pump inhibitor preserves some of the enzymatic activity of these enzymes, which otherwise would be largely destroyed in the acid environment of the stomach.

Overnight feeds and PERT

All fat-containing elemental and polymeric feeds require PERT. The dose is worked out on an individual basis taking the type, fat content and rate of infusion of feed into consideration. If the feed is infused over a long period, only small enzyme doses may be required [28]. This may be partly due to the stimulation of gastric lipase activity [29]. The enzymes are usually given at the beginning and end of the feed [28].

VITAMIN SUPPLEMENTATION

Fat-soluble vitamin deficiency is common in untreated PI patients with CF [30]. Routine vitamin A, D and E supplements should be given to these patients from diagnosis (Table 30.2). Serum levels should be checked annually and doses adjusted accordingly [17,31]. Pancreatic-sufficient patients should have their serum fat-soluble vitamin levels

Table 30.2 Suggested doses of fat-soluble vitamins.

Age	Vitamin A (μg) (IU)	Vitamin D (μg) (IU)	Vitamin E (mg)	Vitamin Kª (mg)
<1 year	400–1500 (1333–5000)	10 (400)	10–50	5
>1 year	1200–3000 (4000–10 000)	10–50 (400–2000)	50–100	5–10
Adults	1200–3000 (4000–10 000)	20–50 (800–2000)	100–200	10

ªVitamin K supplements are currently used if the prothrombin time is increased or there is overt liver disease. However, they may be used routinely in the future due to the role of vitamin K in bone metabolism.

checked annually and supplementation started when levels are low [17].

Vitamin A

Vitamin A is important for vision, integrity and proliferation of epithelial cells and immunity. Low vitamin A levels are associated with poorer clinical status, impaired lung function [32], disturbed night vision and xerophthalmia [33]. Measurement of plasma retinol is unreliable with poor correlation between clinical and biochemical findings. Vitamin A is stored in the liver and plasma levels are unable to detect liver stores. Measurement of retinol binding protein (RBP) will help to interpret plasma vitamin A levels as RBP is the transport protein for vitamin A. Zinc deficiency depresses RBP levels and so zinc supplementation may be necessary if levels are low [34]. The concentration of retinol may also be depressed during acute infection so measurements should be taken during clinical stability [35]. Vitamin A is potentially toxic [36] and high intakes have also been associated with reduced bone mineral density [37], so doses should be increased with caution.

Vitamin D

Clinical deficiency of vitamin D is rare although low plasma 25-hydroxy-vitamin D levels have been reported [38]. Causes include malabsorption, poor dietary intakes, insufficient sunlight exposure and possible deficiency of vitamin D-binding protein. Plasma 25-hydroxy-vitamin D is a good indicator of vitamin D status although there is a wide seasonal variation [38]. Low vitamin D levels lead to reduced calcification of bone contributing to the development of osteopenia and osteoporosis (see Chapter 18) [39].

Vitamin E

Overt clinical symptoms of deficiency (hemolytic anemia, neuromuscular degeneration and retinal and cognitive deficits [40]) are rare. Vitamin E (alpha tocopherol) is, however, a powerful antioxidant that protects lipoprotein and cellular membranes against destruction, so it may have an important role in controlling the progression of lung disease. Serum levels vary according to levels of carrier lipoprotein, so vitamin E/fasting lipid ratio should be determined [17].

Vitamin K

Vitamin K is required for blood clotting and bone health. In addition to fat malabsorption patients with CF are at risk of developing deficiency due to liver disease, bile salt deficiency and antibiotic treatment. Vitamin K is usually only given to patients with abnormal prothrombin times.

However, prothrombin induced in vitamin K absence (PIVKA II) levels have shown vitamin K deficiency is common in most PI patients [41]. Undercarboxylated osteocalcin levels that measure the adequacy of vitamin K status for bone metabolism are also abnormal [42]. These recent findings have questioned the need for, and dose of, routine vitamin K supplementation for all patients.

Essential fatty acids

Biochemical deficiency of essential fatty acids (EFAs) – characterized by low levels of linoleic and α-linolenic acid and omega 3 long-chain polyunsaturated fatty acids such as eicosapentaenoic acid (EPA) and docosahexanoic acid (DHA) – is common in CF [43]. Clinical symptoms of deficiency are rare, but deficiency of EFA increases susceptibility to respiratory infections with *Staphylococcus* and *Pseudomonas* [44]. Deficiency may be partially caused by a defect in fatty acid metabolism related to the CF genotype [43,45]. The dose and type of EFA required is unknown and therefore further work is needed before routine supplementation is recommended [46].

Water-soluble vitamins

In general these vitamins are well absorbed in CF and supplementation is not necessary unless patients have inadequate dietary intakes [17]. Currently the roles of antioxidant vitamins are under investigation. Low levels of vitamin C have been reported in CF [47], and impaired status of vitamin E, glutathione and carotenoids disturb the protective antioxidant screen in CF [48].

PROVIDING NUTRITIONAL SUPPORT

Dietetic advice must take age, nutritional and pancreatic status, financial and family circumstance, religious and cultural dietary beliefs and food preferences into account. Most nutritional management guidelines recommend a staged intervention approach to nutritional support [17,40,48]. Increasing the energy content of the normal diet, oral calorie supplementation, behavioral interventions, enteral tube feeding and parenteral nutrition have all been shown to improve weight gain in patients with CF [4].

Feeding infants, toddlers and young children

An increasing number of infants are being diagnosed by neonatal screening (NS). Age at diagnosis is a critical determinant of nutritional status [49]. Early diagnosis gives the opportunity to prevent nutritional problems, including failure to thrive, anemia, vitamin deficiencies and hypoalbuminemia.

Most infants thrive on either demand breast-feeding or normal infant formulas [50,51]. Breast-feeding should be encouraged as breast milk contains lipase and beneficial nutritional and growth factors. If infant formula is used, 150–200 mL (100–130 cal) per kilogram per day will support normal growth. If catch-up growth is required, or malabsorption is difficult to control, energy requirements will be higher. Approximately 15% of infants are born with meconium ileus (MI). These infants are nutritionally compromised from birth, especially if surgical resection is required [52], and may benefit from a hydrolyzed protein, medium-chain triglyceride containing feed. Over 50% of the energy content of breast milk or formula is derived from fat and therefore infants with obvious malabsorption should commence PERT on diagnosis of CF. Delayed enzyme therapy will have a devastating effect on nutritional status. The importance of regular growth assessment in the first few months of life cannot be over-emphasized.

Gastroesophageal reflux (GER) is relatively common in infants with CF [53] and can compromise growth and exacerbate respiratory symptoms. Treatments include thickening the feed, using a pre-thickened formula, using motility stimulants and reducing gastric acid [54].

If weight gain is poor, increasing the feed volume, using a high-energy infant formula or additional energy supplementation should be considered. Occasionally failure to thrive may be related to, or exacerbated by, a poor sodium intake. The sodium content of normal infant formula is relatively low (approximately 1.6 mmol/kg body weight for every 200 mL/kg fed). Deficiency should be confirmed by serum levels and urine analysis for sodium content (<10 mmol/L). Supplementation with 1–2 mmol/kg should correct deficiency or prevent deficiency in hot climates. A small percentage of infants may develop cows' milk protein intolerance [55]. This should be treated with a protein hydrolysate formula.

Weaning foods should be introduced at 4–6 months of age and by the end of the first year a normal diet should have been introduced. As the diet becomes more varied the need for enzyme variation according to fat intake becomes greater (see above). Dietary counselling is essential throughout early childhood when long-term feeding habits are being established. As the child gets older, food is often used as an effective tool to obtain parental attention and behavioral food refusal can become a problem [56]. Unless carefully handled, this behavior can persist for a number of years resulting in a poor dietary intake and growth. Attention to the behavioral aspects of feeding has been shown to improve energy intakes [57] (Table 30.3).

Adolescents and adults

Adolescence is a physically and emotionally demanding period associated with increased nutritional requirements due to rapid physical growth, pubertal changes and increased physical activity. It is also a phase of developing

Table 30.3 Management of feeding behavior problems.

- Family meals should be encouraged, so meals become a social event. This will encourage correct feeding behavior
- Distractions should be avoided, such as having the television on at mealtimes
- Food that the child is likely to eat should be offered before trying to increase the variety
- Food should be as attractive as possible
- Small portions should be offered rather than over-facing the child and gentle encouragement should be given
- Ignore food refusal. In the child's eyes any reaction is attention and will encourage the bad behavior
- Praise should be given for 'good' or 'positive' behavior
- Mealtimes should be limited to 30 minutes. Allowing mealtimes to extend rarely results in more food being eaten. After 30 minutes food should be removed without comment
- A second meal should never be made if the first is refused
- Ensure there is a consistent approach from all involved with feeding

independence, autonomy and personal identity. There is a risk of disordered eating behavior in adolescents with chronic illness [58], so early identification and treatment of any eating disturbances in adolescents with CF is required [59]. Adolescence is a time when treatment adherence may need addressing. Coping strategies have been shown to influence the extent of adherence to treatment, with positive/optimistic coping enhancing quality of life and facilitating treatment adherence [60]. The prevalence of malnutrition increases with age [6]. Even in those with a normal BMI, a loss of fat-free mass occurs in those with severe lung disease [61]. Age-related complications of CF (e.g. CF-related diabetes and osteoporosis) lead to increased dietary challenges to maintain optimal nutritional status throughout adulthood.

IMPROVING THE ENERGY CONTENT OF THE DIET

Patients should be encouraged to eat a high-fat diet with the liberal use of high-fat snacks and fried food if weight gain is poor. The addition of butter, olive oil, cheese and cream to foods and small frequent meals and snacks will also help. The increased life expectancy of patients with CF has highlighted the need to ensure that the diet is cardioprotective, so mono- and poly-unsaturated fats and fruit and vegetables should also be encouraged.

USE OF ORAL NUTRITIONAL SUPPLEMENTS

If nutritional status remains poor despite encouraging a high-energy diet, nutritional supplements may be beneficial for some patients [62]. Modular products (e.g. glucose polymers and fat emulsions) supply additional energy to the diet and oral sip feeds can provide a wider variety of nutrients. A Cochrane review has suggested a lack of evidence of the value of these products for patients with CF [63], but this does not mean they are not of benefit to individuals. Supplements should be prescribed on an individual basis depending on the patient's age, preference and requirements. The quantity and timing of supplement intake is important as they should not replace food. Taste fatigue is often reported with long-term supplement use, so altering the flavor and type of supplement periodically may help to prevent this happening.

ENTERAL FEEDING

Nasogastric (NG) or gastrostomy feeding may be considered to provide long-term nutritional support in patients unable to meet their energy requirements. Enteral feeding has been shown to improve weight gain and nutritional status and to stabilize or slow the rate of decline in lung function [5,64]. Early intervention is associated with improved outcomes [5,65]. At present there are no randomized control trials to measure the efficacy of enteral feeding in CF [66].

Patient preference and clinical status determine the route for enteral feeding. Nasogastric feeding is usually considered prior to gastrostomy placement, during a respiratory exacerbation or as a less permanent method of nutritional support. The main disadvantage of NG feeding is that tubes can become dislodged by coughing, so gastrostomy feeding is preferred for long-term nutritional support.

The majority of patients receive nocturnal enteral feeds and are encouraged to continue with a high-energy diet throughout the day. A wide variety of enteral feeds are available and the feed chosen should be appropriate to the patient's nutritional requirements, lifestyle and clinical condition. The majority of patients tolerate a high-energy polymeric feed, but an elemental or semi-elemental feed may be beneficial for some. All feeds require PERT (see above) and it is important to monitor for glucose intolerance as a small dose of insulin may be required to cover the feed [17].

PARENTERAL NUTRITION

Parenteral nutrition is not routinely recommended for patients with CF due to the risk of complications, difficulty of administration and high cost [17]. It can be useful for short-term nutritional support following surgery where enteral nutrition is not possible.

APPETITE STIMULANTS AND ANABOLIC HORMONES

Appetite stimulants have been used to try to improve the appetite in patients with CF. Megestrol acetate has been found to improve weight and respiratory function [67]. Cyproheptadine hydrochloride has also been shown to improve the appetite in patients with CF [68].

The anabolic agents, insulin-like growth factor 1 and early insulin therapy [69], have also been studied in CF but evidence of their value is poor. Growth hormone has been shown to improve weight gain and growth [70,71], and

creatine supplementation has resulted in improved muscle strength, patient well-being and body weight [72]. However, most of the studies examining the use of adjunctive drugs have involved small patient groups and some have resulted in undesirable side-effects. Therefore it is generally agreed that larger clinical trials are required before they are used routinely [17].

NUTRITIONAL CHALLENGES

CF-related diabetes

The aims of treatment of CF-related diabetes (CFRD) are to maintain growth and optimize nutritional status, achieve good blood glucose control and avoid long-term complications [73]. Following diagnosis patients should have a detailed dietary review and be encouraged to continue with a diet high in energy, fat (with emphasis on mono- and polyunsaturated fat) and protein. The intake of salt should not be limited. Refined carbohydrate should not be restricted, but the quantity and distribution may need to be adapted. Regular meals containing similar amounts of refined carbohydrate should be encouraged [74]. Patients receiving supplementary enteral feeds will need to have their insulin modified to optimize overnight glycemic control.

Osteoporosis and bone health

Reduced bone mineral density is of concern, especially in adolescent and adult patients [75]. Multiple risk factors contribute to the development of osteopenia and osteoporosis (see Chapter 18), with poor nutritional status and clinical disease severity being the most strongly linked factors [75]. Delayed puberty, vitamin D, calcium and vitamin K deficiencies and to a lesser extent deficiencies of copper, phosphorus, magnesium, zinc and protein and an excess of vitamin A may also have etiological roles [75,76].

The foundation for good bone health is established during infancy, childhood and adolescence, so there should be a focus on minimizing risk factors during these years. Particular attention should be given to achieving a normal nutritional status, ensuring plasma vitamin D levels are above 30 ng/mL (75 nmol/L) [76] and ensuring a high dietary intake of calcium.

Pregnancy and lactation

Nutritional status before and during pregnancy may be an important determinant of outcome [78]. Women with CF who plan their pregnancies and have pre-conceptional advice have significantly greater maternal weight gain and significantly heavier babies [79,80]. Advice regarding folic acid supplementation [81] and general food safety should be given. Dietary reviews should check nutritional adequacy with particular attention to ensure sufficient protein, calcium and vitamin D intakes.

Nausea, vomiting, GER, altered gastric motility, constipation or diabetes may compromise nutritional status. Careful and close monitoring of nutritional status and individual dietary advice is essential. Nutritional intervention should be considered if there is poor weight gain.

Care should be taken with vitamin A supplementation during pregnancy as high doses are teratogenic. Increased risks of birth defects have been associated with intakes greater than 10 000 IU (3000 μg) daily [82]. Women with CF should take less than this and avoid excessive intakes of liver products because of their high vitamin A content [17].

Mothers with CF can successfully breast-feed [78] as their breast milk contains normal amounts of sodium and protein [83]. Maternal nutritional status should be carefully monitored during breast-feeding. Advice and nutritional support should be given to maintain an adequate dietary intake to meet the increased demands of breast-feeding.

Transplantation

Poor nutritional status has been shown to compromise post-transplant survival [84] and is a risk factor for post-operative complications [85]. A detailed nutritional assessment should be conducted at the time of transplant assessment to optimize nutritional status. Nutritional support should be provided in the acute post-transplant period to maintain nutritional status. Patients also need to be taught about food hygiene and safety and dietary interactions with immunosuppressive drugs. Other nutritional related complications that can occur post-transplant include hypertension, osteoporosis, hyperlipidemia, diabetes, nephrotoxicity [86], increased vitamin A and E levels [87] and GER. Distal intestinal obstructive syndrome is also common in the early postoperative period and early medical intervention is essential [88].

CONCLUSIONS

Regular dietetic input to review nutritional status, growth and dietary intake and to monitor for signs of malabsorption is an integral part of CF care. Upon diagnosis patients should have their nutritional and dietary requirements assessed and this should be reviewed regularly so that nutritional interventions can be tailored to meet changes in clinical, physical and psychosocial needs. The majority of patients with CF can achieve good nutritional status from a diet high in energy and protein. Those who cannot may require nutritional support from the use of oral nutritional supplements or enteral feeding. An improvement in survival has led to more dietary challenges such as CF-related diabetes, pregnancy and osteoporosis, which need regular dietetic support to help prevent a decline in nutritional and clinical status. As good nutritional status has an impact on survival and well-being, it is imperative that dietetic intervention be initiated early and continued throughout life.

REFERENCES

1. Corey M, McLaughlin FS, Williams M, Levison H. A comparison of survival, growth and pulmonary function in patients with cystic fibrosis in Boston and Toronto. *J Clin Epidemiol* 1988; **41**:583–591.

2. Zemel BS, Jawad AF, FitzSimmons S, Stallings VA. Longitudinal relationship between growth, nutritional status and pulmonary function in children with cystic fibrosis: analysis of the Cystic Fibrosis Foundation National Patient Registry. *J Pediatr* 2000; **137**:374–380.

3. de Meer K, Gulmans VA, van Der Laag J. Peripheral muscle weakness and exercise capacity in children with cystic fibrosis. *Am J Respir Crit Care Med* 1999; **159**:748–754.

4. Jelalian E, Stark LJ, Reynolds L, Seifer R. Nutrition intervention for weight gain in cystic fibrosis: a meta analysis. *J Pediatr* 1998; **132**:486–492.

5. Walker SA, Gozal D. Pulmonary function correlates in the prediction of long-term weight gain in cystic fibrosis patients with gastrostomy tube feedings. *J Pediatr Gastroenterol Nutr* 1998; **27**:53–56.

6. Steinkamp G, Wiedemann B for the German CFQA Group. Relationship between nutritional status and lung function in cystic fibrosis: cross-sectional and longitudinal analyses from the German Quality Assurance Project. *Thorax* 2002; **57**:596–601.

7. Sharma R, Florea VG, Bolger AP *et al.* Wasting as an independent predictor of mortality in patients with cystic fibrosis. *Thorax* 2001; **56**:746–750.

8. Beker LT, Russek-Cohen E, Fink RJ. Stature as a prognostic factor in cystic fibrosis survival. *J Am Diet Assoc* 2001; **101**:438–442.

9. Pencharz P, Hill R, Archibald E *et al.* Energy needs and nutritional rehabilitation in undernourished adolescents and young adults with cystic fibrosis. *J Pediatr Gastroenterol Nutr* 1984; **3**(Suppl 1):S147–S153.

10. Bell SC, Bowerman AM, Nixon LE *et al.* Metabolic and inflammatory responses to pulmonary exacerbations in adults with cystic fibrosis. *Eur J Clin Invest* 2000; **30**:553–559.

11. Fried M, Durie P, Tsue LC *et al.* The cystic fibrosis gene and resting energy expenditure. *J Pediatr* 1991; **119**:913–916.

12. Miller M, Ward L, Thomas BJ *et al.* Altered body composition and muscle protein degradation in nutritionally growth-retarded children with cystic fibrosis. *Am J Clin Nutr* 1982; **36**:492–499.

13. Vaisman N, Koren G, Goldstein D *et al.* Pharmacokinetics of inhaled salbutamol in patients with cystic fibrosis verses healthy young adults. *J Pediatr* 1987; **111**:914–917.

14. Littlewood JM, Wolfe SP. Control of malabsorption in cystic fibrosis. *Paediatr Drugs* 2000; **2**:205–222.

15. Kawchak DA, Zhao H, Scanlin TF *et al.* Longitudinal, prospective analysis of dietary intake in children with cystic fibrosis. *J Pediatr* 1996; **129**:119–129.

16. White H, Morton AM, Peckham DG, Conway SP. Dietary intakes in adult patients with cystic fibrosis: do they achieve guidelines? *J Cyst Fibros* 2004; **3**:1–7.

17. UK Cystic Fibrosis Trust Nutrition Working Group. *Nutritional Management of Cystic Fibrosis*. CFT, 2002.

18. Zhang Z, Lai HC. Comparison of the use of body mass index percentiles and percentage of ideal body weight to screen for malnutrition in children with cystic fibrosis. *Am J Clin Nutr* 2004; **80**:982–991.

19. Borowitz D. Update on the evaluation of pancreatic exocrine status in cystic fibrosis. *Curr Opin Pulm Med* 2005; **11**:524–527.

20. Walkowiak J, Nousia-Arvanitakis S, Agguridaki C *et al.* Longitudinal follow-up of exocrine pancreatic function in pancreatic sufficient cystic fibrosis patients using the fecal elastase-1 test. *J Pediatr Gastroenterol Nutr* 2003; **36**:474–478.

21. Smyth RL, van Velzen D, Smyth AR *et al.* Strictures of the ascending colon in cystic fibrosis and high strength pancreatic enzymes. *Lancet* 1994; **343**:85–86.

22. Committee on Safety of Medicines. *Report of the Pancreatic Enzymes Working Party*. London, 1995.

23. Francisco MP, Wagner MH, Sherman JM *et al.* Ranitidine and omeprazole as adjuvant therapy to pancrealipase to improve fat absorption in patients with cystic fibrosis. *J Pediatr Gastroenterol Nutr* 2002; **35**:79–83.

24. Taylor CJ, Hillel PG, Ghosal S *et al.* Gastric emptying and intestinal transit of pancreatic enzyme supplements in cystic fibrosis. *Arch Dis Child* 1999; **80**:149–152.

25. Kerem E, Conway S, Elborn S, Heijerman H for the Consensus Committee. Standards of care for patients with cystic fibrosis: a European consensus. *J Cyst Fibros* 2005; **4**:7–26.

26. Dray X, Bienvenu T, Desmazes-Dufeu N *et al.* Distal intestinal obstruction syndrome in adults with cystic fibrosis. *Clin Gastroenterol Hepatol* 2004; **2**:498–503.

27. Mascarenhas MR. Treatment of gastrointestinal problems in cystic fibrosis. *Curr Treat Options Gastroenterol* 2003; **6**:427–441.

28. Kerrin D, Wolfe S, Brownlee K, Conway S. Overnight tube feeds: are enzymes necessary? *Abstract book, International CF Congress*, Stockholm, 2000, p118.

29. Armand M, Hamosh M, Philpott JR *et al.* Gastric function in children with cystic fibrosis: effect of diet on gastric lipase levels and fat digestion. *J Pediatr Res* 2004; **55**:457–465.

30. Feranchak AP, Sontag MK, Wagener JS *et al.* Prospective long-term study of fat-soluble vitamin status in children with cystic fibrosis identified by newborn screening. *J Pediatr* 1999; **135**:601–610.

31. Yankaskas JR, Marshall BC, Sufian B *et al.* Cystic Fibrosis Adult Care: Consensus Conference Report. *Chest* 2004; **125**:1S–39S.

32. Carr SB, Dinwiddie R. Vitamin A as a predictor for lung function in cystic fibrosis [abstract]. *Pediatr Pulmonol* 1996; **13**(Suppl):317.

33. Campbell DC, Tole DM, Doran RML, Conway SP. Vitamin A deficiency in cystic fibrosis resulting in severe xerophthalmia. *J Hum Nutr Diet* 1998; **11**:529–532.

34. Navarro J, Desquilbet N. Depressed vitamin A and retinol binding protein in cystic fibrosis correlations with zinc deficiency. *Am J Clin Nutr* 1981; **34**:1439–1440.

35. Greer RM, Buntain HM, Lewindon PJ *et al.* Vitamin A levels in patients with CF are influenced by the inflammatory response. *J Cyst Fibros* 2004; **3**:143–149.

36. Eid NS, Shoemaker LR, Samiec TD. Vitamin A in cystic fibrosis: case report and review of the literature. *J Pediatr Gastroenterol Nutr* 1990; **10**:265–269.

37. Genaro P de S, Martini LA. Vitamin A supplementation and risk of skeletal fracture. *Nutr Rev* 2004; **62**(2):65–67.

38. Wolfe SP, Conway SP, Brownlee KG. Seasonal variation in vitamin D levels in children with cystic fibrosis in the United Kingdom. *J Cyst Fibros 24th European CF Conference* 2001, p115.

39. Donovan DS, Papadopoulos A, Staron RB *et al.* Bone mass and vitamin D deficiency in adults with advanced cystic fibrosis lung disease. *Am J Resp Crit Care Med* 1998; **157**:1892–1899.

40. Borowitz D, Baker RD, Stallings V. Consensus report on nutrition for pediatric patients with cystic fibrosis. *J Pediatr Gastroenterol Nutr* 2002; **35**:246–259.

41. Rashid M, Durie PR, Andrew M *et al.* Prevalence of vitamin K deficiency in cystic fibrosis. *Am J Clin Nutr* 1999; **70**:378–382.

42. Conway SP, Wolfe SP, Brownlee KG. Vitamin K status among children with cystic fibrosis and its relationship to bone mineral density and bone turnover. *Pediatrics* 2005; **115**:1325–1331.

43. Strandvik B, Gronowitz E, Enlund F *et al.* Essential fatty acid deficiency in relation to genotype in patients with cystic fibrosis. *J Pediatr* 2001; **139**:650–655.

44. Lloyd-Still JD, Bibus DM, Powers CA *et al.* Essential fatty acid (EFA) and predisposition to lung disease in cystic fibrosis. *Acta Paediatr* 1996; **85**:1426–1432.

45. Freedman SD, Blanco PG, Zaman MN *et al.* Association of cystic fibrosis with abnormalities in fatty acid metabolism. *N Engl J Med* 2004; **350**:560–569.

46. Beckles Willson N, Elliott TM, Everard ML. Omega-3 fatty acids (from fish oils) for cystic fibrosis. *Cochrane Database Syst Rev* 2002, Issue 3, CD002201.

47. Winklhofer-Roob BM, Ellemunter H, Fruhwirth M *et al.* Plasma vitamin C concentration in patients with cystic fibrosis: evidence of associations with lung inflammation. *Am J Clin Nutr* 1997; **65**:1858–1866.

48. Sinaasappel M, Stern M, Littlewood J *et al.* Nutrition in patients with cystic fibrosis: a European consensus. *J Cyst Fibros* 2002; **2**:51–75.

49. Farrell PM, Lai HJ, Kosorok MR *et al.* Evidence of improved outcomes with early diagnosis of cystic fibrosis through neonatal screening: enough is enough! *J Pediatr* 2005; **147**:S30–S36.

50. Holliday K, Allen J, Waters DL *et al.* Growth of human milk fed and formula fed infants with cystic fibrosis. *J Pediatr* 1991; **118**:77–79.

51. Ellis L, Kalnins D, Corey M *et al.* Do infants with cystic fibrosis need a protein hydrolysate formula? A prospective, randomised comparative study. *J Pediatr* 1998; **132**:270–276.

52. Lai HC, Kosorok MR, Laxova A *et al.* Nutritional status of patients with cystic fibrosis with meconium ileus: a comparison with patients without meconium ileus and diagnosed early through neonatal screening. *Pediatrics* 2000; **105**:53–61.

53. Heine RG, Button BM, Olinsky A *et al.* Gastro-oesophageal reflux in infants under 6 months with cystic fibrosis. *Arch Dis Child* 1998; **78**:44–48.

54. Brodizicki J, Trawinska-Bartnicka M, Korzon M. Frequency, consequences and pharmacological treatment of gastroesophageal reflux in children with cystic fibrosis. *Med Sci Monit* 2002; **8**:CR529–537.

55. Hill SM, Phillips AD, Mearns M *et al.* Cows' milk sensitive enteropathy in cystic fibrosis. *Arch Dis Child* 1989; **64**:1251–1255.

56. Duff AJA, Wolfe SP, Dickson C *et al.* Feeding behaviour problems in children with cystic fibrosis in the UK: prevalence and comparison with healthy controls. *J Pediatr Gastroenterol Nutr* 2003, **36**:443–447.

57. Powers SW, Jones JS, Ferguson KS *et al.* Randomized clinical trial of behavioral and nutritional treatment to improve energy intake and growth in toddlers and preschoolers with cystic fibrosis. *Pediatrics* 2005; **116**:1442–1450.

58. Neumark-Sztainer D, Story M, Falkner NH *et al.* Disordered eating among adolescents with chronic illness and disability. *Arch Pediatr Adolesc Med* 1998; **152**:871–878.

59. Shearer JE, Bryon M. The nature and prevalence of eating disorders and eating disturbance in adolescents with cystic fibrosis. *J R Soc Med* 2004; **97**(Suppl 44):36–42.

60. Abbott, J. Coping with cystic fibrosis. *J R Soc Med* 2003; **96**(Suppl 43):42–50.

61. Bolton CE, Ionescu AA, Evans WD *et al.* Altered tissue distribution in adults with cystic fibrosis. *Thorax* 2003; **58**:885–889.

62. Skypala IJ, Ashworth FA, Hodson ME *et al.* Oral nutritional supplements promote significant weight gain in cystic fibrosis patients. *J Hum Nutr Diet* 1998; **11**:95–104.

63. Smyth R, Walters S. Oral calorie supplements for cystic fibrosis. *Cochrane Database Syst Rev* 2000, Issue 2, CD000406.

64. Steinkamp G, von der Hardt H. Improvement of nutritional status and lung function after long-term nocturnal gastrostomy feeding in cystic fibrosis. *J Pediatr* 1994; **124**:244–249.

65. Oliver MR, Heine RG, Hang Ng *et al.* Factors affecting clinical outcome in gastrostomy-fed children with cystic fibrosis. *Pediatr Pulmonol* 2004; **37**:324–329.

66. Conway SP, Morton A, Wolfe S. Enteral tube feeding for cystic fibrosis. *Cochrane Database Syst Rev* 1999, Issue 3, CD001198.

67. Eubanks V, Koppersmith N, Wooldridge N *et al.* Effects of megestrol acetate on weight gain, body composition, and pulmonary function in patients with cystic fibrosis. *J Pediatr* 2002; **140**:439–444.

68. Homnick DN, Marks JH, Hare KL, Bonnema SK. Long-term trial of cyproheptadine as an appetite stimulant in cystic fibrosis. *Pediatr Pulmonol* 2005; **40**:251–256.

69. Ripa P, Robertson I, Cowley D *et al.* The relationship between insulin secretion, the insulin-like growth factor axis and growth in children with cystic fibrosis. *Clin Endocrinol* 2002; **56**:383–389.

70. Hardin DS, Ellis KJ, Dyson M *et al.* Growth hormone improves clinical status in prepubertal children with cystic fibrosis: results of a randomized controlled trial. *J Pediatr* 2001; **139**:636–642.

71. Hardin DS, Rice J, Ahn C *et al.* Growth hormone treatment enhances nutrition and growth in children with cystic fibrosis receiving enteral nutrition. *J Pediatr* 2005; **146**:324–328.

72. Braegger CP, Schlattner U, Wallimann T *et al.* Effects of creatine supplementation in cystic fibrosis: results of a pilot study. *J Cyst Fibros* 2003; **2**:177–182.

73. Moran A. Endocrine complications of cystic fibrosis. *Adol Med* 2002; **13**:145–159.

74. UK Cystic Fibrosis Trust Diabetes Working Group: *Management of Cystic Fibrosis Related Diabetes Mellitus.* Bromley, Kent, CFT, 2004.

75. Conway SP, Morton AM, Oldroyd B *et al.* Osteoporosis and osteopenia in adults and adolescents with cystic fibrosis: prevalence and associated factors. *Thorax* 2000; **55**:798–804.

76. Aris RM, Merkel PA, Bachrach *et al.* Guide to bone health and disease in cystic fibrosis. *J Clin Endocrinol Metab* 2005; **90**:1888–1896.

77. Hecker TM, Aris RM. Management of osteoporosis in adults with cystic fibrosis. *Drugs* 2004; **64**(2):133–147.

78. Odegaad I, Stray-Pedersen B, Hallberg K *et al.* Maternal and fetal morbidity in pregnancies of Norwegian and Swedish women with cystic fibrosis. *Acta Obstet Gynecol Scand* 2002; **81**:698–705.

79. Kotloff RM, FitzSimmons SC, Fiel SB. Fertility and pregnancy in patients with cystic fibrosis. *Clin Chest Med* 1992; **13**:623–635.

80. Morton A, Wolfe S, Conway SP. Dietetic intervention in pregnancy in women with CF – the importance of pre-conceptional counselling. *Israel J Med Sci* 1996; **32**(Suppl):S2.

81. UK Department of Health. *Folic Acid and the Prevention of Neural Tube Defects*: Report from the Expert Advisory Group for Health Professionals. London, Department of Health, 1992.

82. Rothman KJ, Moore LL, Singer MR *et al.* Teratogenicity of high vitamin A intake. *N Engl J Med* 1995; **333**:1369–1373.

83. Gilljam M, Antoniou M, Shin J *et al.* Pregnancy in cystic fibrosis: fetal and maternal outcome. *Chest* 2000; **118**:85–91.

84. Hasse JM. Nutritional assessment and support of organ transplant recipients. *JPEN* 2001; **25**:120–131.

85. Beck CE, Lin A, Robbins C, Dosanjh AK. Improvements in the nutritional and pulmonary profiles of cystic fibrosis patients undergoing bilateral sequential lung and heart-lung transplantation. *Nutr Clin Pract* 1997; **12**:216–221.

86. Maurer JR, Tewari S. Nonpulmonary medical complications in the intermediate and long-term survivor. *Clin Chest Med* 1997; **18**:367–382.

87. Stephenson A, Brotherwood M, Roberts R *et al.* Increased vitamin A and E levels in adult cystic fibrosis patients after lung transplantation. *Transplantation* 2005; **79**:613–615.

88. Gilljam M, Chaparro C, Tullis E *et al.* GI complications after lung transplantation in patients with cystic fibrosis. *Chest* 2003; **123**:37–41.

31

Psychological aspects of cystic fibrosis

ALISTAIR J. A. DUFF AND HELEN OXLEY

INTRODUCTION

Living with cystic fibrosis (CF) can be psychologically stressful for patients and families alike, yet at times, both can exhibit outstanding psychological resilience. Over the past decade there has been a dramatic increase in the number of psychological therapists with defined roles [1], integrated into CF teams.

Until recently, the psychological literature has predominantly focused on children and adolescents and their families, with findings being inconsistent and of little immediate help to patients and their relatives. There have been three broad reasons for this. First, early studies presumed that patients and their families would experience psychopathology, which was then, rather predictably, 'found'. It was not until the late 1980s that studies considered risk for, and resilience to, psychological problems more consistently. Second, methodology often failed to address the impact of mediating variables (e.g. age, gender and disease severity), on the etiology of psychopathology. Finally, it was not until the early 1990s that there was more serious consideration of sampling. The severity of CF determines its visibility, intrusiveness and predictability, factors known to increase the risk of developing associated psychological problems [2]. Individual psychosocial development was often ignored, with little homogeneity of study participants. Even more fatally, reviews often failed to consider the changing context of CF, including the effect of different eras of care.

People with CF born after 1990 now have a median life expectancy of over 40 years [3]. However, increased longevity has been accompanied by an increased burden of care and microbiological segregation and it is only now, with the development of reliable measures [4,5], that the quality of these additional years is being explored. Health status can now be described more meaningfully, with better identification of the effects of clinical interventions on psychological and social aspects of daily living.

This chapter considers psychological aspects of CF within the context of the past 15 years, where parents have been told to expect that their child will live into their mid-40s and to anticipate a viable gene therapy, and where health services have had to adapt to caring for increasing numbers of adults with CF, some of whom have already lived longer than either they or their parents expected.

CHILDREN AND ADOLESCENTS WITH CF

Children and young people with chronic conditions have almost three times the risk of developing emotional and behavioral difficulties when compared to their healthy peers [6], and patients with CF are no exception [7]. Of course, children do not adapt to CF in a vacuum. Their reactions are intrinsically linked to how well their parents cope with the diagnosis and develop effective parenting strategies.

Few studies focus exclusively on infants and pre-school children with CF, many of whom do well. Newborn screening for CF is being increasingly advocated around the world with emerging data suggesting that screened infants have better health outcomes than non-screened (see Chapters 8a and 8b). Although mothers report greater parenting stress after diagnosis and view their children as being more demanding and less adaptable than those of healthy children [8], this does not necessarily interfere with the development of normal infant–mother emotional attachments [9]. However, infants and children with CF deemed to have insecure attachments have been shown to have lower weight-for-height-scores. Pre-school children with CF have also been found to be significantly more likely to experience behavior problems than healthy controls [7]. It seems that parents continue to need guidance on how best to discuss CF and on balancing disease management with normal psychosocial development.

As children with CF go through school, like all children, they face the psychological tasks of establishing autonomy, positive self-esteem and peer relationships. For many, the school-age period is one where CF is well-managed, with relative freedom from recurrent exacerbation. Nonetheless, children continue to undergo numerous treatments, face frequent hospital visits and repeated medical procedures, and become increasingly aware that they are different from others [10]. It is thought that this can contribute to the onset of emotional and behavioral difficulties. In one sample, approximately 60% of mothers of children with CF aged between 7 and 12 years old, and the children themselves, reported adjustment difficulties [11]. Anxiety and oppositional disorders have also been reported in this group [12]. Difficulty with mealtime behavior is one of the most frequently cited difficulties in young children with CF [13]. As mealtime progresses, parents increase their efforts to encourage eating [14], acknowledging that some of these are inappropriate. Another area of concern is children's reactions to painful or distressing medical procedures. Children continue to find 'having a needle' one of the most frightening aspects of attending hospital. In CF, one study found over 30% of children felt 'extremely' or 'very' frightened of venepuncture, especially prior to needle-insertion [15]. Other procedures (e.g. cough swabs and using nebulizers) can also be upsetting for younger children.

Adolescence is a period when, psychologically, individuals are expected to achieve a sense of self-identity and independence from their parents and form 'adult' relationships outside their family. However, as well as contending with feeling different, adolescents with CF may also have to deal with the over-involvement of their parents at a time when developmentally they seek to psychologically 'separate' from them. During periods in hospital they report 'losing ground with their friends' and 'feeling out of the loop' [16]. They try to cope by keeping secrets and hiding differences and relying on peers for companionship and emotional support.

Despite the burden of treatment, there is consistent evidence that adolescents with CF are generally a psychologically well-adapted and well-functioning group, reporting a high QoL [17,18], at least until the disease becomes severe [19]. Severity as determined by lung function has a negative impact on QoL in young people. Females generally report a lower QoL than males, but they are more accurate in their evaluations of health status [20]. Pain management has also been reported as problematic for some young people [21].

Even if CF is well-managed, there are those adolescents who psychologically fare less well. They report more problems in their family relationships particularly, in the parent–teenager ones, than healthy controls. Such difficulties have been associated with poorer psychological adjustment [22], higher levels of psychopathology, particularly depressive symptoms [23], and suboptimal adherence [24].

Family conflict often presents CF team members with moral and ethical dilemmas, as parents strive to 'strike a balance' between teenagers' self-sufficiency, parental wishes and the law, and although difficult and contentious, sometimes these need to be discussed in clinic. Just as parents must allow their child to move on, so must the pediatric team caring for them. Parents need to be supported and encouraged to gradually devolve responsibilities for decision-making and taking prescribed medication. Several ways of implementing transfer of care between pediatric and adult units have been described. None has been proven to be better than others, but those that are planned, efficient and expected by the patient are thought to be the most successful [25].

ADULTS WITH CF

As the number of adults with CF rises, descriptions of their changing lives, achievements and difficulties are emerging. However, there is not yet the same volume of literature as in the pediatric field. Many adults with CF, who make up over 50% of the UK CF population [26], need to also manage jobs, relationships and families. The challenge is to maintain such 'normal life' against ever-increasing treatment regimens, complications and severity of disease. CF remains a life-limiting disease, ending ultimately with deterioration and death. Improvements in prognosis do not preclude adults with CF from negative psychological effects.

Studies of QoL in adults have been extensively reviewed [19,20,27]. Deteriorating lung function has been shown to have a negative impact on CF-related QoL [20], however the majority of the variance in QoL is still unaccounted for [28]. Other factors thought to be important are: subjective perceptions of health, coping style and body image [20,29]. Optimistic coping is associated with better QoL and avoidant coping may help some individuals maintain psychological health (though may also be linked to poor adherence) [30]. Helping adults adapt to new stresses and demands may require novel strategies, when previously relied upon methods of coping become ineffective.

Investigation of the prevalence of psychological problems in adults with CF shows mixed results. Some studies suggest that they function well, displaying no more psychopathology than healthy peers [17,31]. However, this may only be the case in the early stages before the disease becomes severe. While studies are lacking in those more severely affected, where they do exist, a range of psychological problems have been described, including depression, poor self-esteem and relationship difficulties [19].

Chronic illness and depression are strongly linked [32]. In adults with CF, while one study found depression to be no higher than in the general population [31], another found 46% to be clinically depressed [33]. A meta-analysis across illness groups has also found depressive symptoms to be associated with a 3-fold increase in the risk of non-adherence [34], and within the CF population depression is linked with the poorer lung functioning [35]. While not yet properly investigated in CF, risk of suicide and self-harm is generally increased by physical illness, depression and hopelessness.

Anxiety disorders, especially panic attacks, are known to be associated with respiratory disease [36] and are often seen clinically in adults with CF [37]. Although they may have satisfactory body image [38], both disturbed eating attitudes and disturbed eating behaviors are seen in adolescents with CF [39] and might be presumed to continue at least into early adulthood [19]. Low self-esteem and difficulties in interpersonal and sexual relationships have also been reported [19].

There are a number of other important psychosocial issues for adults with CF. Pregnancy and reproduction, transplantation and palliative care are considered separately in this volume (Chapters 20, 21 and 32). Segregation of patients for infection control purposes is increasingly common, and investigations of the psychological consequences are under way. Diagnosis of CF in adulthood has short- and long-term consequences including fear, shock, anger, increased awareness of death, feelings of confusion, intrusion and isolation, and effects on identity, lifestyle and personal relationships and those diagnosed as adults may not receive enough information about their condition [40].

In summary, adults with CF are now the group with the most complex and severe health problems and ordinary life challenges. Details of the psychological difficulties they experience are emerging but much further investigation is needed.

ADHERENCE TO TREATMENT

The positive links between adherence and health status are well known, but partial adherence to prescribed medications remains a worldwide problem. Engaging people with CF in treatment is essential if permanent lung damage and family conflict is to be avoided. Notwithstanding the difficulties of definition and measurement, adherence to CF regimens is generally low [41]. Factors thought to influence adherence across all illness groups are emerging and include: knowledge and interaction with health professionals, individual and developmental factors, regimen characteristics, and the family.

Perceptions of knowledge and compliance vary among children with chronic conditions and their parents, some choosing to suppress information as part of their coping style. Further discrepancy arises from patients and parents having different treatment goals from clinicians. In CF, information-gaps and misunderstandings have been reported in as high as 33% of mothers of school-aged children [42]. While levels of understanding can be influenced by interaction with team members, families can be unwilling to express concerns.

In children with CF, adherence difficulties have been reliably shown to increase from 10 years onwards, peaking at around 16 years [41]. As in other illness groups, composite regimens, adverse side-effects, variable efficacy and the fact that not all treatment components yield immediate benefit, can lead to lower rates of adherence. Particularly low levels have been observed for diet [43], physiotherapy and aerosolized therapies [23,44,45].

Family conflict (particularly parent–teenager), over-involvement and poor communication have long been associated with adherence problems. Problematic family functioning has been shown to have a negative impact on health outcomes in CF [46], and it has been suggested that this is mediated by the family's ability to facilitate optimal adherence (see later). Findings on the effect of increased parental involvement and monitoring of treatment behaviors during adolescence are equivocal but engaging teenagers in discussions is vital if such problems are to be effectively addressed.

For adults with CF, treatment regimens can be more onerous than they are for children and adolescents. Levels of adherence are again variable, depending on regimen, with self-reported rates of 65–80% for pancreatic enzymes and nebulized medication, and 40–50% for vitamin therapy, dietary changes, exercise and physiotherapy [47]. In general, complex and time-consuming treatments are associated with poorer adherence, but as in pediatric groups, there are difficulties in defining and measuring adherence accurately.

Several investigations of the complexities of adherence to treatments in adults with CF have been undertaken [19,27,44]. Adherence seems to be better: when treatments give immediate benefits and choices are available [47], when there is worry about health, a perception of little personal control over this and trust in medical practitioners [48], and when there is good self-efficacy [49]. Social support of patients is important in encouraging treatment adherence [27], and the quality of relationships with healthcare professionals may also influence this. In adults, illness severity does not have a simple linear relationship with adherence. Other demographic factors including financial and employment status and age at diagnosis have not been associated with differences in adherence rates in this population [27], nor has general knowledge about CF, although understanding of specific treatments is thought to be important [44]. While good family functioning is known to be important in the pediatric field, the impact of this on adherence in adults has not yet been shown, although it will remain important for some [44]. When patients are asked reasons for partial or non-adherence, the most common reason given is forgetfulness [47], with other explanations being grouped into health, social, time and emotional reasons [27].

Teams need to embrace the notion that partial adherence is inevitable and normal in patients of all ages. Patient care needs to be placed within the context of their other activities and the need to maintain some kind of 'normal life'. The challenges for health professionals remain: to facilitate open and honest discussions about adherence, to spend time expressing empathy and understanding ambivalence, and to collaborate and negotiate with patients over achieving more optimal patterns of adherence.

THE FAMILY

No matter their age, patients are integral to their family system, having an effect on, and being affected by, their relatives.

Equally, just as CF has a major impact on family functioning, how that family 'works' affects how members adapt to CF.

In the UK, increasing numbers of children are diagnosed as neonates, many following screening (see Chapter 8a). The waiting period between raised immunoreactive trypsin on screening and diagnostic confirmation is psychologically distressing for parents. This, together with missed and late diagnoses, has been recognized as leading to depressive symptoms [50], anxiety, guilt and anger, and reduced trust in doctors [51]. Information after newborn screening needs to go beyond genetic counselling and families will vary in their willingness to acquire CF-related information.

Although psychological adaptation to diagnosis has been likened to a bereavement process with discrete stages of shock, disbelief, anger, adjustment and adaptation, this does not accurately reflect the experience commonly reported by parents. Despite improved longevity and hopes of gene therapy, they continue to worry that they will outlive their child. What seems more fitting in CF populations is the concept of 'chronic sorrow', with oscillating phases of normality and routine, punctuated with intense sadness and mourning.

Following diagnosis, parents face a range of challenges, including obtaining the knowledge and skills to manage the disease, adhering to complex daily treatments and balancing the needs of the child with CF with the rest of the family's. One review found evidence that mothers in particular have increased psychological problems [7], role strain of accomplishing tasks relating to family routines, and illness-specific duties and decreased marital satisfaction resulting from having less time to spend together [52]. Another emphasized the disruption to intra-familial relationships that optimal adherence to treatment regimens can cause [53]. Parents can be either too protective or permissive with their child [54], or too enmeshed with each other [17], and less likely to set limits compared to those of healthy children [54]. Overprotection was again observed in parental responses to recommendations on how to prevent environmental acquisition of microbacteria, where risks were exaggerated or misunderstood, to the detriment of the child's and parent's QoL [55].

Mothers and fathers are thought to cope differently with children who have a chronic condition. While fathers report lower rates of adjustment problems [10], they can experience guilt leading to withdrawal and worry about time spent alone with their partner and not having enough money to meet family needs [56]. However, to date, these findings have not properly been explored in fathers of children with CF.

A meta-analysis concluded that there are modest negative psychological effects on well-siblings of children with chronic conditions, relative to comparison groups or normative data [57]. In CF groups, reactions are intrinsically linked to how their sibling with CF responds to the condition, their own perceptions of this and their parents' responses, all of which vary according to disease progression [58]. Differential treatment of children with CF is perhaps

to be expected given the physical and emotional demands placed on parents who may try to protect well-siblings by deliberately not talking about certain aspects of CF.

Family dysfunction and stress have a detrimental impact on CF outcomes. Patterson and co-workers [46] established robust proof that a balanced family coping style, in which members attend to their own needs as well as those of the child with CF, and lower levels of stress, were positively correlated to 10-year lung functioning. Czewski and co-workers [59] linked elements of health status to a range of other family variables, including maternal mental health problems and greater perceived negative impact of the illness on the family. Being a single mother has also been implicated [60]. These associations have important implications for clinical management, particularly in helping parents attend to the family as a whole, and encouraging individual family members and single mothers to attend to their own mental health needs when feeling overwhelmed.

Reciprocal relationships between adults with CF and their families have received little attention. The normal process of gaining independence can be disrupted and, as CF progresses, parents of adult patients can revert to a caring role again, which can be difficult for all. Well-siblings, too, may continue to feel the effects of CF on their lives. Barriers to forming relationships in adulthood have been described in CF, such as lack of independence, fear of moving away from home and embarrassment due to symptoms [19]. Adult relationships may be further affected when the condition becomes more severe, as partners may need to adopt the role of carer. While some adults with CF now have children of their own, there has been little investigation of the psychosocial impact on parents or their offspring. It may be that as illness progresses, caring for children becomes more demanding both practically and emotionally, with consequences for those families and their extended supports. Children of people with CF may themselves become carers, but this remains unexplored.

THE CF TEAM

CF team members may have long, and at times, intense relationships with patients and their relatives. While often rewarding, the experience can also be difficult. Stress can arise from a range of sources, including dealing with difficult clinical situations, patient–team dynamics or conflicts within the CF team.

Strong collaborative relationships between CF caregivers, patients and relatives convey empathy and support, and inspire confidence and trust. However, as patient–professional relationships develop over time, difficulties can arise and issues of maintaining appropriate boundaries and the support needs of the CF team are becoming increasingly recognized.

Difficult patient–team dynamics can emerge quite insidiously (e.g. over-dependence, over-attachment, over-protectiveness or over-involvement). At times, these can make it difficult: to support vulnerable patients or relatives, to handle distressing and sensitive information, to cope when patients physically deteriorate and die, or to tackle any conflict that arises between teams, patients and their families. Disagreement between patients and their CF team may arise in the contexts of adherence (where patients can have different treatment goals from clinicians) and decision-making.

Staff stress and burnout (a syndrome characterized by emotional exhaustion, depersonalization and reduced personal satisfaction) within CF teams has been neglected in the literature despite significant associations between team support and supervision and low burnout [61]. Younger team members with more social problems and anxiety may be more susceptible to unmanageable levels of stress than others [62]. Preventing staff stress and burnout are important tasks. CF teams need to be aware of their own functioning and devote time to addressing problems. Support and supervision seem of particular use in helping team members reflect on, among other things, how personal issues and professional boundaries influence individual practice, not working beyond competencies, and responding to sensitive patient information. How this is achieved will vary between units, but any psychosocial professional working within the team has an integral role to play.

PSYCHOLOGICAL INTERVENTIONS

Psychological interventions are intrinsic to optimizing CF health outcomes by improving adaptation, coping and QoL, ameliorating emotional distress, preventing psychopathology and optimizing patients' levels of self-care. Such work is not the sole responsibility of the psychosocial professional. All team members have much to contribute at all levels of care. Skills can be utilized informally in routine care (e.g. using good communication and active listening skills, demonstrating empathy, and taking account of an individual's needs for information, control, choice and involvement in care). These have been linked to greater patient satisfaction, and increased likelihood of advice being followed [63]. Team members can also undertake specific psychological training (e.g. counselling and motivational interviewing skills), and offer formal emotional support. Good knowledge of the salient features of psychopathology is necessary to ensure patients and relatives receive appropriate early assessment and treatment of problems.

Parental support following diagnosis

Post-diagnosis programs for parents need to offer support in various ways. Many exist, offering a combination of didactic teaching sessions and group and peer interactions. Nutritional knowledge and behavior management was maintained at 3 months after one such initiative, which also contained a mentoring service, focus groups and a series of social events [64]. However, such efforts need to continue beyond the post-diagnosis period and be directed towards the entire family's emotional well-being [65]. It is also important to strike the balance between 'normalizing' emotional reactions and screening for psychological problems. For parents this needs to involve assessment of, among other things, insecure attachments, depression, 'flashbacks' (and other distressing imagery), anxiety, parenting stress and family functioning [66].

Behavioral problems

Anxiety can alter the way in which parents bring up their children, with unwanted behaviors being unwittingly reinforced. Many CF treatment-related difficulties can often be ameliorated by behavioral strategies. An important example of this is the effect of parental anxiety about nutritional intake on mealtimes. Children with CF often display behavior that is incompatible with eating which is inadvertently attended to by their parents. Joint behavioral and dietetic interventions are successful in modifying these actions [67].

Other applications of behavior therapy in CF include improving adherence to specific treatments such as physiotherapy and nebulizer use in younger children, and reducing anxiety and increasing coping strategies in adolescents [68]. It is particularly useful for effectively addressing problems in clinical settings, most notably procedure-related distress where management involves combining relaxation training, graded exposure (to the feared procedure) and positive reinforcement. This is especially important to consider in younger children with CF, given the frequency of venepuncture and cough swabs. Teams need to assess previous experience, allow children to participate in the procedure when appropriate, encourage distraction and allow plenty of time to rehearse anxiety-provoking treatments. Such techniques have been extensively reviewed [69].

Psycho-education for children and families

Given that there are often large gaps and misconceptions in patients' and relatives' CF knowledge [42,70], teams need to implement education programs that inform, motivate and support people with CF and their families. While there is a plethora of CF information available, what seems essential is individualizing educational approaches by assessing what patients and their families want to know and at what times [71]. Evaluations of education programs in CF are scant, despite suggestions that these can improve treatment adherence in respiratory conditions [72]. CD-ROM technology can facilitate more age-appropriate, interactive and exciting education techniques and overcome issues of time-consuming and resource-heavy education strategies. Two such programs exist, with early evaluation showing much promise [73,74].

Adolescents

Few interventions have been described that specifically target adolescents with CF. Interventions that focus on enhancing peer support in other chronic conditions can have positive effects on disease management. Including healthy peers in treatment has increased peer knowledge, decreased parental report of child–parent illness-related conflict, and improved parental perceptions of adherence [75]. In CF, this type of support could be crucial, given contemporary segregation guidelines. Psychopathology, particularly anxiety and depression, can of course be found in teenagers with CF. While the psychological treatment of such problems is akin to that recommended for adult patients, some adjustments need to be made (e.g. specific guidelines for the treatment of depression in young people have recently been published in the UK [76]). However, it is family-based interventions that may yield the most effective strategies in helping teenagers.

Family

Psychological approaches have long acknowledged the importance of involving the entire family in therapy. Systemic family therapy addresses ways family members have a reciprocal effect on each other, communicate, and function together and there is an emerging body of literature that supports such conceptualization of problems and treatment [77]. Negotiating responsibility and improving communication between adolescents and parents are key tasks of such interventions, and continual monitoring, feedback and reinforcement of these factors as well as others are important.

Adults

Although there is little published on the efficacy of psychological interventions with adult CF patients, substantial evaluation in other illness groups has taken place, especially in the areas of adherence and psychological problems. To bring about changes in adherence to long-term treatments, complex combinations of psychological approaches may be required [78]. Cohesive families and good social support, especially practical help, are also associated with better adherence [79]. Work on individuals' motivation to adhere has brought about behavioral change in adults with other illnesses [80]. This can be delivered by trained non-psychologists and shows promise in CF groups [45].

While prevalence of psychological problems among adults with CF is as yet uncertain, such difficulties are known to occur in this group. Early recognition of psychopathology by CF team members is important (e.g. at annual review) and psychometric measures may be useful adjuncts to clinical assessment, particularly the Hospital Anxiety and Depression Scale [81]. Where the need is for increased support, other team members may fulfil this role. When significant psychological problems such as anxiety (e.g. panic attacks, excessive worry, phobias, obsessional disorders), depression, risk of self-harm, or low self-esteem are identified, referral to a psychological therapist for treatment may be required. Cognitive behavior therapy (CBT) has a strong evidence base in ameliorating such problems in chronic illness groups [82]. It has been recommended as a first-line treatment for, among other problems, depression and anxiety disorders and detailed guidelines for this (and adjunctive pharmacological treatment) are available [83,84]. Descriptions of how CBT can be applied to CF populations are also readily obtainable [37, 85]. Related psychological approaches (e.g. solution-focused therapy and brief problem-solving), hold promise for CF populations as do other psychotherapeutic interventions, such as psychodynamic approaches. However, these remain unevaluated.

CONCLUSIONS

Although patients with CF have increased longevity, the challenge for medical teams is to ensure their QoL is equally enhanced. New treatments present new psychosocial challenges for patients and their families as their burden of care rises. We know that risk factors associated with the development of psychological problems are mother–child insecure attachments, parenting stress, marital dissatisfaction, parent–teen conflict and family dysfunction. We also know that siblings of children with CF experience negative psychological affects. Coping and adaptation are influenced by many psychological factors.

While effective psychological interventions exist, there is only limited evidence demonstrating efficacy in CF populations. Enough is known about these in other illness groups to guide us in what may be helpful. Some psychological interventions need not remain the monopoly of psychosocial professionals. Together we can support parents after diagnosis, screen for psychopathology, manage feeding behavior problems and procedural distress. We can optimize the way in which children, adults and their families obtain and use information. The entire team can use a range of 'everyday' psychological skills to establish and nurture collaborative relationships, which lead to honesty and trust in communicating, and consequently, effective emotional support.

Joint work between pediatric and adult teams results in successful transition to adult services. Individual psychotherapy is effective in tackling psychopathology, and psychological therapists working in CF teams have key roles in implementing and evaluating interventions, targeting those thought to be most vulnerable, and working with other team members to consider how psychological care can be effectively and pragmatically incorporated into routine management.

There are many psychosocial aspects of CF that we are only beginning to understand. The effects of family functioning on health outcomes are emerging, particularly with regard to adherence. Parent–child conflict has consistently emerged as a key factor in the establishment and maintenance of adherence difficulties. Health beliefs and illness perceptions are also emerging as important to adherence, and coping strategies associated with more positive health outcomes and successful psychological adaptation must be explored further. Motivational interviewing and active peer support is gaining ground in other illness groups and needs to be evaluated more thoroughly in CF populations.

Yet in concluding, even when there is only partial adherence to treatment, we must acknowledge and salute the tremendous efforts made by patients and their families, many of whom lead normal lives and maintain hope in the face of substantial challenges.

REFERENCES

1. Kerem E, Conway SP, Elborn S, Heijerman HH. Standards of care for patients with cystic fibrosis: a European consensus. *J Cyst Fibros* 2005; **4**:7–26.

2. Pless IB, Nolan T. Revision, replication and neglect: research on maladjustment in chronic illness. *J Child Psychol Psychiat* 1991; **32**:347–365.

3. Frederiksen B, Laang S, Koch C, Hoiby N. Improved survival in the Danish center-treated cystic fibrosis patients: results of aggressive treatment. *Pediatr Pulmonol* 1996; **21**:153–158.

4. Gee L, Abbott J, Conway SP *et al.* Development and validation of a disease specific health related quality of life measure for adults and adolescents with cystic fibrosis. *Thorax* 2000; **55**:946–954.

5. Modi AC, Quittner AL. Validation of a disease-specific measure of health-related quality of life for children with cystic fibrosis. *J Pediatr Psychol* 2003; **28**:535–546.

6. Cadman D, Boyle M, Szatmari P, Offord DR. Chronic illness, disability and mental and social well-being: findings of the Ontario Child Health Study. *Pediatrics* 1987; **79**:805–813.

7. Berge JM, Patterson JM. Cystic fibrosis and the family: a review and critique of the literature. *Fam Syst Hlth* 2004; **22**:74–100.

8. Quittner AL, DiGirolamo AM, Michel M, Eigen H. Parental response to cystic fibrosis: a contextual analysis of the diagnosis phase. *J Pediatr Psychol* 1992; **17**:683–704.

9. van Ijzendoorn MH, Goldberg S, Kroonenberg PM, Frenkel O. The relative effects of maternal and child problems on the quality of attachment; a meta-analysis of attachment in clinical samples. *Child Dev* 1992; **63**:840–858.

10. Thompson RJ, Gustafson KE. *Adaptation to Chronic Childhood Illness.* Washington, DC, American Psychological Association, 1996.

11. Thompson RJ, Gustafson KE, Hamlett KW, Spock A. Psychological adjustment of children with cystic fibrosis: the role of child cognitive processes and maternal adjustment. *J Pediatr Psychol* 1992; **17**:741–755.

12. Thompson RJ, Gustafson KE, Hamlett KW, Spock A. Stress, coping and family functioning in the psychological adjustment of mothers of children and adolescents with cystic fibrosis. *J Pediatr Psychol* 1992; **17**:573–585.

13. Stark LJ, Jelalian E, Powers SW *et al.* Parent and child mealtime behavior in families of children with cystic fibrosis. *J Pediatrics* 2000; **136**:195–200.

14. Stark LJ, Opipari LC, Jelalian E *et al.* Child behaviour and parent management strategies at mealtimes in families with a school-age child with cystic fibrosis. *Health Psychol* 2005; **24**:274–280.

15. Duff AJA, Brownlee KG. The management of emotional distress during venepuncture. *Netherlands J Med* 1999; **54**(Suppl):S8.

16. D'Auria JP, Christian JP, Henderson ZG, Haynes B. The company they keep: the influence of peer relationships on adjustment to cystic fibrosis during adolescence. *J Pediatr Nurs* 2000; **15**:175–182.

17. Blair C, Cull A, Freeman CP. Psychosocial functioning of young adults with cystic fibrosis and their families. *Thorax* 1994; **49**:798–802.

18. Szyndler JE, Towns SJ, van Asperen PP, McKay KO. Psychological and family functioning and quality of life in adolescents with cystic fibrosis. *J Cyst Fibros* 2005; **4**:135–144.

19. Pfeffer PE, Pfeffer JM, Hodson ME. The psychosocial and psychiatric side of cystic fibrosis in adolescents and adults. *J Cyst Fibros* 2003; **2**:61–68.

20. Gee L, Abbott J, Conway SP *et al.* Quality of life in cystic fibrosis: the impact of gender, general health perceptions and disease severity. *J Cyst Fibros* 2003; **2**:206–213.

21. Hubbard PA, Broome ME, Antia LA. Pain, coping and disability in adolescents and young adults with cystic fibrosis: a web-based study. *Ped Nursing* 2005; **31**:82–86.

22. Graetz BW, Shute RH, Sawyer MG. An Australian study of adolescents with cystic fibrosis: perceived supportive and non supportive behaviours from families and friends and psychological adjustment. *J Adol Health* 2000; **26**:64–69.

23. DiGirolamo AM, Quittner AL, Ackerman V, Stevens J. Identification and assessment of ongoing stressors in adolescents with a chronic illness: an application of the Behavior Analytic Model. *J Clin Child Psychol* 1997; **26**:53–66.

24. DeLambo KE, Ievers-Landis CE, Drotar D, Quittner AL. Association of observed family relationship quality and problem-solving skills with treatment adherence in older children and adolescents with cystic fibrosis. *J Pediatr Psychol* 2004; **29**:343–353.

25. Conway SP. Transition from paediatric to adult-orientated care for adolescents with cystic fibrosis. *Disabil Rehab* 1998; **20**:209–216.

26. Cystic Fibrosis Trust. *UK CF Database Annual Data Report.* Bromley, CF Trust, 2003.

27. Abbott J, Gee L. Contemporary psychosocial issues in cystic fibrosis: treatment adherence and quality of life. *Disabil Rehab* 1998; **20**:262–271.

28. Gee L, Abbott J, Hart A *et al.* Associations between clinical variables and quality of life in adults with cystic fibrosis. *J Cyst Fibros* 2005; **4**:59–66.

29. Staab D, Wenninger K, Gebert N et al. Quality of life in patients with cystic fibrosis and their parents: what is important besides disease severity? Thorax 1998; 53:727–731.

30. Abbott J. Coping with cystic fibrosis. J R Soc Med 2003; 96(Suppl):42–50.

31. Anderson DL, Flume PA, Hardy KK. Psychological functioning of adults with cystic fibrosis. Chest 2001; 119:1079–1084.

32. Reid S, Henry JA. Deliberate self-harm. Prim Care Psychiat 2001; 8:1–7.

33. Burker EJ, Sedway J, Carone S. Psychological and educational factors: better predictors of work status than FEV$_1$ in adults with cystic fibrosis. Pediatr Pulmonol 2004; 38:413–418.

34. DiMatteo MR, Lepper HS, Croghan TW. Depression is a risk factor for non-compliance with medical treatment: meta-analysis of the effects of anxiety and depression on patient adherence. Arch Int Med 2000; 160:2101–2107.

35. Riekert KA, Bartlett SJ, Boyle MP, Rand CS. The relationship between depression, disease severity and quality of life in adults with cystic fibrosis. Am J Resp Crit Care Med 2004; 169:A392.

36. Goodwin RD, Pine DS. Respiratory disease and panic attacks among adult in the United States. Chest 2002; 2:645–650.

37. Oxley H, Webb AK. How a clinical psychologist manages the problems of adults with cystic fibrosis. J R Soc Med 2005; 98(Suppl):37–46.

38. Abbott J, Conway S, Etherington C et al. Perceived body image and eating behaviour in young adults with cystic fibrosis and their healthy peers. J Behav Med 2000; 23:501–517.

39. Shearer JE, Bryon M. The nature and prevalence of eating disorders and eating disturbance in adolescents with cystic fibrosis. J R Soc Med 2004; 97(Suppl):36–42.

40. Widerman E. Knowledge, interests and educational needs of adults diagnosed with cystic fibrosis after age 18. J Cyst Fibros 2003; 2:97–104.

41. Quittner AL, Drotar D, Ievers-Landis CE et al. Adherence to medical treatments in adolescents with cystic fibrosis: the development and evaluation of family-based interventions. In: Drotar D (ed.) Promoting Adherence to Medical Treatment in Chronic Childhood Illness: Concepts, Methods and Interventions. Mahwah, NJ, Lawrence Erlbaum Associates, 2000, pp383–407.

42. Ievers-Landis CE, Brown RT, Drotar D et al. Knowledge of physician prescription and adherence to treatment among children with cystic fibrosis and their mothers. J Dev Behav Pediatr 1999; 2:335–343.

43. Stark LJ, Jelalian E, Miller DL. Cystic fibrosis. In: Roberts MC (ed.) Handbook of Pediatric Psychology, 2nd edn. New York, Guilford Press, 1995, 241–262.

44. Kettler LJ, Sawyer SM, Winefield HR, Greville HW. Determinants of adherence in adults with cystic fibrosis. Thorax 2002; 57:459–464.

45. Quinn J, Latchford G, Duff AJA et al. Measuring, predicting and improving adherence to inhalation therapy in patients with CF: a randomised controlled study of motivational interviewing. Pediatr Pulmonol 2004; Suppl 27:360.

46. Patterson JM, Budd J, Goetz DR, Warwick WJ. Family correlates of a 10-year pulmonary health trend in cystic fibrosis. Pediatrics 1993; 91:383–389.

47. Abbott J, Dodd M, Bilton D, Webb AK. Treatment compliance in adults with cystic fibrosis. Thorax 1994; 49:115–120.

48. Abbott J, Dodd M, Webb AK. Health perceptions and treatment adherence in adults with cystic fibrosis. Thorax 1996; 51:1233–1238.

49. Parcel G, Swank PR, Mariotto M, Bartholomew L. Self-management of cystic fibrosis: a structural model for educational and behavioural variables. Soc Sci Med 1994; 38:1307–1315.

50. Tluczek A, Koscik RL, Farell PM, Rock MJ. Psychosocial risk associated with newborn screening for cystic fibrosis: parents' experience while awaiting the sweat-test appointment. Pediatrics 2005; 115:1692–1703.

51. Kharrazi M, Kharrazi LD. Delayed diagnosis of cystic fibrosis and the family perspective. J Pediatr 2005; 147(Suppl):S21–S25.

52. Quittner AL, Espelage DL, Opipari LC et al. Role strain in couples with and without a child with a chronic illness: associations with marital satisfaction, intimacy and daily mood. Health Psychol 1998; 17:112–124.

53. Ievers CE, Drotar D. Family and parental functioning in cystic fibrosis. J Dev Behav Pediatr 1996; 17:48–55.

54. Ievers CE, Drotar D, Dahms WT et al. Maternal child-rearing behaviour in three groups: cystic fibrosis, insulin-dependent diabetes mellitus and healthy children. J Pediatr Psychol 1994; 19:681–687.

55. Ullrich G, Wiedau-Gors S, Steinkamp G et al. Parental fears of Pseudomonas infection and measures to prevent its acquisition. J Cyst Fibros 2002; 1:122–130.

56. Heaman DJ. Perceived stressors and coping strategies of parents who have children with developmental disabilities: a comparison of mothers with fathers. J Pediatr Nurs 1995; 10:311–320.

57. Sharpe D, Rossiter L. Siblings of children with a chronic illness: a meta-analysis. J Pediatr Psychol 2002; 27:699–710.

58. Bluebond-Langer M. Living with cystic fibrosis: the well sibling's perspective. Med Anthropol Quart 1991; 5:133–152.

59. Czyewski DL, Mariotto MJ, Bartholomew K et al. Measurement of quality of well being in a children and adolescent cystic fibrosis population. Med Care 1994; 32:965–972.

60. Macpherson C, Redmon A, Leavy A, McMullan M. A review of cystic fibrosis children born to single mothers. Acta Paediatr 1998; 87:397–400.

61. Coady CC, Kent VD, Davis PW. Burnout among social workers working with patients with cystic fibrosis. Health Social Work 1990; 15:116–124.

62. Carr A, Roseingrave P, Fitzgerald MX. Factors associated with stress responses in staff caring for patients with cystic fibrosis. Irish J Psychol 1996; 17:241–250.

63. Roter DL, Hall JA, Barker LR et al. Improving physician's interviewing skills and reducing patients' emotional distress. Arch Int Med 1995; 155:1877–1884.

64. Haberman D, McDonald CM. Support systems for parents of children with CF. *Pediatr Pulmonol* 2005; Suppl 27:136–137.

65. Bryon M. Psychological interventions. In: Bush A *et al.* (eds) *Cystic Fibrosis in the 21st Century: Progress in Respiratory Research.* Basel, Karger, 2006, pp 309–313.

66. Duff AJA. Psychological interventions in cystic fibrosis and asthma. *Pediatr Resp Rev* 2001; **2**:350–357.

67. Stark LJ, Jelalian E, McGrath AM, Mackner L. Behavioral approaches in cystic fibrosis: applications to feeding and eating. In: Bluebond-Langner M *et al.* (eds) *Psychosocial Aspects of Cystic Fibrosis.* London, Arnold, 2001, pp348–360.

68. Bryon M. Behavior therapy and cognitive-behavior therapy. In: Bluebond-Langner M *et al.* (eds) *Psychosocial Aspects of Cystic Fibrosis.* London, Arnold, 2001, pp318–328.

69. Duff AJA. Incorporating psychological approaches into routine paediatric venepuncture. *Arch Dis Child* 2003; **88**:931–937.

70. Conway SP, Pond MN, Watson A, Hammett T. Knowledge of adult patients with CF about their illness. *Thorax* 1996; **51**:34–38.

71. McMullen AH. Health education. In: Bluebond-Langner M *et al.* (eds) *Psychosocial Aspects of Cystic Fibrosis.* London, Arnold, 2001, pp268–295.

72. Lehrer PM, Sargunaraj D, Hochron S. Psychological approaches to the treatment of asthma. *J Consult Clin Psychol* 1992; **60**:639–643.

73. Davis MA, Quittner AL, Stack CM, Yang MCK. Controlled evaluation of the STARBRIGHT CD-ROM program for children and adolescents with cystic fibrosis. *J Pediatr Psychol* 2004; **29**:259–267.

74. Duff AJA, Ball R, Wolfe SP *et al.* BETTERLAND: an interactive CD-ROM guide for children with cystic fibrosis. *Paediatr Nurs* 2006; **18**:30–33.

75. Greco P, Pendley JS, McDonell K, Reeves G. A peer group intervention for adolescents with type I diabetes and their best friends. *J Pediatr Psychol* 2001; **26**:485–490.

76. National Institute for Clinical Excellence. *Depression in Children and Young People: Identification and Management of Depression in Primary, Community and Secondary Care* (Clinical Guideline 28). London, NICE, 2005.

77. Kazak AE, Simms S, Rourke MT. Family systems practice in pediatric psychology. *J Pediatr Psychol* 2002; **27**:133–144.

78. Haynes RB, Yao X, Degani *et al.* Interventions to enhance medication adherence. *Cochrane Database System Rev* 2005, Issue 4. CD000011.

79. DiMatteo MR. Social support and patient adherence to medical treatment: a meta-analysis. *Health Psychol* 2004; **23**:207–218.

80. Bundy C. Changing behaviour: using motivational interviewing techniques. *J R Soc Med* 2004; **97**(Suppl):43–47.

81. Zigmond AS, Snaith RP. The Hospital Anxiety and Depression Scale. *Acta Psychiatr Scand* 1983; **67**:361–370.

82. White CA. *Cognitive Behaviour Therapy for Chronic Medical Problems: A Guide to Assessment and Treatment in Practice.* Chichester, Wiley, 2001.

83. National Institute for Clinical Excellence. *Depression: Management of Depression in Primary and Secondary Care.* London, NICE, 2004.

84. National Institute for Clinical Excellence. *Anxiety: Management of Anxiety (panic disorder, with or without agoraphobia, and generalised anxiety disorder) in Adults in Primary, Secondary and Community Care.* London, NICE 2004.

85. Heslop K. Cognitive behavioural therapy in cystic fibrosis. *J Roy Soc Med* 2006; **99**(Suppl 46):27–29.

32

Palliative care in cystic fibrosis

CATHERINE E. URCH AND MARGARET E. HODSON

INTRODUCTION

The modern 'palliative care' movement in the UK has been almost exclusively associated with oncology, and care in specialist hospices, when it was founded in the 1960s by Dame Cicely Saunders, but over the last 45 years specialist palliative care has developed and adapted [1]. There are now over 200 hospices throughout the UK, and thousands around the world. More importantly the specialty has been recognized in every country and the need for palliative care acknowledged for a wide range of life-limiting diseases. Over the last decade there has been a more radical acknowledgment, both from within the speciality of palliative care and from the rest of medicine, that there is a need for specialist palliative care outside oncology [2,3]. How this is developed and delivered is still being reviewed and adapted. It is apparent that excellent care (physical, psychological, emotional) from the cystic fibrosis (CF) teams deliver high-quality general palliative care [4,5].

The aim of this chapter is to develop some ideas around the following questions:

- Is there a need for palliative care in CF?
- Should this be delivered by the CF team, or specialist palliative care, or both?
- Does the possibility of transplantation preclude much of the work of specialist palliative care, or is holding the duality of death and life possible?
- How should we approach symptom control in the final stages?
- Who should be involved with spirituality and bereavement issues?

IS THERE A NEED FOR PALLIATIVE CARE IN CF?

The huge medical advances over the last two decades have altered the quality and quantity of life of most people with cystic fibrosis This has been transformed from a disease with death in infancy or childhood, to one where a pediatric death is now rare and the vast majority of patients proceed to adulthood and continue to have a good quality of life [6]. Unfortunately the disease at present is still progressive and fatal. Over time the respiratory secretions, infections, and potential liver, pancreatic and gut complications will lead to death. The commonest cause of death is respiratory failure, preceded by increasingly distressing symptoms of breathlessness, anxiety and sputum production. Lung transplantation has clearly altered the outlook of progressive respiratory failure from one of death to one tinged with hope of renewed quality of life. However, life while waiting for transplantation is difficult, with increasing illness, distress and approaching death, while trying to fight and remain hopeful about a transplant. With the limitation on organ availability, up to 50% of patients on a transplant list will die waiting, and so the hope of a transplant should not obscure effective terminal care [7–10].

The average life expectancy is around 30 years of age, which masks the range of adults that can be cared for, and the vastly different needs at different ages. Cystic fibrosis teams (whether pediatric or adult) have developed a wide range of skills to care holistically for their patients to death [5]. The active nature of treatment to death may suggest there is no role for palliative care. However, as palliative care is defined as 'the holistic care of patients and families at any stage of their disease pathway, without effecting a cure' [11]), there is a role for palliative care and indeed everyone providing care to the CF patient is delivering general palliative or supportive care.

The needs of patients with CF cover all boundaries – physical, emotional, spiritual, psychological, family dynamics – so the teams caring from them should be practising holistic and palliative care [12]. In non-curative chronic conditions care is usually delivered within multidisciplinary teams, and guidelines for chronic life-limiting conditions raise the need for integrated specialist input at the terminal phase and improved care of the dying [13]. Cystic fibrosis multidisciplinary teams already exist as microcosms of general palliative care. Thus the question 'Is palliative care needed?' is already answered in the affirmative and is often delivered.

SPECIALIST PALLIATIVE CARE IN ADDITION TO GENERAL PALLIATIVE CARE

The more interesting question is whether there is a need for specialist palliative care and how this could be delivered. Core specialist palliative care teams most commonly consist of doctors trained in palliative medicine and nurse specialists (delivering specialist palliative care), although the extended teams may include dietitians, psychologists, bereavement councillors, rehabilitation therapists, speech and language therapists, chaplains and social workers. Specialist palliative care focuses on holistic aspects of the terminal phase. This includes raising awareness, open communication and symptom control, and bringing expertise in terminal care from other areas, while working in close collaboration with the CF team, who continue to have a wider role in the active and long-term care of the patient. Specialist palliative care is delivered in nearly every country within the community and hospital settings, but for the vast majority of patients with CF the terminal phase and death occurs in hospital. The role of the specialist palliative care team in hospital is one of collaboration with the CF team, and not one of 'taking over' patient care [14]. This acknowledges many things:

- the patient not feeling abandoned by a team he or she knows and trusts;
- the patient still being able to access the necessary medical/surgical care;
- the educational/collaborative approach of specialist palliative care;
- acknowledgment of the often high level of general palliative care delivered by CF teams;
- specialist palliative care delivering niche ideas/support while not taking over;
- the continuity of the lead clinician (CF consultant) coordinating the care plan.

Specialist palliative care is commonly involved when there are issues around discussion of end of life (including preparation of children and siblings), changing gear, terminal care, symptom control in the terminal phase, family support, involving community support, major life decisions (e.g. quality versus quantity discussions), and supporting bereavement follow-up [15].

TEAM WORKING

There has been a paradigm shift in delivery of best patient care from the paternalistic, single consultant delivering all,

to one of a multidisciplinary team, each member of which delivers a specialist aspect, coordinated and led by the lead consultant. This way of working does not suit all temperaments, and requires a high level of effective communication and trust. Specialist palliative care should form one aspect of the team, adapting locally to the needs and the gaps in the CF team and will be different from the perceived traditional role (one of taking over), to one of raising questions, discussion and education within the team, supporting the CF team, and terminal care [16]. Many of the barriers faced by specialist palliative care in CF are the preconceptions of what specialist palliative care will do; for example, the concept of stopping all acute interventions and the association with instant death (often a consequence of late referral). Early discussion and involvement of specialist palliative care should increase the quality of life and enhance the well-being of dying patients, not precipitate their death [17].

THE TERMINAL PHASE

Acknowledgment and preparation

Caring for many patients with CF in the last year or two of life and in the dying phase is complicated for some by the hope of transplantation [10]. For patients and the team this can be a period of intense uncertainty, with many conflicting emotions and fears [8,10]. Cystic fibrosis is unique in that from childhood patients will be accumulating knowledge about the eventual fatal outcome. By adolescence many will have already had to confront living with dying and developed coping strategies [18]. In addition patients are acutely aware that transplantation discussions are an explicit acknowledgment of the progression of the illness. Many teams take the opportunity that transplantation discussions afford to openly discuss resuscitation and intensive care support, living with uncertainty, and explore aspects and wishes around further deterioration or even death.

Patients will have known friends or siblings who have died from CF [19], and perhaps others for whom transplantation has been successful. Patients usually have an extensive knowledge from non-medical sources; this should be built on and explored by the CF team and not ignored [20,21]. As with all sensitive discussions there is a concern that explicitly discussing resuscitation and death will somehow hasten it, or confuse the patient into thinking that the team is giving up. Evidence from other specialties suggest that open communication about prognosis, while inducing some short-term anxiety, allows for greater participation and acceptance [22–24]. Discussion can lead to the ability for advance planning and optimization of care at the end of life [25]. If the team does not raise these issues early and in a clear manner then the patient will get the message that his or her fears are of no interest. The patient may imagine the worst, have no access to specialist help, and this in turn may increase fear and diminish the ability to cope independently. Leaving discussions about resuscitation, place of death,

Table 32.1 Domains that require discussion during the terminal phase in order to allow optimization of care of the dying.[a]

Insight:
- Prognosis is limited
- Recognition that death may be imminent
- Transplantation possibility (including who, when and where information given and updated)

Preferred language

Level of discussion and involvement in decisions desired

Religious/spiritual needs – including identifying support

Relationships/sexuality (including family tree, key dynamics)

Legacy

Reflection and meaning of their life, legacy for future

Memory boxes

Wills, etc.

Resolution of unfinished business

Preferred place of care/death

Advanced planning or wishes for care around death

Resuscitation status – including transfer to intensive care, ward support, non-invasive ventilatory support

When death is predicted:
- Recognition of a change in focus of care
- Review appropriateness and frequency of investigations
- Review appropriateness and timing of nursing interventions
- Review drug chart – appropriateness of medications, route of medication
- Review and assessment of specific symptoms, i.e. shortness of breath, distress, pain
- Medications for symptom control prescribed as required or regularly
- Patient, family, and team aware
- Family to stay
- Referral to specialist palliative care considered – do early if already known
- Financial care of children

[a]There needs to be discussion with the patient, family and team, and this must be documented to avoid unnecessary repetition and to facilitate interdisciplinary care.
Modified from [50].

fears around dying, saying good-byes, too close to the end becomes an exhausting self-fulfilling prophecy (Table 32.1). The emotional work by the practitioner and patient is greater closer to death, and the death itself may be less satisfactory as there is too little time and energy to prepare [5].

It is difficult to support the patient during the terminal phase [26]. The person is physically unwell, with bouts of respiratory failure, any one of which could be fatal. It is important to maintain clear and open communication, acknowledging the individual patient's hopes and fears [27]. The balance between the necessary interventions and discomfort to the patient and the wish to achieve good symptom control can be difficult [28]. Many drugs that relieve the sensation of breathlessness or pain may also be sedating, and getting the dose correct to minimize side-effects can take time, patience and experience. Other non-drug interventions, such as non-invasive ventilatory support, may be more

effective and timely [29]. Support for the team and the patient's family is vital [5]. As time progresses and the patient becomes more unwell, divisions within the team (such as 'Is the patient dying or not?') need to be discussed and resolved.

The time before death is particularly hard for patients and family, even if this has been discussed and planned for. Patients may not feel ready, may have worries over children, siblings, family and friends. Many are scared of dying awake, suffocating or in pain. These fears need to be openly addressed and managed with patients and their families. Some patients will be called for a transplant during this phase, but the emotional 'work' done in preparation for death is not wasted – rather put aside for another time. Many patients with support appear to be able to work through this preparation 'for the worst' while maintaining 'hope for the best'. Specialist palliative care can assist in holding this rather unique duality [30].

Dying while on the transplant list

Perhaps one of the most difficult situations is when a patient on the transplant list is reaching the final days of life [7]. Acceptance on the list usually brings elation and hope, but over time the patient's health will deteriorate, with life-threatening exacerbations, continuous oxygen and perhaps non-invasive ventilation, bringing fear and the inevitable wondering 'Will there be a transplant organ in time for me?'. Once there is gross respiratory and/or other organ failure there is little hope for a successful transplant. Throughout the terminal phase and the eventual dying period, it is essential to consider and discuss good symptom control (Table 32.2) and the implications of treatments. However, hopes for a transplant should not override the need for good symptom control at every stage as opioids for pain and breathlessness can be reversed with naloxone and benzodiazepines with flumazinal, if a transplant becomes available. The discussions and deliberations around symptom control alongside active treatment are difficult but should be tackled on a regular basis with the whole multidisciplinary team, patient and family. Dying while waiting for a transplant is unfortunately not rare, but patients still require good and effective terminal care and a peaceful death.

Symptom control

During the terminal phase, and especially in the dying phase, the number of symptoms that require purely symptomatic control increases [31]. Most patients and especially families view a death as 'good' if it is peaceful, with good symptom control, no agitation, and the struggle for breath minimized (see Table 32.2).

The majority of patients dying from CF die from respiratory failure complicating infection, hemoptysis or pneumothorax. The predominant symptoms noted in a

Table 32.2 Specific symptom control for adult terminal care in cystic fibrosis. If symptoms persist or are not listed refer for specialist advice (see notes).

Symptom	Non-pharmacological	Pharmacological	Other
Breathlessness	• Optimization of ventilatory support • Oxygen • Controlled breathing pattern • Physiotherapy to clear secretions • Humidification • Aspirate effusions • Optimize pillow at sitting position • Relaxation	• Antibiotics (if appropriate) • Opioids – systemic not nebulized in terminal care • Morphine sulphate 2.5–5 mg (opioid naive) p.o., p.r.n., 4-hourly. Morphine sulphate 2.5 mg (opioid naive) p.o., p.r.n., or 10 mg+ via syringe driver over 24 hours • Titrate dose with effect • No ceiling dose • Alter routine as needed • Benzodiazepines – see below • Treat cardiac causes	• Calm environment • Reassurance of family/patient not allowed to die with suffocation • Familiar staff
Pain	• Optimization of mattress/pillows • Positioning • Massage • Acupuncture • TENS	• Assessment – cause, duration, precipitating and relieving features • WHO ladder plus adjuvants, e.g. (a) non-opioids, (b) weak opioids, (c) opioids Systemic p.o., s.c., transdermal. Dose: start equivalent of p.o. morphine sulphate 2.5–5 mg 2.5–5 mg p.r.n. and 4-hourly, titrate to effect. Seek advice for uncontrolled pain or opioid switch • Syringe driver 10–20 mg morphine sulphate (or equivalent 24-hour dose) over 24 hours may be needed • Remember anti-emetics (cyclizine 25–50 mg t.d.s., or metoclopramide 10 mg t.d.s., both p.o. or s.c.) if naive and laxatives • NSAIDs beware of contraindications • Neuropathic adjuvants (specialist advice)	• Reassure will not allow death in pain • Myths of opioids (a) no dependence if used for analgesia or breathlessness; (b) with correct dosing does not hasten death Effective analgesia enhances quality and quantity of life
Anxiety/panic episodes	• Psychological support • Relaxation techniques • Complementary therapies, e.g. reflexology, aromatherapy, music, TV	• Short acting benzodiazepines p.r.n.: lorazepam 0.5 mg s.l. midazolam 1.25–2.5 mg s.c. or diazepam 2–5 mg p.r.n. to t.d.s. • Phenothiazines: levomepromazine (12.5–25 mg p.o. or s.c., o.d.) chlorpromazine 25 mg p.o., b.d. Butyrophenones: haloperidol 1.5–5 mg p.o. or s.c., o.d. to b.d. • Anti-depressants (seek advice)	• Calm environment • Teach family and nurses relaxation
Terminal agitation		• Benzodiazepine: midazolam 1.25–2.5 mg s.c., p.r.n., then 10 mg+ over 24 hours in syringe driver • Phenothiazines: levomepromazine 6.25–12.5 mg s.c., p.r.n., then 25 mg+ over 24 hours in a syringe driver (seek advice)	• Reverse underlying cause if possible
Fatigue	• Paced moving • Avoid unnecessary disturbances	• No evidence that any medication reverses • Steroids may give a temporary boost to mood, increase fluid retention; no long-term benefit	• Paced visiting, few people, short duration • Allow rest
Anorexia/cachexia	• No intervention during terminal phase	• Steroids (temporary effect if any) • Alcohol/aperitif	• All interventions aimed earlier at prevention
Reduced communication	• Non-verbal, i.e. touch • Hearing thought to be preserved until late		• Reassurance normal part of dying, with reduced consciousness

Notes

1. Subcutaneous route of drug delivery is equivalent to intravenous. A syringe driver can deliver drugs evenly over a 24-hour period. The hourly rate is one twenty-fourth (about 4%) of the total dose.

2. For *pediatric* terminal care, seek specialist advice. Drugs for pain, breathlessness, and agitation remain the same but dosing schedules will vary according to body weight and age. The principle of achieving good symptom control and effecting a peaceful death remains identical to adult care.

3. All opioids are discussed in morphine sulphate. Use conversion tables to find equivalent dose for alternative opioids.

o.d., once daily; b.d., twice daily; t.d.s., three times daily; p.r.n., as required; p.o., oral; s.c., subcutaneous; s.l., sublingual. NSAIDS, non-steroidal anti-inflammatory drugs; TENS, transcutaneous electrical nerve stimulation.

retrospective review of patients indicated that breathlessness and anxiety/fear and fatigue occurred in the vast majority of patients [32]. Pain is a less common symptom when compared to breathlessness, but should be specifically enquired about. Other symptoms common in other diseases such as: nausea, vomiting and seizures rarely occurred. The need for regular assessment and evaluation of symptomatic intervention is paramount [33]. The aim of good symptomatic palliation is to utilize any treatment domain that minimizes the symptoms, increases the quality of life and ideally would not in itself alter the prognosis. Thus, for example, to ameliorate anxiety, the role for early and effective psychological and specialist palliative care support to explore fears and anxieties, develop coping strategies and aid independence are key and should be employed before prescribing drugs such as anxiolytics or antidepressants. Similarly, breathlessness is best ameliorated with physiotherapy, assisted ventilation and controlled breathing strategies before medication [29,34]. Breathlessness is a major symptom and reports of the efficacy of systemic opioids suggest that these should be used earlier in the terminal phase [35].

Terminal care

Understanding the dying process is important in order to employ the rational use of medication for symptom control, to be able to discuss probable scenarios with the family, and to pre-empt problems [31].Towards the end of life often all the non-medical modalities will have been explored and drugs are needed to relieve symptoms. Again the aim is always the use the minimum dose, employing polypharmacy for additive effect, to achieve symptomatic control but not to hasten death [36]. It must be remembered that all drugs commonly used do not preclude transplantation or continued active therapy and can be stopped if no longer needed. Specific discussions around the appropriateness of discontinuation of acute treatment and investigations are necessary to ensure a balance of acknowledgment of imminent death and hope for reversal. Discussion around continuation or cessation of assisted ventilation should be on the basis of symptom control and comfort, although relatives may need warning that mechanical ventilation will continue after death (until the machine is removed) [37]. Fear of death is common and may require exploration – explanation of what is happening, but equally a silent, reassuring presence is therapeutic [38]. Keeping the focus on the patient and family allows for a more individual exploration of their psychosocial, emotional, physical and spiritual needs [37].

Opioids are the mainstay of treatment for pain and breathlessness in the dying phase [33]. However, the definition of the dying phase is difficult in CF and may extend from hours to months. In one study, 86% of patients had between 5 and 30 mg morphine hourly for more than 1 month, while continuing on antibiotics (75%) and acute preventative treatments (72%) to within 12 hours of death [39]. Other symptoms that occur commonly include terminal agitation, fatigue, altered consciousness with reduced communication, all of which require specific evaluation and, where possible, control (see Table 32.2).

Most important throughout this phase is the level and quality of communication. It is tempting with seriously ill or dying, especially young, people not to engage them directly in decision-making but use spouses or parents as a proxy [40]. While this may circumvent short-term difficult conversations, it nearly always leads to a fracturing of trust, miscommunication and even later guilt by the bereaved over decisions taken. All competent adults have the right to be spoken to about events and decisions regarding their bodies and lives. Families are close proxies, especially where they have been involved as caregivers, but they should not displace the patient unless very clear explicit instructions have been given [41]. Ideally communication about the patient's views on life and death, how and where he or she wishes to be cared for, and fears about living and dying should all have been explored long before the final event [42]. It is easier to address these when the patient is ill, in the terminal phase, but not acutely facing the possibility of death. Again a community support nurse, or other member of the team, may be the most appropriate person to explore these issues over time, rather than the specialist palliative care member. However, often the team need support and education and there will always be the more complex family interactions and personalities that may require more direct specialist intervention.

Open team communication and agreement is also vital. Predicting death can be very difficult in patients with CF as any acute infective exacerbation could be fatal, and again death may be sudden and unpredicted. Where possible the level of symptom control, sedation and possible consequences of any intervention must be agreed within the team and with the patient [5]. Thus, the inadequate control of breathlessness, leaving the patient to die with the fear and sensation of suffocation is equally an act of commission (not omission) as sedation [36]. The needs and fears of the team need to be explored and addressed so that they do not hinder effective care of the dying patient. It must be remembered that there is little if any evidence that drugs such as opioids and benzodiazepines used in appropriate doses alter the expected prognosis [33]. Rather it is a question of how the patient will live and die, rather than when. Medicine and people are unpredictable, and prognostication is an art not a science, and everyone will have anecdotes of patients who recover against all expectations, as well as those who died with uncontrolled distress unexpectedly.

The physical and emotional care of the family is important, including provision for them to stay and personalize the room. The environment should be tailored to the patient and family's wishes wherever possible, and their time together without repeated interruptions should be acknowledged. Staying with ill and dying patients is exhausting and this needs to be discussed and a shift pattern within the family encouraged if possible, so as not to exhausted themselves. The direction and aim of care must be clearly communicated.

Terminal care of the adult CF patient

In addition to the general terminal care advice above, the CF patient has specific needs. Physiotherapy can be vital for symptom control (breathlessness and sputum accumulation) and maintaining continuity of care. However, the program should be discussed and tailored to the patient's needs. Continuation of non-invasive ventilation needs to be discussed, and it may be more appropriate to return to an oxygen mask for palliation. Non-invasive saturation checks may be useful as hypoxia can make the patient very restless and uncomfortable, whereas to a certain extent carbon dioxide retention can help the patient to feel drowsy. By this stage 'do not resuscitate' orders should be in place and clear advice in the notes as to the level of intervention (for example changing antibiotics, not for intubation, etc.).

Patients should be given the opportunity to talk and, if possible, for a few minutes most days with staff in the absence of their relatives. They can then often express feelings which would be difficult in front of those who love them. A skilled psychologist, CF nurse specialist, or specialist palliative care practitioner can be particularly helpful at this stage of the patient's disease.

Terminal care in pediatric CF patients

It is inevitable that dealing with end-of-life issues has become secondary to the daily care of a child with CF, so pediatric teams may have lost some of their previously held skills. This is not necessarily a problem as many hospitals provide a palliative care service, but the CF team needs to individualize that service for each child. Individualizing aspects of care are skills used on a daily basis by all CF teams; close communication and honesty within the team can help redirect those skills towards managing the terminal stages of the disease.

Most people with CF know that they are dying – child or adult. Parents want to protect their child (however old) from this knowledge and children will often try to protect their parents from this discussion [43]. This collusion of silence can result in parents and child knowing what is happening but unable to talk about it for fear of upsetting each other. Support and encouragement from the CF team will allow these discussions to take place, allowing not only the family to say good-bye but also enabling the CF team to practically and medically manage the terminal stages in a manner most appropriate to the child and family.

Specific symptom control and terminal care issues are the same as in adults and the aim should be to minimize symptoms, enhance the life left and achieve a peaceful death. Table 32.2 offers advice for adult symptom control,

and while the drugs and philosophy remain the same, specialist advise should be sought as dosing schedules will be dependent on the weight and age of the child.

Chapter 28 has further discussion on end-stage management and bereavement.

PLACE OF DEATH

There is little evidence about the preferred place of care and death of patients with CF. Mitchel and co-workers [44] noted that 82% of patients died in hospital, 15% on an intensive care unit. These figures are unsurprising given the degree of active treatment up to death, that in many countries would be impossible to deliver at such a high level of care at home [39]. However, some patients do have strong views about whether they wish to be cared for at home or hospital; where possible these should be explored and delivered [45]. In the UK and many countries community specialist palliative care nurses would take on the lead coordination of care of the dying at home. They are used to supporting families, aware of the implications for siblings (who may have CF) and are skilled in using medication primarily to relieve symptoms, rather than waiting for the 'last 24 hours'.

In hospital, the division between terminal care and acute care is often more blurred. While the principles of good symptom control should be applied at any stage, and the patient's wishes held paramount, reviews of terminal care in hospitals reveals a high level of inadequate symptom control and lack of involvement of specialist help [46–48]. The development of 'end of life care pathways' has been with a view to improving the care of all dying patients in hospital and elsewhere [49,50]. While many of these do not easily fit with the specific needs of the CF population, further development may allow the use of specialist pathway to enhance the understanding of the needs of dying patients [51,52]. Important areas such as patient assessment, symptom control, goal planning and complex family dynamics can be explored, managed and documented to facilitate team-working [42].

SPIRITUAL CARE

All human beings have a spiritual aspect of their being. In some this may mean following a recognized religion, in others it is just a search for a metaphysical meaning to help them to find a purpose in living with a life-threatening disease. In our Western society, materialism has taken over the outlook of many people; but when patients and families find themselves faced with the prospect of an early death this focuses their thoughts on issues that really matter. Many young adults in the terminal phase of their disease focus not on themselves but on how those who love them will cope when they are gone. Others want to explore the issues of 'What happens after death?'. The CF team should work closely with the chaplaincy team which, although usually led by a Christian minister, often includes trained lay workers. In addition the chaplaincy team will have contacts with other religions, and have skills in helping people discuss spiritual issues, religious or otherwise.

The chaplaincy team will make sure there are Christian services on Sundays and other specific festivals; they will take communion to those who wish, perform urgent baptisms and sometimes conduct funerals when the family has no minister of their own. The provision of an appropriate small library on spiritual issues is helpful. The chaplaincy team in a stressful situation can provide a listening ear for patients, relatives and staff and help those who wish to find hope in a seemingly hopeless situation. When a member of the CF team is asked 'What will happen when I die?' or 'Is there a God?' it is very helpful to have the help of well-trained and caring professionals who have thought about these issues. Reflection on these issues is important for team members, so they can help the patients and families and avoid burnout themselves.

Lay members of the chaplaincy team are often young and can get alongside the patients as friends, spending extra time with those who receive few visitors. Parents and spouses of very sick patients often appreciate someone other than the CF clinical team with whom they can discuss their worries.

BEREAVEMENT AND LOOKING BACK

The Kubler-Ross stages to acceptance of death are well known [53], along with the classical bereavement pathway [54]. Preparation for death, acknowledgment, ability to say good-byes, and ability to talk about future plans before death are all known to ease bereavement [55]. Many relatives begin the bereavement journey even before death [56]. Likewise, sudden, unexpected death, with no preparation is more likely to lead to a protracted and difficult bereavement. Many teams use bereavement tools to try to identify those at high risk [57–59], and some teams will be able to run a formal bereavement service. Most teams will have informal bereavement follow-up with annual reunion or memorials, or contact by team members. In our hospital, the chaplaincy team organizes an annual service of Thanksgiving and Remembrance for the lives of patients who have died. This event is much appreciated by friends, families and staff. Bereavement services may not alter the underlying pathway of the bereaved, although they do allow identification of those who need formal psychological or psychiatric intervention [58].

Although parents and spouses will all have been aware of early death in CF, coming to terms with the death of a loved one will always be painful and difficult. A death also has ramifications for siblings and friends, all of whom may need to be able to discuss how the death has affected their attitude to CF, treatment, transplantation and the team.

It is important to acknowledge the grief and loss of a patient to the CF team who may have cared for the individual

for years. As many patients are young when they die, many teams members may be able to identify readily with the patients – which increases their emotional response, and may also inhibit them from acknowledging the need for appropriate terminal care. The CF teams' needs for debriefing and discussion about deaths that have occurred are an important protection for them, and a learning point for next time. In addition especially vulnerable team members need to be identified and supported. Cystic fibrosis team cohesion and open communication about the care of a patient who is dying is vital to ensure that clear treatment plans are carried out, no conflicting or confusing messages are delivered to the patient, and all practitioners caring for the patient feel supported and involved. Specialist palliative care may have a role in aiding these discussions and being a sounding board for the various viewpoints within the team.

CONCLUSIONS

Patients with cystic fibrosis live with the knowledge of death, and perhaps with the hope for life post-transplant. They need complex support all the way through their life, including death. While rightly the predominant focus must be on extending the quality and quantity of life, we must pay heed to the needs of the patient in the terminal and later dying phase. Prognosis can be difficult but not impossible in this condition, and the period surrounding transplantation consideration is an ideal opportunity to begin to consider concepts of palliation.

The role of specialist palliative care is one of support and part of the highly skilled multidisciplinary team. Areas around discussion of direction of care, symptom control, family dynamics, communication issues and specific terminal care will complement and enhance other team skills. Familiarization with polypharmacy in the dying phase, manipulation of symptoms and the importance of care of the living and dying are key components that may be needed by many teams. The model of specialist palliative care should be less a traditional 'either/or' one, rather one of collaboration and part of the team structure.

REFERENCES

1. Saunders C. The evolution of palliative care hospices: a global network. *Pharos Alpha Omega Alpha Honor Med Soc* 2003; **66**(3):4–7.
2. Horne G, Payne S. Removing the boundaries: palliative care for patients with heart failure. *Palliat Med* 2004; **18**:291–296.
3. Traue DC, Ross JR. Palliative care in non-malignant diseases. *J R Soc Med* 2005; **98**:503–506.
4. Baggs JG, Norton SA, Schmitt MH, Sellers CR. The dying patient in the ICU: role of the interdisciplinary team. *Crit Care Clin* 2004; **20**:525–540, xi.

5. Chapman E, Landy A, Lyon A et al. End of life care for adult cystic fibrosis patients: facilitating a good enough death. J Cyst Fibros 2005; 4(4):249–257.

6. Yankaskas JR, Marshall BC, Sufian B et al. Cystic fibrosis adult care: consensus conference report. Chest 2004; 125(Suppl 1):1S–39S.

7. Warner JO. Heart–lung transplantation: all the facts. Arch Dis Child 1991; 66:1013–1016; discussion 1016–1017.

8. De Meester J, Smits JM, Persijn GG, Haverich A. Lung transplant waiting list: differential outcome of type of end-stage lung disease, one year after registration. J Heart Lung Transplant 1999; 18:563–571.

9. Grady D. Healthy give organs to dying, raising issues of risk and ethics. New York Times June 24, 2001; A1,A16.

10. Lowton K. 'Double or quits': perceptions and management of organ transplantation by adults with cystic fibrosis. Soc Sci Med 2003; 56:1355–1367.

11. Selecky PA, Eliasson CA, Hall RI et al. Palliative and end-of-life care for patients with cardiopulmonary diseases: American College of Chest Physicians position statement. Chest 2005; 128:3599–3610.

12. Shuttleworth A. Palliative care for people with end-stage non-malignant lung disease. Nurs Times 2005; 101(6):48–49.

13. Mast KR, Salama M, Silverman GK, Arnold RM. End-of-life content in treatment guidelines for life-limiting diseases. J Palliat Med 2004; 7(6):754–773.

14. O'Mahony S, Blank AE, Zallman L, Selwyn PA. The benefits of a hospital-based inpatient palliative care consultation service: preliminary outcome data. J Palliat Med 2005; 8:1033–1039.

15. Hallenbeck J. Palliative care in the final days of life: 'they were expecting it at any time'. J Am Med Assoc 2005; 293:2265–2271.

16. Oakley C, Pennington K, Mulford P. Perceptions of the role of the hospital palliative care team. Nurs Times 2005; 101(37):38–42.

17. Olthuis G, Dekkers W. Quality of life considered as well-being: views from philosophy and palliative care practice. Theor Med Bioeth 2005; 26:307–337.

18. Lowton K, Gabe J. Life on a slippery slope: perceptions of health in adults with cystic fibrosis. Sociol Health Illn 2003; 25:289–319.

19. O'Brien JM, Goodenow C, Espin O. Adolescents' reactions to the death of a peer. Adolescence 1991; 26:431–440.

20. Dickerson SS, Boehmke M, Ogle C, Brown JK. Seeking and managing hope: patients' experiences using the Internet for cancer care. Oncol Nurs Forum 2006; 33(1):E8–E17.

21. Kivits J. Informed patients and the internet: a mediated context for consultations with health professionals. J Health Psychol 2006; 11:269–282.

22. Karasz A, Dyche L, Selwyn P. Physicians' experiences of caring for late-stage HIV patients in the post-HAART era: challenges and adaptations. Soc Sci Med 2003; 57:1609–1620.

23. Vigano A, Donaldson N, Higginson IJ et al. Quality of life and survival prediction in terminal cancer patients: a multicenter study. Cancer 2004; 101:1090–1098.

24. Koenigsmann M, Koehler K, Regner A et al. Facing mortality: a qualitative in-depth interview study on illness perception, lay theories and coping strategies of adult patients with acute leukemia 1 week after diagnosis. Leuk Res 2006; Feb 1 [Epub ahead of print].

25. Tonelli MR. End-of-life care in cystic fibrosis. Curr Opin Pulm Med 1998; 4:332–336.

26. Block SD, Billings JA. Learning from the dying. N Engl J Med 2005; 353:1313–1315.

27. Kaplan KO. 'Footprints on the sands of time'. Death Stud 2005; 29:759–767.

28. Barbato MP. Caring for the dying patient. Intern Med J 2005; 35:636–637.

29. Madden BP, Kariyawasam H, Siddiqi AJ et al. Noninvasive ventilation in cystic fibrosis patients with acute or chronic respiratory failure. Eur Respir J 2002; 19:310–313.

30. Ferrin M, Happ MB, Kagan SH. Palliative care and lung transplantation: conflict or continuum? Am J Nurs 2001; 101(2):61–66.

31. Moneymaker KA. Understanding the dying process: transitions during final days to hours. J Palliat Med 2005; 8:1079.

32. Plonk WM, Arnold RM. Terminal care: the last weeks of life. J Palliat Med 2005; 8:1042–1054.

33. Campbell ML. Terminal dyspnea and respiratory distress. Crit Care Clin 2004; 20:403–417, viii–ix.

34. Luce JM, Luce JA. Perspectives on care at the close of life. Management of dyspnea in patients with far-advanced lung disease: 'once I lose it, it's kind of hard to catch it...' J Am Med Assoc 2001; 285:1331–1337.

35. Cohen SP, Dawson TC. Nebulized morphine as a treatment for dyspnea in a child with cystic fibrosis. Pediatrics 2002; 110(3):e38.

36. Levy MH, Cohen SD. Sedation for the relief of refractory symptoms in the imminently dying: a fine intentional line. Semin Oncol 2005; 32:237–246.

37. Robinson W. Palliative care in cystic fibrosis. J Palliat Med 2000; 3:187–192.

38. Penson RT, Partridge RA, Shah MA et al. Fear of death. Oncologist 2005; 10:160–169.

39. Robinson WM, Ravilly S, Berde C, Wohl ME. End-of-life care in cystic fibrosis. Pediatrics 1997; 100(2 Pt 1):205–209.

40. Kuhl DR, Wilensky P. Decision making at the end of life: a model using an ethical grid and principles of group process. J Palliat Med 1999; 2:75–86.

41. Lowton K. Parents and partners: lay carers' perceptions of their role in the treatment and care of adults with cystic fibrosis. J Adv Nurs 2002; 39:174–181.

42. Della Santina C, Bernstein RH. Whole-patient assessment, goal planning, and inflection points: their role in achieving quality end-of-life care. Clin Geriatr Med 2004; 20:595–620, v.

43. Chapman JA, Goodall J. Helping a child to live whilst dying. Lancet 1980; 1:753–756.

44. Mitchell I, Nakielna E, Tullis E, Adair C. Cystic fibrosis: end-stage care in Canada. Chest 2000; 118:80–84.

45. Westwood AT. Terminal care in cystic fibrosis: hospital versus home? Pediatrics 1998; 102(2 Pt 1):436; author reply 436–437.

46. Bookbinder M, Blank AE, Arney E et al. Improving end-of-life care: development and pilot-test of a clinical pathway. J Pain Sympt Manage 2005; 29:529–543.

47. Toscani F, Di Giulio P, Brunelli C *et al.* How people die in hospital general wards: a descriptive study. *J Pain Sympt Manage* 2005; **30**:33–40.

48. White DB, Luce JM. Palliative care in the intensive care unit: barriers, advances, and unmet needs. *Crit Care Clin* 2004; **20**:329–343, vii.

49. Edmonds P, Rogers A. 'If only someone had told me...': a review of the care of patients dying in hospital. *Clin Med* 2003; **3**:149–152.

50. Ellershaw JE, Murphy D. The Liverpool Care Pathway (LCP) influencing the UK national agenda on care of the dying. *Int J Palliat Nurs* 2005; **11**(3):132–134.

51. Emanuel L, Alexander C, Arnold RM *et al.* Integrating palliative care into disease management guidelines. *J Palliat Med* 2004; **7**:774–783.

52. Mirando S, Davies PD, Lipp A. Introducing an integrated care pathway for the last days of life. *Palliat Med* 2005; **19**(1):33–39.

53. Carr J. The dying process: a psychological continuum. A refinement of Kubler-Ross' five-stage theory. *Am J Hosp Care* 1986; **3**(4):34–38.

54. Bruce CA. The grief process for patient, family, and physician. *J Am Osteopath Assoc* 2002; **102**(9 Suppl 3):S28–S32.

55. Hudson PL, Aranda S, Hayman-White K. A psycho-educational intervention for family caregivers of patients receiving palliative care: a randomized controlled trial. *J Pain Sympt Manage* 2005; **30**:329–341.

56. Billings JA, Kolton E. Family satisfaction and bereavement care following death in the hospital. *J Palliat Med* 1999; **2**:33–49.

57. Jordan JR, Baker J, Matteis M *et al.* The grief evaluation measure (GEM): an initial validation study. *Death Stud* 2005; **29**:301–332.

58. Kendler KS, Hettema JM, Butera F *et al.* Life event dimensions of loss, humiliation, entrapment, and danger in the prediction of onsets of major depression and generalized anxiety. *Arch Gen Psychiatry* 2003; **60**:789–796.

59. Kristjanson LJ, Cousins K, Smith J, Lewin G. Evaluation of the Bereavement Risk Index (BRI): a community hospice care protocol. *Int J Palliat Nurs* 2005; **11**:610, 612–618.

PART 7

CYSTIC FIBROSIS: THE FUTURE

33a   Gene and stem cell therapy   453
       Uta Griesenbach and Eric W. F. W. Alton
33b   Non-gene therapy treatments: what will they deliver?   463
       Adam Jaffé and Pierre Barker
34   The future: how will management change?   471
       Andrew Bush and Duncan Geddes

33a

Gene and stem cell therapy

UTA GRIESENBACH AND ERIC W. F. W. ALTON

On behalf of the UK CF Gene Therapy Consortium

INTRODUCTION

The cloning of the cystic fibrosis (CF) gene – the cystic fibrosis transmembrane conductance regulator (CFTR) – in 1989 opened the door for CF gene therapy. Proof-of-principle for *CFTR* gene transfer was quickly established *in vitro* and in animal models [1,2]. The first clinical trials in CF patients were carried out in 1993 and to date 25 trials have been completed incorporating approximately 450 CF patients. These included viral and non-viral gene transfer to both the nasal and bronchial airway epithelium. In general, gene transfer is well tolerated and proof-of-principle for *CFTR* gene transfer (as measured by vector-specific mRNA or CFTR-mediated chloride transport) has been established in some but not all studies. An example is shown in Fig. 33.1. Chloride transport in the lung was measured before and after gene therapy in active- and placebo-treated CF patients. In the active group chloride transport was restored to about 20% of non-CF values. It is currently unclear, however, if this level of gene transfer would translate into clinical benefit.

Despite the theoretical ease of non-invasive access to the lung, gene transfer into the airway epithelium of man has been comparatively inefficient. It is apparent that airway epithelial cells have evolved effective barriers (see later) to prevent uptake of foreign particles, including gene transfer agents. With few exceptions most CF gene therapy trials carried out so far have been designed as phase I/II safety trials, with some limited inclusion of molecular (mRNA) or functional (chloride channel transport) end-point assays. However, it is still unclear whether gene transfer efficiency using currently available vectors is sufficient to change more clinically relevant end-point assays such as lung function, inflammation or bacterial colonization (for further discussion see Chapter 26). Thus, in parallel to further improvements in the efficiency of existing and novel gene transfer agents (GTAs), it is also important to assess if one of the current vectors is capable of changing clinically

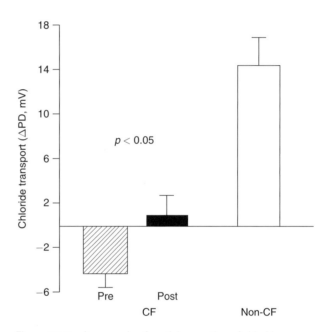

Figure 33.1 An example of partial correction of chloride transport across the airway epithelium of CF patients after gene transfer to the lung. Chloride transport is measured as a change in potential difference (PD) after perfusion with a low chloride-containing solution, which generates a driving force for chloride transport. PD is measured before (Pre) and after (Post) gene transfer. Chloride transport in non-CF subjects is shown as a reference value. Adapted from [62].

relevant features of the CF phenotype. Considering the large number of available viral and non-viral GTAs, careful selection of a vector is crucial. In our view suitable GTAs have to satisfy the following criteria:

- gene transfer efficiency into airway epithelial cells;
- repeatedly administrable without provoking an immune response;
- stable in a clinically used nebulizer;

- low toxicity;
- good manufacturing practices (GMP) available for the vector.

In this review we will highlight GTAs that fulfil these criteria.

CURRENTLY AVAILABLE NON-VIRAL GENE TRANSFER AGENT

DOES THE BEST CURRENTLY AVAILABLE NON-VIRAL GENE TRANSFER AGENT CHANGE CLINICALLY RELEVANT END-POINTS?

As mentioned above, it is currently uncertain whether existing GTAs, which partially restore chloride transport, are sufficient to improve clinically relevant end-points. To address this, the UK CF Gene Therapy Consortium (www.cfgenetherapy.org.uk) has recently completed a large pre-clinical program in mice and sheep to identify the most efficient, currently available non-viral gene transfer agent. Detection of vector-specific human *CFTR* mRNA was the most robust end-point. Based on the milder lung disease in CF patients with low-level residual CFTR function, it is generally anticipated that expression of approximately 5% of endogenous mRNA levels may be sufficient to ameliorate CF lung disease. It is worth noting that sheep transfected with a human CFTR plasmid, complexed with GL67, produced at least equal amounts of human CFTR in airway epithelial cells when compared to endogenous ovine *CFTR* mRNA (UK CF Gene Therapy Consortium, unpublished data). On the back of these data the fifty or so Consortium scientists and clinicians are preparing for a clinical trial program due to start in 2006. The most relevant clinical trial end-point would be a change in FEV_1, or even better in survival. However, trials would have to run for years and decades, respectively, to determine changes in these end-points. In contrast, detection of vector-specific mRNA and changes in PD have the potential to alter rapidly even a few days after gene transfer, which is the reason why these assays have been the primary end-points in most trials so far. It is unlikely that clinically relevant end-points, such as inflammation and infection, change rapidly after one administration of the GTA. In our view, this will require repeated administration, over perhaps a minimum of 6 months (for further discussion see Chapter 26) and require the inclusion of sufficient numbers of patients to be powered to detect changes in clinically relevant assays. Thus, a trial to assess efficacy of the most potent current non-viral GTA will be expensive and will require a significant commitment from patients and all concerned.

EXTRA- AND INTRACELLULAR BARRIERS TO LUNG GENE TRANSFER

In non-CF individuals, CFTR is expressed in serous cells in the submucosal glands and in ciliated airway epithelial cells

(AEC) [3]. It is currently unclear which of these cell types are the main target for CF gene therapy. However, given that CF, at least in the early stages, presents as a small airway disease, airway epithelial cells are likely to be important. Before the gene transfer agent (GTA) can reach the surface of the epithelial cells a number of extracellular physical and immunological barriers have to be overcome (reviewed in [4]). Briefly, the airway epithelium in the lung is generally covered by a thin mucus layer (Fig. 33.2), whose main role it is to trap invading foreign particles. It has been shown that mucus significantly reduces transfection efficiency of most viral and non-viral gene transfer agents. However, transfection efficiency could be increased through pre-treatment with mucolytics or the anticholinergic drug glycopyrrolate *in vitro* and *in vivo* [5].

In CF individuals, particularly at later stages in the disease, the airways are also filled with sticky sputum, consisting of inflammatory cells, cell debris, mucus and DNA, which not only constitutes an additional extracellular barrier to gene transfer, but also causes airflow obstruction and so interferes with aerosol distribution. Gene therapy is, therefore, most likely to be efficient and beneficial in young children, with well-preserved airways. Close communication with appropriate regulatory agencies and parents is necessary to ensure inclusion of children in clinical trials as early as possible. In addition, it may be advisable to 'clean-up' the lungs of CF patients in general with physiotherapy, intravenous antibiotics and possibly DNAse treatment before nebulization of the GTA.

It is likely that cilia also hinder access of GTAs to the apical surface of epithelial cells, while mucociliary clearance (MCC) may also reduce contact time of the GTAs with the cell membrane. In support of this, it has recently

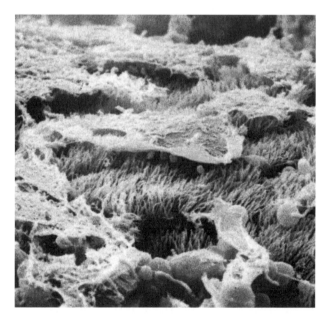

Figure 33.2 Ciliated airway epithelial cells partially covered in mucus. Courtesy of Professor Peter Jeffery, Imperial College London.

been shown that administration of methyl-cellulose, which inhibits MCC, increased viral gene transfer to the airway epithelium *in vivo* [6].

The pharmacological interventions described above have reached early stages of pre-clinical research and will have to be assessed in larger animal models such as sheep using clinically applicable delivery techniques, before they can be used in clinical trials.

NEW STRATEGIES TO IMPROVE NON-VIRAL AIRWAY GENE TRANSFER

In general, non-viral GTAs (lipids and polymers used to condense the plasmid DNA) appear to be less efficient than viral vectors, but are less likely to be toxic. Most importantly, however, they are less likely to induce an immune response, thereby allowing for repeat administration, crucial for the treatment of a chronic, life-long disease such as CF. Clearly, it will be important to check the repeatability of effect of any non-viral GTA on a case-by-case basis.

Improving the efficiency of non-viral gene transfer to airway epithelial cells has been a major focus, with a variety of strategies being followed. Several groups are modifying polyplexes such as polylysine and polyethylenimine (PEI) by adding sugars, based on the rationale that airway epithelial cells express lectins, which selectively bind and internalize glycoconjugates. Although glycoconjugates containing lactose have been efficient in cell culture studies *in vitro* [7,8], their efficacy and safety *in vivo* remains to be demonstrated.

Direct targeting of non-viral GTAs to receptors expressed on the apical surface of AEC by incorporating ligands into the formulation may improve transfection efficacy (Fig. 33.3). Proof-of-principle for this concept has been demonstrated by targeting the serpin enzyme complex receptor (Sec-R) [9]. This receptor is responsible for the uptake into the cell of serine proteases bound to their inhibitors. The receptor recognizes a conserved five-amino-acid binding motif, but tolerates large variation in the attached cargo. Sec-R-directed complexes are prepared by condensing plasmid DNA with a covalent conjugate of a peptide receptor ligand (17 amino acids) and polylysine. Ziady and co-workers have recently demonstrated partial correction of the chloride transport defect in the nasal epithelium of CF knockout mice following administration of Sec-R ligand complexed to a CFTR plasmid [9]. However, formulation and stability problems have so far prevented phase I clinical trials. Peptides resembling integrin-binding domains have also been linked to plasmid DNA and have been shown to transfect airway epithelium of pigs when delivered at bronchoscopy [10]. It remains to be established if anti-peptide immune responses will interfere with using peptide-carrying non-viral formulations for chronic diseases, but the risk of immune responses against the peptide can be minimized by using conserved human peptide sequences. Importantly, traditionally used animal

models may not be suitable to evaluate efficiency or repeat administration of human peptide formulation, if the chosen sequence is not conserved within the animal model.

Another nanoparticle formulation, consisting of a single plasmid molecule compacted with polyethyleneglycol (PEG)-substituted polylysine (polymer of 30 lysines) has been developed. In non-dividing cells the nuclear membrane appears to be an important barrier to gene transfer and one reason why Sec-R ligand polylysine complexes transfect airway cells efficiently might be their small size. With a diameter of 18–25 nm these nanoparticles may be able to enter the nucleus via passive diffusion through the nuclear pore complex, which has a cut-off size of about 25 nm. This was recently assessed in a human nose trial [8]. Plasmid DNA carrying the *CFTR* cDNA under the control of a commonly used immediate-early cytomegalovirus (CMV) promoter/enhancer was compacted with polyethylene glycol-substituted 30-mer polylysine and was slowly perfused on to the nasal epithelium. The study was mainly designed as a phase I dose-escalation safety study (12 subjects), but efficacy end-points were also assessed. Although initially planned as a within-subject placebo-controlled study, administration of the active compound into one nostril led to cross-contamination on the contralateral side, and thus the placebo control was not evaluable. Vector-specific mRNA could not be detected, but chloride transport was

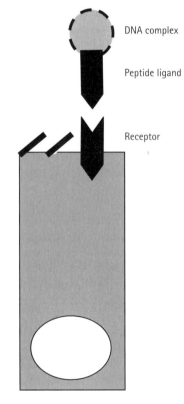

DNA complex

Peptide ligand

Receptor

Figure 33.3 Schematic presentation of receptor-mediated uptake of non-viral gene transfer agents. After identification of a suitable receptor expressed at the apical membrane of airway epithelial cells, a corresponding peptide ligand is added to the DNA complex.

increased in 8 out of 12 patients when compared to pre-treatment values, although the protocols used for nasal potential difference measurements may have been suboptimal. A follow-on study looking at single-dose aerosolization of DNA nanoparticles into CF lungs is currently planned.

The addition of physical energy is an interesting approach to increase non-viral gene transfer. Exposure to an electric field (electroporation), which causes transient permeability of the cell membrane, has been successful in various organs, but for technical reasons may not be suitable for lung transfection. Exposure of cells to ultrasound (sonoporation) also leads to formation of transient holes in the cell membrane (cavitation) [12] and may be useful for lung gene transfer. Mixing of GTAs with iron oxide particles gives them the capacity to move within a magnetic field (Fig. 33.4). Magnet-enhanced gene transfer (magnetofection) relies on these particles being efficiently pulled on to the cell surface thereby increasing contact time. Proof-of-principle has been clearly established *in vitro* [13] and we are currently evaluating magnetofection for airway gene transfer *in vivo*. In particular, oscillating magnets may help to 'pull' magnetic DNA through CF sputum (Jon Dobson, personal communication). Importantly, from a translational viewpoint, both ultrasound and magnets may be efficient when applied externally on to the chest cavity.

In addition to the DNA condensing GTA (lipid or polymer) the plasmid DNA is a crucial component of the complex. Several groups are improving the plasmids for non-viral gene transfer. Certain nucleotide sequences (CpG motifs) are pro-inflammatory in animals and humans after production of plasmid DNA in bacteria. Reduction of CpG motif number reduces inflammation [14,15] and it is, therefore, desirable, albeit difficult, to remove all CpG motifs from the plasmid DNA.

Promoters are regulatory elements that in part determine the duration of gene expression after transfection. Gill and co-workers [16] have studied the effect of different promoters on persistence of lung gene expression by comparing the

frequently used cytomegalovirus (CMV) promoter to the constitutive endogenous polyubiquitin C (UbC) and elongation factor 1α (EF1α) promoters. Although both eukaryotic endogenous promoters lead to about 10-fold less transgene expression at day 2, duration of gene expression was significantly improved when 'naked' pDNA was administered to the lung (CMV: <1 week; UbC: >16 weeks) and UbC-mediated gene expression reached CMV day-2 levels approximately 4 weeks after transfection. Similar results were reported by Yew and colleagues using the ubiquitin B (UbB) promoter [17]. Promoter silencing is likely to contribute to these results and it has previously been demonstrated that the CMV promoter is silenced by TNFα and INFγ, which are both up-regulated after gene transfer and in the CF lung itself. However, it is currently unknown why the EF1α and UbC promoters are more resistant to gene silencing.

In summary, technologies to improve non-viral gene transfer to the lung are constantly being developed. In parallel, the understanding of how plasmid DNA is taken up by primary airway epithelial cells, its movement through the cytoplasm and subsequently into the nucleus will be further studied by us and others, and this knowledge may lead to significant improvements in non-viral gene transfer.

THE ROLE OF ADENOVIRAL VECTORS

CURRENTLY ADENOVIRAL VECTORS DO NOT HOLD GREAT PROMISE FOR CF GENE THERAPY

Despite encouraging results in nasal and pulmonary tissues of pre-clinical models [18,19] and being well-tolerated at low to intermediate doses in humans [20], adenovirus-mediated gene transfer in the absence of epithelial damage has been inefficient in CF patients [21]. This is mainly due to the absence of the coxsackie-adenovirus receptor (CAR) on the apical surface of the majority of human airway epithelial cells (AECs) [22] and highlights the important differences in receptor distribution in animal models and humans.

In addition to problems with low transfection efficiency, the use of adenovirus (Ad) for a chronic disease like CF is limited due to effective cellular and humoral immune responses against the virus. Thus, Harvey and co-workers [23] delivered three doses of Ad-CFTR to the lungs of CF patients 3 months apart and demonstrated that after the third administration vector-specific *CFTR* mRNA was no longer detectable. Similar results have been obtained in animal models. Helper-dependent ('gutted') adenoviral vectors, which are depleted of all viral genes, are less immunostimulatory and have improved safety profiles compared to first- and second-generation viruses, which have only a subset of viral genes deleted. Recently, it was shown that helper-dependant adenovirus combined with the epithelial cell-specific cytokeratin 18 (K18) promoter, leads to reduced inflammation and more prolonged expression in murine airways [24], but there is currently

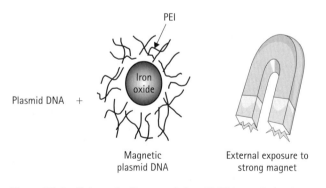

Figure 33.4 Schematic diagram of plasmid DNA coupled to iron oxide particles. Plasmid DNA is bound to polyethylenimine (PEI)-coated iron oxide particles via charge interaction. The magnetic DNA-loaded particles can be pulled on to the cell surface using strong magnets. Courtesy of Stefania Xenariou, Department of Gene Therapy, Imperial College London.

no evidence that 'gutted' adenovirus can be repeatedly administered.

Despite the limitations for human use, adenoviral vectors have proven useful for pre-clinical proof-of-principle studies. Two studies have recently shown that adenovirus-mediated CFTR expression may, to a degree, protect CF mice from the effects of bacteria-induced lung inflammation [25,26].

However, a study by Tosi and colleagues [27] raised concerns that anti-adenovirus immune responses (cytotoxic T lymphocyte responses and MHC class I antigen presentation) may be further enhanced if the host has a pre-existing *Pseudomonas* infection. These data further highlight potential problems for adenoviral vectors in CF gene therapy, and the use of adenoviral vectors for CF gene therapy is likely to be restricted to pre-clinical proof-of-principle studies, until the problems of repeat administration can be overcome.

ADENO–ASSOCIATED VIRUS (AAV) VECTORS

AAV IS CURRENTLY THE MOST COMMONLY USED VECTOR FOR CF GENE THERAPY, BUT REPEATED ADMINISTRATION REMAINS AN UNRESOLVED PROBLEM

Adeno-associated virus (AAV) vectors have attracted much interest due to their good safety profile, broad tissue tropism, long duration of expression, and suggestion of their superior escape from immune system surveillance compared with other viruses. One concern is the limited packaging capacity of the virus, which only barely holds the CFTR gene (4.7 kb). Several clinical trials have been carried out in the nose, sinus and lungs of CF patients, all using the AAV2-based vector TgAAV-CFTR (Targeted Genetics Corp.), which uses the weak AAV long terminal repeat (LTR) promoter to drive expression. Most recently Moss and co-workers [28] published a phase II trial assessing the safety and efficacy of repeated administration (three doses 1 month apart) of AAV2. Viral shedding and increases in neutralizing antibodies were noted, but virus administration was safe. Importantly, a significant reduction in sputum interleukin-8 (a pro-inflammatory cytokine) and a small improvement in lung function (FEV_1) was seen after the first, but not second or third administrations. On the basis of these studies, Targeted Genetics Corporation initiated a large repeat-administration study (100 subjects), sufficiently powered to detect significant changes in lung function. However, recently the company announced that the trial had not met its primary outcome measure and, therefore, the CF program had been discontinued. There may be several reasons for these disappointing results:

- AAV2 may be too inefficient in transducing airway epithelial cells via the apical membrane.
- The LTR promoter used to drive CFTR expression may be too weak.

- Repeat administration of AAV2 to the lung is not possible due to the development of an anti-viral immune response.

Research aimed at addressing these potential limitations of AAV is actively being pursued (see later).

AAV serotype 2 was the first AAV-based vector assessed for lung transfection. More recently AAV2 with capsids from serotypes 1, 5 and 6 (AAV2 genome plus AAV1, 5 or 6 capsids) have been evaluated for lung gene therapy and appear to be more efficient in transducing airway epithelial cells than AAV2 [29,30]. To search for potent AAV vectors with enhanced performance profiles, molecular techniques were employed for the detection and isolation of endogenous AAVs from a variety of human and non-human primate (NHP) tissues [31]. Ten novel provirus sequences were identified, but it remains to be established whether these viruses are suitable for gene therapy applications. Recently, the atomic structure of AAV2 has been identified, which should enable rational engineering of vector capsids for specific cell targeting [32]. Shi and co-workers [33] have already identified specific regions within the capsid protein that can tolerate the insertion of small exogenous peptides and have made an attempt at incorporating integrin-targeting peptides into this region.

Strategies to overcome the AAV packaging problem, thereby allowing incorporation of stronger promoters in addition to the large CFTR gene, have been developed, including approaches based on trans-splicing [34] and homologous recombination [35]. The basic principle of these techniques is to split the therapeutic cDNA and required promoter elements, and package them into two viruses, which when transfecting the same cell may recombine and generate a full-length therapeutic gene. One would speculate that both of these strategies would lead to reduced transfection efficiency, when compared with administration of one intact virus to the lung. However, surprisingly, Halbert and co-workers [35] have demonstrated that AAV2/6 (ITR from AAV2 and capsid from AAV6) recombination-dependent vectors transduced lung cells in mice almost as efficiently as intact vector, with 10% of AECs being positive.

It has been postulated that AAV may not infect antigen-presenting dendritic cells and thereby avoid activation of the host immune system. However, the feasibility of repeated AAV administration is still unresolved. The results of repeat administration have been reported to vary greatly and may depend on the host, delivery route and AAV serotype tested [36–38]. Although the unsuccessful AAV2 repeat administration trial (see above) may argue for problems with repeat administration, Auricchio and co-workers [37,39] have shown that AAV2/5 can be re-administered once to the mouse lung 5 months after the first delivery [39]. More recently, Fischer and co-workers [40] reported successful re-administration of AAV2 (three doses) into rhesus macaques. However, although some low level of GFP reporter gene expression was detected by RT-PCR and via immunohistochemistry, it is unclear how expression levels compared to one-time administration levels. Importantly, repeated AAV2 administration caused an increase in AAV2-neutralizing antibodies, but did not induce lung inflammation. Finally, Halbert and co-workers [41] showed efficient and persistent (18 months) AAV6-mediated reporter gene expression in a rat model. Although the work is currently unpublished, the authors claimed that repeated administration after 18 months resulted in significant gene expression (50% of first-dose levels in three rats). Based on these data, Dusty Miller's group is planning a nose trial in which the AAV6/2 vector holds an easily detectable marker gene, rather than the therapeutic *CFTR* gene [35].

Finally, in addition to alterations to the AAV itself pharmacological interventions may improve AAV transfection. Proteasome inhibitors, for example, have been shown to increase AAV2 and AAV5/2 transfection *in vitro* [42], probably via increasing their chances of transit to the nucleus.

SENDAI VIRUS VECTOR

SENDAI VIRUS IS ARGUABLY THE MOST EFFICIENT VECTOR FOR AIRWAY GENE TRANSFER BUT CANNOT BE ADMINISTERED REPEATEDLY

Sendai virus (SeV) transduces airway epithelial cells rapidly and very efficiently (Fig. 33.5) and is currently the most efficient vector for airway gene transfer. In contrast to adenovirus and AAV, SeV is an RNA virus, which does not go through a DNA intermediate and does not enter the nucleus. In addition SeV uses sialic acid and cholesterol for cell entry, both of which are abundantly expressed on the apical surface of AECs, a prerequisite for efficient airway transfection. First-generation recombinant SeV carrying *CFTR* cDNA can produce functional CFTR chloride channels *in vitro* and after transfection of the nasal epithelium in CF knockout mice.

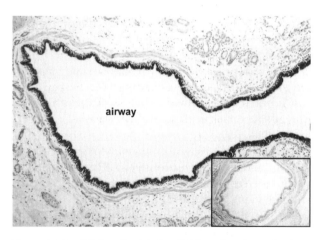

Figure 33.5 Efficient Sendai virus (SeV)-mediated transfection of airway epithelial cells in an animal model. Ferrets were transduced with SeV carrying a β-galactosidase reporter gene, which turn transduced cells blue. Insert shows untransduced control for comparison. *See also Plate 33.5.*

Ferrari and co-workers [43] showed that the potentially safer, second-generation transmission-incompetent SeVs maintain this high transfection efficiency. However, SeV-mediated expression is transient and, therefore, requires repeat administration. Unfortunately, as for other viruses, this is inefficient, and attempts at inducing tolerance against immunodominant SeV peptides were unsuccessful [44].

Although SeV may be useful for acute diseases that require only transient gene expression, in the context of CF the use of SeV will be, as for adenovirus, restricted to pre-clinical proof-of-principle studies, until repeat administration problems can be solved.

GENE REPAIR TRANS–SPLICING TECHNOLOGIES

INEFFICIENCY, AND CONCERNS ABOUT ACCURACY, LIMITS THE SUCCESS OF GENE REPAIR TRANS-SPLICING TECHNOLOGIES

Both gene repair and splicosome-mediated trans-splicing (the post-transcriptional repair of mRNA – Fig. 33.6) have the theoretical advantage that 'corrected' *CFTR* gene expression is under the control of the endogenous *CFTR* promoter. However, despite initial enthusiasm and a flurry of papers, in recent years the number of publications has reduced. Efficiency is the most important bottleneck for oligonucleotide-based gene repair. Thus, De Semir and co-workers

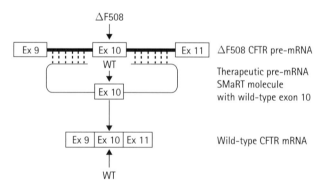

Figure 33.6 Schematic presentation of splicosome-mediated mRNA trans-splicing (SMaRT). Splicing of messenger RNA precursors (pre-mRNAs) is a requisite step in the generation of mRNAs and is carried out in the nucleus by spliceosomes. Components of the spliceosome recognize the exon–intron boundaries at the 5′ and 3′ splice sites, excise the intron and ligate the adjoining exons (Ex). Splicing between two independently transcribed pre-mRNAs is termed trans-splicing. Intronn Inc. has developed mRNA molecules that promote trans-splicing after binding to homologous regions of endogenous mRNA. Trans-splicing happens because the therapeutic mRNA molecules carry strong splicing signals. The wild-type exon 10 in a therapeutic *CFTR* SMaRT molecule replaces the Δ*F508* exon 10 in the mutant *CFTR* mRNA. Dashed lines indicate intronic regions where trans-splicing takes place.

[45] confirmed previously published data showing that gene repair, even in cell-free extracts of CF airway epithelial cells, is very inefficient.

Although proof-of-principle for AAV-based splicosome-mediated trans-splicing in cell lines looks encouraging [46], replication of the technology in lung *in vivo* has not been published yet. Low transfection efficiency may in part be responsible, while it is currently unclear how much 'inappropriate' gene repair and trans-splicing occurs, mainly because current assays are insufficient to address these questions. Thus, in the short-term it is unlikely these strategies will lead to clinical trials.

RNA INTERFERENCE AND ANTISENSE THERAPY

Antisense or RNAi-mediated gene silencing may provide novel opportunities for the treatment of cystic fibrosis. There are several candidate proteins whose inhibition may attenuate CF lung disease. A reduction in the transcription factor nuclear factor kappa B (NFκB) [47], which regulates many pro-inflammatory cytokines, may be beneficial. Second, Lambert and co-workers [48] have recently demonstrated that antisense inhibition of the ER-membrane protein BAP31 increases trafficking of *F508del* protein to the cell surface and restores chloride secretion in a variety of cell types *in vitro*. However, redundancy in these pathways and importantly the central role of these proteins in the cell will make them difficult targets. In contrast, the epithelial sodium channel (ENaC) which is up-regulated in CF and contributes significantly to the imbalanced water movement in the CF lung, may provide a more specific target for gene silencing. The importance of ENaC as a therapeutic target is also highlighted in studies by Mall and co-workers [49] showing the ENaC overexpressing transgenic mice develop CF-like lung disease, and by Sheridan and co-workers [50] showing that CF-like lung disease in some subjects is due to ENaC mutations. We have recently shown that, although antisense and small inhibitory RNA (siRNA) significantly reduced the mRNA of target proteins in the airway epithelium, this was too inefficient to translate into a reduction in protein. Inefficient uptake of the silencing oligonucleotides into the airway epithelium was the likely cause [51]. However, with further improvements in non-viral gene transfer, gene silencing may become a realistic treatment option.

THE RELEVANCE OF FETAL GENE THERAPY

Although proof-of principle for fetal lung gene transfer has been demonstrated [52], it is currently difficult to see a clear clinical application. Unless the hypothesis that the absence of CFTR *in utero* causes significant and irreparable developmental defects proves correct, in-utero gene transfer, particularly using integrating long-lasting vectors, will

most likely be considered too risky. The proposed role for CFTR during in-utero development continues to be discussed. Thus, Cohen and co-workers [53] transiently shut down CFTR expression in rat fetuses with antisense-CFTR and reported the postnatal development of pathological changes including lung fibrosis and inflammation. The authors hypothesized that in the lung CFTR is involved in regulating differentiation of secretory cells, which when disturbed leads to inflammation reminiscent of CF lung disease.

STEM CELL THERAPY IN THE CONTEXT OF CF

Stem cell therapy in the context of cystic fibrosis encompasses several different strategies.

Intravenous injection of 'corrected' bone–marrow–derived stem cells

Ex-vivo transfection of bone-marrow-derived stem cells (BMSCs) with integrating retro- and lentiviral vectors is a well-established, efficient technique. In combination with the concept that bone-marrow-derived hematopoetic or mesenchymal stem cells may have the capacity to differentiate into airway epithelial cells [54,55], some groups have speculated that this strategy may have applications for the treatment of CF. Using slightly different models, both groups suggested that BMSCs were able to adopt properties of alveolar and respiratory epithelium. The frequency of trans-differentiation appeared to be higher in alveolar than in respiratory epithelium and seemed to be enhanced when the airway epithelium was damaged. However, subsequent to these papers intensive discussion and further studies have questioned these data. Importantly, Kotton and co-workers [56] were unable to reproduce their original findings in a follow-up study using a different technique to identify bone-marrow-derived pneumocytes. This highlights the significant technical problems associated with conclusive identification of bone-marrow-derived alveolar and airway epithelial cells. However, after careful optimization of the detection techniques, Macpherson and colleagues [57] maintain that approximately 1% of tracheal epithelial cells are bone-marrow-derived after detergent damage.

In our view, *ex-vivo* transfection and systemic re-administration of BMSCs currently does not hold great promise for CF for a number of reasons:

- Data on trans-differentiation in the lung is conflicting.
- Myelo-ablation and extensive damage of the lung with bleomycin or detergents appear to be a prerequisite for engraftment, neither of which are likely to be clinically applicable.
- In reports that provided evidence of engraftment and differentiation, the frequency in airways is very low (<1%).

Topical administration of ex-vivo corrected stem cells to the lung

In addition to systemic re-administration of ex-vivo corrected BMSCs, topical administration of stem cells directly into the lung might be feasible. This suggestion is very speculative and to the best of our knowledge has not been assessed even in pre-clinical models. Although interesting, the strategy has several major drawbacks including:

- To encourage 'seeding' of stem cells in the airways, existing surface epithelium will likely have to be damaged.
- Delivery into small airways will be difficult.
- Uncontrolled differentiation and proliferation of BMSC in the lung might be toxic.

Targeting of resident airway stem cells with integrating viral vectors

It has been well documented that certain cell types in the mouse lung have stem/progenitor cell properties, although complementary data in humans do not yet exist. Different cell types are likely to be responsible for regeneration in the different regions of the lung [58]. Thus, type 2 pneumocytes are able to differentiate into type 1 cells and reconstitute the alveolar epithelium, certain cells in the bronchoalveolar duct junctions are able to differentiate into alveolar and airway epithelium [59] and subpopulations of Clara cells have a regenerative capacity in the airways.

In contrast to SeV, RNA-based lentiviruses enter the nucleus. The virus stably integrates into the genome of transduced cells and expression is, therefore, likely to last for the lifetime of the cell. Lentiviruses are particularly interesting for the transfection of resident lung stem or progenitor cells and will be discussed below.

Transfection of resident stem/progenitor cells with an integrating lentivirus carrying CFTR will lead to transmission of the gene to daughter cells and may lead to repopulation of the lung with CFTR-expressing cells.

Several groups, including our own, are attempting to generate lentiviral vectors for efficient and persistent gene expression in airway epithelium. An important factor is the incorporation of viral envelope proteins suitable for uptake via the apical membrane. Lentiviruses pseudotyped with Ebola virus [60] and baculovirus GP64 envelope glycoproteins [61] have been shown to enter AEC via the apical membrane and lead to persistent expression (50 weeks). In collaboration with the DNAVEC Corporation, Japan, we have developed a simian immunodeficiency virus pseudotyped with the Sendai virus membrane proteins F (fusion protein) and HN (hemagluttinin–neuraminidase), which are responsible for efficient uptake of SeV into airway epithelial cells. Importantly, unless lentiviral vectors are able to hit airway stem cells efficiently they will likely need to be re-administered and, therefore, may face the same immune-response problems as other viral vectors. Studies are currently under way to assess the feasibility of repeated administration of lentiviral vectors into airways in several groups, including our own, and further data are needed before the relevance of lentiviruses for CF gene therapy can be decided. In addition, the safety profile of virus insertion into the genome of airway epithelial cells has to be carefully monitored.

CONCLUSIONS

Over the last decade it became apparent that gene transfer to the airway epithelial cells is difficult. This is perhaps unsurprising given that the lung has evolved to keep foreign particles out. However, significant progress in the development of viral and non-viral formulation is continuously being made. The major obstacle for viral gene transfer agents is the effective immune surveillance mechanisms in the lung, which prevents repeated administration. Until strategies to overcome the immune system have been identified, the use of viral vectors for CF gene therapy is likely to be restricted to 'single hit' resident stem cell transfection and pre-clinical proof-of-principle studies.

The key question in the context of non-viral vectors is that of efficacy, and the repeat dose-trial to be undertaken by the UK CF Gene Therapy Consortium using clinically relevant surrogate end-points should address whether sufficient transfection efficiency can be achieved by these vectors.

ACKNOWLEDGMENTS

We thank Lucinda Somerton for help with preparation of the manuscript, all our colleagues in the UK CF Gene Therapy Consortium and the Cystic Fibrosis Trust for funding our research.

REFERENCES

1. Alton EW, Middleton PG, Caplen NJ *et al.* Non-invasive liposome-mediated gene delivery can correct the ion transport defect in cystic fibrosis mutant mice. *Nat Genet* 1993; 5:135–131.

2. Drumm ML, Pope HA, Cliff WH *et al.* Correction of the cystic fibrosis defect *in vitro* by retrovirus-mediated gene transfer. *Cell* 1990; 62:1227–1233.

3. Engelhardt JF, Zepeda M, Cohn JA *et al.* Expression of the cystic fibrosis gene in adult human lung. *J Clin Invest* 1994; 93:737–749.

4. Ferrari S, Griesenbach U, Geddes DM, Alton E. Immunological hurdles to lung gene therapy. *Clin Exp Immunol* 2003; 132(1):1–8.

5. Ferrari S, Geddes DM, Alton EW. Barriers to and new approaches for gene therapy and gene delivery in cystic fibrosis. *Adv Drug Deliv Rev* 2002; **54**:1373–1393.

6. Sinn PL, Shah AJ, Donovan MD, McCray PB. Viscoelastic gel formulations enhance airway epithelial gene transfer with viral vectors. *Am J Respir Cell Mol Biol* 2005; **32**:404–410.

7. Fajac I, Thevenot G, Bedouet L *et al.* Uptake of plasmid/glycosylated polymer complexes and gene transfer efficiency in differentiated airway epithelial cells. *J Gene Med* 2003; **5**:38–48.

8. Klink D, Yu QC, Glick MC, Scanlin T. Lactosylated poly-L-lysine targets a potential lactose receptor in cystic fibrosis and non-cystic fibrosis airway epithelial cells. *Mol Ther* 2003; **7**:73–80.

9. Ziady AG, Kelley TJ, Milliken E *et al.* Functional evidence of CFTR gene transfer in nasal epithelium of cystic fibrosis mice *in vivo* following luminal application of DNA complexes targeted to the serpin-enzyme complex receptor. *Mol Ther* 2002; **5**:413–419.

10. Cunningham S, Meng O *et al.* Evaluation of a porcine model for pulmonary gene transfer using a novel synthetic vector. *J Gene Med* 2002; **4**:438–446.

11. Konstan MW, Davis PB, Wagener JS *et al.* Compacted DNA nanoparticles administered to the nasal mucosa of cystic fibrosis subjects are safe and demonstrate partial to complete cystic fibrosis transmembrane regulator reconstitution. *Hum Gene Ther* 2004; **15**:1255–1269.

12. Mehier-Humbert S, Bettinger T, Yan F, Guy RH. Plasma membrane poration induced by ultrasound exposure: implication for drug delivery. *J Control Release* 2005; **104**:213–222.

13. Krotz F, de Wit C, Sohn HY *et al.* Magnetofection: a highly efficient tool for antisense oligonucleotide delivery *in vitro* and *in vivo*. *Mol Ther* 2003; **7**(5 Pt 1):700–710.

14. Yew NS, Zhao H, Wu IH *et al.* Reduced inflammatory response to plasmid DNA vectors by elimination and inhibition of immunostimulatory CpG motifs. *Mol Ther* 2000; **1**:255–262.

15. Krieg AM. CpG motifs in bacterial DNA and their immune effects. *Annu Rev Immunol* 2002; **20**:709–760.

16. Gill DR, Smyth SE, Goddard CA *et al.* Increased persistence of lung gene expression using plasmids containing the ubiquitin C or elongation factor 1alpha promoter. *Gene Ther* 2001; **20**:1539–1546.

17. Yew NS, Przybylska M, Ziegler RJ *et al.* High and sustained transgene expression *in vivo* from plasmid vectors containing a hybrid ubiquitin promoter. *Mol Ther* 2001; **4**:75–82.

18. Katkin JP, Gilbert BE, Langston C *et al.* Aerosol delivery of a beta-galactosidase adenoviral vector to the lungs of rodents. *Hum Gene Ther* 1995; **6**:985–995.

19. Scaria A, St George JA, Jiang C *et al.* Adenovirus-mediated persistent cystic fibrosis transmembrane conductance regulator expression in mouse airway epithelium. *J Virol* 1998; **72**:7302–7309.

20. Harvey BG, Maroni J, O'Donoghue KA. Safety of local delivery of low- and intermediate-dose adenovirus gene transfer vectors to individuals with a spectrum of morbid conditions. *Hum Gene Ther* 2002; **13**:15–63.

21. Joseph PM, O'Sullivan BP, Lapey A *et al.* Aerosol and lobar administration of a recombinant adenovirus to individuals with cystic fibrosis. I: Methods, safety, and clinical implications. *Hum Gene Ther* 2001; **12**:1369–1382.

22. Walters RW, Grunst T, Bergelson JM *et al.* Basolateral localization of fiber receptors limits adenovirus infection from the apical surface of airway epithelia. *J Biol Chem* 1992; **274**:10219–10226.

23. Harvey BG, Leopold PL, Hackett NR *et al.* Airway epithelial CFTR mRNA expression in cystic fibrosis patients after repetitive administration of a recombinant adenovirus. *J Clin Invest* 1999; **104**:1245–1255.

24. Toietta G, Koehler DR, Finegold MJ *et al.* Reduced inflammation and improved airway expression using helper-dependent adenoviral vectors with a K18 promoter. *Mol Ther* 2003; **7**:649–658.

25. Koehler DR, Sajjan U, Chow YH *et al.* Protection of Cftr knockout mice from acute lung infection by a helper-dependent adenoviral vector expressing Cftr in airway epithelia. *Proc Natl Acad Sci USA* 2003; **100**:15364–15369.

26. Van Heeckeren AM, Schluchter MD, Xue W, Davis PB. Response to acute lung infection with mucoid *Pseudomonas aeruginosa* in cystic fibrosis mice. *Am J Respir Crit Care Med* 2006; **1**:288–296.

27. Tosi MF, van Heeckeren A, Ferkol TW *et al.* Effect of *Pseudomonas*-induced chronic lung inflammation on specific cytotoxic T-cell responses to adenoviral vectors in mice. *Gene Ther* 2004; **11**:1427–1433.

28. Moss RB, Rodman D, Spencer LT *et al.* Repeated adeno-associated virus serotype 2 aerosol-mediated cystic fibrosis transmembrane regulator gene transfer to the lungs of patients with cystic fibrosis: a multicenter, double-blind, placebo-controlled trial. *Chest* 2004; **125**:509–521.

29. Sirninger J, Muller C, Braag S *et al.* Functional characterization of a recombinant adeno-associated virus 5-pseudotyped cystic fibrosis transmembrane conductance regulator vector. *Hum Gene Ther* 2004; **15**:832–841.

30. Virella-Lowell I, Zusman B, Foust K *et al.* Enhancing rAAV vector expression in the lung. *J Gene Med* 2005; **7**:842–850.

31. Gao G, Vandenberghe LH, Wilson JM. New recombinant serotypes of AAV vectors. *Curr Gene Ther* 2005; **5**:285–297.

32. Xie Q, Bu W, Bhatia S *et al.* The atomic structure of adeno-associated virus (AAV-2), a vector for human gene therapy. *Proc Natl Acad Sci USA* 2002; **99**:10405–10410.

33. Shi W, Bartlett JS. RGD inclusion in VP3 provides adeno-associated virus type 2 (AAV2)-based vectors with a heparan sulfate-independent cell entry mechanism. *Mol Ther* 2003; **7**:515–525.

34. Duan D, Yue Y, Engelhardt JF. Expanding AAV packaging capacity with trans-splicing or overlapping vectors: a quantitative comparison. *Mol Ther* 2001; **4**:383–391.

35. Halbert CL, Allen JM, Miller AD. Efficient mouse airway transduction following recombination between AAV vectors

carrying parts of a larger gene. *Nat Biotechnol* 2002;
20:697–701.

36. Beck SE, Jones LA, Chesnut K *et al.* Repeated delivery of
adeno-associated virus vectors to the rabbit airway.
J Virol 1999; 73:9446–9455.

37. Halbert CL, Standaert TA, Aitken ML. Transduction by adeno-
associated virus vectors in the rabbit airway: efficiency,
persistence, and readministration. *J Virol* 1997;
71:5932–5941.

38. Halbert CL, Rutledge EA, Allen JM *et al.* Repeat transduction
in the mouse lung by using adeno-associated virus vectors
with different serotypes. *J Virol* 2000; 74:1524–1532.

39. Auricchio A, O'Connor E, Weiner D *et al.* Noninvasive gene
transfer to the lung for systemic delivery of therapeutic
proteins. *J Clin Invest* 2002; 110:499–504.

40. Fischer AC, Beck SE, Smith CI *et al.* Successful transgene
expression with serial doses of aerosolized rAAV2 vectors in
rhesus macaques. *Mol Ther* 2003; 8:918–926.

41. Halbert C, Liggit D, Miller AD. Biosafety study of an adeno-
associated virus 6 vector in rats. *Pediatr Pulmonol* 2005;
(Suppl 28):277–278.

42. Yan Z, Zak R, Zhang Y *et al.* Distinct classes of proteasome-
modulating agents cooperatively augment recombinant
adeno-associated virus type 2 and type 5-mediated
transduction from the apical surfaces of human airway
epithelia. *J Virol* 2004; 78:2863–2874.

43. Ferrari S, Griesenbach U, Shiraki-Iida T *et al.* A defective
nontransmissible recombinant Sendai virus mediates efficient
gene transfer to airway epithelium in vivo. *Gene Ther* 2004;
11:1659–1664.

44. Griesenbach U, Boyton RJ, Somerton L *et al.* Effect of
tolerance induction to immunodominant T-cell epitopes of
Sendai virus on gene expression following repeat
administration to lung. *Gene Ther* 2006; 13:449–456.

45. De Semir D, Nadal M, Gonzalez JR *et al.* Suitability of
oligonucleotide-mediated cystic fibrosis gene repair in
airway epithelial cells. *J Gene Med* 2003; 5:625–639.

46. Liu X, Luo M, Zhang LN *et al.* Spliceosome-mediated RNA
trans-splicing with recombinant adeno-associated virus
partially restores cystic fibrosis transmembrane conductance
regulator function to polarized human cystic fibrosis airway
epithelial cells. *Hum Gene Ther* 2005; 16:1116–1123.

47. Barnes PJ. Nuclear factor kappa B. *Int J Biochem Cell Biol*
1997; 29:867–870.

48. Lambert G, Becker B, Schreiber R *et al.* Control of cystic
fibrosis transmembrane conductance regulator expression
by BAP31. *J Biol Chem* 2001; 27:20340–20345.

49. Mall M, Grubb BR, Harkema JR *et al.* Increased airway
epithelial Na+ absorption produces cystic fibrosis-like lung
disease in mice. *Nat Med* 2004; 10:487–493.

50. Sheridan MB, Fong P, Groman JD *et al.* Mutations in the
beta-subunit of the epithelial Na+ channel in patients with
a cystic fibrosis-like syndrome. *Hum Mol Genet* 2005;
14:3493–3498.

51. Griesenbach U, Wasowicz MY, Smith SN *et al.* Endpoint assay
development and validation of non-viral gene transfer agents
in CF mice. *Pediatr Pulmonol Suppl* 2005: 28:270.

52. Peebles D, Gregory LG, David A *et al.* Widespread and
efficient marker gene expression in the airway epithelia
of fetal sheep after minimally invasive tracheal application
of recombinant adenovirus in utero. *Gene Ther* 2004:
11:70–78.

53. Cohen JC, Larson JE. Pathophysiologic consequences
following inhibition of a CFTR-dependent developmental
cascade in the lung. *BMC Dev Biol* 2005; 5(1):2.

54. Kotton DN, Ma BY, Cardoso WV *et al.* Bone marrow-derived
cells as progenitors of lung alveolar epithelium. *Development*
2001; 128:5181–5188.

55. Krause DS, Theise ND, Collector MI *et al.* Multi-organ, multi-
lineage engraftment by a single bone marrow-derived stem
cell. *Cell* 2001; 105:369–377.

56. Kotton DN, Fabian AJ, Mulligan RC. Failure of bone marrow
to reconstitute lung epithelium. *Am J Respir Cell Mol Biol*
2005; 33:328–334.

57. Macpherson H, Keir P, Webb S *et al.* Bone marrow-derived SP
cells can contribute to the respiratory tract of mice *in vivo*.
J Cell Sci 2005; 118:2441–2450.

58. Bishop AE. Pulmonary epithelial stem cells. *Cell Prolif* 2004;
37:89–96.

59. Kim CF, Jackson EL, Woolfenden AE. Identification of
bronchioalveolar stem cells in normal lung and lung cancer.
Cell 2005; 121:823–835.

60. Medina MF, Kobinger GP, Rux J *et al.* Lentiviral vectors
pseudotyped with minimal filovirus envelopes increased gene
transfer in murine lung. *Mol Ther* 2003; 8:777–789.

61. Sinn PL, Shah AJ, Donovan MD, McCray PB. Viscoelastic gel
formulations enhance airway epithelial gene transfer with
viral vectors. *Am J Respir Cell Mol Biol* 2005; 32:404–410.

62. Alton EW, Stern M, Farley R *et al.* Cationic lipid-mediated
CFTR gene transfer to the lungs and nose of patients with
cystic fibrosis: a double-blind placebo-controlled trial.
Lancet 1999; 20:947–954.

33b

Non-gene therapy treatments:
what will they deliver?

ADAM JAFFÉ AND PIERRE BARKER

INTRODUCTION

As discussed in Chapter 33a, there are many hurdles to overcome before gene therapy enters the clinic as a treatment. Scientists continue to pursue other therapeutic strategies in the hope of translating basic scientific knowledge into real treatments. With the advent of more sophisticated and cheaper molecular techniques, our understanding of the pathophysiology of cystic fibrosis (CF) and how the defective CF transmembrane conductance regulator protein results in disease has increased dramatically since the cloning of the gene in 1989 [63,64] (Fig. 33.7). This understanding has provided the scientific basis for the development of pharmacological agents that are targeted at an array of defects that result from mutations in CFTR. These strategies and their therapeutic potential are discussed in this chapter.

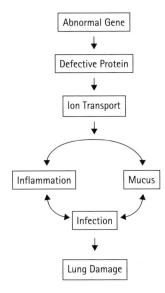

Figure 33.7 Pathophysiology of CF lung disease.

BASIC SCIENCE STRATEGIES IN CF

Protein rescue therapy

The molecular biology of specific mutations has been discussed in detail in Chapter 3. The approaches to overcome defective CFTR protein production, abnormal intracellular processing and the incapacity of CFTR to normally regulate ion channels and other proteins are excellent examples of how basic science can be translated into future therapeutic agents [65].

PHYSIOLOGICAL DRUG SELECTION

Agents that promote CFTR trafficking have exploited the nascent potential of *F508del* to produce functional CFTR protein. It has emerged that the misfolded *F508del* CFTR is retained in the endoplasmic reticulum (ER) by molecular chaperones and subsequently degraded by proteolysis to prevent accumulation of toxic polypeptides. These chaperones are calcium-binding proteins and therefore inhibition of the ER calcium pump with a reduction of calcium concentration may help *F508del* escape, permitting it to travel to the apical surface of the cell. This rational was behind a study which showed in-vitro correction of CFTR defects by the Ca-adenosine triphosphatase pump inhibitor curcumin, a constituent of turmeric, and correction of ion transport abnormalities in *F508del* CF mice [66]. In response to the study many patients began consuming curcumin as part of their diet. However, this compound has been found to be ineffective in extensive in-vitro studies by other groups [67] and subsequent work by the original group demonstrated no effect on ion transport in humans with CF. These studies are a timely reminder of the caution with which new findings purporting to correct CFTR defects should be published, and the responsibility that CF researchers have to

CF patients and their families who are desperately hoping for a cure [68].

Studies of CFTR kinetics have indicated that not only is *F508del* CFTR degraded within the ER, but it is 20 times less stable than wild-type CFTR [69]. Therefore, small molecule drugs capable of increasing CFTR activation kinetics may overcome these problems. There are many examples in recent years that exemplify the translation of these scientific observations into clinical trials. In tissue culture studies of *F508del* cells, sodium-4 phenylbutyrate increased fully mature glycosylated protein with associated improvement of chloride secretory responses to forskolin [70]. Subsequent phase I/II trials demonstrated safety and provided proof-of-principle that up-regulation of CFTR trafficking improves ion transport in nasal respiratory epithelium of *F508del* subjects [71,72]. The exact mechanisms are unclear but it likely to be due to the effect of sodium-4 phenylbutyrate on CFTR transcription or trafficking. Clinical benefit from this therapy has yet to be demonstrated. 8-cyclopentyl-1,3-dipropylxanthine (CPX), an A_1-adenosine receptor antagonist, has also demonstrated an increase in CFTR trafficking in *F508del* CF airway cells [73], and while its safety has been shown in phase I human studies [74], its efficacy has not yet been demonstrated *in vivo*. Again, the mechanisms by which CPX increases trafficking of *F508del* is not known, but is likely to be due to an increase in synthesis or improvement in folding of the protein. A further example is topical gentamicin, which was found to increase protein trafficking and correct ion transport in those patients with *CFTR* stop-mutations [75]. Whether a sufficient dose can be delivered to humans to overcome the stop-mutation defect and effect a clinical change remains to be seen.

These protein rescue studies highlight the challenges in translating molecular and animal effects into clinical benefit. To date, none has shown therapeutic benefit, but hopefully a better understanding of CFTR processing in wild-type and CF cells will aid the development of specific pharmacological therapies [69].

HIGH-THROUGHPUT SCREENING

F508del was initially thought to be a trafficking mutant, but as discussed, researchers have reported defects in folding, stability and activation for this protein. It is clear that if a drug is to be successful it must overcome these three abnormalities. While there are many good examples of how basic science knowledge has translated into clinical studies, there has been a recognition of the need to identify other potential small molecules for the treatment of CF through the development of high-throughput screening programs [64]. These automated facilities screen up to 10 000 chemicals per day. A high-throughput screening program is one of the core activities of the Therapeutic Development Network (TDN) sponsored by the Cystic Fibrosis Foundation and has proved a valuable strategy for pre-clinical drug discovery (Fig. 33.8) [76]. Current studies have focused on cellular reporters which identify c-AMP-dependent transmembrane

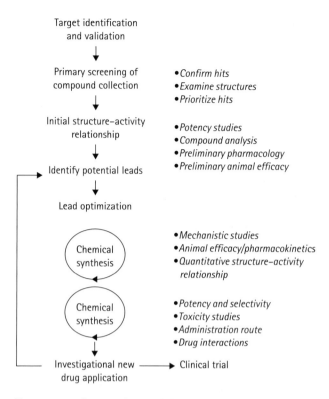

Figure 33.8   Strategy for preclinical drug discovery. Adapted and used with permission from [76].

halide secretion in response to CFTR activation and correctors of channel gating, as occurs in *F508del* and *G551D*. Screening of thousands of small molecule analogues identified phenylglycine and sulfonamide compounds which may have a future role in CF patients with mutations which result in abnormalities of channel gating [77]. Other successful outcomes from this program include the discovery of small molecular analogues of aminoarylthiazoles, quinazolinyl-amino-pyrimidinones and bis-amino-methylbithiazoles which correct defective cellular processing of CFTR and increase stability at the cell surface [78]. The CF mouse provides an invaluable model for assessing the effects of these compounds on functional abnormalities of the nasal epithelium and gastrointestinal tract. Although this approach greatly accelerates drug discovery, these promising compounds will need to follow the usual safety and efficacy studies in animals and humans before realizing their potential as therapeutic agents for CF.

In addition to providing potential therapeutic agents, this program has identified molecules capable of providing further insight into the pathophysiological processes in CF. Examples are the identification of CFTR inhibitors, which proved useful in assessing the role of CFTR in submucosal fluid secretion in non-CF airways [79]. These inhibitors may potentially be useful as probes of CFTR pore structure or in creating CF animal models [80]. It is hoped that future classes of chemicals will be discovered capable of rescuing abnormal CFTR with demonstrable clinical benefit.

PHARMACOGENOMICS

The development of powerful molecular techniques such as genomics and proteomics has enabled us to study the effect of drugs on gene and protein expression as highlighted by the effect of digitoxin on CF cells [81]. The application of digitoxin to cultured CF epithelial cells suppressed interleukin (IL)-8 secretion by blocking phosphorylation of the inhibitor of nucleotide factor (NF) κB. Significant overlap of gene expression and transcription by digitoxin were seen when compared to CF cells treated with gene therapy, suggesting that digitoxin could be a useful drug for the inhibition of IL-8, a cytokine involved in the inflammatory process in CF. Thus the application of pharmacogenomics is likely to be very useful in future drug discoveries in CF and may lead to the development of therapies tailored to the individual.

STRUCTURE–BASED DRUG DESIGN

An important scientific breakthrough has been the determination of the three-dimensional structure of CFTR using electron crystallography [82]. CFTR crystallizes as a monomer and exists in different forms with either a single or double-barrelled central cavity. It has a shallow extracellular cavity with a deep, wide intracellular cavity. Furthermore, the detailed identification of the structure of the nucleotide binding domain [63] has revealed only mild but important structural differences between wild-type and *F508del* [83,84]. These studies suggest that the primary defect of *F508del* is due to abnormal interdomain interactions rather than problems with protein folding. This raises the possibility of developing a small molecule which could reinforce interdomain interactions in CFTR and thus correct the *F508del* mutation. This increase in structural knowledge, together with our greater understanding of the function of CFTR, may herald the development of chemicals aimed at structure-guided drugs designed to overcome structural abnormalities in CFTR.

Ion transport and mucociliary clearance

Principally, CFTR functions as a chloride (Cl) channel although its role in regulation of sodium (Na) transport is equally important in the pathogenesis of CF. The principal therapeutic strategies for circumventing mutated CFTR effect on ion transport are stimulation of alternative Cl channels and fluid secretion, blocking overactive Na channels and stimulating ciliary beat frequency to increase mucociliary clearance.

CFTR's role in the regulation of the amiloride-sensitive sodium channel (ENaC) has been a major target for therapeutic intervention. Initial studies aimed at blocking the sodium channel with amiloride showed short-term slowing of decline in lung function [85] but a subsequent study failed to demonstrate more long-term clinical benefit, possibly due to amiloride's short half-life [86]. Drugs with a longer duration of action such as benzamil may be a candidate for aerosolized therapy in CF [87]. However, as it is rapidly absorbed from mucous membranes its use is limited. The development of more potent, less absorbable, third-generation Na channel blockers provide a potential therapy in CF. One such candidate is a derivative of the intracellular signalling molecule D-*myo*-inositol 3,4,5,6-tetrakisphosphate, which inhibits sodium and fluid absorption across the CF airway epithelium *in vitro* [88]. While these approaches offer ways of modifying ion transport, it is still unknown how much ion transport correction is required for clinical improvement. The recent generation of a mouse model which over-expresses ENaC suggests that sodium absorption is a key factor in the development of airway disease [89]. Despite normal chloride secretion in the murine airway, hyperabsorption of sodium led to lung disease with impaired mucociliary clearance, neutrophilic inflammation and delayed bacterial clearance, similar to that seen in CF. This suggests that future efforts to manipulate ion channels in CF should be concentrated on inhibition of ENaC.

Another therapeutic approach is to increase mucociliary clearance by manipulation of ion transport and water using specific agonists of the purinergic receptor P2Y2. The natural ligand of P2Y2 receptors is uridine triphosphate (UTP), which stimulates chloride and fluid transport via a non-CFTR mechanism and thus has the potential to rehydrate the airway surface liquid and increase mucociliary clearance. A phase I/II clinical trial sponsored by the CF Foundation TDN demonstrated that inhaled denufosol tetrasodium (INS37217, Inspire Therapeutics), a selective P2Y2 agonist, was tolerated in most patients with moderately severe lung disease [90].

Short-term clinical improvement has been seen in studies using mannitol [91] which acts as an osmotic agent on the airway surface liquid layer and increases mucociliary clearance. Its potential as a dry powdered inhaled therapy as an alternative or adjunct to recombinant human DNase (Pulmozyme) is under evaluation. Using a similar principle, two studies have shown that inhaled hypertonic saline increases mucus clearance with demonstrable clinical benefit [92,93]. This is now being used as a treatment adjunct in many CF centers. Osmotic agents offer an inexpensive, safe addition to current treatments for CF, although their long-term value remains undefined. Future work will identify the most effective agent to improve mucus clearance in addition to the most efficient delivery system to the lower airway.

Inflammation

Inflammation is central to the disease process and ultimately the repeated cycles of inflammation and infection result in lung destruction (see Fig. 33.7). It is no surprise, therefore, that successful anti-inflammatory therapy with drugs such as steroids, ibuprofen and azithromycin result in clinical improvement as discussed in detail in other chapters.

Scientific observations have led to the development of other potential anti-inflammatory therapies in CF. Glutathione (GTH), an antioxidant that modulates inflammation via gene transcription, was decreased in the bronchoalveolar lavage (BAL) fluid of patients with CF [94]. It is proposed that this effect may be due either to the high oxidative burden in CF or reduced CFTR-dependent glutathione transport. Preliminary clinical studies of inhaled GTH demonstrated a short-term increase in lung function and some evidence that exogenous GTH may modulate harmful inflammatory and oxidative responses in the CF airway (increased lymphocytes and suppression of prostaglandin E_2 in the BAL fluid) [94,95]. N-acetyl-cysteine repletes glutathione stores and there is developing interest in using either inhaled or oral N-acetyl-cysteine as an anti-inflammatory agent.

Another potential therapeutic anti-inflammatory strategy is the use of lipoxins, which are anti-inflammatory lipid mediators active against many components of neutrophil inflammation. Karp and co-workers [96] demonstrated that lipoxins were reduced in BAL fluid of CF patients and showed improvement in a mouse model of lung disease following administration of a lipoxin analogue, suggesting that lipoxin may have a therapeutic role in CF. The lipid-lowering statins are a class of drug with anti-inflammatory properties and the effects of simvastatin in CF are being evaluated as part of the Cystic Fibrosis Foundation therapeutics pipeline. Other potential future therapies include aerosolized delivery of α_1-antitrypsin [97] and secretory leukoprotease inhibitor (SLPI) [98] which protect lung tissue from destruction by neutrophil elastase. Further work is needed to establish their efficacy.

An anti-inflammatory protein, annexin A1, may be important in the regulation of inflammation in CF. Using a proteomic approach investigators have demonstrated a reduction of annexin A1 both in CF mouse tissue and human nasal epithelial cells [99]. These preliminary results suggest that annexin A1 is involved in CF pathogenesis and deserves further attention, which may herald a novel therapy. Similarly, following the discovery that peroxisome proliferator-activated receptor-gamma (PPARγ) is involved in the inflammatory process, work has focused on modulating this receptor in an attempt to control inflammation.

Our increase in the basic science knowledge of the inflammatory pathways in CF has resulted in the identification of many potential anti-inflammatory therapeutic targets. Translating this basic science knowledge into clinical improvement is fraught with difficulties. An important example is that of a phase II clinical trial of BIIL 284 BS, a leukotriene B4 (LTB4) antagonist [100]. LTB_4 is a potent neutrophilic chemoattractant and thus the rationale behind the study was to block the neutrophilic inflammation seen in CF. The trial was subsequently terminated on the recommendation of the CF Foundation's data safety monitoring board due to an increase in the number of pulmonary infective exacerbations in the treatment arm. It is unclear why this occurred, but it is plausible that the antineutrophil effect rendered the patients vulnerable to uncontrolled infections. Important lessons can be learnt from this study; future anti-inflammatory developments need to address the balance of inflammation that affords protection from infection, against inflammation which results in lung parenchymal destruction. Drugs such as macrolides, which possess both anti-inflammatory and antibacterial properties, may provide this balance [101]. A better understanding of the various molecular pathways involved in the anti-inflammatory effects of macrolides may provide the key to the development of novel comprehensive therapies in CF.

Infection

The increase in survival of patients with CF over the past decades has largely been attributed to aggressive antibiotic use. One of the greatest future challenges is developing more potent antibiotics in response to emerging resistance strains of bacteria such as *Pseudomonas aeruginosa* or *Burkholderia cepacia*. One such example is nebulized aztreonam which is undergoing clinical trials. The development of more efficient nebulizers using technologies such as vibrating meshes and dry-powder devices will reduce the burden of care and enhance delivery to the lower airway. Novel approaches such as delivery of liposomal amikacin (SLIT amikacin) or dry-powdered ciprofloxacin [102] may result in sustained prolonged local release in the airway with enhanced antibacterial activity.

Another anti-infective approach is the development of *Pseudomonas* polyvalent vaccines [103]. Preliminary results are very encouraging and the efficacy and safety results of large European and American phase III studies are awaited. Another novel approach against *Pseudomonas* is the use of immunotherapy with specific egg-yolk antibodies (IgY) which may prevent the acquisition of *Pseudomonas* and be an alternative to antibiotics. Preliminary work in patients who gargled the solution following the first colonization with *Pseudomonas* suggested that chronic infection could be delayed [104]. The pharmaceutical industry will continue to react to the emerging strains of pathogens which cause lung diseases in CF, as well as looking at novel more effective delivery mechanisms.

Lung damage

The parenchymal lung damage in CF is irreversible. Ultimately many patients will require a lung transplant. The life expectancy following transplantation is increasing largely due to the development of improved anti-rejection strategies. The use of azithromycin has been shown to have an effect on chronic rejection and bronchiolitis obliterans syndrome [105]. Another advance has been the discovery that treatment with inhaled ciclosporin caused decreased rejection and increased survival after lung transplant [106]. The challenge over the next few years is to understand the mechanisms of rejection and develop targeted therapies.

FUTURE CHALLENGES OF TRANSLATIONAL RESEARCH

There are many diverse potential therapeutic approaches to the treatment of CF lung disease. In an attempt to accelerate and facilitate drug discovery, the National Heart, Lung and Blood Institute (NHLBI) recently published a report that offers a systematic approach to investigating the processes and proteins that affect CFTR [64]. They highlighted the need to develop improved molecular techniques to increase our understanding of CFTR interactions with other proteins and to assist the development of high-throughput methods of evaluating novel drugs such as the TDN.

The NHLBI report also highlighted the need to develop realistic models of CF including both cellular and animal models. While the creation of the CF mouse heralded a greater understanding of the pathophysiology of CF, and presented an opportunity to assess *in vivo* the effects of drugs on ion transport, the mice do not suffer from CF lung disease. The development of the mouse with airway-specific overexpression of epithelial ENaC is a step forward to the creation of an animal model which resembles CF lung disease [89]. The creation of a CF large-animal model such as a sheep or pig will enable assessment of topical delivery of therapeutic agents and will provide a model that more closely resembles the human with CF.

To this end collaboration is essential. There are 60 000 patients with CF worldwide. Examples of successful collaboration include the Cystic Fibrosis Foundation TDN which has developed an efficient clinical trials network to test drugs in its therapeutics pipeline. The importance of collaboration is further highlighted by the potential to develop therapies that target genes or gene products other than CFTR that modify the CF phenotype. The literature is littered with many studies claiming to have identified potential modifier genes. The small numbers of subjects involved in most of these studies raises the possibility that results may not be subsequently confirmed in larger sample sizes. A recent report from the Gene Modifier Study group, in which 1300 patients from 44 sites were studied, was unable to confirm the effect of previously identified modifier genes but did confirm that tissue growth factor (TGF) β1 is a modifier gene for the CF phenotype [107]. This observation potentially opens the door to the development of specific therapies aimed at manipulating the effects of TGFβ expression.

While the discovery of drugs remains a huge challenge in the field of CF, this pales into insignificance when one considers the challenges of translating these drugs into clinical use [108]. Once a candidate drug is identified it needs to progress through pre-clinical, clinical and regulatory approval, which may take up to 15 years. Given that patients and their families are desperate for new drugs, they often find this an exasperatingly slow process. In addition, the cost of bringing a new drug to market is on average £450 (US$760) million, way beyond any academic budget. Thus the formation of partnerships with pharmaceutical companies is crucial. However, with relatively few patients worldwide, there is very little incentive for these companies to develop new drugs for patients with CF. Fortunately, political pressure and the creation of political structures such as the US Orphan Drug act of 1983 and European Parliament legislation on orphan drug development in 1999 have given financial incentives for drug companies to develop new therapies. Two such successful examples are recombinant human DNase (Pulmozyme) and high-dose inhaled tobramycin (TOBI).

A further challenge for translational clinical research is the identification of clinical outcome measures likely to be meaningful considering the limited number of potential subjects for recruitment into trials. Ultimately, the most important outcome measures are long-term lung function and life expectancy. However, in order to study the latter, a trial will need to be conducted over a 30-year period, an impractical constraint for any study of new therapies. Davis and co-workers [109] estimated that over 1000 CF patients would need to be recruited over a 1-year period in order to detect an arrest in the expected rate of decline of lung function (FEV_1) in this patient population. Fewer subjects would be required if the patients were young with mild pulmonary disease as these patients are more likely to have a faster FEV_1 decline [109]. Thus children with limited lung damage would be the most appropriate subjects to demonstrate an inhibition in FEV_1 decline. The advantages of studying this young patient population needs to be balanced against the moral and ethical concerns surrounding the use of children in trials, particularly with regard to gene therapy [110]. To circumvent these challenges, there has been much interest in the development of surrogate end-points that reflect the effects of the disease process (e.g. airway inflammation, infective exacerbations, radiographic changes, quality-of-life index), or the underlying disease process itself (e.g. nasal potential difference, mucociliary clearance, *Pseudomonas* adherence, molecular markers). The challenge is to extrapolate each of these surrogate study end-points into a prediction of life expectancy or long-term lung function. In addition, individual surrogate measures may have complex interdependencies with other CFTR functions or effects. For example, it is known that approximately 6–10% of correction of CF cells results in the restoration of chloride secretion [111], but we are uncertain whether the correction of chloride secretion alone without concurrent inhibition of sodium absorption will be sufficient to exert a clinical effect. Likewise, it is not known how protein expression and other surrogate markers reflect functional changes required to correct the effects of mutated CFTR. These uncertainties remain a major hurdle to the advancement of therapeutic development in CF. A greater understanding of the clinical picture in CF in the future will help address many of these issues.

The pace of scientific discovery and therapeutic development for CF has accelerated dramatically in two decades, and this has been reflected in a marked improvement in average life expectancy during this time. However, we are now faced with the harsh reality that, despite a huge and sustained scientific effort to develop novel therapeutic interventions, CF still reduces average life expectancy by more than half. As the life expectancy continues to improve, if the cure from gene or stem cell therapy does not materialize, perhaps our goal will be that patients with CF die with their disease but not as a consequence of it.

REFERENCES

63. Boucher RC. New concepts of the pathogenesis of cystic fibrosis lung disease. *Eur Respir J* 2004; 23:146–158.

64. Guggino WB, Banks-Schlegel SP. Macromolecular interactions and ion transport in cystic fibrosis. *Am J Respir Crit Care Med* 2004; 170:815–820.

65. Kerem E. Pharmacological induction of CFTR function in patients with cystic fibrosis: mutation-specific therapy. *Pediatr Pulmonol* 2005; 40:183–196.

66. Egan ME, Pearson M, Weiner SA *et al.* Curcumin, a major constituent of turmeric, corrects cystic fibrosis defects. *Science* 2004; 304:600–602.

67. Song Y, Sonawane ND, Salinas D *et al.* Evidence against the rescue of defective Delta F508-CFTR cellular processing by curcumin in cell culture and mouse models. *J Biol Chem* 2004; 279:40629–40633.

68. Davies J, Bush A. Primum non nocere: does the current research publication system (or the lay press) harm our patients? *Am J Respir Crit Care Med* 2005; 171:937–938.

69. Gelman MS, Kopito RR. Rescuing protein conformation: prospects for pharmacological therapy in cystic fibrosis. *J Clin Invest* 2002; 110:1591–1597.

70. Rubenstein RC, Egan ME, Zeitlin PL. In-vitro pharmacologic restoration of CFTR-mediated chloride transport with sodium 4-phenylbutyrate in cystic fibrosis epithelial cells containing delta F508-CFTR. *J Clin Invest* 1997; 100:2457–2465.

71. Rubinstein RC, Zeitlin PL. A pilot clinical trial of oral sodium 4-phenylbutyrate (buphenyl) in delta F508-homozygous cystic fibrosis patients. *Am J Respir Crit Care Med* 1998; 157:484–490.

72. Zeitlin PL, Diener-West M, Rubenstein RC *et al.* Evidence of CFTR function in cystic fibrosis after systemic administration of 4-phenylbutyrate. *Mol Ther* 2002; 6:119–126.

73. Eidelman O, Zhang J, Srivastava M, Pollard HB. Cystic fibrosis and the use of pharmacogenomics to determine surrogate endpoints for drug discovery. *Am J Pharmacogen* 2001; 1:223–238.

74. McCarty NA, Standaert TA, Teresi M *et al.* A phase I randomized, multicenter trial of CPX in adult subjects with mild cystic fibrosis. *Pediatr Pulmonol* 2002; 33:90–98.

75. Wilschanski M, Yahav Y, Yaacov Y *et al.* Gentamicin-induced correction of CFTR function in patients with cystic fibrosis and CFTR stop mutations. *N Engl J Med* 2003; 349:1433–1441.

76. Verkman AS. Drug discovery in academia. *Am J Physiology* 2004; 286:C465–C474.

77. Pedemonte N, Sonawane ND, Taddei A *et al.* Phenylglycine and sulfonamide correctors of defective delta F508 and G551D cystic fibrosis transmembrane conductance regulator chloride-channel gating. *Mol Pharmacol* 2005; 67:1797–1807.

78. Pedemonte N, Lukacs GL, Du K *et al.* Small-molecule correctors of defective Delta F508-CFTR cellular processing identified by high-throughput screening. *J Clin Invest* 2005; 115:2564–2571.

79. Song Y, Salinas D, Nielson DW, Verkman AS. Hyperacidity of secreted fluid from submucosal glands in early cystic fibrosis. *Am J Physiol* 2006; 290:C741–C749.

80. Muanprasat C, Sonawane N D, Salinas D *et al.* Discovery of glycine hydrazide pore-occluding CFTR inhibitors: mechanism, structure-activity analysis, and in vivo efficacy. *J Gen Physiol* 2004; 124:125–137.

81. Srivastava M, Eidelman O, Zhang J *et al.* Digitoxin mimics gene therapy with CFTR and suppresses hypersecretion of IL-8 from cystic fibrosis lung epithelial cells. *Proc Natl Acad Sci USA* 2004; 101:7693–7698.

82. Rosenberg MF, Kamis AB, Aleksandrov LA *et al.* Purification and crystallization of the cystic fibrosis transmembrane conductance regulator (CFTR). *J Biol Chem* 2004; 279:39051–39057.

83. Lewis HA, Buchanan SG, Burley SK *et al.* Structure of nucleotide-binding domain 1 of the cystic fibrosis transmembrane conductance regulator. *Eur Mol Biol Organiz J* 2004; 23:282–293.

84. Lewis HA, Zhao X, Wang C *et al.* Impact of the delta F508 mutation in first nucleotide-binding domain of human cystic fibrosis transmembrane conductance regulator on domain folding and structure. *J Biol Chem* 2005; 280:1346–1353.

85. Knowles MR, Church NL, Waltner WE *et al.* A pilot study of aerosolized amiloride for the treatment of lung disease in cystic fibrosis. *N Engl J Med* 1990; 322:1189–1194.

86. Graham A, Hasani A, Alton EWFW *et al.* No added benefit from nebulized amiloride in patients with cystic fibrosis. *Eur Respir J* 1993; 6:1243–1248.

87. Hofmann T, Stutts MJ, Ziersh A *et al.* Effects of topically delivered benzamil and amiloride on nasal potential difference in cystic fibrosis. *Am J Respir Crit Care Med* 1998; 157:1844–1849.

88. Moody M, Pennington C, Schultz C *et al.* Inositol polyphosphate derivative inhibits Na+ transport and improves fluid dynamics in cystic fibrosis airway epithelia. *Am J Physiol* 2005; 289:C512–C520.

89. Mall M, Grubb BR, Harkema JR *et al.* Increased airway epithelial Na+ absorption produces cystic fibrosis-like lung disease in mice. *Nat Med* 2004; 10:487–493.

90. Deterding R, Retsch-Bogart G, Milgram L *et al.* Safety and tolerability of denufosol tetrasodium inhalation solution, a novel P2Y2 receptor agonist: results of a phase 1/phase 2 multicenter study in mild to moderate cystic fibrosis. *Pediatr Pulmonol* 2005; 39:339–348.

91. Robinson M, Daviskas E, Eberl S *et al.* The effect of inhaled mannitol on bronchial mucus clearance in cystic fibrosis patients: a pilot study. *Eur Respir J* 1999; **14**:678–685.

92. Elkins MR, Robinson M, Rose BR *et al.* A controlled trial of long-term inhaled hypertonic saline in patients with cystic fibrosis. *N Engl J Med* 2006; **354**:229–240.

93. Donaldson SH, Bennett WD, Zeman KL *et al.* Mucus clearance and lung function in cystic fibrosis with hypertonic saline. *N Engl J Med* 2006; **354**:241–250.

94. Griese M, Ramakers J, Krasselt A *et al.* Improvement of alveolar glutathione and lung function but not oxidative state in cystic fibrosis. *Am J Respir Crit Care Med* 2004; **169**:822–828.

95. Hartl D, Starosta V, Maier K *et al.* Inhaled glutathione decreases PGE2 and increases lymphocytes in cystic fibrosis lungs. *Free Rad Biol Med* 2005; **39**:463–472.

96. Karp, CL, Flick LM, Park KW *et al.* Defective lipoxin-mediated anti-inflammatory activity in the cystic fibrosis airway. *Nat Immunol* 2004; **5**:388–392.

97. Martin SL, Downey D, Bilton D *et al.* Safety and efficacy of recombinant alpha(1)-antitrypsin therapy in cystic fibrosis. *Pediatr Pulmonol* 2006; **41**:177–183.

98. Taggart CC, Cryan SA, Weldon S *et al.* Secretory leucoprotease inhibitor binds to NF-kappaB binding sites in monocytes and inhibits p65 binding. *J Exper Med* 2005; **202**:1659–1668.

99. Bensalem N, Ventura AP, Vallee B *et al.* Down-regulation of the anti-inflammatory protein annexin A1 in cystic fibrosis knockout mice and patients. *Mol Cell Proteom* 2005; **4**:1591–1601.

100. Konstan MW, Doring G, Lands L *et al.* Results of a phase II clinical trial of BIIL 284 BS (an LTB4 receptor antagonist) for the treatment of CF lung disease. *Pediatr Pulmonol* 2005; Suppl 28:125–126.

101. Jaffe A, Bush A. Macrolides in cystic fibrosis. In: Rubin BK, Tamaoki J (eds) *Antibiotics as Anti-Inflammatory and Immunomodulatory Agents.* Basel, Birkhäuser Verlag, 2005, 167–191.

102. Sweeney LG, Wang Z, Loebenberg R *et al.* Spray freeze-dried liposomal ciprofloxacin powder for inhaled aerosol drug delivery. *Int J Pharmaceut* 2005; **305**:180–185.

103. Lang AB, Rudeberg A, Schoni M *et al.* Vaccination of cystic fibrosis patients against *Pseudomonas aeruginosa* reduces the proportion of patients infected and delays time to infection. *Pediatr Infect Dis J* 2004; **23**:504–510.

104. Kollberg H, Carlander D, Olesen H *et al.* Oral administration of specific yolk antibodies (IgY) may prevent *Pseudomonas aeruginosa* infections in patients with cystic fibrosis: a phase I feasibility study. *Pediatr Pulmonol* 2003; **35**:433–440.

105. Gerhardt SG, McDyer JF, Girgis RE *et al.* Maintenance azithromycin therapy for bronchiolitis obliterans syndrome: results of a pilot study. *Am J Respir Crit Care Med* 2003; **168**:121–125.

106. Iacono AT, Johnson BA, Grgurich WF *et al.* A randomized trial of inhaled cyclosporine in lung-transplant recipients. *N Engl J Med* 2006; **354**:141–150.

107. Drumm ML, Konstan MW, Schluchter MD *et al.* Genetic modifiers of lung disease in cystic fibrosis. *N Engl J Med* 2005; **353**:1443–1453.

108. Brennan AL, Geddes DM. Bringing new treatments to the bedside in cystic fibrosis. *Pediatr Pulmonol* 2004; **37**:87–98.

109. Davis PB, Byard PJ, Konstan MW. Identifying treatments that halt progression of pulmonary disease in cystic fibrosis. *Pediatr Res* 1997; **41**:161–165.

110. Jaffe A, Prasad SA, Larcher V, Hart S. Gene therapy for children with cystic fibrosis: who has the right to choose? *J Med Ethics* 2006; **32**:361–364.

111. Johnson LG, Olsen JC, Sarkadi B *et al.* Efficiency of gene transfer for restoration of normal airway epithelial function in cystic fibrosis. *Nat Genet* 1992; **2**:21–25.

The future: how will management change?

ANDREW BUSH AND DUNCAN GEDDES

INTRODUCTION

Early diagnosis through screening, and advances in treatment, have improved survival in cystic fibrosis (CF). The typical scrawny, ill, infected infant who will die as a teenager is thankfully rare; the typical 'patient' is now a fit individual, who has only ever had minimal if any symptoms, who happens to have a problem called 'CF'. Cystic fibrosis was thought to be a disease of the lungs and digestive tract; almost paradoxically, the scope has expanded to that of a multisystem disease, as individuals have lived longer. This has two obvious consequences. First, fit individuals probably do not want to spend many hours of precious time every day doing treatment, or long hours being assessed in the clinic. Second, we need to consider much longer-term, multisystem complications both of the disease and its treatment. It seems likely that the focus will shift from disease management to prevention of complications.

On the other hand, modern sophisticated investigations have revealed functional abnormalities in even young, apparently well patients. Obviously it is important not to over-interpret minor changes, but recent work has painted a picture that is not all rosy. What is a 'well' CF patient? Even babies apparently without any apparent respiratory disease have evidence of airflow obstruction [1,2], and ongoing airway inflammation [3]. Their lung function appears to track through the pre-school years, so perhaps very early on may be a window where really intensive therapy will bear dividends [4,5].

Finally, we should also acknowledge that despite modern therapies, some patients do very badly indeed, dying before adult life; there remains a need to devise and test rescue therapies, holding the difficult balance between finding a cure, and improving survival and quality of life for those whose disease has likely progressed beyond the point when a cure is possible.

DIAGNOSIS AND PREVENTION

Traditionally CF was diagnosed by clinical suspicion and confirmed by a sweat test. Now with genetic testing and newborn screening, milder versions of CF are increasingly recognized. This has two consequences. First the spectrum of CF has extended to include lone infertility, sinus and pancreatic disease and even complete normality. Second, there have been apparent increases in numbers with CF and in overall survival. These trends are likely to continue and the diagnostic classification will become more complicated. Very sophisticated diagnostic testing may throw up 'abnormalities' in the CF gene which may be of little practical significance. The concepts of 'pre-CF' [6] and a CF gene-related disorder [7] are becoming increasingly useful and avoid burdening people who have an excellent prognosis with an inappropriate label. This will be increasingly important to ensure that insurance, employment and life planning are not compromised by over-pessimistic diagnostic labelling.

Prevention of CF is theoretically possible by a combination of genetic screening for carriers, pre-natal diagnosis and offering the option of termination of affected pregnancies. The only real experience of this was the Edinburgh study of the 1990s [8] in which a large majority of couples with a CF pregnancy opted for termination and the incidence of CF fell. Although this demonstrated that prevention was possible it did not lead to similar programs and no country has pursued a policy of prevention. Since then the survival has improved and public opinion has moved somewhat away from terminating pregnancy. This combination makes a program of prevention less likely and at present there is no prospect of reducing the incidence of CF.

NEW TREATMENTS

General considerations

There is an increasing and right call for rigorous clinical trials before new treatments are introduced. However, this brings its own problems. There are only limited numbers of patients who can enter trials, and already huge numbers of potential therapies. We need somehow to prioritize what are the really important questions, and maximize efficiency in testing them. Ways of maximizing efficiency include:

- Multicenter collaboration in a properly resourced program of clinical trials. Clinical trials use scarce resources, including professional time, and these need to be funded.
- Following the example of pediatric oncology in particular, and ensuring that all eligible patients are enrolled in clinical trials. Newborn screening in particular offers a great opportunity for trials of early treatment.
- Minimizing the numbers enrolled by use of factorial design, and aiming to show equivalence of effect of a more convenient treatment, rather than necessarily always attempting to show superiority.

Outcome measures

The choice of end-points will be important; mortality is no longer appropriate, as the survival curves have flattened out, so surrogates are inevitable. As far as the lung is concerned, spirometry is often so stable that rate of change of, for example, FEV_1 as an end-point requires large numbers studied for a long time [9]. More sophisticated lung function testing may help (for example, indices of gas exchange such as lung clearance index [10,11]), but may detect minor and irrelevant changes. Biomarkers of disease may also be of use; but would the reduction of a single inflammatory mediator be accepted as beneficial? Which mediator is truly important? There is no doubt that as our patients are in better health, the detection of benefit will become harder, and this is an ongoing research area.

Ethics and safety

There are many ethical and practical issues related to research in children [12]. In particular, the selection of the timing of the introduction of new treatments and balancing possible risks and benefits especially as disease modifying treatments are likely to work best if given early. The tragic cases of lymphoproliferative disease in children treated with gene

therapy for severe immunodeficiency highlight the potential problems [13]. In some ways the increased longevity of CF patients militates against therapeutic research. An early death in a baby who would have been dead within months is a tragedy, but much worse if instead the projected median survival is 40 years. So we need to find ways of delineating a higher risk young population in whom therapeutic trials are more justified; and we need to address the ethical issues around how early a child can take part in trials of a novel approach like gene therapy. At what point can we say that a treatment is so likely to be efficacious that it would be unfair discrimination to deny it to a 6-year-old, particularly if, as is likely, invasive techniques such as bronchoscopy are needed to determine efficacy [14]? The ideal is that therapeutic efficacy is demonstrated in adults, and non-invasive end-points discovered, before application to children. But what if the nature of the disease, or the changes of normal lung development, mean that a treatment is only efficacious if applied early? How do we avoid missing detecting such a therapy, while remaining ethical? CF patients, parents, care givers and researchers must reach a consensus which facilitates the development of new treatments while minimizing risk.

Reducing the burden of treatment

The two most time-consuming parts of management are aerosol therapy and airway clearance. 'Intelligent' nebulizers, which are breath-activated, are reducing treatment time for a single nebulized agent to less than two minutes, and are thus becoming serious competitors to dry-powder devices. The benefits of nebulized therapy (antibiotics, rhDNase) are undoubted; but they need to be given more quickly and efficiently, without loss of therapeutic efficacy. Reducing the burden and cost of treatment may become as important as developing new compounds but funding this type of research will be difficult.

Devising and testing novel rescue therapies

Infection is the key determinant of decline in CF and antibiotics are the mainstay of treatment. Inevitably bacteria become resistant to antibiotics and with longer survival and more courses of antibiotics this problem will increase. There is therefore a clear need for more powerful, and safer, antibiotics. Possibly increased knowledge of natural antibacterial polypeptides, such as β-defensins, may allow novel agents to be identified. The benefits of macrolides have been well documented [15–17]; but we do not know which of the extensive properties ascribed to this fascinating class of compounds is the key cause of benefit. Macrolides are ubiquitous in the plant and animal kingdom, with around 2000 different compounds described. If only we could know what properties we really needed, perhaps 'designer' macrolides could be used to enhance therapeutic benefit in those failing conventional therapy.

Despite every effort, most patients eventually need a lung transplant if they are to survive. Tragically, in many cases, organs will not become available. New approaches will be needed; much current research is directed at developing transgenic pigs as a source of donor organs. Perhaps more futuristically, as more is known about normal lung development, strategies to regenerate normal lung, perhaps using retinoids, or even to grow new lungs *in vitro* may become practical.

Nutritional failure is still all too common. Some high-profile international sportsmen have set a very bad example of manipulating anabolism. But could this bad knowledge be put to good purposes? Will we in the future use anabolic hormones and designer steroids, combined with intensive calorific support, to improve the nutrition of CF patients who are spiraling downhill in cycles of recurrent infection and weight loss? Safety issues are paramount, and the risks have been highlighted by the sad deaths of young athletes; but perhaps this route should be explored when conventional methods have failed.

NEW COMPLICATIONS

Cystic fibrosis is no longer a lung and digestive disease, but has become a truly multisystem illness. There are two aspects of increased longevity to consider: first, survival allowing the development of new complications; and second, intensive treatments that may bring an epidemic of iatrogenic disease. This last makes it all the more essential that treatment is targeted precisely.

Bone disease

The etiological factors involved in bone disease have been reviewed in Chapter 18. Some risk factors are already treated energetically on their own merits. For example, we already treat infection and inflammation aggressively, and recommend vitamin D and calcium supplements. However, as a result of an appreciation of impending CF bone disease, many clinics now routinely advise oral Vitamin K supplementation. We need to redouble our efforts to persuade children to take part in weight-bearing exercise; pubertal status should be monitored, and any excessive delay should be treated. In the future it may be possible to block pro-inflammatory cytokines in the systemic circulation.

Diabetes and insulin deficiency

In the majority of patients, the exocrine pancreas is irretrievably damaged at birth. Endocrine pancreatic function is normal or at least adequate at birth, but in as many as a third of adults, endocrine pancreatic insufficiency manifested by

insulin deficiency supervenes. We need to develop strategies to preserve endocrine pancreatic function; and if this fails, develop ways of recognizing insulin deficiency before the pre-diabetic period of insidious deterioration of lung function and nutritional status becomes evident. One possible strategy might be to reduce the pro-inflammatory drive on the pancreas of intestinal hormones produced in response to an abnormally low pH, by an aggressive use of proton pump inhibitors. It is well known that prior to the diagnosis of overt diabetes, a period of decline due to insulin deficiency is usual. It is clear that the oral glucose tolerance test is not the ideal way of detecting insulin deficiency, and ways of conveniently and cheaply monitoring home blood glucose continuously over a period of days is necessary. Perhaps the future will include early treatment with inhaled insulin to preserve a good clinical status. Similarly we need to ensure that treatment is adequate to prevent long-term vascular complications.

Other new complications

There are some manifestations of CF that are clearly important, but it is not clear how they should be prevented. One example is liver disease. This is clearly important for a minority of people with CF, but as lung problems (hopefully) recede, death from liver disease may become more frequent. There is a really pitiful paucity of information on how best to detect liver disease in CF, and what to do when it has been detected. One can but contrast the increasingly large number of big trials of lung treatments (prednisolone, ibuprofen, rhDNase, TOBI, azithromycin) with the absence of anything substantial in the field of hepatology. We need better detection strategies for liver disease, and evidence-based early intervention.

Iatrogenic disease

We have used antibiotics very liberally, and it is likely that this has been a major factor in increased longevity. However, there is a threefold price to be paid: antibiotic allergy, emergence of new resistant Gram-negative organisms, and subtle toxicity, in particular to the eighth cranial nerve and the kidney.

Antibiotic allergy is common in CF, with reported prevalence being close to 33% [18,19]. In the Danish clinic, where intravenous antibiotics are used liberally, 121 patients who received a total of 2793 courses of intravenous antibiotics were studied; 62% of patients were reported to have had an allergic reaction, which occurred in 4.5% of the courses [19]. Such problems and the need for desensitization are likely to increase.

Another likely iatrogenic complication of heavy antibiotic use is the emergence of new Gram-negative infections. In a 12-center study of 1419 patients, the emergence of resistant organisms such as *Burkoldheria cepacia* and *Stenotrophomonas maltophilia* were linked with use of antibiotics [20]. Association is not the same as causality, but database and case–control studies have linked the emergence of *S. maltophilia* with intravenous and nebulized antibiotic use [21,22]. Indeed, the large number of different bacteria present in the CF lungs is becoming increasingly recognized. There are likely to be improved methods of detection and of antibiotic sensitively testing to improve the precision of antibiotic prescribing.

Finally, cumulative antibiotic toxicity becomes a problem as the years go by. In one study, prolonged use of nebulized gentamicin was associated with subtle defects in renal tubular and eighth cranial nerve function [23]. In a recent paper [24], the effects of repeated courses of intravenous aminoglycosides on renal function were studied. Some of these adult patients had more than 120 courses in their lifespan! Nearly half had a reduction in glomerular filtration rate (GFR), of whom in around 20% it was less than 60 mL/1.73 m^2 per minute. GFR correlated highly significantly inversely with number of courses given. With that handy diagnostic instrument, the retrospectoscope, were all these courses really necessary?

Increased longevity

From the world of asthma, middle-aged adults who had 'wheezy bronchitis' as children, presumed to be on the basis of developmental reductions in airway caliber, and who 'recovered' completely in later childhood, are now showing an accelerated decline in lung function [25]. We may need to switch our focus to preventing accelerated lung aging (if it exists) in this population also. It seems clear that very early on it is possible to detect decrements in lung function, even in those with no apparent respiratory disease, and that these decrements track through the pre-school years. Maybe we need to intervene particularly aggressively in the very early years of CF, to ensure good long-term lung health, and this will be increasingly important as survival increases.

The current focus is on the prevention of the healthy newborn lungs and nutritional state from deteriorating and leading to premature death. But if we win that battle, will there be an epidemic of premature aging in the CF population? We have advised a high-fat diet with impunity and enormous current clinical benefit, and currently hypercholesterolemia is never seen in CF. This may change as we make fat absorption more efficient. In 20 years time will there be sessions on 'The cardiology of CF' in the big meetings?

The ugly specter of an increased risk of epithelial cell cancer has already raised its head, albeit only as a rare entity. We know that ongoing inflammation is present in the lungs, and at least some components of the high-fat diet may be systemically pro-inflammatory. We may need to be alert to a potential rise in cancer deaths in the CF population.

NEW PATTERNS OF CARE

General considerations

The recurring theme of this chapter, maximizing benefit while minimizing inconvenience, is important in this section also. Issues include balancing the benefits and inconvenience of hospital and home care; and those of the conventional outpatient consultation as opposed to using modern information technology such as telemedicine, or email. Who will then take responsibility – healthcare professional or expert patient? The patient is usually right – but not invariably – and poor perception of symptoms is well known in the context of asthma. As survival improves the disease will be seen as less threatening and the combination of complacency and the less-than-expert patient may lead to deteriorating standards of care and variable adherence to treatment. Ultimately, of course, the individual adult is responsible for his or her care, enlisting such professional aid when desired. The issues are different for children. Adult patients have the right to neglect themselves, but parents and professionals owe a duty of care to children. It will be a challenge to ensure that an e-barrier does not arise to prevent appropriate management of dependant children.

Psychological problems may shift away from anxiety about death felt by parents and child towards the less dramatic difficulties of coping with, and accepting, a chronic illness. Nevertheless CF remains a lethal disease and the burden of the terminal phase will fall progressively on older patients and their partners, some of whom may be less well prepared than CF parents over the past 30 years. Psychological and coping issues will alter but not diminish and the need for psychological and occasional psychiatric help may actually increase.

Outpatient review

The conventional outpatient review involves travel for the patient and sometimes a carer or partner, and prolonged waits in a hospital. There are additional, small risks of acquiring a nosocomial infection, or a pathogen from another CF patient. The alternative options are the use of Internet and telephone technology, and home visits from members of the CF team. Each has promises, but each also has its problems. If we are to use the Internet, we need to decide what are the really important features of physical examination, which will be lost. History-taking should be straightforward, but discussing sensitive issues, or breaking bad news, may not be done best by email. Home visits are welcomed by many patients, and allow unhurried assessment in a non-threatening environment. However, they are very resource-intensive and time-consuming, and increasingly difficult to fund. It might be argued that much could be taken over by the local team; but unless they are trained in CF, and have very close links with the regional center, there is a risk of loss of quality of care.

It is likely that different patterns of care will in the future be best for different patients, and at different stages of CF. Home intravenous antibiotics are at least as good as hospital care for a proportion of patients, but they need to be highly selected. Home care for all is clearly wrong. The challenge of the team will be to work with patients to deliver the best package of care, tailored to the need of the individual CF patient.

Annual review

The annual assessment traditionally has provided the means of taking stock of how the CF patient is progressing. With the increasing appreciation that CF is a multisystem disease, the length and complexity of the process is increasing, and there becomes a risk that we obsess on process without considering outcome. Clearly, this sort of assessment has paid rich dividends in the past, and it is difficult to deny that the approach of intensive investigation and treatment, when compared in particular to a casual, nihilistic attitude, has brought dividends in terms of prolonging survival. However, perhaps the time has come when we need a more selective consideration of who needs what, so the benefits of the old approach can be retained, while restricting testing to those who really need it.

MONITORING

Clearly, the lessons of history for the older CF physician include absolutely to beware of complacency. But it is also quite clear that we need to work to minimize the demands made on the well patient, while continuing to maintain vigilance. The completely well child will simply not do 30 minutes of postural drainage twice daily. Furthermore, there is a precedent for reining in on the 'more is better' approach; the morbidity of fibrosing colonopathy could have been avoided by more cautious use of pancreatic enzymes. A clear challenge will be to maximize the long-term benefit from a minimum management package, in terms of time spent on treatment, intervals between treatment episodes, and number and complexity of interventions. Perhaps in the future the analogy will be with hypertension; the CF patient will be in no immediate danger, but will be taking treatments in order to prevent future complications. Any side-effect of treatment will become unacceptable. Monitoring of treatment, and timing of interventions such as a course of antibiotics, will likely require surrogate markers. There is precedent for this in the current treatment of asthma; intensification of treatment for an asymptomatic increase in exhaled nitric oxide or sputum eosinophil count, or worsening of bronchial hyper-reactivity, has been shown to optimize asthma control, as compared to a symptom- or peak-flow-based approach.

The ultimate aim would be for CF be relegated to the status of what mere carriage of one CFTR mutation is today, namely to cease to be a disease, but to become a risk factor for, for example, pancreatitis, sinusitis or bronchiectasis. This is still some distance off!

SUMMARY AND CONCLUSIONS

The history of cystic fibrosis is one of constant surprises; as one complication is dealt with, so another arises. The disease has metamorphosed from a simple, severe, two-system illness to a complex multisystem series of problems. CFTR exists in tissues that are generally thought to be non-diseased, like the heart, the kidney, and the red blood cell [26]; how long before these batteries are unmasked? It is likely that combination of the defect in a multifunctional protein, CFTR, and the frenetic activities of the medical team, combined over many decades, will produce many more facets to CF. Only a foolish person they could predict even the chapter headings in this or a similar volume in 20 years' time.

REFERENCES

1. Ranganathan S, Dezateux C, Bush A *et al.* Airway function in infants newly diagnosed with cystic fibrosis [research letter]. *Lancet* 2001; **358**:1964–1965.
2. Ranganathan S, Bush A, Dezateux C *et al.* Relative ability of full and partial forced expiratory maneuvers to identify diminished airway function in infants with cystic fibrosis. *Am J Respir Crit Care Med* 2002; **166**:1350–1357.
3. Khan TZ, Wagener JS, Boat T *et al.* Early pulmonary inflammation in infants with cystic fibrosis. *Am J Respir Crit Care Med* 1995; **151**:1075–1082.
4. Ranganathan SC, Stocks J, Dezateux C *et al.* The evolution of airway function in early childhood following clinical diagnosis of cystic fibrosis. *Am J Respir Crit Care Med* 2004; **169**:928–933.
5. Nielsen KG, Pressler T, Klug B *et al.* Serial lung function and responsiveness in cystic fibrosis during early childhood. *Am J Respir Crit Care Med* 2004; **169**:1209–1216.
6. Bush A, Wallis C. Time to think again: cystic fibrosis is not an 'all or none' disease. *Pediatr Pulmonol* 2000; **30**:139–144.
7. Wallis C. Diagnosing cystic fibrosis: blood, sweat, and tears. *Arch Dis Child* 1997; **76**:85–88.
8. Cunningham S, Marshall T. Influence of five years of antenatal screening on the paediatric cystic fibrosis population in one region. *Arch Dis Child* 1998; **78**:345–348.
9. Davis PB, Byard PJ, Konstan MW. Identifying treatments that halt progression of pulmonary disease in cystic fibrosis. *Pediatr Res* 1997; **41**:161–165.
10. Aurora P, Gustafsson PM, Bush A *et al.* Multiple-breath inert gas washout as a measure of ventilation distribution in children with cystic fibrosis. *Thorax* 2004; **59**:1068–1073.

11. Aurora P, Bush A, Gustafsson P *et al.* Multiple-breath washout as a marker of lung disease in preschool children with cystic fibrosis. *Am J Respir Crit Care Med* 2005; **171**:249–256.

12. McIntosh N, Bates P, Brykczynska G *et al.* Guidelines for the ethical conduct of medical research involving children. *Arch Dis Child* 2000; **82**:177–182.

13. Kimmelman J. Recent developments in gene transfer: risks and ethics. *Br Med J* 2005; **330**:79–82.

14. Davies JC, Davies M, McShane D *et al.* Potential difference measurements in the lower airway of children with and without cystic fibrosis. *Am J Respir Crit Care Med* 2005; **171**:1015–1019.

15. Wolter J, Seeney S, Bell S *et al.* Effect of long-term treatment with azithromycin on disease parameters in cystic fibrosis: a randomized trial. *Thorax* 2002; **57**:212–216.

16. Equi A, Balfour-Lynn I, Bush A, Rosenthal M. Long term azithromycin in children with cystic fibrosis: a randomised, placebo-controlled crossover trial. *Lancet* 2002; **360**:978–984.

17. Saiman S, Marshall BC, Meyer-Hamblett N *et al.* Azithromycin in patients with cystic fibrosis chronically infected with *Pseudomonas aeruginosa*: a randomized controlled trial. *J Am Med Assoc* 2003; **290**:1749–1756.

18. Pleasants RA, Walker TR, Samuelson WM. Allergic reactions to parenteral beta-lactam antibiotics in patients with cystic fibrosis. *Chest* 1994; **106**:1124–1128.

19. Koch C, Hjelt K, Jensen ET *et al.* Retrospective clinical study of hypersensitivity reactions to aztreonam and six other beta-lactam antibiotics in cystic fibrosis patients receiving multiple treatment courses. *Rev Infect Dis* 1991; **13**(Suppl 7):S608–S611.

20. Steinkamp G, Wiedemann B, Rietschel E *et al.* Prospective evaluation of emerging bacteria in cystic fibrosis. *J Cyst Fibros* 2005; **4**:41–48.

21. Marchac V, Equi A, Le Bihan-Benjamin C *et al.* Case–control study of *Stenotrophomonas maltophilia* acquisition in cystic fibrosis patients. *Eur Respir J* 2004; **23**:98–102.

22. Talmaciu I, Varlotta L, Mortensen J, Schidlow D. Risk factors for emergence of *Stenotrophomonas maltophilia* in cystic fibrosis. *Pediatr Pulmonol* 2000; **30**:10–15.

23. Ring E, Eber E, Erwa W, Zach M. Urinary *N*-acetyl-beta-D-glucosaminidase activity in patients with cystic fibrosis on long-term gentamicin inhalation. *Arch Dis Child* 1998; **78**:540–543.

24. Al-Aloul M, Miller H, Alapati S *et al.* Renal impairment in cystic fibrosis patients due to repeated intravenous aminoglycoside use. *Pediatr Pulmonol* 2005; **39**:15–30.

25. Edwards CA, Osman LM, Godden DJ, Douglas JG. Wheezy bronchitis in childhood: a distinct clinical entity with lifelong significance. *Chest* 2003; **124**:18–24.

26. Larson JE, Cohen JC. Developmental paradigm for early features of cystic fibrosis. *Pediatr Pulmonol* 2005; **40**:371–377.

APPENDICES

---

1 Transition form   479
   Susan Madge and Jacqueline Francis
2 Practical nursing care required by the cystic fibrosis patient and its delivery   483
   Frances Duncan-Skingle and Tracey Catling

Appendix 1

Transition form

SUSAN MADGE AND JACQUELINE FRANCIS

TRANSITION

Patient name:	Age:	DOB:		
Referring consultant:	Hosp. no. (referring hospital):			
			Yes/No	**Date**
TRANSITION Has transition been discussed with the patient? Has transition been discussed with parents/care giver? Any concerns?				
Has information about and invitation to Transition Clinic been received?				
Agreed date of Transition Clinic?				
Have family and patient visited the adult ward? If 'no', reasons:				
FERTILITY Discussed? Yes ❏ No ❏ Contraception advice given? Yes ❏ No ❏				
TRANSPLANTATION Discussed? Yes ❏ No ❏ Details of discussion:				
DIAGNOSIS Date of diagnosis: Presentation at diagnosis: **Genotype:** **Sweat test results:** left arm/right arm 1. Sodium mmol/L 2. Chloride mmol/L				

CURRENT CLINICAL STATUS
Date of measurements:

Height: Weight: BMI:

Lung function: FEV$_1$:   (%)   FVC: (%)   SaO$_2$:   %

| Portacath: | Date: | Type: |

Gastrostomy: Date: Type:
Feeding regimen:

Appetite:
Pancreatic sufficient: Enzyme treatment:

	Yes/No	Date
ORGANISMS *Staphylococcus aureus* *Haemophilus influenzae* *Pseudomonas aeruginosa* *Strenotrophomonas maltophilia* *Burkholderia cepacia* complex – type: MRSA Atypical mycobacteria – type: Other		

HOSPITALIZATION
How many times in the last year?
Reasons for admission:

DRUG THERAPY

ALLERGIES AND REACTIONS

PHYSIOTHERAPY
Type:

Frequency:

Adherence:

COMPLICATIONS	DETAILS
Oxygen therapy Hemoptysis Pneumothorax ABPA DIOS Liver disease Varices CF-related diabetes Arthropathy Other associated conditions	

FAMILY BACKGROUND

Parents' names:

Siblings' names and ages:

CF-siblings' names and ages:

CF in extended family – state relationship, names and ages:

Ethic origin: Religion:

SOCIAL SUPPORT

Disability Living Allowance: Yes ☐   No ☐   Rate:

Mobility: Yes ☐   No ☐

EMPLOYMENT (Saturday/part-time/weekend/full-time)

EDUCATION

Sixth Form (GCSEs, A Levels, GVNQ):

College/University:

Career interest:

Special educational needs:

HOME CARE

RBH (joint visit with adult CNS?):

Referring hospital (joint visit with adult CNS?):

Primary Care Team:

Contact person and telephone number:

OTHER COMMENTS

Completed by: Date:

ALL ABOUT ME – please introduce yourself to the adult team

Appendix 2

Practical nursing care required by the cystic fibrosis patient and its delivery

FRANCES DUNCAN-SKINGLE AND TRACEY CATLING

Many cystic fibrosis units will have established their own consensus guidelines for the patient's clinical care and management. The employing authority accepts liability and responsibility for the professional functions undertaken on behalf of the organization by nurses. Where this includes an 'extended role of the nurse' these functions should be clearly laid out with guidelines and policy procedures that are agreed by the Hospital Board.

In the UK, under the Code of Conduct (Nursing and Midwifery Council, *Code of Professional Conduct: standards for conduct, performance and ethics*, July 2004), it is the aim of the nursing profession to give the highest standard of care possible to patients. This means patients should not be placed in jeopardy and that a nurse does not undertake any procedure where adequate training instruction and assessment has not been given. The nurse must recognize their own limitations in competence and should not delegate to junior colleagues tasks and responsibilities beyond their knowledge and skills. Patients with CF require the input of other members of the multidisciplinary team and it is part of the nurse's responsibility to refer them as appropriate, to ensure that the patients receive the best possible care.

The following tables list some of the basic nursing care required by the CF patients and its delivery.

Table 1 General nursing care.

Problems	Aims/actions	Outcome/actions
Treatment of chest infections; ineffective airway clearance due to increased pulmonary secretions	Infection control standards and unit guidelines must be strictly adhered to Reduce symptoms caused by an infective exacerbation	• Inform and educate patients on their microbiological status. This will encourage confidence • Encourage and refer to physiotherapy • Bronchodilators may be given before physiotherapy if prescribed • Monitor mobility and breathlessness. If breathless, assist in positioning patient comfortably and encourage mobilization when able. Encourage good posture • Report changes in the amount, quality and color of sputum • Provide mouthwash if sputum is foul tasting, after nebulized antibiotics and after steroid inhalers • Give prescribed nebulized therapy in the order prescribed • Give oxygen therapy as prescribed • Assess respiratory status regularly, i.e. respiratory rate, pulmonary function tests, oxygen saturation
Effective and safe handling of intravenous therapy	Minimize the problems associated with intravenous therapy	• Observe cannula site before each infusion • Ensure cannulae or Huber needle, if implantable port used, is secure [1] • Administer antibiotics as prescribed. In young children and adolescents local anesthetic cream placed on proposed venepuncture site 1 hour prior to insertion of cannula is advisable

(Continued)

Table 1   (Continued)

Problems	Aims/actions	Outcome/actions
		• Check site regularly for signs of phlebitis • Follow correct procedure for i.v. drug administration • Check aminoglycoside levels and ensure appropriate dose is given, getting the prescription dose changed if necessary • Observe the patient for side-effects and report if any occur and/or stop infusion
	Promote self-administration of intravenous drugs	• Teach the patient how to reconstitute i.v. drugs and the method of delivery. • Teach safety aspects on the care of the line or port, the handling and administration of drugs ensuring aseptic techniques are used to reduce the risk of infection • Understand the interactions of drugs and what to observe in the event of possible side-effects • Assess competency of either patient and/or carer according to local standards/guidelines. They should be reassessed with every course of intravenous antibiotics prescribed • Advise on disposal of sharps • Provide emergency contact telephone numbers if having i.v. treatment at home • Provide details of home-care services, if appropriate
Malabsorption of food	Ensure steatorrhea is adequately controlled	• Refer to dietitian for review of pancreatic enzyme replacement therapy • Ensure pancreatic enzymes are taken with all meals and snacks (small babies may require a medium such as fruit pureé to take their enzymes) • Monitor bowel actions and report any changes
Poor dietary intake	Ensure patients' calorie intake is sufficient for their. energy expenditure	• Refer to dietitian to assess nutritional status • Monitor weekly weight and report any loss • Monitor dietary input and advise according to dietetic recommendations • Identify any factors that may affect nutritional status, e.g. breathlessness, nausea, and assist as necessary • Encourage use of supplements if prescribed
	Provide care if alternative feeding methods used in accordance with local hospital policy	*Nasogastric feeding* • Ensure tube is correctly positioned • Teach patient to pass own tube if appropriate • Check that feed is correct for patient • Monitor flow rates of feed so that the correct amount is delivered over the prescribed time *Percutaneous endoscopic gastrostomy feeding tube* [2]: New stoma: • Observe site, re-dress daily with a clean, dry dressing. After 2 weeks patient will be able to bathe fully and to swim. Attention should be paid to drying the stoma carefully otherwise soreness may occur • Teach patient how to care for stoma site • Observe patient for discomfort and bloating during and after administration of feed • Give prescribed antiemetic as necessary • Ensure correct amount of feed is given over the prescribed period • Feeds should always be administered and controlled with a feeding pump *Total parenteral nutrition* (TPN): • Ensure scrupulous attention to intravenous site and keep manipulations to the feeding line at a minimum. If possible use a dedicated feeding line • Carefully monitor vital signs in order to detect infection or reactions to TPN including blood glucose levels • Check intravenous drugs against the prescribed regimen • Observe the TPN for any changes, e.g. separation, creaming, color

Table 2 Nursing activities required for specific complications.

Problems	Aims	Outcome/actions
Poor venous access	Ensure venepuncture is as pain-free as possible and avoid damage to the venous system	• Observe cannula site before each infusion • Ensure that antibiotics are sufficiently diluted to reduce irritation in vein • Promptly remove cannula if problems occur, to reduce risk of damage to veins • Advise patient of other methods of venous access, e.g. long intravenous line, Hickman line, totally implantable venous access system (Port) • Educate patient on how to use various venous access systems and their individual flushing regimens • Use of aids to extend the life of cannulas
Hemoptysis	Help allay fears Promote cessation of bleeding	• Give reassurance • Refer to physiotherapy for advice on airway clearance • Observe amount and type of hemoptysis • Report any increase and frequency • If embolization of bronchial artery is necessary, regular temperature, pulse, respiration, blood pressure, pedal pulses and leg color will need to be observed, as well as leg movements. Pressure maintained on access site and analgesia given as required
Pneumothorax	Relieve breathlessness and promote healing of air leak	• Report sudden onset of breathlessness or chest pain. Be aware of implications. Reassure the patient • Care of patient with chest drain, observe drainage from the chest drain. Report any change in the amount or color of fluid in the drainage bottle • Observe insertion site daily, change bottle and report to the medical team if the drain stops bubbling • Teach patient about chest drain safety • Give analgesia as required • Promote mobility if possible • If suction is required, ensure correct settings are maintained
Diabetes [3,4] and CF-related diabetes (CFRD)	Control and monitor hyperglycemia	• Record blood glucose levels at regular intervals in accordance with local hospital policy • Give insulin or oral hypoglycemic agent as per prescribed regimen • Monitor symptoms of hyperglycemia, e.g. weight and weight loss, polyuria and polydipsia • Educate the patient about their diabetes, hypo- and hyperglycemic episodes and self-administration of insulin • Educate the patient on how to monitor blood glucose levels • Educate the patient on the care of their skin, nails, eyes and feet • Remember that steroids may cause hypoglycemia, so careful monitoring is required during treatment • Diabetic annual assessment is necessary to prevent and control retinopathy [5,6]
Meconium ileus equivalent (MIE) or distal ileus obstructive syndrome (DIOS) [7]	Promote return to previous bowel habits	• Give prescribed laxatives and enemas • Monitor bowel movements, frequency and type • Observe for dehydration and abdominal distension • Administer prescribed intravenous fluids if nil by mouth • Give appropriate analgesia and antiemetic if required
Possible need for ventilatory assistance via non-invasive ventilation (NIV) [8]	Reduce anxiety of patient and relative, and promote good compliance with equipment by working with the multidisciplinary team	• Reassure the patient who will be very anxious • Ensure that the patient understands and consents • Educate patient about safety issues, e.g. no drinking and eating while using NIV due to a possible increased risk of aspiration • Ensure that the patient and relatives know how to disconnect from the machine if necessary • Advise on the meaning of the alarms and significance of the different tones • Observe and record length of time on and off NIV

(Continued)

Table 2   (Continued)

Problems	Aims	Outcome/actions
		• Promote good skin care around mask area. Keep clean and dry. Ensure bridge of nose is relieved of pressure as much as possible. Pressure-relieving agents may be employed
		• Provide backup support and contact emergency telephone numbers in case of machine failure
Coping with the terminal stages of cystic fibrosis	Relieve symptoms	• Try to identify the patient's wishes prior to the terminal stage. Be aware of any advanced directives
		• A patient may wish to die at home. Establish the support systems available and ensure they are all in place. Refer to palliative care team if there is one available
		• Encourage patients, relatives and staff to communicate with each other
		• Allow patients and relatives time and space to be alone
		• Help them to listen to each other's needs
		• Be prepared to answer questions honestly
		• Help patients to maintain independence for as long as possible
		• Alleviate feelings of isolation, anxiety and fear
		• Control symptoms of breathlessness, pain and any other symptoms that may occur, to ensure that a comfortable, dignified death is achieved. The use of opiates may be helpful
		• Provide support for family and friends prior to and following death [9]
		• Provide bereavement follow-up support

REFERENCES

1. Kariyawasam HH, Pepper JR, Hodson ME *et al.* Experience of totally implantable venous access devices (TIV ADs) in adults with cystic fibrosis over a 13-year period. *Respir Med* 2000; 94:1161–1165.

2. Williams SG, Ashworth F, McAlweenie A *et al.* Percutaneous endoscopic gastrostomy feeding in patients with cystic fibrosis. *Gut* 1999; 44:87–90.

3. Marshall BC, Butler SM, Stoddard M *et al.* Epidemiology of cystic fibrosis-related diabetes. *J Pediatr* 2005; 146:681–687.

4. Milla CE, Billings J, Moran A. Diabetes is associated with dramatically decreased survival in female but not male subjects with cystic fibrosis. *Diabetes Care* 2005; 28:2141–2144.

5. Scott AI, Clarke BE, Healy H *et al.* Microvascular complications in cystic fibrosis-related diabetes mellitus: a case report. *JOP* 2000; 1:208–210.

6. Yung B, Landers A, Mathalone B *et al.* Diabetic retinopathy in adult patients with cystic fibrosis-related diabetes. *Respir Med* 1998; 92:871–872.

7. Shidrawi RG, Murugan N, Westaby D *et al.* Emergency colonoscopy for distal intestinal obstruction syndrome in cystic fibrosis patients. *Gut* 2002; 51:285–286.

8. Hill AT, Edenborough FP, Cayton RM *et al.* Long-term nasal intermittent positive pressure ventilation in patients with cystic fibrosis and hypercapnic respiratory failure (1991–96). *Respir Med* 1998; 92:523–526.

9. Farber SJ, Egnew TR, Herman-Bertsch JL *et al.* Issues in end-of-life care: patient, caregiver, and clinician perceptions. *J Palliat Med* 2003; 6:19–31.

Index

Notes: **bold page numbers** are used for figures, *italic page numbers* are used for tables

25-OHD *see* hydroxyvitamin D

AAV *see* adeno-associated virus
ABPA *see* allergic bronchopulmonary
    aspergillosis
Acapella® 412, **412**, 413
ACBT *see* active cycle of breathing
    techniques
N-acetyl-cysteine (NAC) 165, 217, 377
Achromobacter xylosoxidans 146
acid resistant pancreatic enzymes 9,
    11, 211
acid suppressants 212, 215
acrodermatitis enteropathica-like
    eruptions 270
active cycle of breathing techniques
    (ACBT) 409–10, **409**, **410**
ACTs *see* airway clearance techniques
acute pulmonary exacerbations 138–9,
    138, 141, 144, 345, 378
acute rejection of lung grafts 297, 298
AC/VT *see* assist control/volume-
    targeted ventilation
AD *see* autogenic drainage
adaptive aerosol delivery (ADD) devices
    187, *187*
adeno-associated virus (AAV) vectors
    457–8
adenoviral vectors 456–7
ADH *see* antidiuretic hormone
adherence *see* compliance
adhesion of bacteria 70, 377
adjuvant therapy 212
adolescents
    infection risks 403
    lung transplants 301
    nursing care 401, 402–3, *402*
    nutritional support 425–6
    physiological monitoring 345–51
    psychological aspects 91, 287, 431–2,
      436

puberty 253–9, 265, 473
    sexual/reproductive health information
      280, 281, 283
    transition to adult care 393–5, *394*,
      402–3, 479–82
adoption 281
β-adrenergic agonists 168
β-adrenergic receptor (*β*-AR) genes 83
adult respiratory distress syndrome
    (ARDS) 296, *296*
adults
    care history 8, 12
    complications 33–4, **33**
    lung function 29, **29**, **30**
    nursing care 403
    nutritional status 32–3, **32**
    nutritional support 425–6
    physiological monitoring 345–51
    psychological aspects 432–3, 436
    social and demographic features 34–5,
      34, **35**
    terminal care 446
    transition from pediatric care 393–5,
      394, 402–3, 479–82
advanced disease *see* end-stage disease
adverse effects
    antibiotics 6, 7
    drugs in pregnancy *286*
    immunosuppression 297, *297*, 301
    oral therapies 193, *194*
    pancreatic enzyme replacement
      therapy 212–13
advocacy 390, 404
AEP *see* aquagenic wrinkling of the palms
aerobic fitness 353, **353**
aerobic testing 354–6
aerobic training 363–4, *364*, **364**
aerosol therapies *see* inhaled therapies
AFS *see* allergic fungal sinusitis
age
    bone mineral density changes **262**, 263

CF patient distribution 27, **27**, 403
    at death 26, **87**
    at diagnosis 27–8, **28**
    lung function effects 29–30, **30**
    prognostic indicators 37
    at puberty 253–4, 255–6, 257–8
    respiratory infection rate effects 31, **31**
air pollution 89
air trapping **339**, **340**
air travel 168–9, 195–6
airway clearance techniques (ACTs)
    366, 407, 409–15
    see also physiotherapy
airway gland secretion 74
airway obstruction 137, 323–4
airway surface liquid (ASL) 60–2, **61**,
    72, 73–4
Alcaligenes xylosoxidans see
    Achromobacter xylosoxidans
Allan diet 9
allergic bronchopulmonary aspergillosis
    (ABPA) 148–51, *149*, **150**
    clinical features 149
    diagnosis 149–50, *149*
    epidemiology/risk factors 148–9
    historical view 7
    lobar collapse 162
    lung function decline study 347–8, **348**
    pathophysiology 148
    prognosis 151
    screening 150
    sinonasal disease 201
    treatment 150–1
allergic fungal sinusitis (AFS) 200–1
allergy to antibiotics 139
α₁-proteinase inhibitor 73, **73**
alpha-cell function impairment 243
altitude 168–9, 195–6
alveolar hypoventilation 177–8
amenorrhea 282
American Thoracic Society 321

aminoglycosides 54–5, 139, 271, 272
anabolic agents 255, 257, 426
anaerobic cultures 125
anaerobic exercise testing 356–7, **356**, *357*, **357**
anaerobic training 365
anaesthesia 333
analytical studies 311, *311*
Anderson, Dorothy 3–4, **4**, 5
animal models 70, 328, 464, 467
annual reviews 248, 392–3, *392–3*, 475
anomosia 201
anorexia 444
anovulatory females 282, 284
antacids *see* acid suppressants
antenatal care 285
antenatal diagnosis 10, 12, 285
antibiotics
    adverse effects 6, 7
    allergies 139
    aspergillosis role 148–9
    Burkholderia cepacia complex 143
    choice 139
    course number as treatment success indicator 378
    fungal infection role 148–9, 151
    general principles of treatment 138–9
    historical use 5, 6, 7, 8–9, 10–11
    inhaled 10–11, 138, 142, 148–9, 191–2
    intravenous 11, 138–9, 141, 194–5, *195*
    macrolides 139, 140, 166–7, *167*
    methicillin-resistant *Staphylococcus aureus* 144–5
    methicillin-sensitive *Staphylococcus aureus* 144
    non-tuberculous mycobacterial infection 146
    oral contraceptive pill 283
    oral therapy 194
    in pregnancy 285, 286
    prophylaxis 8–9, 138, 148, 296, 297–8
    Pseudomonas aeruginosa 138, 139, 141–2, 333
    renal impairment 271, 272
    resistance 6, 128, 139, 143, 144–5
    sinonasal disease 204
    Stenotrophomonas maltophilia 145–6
    susceptibility testing 127–8
    synergy testing 128
    transplantation patients 296, 297–8
    vaginal yeast infection 284
    young children 333
antibody-based assays 376
antibody production 72
antidiuretic hormone (ADH) 273–4
antifungal agents 148, 150, 296, 297–8

antigen presentation 82–3
anti-inflammatory therapy 165–8, 194, 203
antimicrobial peptides 72
antimicrobial susceptibility testing 127–8
antiproteases 82
antisense oligonucleotide therapy 56, 459
antiviral strategies 147–8
    see also vaccinations
anxiety 442–3, 444, 445
apical cell membrane 49, 50, 60
appendiceal disease 218
appetite stimulants 426
aquagenic wrinkling of the palms (AEP) 270
ARDS *see* adult respiratory distress syndrome
arthralgias 269
arthritis 269, 270, 271
arthropathies 270–1
ascites 232–3
ASL *see* airway surface liquid
Aspergillus spp 148–51
    A. clavitus 148
    A. flavus 148
    A. fumigatus 148, 149
    A. nidulans 148
    A. niger 148
    A. terreus 148
    clinical epidemiology 31, **32**
    sinonasal disease 200–1
    see also allergic bronchopulmonary aspergillosis
assist control/volume-targeted ventilation (AC/VT) 178, **178**, 181, 182
assisted reproduction 281, 282, 287
asthma 87, 166, 474
asynchronous ventilation technique 408
atopy 149, 166, 201
atypical CFTR mutations 53
atypical (non-classic) cystic fibrosis
    additional investigations 105
    genotypes 12, 21, 53, 81
    historic view 8
    late diagnosis 27–8
    pathophysiology 64
    phenotypes *103*, 104
    polymorphisms 56–7
atypical respiratory symptoms 334
autogenic drainage (AD) 410–11, **411**
autoimmune processes 242
azithromycin (AZM) 166–7, *167*
azoospermia 105, 254, 279–82
    see also congenital bilateral absence of the vas deferens

bacterial antimicrobial susceptibility testing 127–8
bacterial binding 62–3, 70, 71
bacterial defence mechanisms 60
bacterial infections
    diarrheal diseases 22, 40–1, 64, 212, 219–20
    emerging pathogens 123
    Haemophilus influenzae 31, **31**, **32**, 145, 199, 204
    identification of species **125–7**, **142**
    mycobacteria 31, 126, 146
    Mycobacterium avium complex 146
    paranasal sinuses 199, 200
    Stenotrophomonas maltophilia 32, 145–6
    see also antibiotics; *Burkholderia cepacia* complex; microbiology; *Pseudomonas aeruginosa*; respiratory infections; *Staphylococcus aureus*
bacterial load quantification 377–8
BAL *see* bronchoalveolar lavage
Balke protocol 354, *355*
balloon tamponade 232
banding ligation 231, **232**
BCEs *see* bicarbonate/chloride exchangers
behavioral aspects *425*, 431–7
benefit systems 390
bereavement 405, 447
best practice 129, 130, 400, *401*, *402*, *404*
β-adrenergic agonists 168
β-adrenergic receptor (β-AR) genes 83
beta-cell function impairment 242–3
bicarbonate/chloride exchangers (BCEs) 63–4, **63**
bicarbonate ion transport 62, 63–4, **63**, 64
bile acids 211, 226, 229
bilevel positive airway pressure ventilation (BiPAP) 178–9, 181
biliary disease 64–5, 225–6, 233, **234**, 235
biofilms 72, 127–8, 140
biopsies 301, 376
BiPAP *see* bilevel positive airway pressure ventilation
birth prevalence 21, 23, *24*
bisphosphates in bone 266–7
blood analysis
    glucose tests 246
    immunoreactive trypsin tests 7, 9, 111, 112, 113
    new treatment assessment 379
BM *see* Boehringer–Mannheim
BMD *see* bone mineral density

BMI *see* body mass index
BMSCs *see* bone-marrow-derived
  stem cells
body image 91, 287, 369
body mass index (BMI) 32–3, *32*, 422
Boehringer–Mannheim (BM)
  meconium test 7
bone disease *see* cystic-fibrosis-related
  low bone mineral density
bone-marrow-derived stem cells
  (BMSCs) 459
bone maturation 254, 257
bone mineral density (BMD) 261–8
  see also cystic-fibrosis-related low bone
    mineral density
BOS *see* bronchiolitis obliterans
  syndrome
breast feeding 120, 285, 287, 425, 427
breath-actuated pressurized metered-dose
  inhalers 191
breath-enhanced nebulizers *187*,
  188, 189
breathing *see* ventilation
breathlessness 366–7, 444
bronchial responsiveness 351
bronchial stenosis in transplanted
  lungs 298
bronchiectasis **339**
bronchiolitis obliterans syndrome (BOS)
  298, 299–300, *300*
bronchoalveolar lavage (BAL)
  bronchoscopy techniques 333
  forced oscillation technique 329
  neonates 70
  neutrophils 70, 73–4
  new treatment assessment 379
  oropharyngeal culture comparison
    332–3
  usefulness 124
  young children 332–3
bronchodilators 6, 167–8, 192
bronchoscopy 331–4, *334*
Bruce protocol 354–5, *355*
Burkholderia cepacia complex
  acquisition factors 89
  antibiotics 143
  B. cenocepacia 127, 142–3, *142*, 144
  B. dolorosa 127, 142, *142*
  B. multivorans 127, 142, *142*, 143
  B. vietnamiensis 127, 142, *142*
  cepacia syndrome 142, 143, **143**
  chronic infection 143
  clinical consequences 142–3
  clinical epidemiology 31–2, *31*, **31**, **32**
  culture media 125, *125*
  genomovars 123, 126–7, *127*, 142–3,
    142, 144

historical view 12
infection control 143–4
microbiological identification 126–7,
  142
pathogenicity 142–3
prognostic indicators 38
respiratory exacerbations 143
transmissibility 142
treatment 143
burnout 396–7, 435

CAL *see* CFTR-associated ligand
calcineurin inhibitors 296, 297, 299
calcium 265, 266
Canada 7, 23, *24*
cancer
  clinical epidemiology 34
  gastrointestinal malignancy 221
  hepatobiliary malignancy 235
  lung transplants 299, 301
  pancreatic malignancy 235
Candida albicans 149, 151, 193, 194,
  200
cardiac complications 163, **163**, 169
cardiopulmonary fitness 353, **353**,
  363–5
cardiovascular response to exercise 361,
  370
care
  future patterns 474–5
  nursing 389, 392, 396, 399–405, 483,
    483–4, *485*–6
'care by parent' units 118
care centers *see* specialist CF centers
Care Teaching and Research Center
  Program 6
carriers *see* heterozygous condition
cascade-impactor measurement 185–6,
  186
case–control studies 312
cathepsin G 73, 74
catheters for intravenous therapies 194
Caucasian populations 22, 23, *24*, *52*
CBAVD *see* congenital bilateral absence
  of the vas deferens
CBT *see* cognitive behavior therapy
CCK *see* cholecystokinin
celiac disease/syndrome 3, 7, 220–1
cell-cycle inhibitors 296, 297
centers of care *see* specialist CF centers
cepacia syndrome 142, 143, **143**
cervical mucus abnormalities 282
CFALD *see* cystic-fibrosis-associated
  liver disease
CFF *see* Cystic Fibrosis Foundation
CF mouse 464, 467
CFQ *see* Cystic Fibrosis Questionnaire

CFRD *see* cystic-fibrosis-related diabetes
CFTR-associated ligand (CAL) 49
CFTR association of non CF disorders
  56–7, 104–5, 282
CFTR gene
  CBAVD 65, 81, 282
  cloning 453
  fetal gene therapy 459
  mRNA assay 375–6
  mutations *103*
    carrier identification 113
    classifications 51–7, *54*, **54**, *55*,
      59–60, 81–2, 242
    diagnosis 99, 102–4
    double 103–4, 112
    heterozygotes 22–3, *22*, 40–1, 64,
      113
    newborn screening 111
    origins 22, **22**
    phenotype relationship 52–3
    sequence variations 51, *53*
    specific populations 21–2, 51, *52*
  polymorphisms *53*, 56–7, 81, 282
  premature termination codons 53–5
  repair technologies 458–9
  reproductive disorders 65, 81, 282
  selective advantage 22, 40–1, 64, 219
  stem cell therapie 459–60
  structure 49, **50**
  transfer therapies 453–60, **453**, **455**,
    456, **458**
CFTR protein
  activator therapy 55–6
  antibody-based assays **376**
  bacterial attachment role 62–3
  bacterial endocytosis role 71
  bicarbonate transport effects 62,
    63–4, **63**
  bone mineral density 266
  chloride ion transport effects 62
  C-terminal deletion 49–50
  domains 49, 51–2
  endocytic recycling 50
  functions 49
  gastrointestinal disease 209
  intrahepatic bile ducts 225–6
  ion channel functions 49, 50–1, **51**,
    376–7
  kidneys 271
  liver pathophysiology 64
  lung pathophysiology 62–3
  mutant form accumulation 60
  non-gene therapy treatments 463–8
  pancreatic pathophysiology 63–4, **63**
  PDZ-mediated protein–protein
    interactions 49–50
  processing 49–51, **51**, **54**, 55, 81

CFTR protein (*Continued*)
  protein–protein interactions 49–51, **51**
  reduced levels **54**, 56
  regulation 49, **54**, 55–6
  sodium ion transport effects 62
  structure 49
  synthesis disruption mutations 53–5, **54**
  tissue sensitivity variation to loss of
    function 81
CFTR-related non-CF disorders 56–7,
  81, 104–5, 282
chaperones 49
checkerboard assay 128
chest radiography 333, 337, 338, **339**,
  380
chest wall stiffness 416
children
  aerosol therapies 186, 191
  bone mineral density 262, 263, 266,
    267
  complications 33–4, **33**
  growth 32, **32**, 253–9
  liver disease 225
  lung functio 29, **29**, *30*, **30**, **300–1**
  lung transplantation 291, **293**, 300–1
  metabolic alkalosis 273
  nursing care 401–2
  nutritional status 32, **32**
  pancreatic insufficiency 211–12
  parental/family factors 87–91
  pediatric to adult care transition
    393–5, *394*, 402–3, 479–82
  physiological monitoring 345–51
  psychological aspects of CF 431–2
  quality of life assessment 294
  terminal care 446
  vitamin deficiencies 211
  see also adolescents; infants; neonates
chloride transport
  ASL effects 61–2, *61*
  assays 376–7
  CFTR gene transfer 453, **453**
  chloride channel proteins/CFTR
    interactions 50–1, **51**
  class II/IV mutations **54**, 55–6
  gastrointestinal tract 64
  metabolic alkalosis 273, **273**
  nucleotide response 62
  pancreas 64
  sweat glands 64, **64**, 100–2, **102**,
    376–7
cholecystokinin (CCK)–secretin test
  211
cholelithiasis 65
cholera resistance 64
cholestatic liver enzymes 64
Chrispin–Norman scoring system 338

chronic obstructive pulmonary disease
  175
ciclosporin A 168
ciliated cells *see* epithelial cells;
  mucociliary clearance; periciliary
  liquid
cirrhosis 6, 64–5, 225–6, 227
  see also cystic-fibrosis-associated liver
  disease
cisapride 216, 218
classification
  CFTR mutations 51–7, *54*, **54**, *55*,
    59–60, 81–2, 234, 242
  phenotypes *103*, 104–5
Cleveland treatment program 6
clinical care *see* specialist CF centers
clinical epidemiology
  age distribution 27, **27**
  complications 33–4, **33**
  definition 21
  diagnosis 27–9, **28**, **29**
  evidence-based medicine 21, 40
  growth and nutritional status 32–3, **32**
  lung function 29–32, **29**, *30*, **30**, *31*, **31**
  medical care provision 39–40
  prognostic indicators 35, 37–9
  respiratory infections 30–2, **30**, **31**
  survival 25–7
clinical microbiology laboratory 123–31
clinical nurse specialist (CNS) 120,
  399–400, 403
clinical outcome measures
  future developments 472
  new treatments 375–81
  translational research 467
  transplantation 299–300
clinical presentation 29, **29**, 99–100, *100*
  bronchoscopy in young children 333
  CF-related diabetes 244–5
  distal intestinal obstruction syndrome
    217, **217**
  gastroesophageal reflux 215
  liver disease 227–9, **228**, **229**
  meconium ileus 213
  pancreatic insufficiency 211
clinical trials 55, 109–10, 311–12, *311*,
  375–81
clinics *see* specialist CF centers
Clostridium difficile 219–20
CMV *see* cytomegalovirus
CNS *see* clinical nurse specialist
coagulation factors 159
cognitive behavior therapy (CBT) 436
cohort analyses 312
cohort effects 29, 30, 32
cohort survival curves 26–7
coincident asthma 166

colistin 139, 142, 149
colomycin 191–2
colonoscopy 217
common bile duct obstruction 227
communication
  bereavement support 447
  microbiological surveillance 130
  newsgiving 117–19, 401
  parents of newly diagnosed newborns
    117–19, *119*
  sexual/reproductive health 280–1, 283,
    287
  terminal care 442–3, *443*, 445, 446
  see also information provision
community CF team *119*, 121, 397
compliance
  adolescents 301, 425
  dietary recommendations 90
  immunosuppression therapy 297
  inhaled therapies 193
  medical regimens 90, 92
  pancreatic enzyme replacement
    therapy 212
  parental stress relationship 90
  PERT therapy 423
  physiotherapy regimens 417
  post-transplant 301
  psychological aspects 433
complications
  of CF-related diabetes 244, *244*
  clinical epidemiology 33–4, **33**
  gallstone disease 233
  gastrointestinal tract 213–21
  high altitude 168–9
  of liver disease 231–3
  new types 473
  non-infectious respiratory conditions
    159–63
  steroid side-effects 165, 166
  surgical patients 169–70, 205–6
  system disorders 269–77
  TIVADs 195
  transplantation 296, 298–300, *299*
composite models of survival prediction
  349–51, **350**
computed tomography (CT)
  early lung structural changes 324
  high resolution 301, 339–41, **339**, **340**
  new treatment assessment 380
  post-transplant children 301
  research program enrolment 121
  sinonasal disease 201–2
  younger children 337, 338–41,
    339, **340**
computerized checks on observational
  data quality 315
conductivity sweat test 102

confirmatory tests of CF diagnosis 100–3
confounding variables 312
congenital bilateral absence of the vas
  deferens (CBAVD) 12, 65, 81, 105,
  279, 282
consensus statement 99–100
consistency checks 315
constipation 169, 170, 218, 423
contact spread *see* cross-infection
continuous glucose monitoring 246
continuous positive airway pressure
  ventilation (CPAP) 178, 179, 181
contraception 280, 283
controlled ventilation technique 341
Cornet® 412, **412**, 413
Cor pulmonale 162
corticosteroids
  allergic bronchopulmonary
    aspergillosis 149, 150
  growth effects 255
  history 8, 11
  inhaled 149, 150, 166, 192–3
  low bone mineral density 265
  sinonasal disease 204
coughing
  exercise stimulation 366
  flow/volume loop 408, **408**
  hemoptysis 159
  neurological problems 274
  surgical patients 170
  urinary incontinence 283–4
cough swabs/plates 124, 332–3
CPAP *see* continuous positive airway
  pressure ventilation
Crohn's disease 220
cross-infection 128–30
  adolescents 403
  Burkholderia cepacia complex 31–2,
    144
  historical view **9, 12**
  Pseudomonas aeruginosa 140
crude mortality rates 25
CT *see* computed tomography
C-terminal deletion 49–50
current survival curves 26
cutaneous vasculitis 269–70, **269**
cystic duct conditions 233
cystic-fibrosis-associated liver disease
  (CFALD)
  clinical epidemiology 33, **33**
  clinical features 227–9, **228, 229**
  complications 231–3
  diabetologists role 391
  epidemiology **33**, 34
  gestational diabetes 248
  historical view 6, 8, 11
  liver function tests 227

management 229–33
modifier genes 83
older children/adults 348–9, **349**
pathophysiology 63, 64–5, 225–7,
  225, 226
post-transplant 297, 299
prevalence 225
risk factors 226–7
transplantation 230
treatment history 11
type I/type II comparison 242, 243
variceal bleeding 231–2, **232**
cystic fibrosis centers *see* specialist CF
  centers
Cystic Fibrosis Foundation (CFF) 6, 7,
  9–10, 111
Cystic Fibrosis Foundation Consensus
  Panel 99
Cystic Fibrosis Questionnaire (CFQ) 368
cystic-fibrosis-related diabetes (CFRD)
  241–51
  clinical features 244–5
  complications 244
  diagnosis 245–6, *245*
  etiology 242
  gender differences 244, 245, 349, **349**
  growth effects 254, 258
  incidence 242
  insulin deficiency 473
  nursing care *485*
  nutritional management 426
  older children/adults 348–9, **349**
  pathophysiology 63
  prevalence 241–2, *242*
  treatment 246–8
cystic-fibrosis-related low bone mineral
  density 261–8, *261*
  bisphosphate therapy 266–7
  calcium 265, 266
  clinical relevance 263–4
  epidemiology 34
  etiology 264–6, 426
  exercise benefits 368
  histomorphology 263, **263**
  management 266–7, 426, 473
  prevalence 34, 262–3
  puberty 256, 473
  risk factors *261*, 264–5, 426
  testing 261–2, 266
  vitamin/mineral supplementation
    264–5, 266, 473
cystic fibrosis teams, psychological
  aspects 434–5
cystic fibrosis transmembrane regulator
  see CFTR gene; CFTR protein
Cystic Fibrosis Trust 7, 8, 10
Cystic Fibrosis Worldwide, history 7

cytokines
  growth factor interactions 254
  immunosuppression 296
  infection relationship 70, 75
  modifier genes 82
  sputum levels in new treatment
    assessment 378
cytomegalovirus (CMV)
    promoter/enhancer 455, 456
cytotoxic agents 168

data collection 9–10, 21, 111, 311–18
data managers 391
dead space 361–2
death
  adolescents 403
  age at **87**
  dying process 445–6
  palliative care 296, 441–60
  place of 446
  terminal care 404–5, 416, 442–3, *443*,
    444, 445–6, *486*
  see also mortality
decongestants 203
defensins (antimicrobial peptides) 72
definition of CF **23**, 27
dehydration 218
delayed puberty 253–4, 255–8, *258*, 265
deletion–insertion polymorphisms
  (DIPs) 82
demographic features 34–5, **34, 35**, 91–2
depression 432
descriptive studies *311*
diabetes mellitus
  type I/II 242, 243
  see also cystic-fibrosis-related diabetes
diabetologists 391
diagnosis
  adults 433
  age at diagnosis 27–8
  allergic bronchopulmonary
    aspergillosis 149–50, *149*
  CF-related diabetes 245–6, *245*
  children 435
  clinical presentation 29, **29**
  criteria 99–106, *100*
  definition of CF **23**, 27
  future developments 471–5
  gastroesophageal reflux 215
  gender differences 91
  genetic 99, 102–3
  induced sputum testing 165
  meconium ileus 213
  newborn screening 7, 12, 28–9,
    109–14, 117–21
  nursing care *401*
  pre-natal 10, 12, 285

diarrheal diseases
  CFTR mutation protection 22, 40–1, 64, 219
  Clostridium difficile 219–20
  giardiasis 212, 220
  inflammatory bowel disease 220
diet 421–7
  celiac disease 221
  CF-related diabetes 247
  disease course variation 90
  fat intake 9, 425, 474
  general nursing care *484*
  historical view 9, 11
  lactose intolerance 221
  low bone mineral density 264–5, 266, 426, 473
  malabsorption 211–13, 421, 422–3, *484*
dietitians *119*, 120, 389, 392, 396
diffuse panbronchiolitis 139, 166
DIOS *see* distal intestinal obstruction syndrome
DIPs *see* deletion–insertion polymorphisms
di Sant'Agnese, Paul 5, 6, 7, 8
discharge planning 393
discussions *see* communication; information provision
disinfection methods 130
distal intestinal obstruction syndrome (DIOS) 209, *209*, 216–18
  clinical features 217, **217**
  diet 423
  historical view 6
  pathophysiology 64, 216, **216**
  prevalence 216–17
  therapy 217–18
dithiothreitol (DTT) 125, 379
DNA gene therapy 453–9
DNA panels 113
DNase *see* rhDNase
donor issues in transplantation 294–5
dornase alfa (rhDNase; pulmozyme) 163–4, 167, 192, 204, 407
DPIs *see* dry-powder inhalers
driving 248–9
droplet spread infection control 129, 130
drugs *see* antibiotics; corticosteroids; medical therapies
dry-powder inhalers (DPIs) 186, *187*, 191
DTT *see* dithiothreitol
dual energy X-ray absorptiometry (DXA) 261–2, 266
dying process 445–6

EA *see* episodic arthritis
early disease 321–3, 333, 337–8

ear nose and throat (ENT) specialists 391
EBC *see* exhaled breath condensate
EBV *see* Epstein–Barr virus
education *see* communication; information provision
educational attainment
  parents 88, 90, 92
  patients 35, **35**
elastase 70, 73–4, **74**
elastic properties of infant lung 324
electrical transepithelial potential 64
electrolyte disorders 273–4, **273**
electrolyte fluxes *see* ion transport
electron crystallography 465
embolization for hemoptysis 160, **160**
emerging pathogens 123
emotional support 405
employment rates 35, **35**, **36**
ENaC (epithelial sodium channel protein) 50, 62, 459
encephalopathy 233
end of life *see* death; end-stage disease
endocrine pancreatic function *see* cystic-fibrosis-related diabetes
endocytosis 50, 71
endoscopic retrograde cholangiography (ERCP) 228, **229**
endoscopy 201, 204–5, *205*, 231–2, **232**
end-stage disease 162–3, **162**
  lung transplantation 291–307
  nursing care 404–5, *404*
  palliative care 296, 441–60
  terminal care 404–5, 416, 442–3, *443*, *444*, 445–6, *486*
energy content of diet 421–2, 425
eNO *see* exhaled nitric oxide
ENT *see* ear nose and throat
enteral feeding 11, 212, 426
enteric infections 219–20
  see also diarrheal diseases
environment
  Aspergillus exposure 151
  Burkholderia cepacia exposure 143–4
  disease course variation 87–91, **88**, 104
  Stenotrophomonas maltophilia exposure 145
environmental tobacco smoke (ETS) 89, 91, 325
enzyme therapy *see* pancreatic enzyme replacement therapy
Epidemiological Registry of Cystic Fibrosis (ERCF) 314–15
Epidemiologic Study of Cystic Fibrosis (ESCF) 317, 318
epidemiology 21–41

age distribution 27–9
allergic bronchopulmonary aspergillosis 148–9
CF definition problems **23**
clinical features 29–34
incidence/prevalence 21–5, *22*, *24*
medical care provision 39–40
microbiology 123
older children/adults 346–8, *347*, *348*
patient registries 313–14
prognosis 35, 37–9
social/demographic features 34–5, *36*
survival 25–7
episodic arthritis (EA) 270
epithelial cells
  airway 60–3
    bacterial binding 70, *71*
    bacterial endocytosis/intracellular killing 71
    damage facilitating bacterial adhesion 70
    ENaC protein 50, 62, 459
    gene transfer 454, **454**
    inflammation control 69
    membrane composition 70
    O_2 consumption 62
    oxygen use 72
  biliary/gallbladder 64
  historical view 12
  pancreas 63, **63**
  pathophysiology 59–68
Epstein–Barr virus (EBV) 301
equal pressure point (EPP) 408, 410
equivocal CF *see* atypical (non-classic) cystic fibrosis
ERCF *see* Epidemiological Registry of Cystic Fibrosis
ERCP *see* endoscopic retrograde cholangiography
erythromycin 166
ESCF *see* Epidemiologic Study of Cystic Fibrosis
Escherichia coli 64
esophageal varices 231–2, **232**
essential fatty acids 9, 424
ethics 472
ethinylestradiol 258
ethnicity 21, 23, *24*, 91–2
ETS *see* environmental tobacco smoke
European CF Consensus Committee 338
European Cystic Fibrosis Society 7
European Respiratory Society 321
evidence-based medicine 21, 40, 92–3, 109–11, 416–17
evolution of airway function 323
exercise

airway clearance 415
benefits 363–70, **364**
bone mineral density 265, 266
capacity measurement 354
CF-related diabetes 248
field tests 357–9
gender differences 91
hypoventilation 177–8
maximal aerobic testing 354–6
metabolic alkalosis 273
new treatment assessment 381
oxygen uptake 354–7
schedules 369–70, *369*
single bouts 361–2
therapeutic 361–70, *363*, *364*, *369*
tolerance 38
exercise testing (XT) 353–9, *353*, *354*, *355*, *356*, *357*, *358*, 381
exhaled breath condensate (EBC) 379
exhaled nitric oxide (eNO) 75, 83, 203, 301, 379
exocrine insufficiency *see* malabsorption; pancreatic insufficiency
expectorated sputum 123, 124, 164–5
expert model of nursing care 400
extracellular barriers to lung gene transfer 454–5
extrahepatic biliary disease 233, **234**
ex-vivo corrected stem cell administration 460
ex-vivo measurements 376
eye problems 274

F508del mutation
  CF mice 463–4
  distribution in populations 21–2, 51
  frequency 102, *103*
  molecular biology 49, 60
families
  environmental tobacco smoke 89, 91, 325
  newborn screening diagnoses *117–21*
  parental educational attainment 88, 90, 92
  psychological aspects 433–4, 436
  stress 90, **90**
  support following diagnosis of child 435
  terminal care 445–6
fasting blood glucose (FBG) 246
fat digestion *see* malabsorption; pancreatic enzymes; pancreatic insufficiency
fatigue 444, 445
fat-soluble vitamins *see* vitamins
fatty acids 9, 424
FBG *see* fasting blood glucose

fecal testing 7
feeding behavior *425*, 432
female sexual/reproductive health 282–7, *283*, *284*
  contraception 283, 391
  fertility 282–3
  historical view 8
  information 283, 391
  pathophysiology 65
  pregnancy 283, *283*, 284–7, *284*, *286*
  puberty 253–9, *258*, 265, 473
  vaginal yeast infections 284
fertility *see* female sexual/reproductive health; male sexual/reproductive health
fertility specialists 391
fetal gene therapy 459
fetal risks of maternal medication 286
FEV *see* forced expiratory volume
fibrosing colonopathy 209, 211, 219
field exercise testing 357–9
fitness 353–9, 363–5, **364**
flow/volume curves/loops 322, **322**, 408, **408**, **413**
Flutter® 412, **412**, 413, **413**
flying 168–9, 195–6
focal biliary cirrhosis 225–6
forced expiration techniques 408, **408**, 409, **409**, 410, **410**
forced expiratory volume in one second (FEV$_1$)
  BOS 300, *300*
  bronchial responsiveness 351
  children 300
  clinical epidemiology 29–30, **29**, *30*, **30**, *31*, 31
  exercise benefits 365–6
  exercise testing **353**
  longitudinal epidemiological data 346–8, *347*, *348*, **348**
  prognostic indicators 37
  young children 338
forced expiratory volume in 0.5 second (FEV$_{0.5}$) 300
forced expiratory volume in 0.75 second (FEV$_{0.75}$) 322, **322**
forced oscillation technique (FOT) 328–9, **328**
forced volume curve (FVC) 322, **322**, 323, **323**
forskolin 376
frequency of mutations in *CFTR* gene *103*
fungal infections
  allergic bronchopulmonary aspergillosis (ABPA) 7, 148–51, **150**, 162, 201
  lung 31, **32**, 126, 148–51

paranasal sinuses 200–1
prophylactic agents 148, 150, 296, 297–8
future developments in diagnosis/ management 471–5
FVC *see* forced volume curve

G452X mutation 21, 22
G551D mutation 21, 22
gallbladder 64, 65, 233
gallstone disease 233, **234**
gas exchange 361
gastroenterologists 391
gastroesophageal reflux (GER) 214–16, 300
gastrografin 11, 213, 217
gastrointestinal conditions 209–21, *209*
  distal intestinal obstruction syndrome 6, 64, 209, *209*, 216–18, 423
  gastroesophageal reflux 214–16
  historical view 6
  malabsorption 211–13, 421, 422–3, *484*
  malignancy 221
  meconium ileus 6, 83, 213, 218–19, *485*
  meconium plug syndrome 213–14
  modifier genes 83–4
  pH effects 210, 211, 212
  vasculitis 269
  see also diarrheal diseases
GCP *see* Good Clinical Practice
gelatinase, lung damage 74
gender
  diabetes 244, 245, 349, **349**
  disease course variation 91
  liver disease 226–7
  lung function 346
  prognostic indicators 37, 349–51
gendered embodiment 91
gender/sex distinction 91
Gene Modifier Study group 467
general health 87, 92
general nursing care *483–4*
gene repair trans-splicing technologies 457, 458–9, **458**
gene therapy 230–1, 377, 453–9
genetic counselling 117–18, *119*, 121, 285
genetic diagnosis 99, 102–3, *103*
genetic factors
  CF-related diabetes 242
  CFTR mRNA assay 375–6
  disease course variation 87, **88**
  historical view 5, 10, 12
  liver disease 226
  male fertility 12, 65, 81, 279, 282
  mortality rates 25–6
  pancreatic disease 234
  pancreatitis 12, 235

genetic factors (*Continued*)
  pathophysiology 59–60
  predisposition but no clinical sequelae 105
  preimplantation genetic diagnosis 281
  pulmonary hyperinflation in infants 325
  racial differences 91–2
  sex differences 91
genetics of *Pseudomonas aeruginosa* 140
gene transfer agents (GTAs) 453–4, 455–6, **455**, **456**
genomovars, *Burkholderia cepacia* complex 123, 126–7, *127*, 142–3, *142*, 144
genotypes
  CFTR mutation classifications 51–7, *54*, **54**, *55*, **55**, 59–60, 81–2, 234, 242
  distribution 21–3, *22*, **22**
  modifier genes 60, 81, 82–4, 104
  phenotype relationship 52–3, 81–5
  prognostic indicators 37
gentamicin 55
GER *see* gastroesophageal reflux
gestational diabetes mellitus 248
GH *see* growth hormone
Giardia duodenalis (giardiasis) 212, 220
Gibson and Cooke technique 101
glucagon response 243
glucocorticoid therapy *see* corticosteroids
glucose absorption 64, 243
glucose tests 246
glutathione 377
glycosylated hemoglobin (HbA$_{1c}$) 245–6
Godfrey protocol 354, *355*
Good Clinical Practice (GCP) 312
growth 253–9
  assessment **256–7**
  clinical epidemiology 32–3, **32**
  epiphyseal closure 265
  factors affecting 254–5
  interventions 255–6, *256*, *258*
  monitoring 422
  post-transplant children 301
  pubertal delay 253–4, *258*
growth hormone (GH) 254–5, *256*
GTAs *see* gene transfer agents
gynecologists 391

habitual physical activity (HPA) 365, 368
  see also exercise
Haemophilus influenzae 31, **31**, **32**, 125, *125*, 145, 199, 204
halide efflux assays 376
hand hygiene 129, 130
harm reduction 111–13, *112*, 472
HbA$_{1c}$ *see* glycosylated hemoglobin

HCO$_3^-$ ion *see* bicarbonate ion
headaches 201, 274
head-down position in physiotherapy 409
healthcare provision variation 39–40, **40**, 92–3
health-related quality of life (HRQoL) 368–9
heart failure 163, **163**, 169
heart rates (HR) 370
heart–lung transplantation 205–6, 291, **292**
heat, exercise effects 362, **362**
height 32–3, *32*, 256, 257, 264
  see also growth
Helicobacter pylori 220
hematemesis 159
hematological problems 274
hemiplegic migraine 274
hemoptysis 159–60, **160**, 416, *485*
hepatic disease *see* cystic-fibrosis-associated liver disease
hepatic glucose production (HGP) 243
hepatic insulin resistance (HIR) 243
hepatobiliary malignancy 235
hepatobiliary pathophysiology 64–5
  see also cystic-fibrosis-associated liver disease
Hering–Breuer inflation reflex 328
heterozygous condition (carriers)
  allergic bronchopulmonary aspergillosis 148
  CBAVD 12, 81, 282
  identification 113
  pancreatitis 12, 235
  phenotype 22–3
  survival advantage 22, 40–1, 64, 219
HGP *see* hepatic glucose production
high-frequency chest compression (HFCC) 413–14, **414**
high-pressure PEP (Hi-PEP) 411, 412
high-resolution computed tomography (HRCT) 301, 339–41, **339**, **340**
high throughput screening 464, **464**
HIR *see* hepatic insulin resistance
histology 203, *203*, 228–9, 263, **263**
history 3–12, 220
HLA *see* human leukocyte antigen
holidays 168–9, 195–6
homecare 395–7, *396*
home intravenous antibiotics 138
homologous recombination 457
hormones
  antidiuretic hormone 273–4
  gastrointestinal tract 211
  growth hormone 254–5, *256*
  sex steroids 255–6, 257–8, *258*, 265

hospital admissions
  home intravenous antibiotics comparison 138
  infection transmission 140, 145
  nursing care 403, 404–5
  pulmonary exacerbations 141
  terminal care 446
host factors 69–72, 82–3
hot conditions, exercise effects 362, **362**
HPA *see* habitual physical activity
HPOA *see* hypertrophic pulmonary arthropathy
HR *see* heart rates
HRCT *see* high-resolution computed tomography
HRQoL *see* health-related quality of life
HS *see* hypertonic saline
huffing 408, **408**, 409, **409**, 410, **410**
human deoxyribonuclease *see* recombinant human deoxyribonuclease-1
human leukocyte antigen (HLA) 82
humoral immune response 72
25-hydroxyvitamin D (25-OHD) 264, *264*, 266
hygiene factors 140
hyperbilirubinbilia 233
hypercapnia 273
hyperglycemia 241, 247
  see also cystic-fibrosis-related diabetes
hypersecretion 407
hypersensitivity 167–8
hypersplenism 233
hypertonic saline (HS) 61, 71, 124, 164–5, 193, 203
hypertrophic pulmonary arthropathy (HPOA) 270–1
hypochloremia 273
hypogonadism 265
hypokalemia 273
hyponatremia 273–4
hypoventilation 176, **177**
hypoxia 162–3, **162**, 169, 195–6

iatrogenic disease 473–4
ibuprofen 167, 194
ICSI *see* intracytoplasmic sperm injection
identification of micro-organism species 125–7, 142
idiopathic pancreatitis 235
IGF-1 *see* insulin-like growth factor
IL-8/IL-10 70
imaging
  infants/pre-school children 337–41
  liver disease 228, **228**
  lung 105, 337–41

new treatment assessment 380
sinonasal disease 201–3
immune response 69–75, 148, 149
see also inflammation; neutrophils
immunizations 75–6, 147, 168, 301
immunoglobulins 168, 378
immunology 69–80, 227, 242, 269
immunoreactive trypsin (IRT) 7, 9, 111, 112, 113
immunosuppression 168, 296, 297, *297*, 301
IMT *see* inspiratory muscle training
incentive spirometry 326
incidence 21–5
incontinence (urinary) 283–4, 367, 415
indications
    bronchoscopy in infants/pre-school children 333–4, *334*
    enteral feeding 425
    exercise testing 353, *353*
    sweat testing 101, 102
    transplantation 291–2, **292**
indicators of new treatment success 375–81
induction of sputum with hypertonic saline 124, 165
infants
    acrodermatitis enteropathica-like eruptions 270
    airway clearance 415
    bronchoscopy 331–4
    growth 253
    lung clearance index 346
    lung function 321–9, 380
    lung imaging 337–41
    new treatment assessment 380
    nursing care 401
    nutritional support 424–5
    pancreatic insufficiency 211, 212, 213
    weight–sweat test influence 101, **101**
    see also neonates
infection control 128–31, *129, 130*
    adolescents 403
    Burkholderia cepacia complex 31–2, 143–4
    historical view 9, 12
    Pseudomonas aeruginosa 140
    strategies 129–30
infections
    diarrheal diseases 40–1, 64, 212, 219–20
    sinonasal disease 199–208
    vaginal yeast 284
    venous access devices 151
    viral 75–6, 147, 168, 301
    see also respiratory infections

infertility 12, 65, 81, 279–82
    see also female sexual/reproductive health; male sexual/reproductive health
inflammation
    anti-inflammatory therapies 165–8, 194, 203
    benefits 165
    bronchiolitis obliterans syndrome 300
    cytokine/growth factor interactions 254
    early lung infection 324
    gastrointestinal tract 210
    hypertonic saline 164
    infants/pre-school children 331–2
    lung damage 137–8
    modifier genes 82
    mucin secretion 62
    neutrophil activation 73–4
    new treatment assessment 378–9
    non-gene therapy treatments 465–6
    respiratory infection relationship 69–70, 137, 324
    transplanted lungs 298
inflammatory bowel disease 220, 254
influenza immunization 147
information provision
    adolescent nursing care 402
    newly diagnosed patient families 118–21, *119*
    physiotherapist advice 417
    sexual/reproductive health 280–1, 283, 287
    terminal care 404
inhaled therapies 185–93
    antibiotics 10–11, 138, 142, 148–9, 191–2
    bronchodilators 192
    corticosteroids 149, 150, 166, 192–3
    delivery systems 186
    drug types 191–3
    dry-powder inhalers *187*, 191
    hypertonic saline 61, 164–5, 193
    mannitol 165
    mucolytics 193
    nebulizers 185, 186–90, *187*
    oxygen 195–6
    particle deposition 185–6, **186**
    pressurized metered-dose inhalers 186, *187*, 190–1, 192
inheritance, *see also* genetic...
innate immune response 69–75
inspiratory muscle training (IMT) 365, 366
inspissated secretions 64, 65, 209
insulin
    clearance rate 243
    deficiency 241, **241**, 242–3, 473

growth effects 254, 255, 258
    replacement therapy 247–8
    resistance 241, 243, 255
    see also cystic-fibrosis-related diabetes
insulin-like growth factor 1 (IGF-1) 254
intensity of exercise 370
international organizations 7
intestinal disease *see* gastrointestinal conditions
intestinal electrolyte/fluid transport 209, **210**, 216
intestinal lavage 217, 218
intestinal motility 210, 216
intestinal obstruction *see* distal intestinal obstruction syndrome; meconium ileus
intestinal permeability 210
intestinal volvulus 218–19
intestinal wall thickness increases 210
intracellular bacterial killing 71
intracellular barriers to gene transfer 454–5
intracytoplasmic sperm injection (ICSI) 281
intrahepatic bile duct plugging 225–6
intrapulmonary percussive ventilation (IPV) 414–15
intrauterine insemination 282
intravenous (IV) therapies 194–5
    antibiotics 11, 138–9, 141, 194–5
    immunoglobulin infusions 168
    nursing care *484, 485*
    regimes 141
    venous access 11, 151, 194–5, **194**, *195, 485*
intussusception 218
invasive ventilation 295–6
ion-channel-related drugs 377
iontophoresis 100–2
ion transport
    airway surface liquid volume 61–2, **61**
    CF derangement processes 62, 63–4
    gastrointestinal tract 64, 209, **210**, 216
    lung 61–2, **61**
    non-gene therapy treatments 465
    pancreas 63–4, **63**
    systemic electrolyte disorders 273–4, **273**
ion transporter proteins 50–1, **51**
IPV *see* intrapulmonary percussive ventilation
iron deficiency 274
iron oxide particles 456, **456**
IRT *see* immunoreactive trypsin
isolated populations 22, 51, *52*
isoproterenol 376

isotonic saline 203
IV *see* intravenous therapies

jaundice 231
jet nebulizers *187*, 188–9
joints 269, 270–1
journal publications 110, *110*

kidneys
    malformations 282
    nephrolithiasis 271–2, **272**
    nephrotic syndrome 271, 272
    nephrotoxins 271, 272, *297*, 299,
        299, 301
    transplant complications *297*, 299,
        299, 301
    vasculitis 269
Kubler-Ross stages of acceptance 447

laboratories 123–31, 391, 392–3
lactose intolerance 221
laparotomy 217
LCI *see* lung clearance index
LFFOT *see* low frequency forced
        oscillation technique
life expectancy *see* mortality; survival
lipopolysaccharide (LPS) 76, 140
liver
    function tests 227
    hepatic glucose production/insulin
        resistance 243
    hepatobiliary malignancy 235
    see also cystic-fibrosis-associated liver
        disease
lobar collapse 162
logic checks 315
longevity *see* survival
longitudinal studies 315, 346–8, **348**
LOS *see* lower esophageal sphincter
low bone mineral density *see* cystic-
        fibrosis-related low bone mineral
        density
low-dose HRCT 340
lower airways *see* inflammation;
        respiratory infections
lower esophageal sphincter (LOS) 214,
        215, 216
low frequency forced oscillation tech-
        nique (LFFOT) 328
low-grade rejection of lung grafts 298
LPS *see* lipopolysaccharide
lung
    aerosol drug deposition 185–6, **186**
    airway gland secretion 74
    airway obstruction 137, 323–4
    airway surface liquid 60–2, **61**, 72,
        73–4

bacterial defence mechanisms 60
β-adrenergic receptor gene effects 83
bronchoalveolar lavage 70, 73–4, 124,
        329, 332–3, 379
drug delivery 185–98
elastic properties in infants 324
function
    atypical phenotype 106
    CFTR mutation class relationship
        60, 81–2
    clinical epidemiology 29–32, **29**, *30*,
        30, *31*, **31**
    decline with age 29–30, **30**
    exercise benefit 365–6
    growth relationship 253, *256*
    historical view 6–7
    infants/pre-school children 321–9,
        338
    modifier genes 82
    older children/adults 345–51
    pregnancy relationship 284, 285
    prognostic indicators 37–8
    testing 141, 338
    see also forced expiratory volume…
hemoptysis 159–60, **160**
imaging 105, 337–41
lobar collapse 162
mechanics 175–83, 361–2, **362**
pathophysiology 60–3
pneumothorax 160–2, **161**
pulmonary exacerbations 138–9, *138*,
        141, 144, 345, 378
pulmonary hyperinflation 325
respiratory failure 162–3
work of breathing 175–6, **175**
see also inflammation; respiratory
        infection; transplantation;
        ventilation
lung clearance index (LCI) 346, 380–1
lymphoproliferative disease (post-
        transplant) 201, 299, 301
lysosomal enzymes 70, 72, 73
see also proteases

MAC *see* *Mycobacterium avium* complex
macrolides 139, 140, 166–7, *167*, 300
magnetic resonance imaging (MRI)
        202–3, 341
major histocompatibility complexes
        (MHCs) 82
malabsorption 211–13, 421, 422–3, *484*
    see also pancreatic enzyme replacement
        therapy; pancreatic insufficiency
male sexual/reproductive health 279–82
    congenital bilateral absence of the vas
        deferens 12, 65, 81, 105, 279, 282
    historical view 8, 12

information 280–1, 391–2
    pathophysiology 65
    puberty 253–9, *258*, 265, 473
    reproductive options 281–2, 287,
        391–2
malignancy
    gastrointestinal malignancy 221
    hepatobiliary malignancy 235
    lung transplants 299, 301
    pancreatic malignancy 235
mannitol inhalation 165
mannose-binding lectin (MBL) 82–3
mass median aerodynamic diameter
        (MMAD) 185–6, 188, 189, 191
maternal educational attainment 88,
        90, 92
Matthews, Leroy 6
maximal aerobic/anaerobic testing
        354–6
maximal expiratory flow (MEF) 321
maximum oxygen uptake ($VO_{2\,max}$)
        354, *356*
MBL *see* mannose-binding lectin
MBW *see* multiple breath washout
MCBT *see* multiple combination bacte-
        ricidal testing
MCC *see* mucociliary clearance
meconium ileus (MI)
    clinical presentation 213
    diagnosis 213
    historical view 3, 6, 11
    liver disease risk 226
    modifier genes 83
    nursing care *485*
    pathophysiology 213
    therapy 213
    volvulus 218–19
meconium plug syndrome 213–14
median age at death 26
median survival ages 10, 26
Medicaid patients 38, 88, 350
medical care provision variation 39–40,
        40, 92–3
medical history 354, *354*
medical teams 387, 389
medical therapies
    aerosols 185–93, **186**, **188**, **190**
    antifungal agents 148, 150, 296, 297–8
    anti-inflammatory therapy 165–8,
        194, 203
    antiviral strategies 147–8
    bronchodilators 6, 167–8, 192
    burden reduction 472
    cytotoxic agents 168
    distal intestinal obstruction syndrome
        217–18
    drug delivery 185–98

drug interactions 169–70
gastroesophageal reflux 215–16
immunoglobulin infusions 168
intravenous access 11, 151, 194–5,
    194, *195*, *485*
molecular biology 54–6
novel therapies 168
oral 11, 150, 151, 165–6, 193–4,
    246–7
pharmacological adjuncts to mucus
    clearance 163–5
in pregnancy 285, 286
protein rescue therapy 463–5, 472–3
sinonasal disease 203–4
see also antibiotics; corticosteroids
MEF *see* maximal expiratory flow
membrane-spanning domains (MSDs)
    49, 51, 53
menstrual irregularity 254, 282
MESA *see* microsurgical epididymal
    sperm aspiration
mesonephric (Wolffian) duct 279
metabolic alkalosis 273
methicillin-resistant *Staphylococcus*
    aureus (MRSA) 144–5
methicillin-sensitive *Staphylococcus*
    aureus (MSSA) 144
MHCs *see* major histocompatibility
    complexes
MI *see* meconium ileus
microbial colonization *see* respiratory
    infections
microbiology
    antimicrobial susceptibility testing
        127–8
    atypical phenotypes 105
    culture media 125, *125*
    identification of species 125–7, 142
    infection control 128–31, *129*, *130*
    lab processing of specimens 123–7
    synergy testing 128
microsurgical epididymal sperm
    aspiration (MESA) 281
microvascular disease 244, *244*
milder disease
    genotypes 12, 21, 53, 81
    historic view 8, 12
    late diagnosis 8, 12, 27–8
    pathophysiology 64
    polymorphisms 56–7
    pregnancy 285
mist tents 7–8
mixed drug inhalation 190, 193
MMAD *see* mass median aerodynamic
    diameter
modifier genes 60, 81, 82–4, 104
molecular assays 375–6

molecular biology 49–58, 209, 225,
    230–1
molecular imaging techniques 341
monitoring
    adults/older children 345–52
    exercise testing 353–9
    future care patterns 475
    growth 422
    young children 321–43
mortality
    age at death **87**
    CF-related diabetes 244
    pregnancy effects 284–5
    rates 25–6
    transplantation criteria 292–4
    see also survival
motility of gastrointestinal tract 210,
    216
motor performance 358–9
mouse models 70, 328, 464, 467
MRI *see* magnetic resonance imaging
mRNA assay 375–6
MRSA *see* methicillin-resistant
    Staphylococcus aureus
MSDs *see* membrane-spanning
    domains
MSSA *see* methicillin-sensitive
    Staphylococcus aureus
mucociliary clearance (MCC)
    airway surface liquid volume
        reduction 60, 62
    factors affecting 407
    hypertonic saline treatment 164
    impairment 70–1
    new treatments assessment 377
    non-gene therapy treatments 465
    nose 199–200
    role 60
mucoid bacterial phenotype 72, 140
mucoid distension of the appendix 218
mucolytic agents 165, 193
mucosal folds of gastrointestinal
    tract 210
mucosal glands 209
mucoviscidosis 5, 7
mucus
    airway clearance physiology 408
    bacterial cell adherence 70–1
    lung environment 62, 72
    pharmacological adjuncts to
        clearance 163–5
    plaques 61, 62
    plugs 334, 338, **339**
multidisciplinary care 93, 387–447
multidisciplinary teams 387–92,
    399–400
multidrug-resistant pathogens 128

multiple breath washout (MBW) 327–8,
    327, 338, 380–1
multiple combination bactericidal
    testing (MCBT) 128
multiple drug inhalation 190, 193
multisystem complications 471
multivariate prognostic models 38–9
muscles 175–82, **175**, **177**, 358, 365–7
mutations *see* CFTR gene, mutations;
    genotypes
mycobacterial infection 31, 126, 146
Mycobacterium abscessus 146
Mycobacterium avium complex
    (MAC) 146

N1300K mutation 22
Na^+/H^+ exchange regulatory factor
    (NHERF) 49–50
Na^+/H exchanger (NHE3) 50
NAC *see* acetyl-cysteine
nasal polyposis 200–6, **200**, **201**, **203**,
    204
nasal saline irrigation 203
nasal/sinus disease 105, 199–208
nasal specialists 391
nasal steroid drops/sprays 204
nasogastric feeding 212
National Committee for Clinical
    Laboratory Standards guidelines
    101
National Cystic Fibrosis Research
    Foundation *see* Cystic Fibrosis
    Foundation
National Heart, Lung and Blood
    Institute (NHLBI) 467
national organizations, history 7, 9–10
National Registry and Epidemiological
    Study of CF 111
NBCs *see* sodium/bicarbonate
    co-transporters
NBDs *see* nucleotide binding domains
NBS *see* newborn screening
nebulizers 185, 186–90, *187*, **188**, **190**
    see also inhaled therapies
neonates
    birth weight/length **253**
    diagnosis 401
    historical view 6
    immune system 69–70
    meconium ileus 6, 83, 213, 218–19, *485*
    meconium plug syndrome 213–14
    neutrophil function 70, 72
    newborn screening 7, 12, 28–9,
        109–14, *112*, 117–21, *119*
    volvulus 218–19
neostingmine 217–18
nephrolithiasis 271–2, **272**

nephrotic syndrome 271, 272
nephrotoxins 271, 272, *297*, 299,
    299, 301
neurological mechanisms of
    breathing 175–6, **175**
neurological problems 274, 298–9
neutrophils
    activation 73–5
    beneficial effects 165
    biofilm effects 140
    cathepsin G 73, 74
    chemotaxis 72, 73
    elastase in airways 70, 73–4, **74**
    function impairment 72
    gelatinase 74
    lung damage 137–8
    macrolide treatment 166
    necrosis 137–8
    neonates 70, 72
    normal lung 69
    phagocytosis impairment 73–4
    proteases 70, 73–4
newborn screening (NBS) 7, 12, 28–9,
    109–14, *112*, 117–21
newborns, *see also* neonates
new database construction 315–18
newsgiving 117–19, 401
New South Wales screening
    program 120
new treatments 168, 375–81, 472
NHE3 *see* Na⁺/H exchanger
NHE3 *see* Na^+/H exchanger
NHERF *see* Na^+/H^+ exchange
    regulatory factor
NHLBI *see* National Heart, Lung and
    Blood Institute
NIPPV *see* non-invasive positive
    pressure ventilation
nitric oxide (NO) 75, 83, 203, 301, 379
nocturnal oxygen therapy 195
non-Caucasian populations 23, *24*, 52
non-CFTR genes *see* modifier genes
non-compliance *see* compliance
non-gene therapy treatments 463–8
non-invasive positive pressure ventilation
    (NIPPV) 178–82, **178**, *179*, 295
non-paternity identification 113
nonsense mutations 102
non-specific (innate) immune response
    69–75
non-steroidal anti-inflammatory agents
    167, 194
non-tuberculous mycobacteria (NTM)
    31, 126, 146
non-viral gene transfer 454, 455–6, **455**,
    456
noscomial transmission *see* infection
    control

nose *see* nasal...
novel therapies 168, 375–81, 472
NTM *see* non-tuberculous mycobacteria
nucleotide binding domains (NBDs) 49,
    51–2, 53
nursing care 389, 392, 396, 399–405,
    400, *401*, *402*, *404*, 483, *483–4*,
    485–6
nutrition 421–7
    historical view 5, 8, 9, 11
    PERT 421, 422–3
    requirements 421–2
    support 424–7
    see also vitamins
nutritional status
    clinical epidemiology 32–3, **32**
    disease course variation factors 90–1
    growth 253
    pancreatic disease pathophysiology 63
    prognostic indicators 38
    pubertal timing 253–4
    surgical patients 169, 170
    urinary incontinence 367, 368

obliterative bronchitis (OB) 299
    see also bronchiolitis obliterans
        syndrome
observational data 311–12, *311*, 313–14
obstetricians 285, 391
obstructions
    airway 137, 323–4
    biliary pathophysiology 64
    distal intestinal obstruction syndrome
        6, 64, 209, *209*, 216–18, 423
    meconium ileus 6, 83, 213, 218–19, *485*
    pancreatic duct 234
    sinus ostial obstruction 199
    vas deferens pathophysiology 65
occupational therapists, care center
    role 390
OCP *see* oral contraceptive pill
ocular problems 274
odds ratio (OR) 312
OGTT *see* oral glucose tolerance test
25-OHD *see* 25-hydroxyvitamin D
older children *see* adolescents
OP *see* oropharyngeal
opioids 445
opsonophagocytosis 73–4
optimal antimicrobial susceptibility
    testing 127
OR *see* odds ratio
oral antibiotics 194
oral anti-inflammatory drugs 194
oral candidiasis 151
oral contraceptive pill (OCP) 283
oral corticosteroids 11, 150, 165–6

oral glucose tolerance test (OGTT) 246
oral health 274
oral hypoglycemic agents 246, 247
oral nutritional supplements 425–6
oral therapies 193–4
oropharyngeal (OP) culture 124, 332–3
oscillating positive expiratory
    pressure 412–13
osmolality sweat test 102
osteomalacia 261, 262, 266
osteoporosis 34, 261, 262, 264, 426
outcomes *see* clinical outcome measures
outpatient review 474–5
overnight feeds 423
oxandrolone 257
oxygen by open delivery 101
oxygen radicals 70, 72, 74–5
oxygen supplementation 168–9, 195–6
oxygen uptake exercise testing 354–6,
    356
oxyhemoglobin saturation (SaO₂)
    356–7, 361–2, **362**

packaging capacity of AAV vectors 457
pain 444, 445
palliative care 296, 441–60
pancreas 234–5
    alpha-cell function 243
    beta-cell function 242–3
    duct secretions 63–4, **63**, 234
    function testing 7, 105
    histology **4**
    islets of Langerhans 234, 243
    malignancy 235
    pathophysiology 63–4, **63**, 234
    polypeptides 243
    see also cystic-fibrosis-related diabetes;
        malabsorption
pancreatic enzyme replacement therapy
    (PERT) 211–12
    adverse effects 212–13
    considerations 421
    enteric coatings 9, 11, 211, 212
    historical view 5, 9, 11
    inadequate therapeutic response 212
    recommendations 422–3, *422*
pancreatic enzymes, pH effects 210,
    211, 212
pancreatic insufficiency 234–5
    clinical presentation 211
    distal intestinal obstruction syndrome
        relationship 216
    genetic factors 81, 234
    history 3–5
    malabsorption 211–13, 421, 422–3, *484*
pancreatic sufficiency
    children 120

exocrine function 211
genotypes 12, 21, 53, 81, 234
pathophysiology 64
prognostic indicators 37
pancreatin *see* pancreatic enzyme
replacement therapy
pancreatitis 9, 64, 234–5, **235**
pancreatitis-associated protein (PAP) 111
pancreozymin–secretin stimulation
tests 7
paracellular permeability of gastrointestinal tract 210
paranasal sinuses 105, 199–208
parenteral nutrition 426
parenting by CF patients 281–2, 284–7,
403
parents
educational attainment 88, 90, 92
environmental tobacco smoke 89, 91,
325
newborn screening diagnoses 117–21,
119
parental target height 256
psychological aspects 90, **90**, 433–4
socioeconomic status 38, 87–93, **88**
support following diagnosis of child
435
see also compliance
partnership model of nursing care 400
passive smoking 89, 91, 325
pathogens *see* bacterial...; fungal
infections; *individual pathogens*;
microbiology; respiratory
infections; viral infections
pathophysiology
CF-related diabetes 242–4
distal intestinal obstruction syndrome
216
epithelial cell biology 59–68
gastroesophageal reflux 214–15
gastrointestinal disease 64, 213, 216
historical view 6–7, 8, 10, 12
liver disease 64–5, 225–7, **225**, **226**
lung disease 60–3
meconium ileus 213
molecular biology 50–1
pancreatic disease 63–4, **63**, 234
reproductive tract disorders 65
respiratory infections 62–3
sinonasal disease 199
sweat gland disorders 64, **64**
patients
data registries 9–10, 21, 111, 313–18,
316, *317*, *318*
individual progress monitoring 313
parenthood options/issues 281, 285,
287

relationship issues 287
sexual/reproductive health
information 280–1, 283, 287
travel 168–9, 195–6
undergoing surgery 169–70
patient-to-patient infection spread *see*
cross-infection
PCL *see* periciliary liquid
PCR *see* polymerase chain reaction
PD&P *see* postural drainage and
percussion
PD *see* potential difference
PDZ-mediated protein–protein interactions 49–50
peak height velocity 253–4
peak oxygen uptake (VO$_{2\,peak}$) 354–6,
356
pediatric *see* adolescents; children;
infants; neonates
PEEP *see* positive end-expiratory pressure
pelvic floor exercises 284, 367
Pendelluft flow 408, 411
PEP *see* positive expiratory pressure
peptic ulceration 220
perceived exertion 357
percutaneous epididymal sperm
aspiration (PESA) 281
periciliary liquid (PCL) 60–1
peripherally inserted central catheters
(PICCs) 194
peripheral muscles 358, 367
PERT *see* pancreatic enzyme replacement therapy
PESA *see* percutaneous epididymal
sperm aspiration
PFT *see* pulmonary function test
PGF *see* primary graft failure
phagocytosis impairment 73–4, **74**
pharmacists, care center role 389
pharmacogenomics 465
pharmacological adjuncts to mucus
clearance 163–5
pH effects
gastrointestinal tract **210**, **211**, **212**
reproductive disorders **65**
physical activity/training *see* exercise
physical examination 354
physical methods of non-viral gene
transfer 456, **456**
physicians 119–20, *119*
physiological drug selection 463–4
physiological monitoring 345–51, 380–1
physiology of airway clearance 408
physiotherapists *119*, 121, 389, 392, 396
physiotherapy
drug inhalation timing **164**, **192**, **193**
exercise relationship **366**

gastroesophageal reflux **214**
history 5, 10
hypoventilation 177
nebulized rhDNase combination 164,
192
neonates *119*, 121
overview 407–17
pharmacological adjuncts 163–5
physiology of airway clearance 408
terminal care 416
urinary incontinence 284, 415
PICCs *see* peripherally inserted central
catheters
pilocarpine sweat tests 5, 101
plasmid DNA 455–6, **456**
pMDIs *see* pressurized metered-dose
inhalers
pneumatosis intestinalis 210
pneumothorax 160–2, **161**, 415, 416,
485
polymerase chain reaction (PCR) 127,
375–6
polymorphisms *53*, 56–7, 81, 82–4,
282
polypeptides 243
polyvalent vaccines 466
population databases 111
population genotype relationships 21–2,
51, *52*
population prevalence 21, 23, 25, *25*
portal systemic shunt 232
portal vascular hypertension 83, 227
positive end-expiratory pressure (PEEP)
179, 181
positive expiratory pressure (PEP)
411–12, **412**, 413, **413**
postoperative care 170
post-transplant lymphoproliferative
disease (PTLD) 201, 299, 301
postural drainage and percussion
(PD&P) 5, 409, 411
potential difference (PD) 62, 106, **106**,
362, 376
poverty *see* socioeconomic status
PPIs *see* proton pump inhibitors
pre-CF condition 105
preclinical drug discovery 464, **464**
pre-diabetic decline 241, *241*, 245
prediction 124, 346–8, *347*, *348*, 349–51,
350
prednisolone 150, 165–6
prednisone 165, 194
pregnancy
assisted reproduction 281, 282, 287
CF-related diabetes 248
CF women 283, *283*, 284–7, *284*, *286*,
403

pregnancy (*Continued*)
    nutritional management 426–7
    physiotherapy 416
preimplantation genetic testing 281
premature termination codons (PTCs)
        53–5
pre-natal diagnosis 10, 12, 285
preoperative care 169–70
prepubertal growth 253
pre-school children *see* infants
presentation *see* clinical presentation
pressure support ventilation (PS) 178,
        178, 181, 182
pressurized metered-dose inhalers
        (pMDIs) 186, *187*, 190–1, 192
preterm deliveries 284, 285
prevalence 21–5
    CF-related diabetes 241–2, *242*
    distal intestinal obstruction syndrome
        216–17
    gastroesophageal reflux disease 214
    gastrointestinal conditions *209*
    low bone mineral density 262–3
    'primary' CF multidisciplinary team
        387, 389–91
primary graft failure (PGF) 296–7, **296**
primary nasal epithelial cell balls 70, **71**
privacy laws 314
professional boundaries 400
prognosis 35, 37–9, 292–4, *294*
progressive renal insufficiency 271, 272
prokinetic drugs 216, 218
promoters for gene therapy 455, 456,
        457
promotor mutations 56
prophylactic antibiotics 8–9, 138, 148,
        296, 297–8
prospectively collected data 312
proteases 70, 72, 73–4, **73, 74**, 82
α_1-proteinase inhibitor 73, **73**
protein rescue therapy 463–5, 472–3
proton pump inhibitors (PPIs)
        212, 215
provision of medical care variation
        39–40, **40**, 92–3
PS *see* pressure support ventilation
pseudo-Bartter syndrome 273
Pseudomonas aeruginosa 139–42
    acquisition factors 89
    acute exacerbation 141
    adherence measurements 377
    anaerobic environment adaptation 72
    antibiotics 127–8, 138–9, 141–2
    biofilm formation 72, 140
    biofilm susceptibility testing 127–8
    bronchoscopy in young children 331–3
    chronic infection 141–2

clinical epidemiology 30–2, *31*, **31, 32**
culture media 125, *125*
diffuse panbronchiolitis 166
endogenous endopthalmitis 274
epithelial cell adhesion 62–3
epithelial cell binding 70, 71
genetics 140
historical view 7, 9, 10–11, 12
host protease release 70
humoral immune response 72
infection control 31, 140
inhaled antibiotics 191–2
initial infection 139, 140, 141
longitudinal studies 346, 348
lung function relationship 30, **31**
microbiology testing **125–7**
mucoid phenotype 72, 140
mucus environment 62
neutrophil elastase use 73
optimal antimicrobial susceptibility
        testing 127
paranasal sinuses 199, 200
patient-to-patient transmission 128–9
phenotype changes 72, 140
polyvalent vaccines 466
population database evidence 111
preventing chronic disease 31, 138,
        139–40
prognostic indicators 38
prophylactic antibiotics 138
species identification 126
sputum/cough swap testing 140–1
time to next positive culture 378
treatment 140–2
vaccination 76, 466
Wisconsin newborn screening project
        109, 110, *110*
Pseudomonas maltophilia see
        Stenotrophomonas maltophilia
psychological aspects of CF 113, 301,
        369, 431–7
psychologists 389, 392
PTCs *see* premature termination codons
PTLD *see* post-transplant lymphoprolif-
        erative disease
puberty 253–9, *258*, 265, 473
publications 110, *110*, *318*
pulmonary, *see also* lung; lung function
pulmonary function test (PFT) 338
pulmonary hyperinflation 325
pulmonary hypertension 64, 162–3
pulmozyme (dornase alfa; rhDNase)
        163–4, 167, 192, 204, 407

quality assurance 312, 313, 314–15
quality of life (QoL)
    CF/normal population comparison

        (QoL) 35, **36**
    exercise benefits **368–9**
    lung transplantation 291, 292, 294,
        300, 301
    new treatment assessment 381
    psychological aspects 432
Quality of Well-Being (QWB) scale 368
quantitative CT 341

RA *see* rheumatoid arthritis
race 21, 23, *24*, 91–2
radiography 333, 337, 338, *339*, 380
    see also computed tomography; dual
        energy X-ray absorptiometry
raised volume rapid thoracoabdominal
        compression (RVRTC) 321–2,
        323, 326
random blood glucose (RBG) 246
randomized controlled trials (RCTs)
        109–10, 311–12, *311*
rapid thoracoabdominal compression
        (RTC) technique 321
rashes 269
RBC *see* random blood glucose
RCTs *see* randomized controlled trials
reactive oxygen species (ROS) 70, 72,
        74–5
read-through of premature termination
        codons 54–5
receptor-mediated uptake of non-viral
        GTAs 455, **455**
recombinant human deoxyribonuclease-1
        (dornase-alfa; rhDNase; pul-
        mozyme) 163–4, 167, 192, 204, 407
recommended practices 129, 130, 400,
        401, 402, 404
recruiting centers for registries 317, *317*
rectal prolapse 219
recurrent acute pancreatitis 9, 235
registries of CF patients 9–10, 21, 111,
        313–18, *316*, *317*, *318*
rejection of lung grafts 297, 298, 466–7
relationship issues 287, 433–4
religion 446–7
renal impairment *see* kidneys
repeat sweat testing 102
repeat transplantation 300
reproductive health *see* female
        sexual/reproductive health; male
        sexual/reproductive health
rescue therapies 463–5, 472–3
research
    bronchoscopy in infants/pre-school
        children 331–2
    CT as clinical research tool 341
    new treatment assessment methods
        375–81

parent information provision 120, 121
program enrolment 121
randomized controlled trials 109–10,
    311–12, *311*
sweat testing 101
resident airway stem cell targeting 460
residential stay centres 118
resistance interrupter (R$_{int}$) technique
    326
resistive inspiratory maneuvers 415
respirable particles in aerosols 185–6
respiratory balance 175–6, **175**
respiratory complications 159–73
respiratory failure 162–3, **162**, 176,
    177–8
respiratory function *see* forced expira-
    tory volume...; lung function
respiratory infections 137–57
    acute rejection of transplant distinc-
        tion 298
    bacterial overview 137–46
    biofilms 72, 140
    bronchoscopy 334
    control 128–31, *129, 130*
        adolescents 403
        Burkholderia cepacia complex 31–2,
            143–4
        historical view 9, 12
        laboratory susceptibility testing 128
        preventative strategies 31–2, 75–6,
            140
        Pseudomonas aeruginosa 140
        strategies 129–30
    cytokines 70, 75
    early markers 324
    epidemiology 30–2, 123
    exposure 89
    fungal 31, **32**, 126, 148–51
    historical view 5, 7, 10–11
    host factors 69–72, 139–40
    humoral immune response 72
    immunology 69–80
    inflammation relationship 69
    microbiology 123–31
    mucoid phenotypes 72, 140
    natural history 137–8
    neutrophils 70, 72, 73–5
    nitric oxide 75, 83
    non-gene therapy treatments 466
    nursing care *483*
    organisms 139–46
    pathophysiology 62–3
    preventative strategies 31–2, 75–6, 140
    prognostic indicators 38
    pulmonary exacerbations 138–9, *138*,
        141, 144, 345, 378
    sources 140

syndrome of inappropriate ADH
    secretion 273–4
transient diabetes 247
treatment outcome measures 377–8
upper respiratory tract 146–8
viral 89, 126, 146–8
young children 331–3, 334
see also individual agents;
respiratory load 175–6, **175**
respiratory muscles 175–82, **175, 177**,
    365–7
respiratory rate in infants 325–6
respiratory symptoms 29, 138, 141
respiratory therapy equipment 130
respiratory tract specimens 123–5
retrospectively collected data 312
retrospective reviews 101
reverse transcriptase polymerase chain
    reaction (RT-PCR) 375–6
rhDNase (dornase alfa; pulmozyme)
    163–4, 167, 192, 204, 407
rheumatoid arthritis (RA) 271
rhinosinusitis 200, 201, 205, 206
    see also sinonasal disease
right ventricular failure 163, **163**, 169
R$_{int}$ *see* resistance interrupter
risk factors
    allergic bronchopulmonary
        aspergillosis 148–9
    CF-associated liver disease 226–7
    CF-related low bone mineral density
        264–5, 426
    low bone mineral density *261*
RNA interference gene therapy 459
roles of specialists 119–21, *119*, 387–92,
    399–400, 403
ROS *see* reactive oxygen species
Royal Children's Hospital, Australia
    119–21
RTC *see* rapid thoracoabdominal
    compression
RT-PCR *see* reverse transcriptase poly-
    merase chain reaction
RVRTC *see* raised volume rapid thora-
    coabdominal compression

safety of therapies 472
    see also adverse effects
saline
    induction of sputum 124, 165
    therapies 61, 71, 164–5, 193, 203
Salmonella enterica 22, 40–1
Salmonella typhi 41
SaO$_2$ *see* oxyhemoglobin saturation
saturated fats 9
Saunders, Dame Cicely 441
'sausage' appendix 218

Scedosporium apiospermum 151
screening
    allergic bronchopulmonary
        aspergillosis 150
    CF-related diabetes 245–6
    high throughput 464, **464**
    newborns 7, 12, 28–9, 109–14, *112*,
        117–21
SDV *see* source data verification
'secondary' CF multidisciplinary
    team 391–2
secretaries 391
secretory immune system 69
secretory leukocyte proteinase inhibitor
    (SLPI) 73
security of data 314
selective media for microbiology speci-
    mens 125–6
self-management *see* compliance
self perception 91, 287, 369
semen analysis 105, 280–1
Sendai virus (SeV) vector 458, **458**
serine proteinase inhibitors 73, **73**
SES *see* socioeconomic status
SeV *see* Sendai virus
sex differences 91
    see also gender
sex/gender distinction 91
sex steroids 255–6, 257–8, *258*, 265
sexual function 280, 287
sexual health *see* female sexual/repro-
    ductive health; male sexual/repro-
    ductive health
sexually transmitted diseases 280, 283
shared care 388
short-circuit current measurements 376
short tandem repeats (STRs) 82
shuttle tests 358
SIADH *see* syndrome of inappropriate
    antidiuretic hormone secretion
siblings 395
side effects *see* adverse effects
single bouts of exercise 361–2
single nucleotide polymorphisms
    (SNPs) 82
sinobronchial allergic mycosis 201
sinonasal disease 105, 199–208
sinus ostial obstruction 199
skin complications 269–70
SLC26 class (SLCA3/SLCA6)
    bicarbonate/chloride exchangers
    63–4, **63**
sleep 176–82, **177**, 193
SLPI *see* secretory leukocyte proteinase
    inhibitor
small intestinal obstruction *see*
    meconium ileus

SMaRT *see* splicosome-mediated mRNA trans-splicing
smoking (passive) 89, 91, 325
SMR *see* standardized mortality ratio
SNPs *see* single nucleotide polymorphisms
social workers 389–90, 392
sociodemographic factors 34–5, **34, 35**, 89–92
socioeconomic status (SES) 38, 87–93, **88**
sodium/bicarbonate co-transporters (NBCs) 63, **63**
sodium butyrate 56
sodium chloride
  induction of sputum 124, 165
  metabolic alkalosis 273
  saline therapies 61, 71, 164–5, 193, 203
sodium transport
  ASL effects 61–2, **61**
  ENaC proteins 50, **51**, 62, 459
  hyperabsorption 62
  pancreas 63
  RNA interference therapy 459
software for database design 316
source data verification (SDV) 315
specialist CF centers 387–97
  clinic management 313
  epidemiology 39–40, **40**
  functions *388*
  historical development 8, 10, 12
  infection spread 140, 144
  multidisciplinary teams 387–92, 399–400
  newly diagnosed patient families 118–21
  nursing care 389, 392, 399
  quality assurance 312, 313, 314–15
  routine monitoring 345
  sexual/reproductive health matters 279–80, 281, 283, 287
  surgical team liaison 169
  terminal care 404–5
  variation in care 39–40, **40**, 92–3
species identification of micro-organisms 125–7, 142
specimens from respiratory tract 123–5
spermatogenesis 279
sperm harvesting techniques 281
sperm in semen analysis 105, 280–1
spiritual care 446–7
spirometry 299, 300–1, 326, 380
splenectomy 233
splenomegaly 233
splicing mutations 56
splicosome-mediated mRNA trans-splicing (SMaRT) 458, **458**

spontaneous ventilation 175–6, **175**
sputum
  expectoration 123, 124, 164–5, 366
  hypertonic saline induction 124, 164–5
  new treatment assessment 378–80
  oropharyngeal culture vs BAL 332–3
  specimen adequacy 123, 379–80
standardized mortality ratio (SMR) 25–6
standards
  data recording for databases 316
  infant lung function tests 321
Staphylococcus aureus 144–5
  biofilm formation 72
  clinical epidemiology 31, **31, 32**
  culture media 125, *125*
  epithelial cell binding 70, **71**
  humoral immune response 72
  methicillin-resistant 144–5
  methicillin-sensitive 144
  oropharyngeal culture vs BAL 332–3
  paranasal sinuses 199, 200, 204
  patient-to-patient transmission 129
  prognostic indicators 38
  prophylactic antibiotics 138
stem cell therapy 459–60
Stenotrophomonas maltophilia 32, 125, *125*, 126, 145–6
step tests 358, *358*
steroids *see* corticosteroids; sex steroids
stool softeners 217
stress 90, **90**, 400 435
STRs *see* short tandem repeats
structural changes in early lung function 324–5, **325**
structure-based drug design 465
submucosal glands 69–70
sunlight exposure 264, 265
supraventricular arrhythmias 163
surgery
  distal intestinal obstruction syndrome 217, 218
  gallstone disease 233
  gastroesophageal reflux 216
  meconium ileus 213
  patient management 169–70
  sinonasal disease 204–6, **204, 205**
  splenomegaly 233
  see also transplantation
surveillance strategies 130–1
survival 25–7
  after lung transplantation **293**, 299, 300
  composite prediction models 349–51
  effects on population prevalence 25
  fitness level **364**
  historical 5, 6, 8–9, 10, 12, 26
  liver disease 227
  lung function 346, *350*

older patients 403, 441, 474
  prognostic indicators 35, 37–9
  transplantation criteria 292–4
  see also mortality
survivor effects in epidemiological study 30, 32
susceptibility testing 128
sweat
  gland disorders 64, **64, 273**, 273
  losses 362
  tests
    epidemiology 27
    historical 3, 5, 7
    indications 101, 102
    newborn screening 111–13
    new treatments assessment 376–7
    physiological basis 64, **64**
    procedure 100–2
    usefulness 99
symptom-limited oxygen uptake *see* peak oxygen uptake
syndrome of inappropriate antidiuretic hormone secretion (SIADH) 273–4
synergy testing of antibiotics 128
system disorders 269–77

T5 polymorphism 282
Targeted Genetics Corporation 457
TDN *see* Therapeutic Development Network
teeth 274
terminal care 404–5, 416, 442–3, *443*, *444*, 445–6, *486*
TESA *see* testicular sperm aspiration
testicular growth 257, **257**
testicular sperm aspiration (TESA) 281
testosterone 265
testosterone esters 258
Therapeutic Development Network (TDN) 464, 467
therapeutic exercise 361–70
thoracic expansion exercises 410, **410**
thrombocytopenia 159
thrombosis 195
thymidine polymorphism in intron 8, 81
tidal breathing 325
tidal volume 361
time effects 104
time to next exacerbation 378
time to next positive culture 378
tissue damage 70, 72
tissue sensitivity variation 81
TIVADs *see* totally implantable venous access devices
TLC *see* total lung capacity
TLOSR *see* transient lower esophageal sphincter relaxation

tobacco smoke 89, 91, 325
tobramycin (Tobi®) 138, 139, 141, 142, 149, 191
topical decongestants 203
total lung capacity (TLC) 366
totally implantable venous access devices (TIVADs) 151, 194–5, **194**, *195*
transbronchial biopsy 301
transcellular permeability of gastrointestinal tract 210
transepithelial potential 64
transient lower esophageal sphincter relaxation (TLOSR) 214, 215
transition form 479–82
transition from pediatric to adult care 393–5, *394*, 402–3, 479–82
translational research 467
transmission of CF pathogens *see* cross-infection; infection control
transplantation 291–302, 466–7
    care center functions 388, 391
    CF-related diabetes 248
    children 291, **293**, 300–1
    complications 296, 298–300, *299*
    contraindications 294, *295*
    donor allocation 294–5
    history 11
    indications 291–2, **292**
    liver disease 230
    low bone mineral density 264, 267
    numbers 291, **292**
    nursing care 404
    nutritional management 427
    outcomes 299–300
    perioperative management 296–7
    physiotherapy 416
    post-operative management 297–300
    post-transplant lymphoproliferative disorder 201
    pregnancy following 285
    preoperative management 295–6
    rejection 297, 298, 466–7
    research areas *302*
    selection 291–4, *294*
    sinus surgery 205–6
    social worker role 390
    terminal phase care 442, 443
trans-splicing 457, 458–9, **458**
travel 168–9, 195–6
treatment adherence *see* compliance
treatment assessment measures 375–81
trypsin tests 7, 9, 111, 112, 113
type I/type II diabetes mellitus 242, *243*
typhoid protection 41

UDCA *see* ursodeoxycholic acid
UK
    Cystic Fibrosis Trust, history 7
    medical care provision 39–40
    mortality rates 25
    pioneers 5, 6
    population prevalence 25
    specialist center history 10
ultrasonic nebulizers 189
upper airways
    sinonasal disease 199–208
    viral infections 146–8
urinary incontinence 283–4, 367, 415
urine analysis 379
urine glucose testing 246
ursodeoxycholic acid (UDCA) 226, 229
US
    adoption of British treatment methods 5, 6
    Cystic Fibrosis Foundation 6, 7
    medical care provision 38
    mortality rates 25–6
    pioneers 3–5
    population prevalence 25

vaccinations 75–6, 147, 168, 301, 466
vaginal yeast infection 284
variable disease expression
    CFTR mutations 52–3, 56, 59–60, 81–2
    CFTR polymorphisms 56–7, 81
    factors 87–96, **88**
    healthcare variation 92–3
    modifier genes 60, 81, 82–4, 104
    sociodemographic factors 87–92
variant CF *see* atypical (non-classic) cystic fibrosis
variceal bleeding 231–2, **232**
vasculitis 269–70, **269**
vas deferens absence 12, 65, 81, 105, 279, 282
venous access 151, 194–5, **194**, *195*, 485
ventilation
    active cycle of breathing techniques 409–10, **410**
    non-invasive positive pressure ventilation 178–82, **178**, *179*
    nursing care *485–6*
    PERT therapy 423
    sleep 176–8, **177**
    spontaneous 175–6, **175**
    work of breathing 175–6, **175**
ventilatory drive 175, 176, **177**
ventilatory muscles 175–82, **175**, **177**, 365–7

The Vest® Airway Clearance System 413–14, **414**
vibrating mesh nebulizers *187*, 189–90, **190**
viral infections
    bacterial infection relationship 147, 148
    post-transplant children 301
    respiratory tract 89, 126, 146–8
    vaccinations 75–6, 147, 168, 301
viral vectors 460
vitamins
    bone mineral density 264–5, *264*, 266
    deficiencies 120, 159, 211, 274
    supplementation 5, 11, 120, 264, 266, 423–6, *423*
    vitamin A 3, 4, 5, 120, 274, 423–4, *423*
    vitamin D 120, 264–5, *264*, 266, 423–4, *423*
    vitamin E 120, 274, 423–4, *423*
    vitamin K 265, 266, 423–4, *423*
    water-soluble 424
VO$_2$ $_{max}$ *see* maximum oxygen uptake
VO$_2$ $_{peak}$ *see* peak oxygen uptake
volume-targeted ventilation *see* assist control/volume-targeted ventilation
volumetric CT 340–1
volvulus 218–19

W1282X mutation 22
walking tests 357–8, *357*
WAnT *see* Wingate anaerobic test
water intake 362, **362**
water-soluble vitamins 424
weight 32–3, **32**, 381
weight bearing exercise 265, 266
Wingate anaerobic test (WAnT) 356
Wisconsin newborn screening project 110–11, *110*
Wolffian (mesonephric) duct 279

Xanthamonas maltophilia see Stenotrophomonas maltophilia
X-rays
    chest radiography 333, 337, 338, **339**, 380
    dual energy X-ray absorptiometry 261–2, 266
    see also computed tomography
XT *see* exercise testing

young children *see* infants; neonates

Z-scores 322, **323**, 326